Berman's Pediatric Decision Making

Berman's Pediatric Decision Making

Fifth Edition

Lalit Bajaj, MD, MPH
Associate Professor of Pediatrics, University of Colorado School of Medicine;
Research Director, Section of Emergency Medicine, Children's Hospital Colorado, Aurora, Colorado

Simon J. Hambidge, MD, PhD
Director of General Pediatrics, Denver Health, Denver; Professor of Pediatrics, University of Colorado School of Medicine, Aurora, Colorado

Gwendolyn Kerby, MD
Associate Professor of Pediatrics, University of Colorado School of Medicine;
Medical Director, Pulmonary Clinic, Children's Hospital Colorado, Aurora, Colorado

Ann-Christine Nyquist, MD, MSPH
Associate Professor of Pediatrics, Associate Dean, Diversity and Inclusion, University of Colorado School of Medicine;
Associate Professor, Community and Behavioral Health, Colorado School of Public Health; Medical Director, Infection Prevention and Control, Children's Hospital Colorado, Aurora, Colorado

ELSEVIER
MOSBY

ELSEVIER
MOSBY

1600 John F. Kennedy Blvd.
Ste 1800
Philadelphia, PA 19103-2899

BERMAN'S PEDIATRIC DECISION MAKING, FIFTH EDITION ISBN: 978-0-323-05405-8

Library of Congress Cataloging-in-Publication Data

Berman's pediatric decision making / [edited by] Lalit Bajaj . . . [et al.]. -- 5th ed.
p. ; cm.
Pediatric decision making
Rev. ed. of: Pediatric decision making / Stephen Berman. 4th ed. c2003.
Includes bibliographical references.
ISBN 978-0-323-05405-8 (pbk.)
1. Pediatrics -- Decision making. I. Bajaj, Lalit. II. Berman, Stephen. III. Berman, Stephen. Pediatric decision making. IV. Title: Pediatric decision making.
[DNLM: 1. Pediatrics. 2. Decision Making. 3. Diagnosis. WS 200]
RJ47.B47 2011
618.92 -- dc23

2011018488

Editor: Judith Fletcher
Developmental Editor: Joanie Milnes
Editorial Assistant: Jackie Wechsler
Publishing Services Manager: Anne Altepeter
Senior Project Manager: Doug Turner
Designer: Steven Stave

Printed in the United States of America

Last digit is the print number: 9 8 7 6 5 4 3 2 1

Preface

The fifth edition of *Pediatric Decision Making* marks a major editorial transition for this ground-breaking textbook of algorithms. I turn the editorial duties over to four outstanding clinicians for this edition, the first to be published in the twenty-first century. I have worked closely with these pediatricians for many years (and with some since residency), and as their careers have matured I have grown to greatly admire and respect their knowledge, clinical skills, and teaching abilities. I am sure that this and future editions will be creative and innovative, providing clinicians with a valuable resource to help them provide the very best care for children.

As a pediatrician for 39 years, I have been fortunate to have had the opportunity to create and edit this book. I have a career and work that I love and a wonderful supportive family—my wife, Elaine, and sons, Seth and Ben. As I reflect on why pediatrics has been so personally fulfilling and meaningful, I realize the importance of having strong personal relationships with patients and their families. These relationships take time to mature. Caring for children continuously over a long time, referred to as "continuity of care," allows pediatricians to share many intense moments of sorrow and joy with our patients and their families.

As my clinical experience and expertise increased over the years, my approach to patients and their families began to change. I realized the need to balance both art and science in caring for children. While science strives to be as objective as possible, art remains intuitive. While science relies on technology, art relies on communication and empathy. While the art of medicine recognizes the value of helping, the science of medicine strives to find cures. Art touches people by sharing feelings and emotion. Art builds an intangible bridge that connects people and makes us aware of the shared elements of the human existence. The art of pediatric practice helps a dying patient live every day to the fullest, enjoying life by being with loved ones. Science requires a thorough understanding of the scientific method and how observations generate hypotheses that can be tested by experiments or trials. Science is about defining, counting, measuring, and then analyzing. Practicing pediatrics is about using science and technology in conjunction with the art of pediatric care to prevent disease, save lives, heal children, and help families cope.

In a textbook of algorithms, it is difficult to demonstrate how to communicate with patients and families, and thus to teach "the art of pediatrics." Therefore, I tried to do this with a different type of book, entitled *Getting it Right for Children: Stories of Pediatric Care and Advocacy,* published by the American Academy of Pediatrics. I learned that successful advocacy involves storytelling that reaches out and touches readers combined with data that provide the evidence needed to make good policy decisions.

While I could not incorporate as much of the art of pediatrics into *Pediatric Decision Making* as I would have liked, I hope that this next generation of editors will have more success. I am sure that they will integrate the rapid advances in our understanding of genetics, pathophysiology and treatment of disease, and technology into this book in ways that will be understandable and useful to clinicians. I thank them for accepting this role and appreciate the opportunity I have to continue to work with them and other members of our Department of Pediatrics at The Children's Hospital on a regular basis.

Stephen Berman, MD

Contributors

Mark J. Abzug, MD
Professor of Pediatrics, Infectious Diseases, University of Colorado Denver School of Medicine; Professor of Pediatrics, The Children's Hospital, Aurora, Colorado

Edythe Albano, MD
Associate Professor of Pediatrics, University of Colorado, Denver, Colorado; Clinical Director Oncology, The Children's Hospital, Aurora, Colorado

Nimisha Amin, MD
Pediatric Nephrologist, Private Practice, Bakersfield, California

Mark E. Anderson, MD
Staff Physician and Team Leader, Kid's Care Clinic at Denver Health Medical Center; Director and PI, Rocky Mountain Region Pediatric Environmental Health Specialty Unit (PEHSU); Associate Professor of Pediatrics, University of Colorado School of Medicine, Aurora, Colorado

Marsha S. Anderson, MD
Associate Professor of Pediatrics, University of Colorado School of Medicine, Section of Pediatric Infectious Diseases, The Children's Hospital, Aurora, Colorado

Susan D. Apkon, MD
Director, Rehabilitation Medicine, Seattle Children's Hospital; Associate Professor, Department of Rehabilitation Medicine, University of Washington, Seattle, Washington

Jennifer Armstrong-Wells, MD, MPH
Assistant Professor, Pediatrics, Section of Neurology, University of Colorado, Aurora, Colorado; Assistant Adjunct Professor, Neurology, University of California, San Francisco, California

Daniel Arndt, MD, MA
Assistant Professor, Pediatrics, Michigan State University School of Medicine; Director, Pediatric Epilepsy Program, DeVos Children's Hospital, Grand Rapids, Michigan

Donald H. Arnold, MD, MPH
Associate Professor, Department of Pediatrics, Division of Emergency Medicine, Center for Asthma and Environmental Research, Vanderbilt University School of Medicine, Nashville, Tennessee

Lalit Bajaj, MD, MPH
Associate Professor of Pediatrics, University of Colorado School of Medicine; Research Director, Section of Emergency Medicine, Children's Hospital Colorado, Aurora, Colorado

Christopher D. Baker, MD
Assistant Professor, Pediatrics, Section of Pulmonary Medicine, University of Colorado School of Medicine, The Children's Hospital, Aurora, Colorado

Vivek Balasubramaniam, MD
Associate Professor of Pediatrics, University of Colorado, Denver; The Children's Hospital, Aurora, Colorado

Jennifer M. Barker, MD
Assistant Professor of Pediatrics, Division of Pediatric Endocrinology, The Children's Hospital, Aurora, Colorado

Barrett H. Barnes, MD
Assistant Professor of Pediatrics, Department of Pediatrics, Section of Pediatric Gastroenterology, Hepatology, and Nutrition, University of Virginia, UVA Children's Hospital, Charlottesville, Virginia

James S. Barry, MD
Assistant Professor, Department of Pediatrics, Medical Division, University of Colorado Hospital NICU, University of Colorado School of Medicine, Aurora, Colorado

Stephen Berman, MD
Professor of Pediatrics, University of Colorado School of Medicine; Chair, Children's Hospital; Academic, General Pediatrics; Past President, American Academy of Pediatrics, Aurora, Colorado

Timothy J. Bernard, MD
Assistant Professor, Pediatric Neurology, University of Colorado School of Medicine, The Children's Hospital, Aurora, Colorado

Robert Brayden, MD
Professor of Pediatrics, University of Colorado School of Medicine, The Children's Hospital, Aurora, Colorado

Alison Brent, MD
Associate Professor of Pediatrics, University of Colorado Health and Sciences Center, Denver, Colorado

Joanna M. Burch, MD
Associate Professor of Dermatology and Pediatrics, The Children's Hospital, Aurora, Colorado

Arelis Burgos-Zavoda, MD
Assistant Professor of Pediatrics and Dermatology, University of Colorado Hospital; Assistant Professor of Dermatology, The Children's Hospital, Aurora; Assistant Professor of Dermatology, Denver Health Medical Center, Denver, Colorado

Jeffrey B. Campbell, MD
Associate Professor, Department of Surgery, Division of Urology, University of Colorado School of Medicine; Department of Pediatric Urology, The Children's Hospital, Aurora, Colorado

William Campbell, MD
Assistant Professor of Pediatrics, University of Colorado School of Medicine; Physician Advisor; Early Intervention Colorado, Denver, Colorado; Developmental-Behavioral Pediatrician, Child Development Unit, The Children's Hospital, Aurora, Colorado

Kelly Casperson, MD
Urology Resident, Department of Surgery, Division of Urology, University of Colorado School of Medicine; Department of Pediatric Urology, The Children's Hospital, Aurora, Colorado

Betsey Chambers, MD
Pediatrician, Newborn Nursery, Denver Health Hospital, Denver, Colorado

Maida Lynn Chen, MD
Assistant Professor of Pediatrics, Pulmonary and Sleep Medicine Division, University of Washington School of Medicine; Associate Director, Pediatric Sleep Disorders Program, Seattle Children's Hospital, Seattle, Washington

Marc Chester, MD
Pediatric Pulmonologist, The Pediatric Lung Center, Fairfax, Virginia

Antonia Chiesa, MD
Senior Instructor, Department of Pediatrics, University of Colorado School of Medicine; Kempe Child Protection Team, The Children's Hospital, Aurora, Colorado

Jason Child, PharmD
University of Colorado School of Medicine, Aurora, Colorado

Abigail Collins, MD
Instructor of Pediatrics and Neurology, Director of Pediatric Movement Disorders, The Children's Hospital, Aurora, Colorado

Steven Colson, MD
Fellow, Department of Pediatrics, Section of Pediatric Gastroenterology, Hepatology and Nutrition, The Children's Hospital, University of Colorado School of Medicine, Aurora, Colorado

Mary N. Cook, MD
Clinical Director, Department of Psychiatry and Behavioral Sciences; Medical Director, Outpatient Services, The Children's Hospital; Assistant Professor, Psychiatry, University of Colorado School of Medicine, Aurora, Colorado

Julie-Ann Crewalk, MD
Fellow in Pediatric Infectious Diseases, Children's National Medical Center, Washington, DC

Donna Curtis, MD, MPH
Fellow, Pediatric Infectious Diseases, University of Colorado School of Medicine, Aurora, Colorado

Jesse Davidson, MD
Fellow, Pediatric Cardiology and Critical Care, The Children's Hospital, Aurora, Colorado

Roberta L. DeBiasi, MD
Associate Professor of Pediatrics, George Washington University School of Medicine; Faculty, Division of Pediatric Infectious Disease, Children's National Medical Center, Washington, DC

Robin R. Deterding, MD
Professor of Pediatric Pulmonary Medicine and Medical Director, Breathing Institute, The Children's Hospital; Director, Children's Interstitial Lung Disease Research Network, The Children's Hospital, University of Colorado, School of Medicine, Aurora, Colorado

Samuel R. Dominguez, MD, PhD
Assistant Professor, Pediatric Infectious Diseases, University of Colorado School of Medicine, Aurora, Colorado

Ellen Roy Elias, MD
Director, Special Care Clinic; Professor, Department of Pediatrics and Genetics, The Children's Hospital, Aurora, Colorado

Kathryn D. Emery, MD
Associate Professor of Pediatrics, University of Colorado School of Medicine, Aurora, Colorado

Monica J. Federico, MD
Assistant Director of Pediatrics, The Children's Hospital, University of Colorado Health Sciences Center, Denver, Colorado

Steven G. Federico, MD
Director, School-Based Health/Denver Health; Associate Professor, General Pediatrics, University of Colorado School of Medicine, Aurora, Colorado

Catherine C. Ferguson, MD
University of Colorado School of Medicine, Aurora, Colorado

David Fox, MD
Assistant Professor, Department of General Pediatrics, The Children's Hospital, University of Colorado School of Medicine, Aurora, Colorado

Julia Fuzak, MD
Clinical Instructor, Department of Pediatrics, Section of Emergency Medicine, The Children's Hospital, University of Colorado School of Medicine, Aurora, Colorado

Kelly K. Gajewski, MD
Assistant Professor of Clinical Pediatrics, Louisiana State University Health Sciences Center, New Orleans, Louisiana

Renata C. Gallagher, MD, PhD
Assistant Professor, Clinical Genetics and Metabolism, Department of Pediatrics, University of Colorado School of Medicine, Aurora, Colorado

Jason Gien, MD
Assistant Professor, University of Colorado Hospital, University of Colorado School of Medicine, Aurora, Colorado

Christine Gilroy, MD, MSPH
Associate Professor, Division of General Internal Medicine, University of Colorado Health Sciences Center, Denver, Colorado

Mary P. Glodé, MD
Professor of Pediatrics and Head, Section of Pediatric Infectious Disease, The Children's Hospital, University of Colorado School of Medicine, Aurora, Colorado

Neil A. Goldenberg, MD, PhD
Associate Professor of Pediatrics and Medicine (Hematology); Associate Center Director; Director, Clinical Research, Mountain States Regional Hemophilia and Thrombosis Center, University of Colorado, Denver, Colorado; Director, Medical Affairs and Venous Thromboembolism Trials, CPC Clinical Research; Co-Director, Pediatric Thrombosis and Stroke Programs, The Children's Hospital, Aurora, Colorado

Edward Goldson, MD
Professor of Pediatrics, University of Colorado School of Medicine, Aurora, Colorado

Carol L. Greene, MD
Professor of Pediatrics, University of Maryland School of Medicine, Baltimore, Maryland

Joseph Grubenhoff, MD
Assistant Professor of Pediatrics, Section of Emergency Medicine, University of Colorado School of Medicine, Aurora, Colorado

Mindy L. Grunzke, MD
The Children's Hospital, University of Colorado School of Medicine, Aurora, Colorado

Sameer Gupta, MD
Assistant Professor of Pediatrics, Division of Pediatric Critical Care, University of Minnesota Medical School, Minneapolis, Minnesota

Greg Gutierrez, MD
Attending Physician, Denver Health Primary Care Musculoskeletal Clinic; Attending Physician, Denver Health Pediatric Minor Fracture Clinic; Staff, Family Medicine Department, Denver, Colorado

Ann C. Halbower, MD
Associate Professor of Pediatrics, Pulmonary Section, The Children's Hospital, University of Colorado School of Medicine, Aurora, Colorado

Sarah Halstead, MD
Clinical Instructor, Fellow, Pediatric Emergency Medicine, The Children's Hospital, University of Colorado, Aurora, Colorado

Simon J. Hambidge, MD, PhD
Director of General Pediatrics, Denver Health, Denver; Professor of Pediatrics, University of Colorado School of Medicine, Aurora, Colorado

Megan G. Henderson, MD, FAAP
General Pediatrician, Westside Pediatric/Teen Clinic, Denver Health; Instructor of Medicine, University of Colorado Health Sciences, Denver, Colorado

Edward J. Hoffenberg, MD
Professor of Pediatrics; Director, Center for Pediatric Inflammatory Bowel Diseases, The Children's Hospital, University of Colorado School of Medicine, Aurora, Colorado

Christine Waasdorp Hurtado, MD
Assistant Professor, Digestive Health Institute, The Children's Hospital, University of Colorado School of Medicine, Aurora, Colorado

Kyros Ipaktchi, MD
Associate Professor, University of Colorado School of Medicine Aurora, Colorado; Attending Surgeon, Department of Orthopaedics, Denver Health Medical Center, Denver, Colorado

Ed Jernigan, MD
Physician, Children's Neurology, Saint Luke's Regional Medical Center, Boise, Idaho

Joshua A. Kailin, MD
Pediatric Cardiology Fellow, The Children's Hospital, Aurora, Colorado

Beena D. Kamath, MD, MPH
Assistant Professor of Pediatrics, Division of Neonatology and Pulmonary Biology, Cincinnati Children's Hospital Medical Center, Cincinnati, Ohio

Naveen Kanathur, MBBS
Division of Sleep, National Jewish Health Organization, Denver, Colorado

Michael S. Kappy, MD, PhD
Chief, Pediatric Endocrinology, The Children's Hospital; Professor of Pediatrics, University of Colorado School of Medicine, Aurora, Colorado

Paritosh Kaul, MD
Associate Professor of Pediatrics, Section of Adolescent Medicine, Department of Pediatrics, The Children's Hospital, University of Colorado School of Medicine, Aurora, Colorado

Sita Kedia, MD
Clinical Instructor, Child Neurology, General Pediatrics, The Children's Hospital, University of Colorado School of Medicine, Aurora, Colorado

Karen L. Kelminson, MD
Assistant Professor, Department of General Pediatrics, University of Colorado School of Medicine, Aurora, Colorado

Megan Kelsey, MD, MS
Assistant Professor of Pediatric Endocrinology, The Children's Hospital, Aurora, Colorado

Gwendolyn Kerby, MD
Associate Professor of Pediatrics, University of Colorado School of Medicine; Medical Director, Pulmonary Clinic, Children's Hospital Colorado, Aurora, Colorado

Ulrich Klein, DMD, DDS, MS
Professor and Chair, Department of Pediatric Dentistry, The Children's Hospital, University of Colorado School of Dental Medicine, Aurora, Colorado

Kelly Knupp, MD
Assistant Professor of Neurology, Department of Neurology, University of Wisconsin School of Medicine and Public Health, Madison, Wisconsin

Kristine Knuti, MD
Pediatrician, Instructor, Department of Pediatrics, Denver Health, University of Colorado School of Medicine, Aurora, Colorado

Mark G. Koch, DDS, MS
Assistant Professor, Pediatric Dentistry, The Children's Hospital; University of Colorado School of Dental Medicine, Aurora, Colorado

Robert E. Kramer, MD
Associate Professor of Pediatrics, Medical Director of Endoscopy, Digestive Health Institute, Section of Pediatric Gastroenterology, Hepatology and Nutrition, The Children's Hospital, University of Colorado School of Medicine, Aurora, Colorado

Amethyst C. Kurbegov, MD
Assistant Professor of Pediatric Gastrointestinal Diseases, University of Colorado Health Sciences Center, The Children's Hospital, Colorado Springs Satellite Clinic, Colorado Springs, Colorado

Theresa Laguna, MD, MSCS
Assistant Professor of Pediatrics, Department of Pediatrics, Division of Pediatric Pulmonology, University of Minnesota, Minneapolis, Minnesota

Peter A. Lane, MD
Professor Hematology and Oncology, Department of Pediatrics, Emory University School of Medicine, Atlanta, Georgia

Martin J. LaPage, MD
Medical University of South Carolina, Charleston, South Carolina

Meegan Leve, MD
Senior Instructor of Pediatrics, University of Colorado School of Medicine, Aurora, Colorado

Paul Levisohn, MD
Associate Professor of Pediatrics and Neurology, University of Colorado School of Medicine; Neurosciences Institute, The Children's Hospital, Aurora, Colorado

Edwin Liu, MD
Associate Professor, Pediatrics, Digestive Health Institute, The Children's Hospital, University of Colorado School of Medicine, Aurora, Colorado

Brandy Lu, MD
Pediatric Gastroenterology and Hepatology, California Pacific Medical Center; Clinical Instructor–Affiliate, Stanford University School of Medicine, Stanford, California

Cara L. Mack, MD
Associate Professor of Pediatrics, Section of Pediatric Gasteroenterology, Hepatology and Nutrition, The Children's Hospital, University of Colorado Denver School of Medicine, Aurora, Colorado

Jody Ann Maes, MD
Associate Director, Denver Emergency Center for Children, Denver Health Medical Center; Clinical Professor, Department of Pediatrics, University of Colorado School of Medicine, Aurora, Colorado

Patrick Mahar, MD
Assistant Professor, Pediatric Emergency, Department of Pediatrics, Section of Pediatric Emergency Medicine, The Children's Hospital, University of Colorado School of Medicine, Aurora, Colorado

Maria Mandt, MD
Physician, Emergency Medicine, The Children's Hospital, Aurora, Colorado

Suzan Mazor, MD
Assistant Professor, Pediatric Emergency Medicine, Toxicology, Seattle, Washington

Elizabeth J. McFarland, MD
Professor of Pediatrics, The Children's Hospital, Aurora, Colorado

Lora Melnicoe, MD, MPH
University of Colorado School of Medicine, Aurora, Colorado

Paul G. Moe, MD
Professor of Pediatric Neurology, Pediatrics, University of Colorado School of Medicine; Physician, Neurology, The Children's Hospital, Aurora, Colorado

Thomas J. Moon, MD
Department of Pediatric Cardiology, University of Denver, The Children's Hospital, Aurora, Colorado

Joseph Morelli, MD

Vincent Mukkada, MD
Assistant Professor of Pediatrics, (Clinical) Pediatric Gastroenterology, Nutrition, and Liver Diseases; Director, Pediatric Food Allergy Program, Hasbro Children's Hospital/Warren Alpert Medical School, Brown University, Providence, Rhode Island

Rachelle Nuss, MD
Professor of Pediatrics, Department of Hematology and Oncology, The Children's Hospital, Aurora, Colorado

Ann-Christine Nyquist, MD, MSPH
Associate Professor of Pediatrics; Associate Dean, Diversity and Inclusion, University of Colorado School of Medicine; Associate Professor, Community and Behavioral Health, Colorado School of Public Health; Medical Director, Infection Prevention and Control, Children's Hospital Colorado, Aurora, Colorado

Judith A. O'Connor, MD
Physician, The Children's Hospital at Oklahoma University Health Science Center, Oklahoma City, Oklahoma

John W. Ogle, MD
Director of Pediatrics, Denver Health, The Children's Hospital; Professor and Vice Chairman Pediatrics, University of Colorado School of Medicine, Aurora, Colorado

Sean T. O'Leary, MD
Assistant Professor, Pediatric Infectious Diseases, The Children's Hospital, University of Colorado, Aurora, Colorado

Scott C. N. Oliver, MD
Assistant Professor, Department of Ophthalmology, University of Colorado Eye Center, University of Colorado School of Medicine, Aurora, Colorado

Carolyn K. Pan, MD
Resident Physician, Rocky Mountain Lions Eye Institute, Department of Ophthalmology, University of Colorado, Denver, Colorado

Julie A. Panepinto, MD
Associate Professor, Pediatrics, Medical College of Wisconsin, Children's Hospital of Wisconsin, Milwaukee, Wisconsin

Sarah Parker, MD
Assistant Professor, Pediatrics, Section of Pediatric Infectious Diseases, University of Colorado School of Medicine; Assistant Professor, Pediatrics, Section of Pediatric Infectious Diseases, The Children's Hospital, Aurora, Colorado

Julie Parsons, MD
Assistant Professor of Pediatrics and Neurology, University of Colorado School of Medicine, The Children's Hospital, Aurora, Colorado

Roopal Patel, MD, DTMH
Medical Epidemiologist, Division of Parasitic Diseases and Malaria, Centers for Disease Control and Prevention, Atlanta, Georgia

K. Brooke Pengel, MD
Medical Director, Rocky Mountain Youth Sports Medicine Institute; HealthONE; Rocky Mountain Hospital for Children at Presbyterian/St. Luke's Medical Center, Denver, Colorado

John Peterson, MD
Director, Child and Adolescent Psychiatric Services, Denver Health Medical Center; Associate Professor, Department of Psychiatry, University of Colorado School of Medicine, Denver, Colorado

Laura Pickler, MD, MPH
Assistant Professor, Family Medicine and Pediatrics, University of Colorado School of Medicine, Aurora, Colorado

Garrett Pohlman, MD
Division of Urology, University of Colorado School of Medicine, Aurora, Colorado

Steven R. Poole, MD
Vice Chair, Department of Pediatrics; Section Head, Community Pediatrics, University of Colorado School of Medicine, Aurora, Colorado

Lara Rappaport, MD, MPH
Assistant Professor, Pediatric Emergency Medicine, University of Colorado School of Medicine, The Children's Hospital, Aurora, Colorado

John H. Reed, MD, MPH
Assistant Professor, Pediatric Cardiology; Director, Pediatric Electrophysiology, Medical University of South Carolina, Charleston, South Carolina

Jason T. Rhodes, MD
Orthopaedic Surgeon, The Children's Hospital; Assistant Professor, University of Colorado School of Medicine, Aurora, Colorado

Mark Roback, MD
Director, Division of Emergency Medicine, University of Minnesota Amplatz Children's Hospital, Minneapolis, Minnesota

Adam Rosenberg, MD
Professor of Pediatrics; Program Director, Pediatric Residency Program, University of Colorado School of Medicine, Aurora, Colorado

Kelley Roswell, MD
Assistant Professor of Pediatrics and Emergency Medicine, University of Colorado School of Medicine; Assistant Professor, Pediatrics and Emergency Medicine, The Children's Hospital, Aurora, Colorado

Tonia Sabo, MD
Medical Director, Headache Clinic, The Children's Hospital, Aurora, Colorado

Amy E. Sass, MD, MPH
Assistant Professor of Pediatrics, University of Colorado School of Medicine; Pediatrics and Adolescent Medicine, The Children's Hospital, Aurora, Colorado

Michael S. Schaffer, MD
Professor of Pediatrics, Section of Cardiology, University of Colorado School of Medicine, Aurora, Colorado

Gunter H. Scharer, MD
Assistant Professor, Department of Pediatrics, Division of Clinical Genetics and Metabolism, The Children's Hospital, University of Colorado School of Medicine, Aurora, Colorado

Barton D. Schmitt, MD
Professor of Pediatrics, University of Colorado School of Medicine; Medical Director, After Hours Call Center, The Children's Hospital, Aurora, Colorado

Stephen M. Scott, MD, FACOG
Associate Professor, Departments of Obstetrics and Gynecology and Pediatrics, University of Colorado Health Sciences Center, Denver, Colorado

Leo K. Seibold, MD
Resident Physician, Department of Ophthalmology, University of Colorado, Denver, Colorado

Judith C. Shlay, MD, MSPH
Director, Immunization and Travel Clinic, Denver Public Health, Denver Health; Professor, Family Medicine, University of Colorado School of Medicine, Aurora, Colorado

Eric J. Sigel, MD
Associate Professor of Pediatrics, University of Colorado School of Medicine, The Children's Hospital, Aurora, Colorado

Marion R. Sills, MD, MPH
Associate Professor, Department of Pediatrics, University of Colorado School of Medicine, Aurora, Colorado

Eric A. F. Simoes, MBBS, DCH, MD
Professor of Pediatrics, Department of Infectious Diseases, The Children's Hospital, University of Colorado Health and Science Center, Aurora, Colorado

Andrew Sirotnak, MD
Professor of Pediatrics, University of Colorado School of Medicine; Director, Child Protection Team, The Children's Hospital, The Kempe Center for the Prevention and Treatment of Child Abuse and Neglect, Aurora, Colorado

Joseph M. Smith, MD, FAAP
Assistant Clinical Professor, University of Colorado Health Sciences Center, Aurora; Pediatric Clinical Section Head, Platte Valley Medical Center, Brighton, Colorado

Jason Soden, MD
Assistant Professor of Pediatrics, Section of Pediatric Gastroenterology, Hepatology, and Nutrition, The Children's Hospital, University of Colorado School of Medicine, Aurora, Colorado

Jennifer B. Soep, MD
Assistant Professor, Pediatric Rheumatology, University of Colorado School of Medicine, Aurora, Colorado

David M. Spiro, MD, MPH
Associate Professor, Emergency Medicine and Pediatrics, Oregon Health and Science University, Portland, Oregon

Britt Stroud, MD
Physician, Pediatric Neurology Sleep Medicine, Lee Memorial Health System, Fort Meyers, Florida

Henry R. Thompson, MD
Pediatric Gastroenterologist, Pediatric Department Chair, Cystic Fibrosis Center, St. Lukes Children's Hospital; Director, Cystic Fibrosis Center of Idaho, Boise, Idaho

Anne Chun-Hui Tsai, MD, MSc, FAAP, FACMG
Associate Professor, Pediatrics/Genetics, University of Colorado School of Medicine; Attending Physician, Clinical Geneticist, Pediatrics/Genetics, The Children's Hospital, Aurora, Colorado

Sondra Valdez, BSN
Clinical in-Staff Nurse, Cleft Palate Team, The Children's Hospital, Aurora, Colorado

R. Paul Wadwa, MD
Assistant Professor of Pediatrics, Barbara Davis Center for Childhood Diabetes, University of Colorado School of Medicine, Aurora, Colorado

Jeffrey S. Wagener, MD
Professor of Pediatrics, Pediatric Pulmonary, The Children's Hospital, Aurora, Colorado

Michael Walsh, MD
Medical University of South Carolina, Charleston, South Carolina

George S. Wang, MD
Pediatric Emergency Medicine Fellow, Section of Emergency Medicine, The Children's Hospital, University of Colorado School of Medicine, Aurora, Colorado

Joe Wathen, MD
Attending Physician, Emergency Department, University of Colorado Medical Center, Aurora, Colorado

Kathryn Wells, MD, FAAP
Community Pediatrician, Community Health Services, Denver Health; Medical Director, Denver Family Crisis Center, Denver; Assistant Professor of Pediatrics, Department of Pediatrics, University of Colorado School of Medicine, Aurora, Colorado

Andrew White, MD, PhD
Instructor, Pediatric Neurology, University of Colorado School of Medicine, Aurora, Colorado

Anne Wilson, DDS, MS
Associate Professor, Department of Pediatric Dentistry, University of Colorado School of Dental Medicine, The Children's Hospital, Aurora, Colorado

Samantha A. Woodruff, MD
Pediatrician, University of Massachusetts Medical Center, Pediatric Gastroenterology and Nutrition, Worcester, Massachusetts

Carter Wray, MD
Acting Instructor of Neurology, Seattle Children's Hospital, Seattle, Washington

Elizabeth Yeung, MD
Assistant Professor of Pediatrics, Division of Cardiology, The Heart Institute, The Children's Hospital, Cardiac and Vascular Center, Division of Adult Cardiology, University of Colorado Hospital, Aurora, Colorado

Patricia J. Yoon, MD
Associate Professor of Otolaryngology, University of Colorado School of Medicine; Associate Director, The Bill Daniels Center for Children's Hearing, The Children's Hospital, Aurora, Colorado

Janine Young, MD
Clinical Instructor, Department of Pediatrics, Yale University; Pediatrician, Department of Pediatrics, Yale Health Plan, New Haven, Connecticut

Lester Young, MD
Denver, Colorado

Pamela A. Zachar, MD
Instructor of Pediatrics, Neonatal-Perinatal Medicine; Fellow, Dartmouth Hitchcock Medical Center, Norwich, Vermont

Joshua J. Zaritsky, MD, PhD
Assistant Professor of Pediatrics, Division of Nephrology, Mattel Childrens Hospital at UCLA, Los Angeles, California

Lucy Zawadzki, MD
Assistant Professor, Pediatric Neurology, University of Wisconsin; Medical Doctor, Pediatric Neurology, University of Wisconsin Hospital and Clinics, Madison; Medical Doctor, Pediatric Neurology, Aspirus Wausau Hospital, Wausau, Wisconsin

Edith T. Zemanick, MD, MSCS
Assistant Professor of Pediatrics, University of Colorado School of Medicine, Aurora, Colorado

Julie D. Zimbelman, MD
Pediatric Oncologist and Hematologist, Rocky Mountain Pediatric Hematology and Oncology, Denver, Colorado

Contents

EAR/NOSE/THROAT

ENDOCRINE

FEVER

GASTROINTESTINAL

GENITOURINARY

Trauma

Toxicology

SPECIFIC DISORDERS

Adolescent Medicine

Behavioral/Developmental Disorders/Psychiatric Issues

Cardiovascular Disorders

Children with Special Health Care Needs

Dermatology

Gastroenterologic Disorders

Hematologic Disorders

Infectious Diseases

International Pediatrics

Clinical Decision Making

Clinical Decision Making

Stephen Berman, MD

One of the greatest challenges of clinical pediatrics is being able to organize one's knowledge in a way that the appropriate information can be rapidly and accurately accessed and used. Think about all your knowledge as the clothes that you have acquired over many years of study and experience. If you allow all your clothes to lie in one large pile in the middle of your closet, it will not be easy to get dressed quickly with clothes that are appropriate for the weather, work, or a special occasion. However, if your closet is well organized so you can quickly and easily find what you want, dressing rarely presents a problem. Pediatric decision making is designed to help you organize your closet of medical knowledge by better understanding the organizational structure for clinical decision making.

Clinical decision making has three integrated phases: (1) diagnosis, (2) assessment of severity, and (3) management. Appropriate clinical decision making considers the need to make a precise diagnosis as well as the costs associated with inappropriate or indiscriminate use of diagnostic tests. It also assesses the risk for an adverse outcome because of inappropriate management, and the costs and possible harmful effects of therapeutic interventions.

A. All three phases of clinical decision making are based on a well-done history and physical examination. Clinical decision making is often difficult because of the overlap among many types of conditions. A single disorder can produce a wide spectrum of signs and symptoms, and many disorders can produce similar signs and symptoms. The pediatric history should include a review of the present illness. Identify the reasons for the visit, and list the child's current problems. Evaluate the problems with respect to onset, duration, progression, precipitating or exacerbating factors, alleviating factors, and associations with other problems. Determine the functional impairment in relation to eating, play, sleep, other activities, and absence from school. Ask the parents why they brought the child to see you. Does the patient have any allergies to drugs or foods? Is the patient taking any medications? Are the child's immunizations up to date? Has the patient ever been hospitalized or had any serious accidents? The medical history explores the general state of health. Review the birth and developmental history. Elicit a focused review of symptoms, and a relevant family history and socioeconomic profile.

B. During the physical examination, approach the child with gentleness, using a friendly manner and a quiet voice. First observe the child from a distance. If the child has a cold or cough, count respirations and assess for respiratory distress before removing the child's clothing. Note the general appearance. Is the child interactive and consolable? Note the level of activity and playfulness. Look at the skin and note any pallor, erythema, jaundice, cyanosis, and lesions. Check the lymph nodes for size, inflammation, and sensitivity. Examine the head, eyes, ears, nose, mouth, and throat. Use a pneumatic otoscope to assess tympanic membrane mobility and inflammation. Note abnormalities of the neck, such as abnormal position, masses, and swelling of the thyroid glands. Examine the lungs for retractions and tachypnea, and listen for stridor, rhonchi, wheezing, and crepitations. When examining the heart, palpate for heaves or thrills and listen for murmurs, friction rubs, abnormal heart sounds, and uneven rhythm. During the abdominal examination, note tympany, shifting dullness, tenderness, rebound tenderness, palpable organs or masses, fluid waves, and bowel sounds. Examine the male genitalia for hypospadias, phimosis, presence and size of the testes, and swellings or masses. Examine the female genitalia for vaginal discharge, adhesions, hypertrophy of the clitoris, and pubertal changes. Examine the rectum and anus, noting fissures, inflammation or irritation, prolapse, muscle tone, and imperforation of the anus. Examine the musculoskeletal system, noting limitations in full range of motion, point tenderness, any deformities or asymmetry, and gait disturbances. Examine the joints, hands, and feet. Assess the spine and back, noting posture, curvatures, rigidity, webbing of the neck, dimples, and cysts. With the neurologic examination, assess cerebral function, cranial nerves, cerebellar function, the motor system, and the reflexes.

C. Initial nonspecific screening tests often include the complete blood cell count with differential and urinalysis. Subsequent laboratory tests and ancillary studies are based on the findings, history, and physical examination. These tests and studies should establish the pattern of involvement and extent of dysfunction. Information on the pattern of signs, symptoms, and findings from the ancillary tests is useful in identifying the cause of the disorder.

(Continued on page 4)

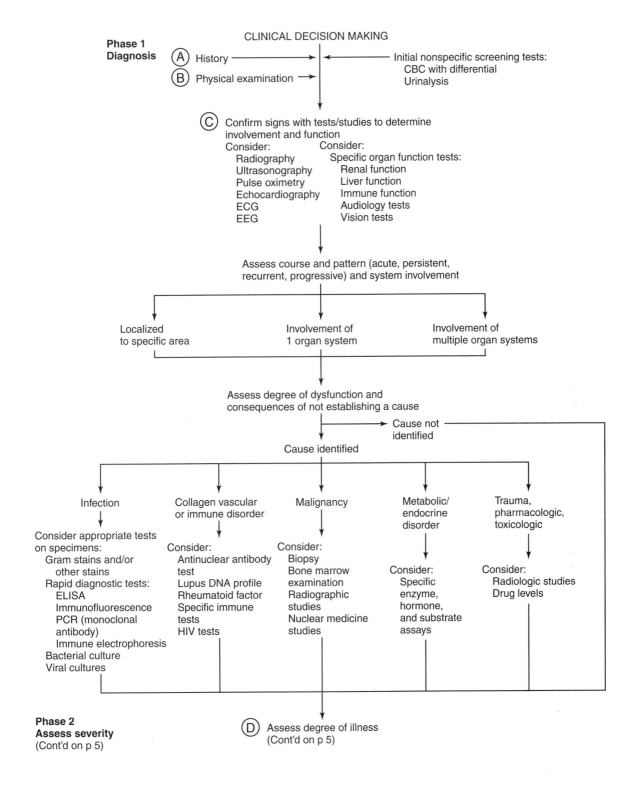

Phase 1
Diagnosis

CLINICAL DECISION MAKING

(A) History →
(B) Physical examination →

← Initial nonspecific screening tests:
- CBC with differential
- Urinalysis

↓

(C) Confirm signs with tests/studies to determine involvement and function

Consider:
- Radiography
- Ultrasonography
- Pulse oximetry
- Echocardiography
- ECG
- EEG

Consider:
- Specific organ function tests:
  - Renal function
  - Liver function
  - Immune function
  - Audiology tests
  - Vision tests

↓

Assess course and pattern (acute, persistent, recurrent, progressive) and system involvement

- Localized to specific area
- Involvement of 1 organ system
- Involvement of multiple organ systems

↓

Assess degree of dysfunction and consequences of not establishing a cause

→ Cause not identified

↓

Cause identified

Infection

Consider appropriate tests on specimens:
- Gram stains and/or other stains
- Rapid diagnostic tests:
  - ELISA
  - Immunofluorescence
  - PCR (monoclonal antibody)
  - Immune electrophoresis
- Bacterial culture
- Viral cultures

Collagen vascular or immune disorder

Consider:
- Antinuclear antibody test
- Lupus DNA profile
- Rheumatoid factor
- Specific immune tests
- HIV tests

Malignancy

Consider:
- Biopsy
- Bone marrow examination
- Radiographic studies
- Nuclear medicine studies

Metabolic/endocrine disorder

Consider:
- Specific enzyme, hormone, and substrate assays

Trauma, pharmacologic, toxicologic

Consider:
- Radiologic studies
- Drug levels

↓

Phase 2
Assess severity
(Cont'd on p 5)

(D) Assess degree of illness
(Cont'd on p 5)

D. The clinical information obtained from the history, physical examination, and laboratory and ancillary tests is used to assess the degree of illness, which classifies patients into four categories. Very severely ill patients require immediate intervention and stabilization to prevent irreversible damage and death or severe morbidity. Severely ill patients require hospital admission for two reasons: (1) to receive therapy not usually available on an outpatient basis, or (2) to have close observation and monitoring because of high risk for a complication or rapid progression of the disease. The ability of parents and others to care for a child at home and the availability of a telephone and transportation, geographic isolation, and weather may also affect the decision for hospitalization. Moderately ill patients require specific treatment in an ambulatory setting. Mildly ill patients have a self-limited condition that will resolve spontaneously. This approach may require some modification to accommodate the substitution of home health care services for hospitalization. Home health care services allow patients to leave the hospital earlier than they would otherwise be permitted.

E. The assessment of severity (degree of illness) links diagnostic decision making with management. The management phase of clinical decision making addresses four questions: (1) Does the patient require immediate therapeutic intervention? (2) What specific therapy is indicated? (3) Where should the patient be managed: a hospital intensive care unit, a hospital ward, or at home? and (4) How should the patient be monitored, and what is the appropriate follow-up? The four management decisions—stabilization, hospitalization, specific treatment, and follow-up—are identified in each algorithm. A very severely ill patient should be hospitalized in an intensive care unit. Stabilization should include respiratory, circulatory, and neurologic support. The goal of stabilization is to maintain tissue oxygenation, especially to the brain and other vital organs. Tissue oxygenation depends on the delivery of oxygen to the tissue. It requires a functioning respiratory system including the airway and lungs, adequate circulatory blood volume, a functioning pump (heart), and adequate oxygen-carrying capacity (hemoglobin). It is therefore essential to maintain the ABCs (airway, breathing, and cardiac functions). In stabilizing a patient, establish an open airway, deliver oxygen, and assess air exchange (breathing). When exchange is inadequate, consider intubation and ventilation. Circulatory support is needed when hypotension or signs of poor perfusion are present. These signs include pale or mottled skin, coolness of the extremities, and capillary refill prolonged beyond 2 seconds. The initial phase of circulatory support is intravenous fluids. Additional pharmacologic treatment may be necessary. Severe anemia or hemorrhage requires the replacement of hemoglobin as well as volume with whole blood or packed blood cell transfusions. Some children with seizures or signs of neurologic dysfunction need neurologic support. This may include the administration of rapid-acting anticonvulsants and the rapid correction of any metabolic disturbance, such as hypoglycemia or electrolyte abnormalities. Always include a plan to monitor and assess the response to therapy. In many circumstances, the follow-up is the most important part of the management plan. Informing the family and patient and introducing shared decision making is an important component of any management plan. Proper education of the patient and family is the essential element in the follow-up plan. It must receive the attention that it deserves.

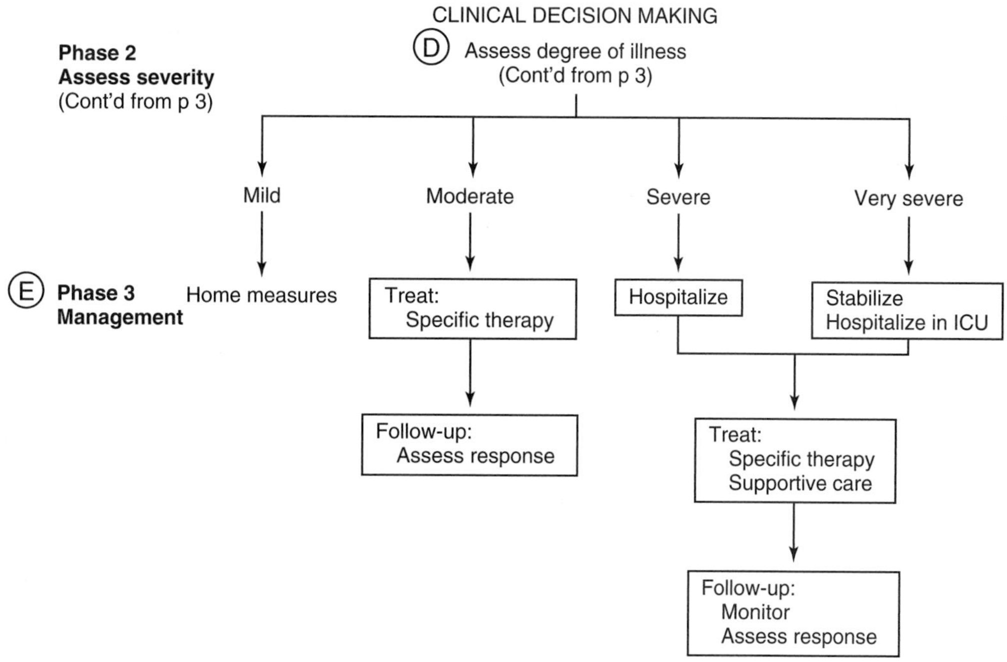
CLINICAL DECISION MAKING
Phase 2
Assess severity
(Cont'd from p 3)
D Assess degree of illness
(Cont'd from p 3)
Mild
Moderate
Severe
Very severe
E Phase 3
Management
Home measures
Treat:
Specific therapy
Hospitalize
Stabilize
Hospitalize in ICU
Follow-up:
Assess response
Treat:
Specific therapy
Supportive care
Follow-up:
Monitor
Assess response

PRESENTING COMPLAINTS

GENERAL

Anaphylaxis
Growth Deficiency/Failure to Thrive
Crying: Acute, Excessive
Generalized Lymphadenopathy
Obesity
Polyuria and Polydipsia
Shock
Syncope

Anaphylaxis

Marion R. Sills, MD, MPH

Anaphylaxis is an acute, potentially life-threatening allergic reaction with varied mechanisms and clinical presentations. Depending on the route of exposure to the inciting agent, symptoms can begin in minutes to hours; reactions within 3 hours of exposure are usually more severe.

A1. and B1. On brief, initial history and physical examination, assess for the following clinical criteria for diagnosing anaphylaxis, which must include one of the following three criteria:

1. Acute onset of illness involving skin/mucosal urticaria, pruritus, or swelling AND at least one of the following:
   a. Respiratory compromise
   b. Hypotension/hypoperfusion
2. Two or more of the following occurring rapidly after exposure to a likely allergen for that patient:
   a. Skin/mucosal urticaria, pruritus, or swelling
   b. Respiratory compromise
   c. Hypotension/hypoperfusion
   d. Persistent gastrointestinal symptoms.
3. Hypotension/hypoperfusion after exposure to a *known* allergen for that patient

A2. When necessary, stabilize the child before obtaining a history. When appropriate, attempt to determine the offending agent and the onset and progression of symptoms. Assess upper airway involvement by asking about pruritus or swelling of lips and tongue, throat tightness, stridor, dysphonia, or dysphagia; lower respiratory tract symptoms by cough, wheezing, dyspnea, or sense of chest tightness; cardiovascular abnormalities by tachycardia, syncope, or dizziness; central nervous system abnormalities by dizziness, syncope, altered mental status, or seizures; gastrointestinal symptoms of nausea, vomiting, abdominal cramps, and diarrhea; and cutaneous symptoms of hives (urticaria) or angioedema of the face or extremities. Note any prior history of atopy, including anaphylaxis, asthma, and eczema or hives. Note any associated chronic conditions, acute illnesses, and medications.

B2. Initially, assess and stabilize airway, breathing, circulation, and level of consciousness before a more detailed physical examination. Assess the upper and lower airway, looking for swelling of lips or tongue, stridor, dysphonia, hypoxia, cough, tachypnea, wheezing, retractions, and poor aeration. Evaluate the cardiovascular system for tachycardia, decreased peripheral perfusion, arrhythmias, and hypotension. Central nervous system signs include altered mental status and seizure activity; either may indicate hypoxia or hypoperfusion.

B3. After first assessing and stabilizing airway, breathing, circulation, and level of consciousness, a more complete physical examination should include examination of the skin for urticaria or angioedema and the gastrointestinal system for abdominal tenderness.

C1. If this primary survey shows any compromise, immediately begin epinephrine, oxygen, and volume replacement. Epinephrine can be given intramuscularly (preferred) or subcutaneously, every 5 minutes to control hypotension and airway edema. Although not evidence based, nebulized, sublingual, intraosseous, and endotracheal routes can also be considered. Administer oxygen to patients with evidence of airway involvement, or who require multiple doses of epinephrine or other β agonists.

C2. Patients with upper airway compromise require immediate airway management. Consider early intubation in patients with rapid onset of symptoms, prior anaphylaxis, and upper airway swelling, because airway edema can progress rapidly, making intubation increasingly difficult. Stridor, hypoxia, and respiratory distress are all late signs of upper airway compromise. If intubation is unsuccessful, consider attempting a cricothyrotomy. Although it has not been specifically studied in this context, some authors recommend concomitant nebulized epinephrine.

C3. Because plasma volume may decline suddenly by 50% in anaphylaxis syndrome, give poorly perfused patients aggressive fluid resuscitation, starting with a rapid saline fluid bolus of 20 ml/kg, repeated as necessary. Patients should be placed in the recumbent position with legs elevated, unless precluded by dyspnea or vomiting. If shock persists, consider a continuous infusion of epinephrine (0.1 μg/kg/min, titrated up to 1.0 μg/kg/min). For patients with persistent hypotension, start vasopressors (see Shock, p. 32).

C4. If response to volume replacement is inadequate, consider administering epinephrine intravenously, either through repeated dosing or via an infusion. Note that intravenous administration of epinephrine increases the risk for arrhythmia, so it should be used only in patients with hypotension who have not responded successfully to intramuscular epinephrine and volume replacement. If response to crystalloid infusion is inadequate, also consider colloid infusion.

C5. For bronchospasm refractory to epinephrine, treat with supplemental oxygen, as well as bronchodilators, such as albuterol and/or ipratropium, and corticosteroids. For patients taking beta-blocking agents, which may attenuate the response to treatment, consider glucagon administration.

C6. Assess the organ systems involved, as well as the degree of severity and progression. The first-line therapies for anaphylaxis are epinephrine, oxygen, and volume replacement. Consider giving an H1-receptor

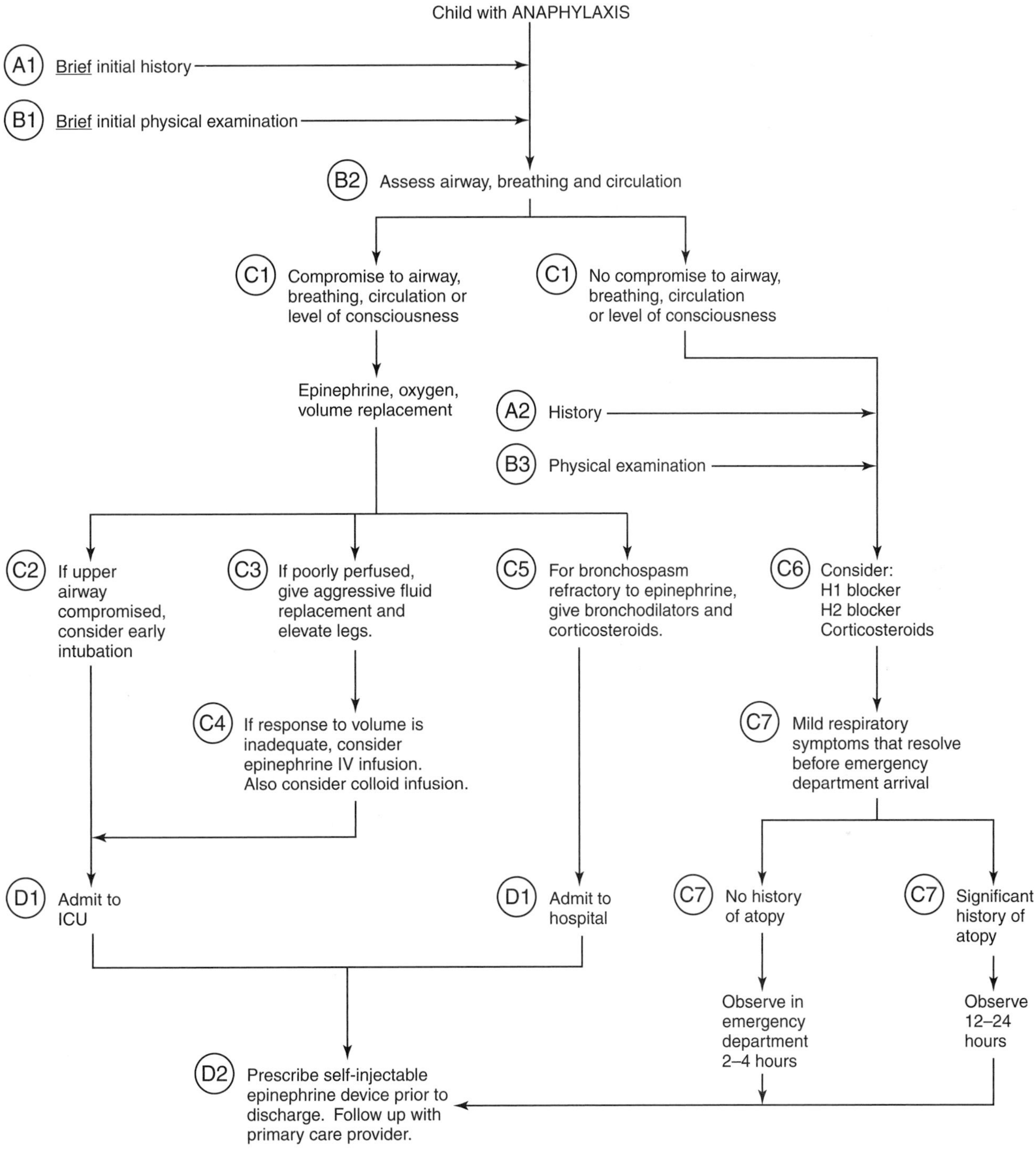
Child with ANAPHYLAXIS
A1 Brief initial history
B1 Brief initial physical examination
B2 Assess airway, breathing and circulation
C1 Compromise to airway, breathing, circulation or level of consciousness
C1 No compromise to airway, breathing, circulation or level of consciousness
Epinephrine, oxygen, volume replacement
A2 History
B3 Physical examination
C2 If upper airway compromised, consider early intubation
C3 If poorly perfused, give aggressive fluid replacement and elevate legs.
C5 For bronchospasm refractory to epinephrine, give bronchodilators and corticosteroids.
C6 Consider: H1 blocker H2 blocker Corticosteroids
C4 If response to volume is inadequate, consider epinephrine IV infusion. Also consider colloid infusion.
C7 Mild respiratory symptoms that resolve before emergency department arrival
D1 Admit to ICU
D1 Admit to hospital
C7 No history of atopy
C7 Significant history of atopy
Observe in emergency department 2–4 hours
Observe 12–24 hours
D2 Prescribe self-injectable epinephrine device prior to discharge. Follow up with primary care provider.

antihistamine, such as diphenhydramine, and an H2-receptor antihistamine, such as cimetidine or ranitidine; these work synergistically with the epinephrine therapy, but are considered second-line therapy to epinephrine, and should never be used alone in the treatment of anaphylaxis. Corticosteroids do not take effect during initial resuscitative efforts; their early use can help reduce the incidence and severity of late-phase reactions (Table 1).

C7. Patients with a history of mild symptoms that have resolved before arrival in the emergency department may be discharged home after a short observation period (2–4 hours). Observe patients with a significant history of atopy (asthma, allergic rhinitis) for 12 to 24 hours because they are at increased risk for a late-phase reaction.

D1. Hospitalize any patient with significant symptoms of laryngeal edema or hypotension. Consider intensive care unit admission for patients requiring more than one dose of epinephrine.

D2. Before discharge, patients diagnosed with anaphylaxis should: (1) be prescribed a self-injectable epinephrine device (one for each location—school, home, child care, etc.) and instructed in its use; (2) receive information regarding avoidance of the precipitating allergen; and (3) be advised to follow up with their primary care provider and consider follow-up evaluation with an allergist.

Table 1. **Drugs Used in the Treatment of Anaphylaxis**

Drug	Dosage
Sympathomimetic Agents	
Epinephrine	Initial treatment: 0.01 mg/kg, IM (maximum: 0.5 mg/dose) q5min Hypoperfused patient: 0.01 mg/kg/dose, IV/IO Continuous infusion: 0.1–1 μg/kg/min, IV/IO Nebulized: 0.5 ml/kg of 1:1000 in 2.5 ml normal saline (maximum: <4 yr, 2.5 ml/dose; ≥4 yr, 5 ml/dose) Nebulized racemic epinephrine: 2.25%, 0.5 ml in 2.5 ml normal saline
Other Inotropic Agent	
Glucagon	Children <20 kg: 0.5 mg/dose, SC/IV/IM q20min (or 0.02–0.03 mg/kg/dose) Children ≥20 kg and adults: 1 mg/dose IM/IV/SC q20min
Histamine-1 Antagonists	
Diphenhydramine	1 mg/kg/dose, PO/IV/IM/IO q6h (maximum: 50 mg/dose)
Hydroxyzine	0.5–1 mg/kg/dose, PO/IM q6h IV/SC administration associated with thrombosis
Histamine-2 Antagonists	
Ranitidine	0.75–1.5 mg/kg/dose, IV/IM/IO q6–8h (maximum: 6 mg/kg/day) 1.5–2.5 mg/kg/dose, PO q8–12h (maximum: 6 mg/kg/day)
Cimetidine	5–10 mg/kg/dose, PO/IV/IM/IO q6–12h (maximum: 2400 mg/day)
Bronchodilators	
Albuterol	Intermittent nebulization <12 yr: 2.5 mg neb q20min ≥12 yr: 5 mg neb q20min Continuous nebulization: 0.5 mg/kg/hr (maximum: 15 mg/hr)
Ipratropium	Intermittent nebulization <12 yr: 250 μg neb q20min ≥12 yr: 500 μg neb q20min
Corticosteroids	
Dexamethasone	0.3–0.6 mg/kg, PO IV/IM (maximum: 10 mg)
Methylprednisolone	Loading dose: 2 mg/kg × 1 Maintenance: 0.5 mg/kg/dose q6h
Prednisone	2 mg/kg/24 hr PO ÷ qd–bid (maximum dose: 80 mg)

IM, intramuscularly; *IO*, intraosseous; *IV*, intravenously; *PO*, orally; *SC*, subcutaneously.

References

Krounse JH, Derebery MJ, Chadwick SJ. Managing the allergic patient. New York: Elsevier Inc; 2008.

Lieberman P, Kemp S, Oppenheimer J, et al. The diagnosis and management of anaphylaxis: an updated practice parameter. Joint Task Force on Practice Parameters, Work Group on Diagnosis and Management of Anaphylaxis. J Allergy Clin Immunol 2005;115: S483–S523.

Marx JA. Rosen's emergency medicine: concepts and clinical practice. 6th ed. St. Louis: Mosby; 2008.

Sampson HA, Muñoz-Furlong A, Campbell RL, et al. Second Symposium on the Definition and Management of Anaphylaxis: summary report—Second National Institute of Allergy and Infectious Disease/ Food Allergy and Anaphylaxis Network symposium. J Allergy Clin Immunol 2006;117:391-7.

Waibel KH. Anaphylaxis. Pediatr Rev 2008;29(8):255–63; quiz 263.

Growth Deficiency/ Failure to Thrive

Janine Young, MD

Growth deficiency/failure to thrive (FTT) is not a diagnosis in and of itself but rather a sign of poor growth in infancy based on inadequate weight gain for age and height. There is no universally accepted criteria or name for growth deficiency in infancy; however, the more common definitions used include: (1) a full-term infant younger than 2 years whose weight is below the 3rd to 5th percentile for age at more than one visit (and not small for gestational age or with intrauterine growth retardation), or (2) an infant younger than 2 years whose weight crosses two major percentiles downward on a standard growth chart. In more severe cases of FTT, particularly if chronic, height velocity slows followed by decreasing head circumference growth. In severe cases of malnutrition, weight, height, and head circumference measurements may decline below the 3rd percentile. Significant malnutrition may result in marasmus or kwashiorkor.

A. Given that inadequate caloric intake is the most common cause of FTT, obtain a detailed nutritional history. Determine the frequency and quantity of milk the infant is taking, and whether it is breast milk, formula, or whole milk, depending on age. In a breast-fed newborn, assure proper latch and adequate milk production. If formula-fed, assure proper mixing of formula. In older infants, assure adequate, though not excessive, milk intake, given that by 9 months of age, infants should begin to transition to an increased intake of solid foods. Ask about supplemental beverages at all ages, given that some families may give water, tea, juice, or sugar-laden drinks to even newborns. Determine whether soft solids have been introduced between 4 and 6 months of age, and that solids are advanced and offered at mealtimes after that time. If financial constraints are affecting feeding patterns, refer to the local Woman, Infant, and Children (WIC) program, as well as any other programs available to support the family. Ask about early feeding patterns. Was the infant able to latch to the breast or bottle at birth and did he/she have coordinated sucking and swallowing? Was the infant fussy with feedings or have reflux? There is a critical window to establish normal feeding patterns, and if these patterns are not established within the first year, it is much more difficult to "teach" feeding. If such a history is obtained, it is important to establish early and regular occupational and nutritional therapy, preferably in the home.

Ensure that the infant is fed on a regular basis appropriate for age. For toddlers, advise that they should be fed seated at the table with no distractions (e.g., not in front of the TV) and should be given foods before liquids. Toddlers with FTT should be offered three high-calorie meals and three high-calorie snacks per day, as opposed to "grazing" behavior, where the toddler is snacking on small amounts of food all day, which may suppress appetite.

Obtain a detailed medical history. Is the infant developmentally appropriate for age? Note the frequency of intercurrent acute or chronic illnesses, such as otitis media, severe atopic dermatitis, vomiting, diarrhea, respiratory, or urinary tract infection (though urinary tract infections may be occult in cases of FTT). Are there predisposing medical conditions that may cause inadequate calorie intake, such as cleft lip/palate, micrognathia, cerebral palsy or other central nervous system disorder causing hypotonia or hypertonia? Has there been recent travel to a developing country, which could result in a parasitic infection and inadequate calorie absorption? Or are there increased calorie requirements from chronic or recurrent infections or endocrinopathies? Note: "Nonorganic" FTT stemming from psychosocial stressors can easily lead to "organic" FTT, where the infant acquires dysfunctional feeding patterns and vitamin deficiencies secondary to this decreased intake. Similarly, "organic" FTT can result in increased psychosocial stressors at home and lead to some component of environmental "nonorganic" FTT. Given this continuum, it is essential to address all aspects of feeding, including psychosocial issues and stressors, regardless of whether the infant ultimately is diagnosed with a primary "organic" or "nonorganic" FTT.

Determine whether any medicines, nutritional supplements, or home remedies are being given. Some medications have adverse effects such as anorexia, which may lead to FTT. Ensure that supplements and home remedies given are appropriate.

Explore the family history for such diagnoses as inadequate growth, metabolic disorders, genetic syndromes, and fetal, neonatal, or infant demise.

Determine whether there are psychosocial stressors/environmental issues at home that may affect the feeding schedule and relationship between caregivers and the infant. Assess the mother–child/father–child interaction and level of family functioning. Is the family food insecure? Have there been many missed appointments or inadequate well-child care visits? Are immunizations up to date? Are there any red flags pointing to abuse? If environmental stressors or frank abuse are suspected, have a low threshold to refer to social work or to child protective services to obtain adequate support and interventions as needed.

Patient with GROWTH DEFICIENCY OR FAILURE TO THRIVE*

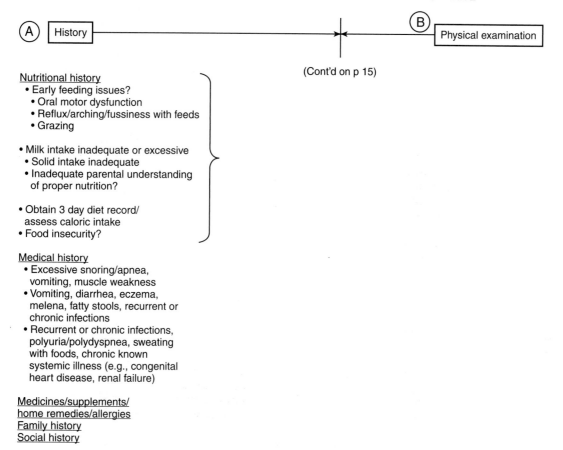

(A) History

(B) Physical examination

(Cont'd on p 15)

<u>Nutritional history</u>
- Early feeding issues?
  - Oral motor dysfunction
  - Reflux/arching/fussiness with feeds
  - Grazing

- Milk intake inadequate or excessive
  - Solid intake inadequate
  - Inadequate parental understanding of proper nutrition?

- Obtain 3 day diet record/ assess caloric intake
- Food insecurity?

<u>Medical history</u>
- Excessive snoring/apnea, vomiting, muscle weakness
- Vomiting, diarrhea, eczema, melena, fatty stools, recurrent or chronic infections
- Recurrent or chronic infections, polyuria/polydyspnea, sweating with foods, chronic known systemic illness (e.g., congenital heart disease, renal failure)

<u>Medicines/supplements/ home remedies/allergies</u>
<u>Family history</u>
<u>Social history</u>

*Failure to thrive has become a legal term indicating neglect or abuse. It should not be used as a diagnosis when neglect or abuse is not evident.

B. A complete physical examination should include evaluation of the child's or infant's developmental status. Ensure that the child/infant is developmentally normal for age. Note signs of neglect or abuse. Note such findings as dysmorphic features, cardiac murmurs, hepatosplenomegaly, hypotonia or hypertonia, lymphadenopathy, among others.

Consider early referral to a nutritionist and occupational therapist well-versed in working with young infants and children. A several-day calorie count may help in working up an infant with FTT. If the calorie counts are adequate, consider organic diagnoses that lead to decreased calorie absorption or increased calorie needs. However, as noted earlier, organic diseases may ultimately lead to inadequate calorie intake, given that chronic poor nutrition and vitamin deficiencies may result in the suppression of appetite.

When organic causes of FTT are of concern, almost any systemic illness may be the culprit. Therefore, working up an infant for FTT should be approached in a stepwise, logical fashion, instead of testing widely.

C. If inadequate calorie intake is suspected as the primary cause of FTT, consider psychosocial/environmental issues such as poverty/food insecurity (e.g., diluting formula), Münchausen syndrome by proxy (medical child abuse), or inadequate understanding of proper nutrition for age. Some infants may have oral motor dysfunction or neurologic dysregulation of hunger leading to early satiety. Cleft lip/palate, micrognathia, adenoid hypertrophy, or vascular rings/slings may lead to oral motor dysfunction and/or mechanical obstruction and inadequate calorie consumption. Cerebral palsy or other central nervous system disorders may lead to hypotonia or hypertonia and uncoordinated feeding patterns. Myopathy, metabolic disorders, lead toxicity, zinc deficiency, and severe iron deficiency anemia may lead to weakness, limiting adequate calorie intake. Hydrocephalus, pyloric stenosis, gastroesophageal reflux, and food allergies may cause vomiting sufficient to cause weight loss.

D. Inadequate calorie absorption should be considered in select cases, including diagnoses such as milk protein intolerance, food allergy, celiac disease, cystic fibrosis, metabolic disorders, immunodeficiencies, inflammatory bowel disease, and parasitic infections.

E. Increased calorie requirements may occur when an infant has a chronic systemic disease causing a hypermetabolic state, such as congenital heart disease, chronic/recurrent infection such as HIV, tuberculosis or urinary tract infections, chronic respiratory diseases, malignancy, endocrine disorders (such as hyperthyroidism or diabetes mellitus), or renal tubular acidosis.

(Continued on page 16)

Patient with GROWTH DEFICIENCY OR FAILURE TO THRIVE*
(Cont'd from p 13)

(C) Inadequate caloric intake

Depending on history, consider:

Oralmotor dysfunction/obstruction
- Cleft lip/palate
- Micrognathia
- Adenoid hypertrophy
- Vascular rings/slings
- Cerebral palsy

Emesis
- Hydrocephalus
- Pyloric stenosis
- GER
- Food allergies

Weakness
- Metabolic disorder
- Myopathy
- Lead intoxication
- Severe anemia

Assess amount of food offered

Inadequate

Assess parents' understanding of nutrition (cont'd on p 17)

Adequate

Adequate caloric intake; assess for organic disease

(D) Inadequate caloric absorption

Consider:
- Milk protein intolerance
- Food allergy
- Celiac disease
- Cystic fibrosis
- Metabolic disorder
- Immunodeficiency
- Inflammatory bowel disease
- Parasitic infection

(E) Increased calorie requirements/hypermetabolic state

Consider:
- Congenital heart disease
- HIV, TB
- Occult UTI
- Malignancy
- Endocrinopathies
- RTA

Assess family function and eating behaviors (cont'd on p 17)

*Failure to thrive has become a legal term indicating neglect or abuse. It should not be used as a diagnosis when neglect or abuse is not evident.

F. If there is concern for organic FTT but no obvious causative factor, consider a "general" laboratory screen for occult illness, including complete blood cell count and differential, metabolic panel (including electrolytes, blood urea nitrogen, creatinine, liver function tests), simultaneous urinalysis (for renal tubular acidosis), erythrocyte sedimentation rate, and/or lead level. Tuberculosis should be considered, especially in immigrant populations.

Unless there are signs and symptoms consistent with a particular organic causative factor for FTT, an extensive laboratory/radiologic workup is not worthwhile. However, if a child does not gain adequate weight after initial nutritional interventions, consider further studies, based on a review of signs and symptoms.

Infants with mild-to-moderate malnutrition should be managed closely as outpatients to document appropriate catch-up growth. Initially, weekly or bimonthly visits are often needed. Once a stable increase in growth over several months is noted, continued regular visits every 2 to 3 months are appropriate to ensure continued progress.

G. A secondary screen for more severe FTT with other specific signs and symptoms could include prealbumin and albumin, free thyroxine, thyroid-stimulating hormone, serum amino acids, urine organic acids, pyruvate, lactate, ammonia, sweat chloride test, HIV, IgA, anti-tissue transglutaminase and anti-endomysial antibodies, immunoglobulins, alkaline phosphatase, calcium, phosphorus, bone age, upper gastrointestinal study/swallow study, or chest radiograph.

Hospitalization of an infant with severe FTT and/or where abuse or neglect is suspected is often necessary to help quickly coordinate services, including gathering input from nutritional and occupational therapists, social workers, and child protective services, as well as obtaining any studies that need to be done while inhouse. A multidisciplinary approach is often key in these cases. However, notably, appropriate or inappropriate weight gain while hospitalized does not help distinguish between organic and nonorganic causes of FTT. Once discharged, home visits by a visiting nurse, nutritionist, and/or occupational therapist provide ongoing support to the family and invaluable insight to clinicians regarding the home environment.

Some general pearls for managing infants with FTT:

1. Consider zinc sulfate supplementation in any infant with FTT, as well as initiating higher calorie formula, breast milk, or whole milk, as appropriate for age.
2. Average daily weight gain for infants and toddlers: 0 to 3 months, 26 to 31 g/day; 3 to 6 months, 17 to 18 g/day; 6 to 9 months, 12 to 13 g/day; 9 to 12 months, 9 to 13 g/day; 12 months to 3 years, 7 to 9 g/day.
3. Increasing calories in formula: 20 kcal/oz: 1 scoop of formula to 2 oz water; 22 kcal/oz: 1 scoop of powdered formula to 1.8 oz water; 24 kcal/oz: 1 scoop of formula to 1.6 oz water.
4. Increasing calories in breast milk: 22 kcal/oz: 4 oz breast milk to 3 ml (¾ tsp) powdered formula; 24 kcal/oz: 4 oz breast milk to 6 ml (1.5 tsp) formula; 26 kcal/oz: 4 oz breast milk to 9 ml (2 tsp) formula.

References

Adedoyin O, Gottlieb B, Frank R, et al. Evaluation of failure to thrive: diagnostic yield of testing for renal tubular acidosis. Pediatrics 2003;112:e463.

Berwick DM, Levy JC, Kleinerman R. Failure to thrive: diagnostic yield of hospitalisation. Arch Dis Child 1982;57:347–51.

Daniel M, Kleis L, Cemeroglu AP. Etiology of failure to thrive in infants and toddlers referred to a pediatric endocrinology outpatient clinic. Clin Pediatr 2008;47:762–5.

Failure to thrive. In: Ronald E. Kleinman, editor. Pediatric nutrition handbook. 6th ed. Elk Grove Village (IL): American Academy of Pediatrics; 2009. p. 601–36.

Frank D. Failure to thrive. In: Developmental and behavioral pediatrics: a handbook for primary care. 2nd ed. Philadelphia: Lippincott Williams & Wilkins; 2004. p. 183.

Heptinstall E, Puckering C, Skuse D, et al. Nutrition and mealtime behaviour in families of growth-retarded children. Hum Nutr Appl Nutr 1987;41A:390–402.

Pediatric feeding and swallowing disorders. In: Ronald E. Kleinman, editor. Pediatric nutrition handbook. 6th ed. Elk Grove Village (IL): American Academy of Pediatrics; 2009. p. 577–99.

Pugliese MT, Wayman-Dawn M, Moses N, Lifshitz F. Parental health beliefs as a cause of nonorganic failure to thrive. Pediatrics 1987;80:175.

Sills RH. Failure to thrive: the role of clinical and laboratory evaluation. Am J Dis Child 1978;132:967.

Smith MM, Lifshitz F. Excess fruit juice consumption as a contributing factor in nonorganic failure to thrive. Pediatrics 1994;93:438–43.

Tolia V. Very early onset nonorganic failure to thrive in infants. J Pediatr Gastroenterol Nutr 1995;20:73–80.

Walravens PA, Hambidge KM, Koepfer DM. Zinc supplementation in infants with a nutritional pattern of failure to thrive: a double-blind, controlled study. Pediatrics 1989;83:532–8.

Weston JA, Colloton M. A legacy of violence in nonorganic failure to thrive. Child Abuse Negl 1993;17:709.

Zenel JA. Failure to thrive: a general pediatrician's perspective. Pediatr Rev 1997:18:371–8.

Patient with GROWTH DEFICIENCY OR FAILURE TO THRIVE*

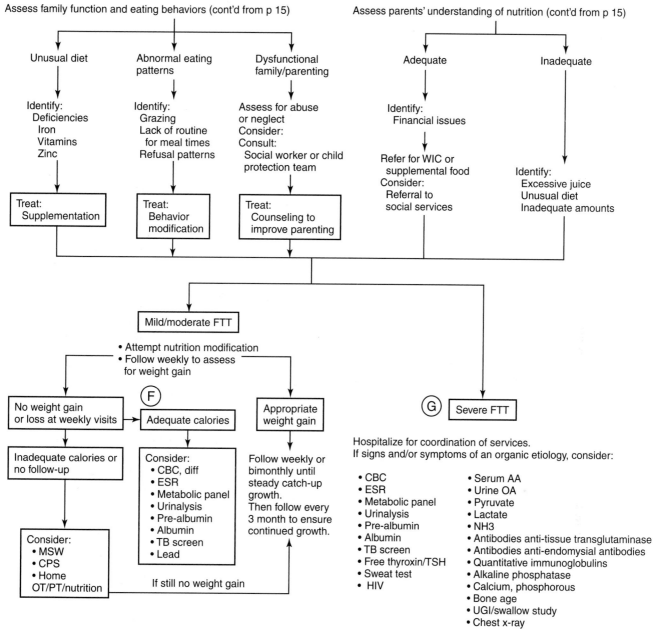

Assess family function and eating behaviors (cont'd from p 15)

- Unusual diet
  - Identify:
    - Deficiencies
      - Iron
      - Vitamins
      - Zinc
  - Treat: Supplementation
- Abnormal eating patterns
  - Identify:
    - Grazing
    - Lack of routine for meal times
    - Refusal patterns
  - Treat: Behavior modification
- Dysfunctional family/parenting
  - Assess for abuse or neglect
  - Consider:
  - Consult:
    - Social worker or child protection team
  - Treat: Counseling to improve parenting

Assess parents' understanding of nutrition (cont'd from p 15)

- Adequate
  - Identify:
    - Financial issues
  - Refer for WIC or supplemental food
  - Consider:
    - Referral to social services
- Inadequate
  - Identify:
    - Excessive juice
    - Unusual diet
    - Inadequate amounts

Mild/moderate FTT

- Attempt nutrition modification
- Follow weekly to assess for weight gain

No weight gain or loss at weekly visits → Adequate calories

Inadequate calories or no follow-up

Consider:
- MSW
- CPS
- Home OT/PT/nutrition

If still no weight gain → Follow weekly or bimonthly until steady catch-up growth.

(F) **Adequate calories**

Consider:
- CBC, diff
- ESR
- Metabolic panel
- Urinalysis
- Pre-albumin
- Albumin
- TB screen
- Lead

Appropriate weight gain

Follow weekly or bimonthly until steady catch-up growth. Then follow every 3 month to ensure continued growth.

(G) **Severe FTT**

Hospitalize for coordination of services.
If signs and/or symptoms of an organic etiology, consider:

- CBC
- ESR
- Metabolic panel
- Urinalysis
- Pre-albumin
- Albumin
- TB screen
- Free thyroxin/TSH
- Sweat test
- HIV
- Serum AA
- Urine OA
- Pyruvate
- Lactate
- NH3
- Antibodies anti-tissue transglutaminase
- Antibodies anti-endomysial antibodies
- Quantitative immunoglobulins
- Alkaline phosphatase
- Calcium, phosphorous
- Bone age
- UGI/swallow study
- Chest x-ray

*Failure to thrive has become a legal term indicating neglect or abuse. It should not be used as a diagnosis when neglect or abuse is not evident.

Crying: Acute, Excessive

Steven R. Poole, MD

DEFINITION

Acute, excessive crying manifests in infants with the sudden onset of crying or fussiness without fever, for which there is no cause that is obvious to the parents. The differential diagnosis includes a variety of harmless causes and a number of serious ones (Tables 1 and 2).

A. In the patient's history, ask about previous episodes, recent immunization, medications, constipation, emesis, diarrhea, blood in the stool, fever, trauma, overstimulation, changes in diet, possible ingestion, the child's location at the onset, and any suspicions the parents may have. The parents' suspicions are correct less than half of the times when they have a strong suspicion. The consolability and time of onset do not appear to correlate with the severity of the cause. History will reveal helpful clues 20% of the time, but will also uncover symptoms that may be unrelated to the correct diagnosis 20% of the time. Therefore, carefully corroborate clues in the history with appropriate physical examination or testing.

B. Physical examination alone will identify a cause approximately 40% of the time. The physical examination must be meticulous and should include assessment of the level of toxicity, complete inspection of every bit of the surface of the infant's body, careful palpation of the body for subtle signs of tenderness, otoscopy, eversion of the eyelids, fluorescein staining of the corneas, complete observation of the oropharynx (consider using a laryngoscope), careful abdominal examination, rectal examination with Hematest of the stool, auscultation of the heart, retinal examination, and careful neurologic and developmental assessment. A bruise, bite, or hair tourniquet may be hiding under clothing. Fractures may present without visible swelling and may be diagnosed only on careful palpation and observation. Corneal abrasion most often causes only crying, without tearing, blepharospasm, or conjunctival redness. Pharyngeal foreign bodies may not be visible without a laryngoscope. Retinal hemorrhages may be the only physical sign of shaking injury or head trauma.

C. When the diagnosis is apparent on physical examination, treat accordingly, keeping in mind that 5% of patients have two causes of fussiness. Follow-up contact should be maintained until crying has ceased. When you suspect a particular diagnosis but are not certain, keep in mind that the differential includes many serious conditions. Therefore, it is dangerous to jump to a diagnosis based only on suspicion. A brief period of observation may be necessary to confirm the suspicion.

D. Many infants have ceased crying by the time they are seen by the physician and the crying does not recur. This syndrome is called *idiopathic acute crying episode.* It must include the following elements: unalarming history, normal findings on physical examination, cessation of crying before the physician is seen, lack of signs of toxicity, and no subsequent episodes. The parents can be reassured, and the infant can be observed at home. However, if the crying resumes, the infant should be re-examined.

E. The cause may not be apparent after the initial history and physical examination of as many as one in three infants with this type of episode. Infants who continue to cry and have no apparent diagnosis on initial examination often have a serious cause requiring specific treatment. Screening tests are of limited value; only urinalysis and urine culture have been shown to be effective. A period of observation lasting 1 to 2 hours with repeated observation and examination (including all of the special examinations described earlier) will often uncover clues to the diagnosis. For many infants, crying is the first symptom of an illness that will manifest other more helpful signs or symptoms in a matter of hours (i.e., gastroenteritis, viral exanthems, enanthems, infectious illnesses, intussusception, encephalitis).

F. Some infants cease crying during the observation. The infant should be observed for a time because many serious causes have temporary asymptomatic periods.

G. For infants who continue to cry or fuss and for whom the diagnosis remains in question, consider additional studies that are both invasive and expensive. Follow clues or instincts in selecting from this list: skeletal radiographs, lumbar puncture, barium enema study, computed tomographic scan of the head, electrolytes and pH, toxicology, electrocardiography or echocardiography, pulse oximetry, and foreign body radiologic series. It is unwise to discharge an infant with acute, excessive, unexplained crying before making a diagnosis. Therefore, many of these infants must be observed longer.

H. Colic includes all of the following: (1) recurrent spells of excessive crying or fussiness, (2) occurrence at predictable times more than 3 days a week, (3) duration of 3 or more hours a day, (4) initiation in the first 3 weeks of life and resolution by 3 to 4 months of age, (5) an infant who is eating well and is developing and growing normally, (6) no other concerning symptoms, and (7) normal findings on physical examination by the physician. Without each of the seven elements described, the diagnosis should not be made. Therefore, it is difficult to make the diagnosis with complete confidence on the first night of colic, and follow-up is needed to confirm it.

I. Soothing techniques include rhythmic motion such as rocking and stroller or car rides; monotonous noise from a radio, tape, or clock; a pacifier; and warm water bottle next to the abdomen. Being carried in a sack may help. Parents may need support for leaving the infant with a baby-sitter for an evening out. The effectiveness of formula changes is unclear. Pharmacologic therapy should be discouraged.

(Continued on page 20)

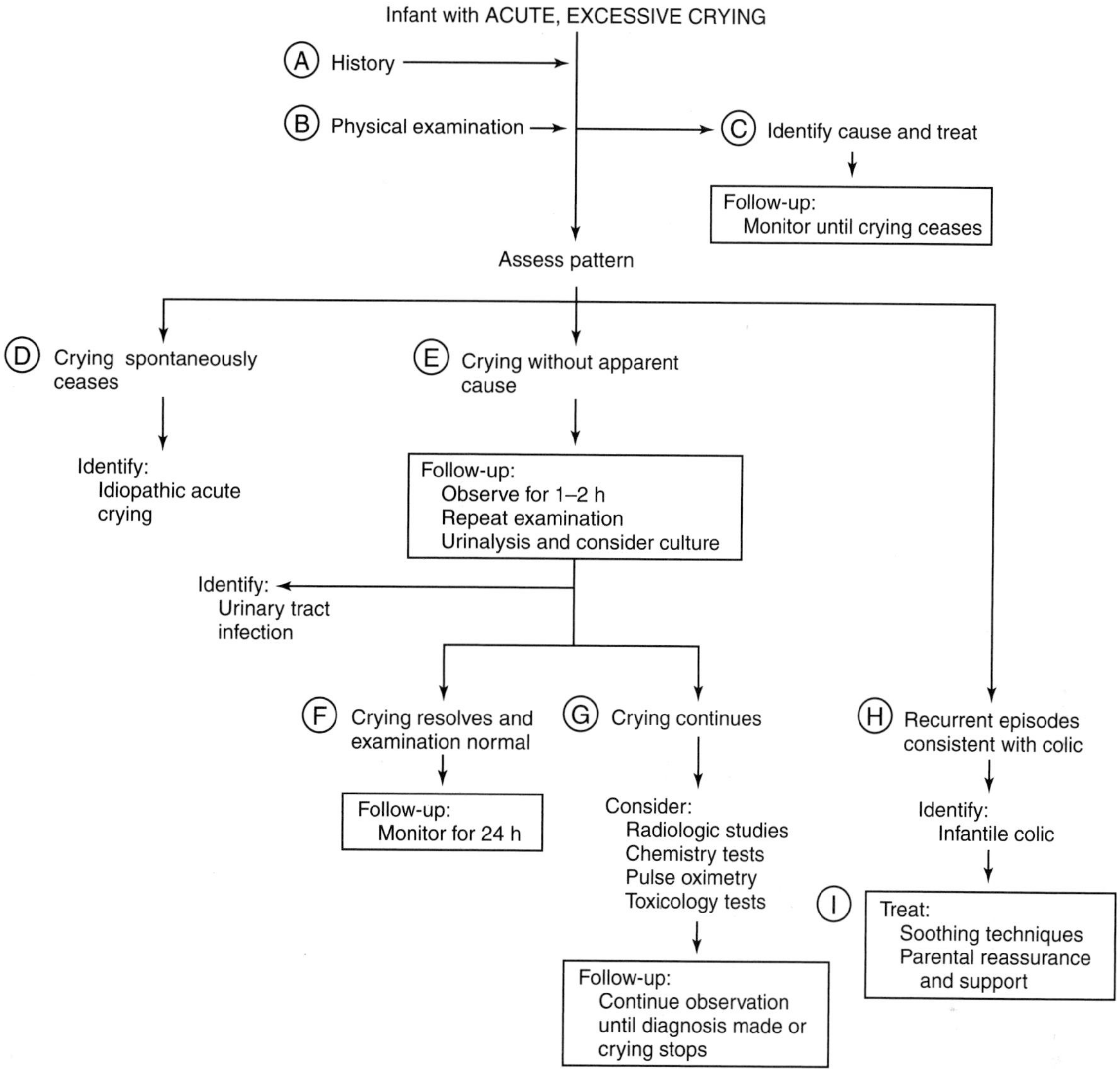
Infant with ACUTE, EXCESSIVE CRYING
A History
B Physical examination
C Identify cause and treat
Follow-up:
Monitor until crying ceases
Assess pattern
D Crying spontaneously ceases
Identify:
Idiopathic acute crying
E Crying without apparent cause
Follow-up:
Observe for 1–2 h
Repeat examination
Urinalysis and consider culture
Identify:
Urinary tract infection
F Crying resolves and examination normal
Follow-up:
Monitor for 24 h
G Crying continues
Consider:
Radiologic studies
Chemistry tests
Pulse oximetry
Toxicology tests
Follow-up:
Continue observation until diagnosis made or crying stops
H Recurrent episodes consistent with colic
Identify:
Infantile colic
I
Treat:
Soothing techniques
Parental reassurance and support

Table 1. **Diagnoses in 56 Infants with an Episode of Unexplained Excessive Crying**

Diagnosis	No. with Diagnosis
Idiopathic	10
Colic	6
Infectious Causes	
Otitis media*	10
Viral illness with anorexia, dehydration*	2
Urinary tract infection*	1
Mild prodrome of gastroenteritis	1
Herpangina*	1
Herpes stomatitis*	1
Trauma	
Corneal abrasion*	3
Foreign body in eye*	1
Foreign body in oropharynx*	1
Tibial fracture*	1
Clavicular fracture*	1
Brown recluse spider bite*	1
Hair tourniquet syndrome (toe)*	1
Gastrointestinal Tract	
Constipation	3
Intussusception*	1
Gastroesophageal reflux and esophagitis*	1
Central Nervous System	
Subdural hematoma*	1
Encephalitis*	1
Pseudotumor cerebri*	1
Drug Reaction or Overdose	
DTP reaction*	1
Inadvertent pseudoephedrine overdose*	1
Behavioral	
Night terrors	1
Overstimulation	1
Cardiovascular	
Supraventricular tachycardia*	2
Metabolic	
Glutaric aciduria, type I*	1
Total	**56**

*Conditions considered serious.

DTP, Diphtheria-tetanus-pertussis vaccine.

From Poole SR. The infant with acute, unexplained crying. Pediatrics 1991;88:450. By permission.

Table 2. **Differential Diagnosis of 200 Infants Younger Than 24 Months with Excessive Crying, by Age Group**

		AGE			
Groups	**Diagnosis**	**<3 Months**	**3–12 Months**	**>12 Months**	**Total (%)**
Infectious diseases n = 63 (31.5%)	Acute otitis media	5	23	3	31 (15.5)
	Gastroenteritis	1	4	3	8
	Herpetic gingivostomatitis	0	1	3	4
	Oral thrush	4	1	0	5
	Roseola infantum	1	3	0	4
	Urinary tract infection	3	3	1	7
	Chickenpox	1	0	0	1
	Conjunctivitis	1	0	1	2
	Bronchiolitis	1	0	0	1
Gastrointestinal diseases n = 80 (40%)	Gastroesophageal reflux	3	0	0	3
	Colic	51	8	0	59 (29.5)
	Constipation	7	3	1	11 (5.5)
	Intussusception	0	5	2	7
Central nervous system n = 4 (2%)	Pseudotumor cerebri	0	2	1	3
	Choroid plexus papilloma	0	1	0	1
Immunologic reactions n = 18 (9%)	DTP vaccine reaction	2	3	1	6
	Food allergy	3	2	14	9 (4.5)
	Drug hypersensitivity	0	1	1	2
	Insect bite	0	1	0	1
Foreign body n = 3 (1.5%)	Eye	0	1	0	1
	Mouth	0	1	0	1
	Truncal	1	0	0	1
Others n = 32 (16%)	Opium withdrawal	0	1	0	1
	Inguinal hernia	4	2	2	8
	Hydrocele	1	1	0	2
	Circumcision site inflammation	1	3	0	4
	Napkin dermatitis	0	2	0	2
	Neuroblastoma	0	0	1	1
	Acute lymphoblastic lymphoma	0	0	2	2
	Endocardial fibroelastosis	1	0	0	1
	Contact dermatitis	0	2	1	3
	Overfeeding	0	2	20	2
	Nasal obstruction	0	2	0	2
	Unknown	1	3	0	4
Total (%)		**92 (46)**	**81 (40.5)**	**27 (13.5)**	**200 (100)**

From Fahimi D, Shamsollahi B, Salamati P, Sotoudeh K. Excessive crying of infancy: a report of 200 cases. Iran J Ped 2007;17(3):222–226. By permission.
DTP, Diphtheria, tetanus, pertussis.

References

Fahimi D, Shamsollahi B, Salamati P, Sotoudeh K. Excessive crying of infancy: a report of 200 cases. Iran J Ped 2007;17(3):222–6.

Nooitgedagt JE, Zwart P, Brand PL. Causes, treatment and clinical outcome in infants admitted because of excessive crying to the pediatric department of the Isala clinics, Zwolle, the Netherlands, 1997–2003. Ned Tijdschr Geneeskd 2005;149(9):472–7.

Poole SR. The infant with acute, unexplained, excessive crying. Pediatrics 1991;88:450.

Generalized Lymphadenopathy

Edythe Albano, MD

DEFINITION

Generalized lymphadenopathy is abnormal enlargement of more than two noncontiguous lymph node regions.

A. In the patient's history, review systemic symptoms such as persistent or recurrent fever (infection, malignant neoplasm, collagen vascular disease), sore throat (infectious mononucleosis), cough (tuberculosis fungal infection, mediastinal mass, or hilar adenopathy), epistaxis or easy bruising (leukemia), limp, or limb pain (juvenile rheumatoid arthritis, leukemia, neuroblastoma), weight loss (infection, malignant neoplasm), and night sweats (lymphomas, particularly Hodgkin disease). Note duration and severity of any systemic symptoms and assess whether they are improving or progressing. Obtain a complete history of travel and animal exposures. Note all recent immunizations and medications (serum sickness, drug reaction, phenytoin-induced lymphadenopathy). Document routine immunizations; inquire about possible exposure to tuberculosis. Identify risk for infection with human immunodeficiency virus (HIV).

B. In the physical examination, note the degree and extent of lymphadenopathy. Record measurements of all lymph nodes of concern for future comparison. Discrete, mobile, nontender lymph nodes are palpable in most healthy children. Small inguinal or high cervical nodes (1.5–2 cm) and occipital, submandibular, or axillary nodes (≤1 cm) are normal. Note thyromegaly (hyperthyroidism), hepatosplenomegaly (malignant neoplasm, storage disease, infection), arthritis (collagen vascular disease, leukemia), or a rash or conjunctivitis (viral exanthem, juvenile rheumatoid arthritis, systemic lupus, Kawasaki disease, leptospirosis, histiocytosis, lymphoma).

C. Atypical lymphocytes are frequently associated with many viral illnesses. A differential count of 20% or more atypical lymphocytes suggests infectious mononucleosis (Epstein–Barr virus), cytomegalovirus infection, viral hepatitis, or drug hypersensitivity.

D. False-negative monospot test results frequently occur early in the course of infectious mononucleosis and are common in very young children with Epstein–Barr virus infection. A positive monospot does not rule out other infections or malignancy. This test result must be interpreted in the context in which it occurs.

E. Parasitic infections that may present with generalized lymphadenopathy include filariasis (tropics, subtropics; vector: mosquito), Leishmania (kala-azar, Oriental sore, chiclero—Latin America, Middle East, India; vector: sandfly), Schistosoma (Asia, Africa, Caribbean, South America; intermediate host: snail), and Trypanosoma (Chagas disease—Latin America; sleeping sickness—Africa; vector: tsetse fly). Consider these when there has been travel to endemic areas or the child lives in such an area. Eosinophilia may be associated with parasitic infection.

F. Children with prolonged fever, unexplained weight loss, persistent cough, known exposure to tuberculosis, or risk factors for HIV are likely to have a serious, treatable illness. Malignant lesions are usually 3 cm or larger, of more than 4 weeks in duration, and often associated with abnormal laboratory and chest radiograph findings. Supraclavicular lymphadenopathy is usually malignant.

G. Anemia, neutropenia, and/or thrombocytopenia accompanying generalized lymphadenopathy suggests a malignant neoplasm, severe infection, or storage disease. Obtain a hematology/oncology consultation before referring patient for a lymph node biopsy to avoid the omission of important special studies (such as electron microscopy, chromosomes, molecular studies, immunohistochemical stains, flow cytometry, as well as fungal and viral cultures). In addition, a bone marrow aspirate and biopsy may yield the diagnosis without a surgical procedure.

References

Leung AK, Robson WL. Childhood cervical lymphadenopathy. J Pediatr Health Care 2004;18:3–7.

Oguz A, Karadeniz C, Temel EA, et al. Evaluation of peripheral lymphadenopathy in children. Pediatr Hematol Oncol 2006;23:549–61.

Twist CJ, Link MP: Assessment of lymphadenopathy in children. Pediatr Clin North Am 2002;49:1009–25.

Yaris N, Cakir M, Sözen E, et al. Analysis of children with peripheral lymphadenopathy. Clin Pediatr (Phila) 2006;45:544–9.

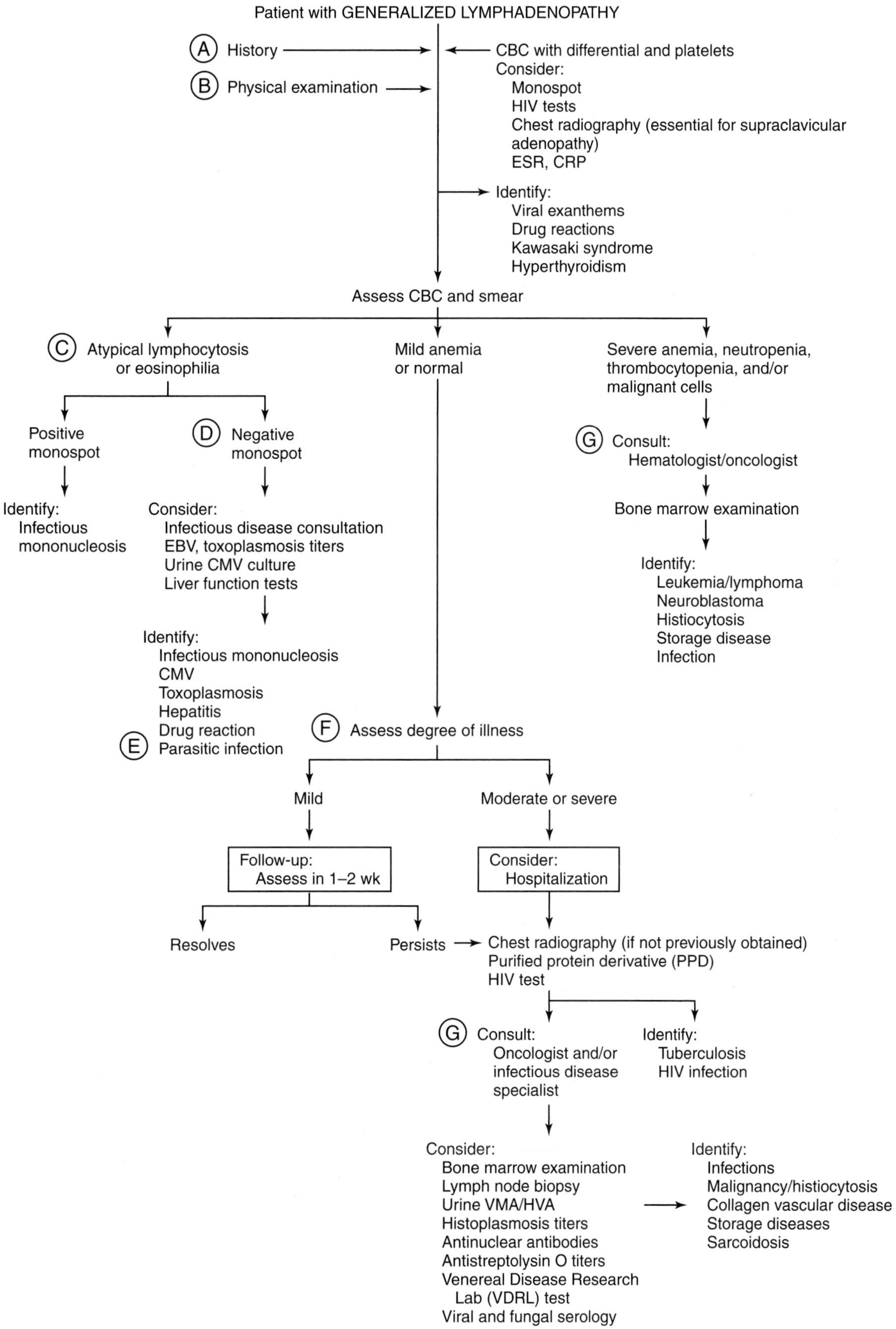
Patient with GENERALIZED LYMPHADENOPATHY
(A) History
(B) Physical examination
CBC with differential and platelets
Consider:
Monospot
HIV tests
Chest radiography (essential for supraclavicular adenopathy)
ESR, CRP
Identify:
Viral exanthems
Drug reactions
Kawasaki syndrome
Hyperthyroidism
Assess CBC and smear
(C) Atypical lymphocytosis or eosinophilia
Positive monospot
Identify:
Infectious mononucleosis
(D) Negative monospot
Consider:
Infectious disease consultation
EBV, toxoplasmosis titers
Urine CMV culture
Liver function tests
Identify:
Infectious mononucleosis
CMV
Toxoplasmosis
Hepatitis
Drug reaction
(E) Parasitic infection
Mild anemia or normal
Severe anemia, neutropenia, thrombocytopenia, and/or malignant cells
(G) Consult:
Hematologist/oncologist
Bone marrow examination
Identify:
Leukemia/lymphoma
Neuroblastoma
Histiocytosis
Storage disease
Infection
(F) Assess degree of illness
Mild
Follow-up:
Assess in 1–2 wk
Resolves
Persists
Moderate or severe
Consider:
Hospitalization
Chest radiography (if not previously obtained)
Purified protein derivative (PPD)
HIV test
(G) Consult:
Oncologist and/or infectious disease specialist
Identify:
Tuberculosis
HIV infection
Consider:
Bone marrow examination
Lymph node biopsy
Urine VMA/HVA
Histoplasmosis titers
Antinuclear antibodies
Antistreptolysin O titers
Venereal Disease Research Lab (VDRL) test
Viral and fungal serology
Identify:
Infections
Malignancy/histiocytosis
Collagen vascular disease
Storage diseases
Sarcoidosis

Obesity

Robert E. Kramer, MD

DEFINITION

Obesity is defined as "an increase in body weight beyond the limitation of skeletal and physical requirement, as a result of an excess accumulation of fat." It has become well recognized that this excess accumulation represents a true disease state with pervasive adverse metabolic consequences. In the pediatric population, the precise diagnostic criteria used to define obesity have been controversial, but recent consensus has defined it to be when a child's body mass index (BMI) equals or exceeds the 95th percentile for age and sex, as plotted on the Centers for Disease Control and Prevention growth charts. A BMI between the 85th and 95th percentile is now defined as "overweight." Most obese children and teens do not have a defined underlying metabolic or genetic cause for their obesity, but rather their obesity results from sustained consumption of calories in excess of their expenditure because of environmental influences. Management strategies, therefore, should focus on identifying and treating comorbid conditions while systematically addressing the environmental factors that contribute to the caloric imbalance.

A. History: A detailed history is vital in the evaluation of the obese child, both to differentiate the rare child with an underlying organic cause of their obesity and to identify the various environmental factors responsible for caloric imbalance. Factors that should alert the clinician to potential organic causative factors would include history of developmental delay, short stature, congenital anomalies, central nervous system trauma or malignancy, prolonged or repeated use of corticosteroids, and atypical antipsychotic therapy. Dietary history should focus on sweetened beverage intake, frequency of meals eaten outside the home, portion sizes, consumption of energy-dense foods, and restrained eating patterns. Activity history should ascertain the daily quantity of all screen time, including television, computer use, and video games, as well as the frequency and duration of any regular physical activity. It is important that family history include history of type 2 diabetes, early myocardial infarction, stroke, hypertension, and dyslipidemia, as well as obesity or need for bariatric surgery, to help assess cardiovascular risk. A detailed social and psychiatric history is important to identify psychosocial factors that may be either a cause or a consequence of obesity. Sleep history is important in the obese child to determine whether signs or symptoms of snoring or sleep apnea are significant enough to warrant a formal sleep study.

B. Physical Examination: Examination should include an accurate weight, height, and blood pressure, obtained without shoes, with only light clothing on, and with an appropriately sized blood pressure cuff, covering 80% of the arm. Adult or thigh cuffs may need to be used for morbidly obese teens. Waist circumference may be helpful as an adjunctive measure of adiposity, which can be tracked over time but is limited by poor interobserver consistency. General examination, with close attention paid to developmental stage, the presence of dysmorphic features, or short stature, may give clues that an underlying chromosomal or genetic syndrome is present. Neck examination for masses or nodules is important in the assessment of possible thyroid disease. The presence of acanthosis nigricans, hyperpigmentation in the folds of the neck or axillae, may be indicator of insulin resistance. Hidradenitis suppurativa, chronic infected papules and abscesses of the skin caused by occlusion of the apocrine sweat glands of the groin and axillae are also important to note. The presence of striae in the abdomen suggests rapid weight gain and, in conjunction with a buffalo hump, may suggest hypercorticism as a cause of obesity. Skin xanthomas, especially on the extensor surfaces, are indicative of severe hyperlipidemia. Abdominal examination for signs of right upper quadrant tenderness or hepatomegaly is helpful in assessing hepatobiliary disease, such as cholelithiasis or nonalcoholic fatty liver disease. The presence of hypogonadism or short digits is suggestive of Prader–Willi syndrome.

C. Comorbidity Screening: Routine laboratory screening for all children with a BMI greater than the 95th percentile has been recommended to assess for many of the common obesity comorbid conditions, such as dyslipidemia, insulin resistance/type 2 diabetes, and nonalcoholic fatty liver disease. This screening can be accomplished with a fasting lipid panel, glucose level, and hepatic profile. The need for further workup or referral to subspecialists can then be determined based on the results of these screenings.

(Continued on page 26)

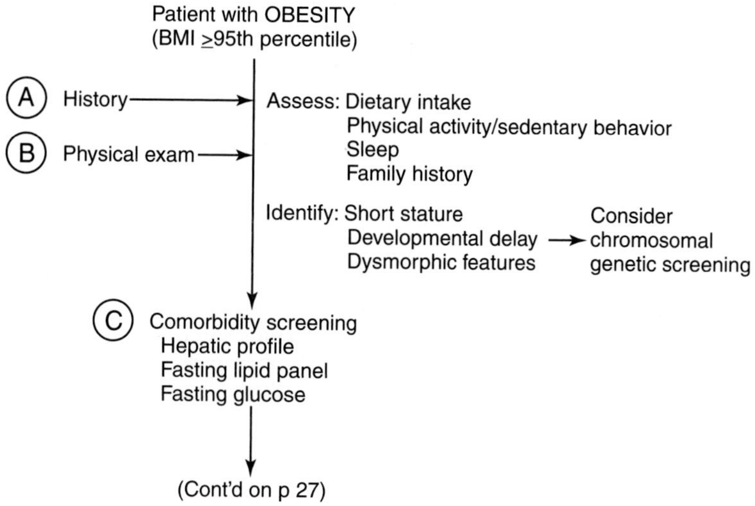
Patient with OBESITY
(BMI ≥95th percentile)
A
History
B
Physical exam
Assess: Dietary intake
Physical activity/sedentary behavior
Sleep
Family history
Identify: Short stature
Developmental delay
Dysmorphic features
Consider
chromosomal
genetic screening
C
Comorbidity screening
Hepatic profile
Fasting lipid panel
Fasting glucose
(Cont'd on p 27)

D. Elevated Blood Pressure: Blood pressure greater than the 95th percentile for a given patient's age, sex, and height is defined as "elevated." (Normative data for blood pressure in children can be found online at: http://www.nhlbi.nih.gov/guidelines/hypertension/child_tbl.htm.) Treatment should not be considered as a result of an isolated elevation in blood pressure. Initial steps should be to ensure that an accurate measure was obtained in the first place, by assessing cuff size and repeating the measure after 10 to 15 minutes. Be aware that automated blood pressure monitors often overestimate blood pressure, so a manual measurement by an experienced caregiver may be required. If there is suspicion of "white coat hypertension," with falsely increased values secondary to anxiety, 24-hour ambulatory blood pressure monitoring may be considered. If true elevation of blood pressure is consistently and reliably observed in a patient, a trial of lifestyle modification and weight loss therapy should still be the initial therapy before advancing to pharmacologic therapy. See Hypertension (p. 84) for further details.

E. Elevated Transaminases: Elevated aspartate aminotransferase (AST) or alanine aminotransferase (ALT) may often be found in the examination of the obese child. Most commonly, this is a manifestation of nonalcoholic fatty liver disease; however, transient elevation from intercurrent infection, as well as other forms of chronic liver disease, must also be considered. Typically, aminotransferases are between one and four times the upper limit of normal, usually with the ALT greater than the AST. Higher elevation should increase suspicion for an alternative cause of liver inflammation and may hasten the need for further evaluation. If alkaline phosphatase, bilirubin, or both are elevated as well, biliary obstruction should be suspected. Repeating a hepatic profile after several weeks to determine whether the elevation persists and obtaining a hepatic ultrasound would be the next steps in evaluation. If the elevation is persistent and the ultrasound does not reveal an obstructive process, further evaluation should be performed to exclude other chronic forms of liver disease in children, such as alpha-1 antitrypsin deficiency, viral hepatitis (hepatitis B and C), autoimmune hepatitis, and Wilson disease. Referral to a pediatric hepatologist should be considered at this point.

F. Elevated Fasting Glucose: Screening for type 2 diabetes and impaired fasting glucose/glucose tolerance is performed with a simple fasting glucose level. A level less than 100 mg/dl is normal, between 100 and 125 mg/dl is defined as impaired fasting glucose, and greater than 125 mg/dl is consistent with a provisional diagnosis of type 2 diabetes. Any significant increase in an obese patient warrants a more complete evaluation with a 2-hour glucose tolerance test. At 2 hours, a glucose level less than 140 mg/dl is normal, between 140 and 200 mg/dl is defined as impaired glucose tolerance, and greater than 200 mg/dl indicates provisional diabetes. Levels in the diabetic range should prompt referral to a pediatric endocrinologist for diabetic teaching and initiation of therapy. Levels in the impairment range indicate a need for a trial of weight loss and lifestyle modification, with close follow-up.

G. Snoring/Disordered Sleep: Obstructive sleep apnea is a common obesity comorbidity with serious cardiovascular consequences. Recent evidence, however, suggests a strong link between quality and quantity of stage 4 sleep and appetite regulation. Sleep apnea may thereby exacerbate obesity, creating a vicious cycle that is difficult to break. Careful assessment of the sleep history of obese patients is vital to identify these patients as early as possible. The history should focus on the presence of snoring, overt apneic episodes, need for head elevation to fall asleep, symptoms of daytime somnolence, and primary or secondary insomnia. Bedtime patterns and total hours of sleep are also important to obtain. Physical examination should assess the degree of tonsillar hypertrophy and airway obstruction. Patients with identified risk factors of sleep apnea should be referred for a polysomnogram to identify obstructive sleep apnea and other sleep disorders. If apnea is identified, consideration may be given to nighttime continuous positive airway pressure therapy, tonsillectomy/adenoidectomy, or both.

H. Low-Density Lipoprotein (LDL) Elevation: Dyslipidemia is another common obesity comorbidity, with important long-term cardiovascular implications. Current guidelines for treatment primarily focus on management of elevated LDL cholesterol levels, although in the obese pediatric population, elevated triglycerides and decreased high-density lipoprotein (HDL) cholesterol is the predominant pattern. An LDL level greater than 130 mg/dl is considered elevated. Initial treatment centers around a low-fat/low-cholesterol diet (<7% of calories from saturated fat, <200 mg cholesterol per day) and increased physical activity with weight loss over a 6- to 12-month period. Levels should then be reassessed. Elevated LDL more than 190 mg/dl in children 8 and older (or >160 mg/dl with a family history of early heart disease or with greater than two risk factors) should prompt consideration of pharmacologic treatment with lipid-lowering medications, either before or after a trial of diet and activity modification. "Statin" drugs, which inhibit HMG coenzyme A reductase in cholesterol synthesis, have been fairly well studied for use in children as young as 8 and are generally considered the first-line therapy. Treatment goals should be reduction in LDL to less than 160 mg/dl, or even 110 to 130 mg/dl in those with a strong family history. Serum aminotransferases and creatinine kinase levels can increased by treatment and should be monitored.

(Continued on page 28)

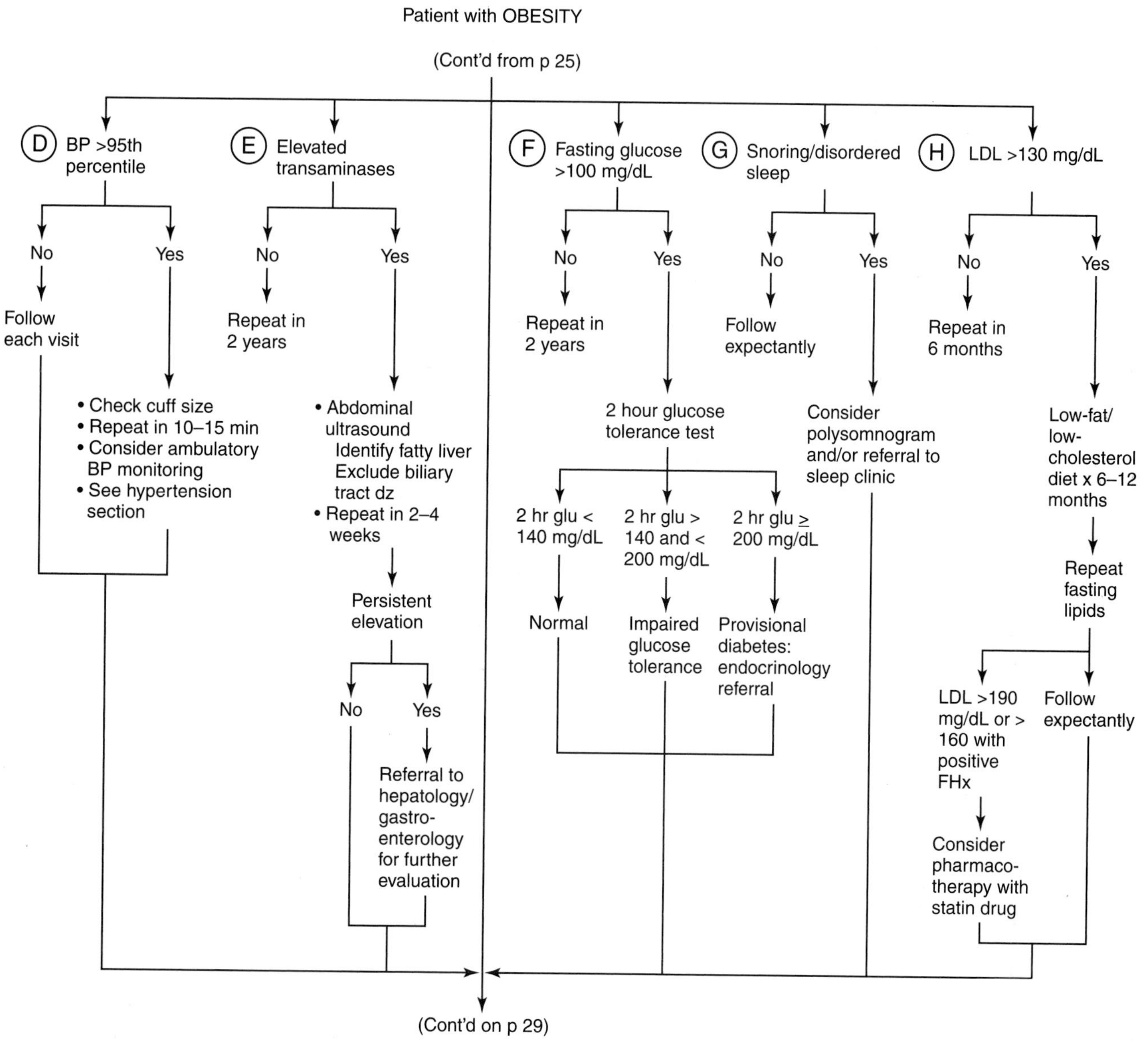
Patient with OBESITY
(Cont'd from p 25)
D BP >95th percentile
No
Follow each visit
Yes
• Check cuff size
• Repeat in 10–15 min
• Consider ambulatory BP monitoring
• See hypertension section
E Elevated transaminases
No
Repeat in 2 years
Yes
• Abdominal ultrasound
Identify fatty liver
Exclude biliary tract dz
• Repeat in 2–4 weeks
Persistent elevation
No
Yes
Referral to hepatology/gastro-enterology for further evaluation
F Fasting glucose >100 mg/dL
No
Repeat in 2 years
Yes
2 hour glucose tolerance test
2 hr glu < 140 mg/dL
Normal
2 hr glu > 140 and < 200 mg/dL
Impaired glucose tolerance
2 hr glu ≥ 200 mg/dL
Provisional diabetes: endocrinology referral
G Snoring/disordered sleep
No
Follow expectantly
Yes
Consider polysomnogram and/or referral to sleep clinic
H LDL >130 mg/dL
No
Repeat in 6 months
Yes
Low-fat/low-cholesterol diet x 6–12 months
Repeat fasting lipids
LDL >190 mg/dL or > 160 with positive FHx
Consider pharmaco-therapy with statin drug
Follow expectantly
(Cont'd on p 29)

I. Stage 1/Prevention Plus: This intervention is designed to be delivered in the primary care setting to obese children by the physician or trained office staff such as a nurse or dietitian. Specific evidence-based lifestyle modification recommendations are made, with a goal of weight maintenance, as linear growth continues, resulting in decreasing BMI. Monthly follow-up is scheduled to reinforce the lifestyle modifications, until reassessment is performed after 3 to 6 months.

J. Stage 2/Structured Weight Management: If BMI remains elevated above the 95th percentile after a sufficient trial of stage 1 intervention, patients are advanced to this stage. This intervention is also designated to be performed in the primary care setting, but with an increased level of parental supervision required. Use of motivational interviewing techniques is helpful to increase readiness for change. A more structured nutritional plan is desirable and, therefore, referral to a dietitian is also beneficial. Increased monitoring of diet and activity through the use of logbooks is encouraged. Monthly visits are maintained and the primary goal remains weight maintenance with decreasing BMI.

K. Stage 3 and 4/Comprehensive Multidisciplinary Program/Tertiary Care Intervention: After 3 to 6 months of stage 2 intervention in the primary care setting, referral to a multidisciplinary pediatric obesity clinic should be considered if BMI remains greater than the 95th percentile. Alternatively, if BMI at the start of treatment is greater than the 99th percentile, it may be appropriate to skip stage 1 and 2 and move straight to stage 3 or 4. These programs emphasize a multidisciplinary approach, encompassing medical, dietary, physical, and psychological therapies, and more frequent visits. Monthly visits in the primary care setting should be maintained. Alternative therapies such as meal replacements, very-low-calorie diet, protein-sparing modified fast, pharmacotherapy, and bariatric surgery may be considered for appropriate candidates.

References

Daniels SR, Greer FR. Committee on Nutrition. Lipid screening and cardiovascular health in childhood. Pediatrics 2008;122:198–208.

Krebs NF, Himes JH, Jacobson D, et al. Assessment of child and adolescent overweight and obesity. Pediatrics 2007;120(suppl 4): S193–S228.

Spear BA, Barlow SE, Ervin C, et al. Recommendations for treatment of child and adolescent overweight and obesity. Pediatrics 2007;120(suppl 4):S254–S288.

U.S. Preventive Services Task Force. Screening for obesity in children and adolescents: U.S. Preventive Services Task Force Recommendation Statement. Pediatrics 2010;125:361–7.

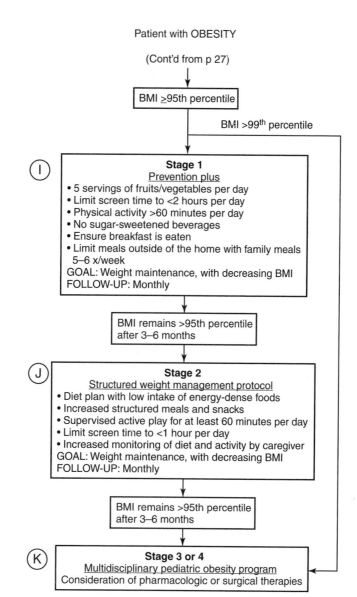

Patient with OBESITY

(Cont'd from p 27)

BMI ≥95th percentile

BMI >99th percentile → Stage 3 or 4

(I) **Stage 1**

Prevention plus

- 5 servings of fruits/vegetables per day
- Limit screen time to <2 hours per day
- Physical activity >60 minutes per day
- No sugar-sweetened beverages
- Ensure breakfast is eaten
- Limit meals outside of the home with family meals 5–6 x/week

GOAL: Weight maintenance, with decreasing BMI
FOLLOW-UP: Monthly

BMI remains >95th percentile after 3–6 months

(J) **Stage 2**

Structured weight management protocol

- Diet plan with low intake of energy-dense foods
- Increased structured meals and snacks
- Supervised active play for at least 60 minutes per day
- Limit screen time to <1 hour per day
- Increased monitoring of diet and activity by caregiver

GOAL: Weight maintenance, with decreasing BMI
FOLLOW-UP: Monthly

BMI remains >95th percentile after 3–6 months

(K) **Stage 3 or 4**

Multidisciplinary pediatric obesity program

Consideration of pharmacologic or surgical therapies

Polyuria and Polydipsia

David Fox, MD

A. Polyuria and polydipsia are not uncommon presenting symptoms for the pediatric patient. In taking a history, it is important to separate cases of true polyuria from those patients with nocturia or frequency. Nocturia implies no actual increase in the total volume of urine in a day, but simply voiding at night. However, nocturia may be the first manifestation of polyuria because the relative fluid restriction during sleep masks the increased urine output during the morning. Similarly, urinary frequency does not imply an increased urinary volume, but simple more frequent and often smaller volume voiding. It is associated with urinary tract infections, as well as dysfunctional voiding seen in toddlers, and is often associated with daytime enuresis. True polyuria is defined as urine output of more than 2 L/m^2/24 hr. Polydipsia is simply an increase in water intake and has a variety of causative factors. For infants, a history of irritability, failure to thrive, and intermittent fevers may suggest diabetes insipidus (DI). In taking the history, it is important to identify any medical history of head trauma or injury, or congenital abnormalities associated with midline brain defects. Surgical history should examine any recent intracranial procedure, specifically trans-sphenoidal pituitary procedures. Family history is important in defining relevant forms of diabetes mellitus and the rare cases of familial DI. Medications should also be documented.

B. Assess vital signs, breathing, circulation, and hydration status. Examine the growth percentiles for any pattern of weight loss or persistent obesity. For children younger than 2, assess the head circumference percentile in the context of past measurements. Note any alterations in mental status, particularly lethargy or focal neurologic signs.

C. In the outpatient setting, when presented with complaints of polyuria and/or polydipsia, a reasonable first test is a urinalysis, which can help guide further management. The urinalysis can provide valuable information, not least of which is whether glucose is present. The presence of glucose is suggestive, though by no means diagnostic, of diabetes mellitus. Further examination of the urinalysis for the presence of ketones will provide further context for any glucosuria.

D. In the context of a patient with polyuria and polydipsia who has glucosuria, diabetes must be considered first and foremost. In its most severe form, diabetes mellitus will present with ketones in the urine and acidosis. Electrolytes and a blood gas should be obtained, and endocrine consultation should focus on fluid management and insulin therapy in the inpatient or intensive care unit setting. For known diabetic patients, outpatient management with a diabetes team is appropriate. For the new diabetic patient, a coherent education plan must be implemented for the family, in conjunction with a diabetes team that may include a dietician, nurse coordinator, and endocrinologist. Steroids, systemic infection, and bodily stress can also present with glucosuria, but typically it is transient and not associated with the metabolic derangements of diabetes mellitus including persistent hyperglycemia.

E. With a negative glucose on urinalysis, if other findings suggest primary urinary tract infection, consider that you are dealing with urinary frequency as opposed to polyuria. For the true polyuric/polydipsic patient without glucose in the urine, DI is likely. It is important then to compare the serum osmolality with the urine osmolality to assess the concentrating ability of the kidney. To do this, one should obtain serum for osmolality and a basic metabolic profile that includes calcium and urine for osmolality and specific gravity. Hypernatremia is expected in the case of DI. DI is likely if the serum osmolality is greater than 300 mOsm/kg and the urine is less than 300 mOsm/kg. Less strict guidelines are appropriate for the postneurosurgical patient, who is at high risk for DI. DI is unlikely if the serum osmolality is less 270 mOsm/kg or the urine is greater than 600 mOsm/kg.

F. DI can be divided into four categories: nephrogenic, central, polydipsic, or gestagenic (pregnancy associated). A water deprivation test can help distinguish central and nephrogenic causes. Central causes vary widely from genetic defects in the vasopressin gene, to damage to the vasopressin neurons, to congenital malformations of the pituitary or hypothalamus (septo-optic dysplasia or holoprosencephaly, for example). Up to 10% of cases are idiopathic. Treatment often involves vasopressin analogs and careful fluid management. Nephrogenic DI often involves removal of the offending agent or disease process. Gestagenic DI is uncommon in pediatrics and resolves after the pregnancy. A diagnosis of DI argues for endocrinology or nephrology consultation.

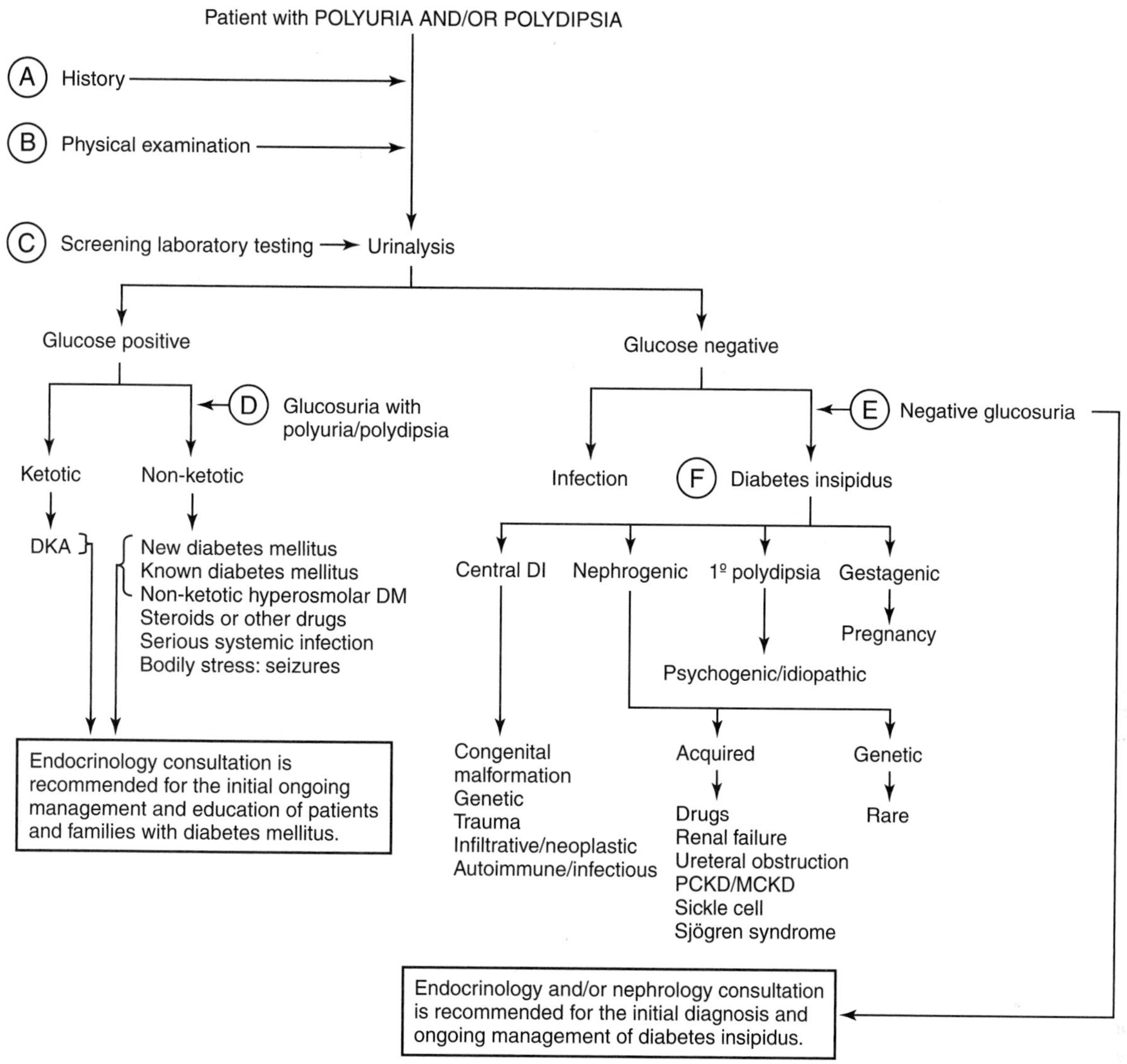
Patient with POLYURIA AND/OR POLYDIPSIA
A History
B Physical examination
C Screening laboratory testing
Urinalysis
Glucose positive
Glucose negative
D Glucosuria with polyuria/polydipsia
E Negative glucosuria
Ketotic
Non-ketotic
Infection
F Diabetes insipidus
DKA
New diabetes mellitus
Known diabetes mellitus
Non-ketotic hyperosmolar DM
Steroids or other drugs
Serious systemic infection
Bodily stress: seizures
Central DI
Nephrogenic
1º polydipsia
Gestagenic
Pregnancy
Psychogenic/idiopathic
Endocrinology consultation is recommended for the initial ongoing management and education of patients and families with diabetes mellitus.
Congenital malformation
Genetic
Trauma
Infiltrative/neoplastic
Autoimmune/infectious
Acquired
Genetic
Drugs
Renal failure
Ureteral obstruction
PCKD/MCKD
Sickle cell
Sjögren syndrome
Rare
Endocrinology and/or nephrology consultation is recommended for the initial diagnosis and ongoing management of diabetes insipidus.

Shock

Sameer Gupta, MD, and Mark Roback, MD

DEFINITION

Shock has been defined in numerous ways over the last two centuries. In 1872, Samuel D. Gross, MD, defined shock as: "A manifestation of the rude unhinging of the machinery of life." In 1895, John Collins Warren, MD, described it as: "This momentary pause in the act of death." Shock is more completely described as a clinical syndrome characterized by disruption of cardiovascular function resulting in inadequate provision of oxygen and nutrients to meet the metabolic demands of tissues. This is best represented by examining the difference between oxygen delivery (Do_2) and oxygen consumption (Vo_2). A shock state results when consumption of oxygen exceeds delivery. Delivery of oxygen can be augmented by improving cardiac output, increasing hemoglobin, and increasing oxygen saturation. Although most therapy is aimed at improving oxygen delivery, work can also be done to decrease consumption. Methods to reduce oxygen consumption include sedation, paralysis, mechanical ventilation, and fever reduction.

SHOCK CLASSIFICATION

Discerning the type of shock present is critical in determining appropriate therapy.

Hypovolemic Shock: Characterized by decreased circulating blood volume caused by dehydration (gastrointestinal and renal losses), hemorrhage, or capillary leak. The diminished blood volume causes a decrease in preload and, thus, a decrease in cardiac output. Hypovolemia is the most common type of shock seen in children.

Distributive Shock: Caused by abnormal regulation of blood flow with decreased systemic vascular resistance leading to poor perfusion of some areas and increased perfusion of others. Examples include septic shock, anaphylactic shock, and neurogenic shock.

Septic Shock: Not truly a class of its own, septic shock is usually classified under distributive shock, although this is not completely accurate. It actually is a combination of hypovolemic shock secondary to dehydration and capillary leak, cardiogenic shock caused by myocardial depression, and distributive shock because of abnormal systemic vascular resistance regulation.

Obstructive Shock: Defined by obstruction of ventricular inflow or outflow. Examples include tension pneumothorax causing a decrease in inflow to the right ventricle, severe pulmonary hypertension or pulmonary embolus reducing right ventricular outflow, cardiac tamponade restricting right ventricular inflow, or critical aortic stenosis causing diminished left ventricular outflow.

Dissociative Shock: Characterized by an inability of the body to deliver or use oxygen. Often, cardiac output is preserved in the initial stages, but at the cellular level, the body is deprived of oxygen and cannot produce the energy needed for metabolism. Examples include carbon monoxide poisoning, severe salicylate toxicity, cyanide poisoning, and methemoglobinemia.

Cardiogenic Shock: A state of decreased perfusion directly related to decreased cardiac output caused by systolic dysfunction, diastolic dysfunction, or arrhythmias. Examples include cardiomyopathy, myocarditis, arrhythmias such as unstable supraventricular tachycardia, and postoperative congenital heart disease.

A. As initial therapy is begun, take a complete history specifically assessing for symptoms of infection (fever, rash), heart failure (swelling, palpitations), possible ingestions, trauma, and pertinent medical history such as immunocompromised states and cardiac disease.

B. The cardiovascular examination will lead to the diagnosis of shock. Early findings of shock include tachycardia and increased systemic vascular resistance, which leads to prolonged capillary refill, decreased intensity of peripheral pulses, and cool extremities. Late findings of shock are low blood pressure for age (hypotension), decreased mental status, and oliguria/anuria. The physical examination findings in warm shock, typically seen in response to sepsis, can differ with bounding pulses, warm extremities, and brisk capillary refill, but warm shock will still be accompanied by hypotension.

C. Begin laboratory evaluation at the time of initial resuscitation and obtain a complete blood cell count with differential, electrolyte panel including ionized calcium, and bedside blood glucose. If the patient has hypotensive/decompensated shock, obtain a lactate level, venous blood gas, and coagulation studies. A mixed venous oxygen saturation (Mvo_2) or systemic venous oxygen saturation (Svo_2) can be used as an indicator of the balance between delivery and consumption. A normal Svo_2 indicates an appropriate balance between oxygen delivery and consumption, whereas a low Svo_2 indicates greater utilization of oxygen than delivery. A high Svo_2 can also be helpful because it can indicate a state of significantly reduced oxygen consumption (sedated and muscle relaxed) or an inability to use oxygen (cyanide poisoning and severe sepsis).

D. Severity of the shock state is noted by differences in physical examination findings and vital signs. Patients with less severe shock or compensated shock will maintain normal for age blood pressures, but still exhibit signs of decreased capillary refill, poor peripheral pulses, and cool extremities. Those patients with more severe or hypotensive shock will demonstrate decreased blood pressures, absent peripheral pulses, weak central pulses, and signs of altered mental status.

(Continued on page 34)

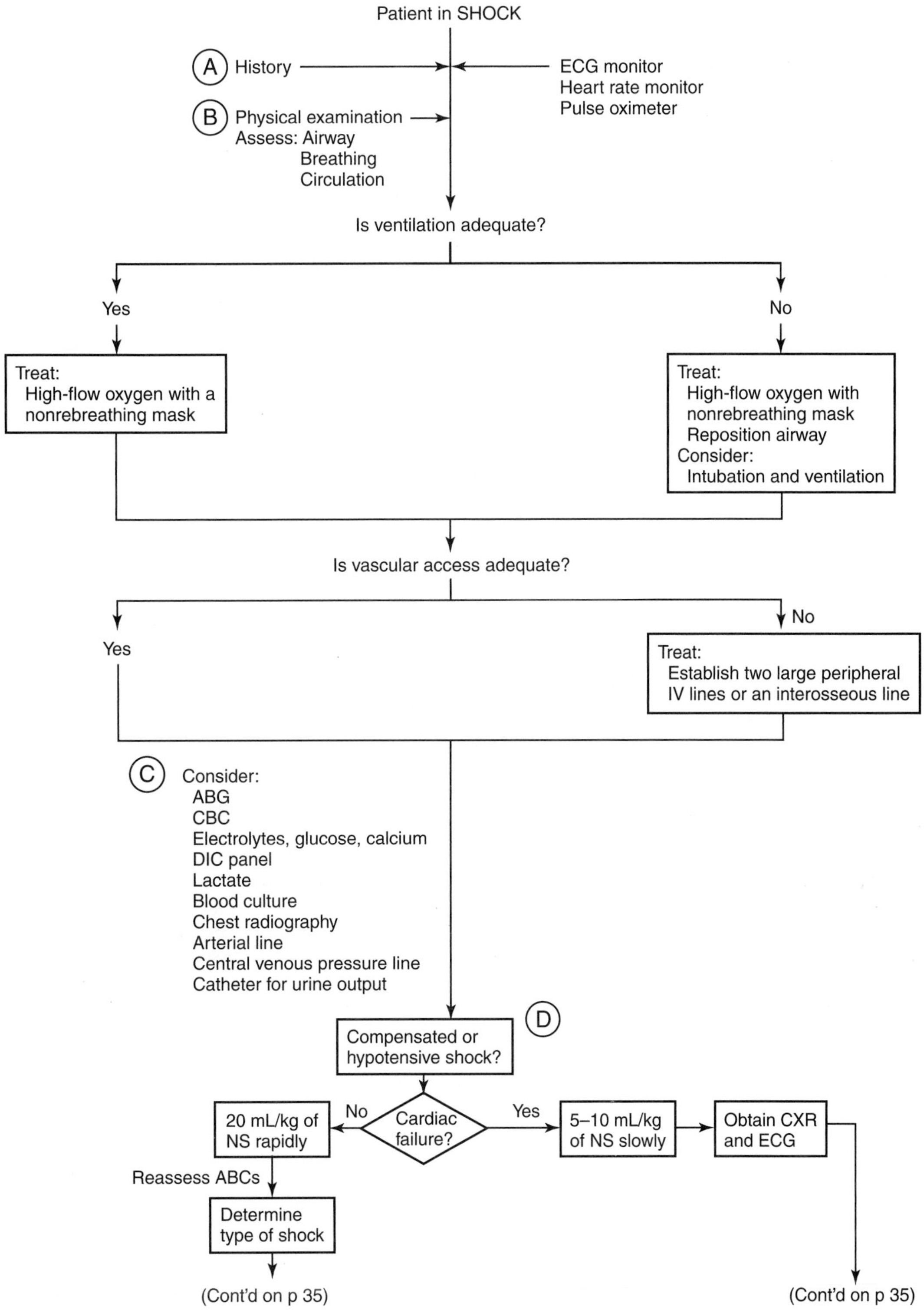

Patient in SHOCK
A History
B Physical examination
Assess: Airway
Breathing
Circulation
ECG monitor
Heart rate monitor
Pulse oximeter
Is ventilation adequate?
Yes
No
Treat:
High-flow oxygen with a nonrebreathing mask
Treat:
High-flow oxygen with nonrebreathing mask
Reposition airway
Consider:
Intubation and ventilation
Is vascular access adequate?
Yes
No
Treat:
Establish two large peripheral IV lines or an interosseous line
C Consider:
ABG
CBC
Electrolytes, glucose, calcium
DIC panel
Lactate
Blood culture
Chest radiography
Arterial line
Central venous pressure line
Catheter for urine output
D
Compensated or hypotensive shock?
Cardiac failure?
No
Yes
20 mL/kg of NS rapidly
Reassess ABCs
Determine type of shock
5–10 mL/kg of NS slowly
Obtain CXR and ECG
(Cont'd on p 35)
(Cont'd on p 35)

MANAGEMENT OF SHOCK

E. Initial shock management begins the same as in any disease process in acutely ill children, with a complete assessment of airway, breathing, and circulation. Next, attach a cardiorespiratory monitor with continuous electrocardiogram (ECG) and continuous pulse oximetry, and make sure to frequently measure blood pressure (every 3–5 minutes). Manage airway and breathing by administering supplemental oxygen (unless the patient has a known congenital cardiac abnormality that precludes the use of oxygen) and providing positive pressure ventilation as needed. If signs of respiratory distress or increased work of breathing exist, obtain a chest radiograph and evaluate for congestive heart failure, pneumonia, pneumothorax, or cardiomegaly.

After the diagnosis of shock is made, initiate treatment by obtaining vascular access (peripheral intravenous or intraosseous line) and rapidly administrating isotonic crystalloid. Initial fluid resuscitation volumes should be 20 ml/kg unless cardiogenic shock is being considered, then start with 5 to 10 ml/kg. The diagnosis of cardiogenic shock is ascertained with a combination of history and physical examination. The history may indicate congenital heart disease or previous diagnosis of cardiac disease, and the physical examination may demonstrate signs of heart failure: gallop rhythm, hepatomegaly, and/or distended neck veins.

After all interventions, rapidly reassess the patient's condition to monitor effectiveness of therapy. Children with shock require frequent re-examination and reevaluation. Treatment after the initial fluid bolus will vary depending on the shock state that is present.

Hypovolemic shock: Determine whether hypovolemia is secondary to fluid loss or hemorrhage. If the patient has not responded to 20 to 40 ml/kg isotonic crystalloid and hemorrhage is suspected, consider administration of packed red blood cells. If there is massive hemorrhage, consider other blood products, such as fresh-frozen plasma and platelets to promote hemostasis. Consult surgical services early for possible operative intervention to stop the bleeding. For hypovolemic shock secondary to fluid losses, other than bleeding, continue with normal saline boluses to restore vascular volume. Once the shock state has been corrected, continue to monitor and replace ongoing fluid losses. Gastrointestinal losses may be associated with metabolic acidosis secondary to bicarbonate loss and, therefore, may necessitate sodium bicarbonate administration in severe cases.

Septic/Distributive Shock: If there is a concern for septic shock, then administer broad-spectrum antibiotics and evaluate the patient to determine a source of the infection. Continue normal saline boluses for correction of perfusion. If the patient has been given between 60 and 100 ml/kg fluid or is starting to demonstrate signs and symptoms of pulmonary edema without resolution of shock, begin vasoactive drug support. Initial pharmacologic support is typically started with dopamine, which will help to improve cardiac output at low doses and increase systemic vascular resistance at higher doses. If the patient does not improve with dopamine, then the patient should be started on an epinephrine infusion for cold shock (cold extremities, prolonged capillary refill, weak peripheral pulses, hypotension) and norepinephrine or vasopressin infusions for warm shock (bounding pulses, brisk capillary refill, warm extremities, hypotension). At this time, consider checking a cortisol level and administering steroids to address the possibility of relative adrenal insufficiency.

Obstructive Shock: Continue with normal saline boluses to overcome the obstruction and improve perfusion. However, definitive therapy of obstructive shock requires correction of the process causing the obstruction. Examples include pericardiocentesis for cardiac tamponade, needle decompression of tension pneumothorax, 100% FiO_2 and nitric oxide for pulmonary hypertension, and prostaglandins for critical aortic stenosis or critical coarctation of the aorta to maintain patency of the ductus arteriosus. Occasionally, inotropic support with epinephrine is needed when ventricular outflow is impeded.

Dissociative Shock: Continue normal saline boluses to help with perfusion. Identify the underlying cause of dissociative shock and treat accordingly. Treat carbon monoxide poisoning with 100% FiO_2 and, in severe cases, hyperbaric oxygen. Methemoglobinemia treatment varies by individual but begins with removal of the causative agent and may include methylene blue in some populations and ascorbic acid for those with G6PD deficiency. Treat cyanide poisoning by decontaminating the skin and gastrointestinal tract, and administering the antidote.

Cardiogenic Shock: After initial normal saline bolus, reassess patient for improvement in perfusion. Evaluate for and treat any arrhythmias that may be present, because the cessation of an arrhythmia may help with resolution of the shock state. Concurrent with treatment, consult pediatric cardiology, as an echocardiogram may be needed to assess cardiac function. Drug therapies that may be useful in improving cardiac function include milrinone, epinephrine, dobutamine, and dopamine (see Table 1). Consider intubation and mechanical ventilation to reduce oxygen consumption and decrease left ventricular afterload.

With all shock states, continue to assess end-organ perfusion throughout treatment. To determine effectiveness of therapy, monitor urine output, assess mental status, and check laboratory values such as blood urea nitrogen, creatinine, lactate, and liver enzymes.

References

Brierley J, Carcillo JA, Choong K, et al. Clinical practice parameters for hemodynamic support of pediatric and neonatal septic shock: 2007 update from the American College of Critical Care Medicine. Crit Care Med 2009;37:666–88.

Russel JA. Management of sepsis. N Engl J Med 2006;355:1699–1713.

American College of Surgeons Committe on Trauma. Shock. In: Advanced Trauma Life Support for doctors student course manual. 7th ed. Chicago: American College of Surgeons; 2004. p. 69–85.

Smith L, Hernan L. Shock states. In: Fuhrman BP, Zimmerman JJ, editors. Pediatric critical care. 3rd ed. Philadelphia: Mosby Elsevier; 2006. p. 394–410.

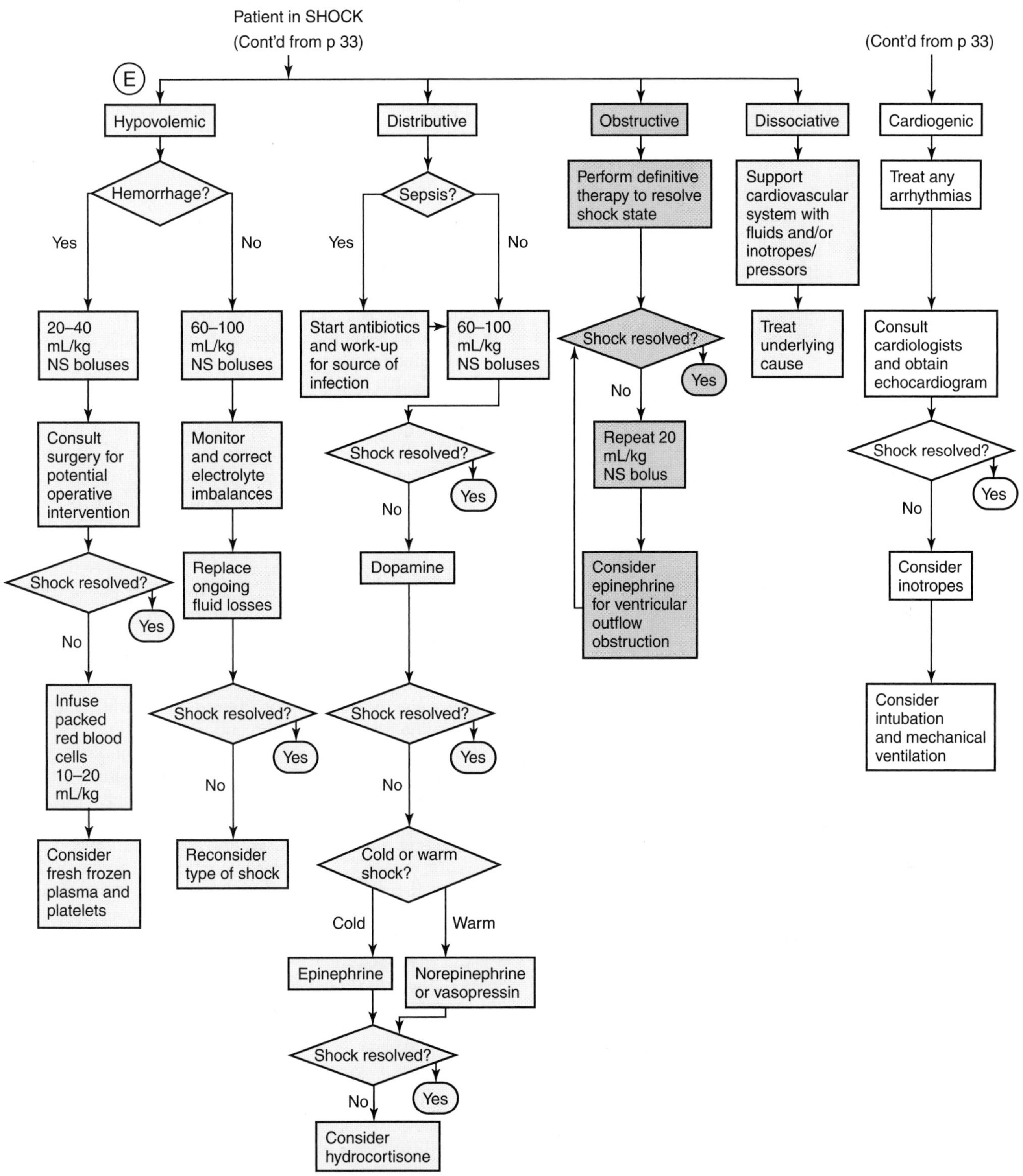
Patient in SHOCK
(Cont'd from p 33)
(Cont'd from p 33)
E
Hypovolemic
Distributive
Obstructive
Dissociative
Cardiogenic
Hemorrhage?
Yes
No
20–40 mL/kg NS boluses
60–100 mL/kg NS boluses
Consult surgery for potential operative intervention
Monitor and correct electrolyte imbalances
Shock resolved?
Yes
No
Replace ongoing fluid losses
Infuse packed red blood cells 10–20 mL/kg
Shock resolved?
Yes
No
Consider fresh frozen plasma and platelets
Reconsider type of shock
Sepsis?
Yes
No
Start antibiotics and work-up for source of infection
60–100 mL/kg NS boluses
Shock resolved?
Yes
No
Dopamine
Shock resolved?
Yes
No
Cold or warm shock?
Cold
Warm
Epinephrine
Norepinephrine or vasopressin
Shock resolved?
Yes
No
Consider hydrocortisone
Perform definitive therapy to resolve shock state
Shock resolved?
Yes
No
Repeat 20 mL/kg NS bolus
Consider epinephrine for ventricular outflow obstruction
Support cardiovascular system with fluids and/or inotropes/ pressors
Treat underlying cause
Treat any arrhythmias
Consult cardiologists and obtain echocardiogram
Shock resolved?
Yes
No
Consider inotropes
Consider intubation and mechanical ventilation

Table 1. **Inotropes and Vasopressors**

Agent	Dosing	Effect
Dopamine	1–20 μg/kg/min	0–5 μg/kg/min: increased splanchnic perfusion 5–10 μg/kg/min: increased chronotropy and inotropy >10 μg/kg/min: increased systemic vascular resistance
Dobutamine	2–20 μg/kg/min	Increased inotropy and chronotropy without much change in SVR
Epinephrine	0.01–5 μg/kg/min	0.01–0.1 μg/kg/min: inotropy, chronotropy 0.1–2 μg/kg/min: inotropy, chronotropy, and increased SVR >2 μg/kg/min: increased SVR
Norepinephrine	0.01–1 μg/kg/min	Increased SVR with small amount of inotropy
Milrinone	0.2–1.0 μg/kg/min	Inotropy and afterload reduction
Vasopressin	Start at 0.0003 U/kg/min	Increased SVR

SVR, systemic vascular resistance.

Syncope

Thomas J. Moon, MD, and Michael S. Schaffer, MD

DEFINITION

Syncope is a transient loss of consciousness and muscle tone with spontaneous recovery. Near syncope or presyncope is a transient alteration in consciousness without a period of unconsciousness.

CAUSATIVE FACTORS

Neurocardiogenic syncope (vasovagal syncope) is the cause of syncope in 80% of pediatric patients presenting to the emergency department. Less common causes of syncope include neurologic (9%), psychogenic (4%), cardiac (2%), breath-holding spell (2%), and intoxication (2%). The cause of syncope in most patients can be correctly identified with a thorough history and physical examination. Ancillary testing is helpful in confirming a suspected diagnosis or ruling out serious pathology, but such testing should only be performed when indicated by the history and physical examination.

A. The history should clarify predisposing conditions such as warm environment, dehydration, intercurrent illness, prolonged fasting, recent head trauma, or menstruation/pregnancy. Events immediately preceding the syncopal event are crucial and include prolonged or sudden standing, position at the time of syncope, exercise, micturition, paroxysm of coughing, sudden strong emotion or stress, and related subjective feelings such as nausea, light-headedness, dizziness, dimming of vision, palpitations, or chest pain. The account from a witness to the event can provide information about loss of tone and/or posture, duration of unconsciousness, convulsions or shaking, loss of bowel or bladder contents, skin color, resuscitative measures, mental status on regaining consciousness and neurologic sequelae. The patient's medical history should identify any cardiac (congenital heart disease, arrhythmias, Kawasaki disease), pulmonary (asthma, pulmonary hypertension), neurologic (seizure disorder, migraines, narcolepsy), or psychiatric (depression, anorexia/bulimia, substance abuse) history. Any previous events of syncope should be discussed together with any pertinent review of symptoms including fatigue, dyspnea on exertion, decreased exercise tolerance, palpitations, edema, chest pain, or snoring. Current medications and other ingested substances need to be reviewed. Finally, a family history should identify relatives with syncope, early or sudden deaths, arrhythmias, hypercholesterolemia, cardiomyopathy, Marfan syndrome, and any history of cardiac, pulmonary, neurologic, or psychiatric disorders.

B. Perform a complete physical examination. The physical examination should include an expanded panel of vital signs including temperature, orthostatic heart rate and blood pressure, four-extremity blood pressure, respiratory rate, and pulse oximetry. Note signs of cardiac disease, respiratory distress, and neurologic disease. Findings that suggest cardiac disease are heart murmur, increased intensity of the second heart sound, tachycardia/bradycardia, clicks, gallop rhythm, friction rub, and decreased femoral pulses. Signs of respiratory distress are tachypnea, retractions, decreased breath sounds, wheezing, rales, and cyanosis. Signs of central nervous system disease include altered mental status, focal neurologic signs, weakness, abnormal tone and reflexes, and abnormal growth and development.

C. Findings on electrocardiography and chest radiography may suggest cardiac disease. Pericarditis and myocarditis related to an infection or vasculitis can cause ST-T segment wave changes and cardiomegaly. Aortic stenosis and idiopathic hypertrophic subaortic stenosis manifest as a systolic heart murmur and left ventricular hypertrophy. Coarctation syndromes cause decreased femoral pulses, decreased lower extremity blood pressure, and left ventricular hypertrophy. Primary pulmonary hypertension and pulmonary stenosis produce right ventricular hypertrophy. Coronary artery disease related to Kawasaki disease, hypercholesterolemia, aberrant left coronary artery, and lesions associated with decreased coronary artery blood flow, such as severe aortic stenosis or idiopathic hypertrophic subaortic stenosis, produce ischemic ST-T segment changes. Arrhythmias such as atrioventricular block, sick sinus syndrome, supraventricular tachycardia, and long QT syndrome are associated with electrocardiographic findings of abnormal conduction pattern.

D. Seizure activity is suggested when a syncopal episode lasts longer than 2 minutes, is followed by confusion or impaired mental status (postictal state), or is associated with incontinence, muscle jerks, or cyanosis. Frequent recurrent episodes also suggest seizures.

(Continued on page 38)

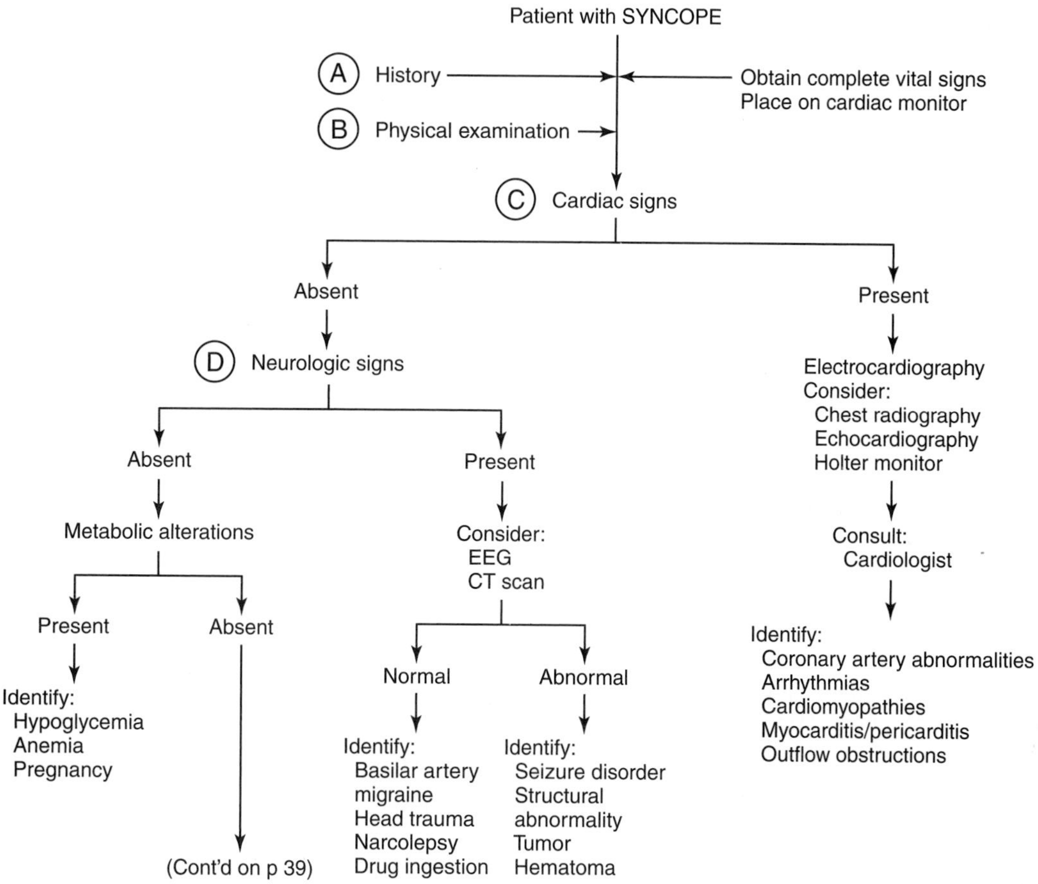
Patient with SYNCOPE
(A) History
Obtain complete vital signs
Place on cardiac monitor
(B) Physical examination
(C) Cardiac signs
Absent
Present
(D) Neurologic signs
Electrocardiography
Consider:
Chest radiography
Echocardiography
Holter monitor
Absent
Present
Metabolic alterations
Consider:
EEG
CT scan
Consult:
Cardiologist
Present
Absent
Normal
Abnormal
Identify:
Coronary artery abnormalities
Arrhythmias
Cardiomyopathies
Myocarditis/pericarditis
Outflow obstructions
Identify:
Hypoglycemia
Anemia
Pregnancy
Identify:
Basilar artery migraine
Head trauma
Narcolepsy
Drug ingestion
Identify:
Seizure disorder
Structural abnormality
Tumor
Hematoma
(Cont'd on p 39)

E. Orthostatic syncope is associated with a decline in blood pressure on standing. Consider documentation of this condition with tilt-table testing. Rarely, syncope may follow micturition when rapid bladder decompression produces postural hypotension and decreased cardiac return. Educate the patient to move slowly from a lying to a standing position. Frequently recurring episodes may be prevented by increasing the patient's intravascular volume. This can be achieved by increasing salt and water intake with or without a salt-retaining oral mineralocorticoid, fludrocortisone. Consider the use of elastic hose to prevent venous pooling.

F. Vasovagal syncope is caused by a sudden decrease in peripheral vascular resistance. It is usually precipitated by sudden fear, anger, or another strong emotion and, similar to orthostatic syncope, may respond to increasing intravascular volume. An alternative treatment approach is to increase the systemic vascular resistance and blood pressure with a peripherally acting α agonist, midodrine.

G. Breath holding occurs in children younger than 6 years and is precipitated by crying, sudden pain, or fear. Loss of tone and consciousness may occasionally be followed by stiffening and clonus, a reflex anoxic seizure. Cyanosis, if present, should precede any abnormal movements. No postictal or confusional state occurs. The prognosis is excellent; spells of breath holding usually resolve by 6 years of age. Treatment is reassuring the parents of the benign nature of the problem. Breath-holding spells may involve an abnormal vagal response to sudden emotion. Historically, ocular compression, attempting to trigger the oculocardiac reflex, was performed during electrocardiographic and electroencephalographic monitoring. This technique is no longer recommended. When breath holding occurs frequently, consider anticholinergic therapy to block vagal effects.

H. Hyperventilation produces reduction in carbon dioxide tension with alkalosis, decreased ionized calcium, and tetany. This syndrome is frequently associated with light-headedness, giddiness, dizziness, paresthesias, and chest pain. In most cases, high anxiety related to life stress or an underlying psychopathologic process is identified.

I. Paroxysmal coughing produced by *Bordetella pertussis* or asthma may decrease cardiac output and cause hypoxia resulting in syncope.

References

Chronister TE. Pediatric neurologist as consultant in evaluation of syncope in infants and children: when to refer. Prog Pediatr Cardiol 2001;13(2):133–8.

Geggel RL. Conditions leading to pediatric cardiology consultation in a tertiary academic hospital. Pediatrics 2004;114:e409–e417.

Goble MM, Benitez C, Baumgardner M, Fenske K. ED management of pediatric syncope: searching for a rationale. Am J Emerg Med 2008;26(1):66–70.

Johnsrude CL. Current approach to pediatric syncope. Pediatr Cardiol 2000;21(6):522–31.

Kapoor WN, Peterson JR, Karpf M. Micturition syncope. JAMA 1985;253:796.

Katz RM. Cough syncope in children with asthma. J Pediatr 1979;77:48.

Khositseth A, Martinez MW, Driscoll DJ, Ackerman MJ. Syncope in children and adolescents and the congenital long QT syndrome. Am J Cardiol 2003;92(6):746–9.

Khurana DS, Valencia I, Kruthiventi S, et al. Usefulness of ocular compression during electroencephalography in distinguishing breath-holding spells and syncope from epileptic seizures. J Child Neurol 2006;21:907–10.

Kuriachan V, Sheldon RS, Platonov M. Evidence-based treatment for vasovagal syncope. Heart Rhythm 2008;5(11):1609–14.

Levine MM. Neurally mediated syncope in children: results of tilt testing, treatment, and long-term follow-up. Pediatr Cardiol 1999;20(5):331–5.

Lewis DA, Dhala A. Syncope in the pediatric patient: the cardiologist's perspective. Pediatr Clin North Am 1999;46:205–19.

Lombroso CT, Lerman P. Breathholding spells. Pediatrics 1967;39: 563–81.

Massin MM, Bourguignont A, Coremans C, et al. Syncope in pediatric patients presenting to an emergency department. J Pediatr 2004;145:223–8.

Massin MM, Malekzadeh-Milani S, Benatar A. Cardiac syncope in pediatric patients. Clin Cardiol 2007;30(2):81–5.

Narchi H. The child who passes out. Pediatr Rev 2000;21(11):384–8.

Ritter S, Tani LY, Etheridge SP, et al. What is the yield of screening echocardiography in pediatric syncope? Pediatrics 2000;105:e58.

Steinberg LA, Knilans TK. Syncope in children: diagnostic tests have a high cost and low yield. J Pediatr 2005;146(3):355–8.

Stephenson JB. Clinical diagnosis of syncope (including so-called breath-holding spells) without electroencephalography or ocular compression. J Child Neurol 2007;22:502–8.

Taggart NW, Haglund CM, Tester DJ, Ackerman MJ. Diagnostic miscues in congenital long-QT syndrome. Circulation 2007;115(20):2613–20.

Woody RC, Kiel EA. Swallowing syncope in a child. Pediatrics 1986;78:507.

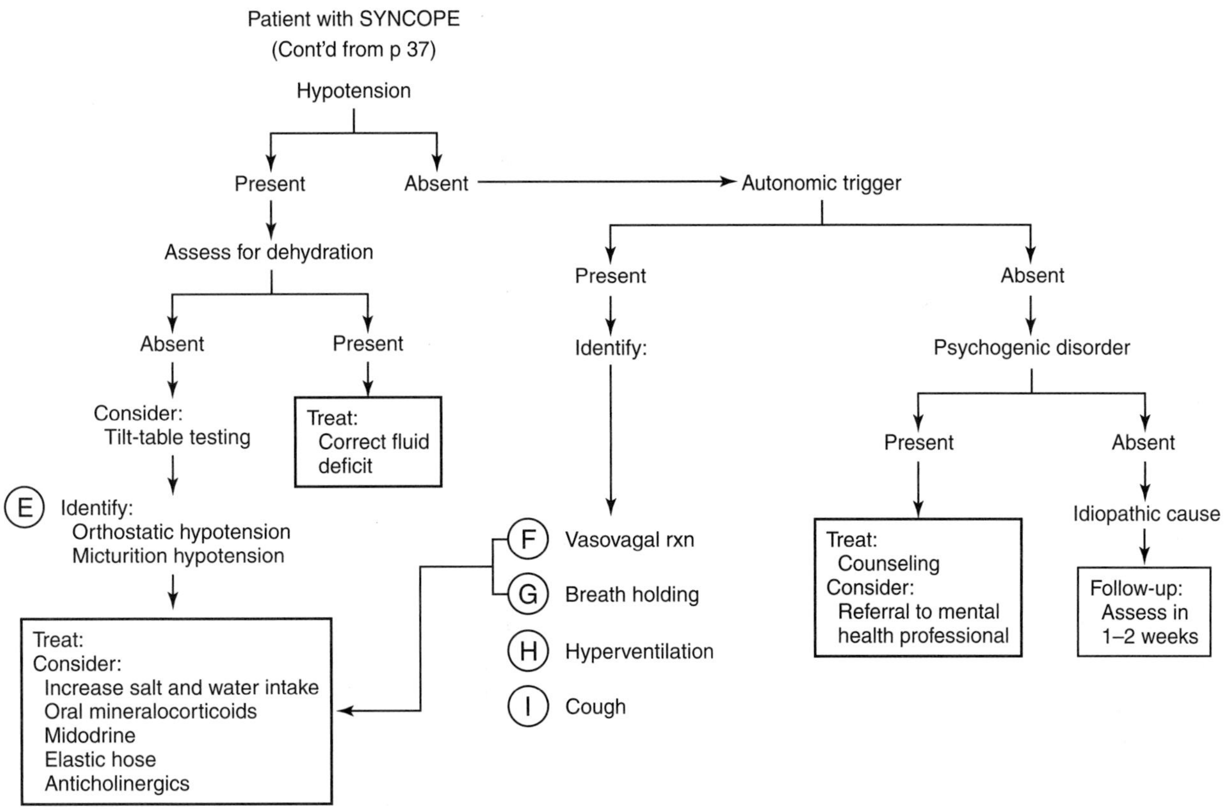
Patient with SYNCOPE
(Cont'd from p 37)
Hypotension
Present
Absent
Autonomic trigger
Assess for dehydration
Absent
Present
Consider:
Tilt-table testing
Treat:
Correct fluid deficit
E
Identify:
Orthostatic hypotension
Micturition hypotension
Treat:
Consider:
Increase salt and water intake
Oral mineralocorticoids
Midodrine
Elastic hose
Anticholinergics
Present
Identify:
F
Vasovagal rxn
G
Breath holding
H
Hyperventilation
I
Cough
Absent
Psychogenic disorder
Present
Treat:
Counseling
Consider:
Referral to mental health professional
Absent
Idiopathic cause
Follow-up:
Assess in 1–2 weeks

Adolescent

Primary and Secondary Amenorrhea

Amy E. Sass, MD, MPH

Primary amenorrhea is the failure to begin menstruation when expected. Age 15 is commonly used as the cutoff for primary amenorrhea because 98% of girls in the U.S. general population achieve menarche by this age. Menarche occurs, on average, 2 years after breast development. Therefore, the absence of secondary sexual characteristics by age 13 may suggest pubertal delay and the potential need for evaluation well before age 15. In the adolescent who has achieved menarche, secondary amenorrhea is defined as the absence of menses for three consecutive cycles in a patient with regular periods or for 6 months in a patient with irregular periods. In evaluating amenorrhea, it is helpful to consider anatomic levels of possible abnormalities from the hypothalamus to the genital tract in a systematic way (Table 1). A stepwise approach using the clinical history, growth charts review, physical examination, and appropriate laboratory studies will allow providers to determine the cause of amenorrhea in most adolescents.

Pregnancy must be considered as a possible causative factor of amenorrhea regardless of history because denial of intercourse among adolescents is common and the patient may not able to disclose sexual activity or abuse. Amenorrhea may be caused by anatomic abnormalities that may not be recognized until puberty (e.g., imperforate hymen and transverse vaginal septum). Chromosomal abnormalities may also present with amenorrhea (e.g., Turner syndrome, androgen insensitivity). If the history or physical examination suggests a specific diagnosis, it is not necessary to wait until a certain age to begin further evaluation.

Functional hypothalamic amenorrhea, a fairly common explanation for young women with amenorrhea, is a diagnosis of exclusion when pregnancy and other pathologic causative agents are not determined. It is characterized by a decrease in hypothalamic gonadotropin-releasing hormone secretion, decreased pulses of gonadotropins, low serum estradiol concentrations, and anovulation. Multiple factors may contribute to the pathogenesis of functional hypothalamic amenorrhea, including malnutrition, eating disorders, vigorous exercise, and stress. Low serum gonadotropin concentration can also be caused by endocrinopathies, chronic diseases that are associated with poor nutrition (celiac disease, inflammatory bowel disease, cystic fibrosis), or central nervous system tumors.

Table 1. **Differential Diagnosis of Amenorrhea by Anatomic Site of Cause**

Hypothalamic-Pituitary Axis
Hypothalamic suppression
Chronic disease
Stress
Malnutrition
Strenuous athletics
Drugs (haloperidol, phenothiazines, atypical antipsychotics)
Central nervous system lesion
Pituitary lesion: adenoma, prolactinoma
Craniopharyngioma, brainstem, or parasellar tumors
Head injury with hypothalamic contusion
Infiltrative process (sarcoidosis)
Vascular disease (hypothalamic vasculitis)
Congenital conditions*
Kallmann syndrome (anosmia)
Ovaries
Gonadal dysgenesis*
Turner syndrome (XO)
Mosaic (XX/XO)
Injury to ovary
Autoimmune disease (oophoritis)
Infection (mumps)
Toxins (alkylating chemotherapeutic agents)
Irradiation
Trauma, torsion (rare)
Polycystic ovary syndrome
Ovarian failure
Uterovaginal Outflow Tract
Müllerian dysgenesis*
Congenital deformity or absence of uterus, uterine tubes, or vagina
Imperforate hymen, transverse vaginal septum, vaginal agenesis, agenesis of the cervix*
Androgen insensitivity syndrome (absent uterus)*
Uterine lining defect
Asherman syndrome (intrauterine synechiae postcurettage or endometritis)
Tuberculosis, brucellosis
Defect in Hormone Synthesis or Action (Virilization may be Present)
Adrenal hyperplasia*
Cushing disease
Adrenal tumor
Ovarian tumor (rare)
Drugs (steroids, ACTH)

*Indicates condition that usually presents as primary amenorrhea.
ACTH, adrenocorticotropic hormone.

A. Establishing a pubertal timeline including age at thelarche, adrenarche, growth spurt, and menarche is helpful in evaluating pubertal development. Although there can be variations in the onset, degree, and timing of these stages, the progression of stages is predictable. Adrenal androgens are largely responsible for axillary and pubic hair; estrogen is responsible for breast development, maturation of the external genitalia, vagina, and uterus, and menstruation. Lack of development suggests pituitary or ovarian failure or gonadal dysgenesis. Relevant components of the medical and surgical histories include the neonatal history, treatment for malignancies, presence of autoimmune disorders or endocrinopathies, and current medications (prescribed and over the counter). Family history includes age at menarche of maternal relatives, familial gynecologic or fertility problems,

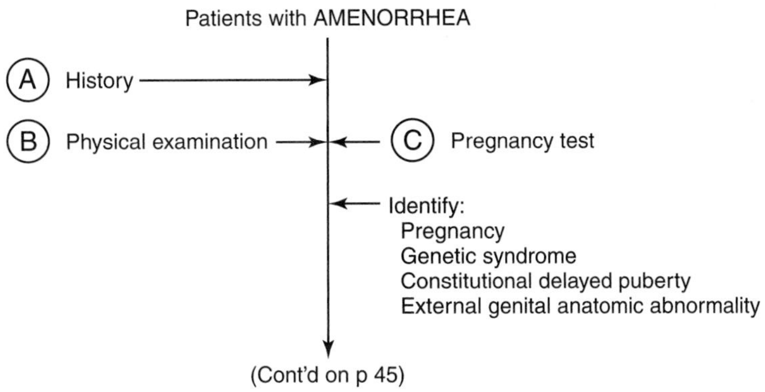
Patients with AMENORRHEA
A History
B Physical examination
C Pregnancy test
Identify:
Pregnancy
Genetic syndrome
Constitutional delayed puberty
External genital anatomic abnormality
(Cont'd on p 45)

autoimmune diseases, or endocrinopathies. A review of systems should focus on symptoms of hypothalamic-pituitary disease such as weight change, headache, visual disturbance, galactorrhea, polyuria, and/or polydipsia. A history of cyclic abdominal and/or pelvic pain in a mature adolescent with amenorrhea may indicate an anatomic abnormality such as an imperforate hymen. Acne and hirsutism are clinical markers of androgen excess. Changes in weight, quality of skin and hair, and stooling pattern may indicate a thyroid problem. A confidential social history should include sexual activity, contraceptive use, the possibility of pregnancy, and use of tobacco, drugs, and alcohol. The patient should also be questioned about major stressors, symptoms of depression and anxiety, changes in weight, and dietary habits, including nutritional intake, any disordered eating or weight-loss behaviors, and extent of physical activity. Growth charts illustrate trends in growth and are useful tools when evaluating amenorrhea. For example, longitudinal growth retardation or failure can occur in the setting of chronic disease states such as inflammatory bowel disease. In conditions associated with inadequate nutrition, patients are typically underweight for height. Patients with chronic disease states that do not affect nutrition status such as acquired hypothyroidism are typically overweight for height.

Table 2. **Components of the Physical Examination for Amenorrhea**

General appearance	Syndromic features (e.g., Turner syndrome), midline facial defects, renal and vertebral anomalies
Anthropometrics	Height, weight, BMI and percentiles for age, vital signs (HR, BP)
Neck	Thyromegaly
Breast	SMR staging, galactorrhea
Abdomen	Masses, tenderness
External genital examination	SMR staging, estrogenization of vaginal mucosa, hymenal patency, clitoromegaly
Internal genital examination	Vaginal length; presence of uterus by digital or bimanual examination
Neurologic	Sense of smell, visual field cuts, papilledema
Skin	Acne, hirsutism, acanthosis nigricans

BMI, body mass index; *BP,* blood pressure; *HR,* heart rate; *SMR,* sexual maturity rating.

B. A thorough physical examination should include the components listed in Table 2. General appearance may reveal syndromic features (e.g., Turner syndrome with webbed neck, shield chest, widely spaced nipples, increased carrying angle of the arms); midline facial defects can be associated with hypothalamic-pituitary axis problems and renal and vertebral anomalies that can be assocaited with Müllerian defects. Anthropometrics may reveal malnutrition or obesity and/or short stature. These data, when evaluated with the historical puberty timeline, sexual maturity rating on physical examination, and comparison with growth charts, can suggest constitutionally delayed puberty if there seems to be a normal progression through puberty, however at a delayed rate. Longitudinal growth failure could suggest an underlying chronic disease. An enlarged thyroid on an examination is suggestive of possible thyroid disease. In addition to determining the sexual maturity rating of the breasts, the presence of galactorrhea can be assessed with gentle compression of the nipple, raising concern for prolactinoma. The abdominal examination may reveal pelvic masses. Important components of the external genital examination include sexual maturity rating, assessment of estrogenization (moist, pink vaginal mucosa vs. thin, red mucosa of hypoestrogenization), hymenal patency, and clitoromegaly (width >5 mm), which can be seen with androgen excess. The length of the vagina can be assessed by insertion of a saline moistened applicator swab into the vagina. The length is reduced (usually <2 cm) with a low-lying transverse vaginal septum or vaginal agenesis. The presence of a uterus can be assessed by a single finger or bimanual examination. If a patient cannot tolerate an internal examination, the presence of the uterus can be assessed by a rectoabdominal examination or ultrasonography. Pelvic magnetic resonance imaging is a more sensitive test to evaluate suspected genital congenital anomalies or an obstructed genital tract. The neurologic examination includes testing the sense of smell (absent in Kallman syndrome), visual field cuts, and an opthalmologic examination to evaluate for papilledema, which might suggest a pituitary or other central nervous system mass. The skin examination includes assessment of acne, hirsutism, or both, which can be found with androgen excess and acanthosis nigricans, indicating insulin resistance.

C. Initial laboratory studies should include a urine pregnancy test, complete blood cell count, thyroid-stimulating hormone (TSH), prolactin, and follicle-stimulating hormone (FSH). If short stature and delayed puberty are present, a bone age should be obtained and karyotype should be considered.

D. For patients with constitutional delayed puberty, it is reasonable to observe the patient clinically every 3 to 6 months to monitor progression to puberty and menarche. For other patients with secondary sexual characteristics, normal physical examination findings including normal external genitalia and uterus, a negative pregnancy test, and normal TSH, prolactin, and FSH, administer a progestin challenge test of medroxyprogesterone acetate, 10 mg by mouth daily for 10 days. The positive response with withdrawal vaginal bleeding, typically 2 to 10 days after completion of the medication, confirms the presence of an estrogen-primed uterus. A negative response suggests a low estrogen state. Further scrutiny of weight and growth charts may reveal weight less than the patient's previous healthy trend and the need for weight gain back to the healthy baseline for resumption of menses. In addition, further assessment of physical activity level and stressors could reveal functional amenorrhea. For patients with appropriate weight and functioning, further consideration of pituitary or other central nervous system lesions and underlying chronic diseases is necessary. Additional laboratory studies including a urinalysis and a chemistry panel (including renal and liver function tests) and erythrocyte sedimentation rate, if not already obtained, can be useful. A neurologic or endocrinologic consultation for brain imaging and additional neuroendocrine studies may also be helpful. Once identified, treating the underlying illnesses will often result in resumption of menses. Bone density also needs to be a consideration for patients with prolonged hypoestrogenemia (>6 months) because they are at risk for development of osteopenia. In addition to resuming and maintaining a healthy weight, these patients should be counseled to have adequate calcium (1300 mg daily) and vitamin D (400 IU daily) intake. Bone densitometry testing can be considered to establish a baseline following 6 months or more amenorrhea.

E. Increased TSH indicates hypothyroidism and low TSH hyperthyroidism. An expanded thyroid panel including total thyroxine (T4) and free T4 can provide additional imformation about thyroid function before a referral to a pediatric endocrinologist and/or treatment.

F. Increased serum prolactin indicates a possible prolactin-secreting tumor. Pregnancy, idiopathic prolactinemia, pituitary adenomas, diseases of the hypothalamus (e.g., craniopharyngioma), hypothyroidism, and medications that are dopamine-receptor antagonists including antipsychotics and gastric motility agents can increase prolactin levels. Prolactin testing is also sensitive and can be increased with nipple stimulation or stress. A mildly elevated test should be repeated before magnetic resonance imaging of the brain for a prolactinoma is performed. Patients with consecutive increased values should be referred to a pediatric endocrinologist.

G. Increased FSH indicates ovarian insufficiency or gonadal dysgenesis, and a karyotype for Turner syndrome/mosaic should be obtained. Autoimmune oophoritis should be assessed by anti-ovarian antibodies if the chromosome analysis is normal. Patients with autoimmune oophoritis are at risk for development of adrenal insufficiency and other autoimmune endocrinopathies such as thyroid and parathyroid disease, diabetes mellitus, myasthenia gravis, and pernicious anemia, and should be referred to a pediatric endocrinologist for further evaluation.

H. Patients with clinical evidence of hyperandrogenemia including hirsutism and acne should have evaluation of adrenal androgens including total and free testosterone and dehydroepiandrosterone sulfate. Polycystic ovary syndrome (PCOS) is the most common endocrine disorder of reproductive-age women. It occurs in up to 6% of adolescents and 12% of adult women. PCOS is characterized by ovarian dysfunction, disordered gonadotropin secretion, and hyperandrogenemia, which causes amenorrhea, hirsutism, and acne. Many adolescents with PCOS are overweight, and the association of PCOS with insulin resistance is well established. Adolescents with PCOS are at increased risk for obesity-related morbidities including type 2 diabetes mellitus, dyslipidemia and cardiovascular disease, low self-esteem, and adult reproductive health problems including infertility and endometrial cancer. Excessively increased testosterone (>200 ng/dl) or dehydroepiandrosterone sulfate (>700 μg/dl) levels, or both, are concerning for an adrenal or ovarian tumor, and pelvic and adrenal imaging to evaluate for possible tumor is necessary. If other causative factors of virilization such as late-onset congenital adrenal hyperplasia (history of premature pubarche, high dehydroepiandrosterone sulfate, clitoromegaly) are suspected, a first morning 17-hydroxyprogesterone should be collected to look for 21-hydroxylase deficiency. Urine cortisol or a dexamethasone suppression test is performed if Cushing syndrome is suspected. If the patient is overweight or has acanthosis nigricans, or both, a fasting insulin test, lipid panel, and 2-hour oral glucose challenge test are recommended. A simple fasting glucose test is less ideal because many women with PCOS have normal fasting glucose results but impaired postprandial tests. Consultation with a pediatric endocrinologist can assist in further evaluation and management of significantly increased androgen levels and endocrinopathies. Encouraging lifestyle changes that will promote weight loss is a primary goal of therapy for PCOS in adolescents. Weight loss is associated with improved menstrual regulation and decreased symptoms of hyperandrogenemia, obesity-related comorbidities, and infertility. Combination estrogen/progesterone hormonal contraceptives improve menstrual regularity by increasing sex hormone–binding globulin, which effectively decreases free androgen exposure. There are no current guidelines for the use of insulin-sensitizing medications such as metformin to treat PCOS in adolescents; however, it can be considered with glucose intolerance.

I. If the physical examination or ultrasound reveals an absent uterus, chromosomal analysis and serum testosterone should be obtained to differentiate between Müllerian dysgenesis and androgen insensitivity. Müllerian dysgenesis, or Mayer-Rokitansky-Küster-Hauser syndrome, is the congenital absence of the vagina with variable uterine development. These women have normal serum testosterone levels. Pelvic

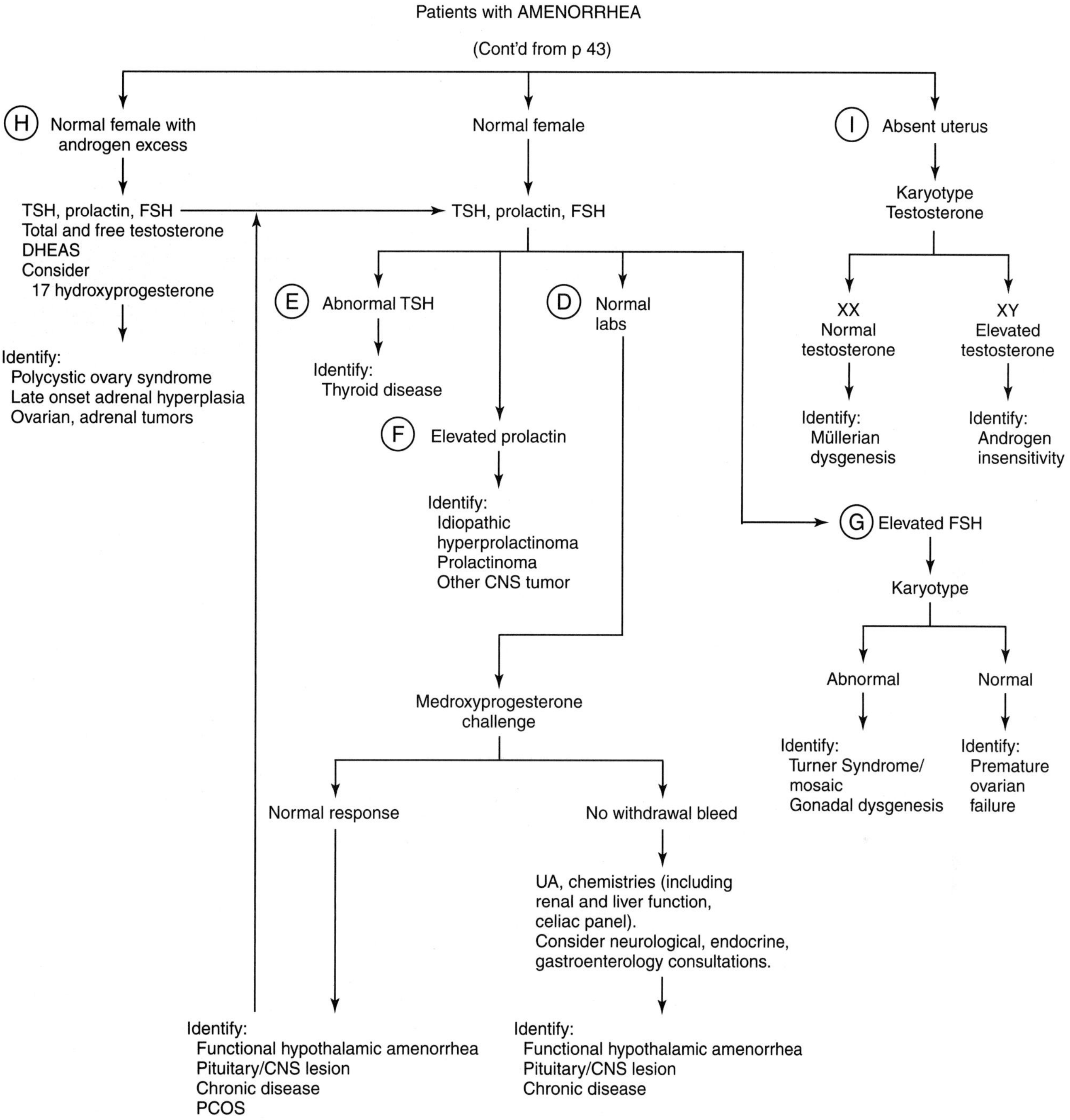
Patients with AMENORRHEA
(Cont'd from p 43)
H Normal female with androgen excess
TSH, prolactin, FSH
Total and free testosterone
DHEAS
Consider
17 hydroxyprogesterone
Identify:
Polycystic ovary syndrome
Late onset adrenal hyperplasia
Ovarian, adrenal tumors
Normal female
TSH, prolactin, FSH
E Abnormal TSH
Identify:
Thyroid disease
D Normal labs
F Elevated prolactin
Identify:
Idiopathic
hyperprolactinoma
Prolactinoma
Other CNS tumor
Medroxyprogesterone challenge
Normal response
No withdrawal bleed
UA, chemistries (including renal and liver function, celiac panel).
Consider neurological, endocrine, gastroenterology consultations.
Identify:
Functional hypothalamic amenorrhea
Pituitary/CNS lesion
Chronic disease
PCOS
Identify:
Functional hypothalamic amenorrhea
Pituitary/CNS lesion
Chronic disease
I Absent uterus
Karyotype
Testosterone
XX
Normal testosterone
XY
Elevated testosterone
Identify:
Müllerian dysgenesis
Identify:
Androgen insensitivity
G Elevated FSH
Karyotype
Abnormal
Normal
Identify:
Turner Syndrome/
mosaic
Gonadal dysgenesis
Identify:
Premature
ovarian
failure

magnetic resonance imaging is helpful to clarify the nature of the vaginal agenesis and to differentiate it from low-lying transverse vaginal septum, agenesis of the uterus and vagina, and imperforate hymen. Renal imaging to rule out associated renal abnormalities is also important. These patients should be referred to a gynecologist with expertise in this area. Individuals with androgen insensitivity are phenotypically female but have an absent upper vagina, uterus, and fallopian tubes, a male karyotype, and increased serum testosterone levels (normal range for male sex). These patients should be referred to a pediatric endocrinologist. Surgical removal of the testes is also necessary to prevent malignant degeneration.

References

Bekx MT, Conor EC, Allen DB. Characteristics of adolescents presenting to a multidisciplinary clinic for polycystic ovarian syndrome. J Pediatr Adolesc Gynecol 2010;23:7–10.

Berlan ED, Emans SJ. Managing polycystic ovary syndrome in adolescent patients. J Pediatr Adolesc Gynecol 2009;22:137–40.

Bloomfield D. Secondary amenorrhea. Pediatr Rev 2006;27:113–14.

Emans SJ, Laufer MR, Goldstein DP. Pediatric and adolescent gynecology. 5th ed. Philadelphia: Lippincott–Raven; 2005.

Kaplan DW, Sass AE. Adolescence. In: Hay Jr WW, Levin MJ, Sondheimer JM, Deterding RR, eds. Current pediatric diagnosis and treatment. ed 20. New York: Lange Medical Books/McGraw Hill; 2011.

Pfeifer AM, Kives S. Polycystic ovary syndrome in the adolescent. Obstet Gynecol Clin North Am 2009;36:129–52.

The Practice Committee of the American Society for Reproductive Medicine. Current evaluation of amenorrhea. Fertil Steril 2008;90:S219–S225.

Breast Pain in Adolescent Girls

Christine Gilroy, MD, MSPH

The prevalence rate of mastalgia has been estimated to be between 47% and 69% in adult women. Young women overestimate the population and personal risk for development of breast cancer, and may interpret breast pain as a symptom of cancer. Although mastalgia is a common and enigmatic problem, the cause and treatment are still poorly defined.

A. History: Initial evaluation should include an estimate of severity of pain and number of days per month that pain is experienced, in addition to how the pain affects the patient's daily activities, sleep, and social and sexual relationships. Retrospective reports of a patient's breast pain are complicated by low-to-moderate validity rates, and prospective daily reports for 2 months using an assessment tool, such as the Cardiff Breast Pain Chart or the McGill Pain Questionnaire, provide more accurate and actionable data. A reproductive history, together with pregnancy risk, is also imperative because breast pain is one of the most common symptoms of early pregnancy. Unilateral or bilateral pain, quality of pain, relation to menstrual cycle, trauma history, and an extensive medication list, including herbal medications and illicit substance use, are important to assess. Any medication that can cause gynecomastia or galactorrhea can also cause mastalgia.

B. Physical Examination: Before having the patient disrobe, observe the fit of the patient's bra, the presence of underwires and their juxtaposition to breast tissue, the impact of the shoulder strap on the shoulder tissue, the general supportiveness of the choice of bra design, and herniation of breast tissue around the bra. Have the patient disrobe and then perform a thorough breast examination in the presence of a chaperone. The breasts should be examined in the upright and supine position. Perform a thorough breast examination, including the skin, all four quadrants, under the areola, pressing all the way to the chest wall and tracking the breast tail into the axilla. The method of the examination (circular vs. vertical strips) is less important than taking time (minimum 3 minutes per breast) to examine as much breast tissue as possible. Check for lymphadenopathy in the axillary, supraclavicular, and cervical areas. The patient should then be placed in the lateral decubitus position, so the breast tissue falls away from the chest wall, and the chest wall should be palpated to determine whether it is the source of discomfort. Identification of focal breast pain over a breast lump should follow the algorithm for evaluation of a breast lump. Evidence of infection should follow with appropriate treatment for mastitis or abscess. If no specific cause of breast pain is identified, pregnancy test should be performed.

C. Chest wall pain comprises a group of conditions with more musculoskeletal causative factors in young women and should be easy to elicit on examination. Causes include costochondritis, Tietze syndrome, trauma, rib clicking or slipping, cervical radiculopathy, shoulder pain, or fibromyalgia. Cardiac or esophageal cause may be considered but are unlikely in adolescents and young women. Treatment may include nonsteroidal anti-inflammatory drugs, injection with corticosteroids and lidocaine, or physical therapy.

(Continued on page 48)

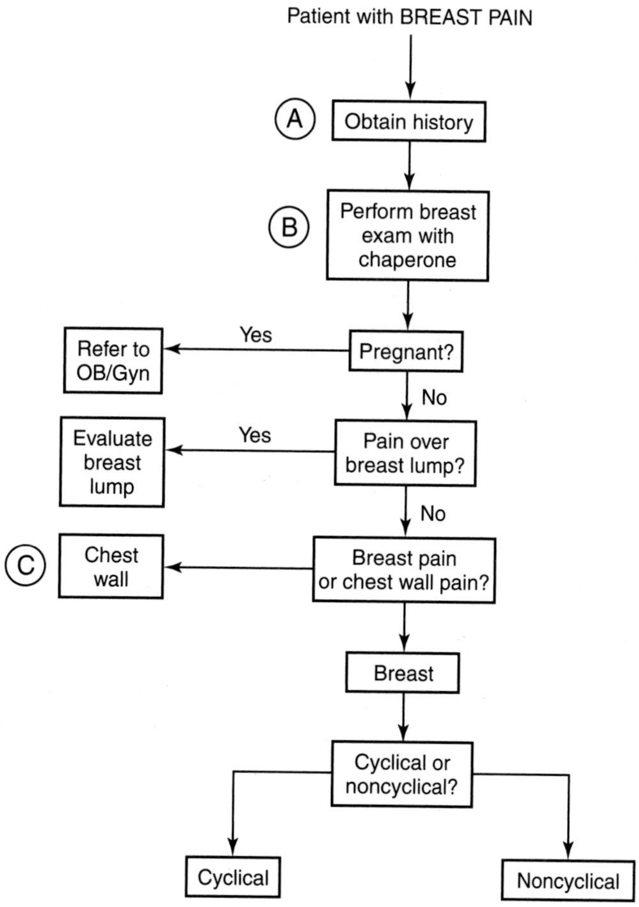

Patient with BREAST PAIN
A
Obtain history
B
Perform breast exam with chaperone
Pregnant?
Yes
Refer to OB/Gyn
No
Pain over breast lump?
Yes
Evaluate breast lump
No
Breast pain or chest wall pain?
C
Chest wall
Breast
Cyclical or noncyclical?
Cyclical
Noncyclical

(Cont'd on p 49)
(Cont'd on p 49)

D. Cyclical mastalgia represents 60% to 70% of mastalgia in young women, with greatest prevalence in women in their 20s and 30s. Pain is usually described as bilateral, "dull," "heavy," or "aching," occurring in the last half of the menstrual cycle, and is relieved with the menses. Most frequently, the pain is located in the upper outer quadrants of the breast. "Normal" or physiologic mastalgia is pain that lasts 1 to 4 days, occurring in the week before menses, and of severity 4 or less out of 10 on a visual analog pain scale. The natural history is of a relapsing course, and remission frequently occurs with hormonal events, such as pregnancy (8%) or menopause (42%), but may occur spontaneously (14%). Earlier age of onset is associated with more persistent duration of pain. Therapy should begin with nonpharmacologic management.

E. Noncyclical mastalgia represents 20% to 30% of breast pain complaints to physicians, occurring more frequently in older women (i.e., 40s to 50s). The pain is often, but not exclusively, unilateral and localized, more often in the inner quadrants, and described as "drawing," "burning," "achy," and "sore." Causes of noncyclical breast pain include pregnancy, trauma, mastitis, thrombophlebitis, tumor or cancer, and medications, which include psychiatric medications, hormones and hormonal contraceptives, and spironolactone. However, most noncyclical breast pain arises for unknown reasons, and it is believed to be anatomically rather than hormonally mediated. Treatment should focus on nonpharmacologic management.

F. Nonpharmacologic Treatment: Recommendations are impacted by the paucity of high-quality data. In one clinical series, 78% of symptomatic women were reassured after normal findings on evaluation and did not want further evaluation. Up to 70% of women wear improperly fitted bras, and given the delicate nature of the supportive Cooper ligaments of the breasts, recommendations should begin with wearing a sports bra during exercise and wearing a properly fitted, soft, supportive bra during the day and night, which improved or relieved pain in 75% of women in a 1976 study. Dietary recommendations are commonly made, as the cost is low and the potential for harm negligible. The effect of decreased methylxanthine consumption is debatable, with positive and negative studies; however, it is relatively easy. Data supporting restriction of dietary fat is more positive, with complete pain relief in 9 of 10 patients enrolled in one study; however, all positive studies required dietary fat restriction to less than 20% of daily caloric intake, which may be difficult to achieve or inappropriate in some patients. Changing the omega 3-6-9 fatty acid balance of fat consumed has been evaluated with evening primrose oil, with mixed results. These studies are confounded by the lack of standardization of herbal content for the evening primrose oil. The risk for harm is low, but the cost substantially greater for this intervention. The recommended dosage of evening primrose oil is 9% gamma-linolenic acid by weight, 3000 mg/day in divided doses. In addition to evening primrose oil, one study of fish oil was negative and studies of flaxseed are of poor quality. The German Commission E has found adequate data to support the prescription of chasteberry for premenstrual syndrome and mastalgia, using a German herbal compound Mastodynon, not available in the United States, with relief occurring twice as frequently than with placebo.

G. Pharmacologic Treatment: Hormonal contraception has been demonstrated to both improve and worsen cyclical mastalgia. Consider starting or adjusting to a 20 microgram estrogen contraceptive pill, or starting depomedroxyprogesterone. Side effects of both medications in adolescents may include inadequate bone mineralization. Oral nonsteroidal anti-inflammatory drugs have not been evaluated for efficacy in mastalgia, but topical nonsteroidal anti-inflammatory drugs have been demonstrated to improve pain in 81% to 92% of patients. For persistent severe pain, which impairs daily activities, other hormonally active therapy should be considered. Danazol and tamoxifen, both of which have good efficacy for mastalgia in older women, have been paired with severe side effects. In addition, neither medication has been studied specifically in adolescents, and may have serious effects on sexual maturation and bone mineral density. Prescription of these agents should not be undertaken without endocrine specialty consultation.

References

Ader DN, Browne MW. Prevalence and impact of cyclic mastalgia in a United States clinic-based sample. Am J Obstet Gynecol 1997;177: 126–32.

Basch E, Bent S, et al. Flax and flaxseed oil: a review by the Natural Standard Research collaboration. J Soc Integr Oncol 2007;5(3): 92–105.

Berenson AB, Odom SC, et al. Physiologic and psychologic symptoms associated with use of injectable contraception and 20 mcg oral contraceptive pills. Am J Obstet Gynecol 2008;199:351.e1–12.

Blommers J, de Lange-De Klerk ES, Kuik DJ, et al. Evening primrose oil and fish oil for severe chronic mastalgia: a randomized, double-blind controlled trial. Am J Obstet Gynecol 2002;187:1389–94.

Davies EL, Gateley CA, Miers M, Mansel RE. The long-term course of mastalgia. J R Soc Med 1998;91:462–4.

Dennehy CE. The use of herbs and dietary supplements in gynecology: an evidence-based review. J Midwifery Women's Health 2006;51: 402–9.

Irving AD, Morrison SL. Effectiveness of topical non-steroidal anti-inflammatory drugs in the management of breast pain. J R Coll Surg Edinb 1998:43:158–9.

Klimberg SV. Etiology and management of breast pain. In: Bland KI, Copeland EM, editors. The breast: Comprehensive management of benign and malignant diseases, ed 2. Philadelphia: WB Saunders; 1998. p. 247–60.

Millet AV, Dirbas FM. Clinical management of breast pain: a review. Obstet Gynecol Surv 2002;57:451–61.

Qureshi S, Sultan N. Topical nonsteroidal anti-inflammatory drugs versus oil of evening primrose in the treatment of mastalgia. Surgeon 2005;3(1)7–10.

Smith RL, Pruthi S, Fitzpatrick LA. Evaluation and management of breast pain. Mayo Clin Proc 2004;79:353–72.

Wilson MC, Sellwood RA. Therapeutic value of a supporting brassiere in mastodynia. BMJ 1976;2:90.

Patient with BREAST PAIN

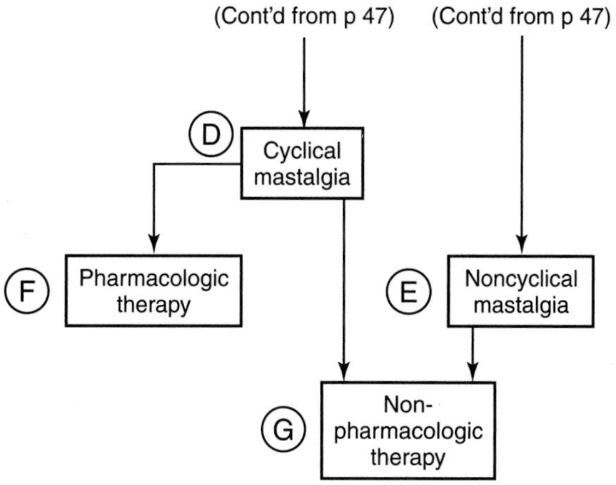
(Cont'd from p 47)
(Cont'd from p 47)
D
Cyclical mastalgia
F
Pharmacologic therapy
E
Noncyclical mastalgia
G
Non-pharmacologic therapy

Breast Lump in Adolescent Girls

Christine Gilroy, MD, MSPH

The primary concern of young women presenting with breast lump is for cancer, despite the absolute rarity of breast cancer in female individuals younger than 25 years. American culture is preoccupied with a fear of breast cancer, to the extent that 80% of women in one study overestimated personal risk for breast cancer by 50% or more. Occasionally, the complaint of a breast lump is "code" for another concern about the breast, including different breast size. A thorough and respectful evaluation, while minimizing potential trauma, are important goals in the evaluation and management of this problem.

A. History: Although breast cancer is rare in adolescents, cases have occurred, and a thorough history is important. Menarche, menstrual history, risk for pregnancy, reproductive history, trauma, history of radiation therapy, family history of breast or ovarian cancer, duration of lump, associated breast pain, cyclical change in lump, and change in size are all important factors to elicit. In those with a strong family history of breast cancer, or known *BRCA1* or *BRCA2* phenotype, or with a history of supradiaphragmatic radiation therapy, imaging and biopsy should be considered at the outset.

B. Physical Examination: First, ask the patient to indicate the area of concern. In the presence of a chaperone, perform a thorough breast examination, including the skin, all four quadrants, and under the areola, pressing all the way to the chest wall and tracking the breast tail into the axilla. The method of the examination (circular vs. vertical strips) is less important than taking time to examine as much breast tissue as possible. Check for lymphadenopathy in the axillary, supraclavicular, and cervical areas. Is the breast tissue homogeneous or "lumpy-bumpy" consistent with fibrocystic change? Is the "lump" in the breast tissue or the axilla? For maximum sensitivity of the clinical breast examination for breast cancer, the examination requires 3 minutes per breast, with particular attention to the nipple, areola, and subareolar complex, where 15% of breast cancers arise.

C. No Lump: Assess for other concerns. Otherwise, have the patient return for evaluation during the luteal phase of menstrual cycle (1 week before menses). The breasts of most (50%–60%) women have a nodular texture that undergoes proliferative changes during the menstrual cycle, with a change in breast volume of up to 15% in the luteal phase. If the lump comes and goes with hormonal stimulation, the patient may be reassured.

D. Axillary Lump: If distinct from the tail of the breast, consider lymphadenitis or hidradenitis. Encourage the patient to discontinue antiperspirant and re-evaluate in 6 weeks. If persistent, consider surgical excision, as lymphoma is possible, and represented 13% of biopsied breast lumps in Neinstein's series in adolscents. If larger, consider ultrasound.

E. Inflammation/Infection: In a series reviewed by Neinstein, infection was the cause of 3.7% of breast lumps in adolescents. If inflammation with lump is seen, consider risk factors for infection, including current lactation or history of lactation, nipple piercing, and nipple trauma. Treat with antibiotics and re-evaluate in 2 weeks. In lactation, coverage of *Staphylococcus aureus* is the goal; for nipple trauma, particularly with piercing, broad coverage of gram-negative bacteria and anaerobes should be considered. If history of breast trauma, consider hematoma with subsequent fat necrosis. If history of pregnancy, consider granulomatosis. If inflammation persists or progresses in spite of therapy, consider inflammatory breast cancer and refer for biopsy.

F. Breast Lump: If a palpable lump is noted or if the patient has a strong family history of breast cancer, known *BRCA1* or *BRCA2*, or history of supradiaphragmatic radiation therapy, refer directly for ultrasound with core biopsy or fine-needle aspiration, or consider magnetic resonance imaging if not easily visualized with ultrasound. Mammography is not indicated in the adolescent patient. A lump 5 cm or more in diameter and/or rapid progression over 3 months or less suggests giant fibroadenoma or phyllodes tumor; in this case, obtain surgical consultation. (Giant fibroadenoma represents 1% and phyllodes tumor 0.4% of breast lesions in adolescents). A smaller lump may be observed briefly in an adolescent. In the patient's chart, carefully document size and location by quadrant and relative to areola. Ask the patient to return during the follicular phase of menstrual cycle (1 week after menses). If lump resolves, reassure the patient. Breast tissue volume can change by 15% under the influence of cyclic hormonal change, resulting in transient, prominent nodularity. If lump persists, refer for ultrasound. In Diehl's series of adolescents with breast mass, 51% of the masses were fibrocystic change, and 47% had improvement or complete resolution over time.

(Continued on page 52)

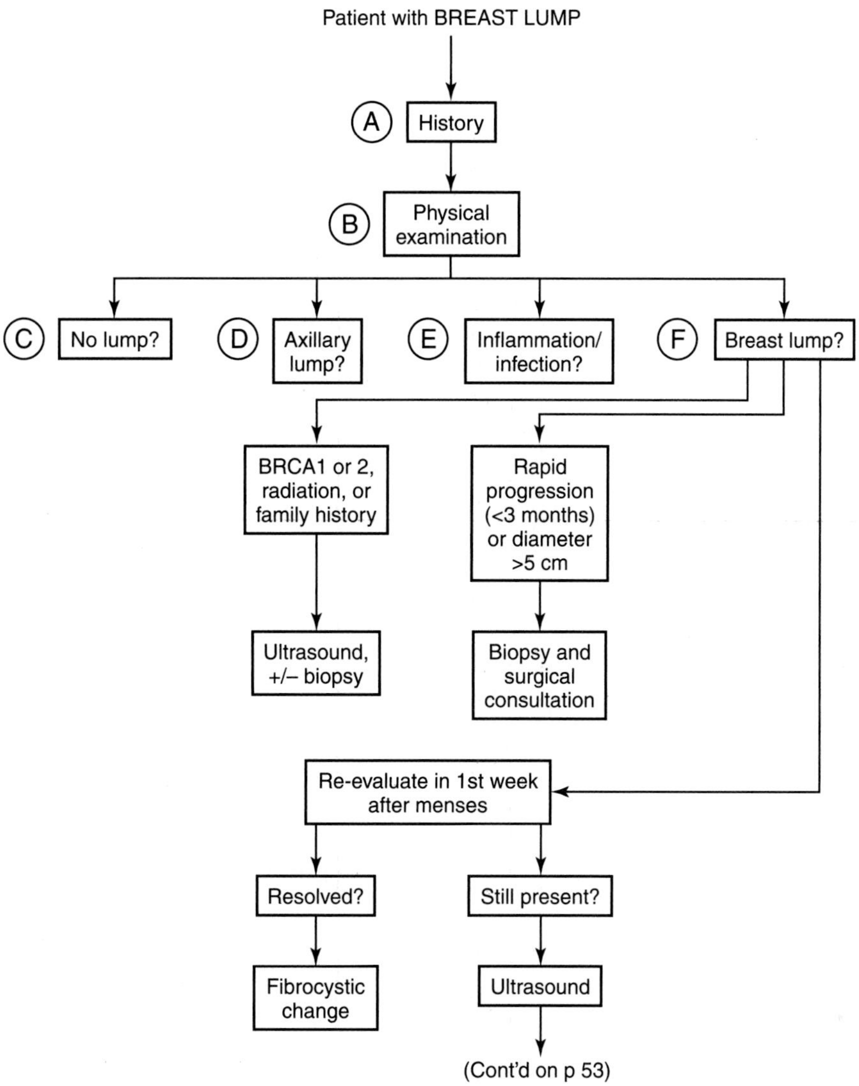
Patient with BREAST LUMP
A
History
B
Physical examination
C
No lump?
D
Axillary lump?
E
Inflammation/ infection?
F
Breast lump?
BRCA1 or 2, radiation, or family history
Rapid progression (<3 months) or diameter >5 cm
Ultrasound, +/– biopsy
Biopsy and surgical consultation
Re-evaluate in 1st week after menses
Resolved?
Still present?
Fibrocystic change
Ultrasound
(Cont'd on p 53)

G. Fibroadenoma represents 50% to 76% of breast masses in young women. In an autopsy series of women in adolescence up to age 25, 15% to 23% were found to have fibroadenoma. On examination, fibroadenomas are rubbery, well demarcated, and mobile within the surrounding breast tissue. They occur most commonly in the upper outer quadrant. Fibroadenomas with benign appearance by ultrasound may be managed conservatively, with sequential examination and ultrasound, and biopsy and surgery are to be avoided to prevent damage to developing breast tissue. About 16% to 37% of fibroadenomas resolve within 1 to 3 years; of the remaining fibroadenomas, 30% to 40% shrink within 5 years, and the rest stop growing when they reach a diameter of 1 to 3 cm. However, in one study of conservative management, only 25% of patients would accept nonoperative management, even when reassured the approach was safe. Fibroadenomas with sonographic appearance concerning for malignancy or growth rate greater than 16% per month should be considered for biopsy or excision.

H. Cysts: Cysts are less common in young women, accounting for 6% to 12% of breast masses in adolescents. Presenting complaints in one series were mastalgia (67%) or breast lump (32%). If subareolar, and associated with pain and inflammation, it likely represents an obstruction of Montgomery tubercles, and treatment consists of oral antibiotics directed at Staphylococcus and nonsteroidal anti-inflammatory drugs, with expected resolution in 7 days. Cysts can be aspirated during ultrasound, and resolution under ultrasound confirms a benign lesion. Complex cysts should be further evaluated to rule out malignancy.

I. Other Masses: Lumps that are not clearly fibroadenomas or cysts by ultrasound require further evaluation with biopsy. The differential is extensive, and the lump is still most likely one of the earlier described lesions. Subareolar masses associated with bloody discharge are most likely intraductalpapillomas, which are not cancer, but are associated with an increased risk for development of cancer. Cancer represents less than 1% of breast disease in adolescents. In Neinstein's series, 38% of cancers were metastases, 31% adenocarcinoma, and 13% were lymphoma. In youths with adenocarcinoma, 30% to 50% have a family history of breast cancer. Biopsy is recommended for evaluation, but the patient and family should be reassured that the likelihood of cancer remains very low.

References

Cant PJ, Maddem MV, et al. Non-operative management of breast masses diagnosed as fibroadenomas. Br J Surg 1995;82(6):792–4.

Chang DS, McGrath MH. Management of benign tumors of the adolescent breast. Plast Reconstr Surg 2007;120:13e–9e.

Chung EM, Cube R, Hall GJ, et al. Breast masses in children and adolescents: radiologic-pathologic correlation. RadioGraphics 2009;29:907–31.

Diehl T, Kaplan DW. Breast masses in adolescent females. J Adol Health Care 1985; 6(5):353–7.

Goehring C, Morabia A. Epidemiology of benign breast disease, with special attention to histologic types. Epidemiol Rev 1997;19:310–27.

Greydanus DE, Matytsina L, Gains M. Breast disorders in children and adolescents. Prim Care Clin Office Pract 2006;33:455–502.

Huneeus A, Shilling A, Horvath E, et al. Retroareolar cysts in the adolescent. J Pediatr Adolesc Gynecol 2003;16:45–9.

Love S, Gelman RS, Silen W. Fibrocystic "disease" of the breast—a nondisease? N Engl J Med 1982;307:1010–4.

Neinstein LS. Breast disease in adolescents and young women. Pediatr Clin North Am 1999;46:607–29.

Neinstein LS. Review of breast masses in adolescents. Adolesc Pediatr Gynecol 1994;7:119.

Nirupama K, De Silva MD, Brandt ML. Disorders of the breast in children and adolescents, part 2: breast masses. J Pediatr Adolesc Gynecol 2006;19:415–8.

Potten CS, Watson RJ, Williams GT, et al. The effect of age and menstrual cycle upon proliferative activity of the normal human breast. Br J Cancer 1988;58:163–70.

Smith BL, Gadd MA, et al. Perception of breast cancer risk among women in breast cancer and primary care settings: correlation with age and family history of breast cancer. Surgery 1996;120(2): 297–303.

Vade A, Lafita V, Ward KA, et al. Role of breast sonography in imaging of adolescents with palpable solid breast masses. Am J Radiol 2008;191:659–63.

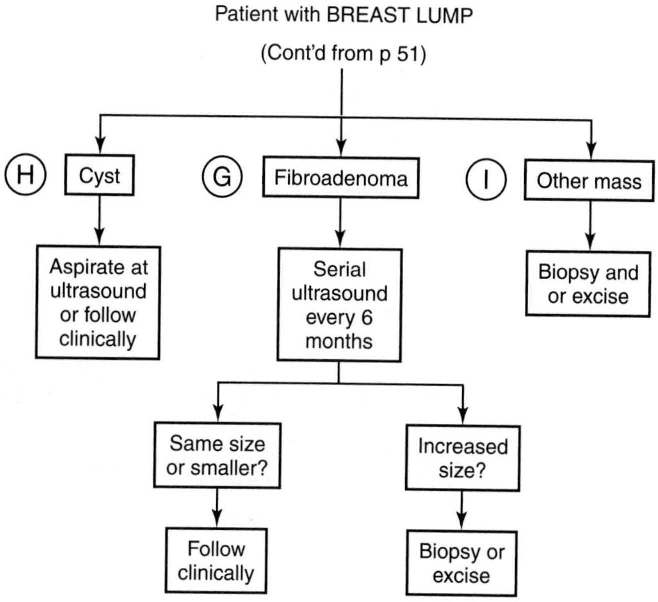
Patient with BREAST LUMP
(Cont'd from p 51)
H
Cyst
G
Fibroadenoma
I
Other mass
Aspirate at ultrasound or follow clinically
Serial ultrasound every 6 months
Biopsy and or excise
Same size or smaller?
Increased size?
Follow clinically
Biopsy or excise

Nipple Discharge in Adolescent Girls

Christine Gilroy, MD, MSPH

Nipple discharge is a less common complaint than breast pain or lump among women of reproductive age. Nipple discharge raises concerns of breast cancer or pituitary tumor, even in adolescence, but these are a rare cause of nipple discharge. A focused evaluation is important because many of the endocrine tests that are ordered in association with nipple discharge have a high rate of false-positive results.

A. History: A detailed history is the most important element in the evaluation of nipple discharge. Reproductive history is the most important, because galactorrhea may continue for a year or more after weaning or the end of pregnancy. In addition, the presence of oligoamenorrhea or amenorrhea with nonlactational galactorrhea significantly increases the likelihood of pituitary prolactinoma. Medical history should focus on thyroid disease, chronic renal disease, herpes zoster, illicit substance use, and a complete list of medications and herbal supplements. Surgical history should pay particular attention to breast or thoracic surgery, and history of nipple or breast piercing. Review of systems should focus on headache, vision changes, constitutional, skin, and gastrointestinal symptoms, and a psychosocial stress and sleep inventory.

B. Pregnancy or Postpartum: During pregnancy, the breasts and Montgomery tubercles may produce a clear discharge. Postpartum, milk production may persist for more than a year after weaning and is not considered galactorrhea. Postpartum milk production can be irritating, and the patient should be advised to minimize nipple stimulation, both as part of sexual interaction and from clothing. The patient may wear a padded, well-fitted bra during the day and night, and may need to add nipple shields to decrease stimulation enough for lactation to stop.

C. Physical Examination: In addition to a thorough breast examination, visual fields should be assessed, as well as the thyroid, skin texture, presence of tremor, and reflexes. It is important to remember that with significant pressure to the nipple, a nipple discharge may be produced in up to 85% of women. The color of the nipple discharge may provide additional information.

D. Areolar Discharge: May arise from the areola, not the nipple, from Montgomery or Morgani tubercles, which may be associated with an underlying mammary lobule. An episodic, thin, clear to brown discharge tends to resolve within 3 to 5 weeks. An associated lump is expected to resolve in 4 months.

(Continued on page 56)

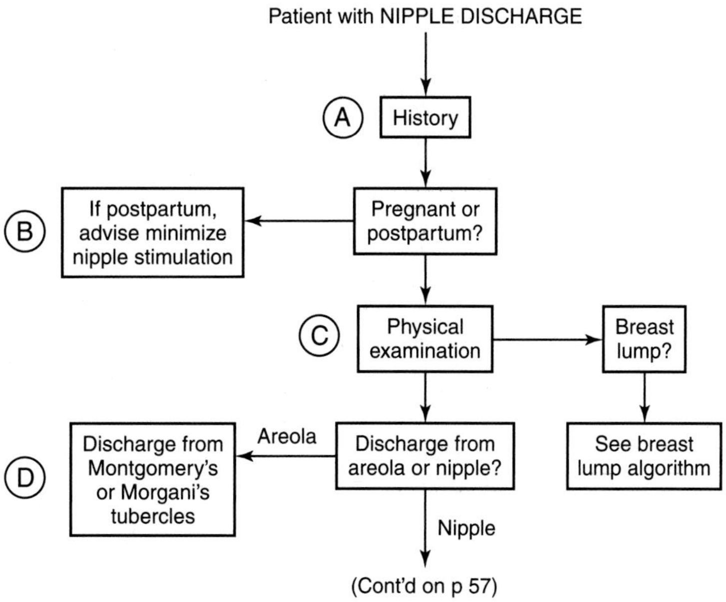
Patient with NIPPLE DISCHARGE
A
History
B
If postpartum, advise minimize nipple stimulation
Pregnant or postpartum?
C
Physical examination
Breast lump?
D
Discharge from Montgomery's or Morgani's tubercles
Areola
Discharge from areola or nipple?
See breast lump algorithm
Nipple
(Cont'd on p 57)

E. Milky Discharge: Milky discharge is consistent with galactorrhea. It is the most common discharge in adolescent girls. In the absence of pregnancy or postpartum state, milky discharge should be evaluated with an initial random prolactin and thyroid-stimulating hormone. Other causes to consider include chest wall or nipple trauma, spinal cord disorders, diffuse brain disease, uremia, hypernephroma, hypogonadism, adrenal tumor, and pituitary disorder.

F. Multicolored or Sticky Discharge: Consistent with ductal ectasia or fibrocystic change. The color most usually described is green or green-black. Ductal ectasia is characterized as the dilatation of subareolar ducts, is associated with fibrocystic change, and may cause noncyclical mastalgia.

G. Purulent Discharge: If there is a question whether discharge is purulent or milky, a wet prep may help differentiate by the presence of white cells. Consistent with mastitis, the most common infecting organism is *Staphylococcus aureus*. Preceding factors may include trauma or ductal ectasia. If nipple piercing is present, consider broader antibiotic coverage.

H. Watery, Serous, or Serosanguineous Discharge: A broad differential is possible, including in order of prevalence in adolescents: fibrocystic change or ductal ectasia, intraductal papilloma, or breast cancer. Intraductal papillomas represented 1.2% of breast lesions in adolescents for which a biopsy was performed and breast cancer represented less than 1% in Neinstein's review. In two series reviewing intraductal papilloma in adolescents, a serosanguineous breast discharge had variable prevalence rate (23%–95%). The incidence of breast cancer is lower. Evaluation should not include cytopathology of the nipple discharge, but instead ultrasound and biopsy of any lump. If no lump is palpated during a thorough (3 minutes per breast) examination, careful clinical monitoring is adequate, unless the risk for breast cancer is high (*BRCA*, primary relative, previous radiation). If the risk for breast cancer is high, referral to a breast clinic or surgeon is appropriate.

I. Abnormal Thyroid-Stimulating Hormone: Hypothyroidism results in increased thyrotropin releasing hormone production, lactotroph stimulation, and decreased physiologic clearance of prolactin. Treat the hypothyroidism adequately (normal thyroid-stimulating hormone for 6–8 weeks) and follow with a repeat prolactin.

J. Normal Serum Prolactin: This does not preclude the presence of galactorrhea, but the history and physical examination should be revisited to exclude the possibility of a ductal source of discharge. If the prolactin level is normal and the discharge is galactorrhea, medications should be reviewed and those associated with galactorrhea should be discontinued. Chest wall injury and nipple stimulation have been associated with persistent galactorrhea, and stimulation should be minimized (remove piercings, try nipple shields). If idiopathic normoprolactinemic galactorrhea persists, consider treating with a dopamine agonist to determine whether this inhibits secretion.

K. Increased Serum Prolactin: Review for medications associated with galactorrhea; discontinue those medications, if present. For those women taking typical antipsychotics or risperidone, switching to olanzapine or quetiapine has been shown to decrease galactorrhea in some without exacerbating psychiatric symptoms. If no galactorrhea-associated medications/illicit drugs/herbals are being taken, repeat a prolactin level. Physiologic conditions that may produce transient increases in prolactin secretion include physical and emotional stress, high-protein midday meal, sleep, orgasm, exercise, menstrual cycle, excessive breast stimulation, pseudopregnancy, and pregnancy. If serum prolactin level is increased again, obtain a fasting morning prolactin level. If this is increased, obtain magnetic resonance imaging of the pituitary. If a pituitary abnormality exists, refer to endocrine specialist. If pituitary is normal, review other causative factors and consider a dopamine agonist (cabergoline) or referral to endocrine specialist for treatment. Women with hyperprolactinemia are at risk for osteoporosis; therefore, a documented and persistent increase in prolactin levels should be treated.

References

Bachman JW. Breast Problems. Primary Care 1988;15:643–64.

Elmore JG, Armstrong K, Lehman CD. Screening for breast cancer. JAMA 2005;293:1245–56.

Falkenberry SS. Nipple discharge. Obstet Gynecol Clin North Am 2002;29:21–9.

Greydanus DE, Matytsina L, Gains M. Breast disorders in children and adolescents. Prim Care Clin Office Pract 2006;33:455–502.

Kinon BJ, Ahl J, et al. Improvement in hyperprolactinemia and reproductive comorbidities in patients with schizophrenia switched from conventional antipsychotics or risperidone to olanzapirne. Psychoneuroendocrinology 2006;31(5)577–88.

Leung AKC, Pacaud D. Diagnosis and treatment of galactorrhea. Am Fam Physician 2004;70:543–50.

Miltenburg DM, Speights VO. Benign breast disease. Obstet Gynecol Clin North Am 2008;35:285–300.

Neinstein LS. Breast disease in adolescents and young women. Pediatr Clin North Am 1999;46:607–29.

Pena KS, Rosenfeld JA. Evaluation and treatment of galactorrhea. Am Fam Physician 2001;63:1763–71.

Roke Y, van Harten PN, Boot AM, Buitelaar JK. Antipsychotic medication in children and adolescents: a descriptive review of the effects on prolactin level and associated side effects. J Child Adolesc Psychopharmacol 2009;19:403–14.

Sobrinho LG. Prolactin, psychological stress and environment in humans: adaptation and maladaptation. Pituitary 2003;6:35–9.

Vartej P, Poiana C, Vartej I. Effects of hyperpolactinemia on osteoporotic fracture risk in premenopausal women. Gynecol Endocrinol 2001;15(1):43–7.

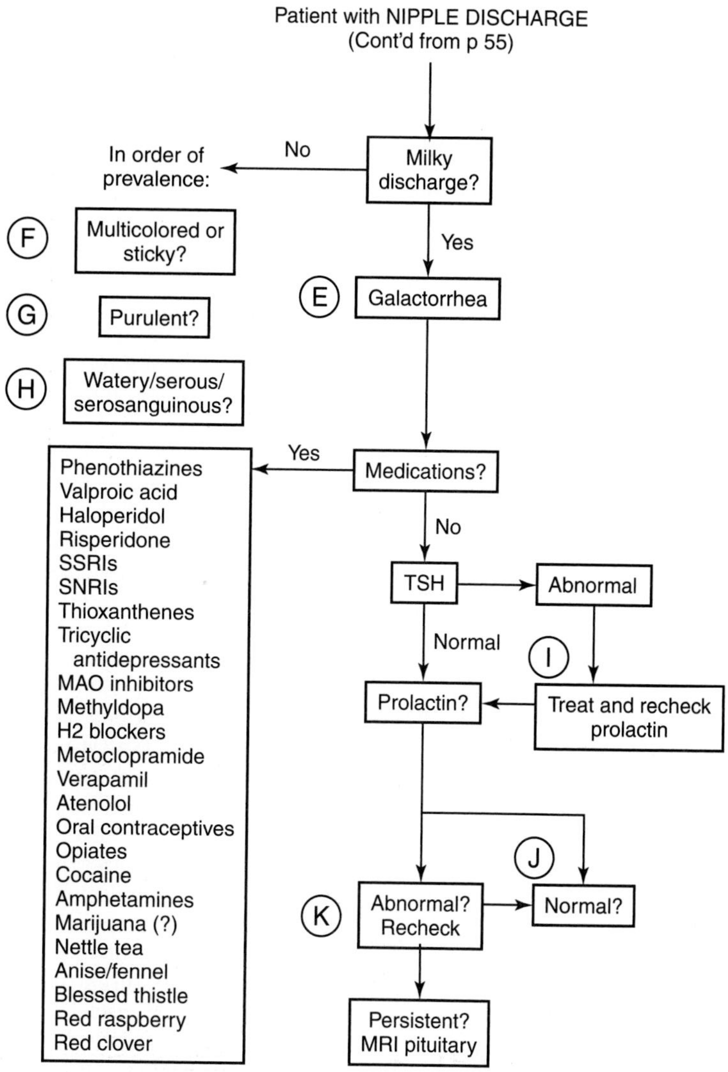

Patient with NIPPLE DISCHARGE
(Cont'd from p 55)
No
Milky discharge?
In order of prevalence:
F
Multicolored or sticky?
G
Purulent?
H
Watery/serous/ serosanguinous?
Yes
E
Galactorrhea
Yes
Medications?
Phenothiazines
Valproic acid
Haloperidol
Risperidone
SSRIs
SNRIs
Thioxanthenes
Tricyclic antidepressants
MAO inhibitors
Methyldopa
H2 blockers
Metoclopramide
Verapamil
Atenolol
Oral contraceptives
Opiates
Cocaine
Amphetamines
Marijuana (?)
Nettle tea
Anise/fennel
Blessed thistle
Red raspberry
Red clover
No
TSH
Abnormal
Normal
I
Prolactin?
Treat and recheck prolactin
J
Normal?
K
Abnormal? Recheck
Persistent? MRI pituitary

Menstrual Problems and Vaginal Bleeding

Stephen M. Scott, MD, FACOG

Menstruation is usually the final sign of female pubertal development providing continued evidence that the brain–ovary pathways have been released from suppression and the ovaries are producing estrogen. Other clinical signs of estrogen production include breast development, maturation of the vaginal mucosa, and accelerated linear growth. Early in puberty, the ovaries make only estrogen and initial menses occur without ovulation. It can take up to 2 years to achieve regular ovulatory cycles. Once ovulation begins, the ovaries also produce progesterone, which provides stabilization of the endometrium in preparation for pregnancy implantation. If pregnancy does not occur, the ovary temporarily halts progesterone and estrogen production. The decline in progesterone levels initiates the process of endometrial shedding. The cycle begins again with increasing levels of estrogen to repair and proliferate the surface lining. Ovulation cycles usually range from 21 to 35 days and bleeding typically lasts from 3 to 7 days. They are often associated with premenstrual symptoms such as cramping.

It is important to understand the underlying hormonal status of a child or adolescent with irregular bleeding to determine the correct cause. An "estrogen-deficient" state is found before puberty or during adolescence when the brain fails to stimulate the ovaries or the ovaries fail to respond to brain signals. Without estrogen, the endometrial lining remains thin and is not a source of bleeding. Anatomic genital lesions should be investigated as the source of bleeding. An "estrogen variation" state occurs when ovaries produce estrogen but fail to ovulate and initiate progesterone production. Anovulation results in thick, disorganized, and fragile endometrium that bleeds irregularly and does not efficiently remove and replenish surface lining. A "progesterone excess" state is usually iatrogenic because of excessive levels of progesterone or progestins, leading to an atrophic lining that is thin, fragile, and may bleed irregularly. It is important to remember that even oral contraceptives with estrogen can lead to progesterone excess. "Progesterone withdrawal" states are usually due to ovulation cycles or cyclic hormonal contraceptive use. When irregular bleeding occurs in this environment, a secondary anatomic genital lesion is the likely cause of bleeding between regular menses.

A. When a pediatric patient has abnormal vaginal bleeding, clinicians should obtain a thorough history and physical examination. Determination of volume status and severity of anemia will determine whether acute treatment is necessary.

B. The presence or absence of estrogen will provide vital clues to the status of the endometrial lining. Breast development, estrogenized genital tissue, or an increased estradiol level indicates the presence of estrogen. If no estrogen stimulation is present, the patient has prepubertal bleeding. Anatomic lesions such as bacterial vulvovaginitis, foreign body, cervicitis, endometritis, urethral prolapse, trauma, urinary tract infections, and neoplasms of genitourinary and gastrointestinal sources should be ruled out and treated.

C. If there are signs of estrogen stimulation, the patient's age will determine the presence of precocious puberty. Precocious puberty is defined as breast development before 8 years of age with progression of bone age and possible menstrual bleeding. It can be divided into central "GnRH-dependent" precocious puberty (CPP) versus peripheral "GnRH-independent" precocious puberty (PPP). Although GnRH stimulation testing is the gold standard in diagnosing CPP, an increased basal leuteinizing hormone level or basal leuteinizing hormone/follicle-stimulating hormone ratio has utility. Suppressed gonadotropin levels suggest PPP. Most cases of CPP are idiopathic, but brains lesions should be ruled out with magnetic resonance imaging. Treatment of CPP usually involves suppression of hypothalamic signaling with GnRH agonists. Surgical removal of pedunculated lesions is an option, but the risk for damage to surrounding normal tissue is too great when tumors are embedded. Causes of PPP include iatrogenic estrogen administration, exogenous ingestion, McCune-Albright syndrome, tumors of the ovaries, and rarely, tumors of the adrenal glands. Exogenous causes of PPP can be diagnosed through a careful history. Ultrasound of the ovaries and adrenal glands for lesions is recommended if no exogenous source is identified. If café-au-lait spots are present, a skeletal survey noting lytic lesions will uncover McCune-Albright syndrome. Removal of the underlying estrogen source is the primary treatment for PPP. Signs of estrogen reversal should be monitored closely to ensure preservation of epiphyseal plates and continued linear growth. Growth hormone levels may be disrupted in the face of CPP caused by a brain lesion. Assessment of growth hormone levels is needed if linear growth stalls after treatment begins.

D. Age-appropriate puberty is present when bleeding begins at 10 years of age or beyond. Pregnancy and its complications should always be ruled out in an age-appropriate patient with abnormal genital bleeding.

(Continued on page 60)

Patient with MENSTRUAL PROBLEMS AND VAGINAL BLEEDING

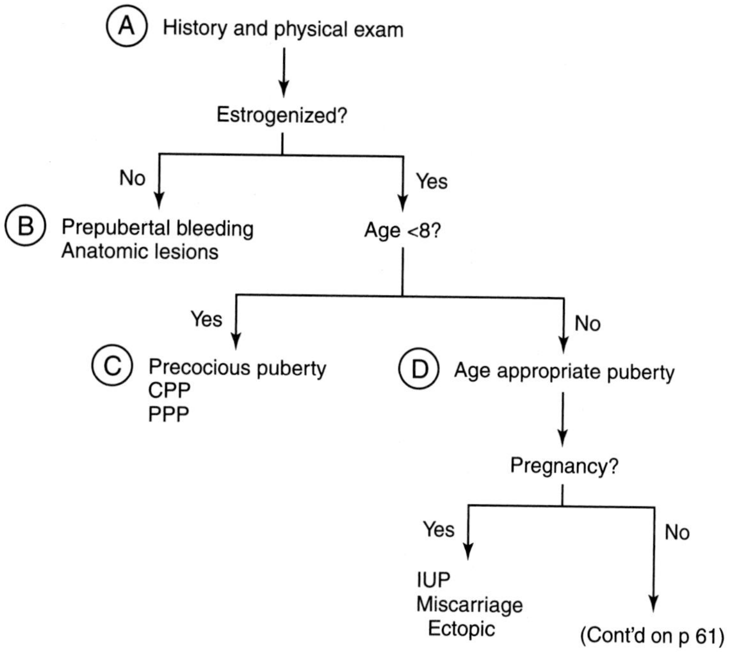
A History and physical exam
Estrogenized?
No
Yes
B Prepubertal bleeding
Anatomic lesions
Age <8?
Yes
No
C Precocious puberty
CPP
PPP
D Age appropriate puberty
Pregnancy?
Yes
No
IUP
Miscarriage
Ectopic
(Cont'd on p 61)

E. Once pregnancy is ruled out, ovulation status will aid in determining the cause of irregular bleeding. Irregular, unpredictable bleeding patterns lacking premenstrual symptoms or cramping generally point to anovulation; however, monthly bleeding patterns do not automatically prove ovulation. A progesterone level of 5 ng/ml or greater, drawn 10 days before the next expected menses, confirms ovulation. If ovulation is confirmed, then anatomic genital lesions are likely creating irregular bleeding between regular progesterone withdrawal cycles. Causative factors include lesions mentioned in prepubertal bleeding.

F. If the patient is anovulatory, then dysfunctional uterine bleeding (DUB) is diagnosed. The presence or absence of androgenizing signs will help to categorize causes of DUB. Obesity, hirsutism, and acne are typical signs of high androgens. Most cases of androgenized DUB are caused by polycystic ovarian syndrome. Other causative factors should be investigated if greater levels of androgens are suspected. Virilizing signs such as clitoromegaly, male pattern baldness, and deepening of the voice should prompt workup for androgen-producing tumors in the ovaries and adrenals, adult-onset congenital adrenal hyperplasia, and Cushing disease.

G. Disruptions of brain–ovary signaling are the causes of DUB in the absence of androgenizing signs. Within the first 2 years from menarche, this may be self-limited and correct on its own. Beyond that time, pathologic causative factors should be suspected. Disruptions of the normal GnRH pulse pattern can be caused by excessive exercise or dieting, stress, increased levels of prolactin from tumors or medications, and hypothyroidism. Pituitary disruptions occur from gland necrosis, infections, or prolactin- versus nonprolactin-secreting tumors. Premature ovarian failure will eventually lead to amenorrhea, but early on may present with irregular bleeding. Premature ovarian failure should be considered if signs of reduced estrogen levels are present such as hot flashes, decreased breast size, vaginal dryness, or vaginal mucosa atrophy. Increases of follicle-stimulating hormone and leuteinizing hormone into the postmenopausal range will confirm ovarian failure and should prompt genetic karyotyping. Blood dyscrasias should be suspected if bleeding is severe enough to require hospitalization or blood transfusion at menarche.

H. Treatment of DUB may range from reassurance to treatment of underlying disorders. Iron and multivitamin supplementation is recommended if anemia is present. Endometrial stabilization is achieved with progesterone or progestin replacement. Unless contraindicated, combined oral contraceptive pills (OCPs) are usually the easiest treatment method to achieve regular cycles. Once endometrial shedding is complete, transition to continuous OCP regimen may result in long-term amenorrhea. At least 6 to 12 months of treatment is recommended, and in many cases, longer term management with OCPs is required. In general, nonsteroidal anti-inflammatory drugs (e.g., ibuprofen) should be considered during placebo days because endometrial shedding may lead to cramping for the first time. Estrogens in OCPs provide an added benefit of suppressing androgen activity in cases of polycystic ovarian syndrome. Patients with polycystic ovarian syndrome may also benefit from hirsutism treatments and early screening and intervention for hyperinsulinemia and type 2 diabetes.

References

Demers C. Gynaecological and obstetric management of women with inherited bleeding disorders. Int J Gynaecol Obstet 2006;95:75–87.

Fahmy JL. The radiological approach to precocious puberty. Br J Radiol 2000;73:560–7.

Houk CP. Adequacy of a single unstimulated luteinizing hormone level to diagnose central precocious puberty in girls. Pediatrics 2009;123:1059–63.

Minjarez DA. Abnormal bleeding in adolescents. Semin Reprod Med 2003;21:363–73.

Scott S. Normal and abnormal puberty. In: Alvero R, editor. Reproductive endocrinology and infertility: the requisites in obstetrics and gynecology. New York: Elsevier Science; 2006.

Stanley T, Misra M. Polycystic ovary syndrome in obese adolescents. Curr Opin Endocrinol Diabetes Obes 2008;15:30–6.

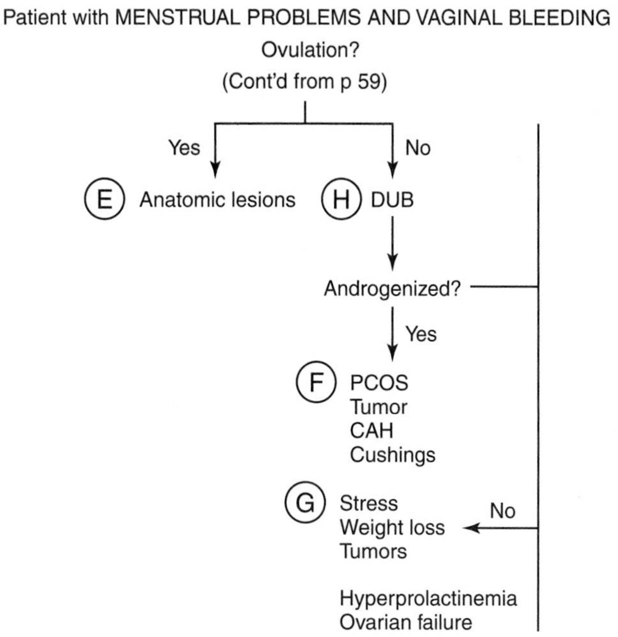
Patient with MENSTRUAL PROBLEMS AND VAGINAL BLEEDING
Ovulation?
(Cont'd from p 59)
Yes
No
E Anatomic lesions
H DUB
Androgenized?
Yes
F PCOS
Tumor
CAH
Cushings
G Stress
Weight loss
Tumors
No
Hyperprolactinemia
Ovarian failure

Sexually Transmitted Infections in Adolescents

Paritosh Kaul, MD

Adolescents are at an increased risk for sexually transmitted infections (STIs) because of various factors. These factors include biological, psychosocial, confidentiality, ethical, and legal issues, as well as lack of access to health care. Adolescents have the greatest rates of STIs compared with other age groups, and half of all STIs diagnosed are among 15- to 24-year-olds. Two thirds (65%) of 12th-grade students have had vaginal intercourse. The adolescent interview is critical to elicit a history of sexuality, sexual activity, and other high-risk behaviors. These areas should be explored with the adolescent alone. The interviewer should be open, nonjudgmental, and ensure confidentiality.

This chapter starts with decision making with vaginal discharge and cervicitis, then pelvic inflammatory disease (PID), and then STIs among adolescent boys.

VULVOVAGINITIS IN THE ADOLESCENT

A. History: In the adolescent with vulvovaginitis, ask about the color, odor, quantity of vaginal discharge, and relation to menstrual period. Candidiasis occurs premenstrually, whereas trichomoniasis occurs during or immediately after the menses. Inquire about sexual activity including change in sex partners, condom use, and history of previous STIs. Ask about medications including contraceptives, antibiotics, steroids, use of soaps, deodorants, and douching. Also ask about history of diabetes mellitus. Explore the possibility of trauma or foreign body.

B. Examination: Carefully inspect the perineum, vulva, vagina, and cervix for erythema, excoriation, swelling, lesions, signs of trauma, and foreign body. Also look for color, texture, adherence, and odor of vaginal discharge. Perform a speculum examination and closely inspect the vagina walls for lesions or anatomic abnormalities (polyp, tumor, and abscess). A bimanual examination should be performed to rule out PID or adnexal masses.

C. Diagnostic Evaluation: Examine the vaginal discharge for pH, "whiff test," and microscopy. Vaginitis caused candidiasis, trichomoniasis, and bacterial vaginosis is described in Table 1. Also, test the vaginal secretions for gonorrhea and chlamydia. A pregnancy test should be performed on all sexually active adolescents.

D. Treatment: Depending on the cause of vulvovaginitis, the treatments are described in Table 2. Sexual partners of adolescents with trichomoniasis need to be notified and treated. Sexual partners of adolescents with bacterial vaginosis do not need treatment.

CERVICITIS

Cervicitis represents an infection of the cervix. It may produce discharge from the cervix and can be confused with vaginitis. Mucopurulent cervicitis is characterized by a mucopurulent discharge from the cervix. Chlamydia and gonorrhea are the most common causative organisms for mucopurulent cervicitis, but often the organisms cannot be identified. Other causative agents include herpes simplex, *Trichomonas vaginalis,* and *Candida albicans*.

A. History: The adolescent may have symptoms of vaginal discharge, dyspareunia, irregular vaginal bleeding, and vaginal itching.

B. Examination: On examination, mucopurulent endocervical discharge, endocervical friability, edema, and erythema of the cervix can be noticed.

C. Diagnostic Evaluation: Ten or more white blood cells (WBCs) per high-power field on a Gram stain specimen is diagnostic of mucopurulent cervicitis. The cervical fluid should be sent for chlamydia and gonorrhea testing. The wet mount should be examined for trichomoniasis, hyphae, and clue cells.

D. Treatment: The treatment for mucopurulent cervicitis is described in Table 3.

PELVIC INFLAMMATORY DISEASE

PID is a polymicrobial infection in which sexually transmitted and/or endogenous vaginal microorganisms spread from the lower genital tract to infect all or some of the pelvic organs. If inadequately treated, serious complications such

Table 1. **Clinical and Microscopic Features of Vulvovaginitis**

Infection	Symptoms	Vaginal Discharge	pH	Whiff Test	Microscopy
Candidiasis	Pruritus, burning, discharge	Thick, adherent, white	4–4.5	Negative	↑ WBC, budding yeast, pseudohyphae
Trichomoniasis	Frothy, foul-smelling discharge, pruritus, dysuria	Purulent, profuse, irritating, frothy, green-yellow	>4.5	Variably positive	↑ WBC, trichomonads
Bacterial vaginosis	Foul-smelling discharge, increased after intercourse	Thin, homogenous, gray-white	>4.5	Positive	>20% clue cells

WBC, white blood cell count.

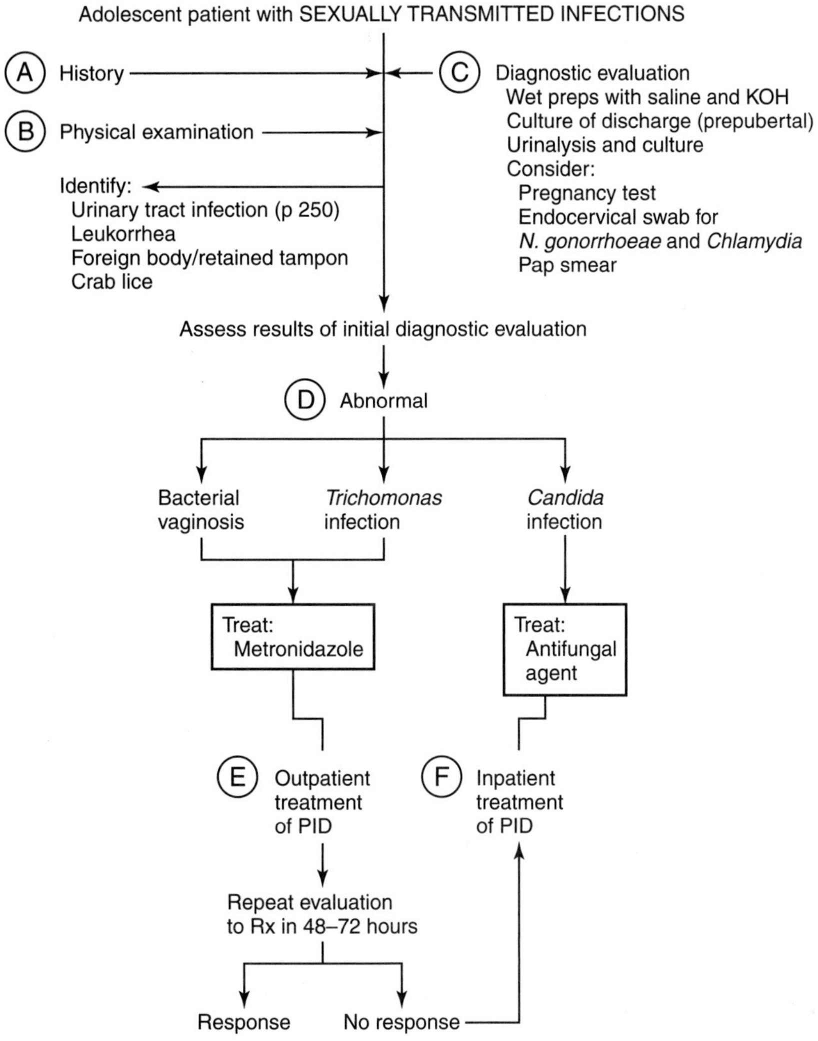
Adolescent patient with SEXUALLY TRANSMITTED INFECTIONS
(A) History
(B) Physical examination
(C) Diagnostic evaluation
Wet preps with saline and KOH
Culture of discharge (prepubertal)
Urinalysis and culture
Consider:
Pregnancy test
Endocervical swab for
N. gonorrhoeae and Chlamydia
Pap smear
Identify:
Urinary tract infection (p 250)
Leukorrhea
Foreign body/retained tampon
Crab lice
Assess results of initial diagnostic evaluation
(D) Abnormal
Bacterial vaginosis
Trichomonas infection
Candida infection
Treat: Metronidazole
Treat: Antifungal agent
(E) Outpatient treatment of PID
(F) Inpatient treatment of PID
Repeat evaluation to Rx in 48–72 hours
Response
No response

as ectopic pregnancy, infertility, and chronic pelvic pain may ensue. PID is a clinical diagnosis and is imprecise. PID is a polymicrobial and is caused by sexually transmitted organisms, especially *Chlamydia trachomatis* and *Neisseria gonorrhoeae*. Other organisms include anaerobes, *Gardnerella vaginalis, Haemophilus influenzae,* enteric Gram-negative rods, and *Streptococcus agalactiae.* In addition, cytomegalovirus (CMV), *Mycoplasma hominis, Ureaplasma urealyticum,* and *Mycoplasma genitalium* might be associated with some cases of PID. In many cases, no organism is associated with PID.

A. History: Any adolescent girl with lower abdominal pain could have PID. History includes sexually activity, vaginal discharge, irregular vaginal bleeding, or dysuria. Systemic signs of anorexia, nausea, vomiting, fever, or malaise are infrequent.

B. Physical Examination: PID is a clinical diagnosis. The Centers for Disease Control and Prevention has defined minimal criteria for PID (see Table 4). Findings may include abdominal pain or right upper quadrant pain, which is seen in Fitz–Hugh–Curtis syndrome.

C. Laboratory Evaluation: Supports but does not make the diagnoses of PID. Testing for gonorrhea and chlamydia should be performed, although negative test results are common. A pregnancy test should be performed to rule out ectopic pregnancy, which can mimic PID. Other optional tests are WBC count, erythrocyte sedimentation rate, or C-reactive protein, which can be increased. In addition, ultrasonography helps to exclude ectopic pregnancy or tubo-ovarian abscess.

D. Diagnosis of PID: As mentioned earlier, PID is an imprecise clinical diagnosis. The minimal criteria for diagnosis of PID are enumerated in Table 4.

E. Outpatient Treatment of PID: The adolescent girl with PID can be treated on an outpatient basis provided there are no criteria for hospitalization as described in Table 5. The patient should return for re-evaluation in 48 to 72 hours to ensure clinical improvement in signs and symptoms. If there is no clinical improvement, the patient will need hospitalization. The outpatient treatment of PID as suggested by Centers for Disease Control and Prevention is described in Table 6. Partner notification, counseling regarding safe sex, risk reduction, and screening for other STIs should also be part of the follow-up visit.

F. Inpatient Treatment of PID: Adolescents who meet criteria for hospitalizations should receive inpatient

Table 2. **Treatment of Vaginitis**

Bacterial Vaginosis

Metronidazole: 500 mg orally twice a day for 7 days
OR
Metronidazole gel: 0.75%, one full applicator (5 g); intravaginally, once a day for 5 days
OR
Clindamycin cream: 2%, one full applicator (5 g); intravaginally at bedtime for 7 days

Trichomoniasis

Metronidazole: 2 g orally in a single dose
OR
Tinidazole: 2 g orally in a single dose

Candidiasis

Clotrimazole: 500 mg vaginal suppository, once; 200 mg vaginal suppository qd × 3 days
Miconazole: 2% cream, apply at bedtime × 7 days
Nystatin: 100,000 units vaginal suppositories once daily × 14 days
Fluconazole: 150 mg orally once

Table 3. **Treatment of Mucopurulent Cervicitis**

Azithromycin 1 g PO once
OR
Doxycycline 100 mg PO bid × 7 days

Consider concurrent treatment for gonococcal infection if prevalence of gonorrhea is high in the patient population under assessment.
PO, orally.

Table 4. **Centers for Disease Control and Prevention Criteria for Diagnosis of Pelvic Inflammatory Disease**

Minimal Clinical Criteria for Diagnosis of Pelvic Inflammatory Disease

Cervical motion tenderness
OR
Uterine or adnexal tenderness

Additional Criteria to Increase Specificity

- Oral temperature >101° F (>38.3° C)
- Abnormal cervical or vaginal mucopurulent discharge
- Presence of abundant numbers of white blood cells on saline microscopy of vaginal secretions
- Increased erythrocyte sedimentation rate
- Increased C-reactive protein
- Laboratory documentation of cervical infection with *Neisseria gonorrhoeae* or *Chlamydia trachomatis*

Table 5. **Criteria for Hospitalization for Pelvic Inflammatory Disease**

- Surgical emergencies (e.g., appendicitis) cannot be excluded.
- The patient is pregnant.
- The patient does not respond clinically to oral antimicrobial therapy.
- The patient is unable to follow or tolerate an outpatient oral regimen.
- The patient has severe illness, nausea and vomiting, or high fever.
- The patient has a tubo-ovarian abscess.

Table 6. **Outpatient Treatment of Pelvic Inflammatory Disease**

Regimen 1

Levofloxacin: 500 mg orally once daily for 14 days*
OR
Ofloxacin: 400 mg orally twice daily for 14 days*
WITH OR WITHOUT
Metronidazole: 500 mg orally twice a day for 14 days

Regimen 2

Ceftriaxone: 250 mg intramuscularly in a single dose
PLUS
Doxycycline: 100 mg orally twice a day for 14 days
WITH OR WITHOUT
Metronidazole: 500 mg orally twice a day for 14 days

Regimen 3

Cefoxitin, 2 g intramuscularly in a single dose, and Probenecid, 1 g orally administered concurrently in a single dose
PLUS
Doxycycline: 100 mg orally twice a day for 14 days
WITH OR WITHOUT
Metronidazole: 500 mg orally twice a day for 14 days

Regimen 4

Other parenteral third-generation cephalosporin (e.g., ceftizoxime or cefotaxime)
PLUS
Doxycycline 100 mg orally twice a day for 14 days
WITH OR WITHOUT
Metronidazole: 500 mg orally twice a day for 14 days

treatment for PID as described in Table 7. The inpatient treatment should continue for 24 hours after clinical improvement of symptoms. Patients may be discharged and advised to complete oral doxycycline for a total of 14 days.

SEXUALLY TRANSMITTED INFECTIONS IN THE MALE SEX

Adolescent boys with STIs are commonly asymptomatic. They may present with symptoms of urethritis or epididymitis. The causes of urethritis in adolescents are given in Table 8.

A. A good sexual history is essential. This should be taken with the adolescent alone, ensuring confidentiality. Inquire from the adolescent about sexual activity, number of sexual partners, dysuria, hematuria, and urethral discharge. The adolescent should be asked about history of previous STI or a partner with a STI. Obtain history of type of sexual activity including oral sex and anal sex (both insertive and penetrative). History of any urologic procedure predisposes to urethritis, whereas history of joint involvement raises the suspicion of disseminated gonococcal infection or Reiter syndrome.

B. Examination should be done with adequate lighting and with the patient in a standing position. Look for penile discharge; if no discharge is present, the penis can be milked a few times to help produce the discharge. Retraction of the foreskin is critical in uncircumcised patients. The penis should be inspected for

Table 7. Inpatient Treatment for Pelvic Inflammatory Disease

Parenteral Regimen 1

Cefotetan: 2 g IV every 12 hours
OR
Cefoxitin: 2 g IV every 6 hours
PLUS
Doxycycline: 100 mg orally or IV every 12 hours
OR

Regimen 2

Clindamycin: 900 mg IV every 8 hours
PLUS
Gentamicin loading dose IV or IM (2 mg/kg of body weight), followed by a maintenance dose (1.5 mg/kg) every 8 hours. Single daily dosing may be substituted.

IM, intramuscularly; *IV,* intravenously.

Table 8. Causes of Urethritis in Adolescents

Principal Bacterial Pathogens

No pathogen identified
Chlamydia trachomatis
Neisseria gonorrhoeae

Other Pathogens

Trichomonas vaginalis
Ureaplasma urealyticum
Mycoplasma genitalium
Mycoplasma hominis
Herpes simplex virus

Table 9. Treatment of Urethritis

Recommended Regimens

Azithromycin: 1 g orally in a single dose
OR
Doxycycline: 100 mg orally twice a day for 7 days

Alternative Regimens

Erythromycin base: 500 mg orally four times a day for 7 days
OR
Erythromycin ethylsuccinate: 800 mg orally four times a day for 7 days
OR
Ofloxacin: 300 mg orally twice a day for 7 days
OR
Levofloxacin: 500 mg orally once daily for 7 days

Table 10. Treatment of Epididymitis

Recommended Regimens

For acute epididymitis most likely caused by gonococcal or chlamydial infection:

Ceftriaxone: 250 mg intramuscularly in a single dose
PLUS
Doxycycline: 100 mg orally twice a day for 10 days

For acute epididymitis most likely caused by enteric organisms or for patients allergic to cephalosporins and/or tetracyclines:

Ofloxacin: 300 mg orally twice a day for 10 days
OR
Levofloxacin: 500 mg orally once daily for 10 days

ulcers or warts. Examine the testes for signs of epididymitis and the anal area for warts or ulcers. The inguinal area should be examined for lymphadenopathy.

C. Urethritis and epididymitis are both diagnosed by one of the following: observation of mucoid or purulent urethral discharge or first-void urine-positive leukocyte esterase or microscopic examination of more than 10 WBCs/high-power field or at least 5 WBCs/high-power field or gram-negative intracellular diplococci on Gram stain. Nucleic acid amplification tests are the most sensitive tests and gold standard for diagnosing gonorrheal or chlamydial infections.

D. Patients who are symptomatic need to be treated for gonorrhea, chlamydia, or both as per Centers for Disease Control and Prevention guidelines. All sexual partners of patients from the past 60 days should be notified. If possible, adolescents should be observed taking treatments. Treatment of urethritis is given in Table 9.

E. Epididymitis presents with unilateral testicular pain and swelling, erythema of the scrotal skin, hydrocele, and involvement of the adjacent testis. Urethritis may or may not be present. Treatment includes bed rest, scrotal elevation, analgesics, nonsteroidal anti-inflammatory drugs, and antibiotics to treat the infection. Differential diagnosis includes testicular torsion, infarction, and torsion of the appendix testis. Treatment is summarized in Table 10.

F. Teens diagnosed with a STI are at greater risk for syphilis, HIV, and other STIs. Counseling should include risk reduction methods such as abstinence, condom use, and alternative sexual behavior.

References

Biggs WS, Williams RM. Common gynecological infections. Prim Care Clin Office Pract 2009;36: 33–51.

Burstein GR, Murray MJ. Diagnosis and management of sexually transmitted diseases among adolescents. Pediatr Rev 2003 Apr;24(4): 119–27.

Centers for Disease Control and Prevention. Sexually transmitted diseases treatment guidelines 2006. MMWR Recomm Rep 2006;55(No. RR-11:[1–94]).

Frenkl TL, Potts J. Sexually transmitted infections. Urol Clin North Am 2008;35:33–46.

Holland-Hall C. Sexually transmitted infections: screening, syndromes and symptoms. Prim Care Clin Office Pract 2006;33: 433–454.

Hollier LM, Workowski K. Treatment of sexually transmitted infections in women. Infect Dis Clin North Am 2008;22:665–91.

Kaul P, Stevens-Simon C, Saproo A, Coupey SM. Trends in illness severity and length of stay in inner-city adolescents hospitalized for pelvic inflammatory disease. J Pediatr Adolesc Gynecol 2008;21:289–93.

Lareau SM, Beigi RH. Pelvic inflammatory disease and tubo-ovarian abscess. Infect Dis Clin North Am 2008;22:693–708.

Shafii T, Burstein GR. An overview of sexually transmitted infections among adolescents. Adolesc Med Clin 2004;15:201–14.

Tracy CR, Steers WD, Costabile R. Diagnosis and management of epididymitis. Urol Clin North Am 2008;35:101–8.

Behavior

Encopresis (Soiling)

Enuresis (Bed Wetting)
Nocturnal and Diurnal

Encopresis (Soiling)

Barton D. Schmitt, MD

Encopresis, or soiling, is the voluntary or involuntary passing of feces into the underwear or other inappropriate site.

A. Most children with encopresis have severe constipation (impaction). They soil themselves several times a day with small amounts of stool. These children periodically have pain with bowel movements, blood on toilet tissue, and a huge stool that clogs the toilet. Some children hold back stools to avoid pain, others because they are locked in a power struggle with the parent. Determine whether the patient uses the toilet for bowel movements, and if public and school toilets are accepted. Because psychogenic factors are common, perform a psychosocial screen of all children with encopresis. Some have had punitive toilet training. Others have resistance as a result of too many reminders, practice runs, lectures, or nagging. For intermittent encopresis of unknown origin, have the parents keep an encopresis diary to help determine the circumstances and triggers.

B. Differentiate retentive from nonretentive encopresis on the basis of impacted stool on abdominal and rectal examination. In impaction, the rectum is distended and packed with claylike stool, and a midline suprapubic mass is usually palpable. Leakage of stool from the bottom of the impaction may occur several times a day (overflow diarrhea). Suspect nonimpacted encopresis when a normal bowel movement is passed into the underwear once or twice a day without any history of constipation. A barium enema is indicated only if the anal canal will not admit a finger or if the rectum is empty on repeated examination. An abdominal radiograph is useful to confirm the diagnosis of impaction in atypical cases or if the patient refuses a rectal examination.

C. Remove the impaction with hyperphosphate enemas. Give one enema per day for 2 or 3 days. Another way to dislodge an impaction is with oral medications. Give high-dosage mineral oil (1 oz per year of age/day with 8 oz/day maximum) or polyethylene glycol (1.5 g/kg/day with 3 capfuls/day maximum) by mouth for 3 or 4 days. After disimpaction, treat the child with a stool softener, such as mineral oil, milk of magnesia, lactulose, or polyethylene glycol for 3 months, until the diameter and tone of the bowel return to normal. Children who hold back stools because of pain or negativism need to be treated with a laxative (e.g., Dulcolax or senna product) in addition to the stool softener. Recommend a diet that includes increased amounts of bran, fresh fruits, and vegetables, and decreased milk products. Instruct the parents that the child should also sit on the toilet three times a day or the program will fail. Some children will not sit on the toilet unless offered incentives. The physician's continued involvement is critical even if the child needs referral to a psychologist or psychiatrist.

D. If the child has no evidence of constipation and the encopresis consists of a normal-sized bowel movement into the underwear once or twice a day, the cause is almost always emotional. If there is no evidence of constipation and the soiling is a small amount, consider poor bowel habits, such as postponing bowel movements (with partial leakage before reaching the toilet), small leakage with gas (e.g., lactose intolerance), partial emptying with sticky stools, or poor wiping.

E. Pediatric counseling, especially for soiling without constipation, involves setting up a new toileting program with the child's active participation, stopping any reminders to sit on the toilet (to remove the power struggle), and giving incentives for the release of any normal-sized stools into the toilet. The parents' main job is to detect any accidents and help the child change as soon as possible. Enemas and medications are not needed in nonretentive encopresis. Refer severely emotionally disturbed children (e.g., those who are depressed, acting out, or older than 6 years and not impacted) for therapy.

References

Abi-Hanna A, Lake AM. Constipation and encopresis in childhood. Pediatr Rev 1998;19:23–31.

Beddali N, van den Berg MM, Dijkgraaf MG, et al. Rectal fecal impaction treatment in childhood constipation: enemas versus high doses oral PEG. Pediatrics 2009;124:e1108–15.

Constipation Guideline Committee of the North American Society for Pediatric Gastroenterology. Evaluation and treatment of constipation in infants and children. J Pediatr Gastroenterol Nutr 2006;43:e1–e13.

Dautenhahn LW, Blumenthal BI. Functional constipation: a radiologist's perspective. Pediatr Ann 1999;28:304–6.

Felt B, Wise CG, Olson A, et al. Guideline for the management of pediatric idiopathic constipation and soiling. Arch Pediatr Adolesc Med 1999;153:380–5.

Lowe JR, Parks BR. Movers and shakers: a clinician's guide to laxatives. Pediatr Ann 1999;28:307–10.

Nowicki JM, Bishop PR. Organic causes of constipation in infants and children. Pediatr Ann 1999;28:293–300.

Schmitt BD. Toilet training: getting it right the first time. Contemp Pediatr 2004;21:105–22.

Schmitt BD. Toilet training problems: underachievers, refusers and stool holders. Contemp Pediatr 2004;21:71–82.

Schum TR, Kolb TM, McAuliffe TL, et al. Sequential acquisition of toilet-training skills: a descriptive study of gender and age differences in normal children. Pediatrics 2002;109:1–7.

Youssef NN, Di Lorenzo C. Childhood constipation: evaluation and treatment. J Clin Gastroenterol 2001;33:199–205.

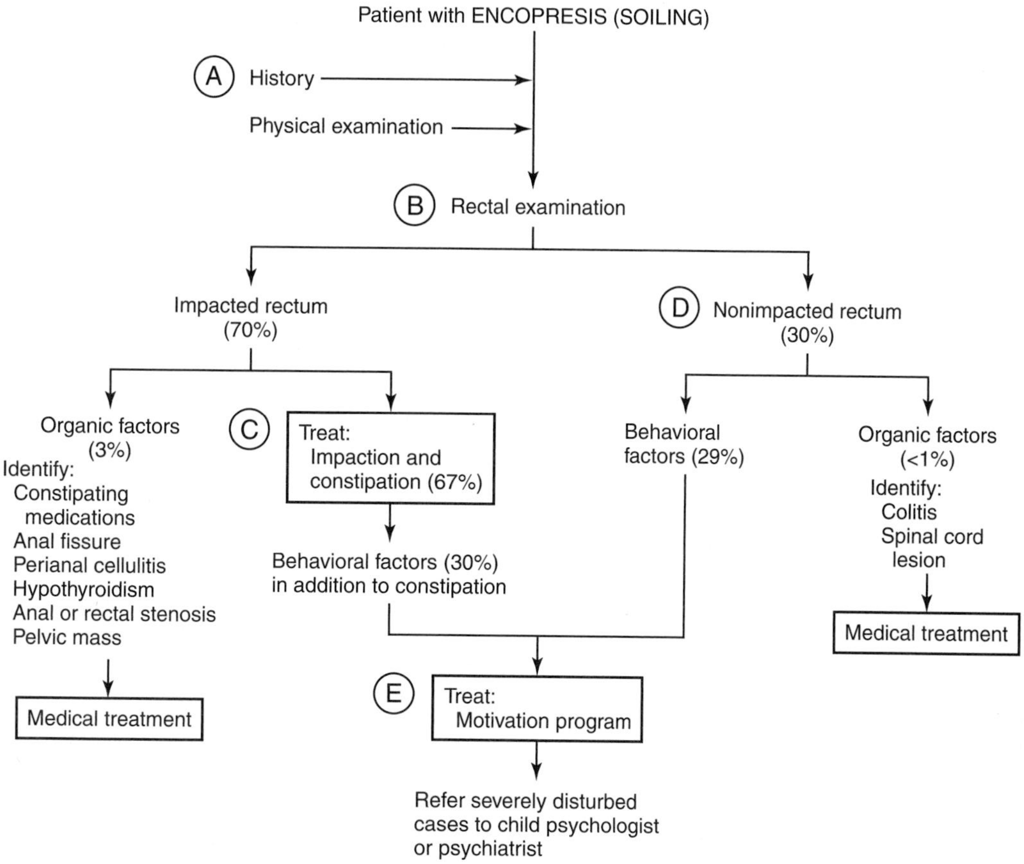
Patient with ENCOPRESIS (SOILING)
A
History
Physical examination
B
Rectal examination
Impacted rectum (70%)
D
Nonimpacted rectum (30%)
Organic factors (3%)
Identify:
Constipating medications
Anal fissure
Perianal cellulitis
Hypothyroidism
Anal or rectal stenosis
Pelvic mass
Medical treatment
C
Treat:
Impaction and constipation (67%)
Behavioral factors (30%) in addition to constipation
Behavioral factors (29%)
Organic factors (<1%)
Identify:
Colitis
Spinal cord lesion
Medical treatment
E
Treat:
Motivation program
Refer severely disturbed cases to child psychologist or psychiatrist

Enuresis (Bed Wetting)
Nocturnal and Diurnal

Barton D. Schmitt, MD

A. Determine the age at onset, pattern (daytime vs. nighttime), and frequency of wetting. Note any dysuria, an abnormal urine stream (dribbling), constipation, soiling, polydipsia, and polyuria. Identify predisposing conditions, such as frequent urinary tract infections, fecal impaction, diabetes mellitus, central nervous system disease or trauma (diabetes insipidus), and severe emotional disturbance (deliberate wetting). Obtain a psychosocial history and identify children who appear to be severely disturbed.

B. Note a distended bladder or fecal impaction. Examine external genitals for vulvitis, labial adhesions, and signs of sexual abuse. Assess the anal sphincter wink, the child's gait, and the ankle deep tendon reflexes. Observe the urine stream. Perform a urinalysis for all patients, with special emphasis on the specific gravity, urine glucose, nitrite, and leukocytes.

C. Suspect an associated urinary tract malformation when an abnormal urine stream, constant wetness (dampness), or recurrent urinary tract infections are present. Radiologic studies, including a voiding cystourethrogram (VCUG) and intravenous pyelography or renal ultrasonography, will identify ectopic ureters, a lower urinary tract obstruction, or a neurogenic bladder.

D. Categorize patients according to the pattern of enuresis. Nocturnal enuresis is common (>10% of 5-year-olds wet their beds); diurnal enuresis is far less common. Nocturnal enuresis is involuntary; diurnal enuresis is commonly voluntary. When both forms are present, treat diurnal enuresis first.

E. Approximately one third of daytime wetters have urgency incontinence (unstable bladder). These children wet themselves while running to the toilet or while trying to undress. They do use the toilet, unlike those with behavioral problems. Most are girls, and they may have a long history of intense bladder spasms; they are embarrassed by their problem, and the family history is commonly positive. Treat these children with stream-interruption exercises (counting to 10 while stopping at midstream); they should work up to interrupting for 1 minute (use an egg timer). Oxybutynin (Ditropan) is also helpful for reducing bladder spasms. Bladder-stretching exercises are contraindicated; they lead to increased wetting.

F. Many daytime wetters deliberately wet themselves to retaliate for the pressures of toilet training. Some have been physically punished; others have been endlessly nagged and reminded. Most have mild oppositional problems and can be treated by the primary physician. Set up a new toilet-training program with the child's active participation using a calendar and incentive system for each dry day. Have the parents discontinue any reminders to use the toilet but continue to remind the youngster to change to dry clothing when wet. Stream-interruption and bladder-stretching exercises are both counterproductive because the child considers them an intrusion. Refer to a child psychiatrist or psychologist those who are depressed, overtly angry, or older than 8 years. Also refer children with pervasive emotional problems.

G. A few children (infrequent voiders) hold back their urine for extended periods (e.g., >8 hours). Some become partial emptiers and have an increased risk for urinary tract infections. Some experience development of trabeculated bladders, vesicoureteral reflux, hydronephrosis, and even renal failure. All of these children need a uroflow study and bladder ultrasound for residual urine. If the results are abnormal, they need referral to a urologist. Most respond to the motivation program described in F. Those with urinary tract infections may require prophylactic antibiotics. Those with vesicoureteral reflux require timed voidings every 3 hours. Younger children may need incentives to comply with timed voidings.

H. More than 75% of nighttime bed-wetters have a small bladder capacity. Normal bladder capacity is 1 oz per year of age plus 2, or 10 ml/kg. Children with small bladders all need to learn to awaken at night to urinate. Portable transistorized enuresis alarms (Potty Pager, Malem, Wet Stop, etc.) are the intervention of choice to achieve this goal. Bladder-stretching exercises can be used, but they cure only 35% of children and yield slow progress. Desmopressin is an effective, safe drug that can be used for overnights and vacations.

I. Children with an increased or normal bladder capacity respond to a program that helps them take responsibility for their symptom. Have the family discontinue any punishment. Dry mornings should result in positive recognition (praise, a calendar, incentives). Wet mornings carry the natural consequence of changing the bed. Fluids are decreased during the 2 hours before bedtime, and the bladder is emptied at bedtime.

References

Austin PF, Ritchey ML. Dysfunctional voiding. Pediatr Rev 2000;21:336–41.

Bennett H. Clinical tips for helping patients overcome bedwetting. Contemp Pediatr 2005;22:92–6.

Fernandes E. The unstable bladder in children. J Pediatr 1991;118:831.

Lawless MR, McElderry DH. Nocturnal enuresis: current concepts. Pediatr Rev 2001;22:399–406.

Monda JM, Husmann DA. Primary nocturnal enuresis: a comparison among observation, imipramine, desmopressin acetate, and bed-wetting alarm systems. J Urol 1995;54:745–8.

Robson WL. Diurnal enuresis. Pediatr Rev 1997;18:407–12.

Schmitt BD. Nocturnal enuresis. Pediatr Rev 1997;18:183–90.

Schulman S, Berry A. Helping the child with daytime wetting stay dry. Contemp Pediatr. 2006;23:64–80.

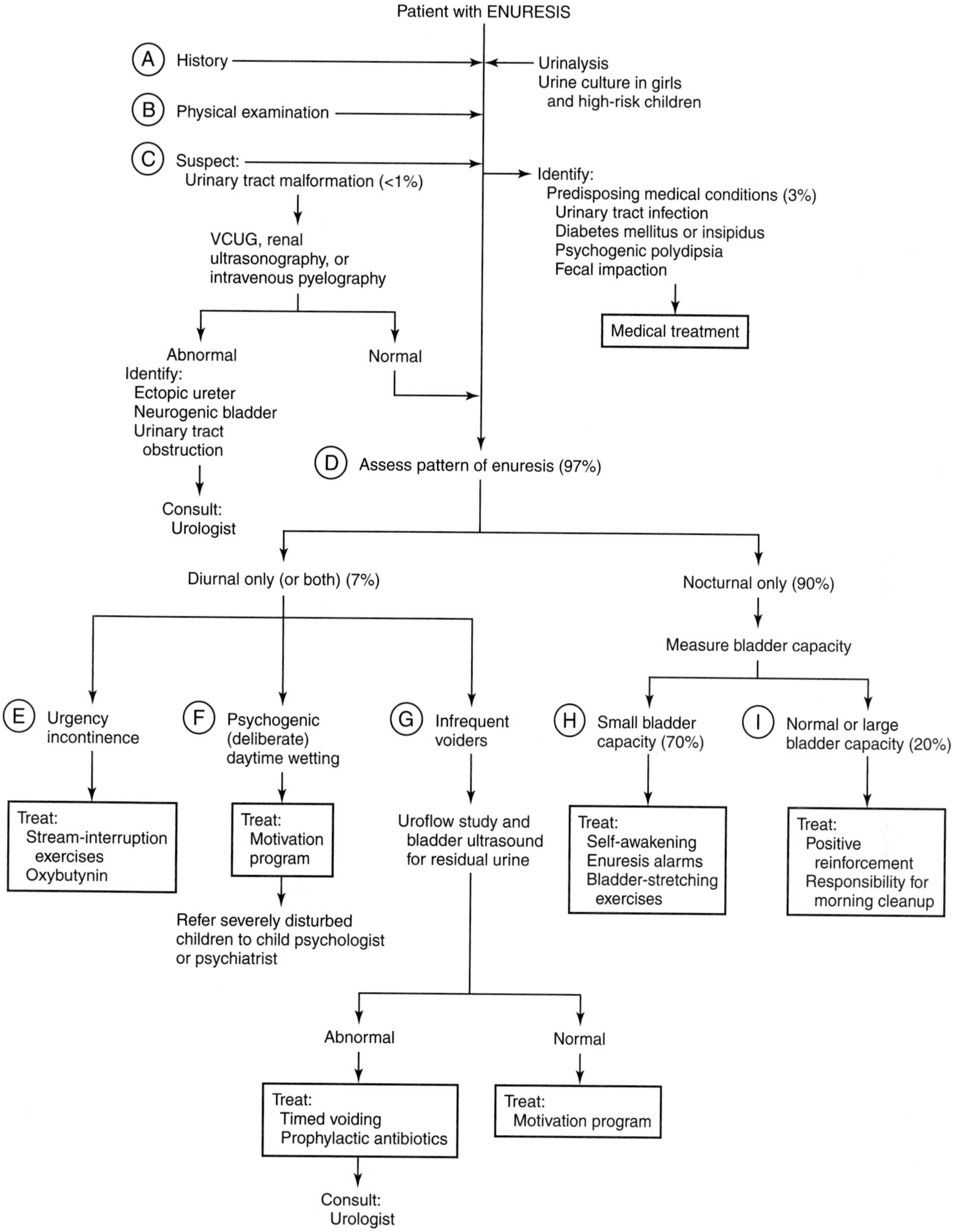
Patient with ENURESIS
A History
B Physical examination
C Suspect:
Urinary tract malformation (<1%)
Urinalysis
Urine culture in girls and high-risk children
Identify:
Predisposing medical conditions (3%)
Urinary tract infection
Diabetes mellitus or insipidus
Psychogenic polydipsia
Fecal impaction
Medical treatment
VCUG, renal ultrasonography, or intravenous pyelography
Abnormal
Identify:
Ectopic ureter
Neurogenic bladder
Urinary tract obstruction
Consult:
Urologist
Normal
D Assess pattern of enuresis (97%)
Diurnal only (or both) (7%)
Nocturnal only (90%)
Measure bladder capacity
E Urgency incontinence
Treat:
Stream-interruption exercises
Oxybutynin
F Psychogenic (deliberate) daytime wetting
Treat:
Motivation program
Refer severely disturbed children to child psychologist or psychiatrist
G Infrequent voiders
Uroflow study and bladder ultrasound for residual urine
Abnormal
Treat:
Timed voiding
Prophylactic antibiotics
Consult:
Urologist
Normal
Treat:
Motivation program
H Small bladder capacity (70%)
Treat:
Self-awakening
Enuresis alarms
Bladder-stretching exercises
I Normal or large bladder capacity (20%)
Treat:
Positive reinforcement
Responsibility for morning cleanup

Cardiovascular

Bradyarrhythmias

Martin J. LaPage, MD, and John H. Reed, MD, MPH

Rarely will a patient have a chief complaint of "bradycardia." Rather, this will be found during the physical examination of a patient with fatigue or syncope, or a patient who is completely asymptomatic. Bradycardia will be defined and evaluated differently depending on the patient's age and the circumstances of presentation. Bradycardia is defined as heart rate less than 2nd percentile for age (Table 1). However, there is wide variation in heart rate at all ages, and it is not uncommon for healthy children to manifest heart rates lower than normal. The following algorithm is oriented toward the evaluation of bradycardia presenting in the outpatient setting.

ASSESS DEGREE OF ILLNESS

Bradycardia with acute hemodynamic compromise should be managed according to Pediatric Advanced Life Support guidelines, including cardiopulmonary resuscitation and administration of epinephrine, atropine, or both.

A. History: Attempt to identify the onset of symptoms. Evidence of congestive heart failure in infants includes poor weight gain and tachypnea especially with feeding. Syncope and easy fatigability are more typical in the older child. Additional symptoms may include chest pain, palpitations, light-headedness, weight gain (edema), or nausea. History of congenital heart disease and cardiac surgery should be recognized, including a history of ablation for arrhythmias. Recent illnesses or exposures may suggest infectious causative agent. Neurologic abnormalities or developmental delay or regression may suggest a metabolic disorder. Consider drug ingestions. Maternal lupus status is an important cause of congenital complete heart block (Table 2).

B. Physical Examination: Focus should be on signs of congestive heart failure: tachypnea, poor perfusion, hepatomegaly, and hypotension. Examine for evidence of congenital heart disease by searching for abnormalities in the heart sounds. Note the regularity of the heart rhythm. Complete examination may suggest an underlying condition such as Lyme disease, rheumatic disease, or a metabolic syndrome.

C. Electrocardiogram (ECG): All suspected bradycardia must be confirmed with electrocardiogram. Evaluation of rhythm is essential for further management. Sinus arrhythmia is a normal variation in heart rate correlating with breathing; it may produce sinus pauses up to 2 to 3 seconds in sleeping individuals. Sinus bradycardia will have a normal, regular PR interval and a 1:1 association of P waves to the QRS complexes. Frequent atrial premature beats may block in the atrioventricular node and cause bradycardia, especially in the neonate; the premature P wave may be concealed in the T wave. Type 1 second-degree heart block (atrioventricular block [AVB]) has progressive lengthening of the PR interval until a completely blocked P wave is seen. Type 2 second-degree AVB shows intermittent blocked P waves without PR prolongation. Complete atrioventricular block demonstrates atrioventricular dissociation and may be missed if the atrial and ventricular rates are similar (isosynchronous).

(Continued on page 76)

Table 1. **Heart Rate by Age**

Age	2nd Percentile	Mean	98th Percentile
1 day	94	122	155
7–30 days	105	150	182
1–3 months	120	150	180
3–6 months	105	142	185
6–12 months	108	132	168
1–3 years	90	120	150
3–5 years	73	110	138
5–8 years	65	100	133
8–12 years	62	90	130
12–16 years	62	85	120

Data from Davignon A, Rautaharju P, Boisselle E, et al. Normal ECG standards for infants and children. Pediatr Cardiol 1979;1:123–31.

Table 2. **Causes of Sinus Bradycardia and Heart Block**

Increased vagal tone	Congenital heart disease
Familial	Endocardial cushion defect
Hypothyroidism	Ebstein anomaly of the tricuspid valve
Hypothermia	Congenitally corrected transposition
Electrolyte abnormalities:	Heterotaxy syndromes
Hypokalemia or hyperkalemia	Surgery/ablation
Hypocalcemia or hypercalcemia	Chest trauma
Hypoglycemia	Maternal connective tissue disease
Hypomagnesemia	Systemic lupus erythematosus
Antiarrhythmic drugs	Sjögren syndrome
Toxic ingestions	Mixed connective tissue disease
Infection:	Fetal myocarditis
Myocarditis	Cardiomyopathy
Endocarditis	Muscular dystrophy
Lyme disease	Kearns-Sayre syndrome
Rocky Mountain spotted fever	Holt-Oram syndrome
Acute rheumatic fever	Long QT syndrome
Chagas disease	18p− syndrome
Diphtheria	Metabolic
Rubella	Carnitine deficiency
Mumps	Glycogen storage disease
Trichinosis	
Human immunodeficiency virus	

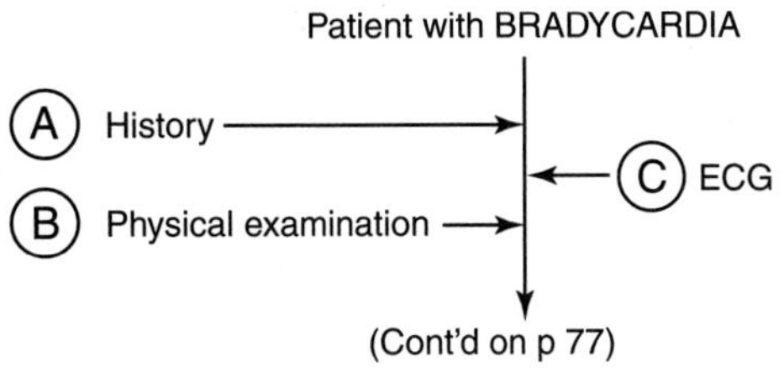
Patient with BRADYCARDIA
A History
B Physical examination
C ECG
(Cont'd on p 77)

D. Sinus Bradycardia: May be a benign finding in an otherwise healthy patient; assure that the patient has an adequate chronotropic response to exercise. Inability to raise heart rate for activity is a sign of sinus node dysfunction and is rare in patients without congenital heart disease. Excessive vagal tone in infants can produce bradycardia associated with apnea or breath-holding spells. Twenty-four-hour Holter monitor should be performed and reviewed by a pediatric cardiologist to evaluate heart rate variability and assess for significant sinus pauses or any AVB.

E. First or Second-Degree AVB: First-degree AVB is not a cause of bradycardia; it is included here only for completeness. Both first- and second-degree type 1 (Wenckebach) AVB may be present in normal children during rest or sleep. Resolution of the block by increasing the heart rate with activity suggests that this is benign. Alternatively, first- or second-degree AVB may be the harbinger of progressive conduction system disease or underlying systemic illness. Type 2 second-degree AVB is suggestive of an underlying conduction abnormality. Evaluation with Holter monitor may uncover higher grade AVB. These findings or progression of heart block over time should prompt pediatric cardiology evaluation.

F. Asymptomatic High-Grade AVB or Complete Heart Block: High-grade AVB is the presence of serially blocked P waves interspersed with normally conducted beats. Previously unrecognized congenital heart disease such as congenitally corrected transposition of the great arteries may present with heart block in the presumed healthy teenager. Consider congenital AVB, which may not be discovered until beyond the neonatal period. Infectious, inflammatory, metabolic, and pharmacologic causative factors should always be considered in new-onset AVB. Hospitalization of the infant with complete heart block is warranted during evaluation. The asymptomatic child or adolescent with complete heart block may be managed as an outpatient. In either case, referral to a pediatric cardiologist is essential.

G. Mild to Moderate Symptoms: Symptoms may not be immediately obvious (see part A). Chest radiograph and echocardiogram can further delineate degree of heart failure or presence of congenital heart disease. Hospitalization should be considered for monitoring and to manage symptoms of heart failure until cause and course of therapy can be determined.

H. Symptomatic High-Grade AVB or Complete Heart Block: Hospitalization with continuous telemetry is warranted in most cases during the evaluation, especially if acute onset of AVB is suspected. Chronic AVB is unlikely to present with more than subtle symptoms. Degree of hemodynamic compromise should be determined including renal function. Suspected causative factors such as infection should be addressed. Supplemental oxygen will relieve some of the demand on the heart. Isoproterenol infusion at 0.05 to 2 μg/kg/min or epinephrine at 0.01 to 1 μg/kg/min can increase ventricular rate to increase cardiac output. Atropine 0.02 mg/kg every 5 minutes may be useful if sinus node dysfunction is suspected.

I. Severe Congestive Heart Failure: Overt evidence of congestive heart failure demands hospitalization and intensive care unit care should be strongly considered. Chronotropic therapy with isoproterenol or epinephrine (see earlier) is typically required. Transcutaneous, transesophageal, or temporary transvenous pacing should be used during stabilization and initial evaluation. Consultation with a pediatric cardiologist is essential.

References

2005 American Heart Association Guidelines for Cardiopulmonary Resuscitation and Emergency Cardiovascular Care: part 12: Pediatric Advanced Life Support. Circulation 2005;112:IV-167–87.

Brodsky M, Wu D, Denes P, et al. Arrhythmias documented by 24 hour continuous electrocardiographic monitoring in 50 male medical students without apparent heart disease. Am J Cardiol 1977;39(3): 390–5.

Davignon A, Rautaharju P, Boisselle E, et al. Normal ECG standards for infants and children. Pediatr Cardiol 1979;1:123–31.

Dickinson DF, Scott O. Ambulatory electrocardiographic monitoring in 100 healthy teenage boys. Br Heart J 1984;51(2):179–83.

Epstein AE, DiMarco JP, Ellenbogen KA, et al. ACC/AHA/HRS 2008 Guidelines for Device-Based Therapy of Cardiac Rhythm Abnormalities: a report of the American College of Cardiology/American Heart Association Task Force on Practice Guidelines (Writing Committee to Revise the ACC/AHA/NASPE 2002 Guideline Update for Implantation of Cardiac Pacemakers and Antiarrhythmia Devices): developed in collaboration with the American Association for Thoracic Surgery and Society of Thoracic Surgeons. Circulation 2008;117:e350–408.

Kannankeril PJ, Fish FA. Disorders of cardiac rhythm and conduction. In: Allen HD, Driscoll DJ, Shaddy RE, Feltes TF, editors. Moss and Adams' heart disease in infants, children, and adolescents, ed 7. Philadelphia: Lippincott Williams & Wilkins; 2007. p. 293–4, 302–6.

Montague TJ, Taylor PG, Stockton R, et al. The spectrum of cardiac rate and rhythm in normal newborns. Pediatr Cardiol 1982;2(1):33–8.

Southhall DP, Johnston F, Shinebourne EA, Johnston PG. 24-hour electrocardiographic study of heart rate and rhythm patterns in population of healthy children. Br Heart J 1981;45(3):281–91.

Patient with BRADYCARDIA

(Cont'd from p 75)

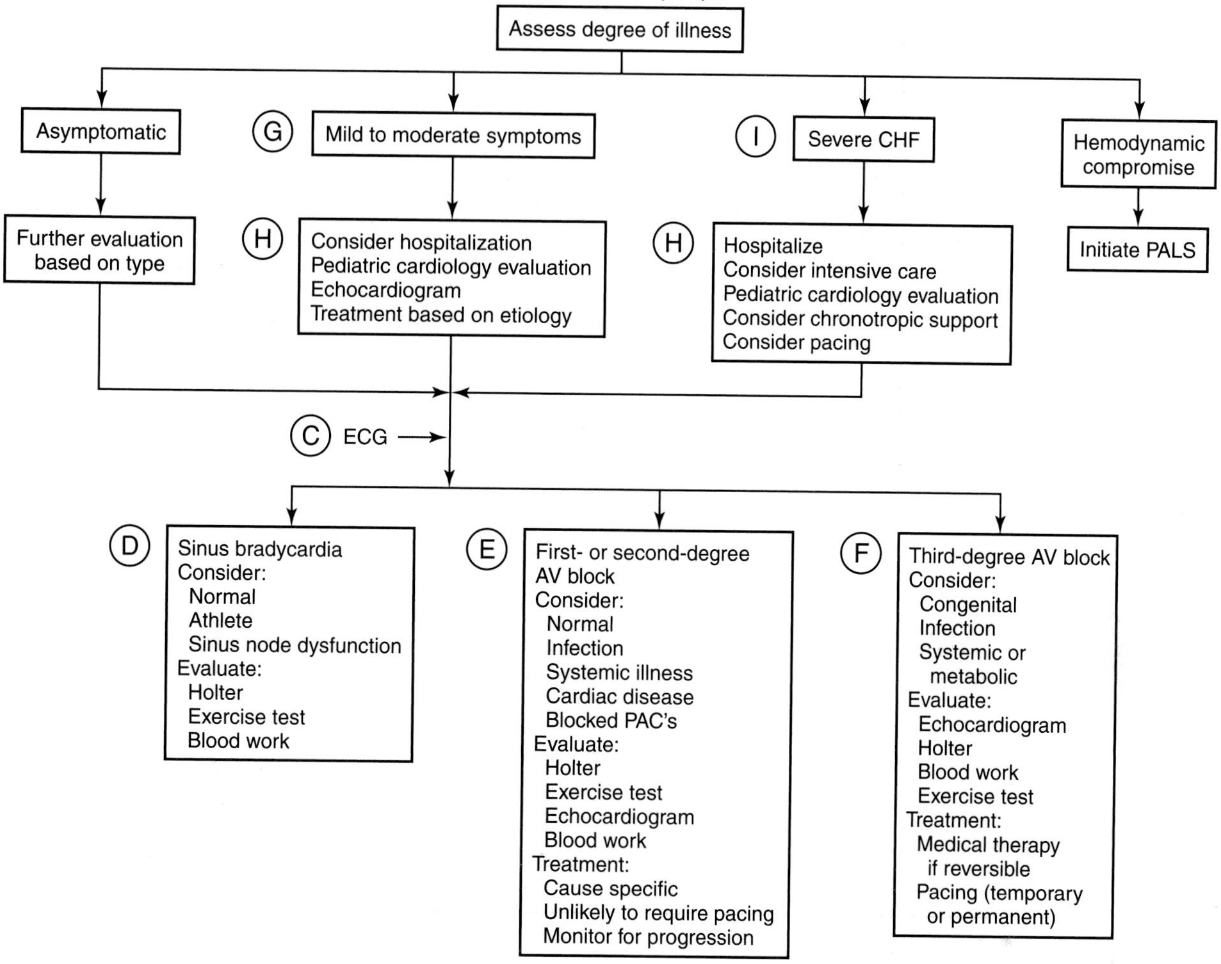
Assess degree of illness
Asymptomatic
Further evaluation based on type
G
Mild to moderate symptoms
H
Consider hospitalization
Pediatric cardiology evaluation
Echocardiogram
Treatment based on etiology
I
Severe CHF
H
Hospitalize
Consider intensive care
Pediatric cardiology evaluation
Consider chronotropic support
Consider pacing
Hemodynamic compromise
Initiate PALS
C
ECG
D
Sinus bradycardia
Consider:
Normal
Athlete
Sinus node dysfunction
Evaluate:
Holter
Exercise test
Blood work
E
First- or second-degree AV block
Consider:
Normal
Infection
Systemic illness
Cardiac disease
Blocked PAC's
Evaluate:
Holter
Exercise test
Echocardiogram
Blood work
Treatment:
Cause specific
Unlikely to require pacing
Monitor for progression
F
Third-degree AV block
Consider:
Congenital
Infection
Systemic or metabolic
Evaluate:
Echocardiogram
Holter
Blood work
Exercise test
Treatment:
Medical therapy if reversible
Pacing (temporary or permanent)

Evaluation of a Child with a Heart Murmur

Michael Walsh, MD, and John H. Reed, MD, MPH

Most children will have a heart murmur at some point in their lives. The challenge to the primary caregiver is to distinguish the pathologic minority of murmurs from the innocent majority. A detailed history and focused cardiovascular examination will aid the clinician in doing so.

A. A thorough history is the first step in the evaluation of a murmur. Prenatal and perinatal history should focus on infections, teratogenic exposures, and gestational diabetes, all of which predispose to structural heart disease. Medical history may reveal diseases or syndromes associated with cardiac abnormalities. Symptoms of organic heart disease vary by lesion and age. The infant may present with inappropriate tachypnea, failure to thrive, or poor feeding, including cyanosis or diaphoresis with feeds. Older children and adolescents may complain of exercise intolerance, exertional chest pain, syncope, orthopnea, or recurrent lower respiratory infections. Family history should identify heart disease or sudden, unexplained death in young family members and genetic disorders, such as Marfan, Noonan, or Turner syndromes.

B. A complete cardiac physical examination should begin with assessment of the vital signs. Tachycardia or tachypnea, decreased oxygen saturation, or alterations in the blood pressure may suggest congenital or acquired heart disease. Alternatively, the increased cardiac output associated with fever may itself cause a murmur. Growth parameters including weight, height, and head circumference are of utmost importance. Delay in all three may indicate a genetic disorder, whereas isolated weight retardation is often seen in congestive heart failure secondary to poor caloric intake and excessive caloric expenditure. Cyanosis can be most easily seen in the tongue because of its vascularity and lack of pigmentation. Precordial inspection may reveal a heave when there is ventricular hypertrophy, and precordial palpation in this setting may find a thrill. The point of maximal impulse, which can indicate abnormal cardiac position or ventricular hypertrophy, should be determined. Pulses should be palpated simultaneously in the upper and lower extremities. Weak or delayed lower extremity pulses could represent aortic coarctation.

C. Cardiac auscultation begins with the normal heart sounds, S1 and S2. The first heart sound represents closure of the mitral and tricuspid valves, and is often single, especially in infancy. The second heart sound represents semilunar (aortic and pulmonary) valve closure and is of particular diagnostic value. The physiologic splitting of S2 that increases with inspiration is a normal finding. A single second heart sound is a concerning finding in neonates, because it can represent a single semilunar valve, transposition of the great arteries, or pulmonary hypertension. A widely split S2 is associated with conditions that prolong right ventricular emptying, most notably the atrial septal defect. The third and fourth heart sounds, S3 and S4, are low-frequency sounds that, if present, will be heard during diastole and create a gallop rhythm. The third heart sound is often a normal finding. The fourth heart sound, in contrast, is always abnormal and is most common in congestive heart failure or cardiomyopathy, or both. A systolic ejection click, which is a loud, high-frequency sound immediately following S1, is often caused by valvar aortic or pulmonary stenosis. Mitral valve prolapse produces a midsystolic click best heard at the apex that may be associated with a late systolic murmur.

D. Characterization of murmurs requires delineation of their timing, location, radiation, intensity, and quality. Murmurs are initially separated according to their timing within the cardiac cycle (systolic, diastolic, or continuous). The location on the precordium where the murmur is best heard gives an important clue to the source of the murmur. The upper right and left sternal borders will be the best place to hear murmurs originating from the aortic and pulmonary valves, respectively. The tricuspid valve is auscultated over the left lower sternal border, whereas the apex is the usual "listening post" for the mitral valve. The radiation of a murmur is related to the path of turbulent blood flow. For example, aortic stenosis causes turbulent flow across the valve and into the ascending aorta and carotids such that the clinician is likely to hear radiation of the murmur from the upper right sternal border to the neck. Similarly, the murmur of pulmonary stenosis radiates to the back and axillae, following the course of the branch pulmonary arteries. The intensity of a murmur should be graded from I to VI (Table 1). Description of the quality and pitch of a murmur takes some degree of experience but is extremely useful in distinguishing innocent murmurs (particularly a Still's murmur) from those that require further evaluation.

E. Most systolic murmurs (those occurring between S1 and S2) may be further divided into systolic ejection murmurs and holosystolic murmurs. Systolic ejection murmurs begin after S1, increase and then decrease in

Table 1. **Grading of Cardiac Murmurs by Intensity**

Grade I	Barely audible (softer than the heart sounds)
Grade II	Soft, but easily audible (about as loud as heart sounds)
Grade III	Moderately loud murmur without a thrill (louder than the heart sounds)
Grade IV	Loud murmur with a thrill
Grade V	Murmur heard with the stethoscope barely touching the chest
Grade VI	Murmur heard with the stethoscope off of the chest

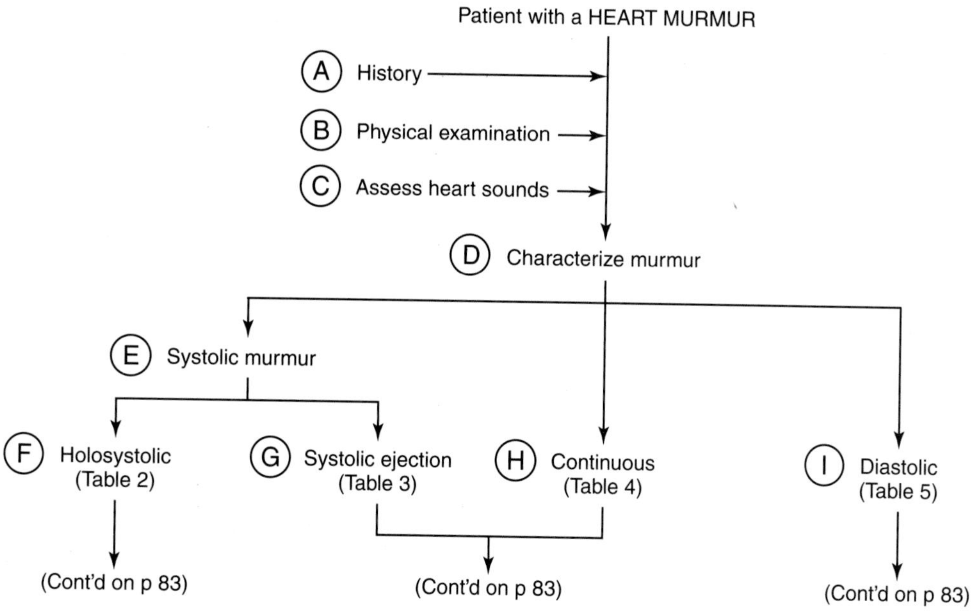
Patient with a HEART MURMUR
(A) History
(B) Physical examination
(C) Assess heart sounds
(D) Characterize murmur
(E) Systolic murmur
(F) Holosystolic (Table 2)
(G) Systolic ejection (Table 3)
(H) Continuous (Table 4)
(I) Diastolic (Table 5)
(Cont'd on p 83)
(Cont'd on p 83)
(Cont'd on p 83)

intensity (crescendo-decrescendo), and end in late systole. Holosystolic murmurs begin with S1 and continue through systole with the same intensity.

F. Holosystolic murmurs (Table 2) are those of the ventricular septal defect (VSD) and atrioventricular valve regurgitation. A VSD may not be heard at birth, because the right ventricular pressure of the neonate is close to that of the left ventricle. As pulmonary vascular resistance declines, the pressure gradient across the ventricular septum increases, causing more shunting and the emergence of the murmur. VSDs are, therefore, often heard for the first time at a well-child visit between 1 and 6 weeks. The murmur of a closing VSD will become louder as the flow across the defect becomes more turbulent. Tricuspid regurgitation is heard best at the left lower sternal border and increases with inspiration. Mitral regurgitation is a blowing pansystolic murmur heard best at the apex with radiation commonly to the left axilla. All holosystolic murmurs are pathologic and warrant further evaluation.

G. Systolic ejection murmurs (Table 3) are usually the result of turbulent blood flow across the ventricular outflow tracts. The murmur of aortic stenosis is loudest at the upper right sternal border and radiates to the neck; that of pulmonary stenosis is most prominent at the upper left sternal border with radiation to the back and axillae. Like other right-heart murmurs, pulmonary stenosis increases with inspiration, which increases venous return to the right side of the heart. Outflow tract obstruction can occur below, above, or at the level of the semilunar valve. An early systolic click suggests valvar obstruction and essentially rules out an innocent flow murmur. Coarctation of the aorta most typically causes a grade I-III/VI murmur heard at the upper left sternal border with radiation to the back. Blood pressure or pulse discrepancy between the upper and lower extremities will support such a diagnosis.

H. Continuous murmurs (Table 4) are heard with a patent ductus arteriosus, arteriovenous fistulas, and surgically created systemic-to-pulmonary shunts. In these situations, there is a pressure gradient in both systole and diastole, producing the continuous flow and murmur. The murmur typically obscures the second heart sound (S2). This distinguishes a continuous murmur from the "to-and-fro" murmur of semilunar valve stenosis and regurgitation. The venous hum is the only innocent continuous murmur. It is a soft, low-pitched murmur heard bilaterally in the upper chest that disappears with supination, turning the neck, or jugular vein compression.

I. Diastolic murmurs (Table 5) are produced by regurgitant semilunar valves or turbulent flow across the atrioventricular valves. Aortic and pulmonary regurgitation occur early in diastole and get softer as the ventricles fill. Aortic regurgitation causes a high-pitched murmur that radiates to the apex. Pulmonary regurgitation is usually medium-pitched and radiates down the left sternal border. Turbulent flow across the AV valves causes a mid-diastolic murmur, which will be low-pitched and best appreciated with the bell of the stethoscope. This can be caused by normal flow across a narrowed valve (mitral and tricuspid stenosis) or excessive flow across a normal valve (as with the increased right atrial volume of an ASD or the excessive pulmonary venous return of a left-to-right shunt).

Table 2. **Holosystolic Murmurs**

Substrate	Diagrammatic Representation	Chief Murmur Characteristics	Associated Findings
Ventricular septal defect	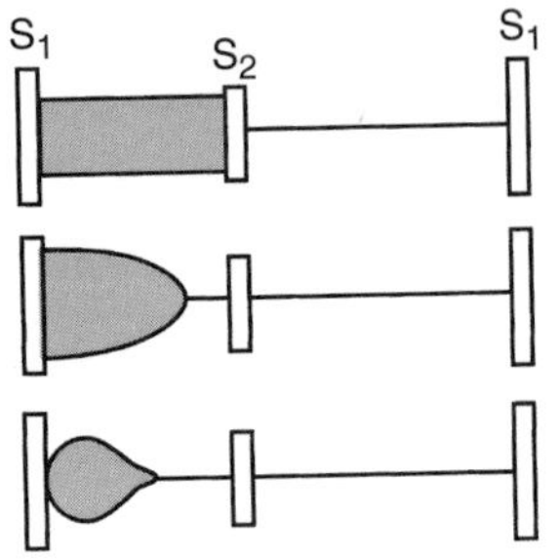S1 S2 S1	Well-localized holosystolic murmur usually at left lower sternal border; thrill may be present; soft	Congenital lesion; common in fetal alcohol syndrome, Down syndrome; precordial hyperactivity may be present
Mitral regurgitation	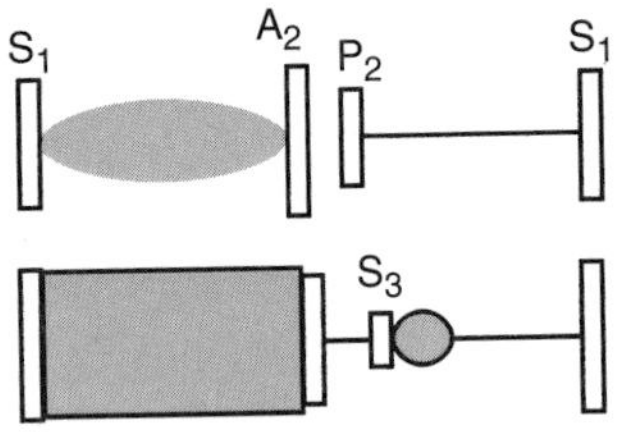S1 A2 P2 S1 S3	Holosystolic murmur at apex, transmits to left axilla; grade III-IV; wide splitting of S2; murmur heard at left axilla	May occur in Marfan syndrome; precordial noise may be present, short rumbles after loud S3 when lying on left side
Tricuspid regurgitation	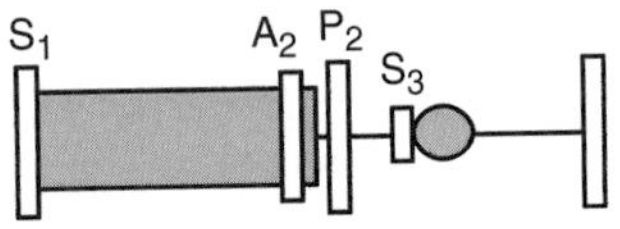S1 A2 P2 S3	Holosystolic murmur to immediate right or left of sternum; grade II-III; wide splitting of S2; short rumbles after loud S3	Seen more often in infants, toddlers; inspiration intensifies murmur and S3

Adapted from Park MK. Pediatric cardiology for practitioners, ed 2. Chicago: Year Book Medical Publishers; 1988. In: Allen HD, Golinko RJ, Williams RG. Heart murmurs in children: when is a workup needed? Contemp Pediatr 1994;11:29.

Table 3. **Systolic Ejection Murmurs**

Substrate	Diagrammatic Representation	Chief Murmur Characteristics	Associated Findings
Pulmonary stenosis	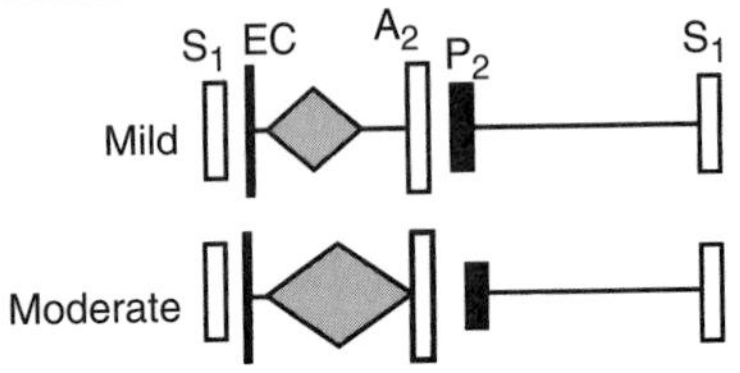S1 EC A2 P2 S1 Mild Moderate	Ejection murmur at upper left sternal border (toward baseline in infants); thrill; ejection click	Congenital lesion; inspiration intensifies murmur; expiration intensifies click
Aortic stenosis	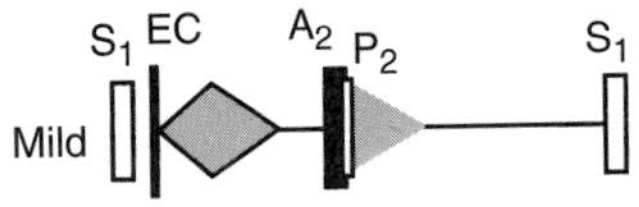S1 EC A2 P2 S1 Mild	Ejection murmur primarily at upper right sternal border but transmits to neck and left lower sternal border; thrill; ejection click	Congenital lesion
Atrial septal defect	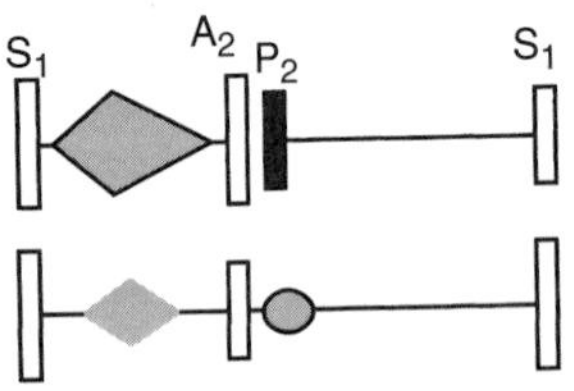S1 A2 P2 S1	Ejection murmur at upper left sternal border; loud S1; widely split, fixed S2; mid-diastolic murmur may be present	Congenital lesion; common in fetal alcohol syndrome; left chest may be enlarged
Coarctation of the aorta	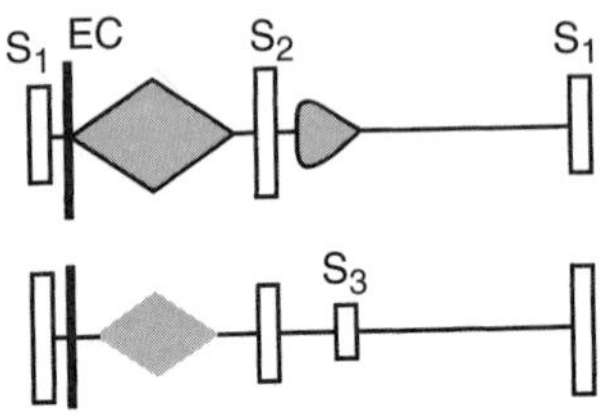S1 EC S2 S1 S3	Sometimes heard in back; thrill; soft; ejection clicks, early diastolic murmurs may be present if associated with bicuspid aortic valve	Arm pulses stronger and earlier than leg pulses; heaving apical impulse may be present

Adapted from Park MK. Pediatric cardiology for practitioners, ed 2. Chicago: Year Book Medical Publishers; 1988. In: Allen HD, Golinko RJ, Williams RG. Heart murmurs in children: when is a workup needed? Contemp Pediatr 1994;11:29.

Table 4. **Continuous Murmurs**

Substrate	Diagrammatic Representation	Chief Murmur Characteristics	Associated Findings
Patent ductus arteriosus	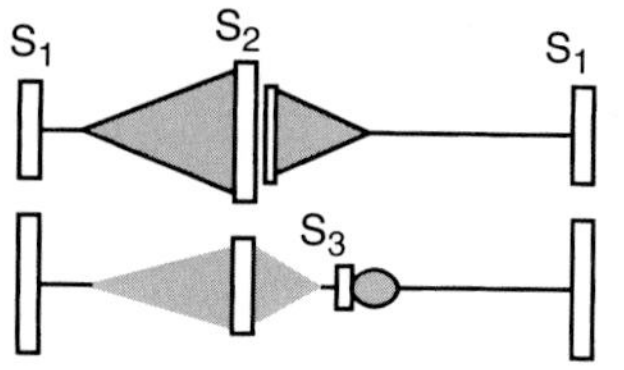 S_1 S_2 S_1 S_3	Continuous murmur along upper left sternal border (seldom continuous in neonates); thrill; grade I-IV; machinery-like	Congenital lesion; often detected at birth, especially in preterm infants, bounding pulses, precordial hyperactivity may be present; murmur intensities on supination

Adapted from Park MK. Pediatric cardiology for practitioners, ed 2. Chicago: Year Book Medical Publishers; 1988. In: Allen HD, Golinko RJ, Williams RG. Heart murmurs in children: when is a workup needed? Contemp Pediatr 1994;11:29.

Table 5. **Diastolic Murmurs**

Substrate	Diagrammatic Representation	Chief Murmur Characteristics	Associated Findings
Mitral stenosis	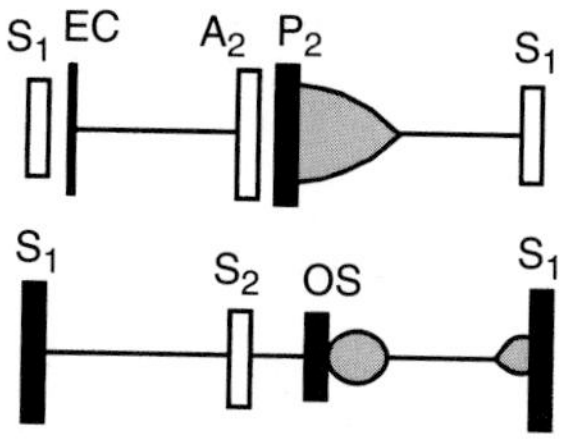 S_1 EC A_2 P_2 S_1 S_1 S_2 OS S_1	Loud S1 at apex; short opening snap and harsh murmur at left lower sternal border usually at mid-diastole; low-pitched presystolic murmur may be present	Seen several years after rheumatic fever; murmur intensified by lying on left side
Aortic regurgitation	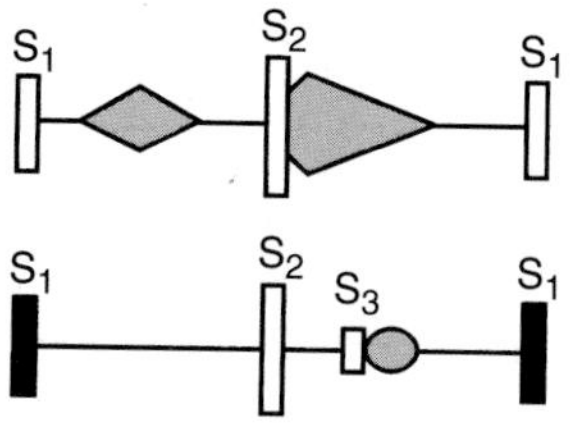 S_1 S_2 S_1 S_1 S_2 S_3 S_1	Early diastolic decrescendo murmur at or left of sternum; blowing; thrill, secondary midsystolic murmur caused by increased flow may be present	May occur in Marfan syndrome; bounding pulses and precordial noise may be present; murmur intensified by sitting, leaning forward, and holding breath
Pulmonary regurgitation	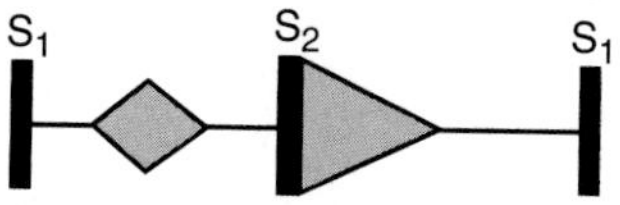 S_1 S_2 S_1	Short, early diastolic murmur and secondary midsystolic murmur caused by increased flow along left sternal border	Usually congenital lesion

Adapted from Park MK. Pediatric cardiology for practitioners, ed 2. Chicago: Year Book Medical Publishers; 1988. In: Allen HD, Golinko RJ, Williams RG. Heart murmurs in children: when is a workup needed? Contemp Pediatr 1994;11:29.

Table 6. **Innocent Heart Murmurs**

Substrate	Diagrammatic Representation	Chief Murmur Characteristics	Associated Findings
Vibratory (Still's) murmur	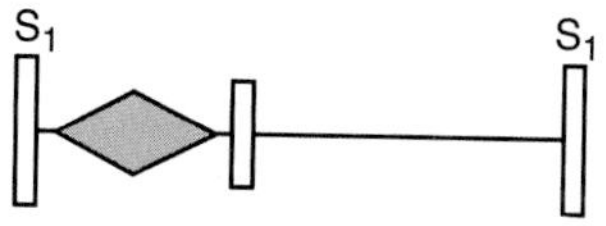 S_1 S_1	Systolic murmur between left lower sternal border and apex; musical quality intensifies on supination	Detected during early school years; murmur
Pulmonary flow murmur	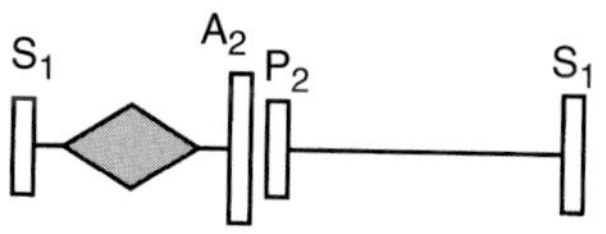 S_1 A_2 P_2 S_1	Systolic murmur at upper left sternal border; soft; in infants, transmits to back and axillae	Present in infants or adolescents; murmur dissipates on supination
Carotid bruit	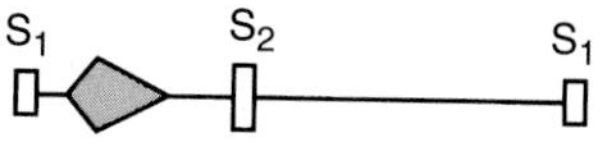 S_1 S_2 S_1	Systolic murmur near the clavicles or over the carotids; soft; faint thrill	Present at any age; murmur disappears on supination
Venous hum	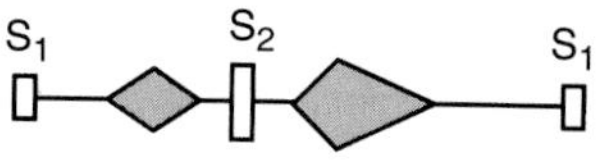 S_1 S_2 S_1	Continuous murmur at clavicles	Detected during early school years; murmur disappears on supination, compression of jugular vein, turning head

Adapted from Park MK. Pediatric cardiology for practitioners, ed 2. Chicago: Year Book Medical Publishers; 1988. In: Allen HD, Golinko RJ, Williams RG. Heart murmurs in children: when is a workup needed? Contemp Pediatr 1994;11:29.

J. An innocent heart murmur (Table 6) must meet the following criteria: (1) The patient must be asymptomatic from a cardiovascular perspective; (2) the cardiac examination should be normal by inspection and palpation; (3) with the exception of the venous hum, the murmur should be heard only during systole; (4) it should not be graded greater than III/VI in intensity; and (5) the specific type of murmur should be suggested by the examination. The most common innocent murmur of childhood is the Still's murmur. This is a low-pitched systolic murmur often described as vibratory or musical in quality that is best heard between the left lower sternal border and the apex when the patient is supine. Common in infancy, the murmurs of peripheral pulmonic stenosis radiate from the left upper sternal border to the axillae and back. It is heard more commonly in premature infants and disappears by 6 months of age. A common murmur in older children and adolescents is the pulmonary flow murmur. It is louder in high-output states, such as fever or anemia, and is best heard over the pulmonary outflow area. Unlike valvar pulmonary stenosis, it has no associated click and will have a normal second heart sound. The venous hum was discussed earlier.

K. Although murmurs can be the initial presentation of congenital or acquired heart disease, the majority of murmurs heard in the outpatient setting will not be associated with any cardiac pathology. The clinician must weigh the suspicion for pathologic heart disease against the cost of cardiology referral. A patient with cardiac symptoms and a murmur should see a pediatric cardiologist as soon as possible. In the evaluation of a murmur, the clinician may consider chest radiography and electrocardiography to further assist in his or her decision making. If the decision is made not to refer, the patient must be observed for the development of symptoms or any changes in the murmur.

References

Allen HD (hon), Phillips JR, Chan DP. History and physical examination. In: Allen HD, editor. Moss and Adams' heart disease in infants, children, and adolescents. 7th ed. Philadelphia: Lippincott Williams & Wilkins; 2008. p. 145–52.

Johnson WH, Moller JH. Pediatric cardiology. Philadelphia: Lippincott Williams & Wilkins; 2001. p. 16–29.

McConnell ME, Adkins SB III, Hannon DW. Heart murmurs in pediatric patients: when do you refer? Am Fam Physician 1999;60:558–65.

Park MK, editor. Pediatric cardiology for practitioners, ed 3. St. Louis: Mosby–Year Book; 1996. p. 18–33.

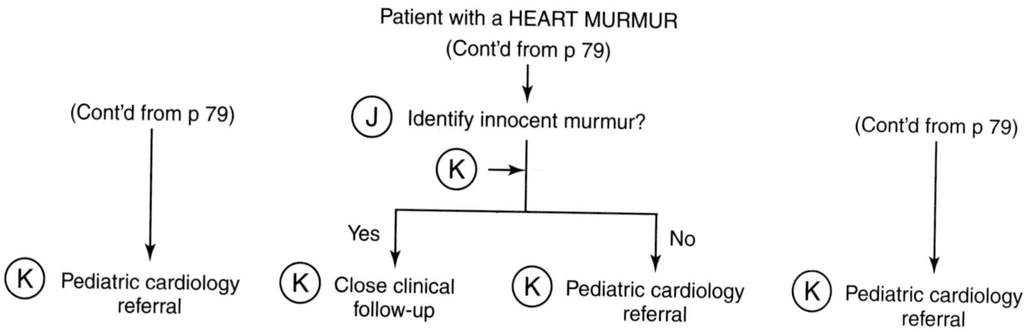
Patient with a HEART MURMUR
(Cont'd from p 79)
J Identify innocent murmur?
K
Yes
No
K Close clinical follow-up
K Pediatric cardiology referral
(Cont'd from p 79)
K Pediatric cardiology referral
(Cont'd from p 79)
K Pediatric cardiology referral

Hypertension

Elizabeth Yeung, MD, and Michael S. Schaffer, MD

Hypertension is systolic or diastolic blood pressure (BP) at or exceeding the 95th percentile for age, sex, and height, as established by the National Heart, Lung, and Blood Institute (the complete chart is available online at: www.nhlbi.nih.gov/guidelines/hypertension/child_tbl.pdf). The elevated BP should be documented on repeat measurements. A thorough history and physical examination must be sought to evaluate for an organic cause for the hypertension, known as *secondary hypertension.* Primary or essential hypertension is less likely in young children than it is in adults, although it is rapidly changing because of the obesity epidemic. Obesity and prematurity are two major risk factors for essential hypertension. Long-standing hypertension is a precursor to adult cardiovascular disease and its sequelae.

A. In the history, ask about family history of cardiac disease including hypertension, heart disease, and stroke. Review medical history for renal disease, including history of urinary tract infections, prematurity at birth, and use of umbilical artery catheter in the newborn. Note full review of systems, including symptoms and signs of undiagnosed renal disorders (polyuria, dysuria, hematuria, and edema), sleep apnea (snoring, daytime somnolence), cardiac symptoms (dyspnea, palpitations, or chest pain), metabolic disorders (including metabolic syndrome), collagen vascular disorders, and current medications. Ask for symptoms of nausea, headache, irritability, failure to thrive, and deteriorating school performance to assess for severity and impact from hypertension.

B. BP and pulses should be taken in all four extremities. The bladder width should be at least 40% of the arm circumference. The bladder length should cover 80% to 100% of the circumference of the arm. Unfortunately, the commonly used electronic devices often have a systematic error with the systolic pressure reading that is spuriously high if the right arm pressure is elevated. The mean arterial pressure is most accurate on these machines. Differential pulses and differential BP with upper extremity pressures higher than the lower pressures are suggestive of a coarctation of the aorta. Lower extremity systolic pressures are usually 10 to 20 points greater than the upper extremity. Perform a thorough ophthalmoscopic examination, looking for arteriovenous nicking, tortuosity, hemorrhage, and papilledema as evidence of long-standing hypertension. Note signs of hypertensive encephalopathy, such as seizures, stroke, altered mental status, and focal neurologic defects. An abdominal bruit suggests renal artery stenosis. Note edema, thyroid size, hirsutism, striae, and other signs of an endocrine disorder.

C. Assess the severity of hypertension (Table 1). Less than 90% for age/height/sex is considered normal. The category of prehypertension is about 90% to 95%. Hypertension is BP greater than 95% documented on three or more occasions. Stage I hypertension is 95% to 99%, and stage II hypertension is defined as greater than 99%. (Because of the small margin between 95% and 99%, stage I is designated as 95% to 5 mm Hg greater than 99%, and stage II is for BP 5 mm Hg greater than 99%). Severely ill patients may have accelerated hypertension with signs of congestive heart failure (infants) or hypertensive encephalopathy. Moderate hypertension usually has no symptoms.

D. Because of the unreliability of commonly used electronic BP measurement devices, the measurements should be validated with a sphygmomanometer. Ambulatory BP monitoring may be helpful in this scenerio. It is a portable device that measures BP repeatedly over 24 hours.

(Continued on page 86)

Table 1. **Severity of Hypertension**

Prehypertension	Hypertension Stage I	Hypertension Stage II
90–95% asymptomatic	≥95–99% + 5 mm Hg mild symptoms	≥99% + 5 mm Hg signs of congestive heart failure or hypertensive encephalopathy

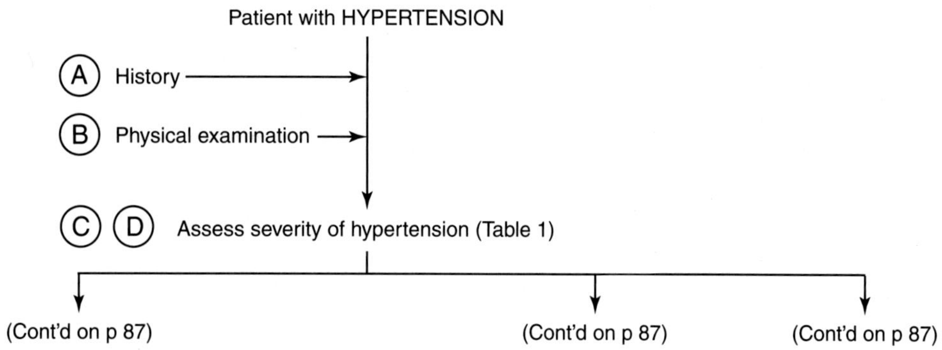
Patient with HYPERTENSION
A History
B Physical examination
C D Assess severity of hypertension (Table 1)
(Cont'd on p 87)
(Cont'd on p 87)
(Cont'd on p 87)

E. All patients with prehypertension or hypertension should be counseled with nonpharmacologic therapy. Nonpharmacologic therapy includes reduced sodium intake, weight reduction for obese patients, exercise, change in lifestyle, and decreased stress. Avoid stimulant medications, sympathomimetics, amphetamines, steroids, oral contraceptives, and decongestants, which may elevate pressures. Discourage cigarette smoking. Participation in dynamic exercise may continue, including competitive sports, unless the BP is greater than the 99th percentile (uncontrolled) or there is demonstrable end-organ damage. Isometric exercise with systemic hypertension is considered by many to be contraindicated until the BP is well controlled.

F. Perform a basic diagnostic evaluation in patients with documented BPs greater than the 95th percentile. In those with BPs between the 90th and 95th percentiles, repeated pressures should be performed in 4 to 6 weeks. The evaluation includes complete blood cell count, urinalysis and urine culture, basic metabolic panel, lipid panel, thyroid function, renal ultrasound, and echocardiography (for baseline left ventricular mass). For the prehypertensive group, the above testing should be directed by history and physical. A lipid panel should be drawn if the patient is obese or there is a positive family history. Referral should be made to subspecialists if a primary cause is found.

G. Pharmacologic therapy may be considered for stage I hypertensive patients if they are symptomatic, have evidence of end-organ damage or diabetes mellitus type 1 or 2, or if the hypertension persists despite lifestyle modifications. Treatment may be considered for prehypertensive patients with chronic kidney disease, diabetes, or left ventricular hypertrophy. First-line medications depend on the cause of the hypertension and include beta-blockers, an angiotensin-converting enzyme inhibitor, a calcium channel blocker, or a diuretic. For dosages, see Table 2.

H. For severe hypertension, consider referring to a pediatric hypertension specialist. Asymptomatic patients should be treated for primary cause if present and started on antihypertensive medication. In symptomatic patients, hospitalization may be required. Patients with severe uncontrolled hypertension may be at risk for encephalopathy. Patients may be treated with a continuous infusion of sodium nitroprusside. When it is used longer than 48 hours or in high dosages, monitor for cyanide toxicity. Esmolol and nicardipine are other agents that may be considered. The goal should be to decrease BP by 25% in the first 8 hours, then normalize it in the next 24 to 48 hours.

I. Intravenous labetalol or hydralazine may be used in less urgent situations, followed by diuretics (unless volume contracted) and other parenteral antihypertensives (beta-blockers, vasodilators). Patients must be monitored closely during administrations.

(Continued on page 88)

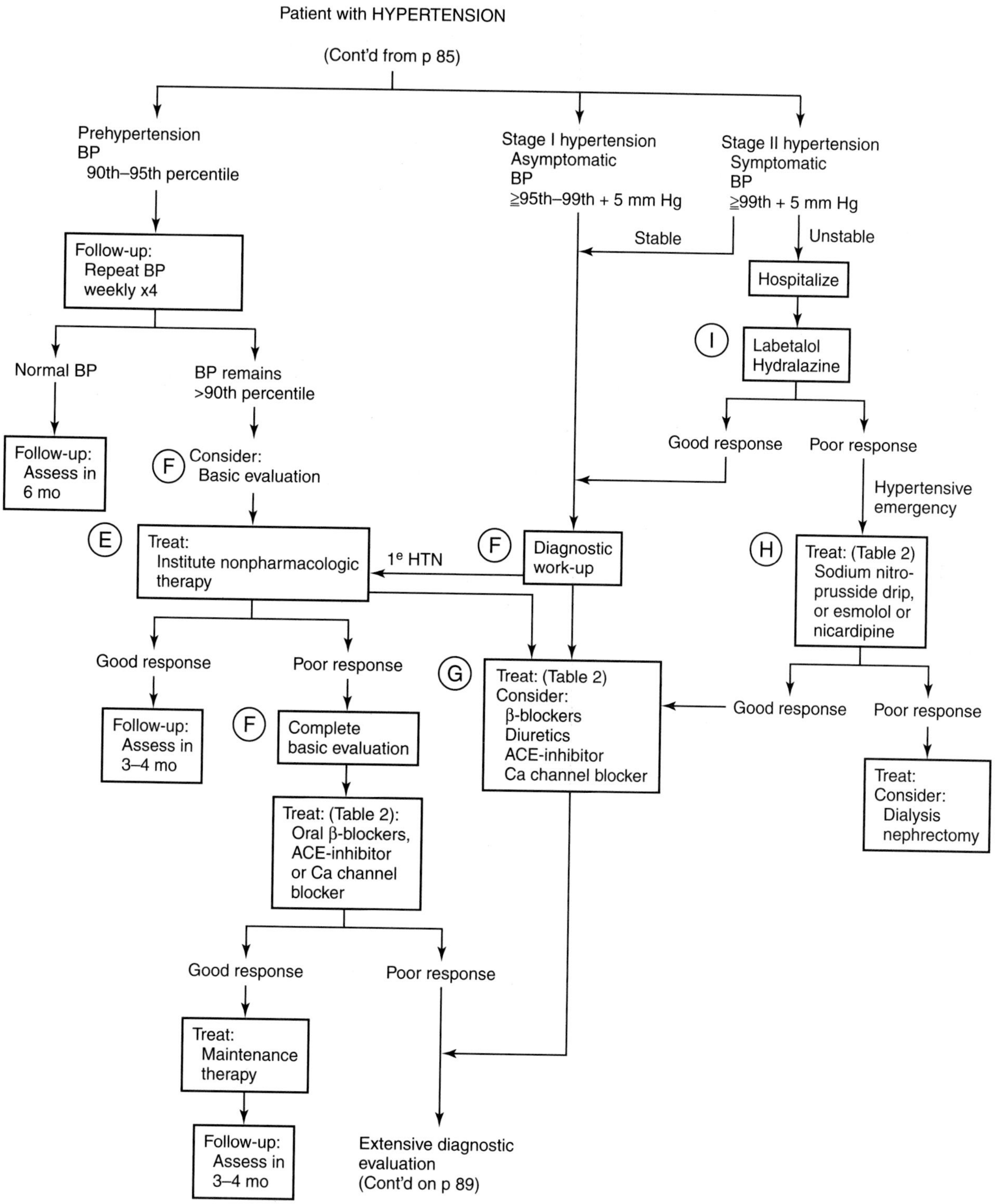
Patient with HYPERTENSION
(Cont'd from p 85)
Prehypertension BP 90th–95th percentile
Stage I hypertension Asymptomatic BP ≧95th–99th + 5 mm Hg
Stage II hypertension Symptomatic BP ≧99th + 5 mm Hg
Stable
Unstable
Follow-up: Repeat BP weekly x4
Hospitalize
I
Labetalol Hydralazine
Normal BP
BP remains >90th percentile
Good response
Poor response
Follow-up: Assess in 6 mo
F
Consider: Basic evaluation
Hypertensive emergency
E
Treat: Institute nonpharmacologic therapy
1e HTN
F
Diagnostic work-up
H
Treat: (Table 2) Sodium nitro-prusside drip, or esmolol or nicardipine
Good response
Poor response
G
Treat: (Table 2) Consider: β-blockers Diuretics ACE-inhibitor Ca channel blocker
Good response
Poor response
Follow-up: Assess in 3–4 mo
F
Complete basic evaluation
Treat: Consider: Dialysis nephrectomy
Treat: (Table 2): Oral β-blockers, ACE-inhibitor or Ca channel blocker
Good response
Poor response
Treat: Maintenance therapy
Follow-up: Assess in 3–4 mo
Extensive diagnostic evaluation
(Cont'd on p 89)

J. Ultimately, the cause of severe hypertension must be dealt with.

Table 2. **Drugs Used in the Treatment of Hypertension in Children**

Drug	Dosage
Severe Hypertension	
Sodium nitroprusside	0.3–0.5 μg/kg/min IV drip, may titrate (maximum: 10 μg/kg/min)
Esmolol	500 μg/kg/min load, followed by continuous infusion and titrate 50–200 μg/kg/min
Nicardipine	0.5–3 μg/kg/min IV infusion
Moderate to Severe Hypertension	
Hydralazine	0.1–0.2 mg/kg/dose IM or IV every 4-6h PRN 0.75–3 mg/kg/24 hr PO every 6–12h
Calcium channel blocker	
Nifedipine	0.25–0.5 mg/kg/dose PO tid or qid
Beta-blocker	
Propranolol	Infants: 0.1–0.25 mg/kg/dose PO qid (maximum: 1 mg/kg/dose) Children: 0.5–2 mg/kg/day divided doses every 6–8 hours (maximum: 60 mg/day) Adolescent: begin 10 mg PO qid, then increase at 1- to 2-wk intervals (maximum adult dose, 320–480 mg/day)
Enalapril	0.05 mg/kg/dose IV every 6h (maximum: 5 mg/dose) Children: 0.1–0.5 mg/kg/24 hr divided 1–2 times/day PO (maximum: 40 mg/24 hr) Adolescent/adult: 2.5–5 mg/day PO; increase to 10–40 mg/day in 1–2 divided doses
Other Common Agents for Outpatient Therapy	
ACE inhibitors	
Captopril	Neonates: 0.05–0.1 mg/kg/dose every 8-24h; titrate up to 0.5 mg/kg/dose Child: begin 0.1 mg/kg/dose tid, increase to maximum of 6 mg/kg/day Adolescent: Begin 25 mg bid or tid; increase at 1- to 2-wk intervals to maximum 150 mg tid
Lisinopril	0.07 mg/kg/day up to 5 mg/day (maximum: 0.6 mg/kg/day or 40 mg/day)
Angiotensin receptor blocker	
Losartan	0.7 mg/kg/day up to 50 mg/day (maximum: 1.4 mg/kg/day or 100 mg/day)
Beta-blocker	
Atenolol	1–1.2 mg/kg/dose in 1–2 doses (maximum: 2 mg/kg/day or 100 mg/day)
Ca channel blocker	
Amlodipine	Children 6–17 years old: 2.5–5 mg daily (10 mg maximum daily in adults)
Central α-agonist	
Clonidine	5–10 μg/kg/day divided bid to tid, may increase to 5–25 μg/kg/day
Diuretics*	
Hydrochlorothiazide	<6 months: up to 3.3 mg/kg/24 hr in 2 divided doses (maximum: 37.5 mg/day) >6 months: 2–2.22 mg/kg/24 hr in 2 divided doses (maximum: 200 mg/day)
Furosemide	1–2 mg/kg/dose PO bid or tid
Spironolactone	1–2 mg/kg/dose PO bid; may use with hydrochlorothiazide or furosemide for potassium sparing

*Monitor electrolytes.
IM, intramuscular; *IV*, intravenous; *PO*, orally; *PRN*, as needed.

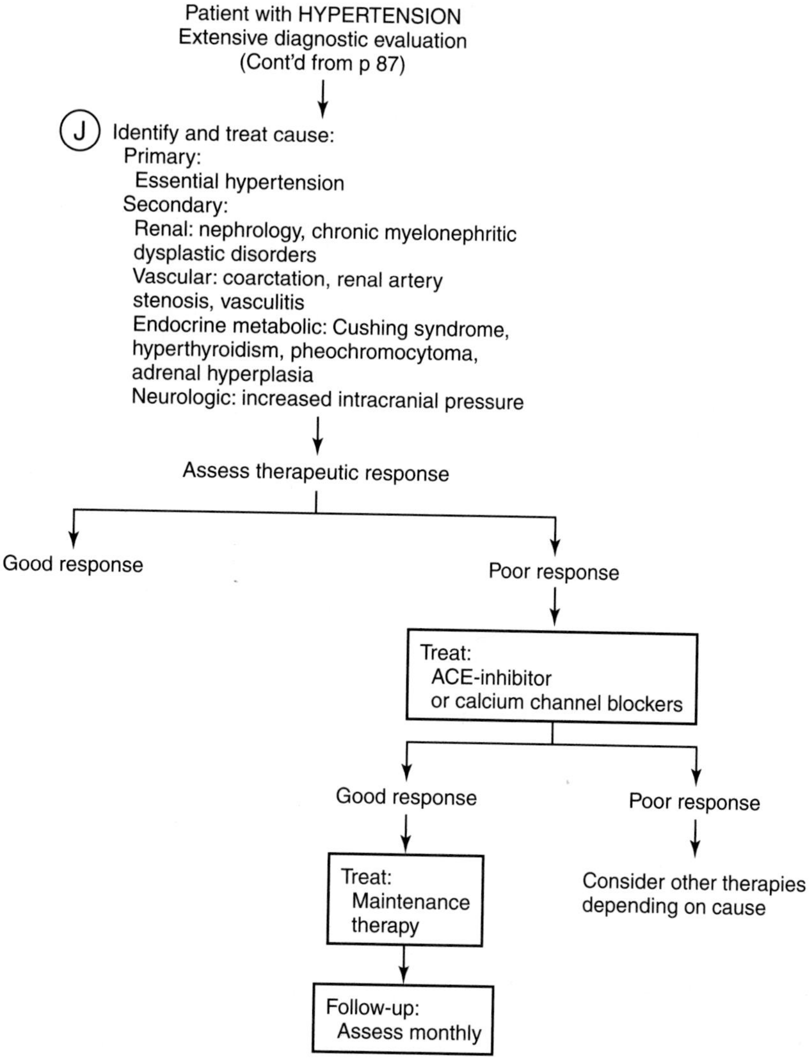
Patient with HYPERTENSION
Extensive diagnostic evaluation
(Cont'd from p 87)
J
Identify and treat cause:
Primary:
Essential hypertension
Secondary:
Renal: nephrology, chronic myelonephritic dysplastic disorders
Vascular: coarctation, renal artery stenosis, vasculitis
Endocrine metabolic: Cushing syndrome, hyperthyroidism, pheochromocytoma, adrenal hyperplasia
Neurologic: increased intracranial pressure
Assess therapeutic response
Good response
Poor response
Treat:
ACE-inhibitor
or calcium channel blockers
Good response
Poor response
Treat:
Maintenance therapy
Consider other therapies depending on cause
Follow-up:
Assess monthly

References

American Academy of Pediatrics, Committee on Sports Medicine and Fitness. Athletic participation by children and adolescents who have systemic hypertension. Pediatrics 1997;99:635.

Bartosh SM, Aronson AJ. Childhood hypertension. An updated etiology, diagnosis, and treatment. Pediatr Clin North Am 1999;46:235.

Constantine, Erika MD, Linakis, James MD. The assessment and management of hypertensive emergencies and urgencies in children. Pediatr Emerg Care 2005; 21(6):391–6.

Fourth report on diagnosis, evaluation and treatment of high blood pressure in children and adolescents. Bethesda (MD): National Heart, Lung, and Blood Institute, National Institutes of Health; May 2004.

Lauer RM, Burns TL, Clarke WR. Assessing children's blood pressure—considerations of age and body size. The Muscatine Study. Pediatrics 1987;75:1081.

Rosner B, Prineas RJ, Loggie JMH, Daniels SR. Blood pressure nomograms for children and adolescents, by height, sex, and age, in the United States. J Pediatr 1993;123:871.

Shalma A, Sinaiko AR. Systemic hypertension. In: Emmanuoilides GC, Riemenschneider TA, Allen HD, Gutgesell HP, editors. Moss and Adams' heart disease in infants, children, and adolescents. Baltimore (MD): Williams & Wilkins; 1995. p. 1641.

Stabouli S, Kotsis V, Zakopoulos N. Ambulatory blood pressure monitoring and target organ damage in pediatrics. J Hypertens 2007;25(10):1979–86

Williams CL, Hayman LL, Daniels SR et al. Cardiovascular health in childhood: a statement for health professionals from the Committee on Atherosclerosis, Hypertension, and Obesity in the Young (AHOY) of the Council on Cardiovascular Disease in the Young, American Heart Association. Circulation 2002; 106:143–60.

Supraventricular Tachycardia

Kelly K. Gajewski, MD, and John H. Reed, MD, MPH

Supraventricular tachycardia (SVT) is the most common symptomatic dysrhythmia in the pediatric population, with an estimated incidence between 1 in 250 and 1 in 25,000 children. Approximately half of pediatric patients with SVT present with their first episode of SVT in the first year of life, usually before 4 months of age. The heart rate is usually between 200 and 300 beats/min in infants and between 180 and 250 beats/min in older children. Greater than 90% of SVT in the pediatric population is from a reentrant rhythm involving the atrioventricular (AV) node or an accessory pathway. This type is characterized by sudden onset and offset, and has little or no variation in heart rate.

Table 1. **Degree of Illness in Supraventricular Tachycardia**

Mild	Moderate	Severe
Asymptomatic and stable	Symptoms of decreased cerebral or coronary artery blood flow or mild congestive heart failure	Shock or hypotension Altered mental status Moderate to severe congestive heart failure

A. The history should focus on precipitating factors, duration, severity, associated symptoms, and mode of offset (abrupt suggesting SVT vs. gradual suggesting an automatic mechanism including sinus tachycardia). Infants are often asymptomatic, but they may present with acute irritability, pallor, tachypnea, feeding difficulty, or even with severe congestive heart failure if the tachycardia has been long-standing. Older children often describe their "heart beeping." Adolescents most commonly complain of palpitations or chest discomfort, but isolated SVT does not cause severe chest pain. Presyncope is not unusual, but frank syncope suggests more significant arrhythmia or heart disease. The symptoms may start at rest or during activity and typically last for minutes but can be as brief as a few seconds or as long as many hours. Identify any conditions predisposing to arrhythmias such as Wolff–Parkinson–White syndrome (WPW), congenital heart disease, infection (myocarditis), fever, or drugs (sympathomimetics, amphetamines). Though SVT is usually sporadic, it is on rare occasion familial.

B. The physical examination should initially focus on hemodynamic compromise. The hypotensive, poorly perfused child should be treated immediately (see later). In the more stable patient, look for signs of congenital heart disease (primarily murmurs) or congestive heart failure (gallop rhythm, pulmonary rales, hepatomegaly, edema) (Table 1).

C. Any suspected arrhythmia should be evaluated with a 12- or 15-lead electrocardiogram. SVT usually presents with narrow QRS complexes either without discernible P waves or with small inverted P waves immediately after the QRS complexes. There is little beat-to-beat variability, and the heart rate generally does not change significantly with stimulation. Although a rapid rhythm with a wide complex may represent SVT with aberrant conduction, consider and treat these findings as ventricular tachycardia until proved otherwise.

D. Vagal maneuvers are the initial treatment of choice for the stable patient with SVT. The increase in vagal tone causes transient AV nodal block, thereby terminating the reentrant circuit. The most effective technique in infants is placing a bag filled with ice slurry over the forehead and bridge of the nose for up to 30 seconds. Other techniques include passing a nasogastric tube, placing a rectal thermometer, applying gentle abdominal pressure, or lifting the feet above the head. Older children and adolescents can be asked to perform a Valsalva maneuver, cough or clear the throat, or stand on their head (with careful assistance). Two commonly taught techniques should be avoided: Application of ocular pressure is contraindicated secondary to possible eye trauma, and carotid massage may interfere with cerebral perfusion.

E. Adenosine is the next therapeutic step in the stable patient. Properly administered, it is extremely effective in the acute treatment of SVT. Like vagal maneuvers, but more effectively, it causes transient AV block terminating any reentrant circuit involving the AV node. Although adenosine typically will not terminate atrial flutter, atrial fibrillation, or ventricular tachycardia, the AV node block caused by adenosine will often help clarify the diagnosis. The dose is 0.1 to 0.2 mg/kg intravenously with a maximum of 12 mg. Adenosine has a very short half-life. Therefore, set up a three-way stopcock and administer a rapid saline bolus immediately after the adenosine dose. In addition to routine blood pressure and heart rate monitoring, a multilead electrocardiographic rhythm strip should be obtained during adenosine administration. The clinician should be prepared to treat the (rare) significant cardiac adverse effects of adenosine. Ventricular fibrillation is the most important; therefore, a defibrillator should be available. More common side effects include flushing, headache, nausea, vomiting, chest pain, dyspnea, and dizziness. The most serious noncardiac adverse effect of adenosine is bronchospasm. In asthmatic children who receive adenosine, be prepared to treat immediate and delayed bronchospasm.

F. Direct current cardioversion is indicated for the hemodynamically unstable patient with SVT. Initial energy should be 0.5 J/kg. Energy can be increased up to 2 J/kg, but cardioversion of SVT rarely requires this much energy and alternate diagnoses should be considered in this setting. The shock should be synchronized to the QRS complex to avoid shock on T wave, which

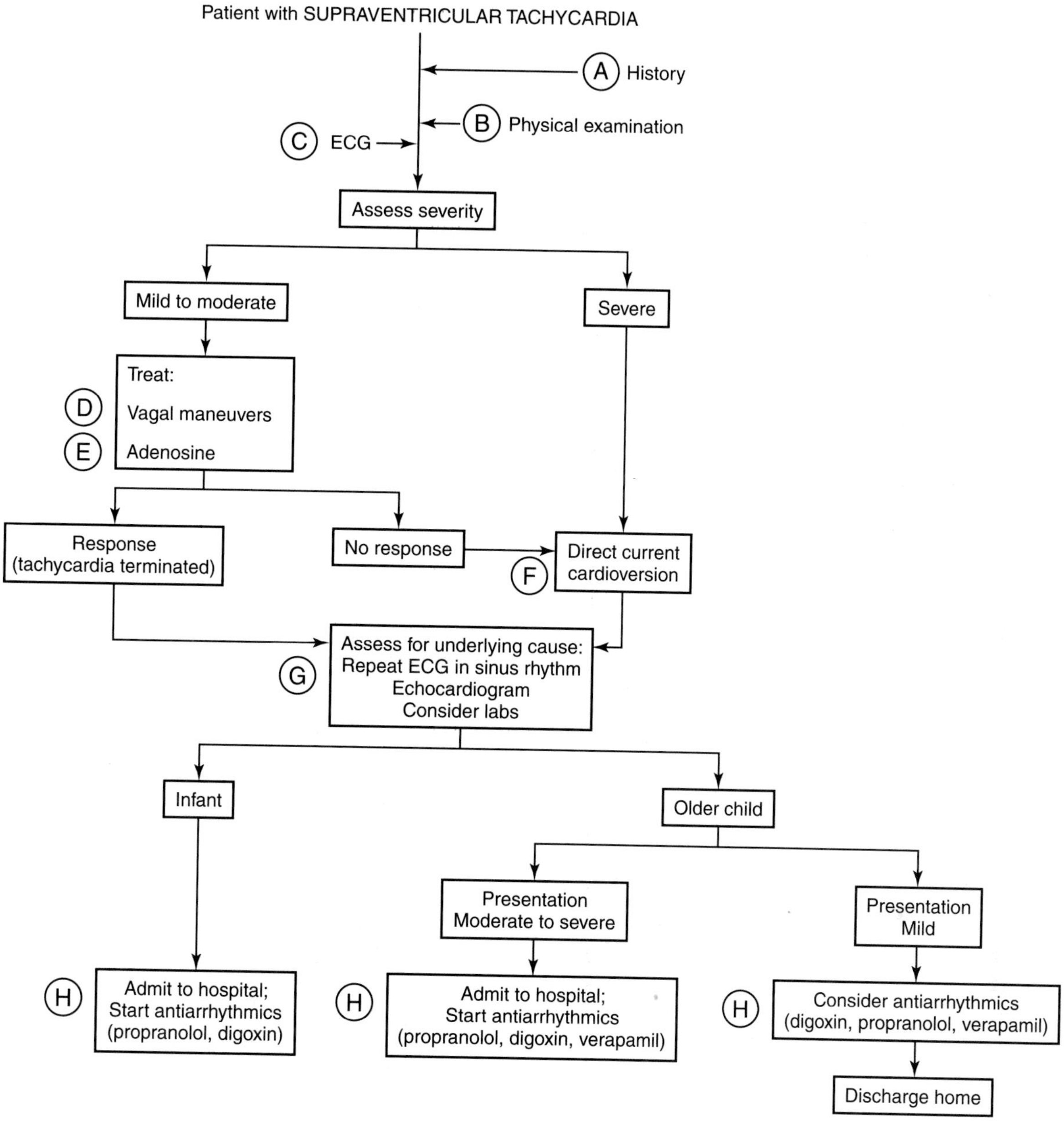
Patient with SUPRAVENTRICULAR TACHYCARDIA
A History
B Physical examination
C ECG
Assess severity
Mild to moderate
Severe
Treat:
D Vagal maneuvers
E Adenosine
Response (tachycardia terminated)
No response
Direct current cardioversion
F
G
Assess for underlying cause: Repeat ECG in sinus rhythm Echocardiogram Consider labs
Infant
Older child
Presentation Moderate to severe
Presentation Mild
H
Admit to hospital; Start antiarrhythmics (propranolol, digoxin)
Admit to hospital; Start antiarrhythmics (propranolol, digoxin, verapamil)
Consider antiarrhythmics (digoxin, propranolol, verapamil)
Discharge home

may induce ventricular fibrillation. If time permits, run a multilead rhythm strip when performing the cardioversion.

G. After conversion to normal sinus rhythm, obtain an electrocardiogram and perform studies to attempt to elucidate a potential cause of the SVT. Look for WPW. In WPW, there is an antegrade-conducting accessory AV connection that together with the atrium, AV node, and ventricle forms the reentrant tachycardia circuit. On electrocardiogram, WPW is manifest by a short PR interval and a delta wave that is a slurred initial portion of the QRS complex. Most patients with SVT have no associated illness, but if one is suggested by the history and physical examination, consider obtaining electrolytes, complete blood cell count, toxicology screen, blood gas, or thyroid function tests. Consider creatine kinase and troponins if myocarditis is suspected. An echocardiogram can help rule out cardiomyopathy or associated congenital heart disease.

H. Preventive oral antiarrhythmic therapy should be considered in infants after an initial episode and older children with recurrent or severe symptoms (Table 2). This should be done in conjunction with pediatric cardiology consultation. The most common first-line drugs in infants include digoxin and propranolol. In older children, atenolol is frequently used. Patients with WPW should not be treated with digoxin because there is a small increase in the risk for sudden cardiac death. Because of their incompletely developed sarcoplasmic reticulum, children younger than 1 year should not be treated with verapamil. In the absence of WPW, infants often do not have recurrences of their tachycardia after 1 year of age. Therefore, their medication is often discontinued at around that time. Patients who are refractory to treatment and those who want to avoid long-term antiarrhythmic medications (generally older than 5 years) should undergo electrophysiologic study and transcatheter ablation of their arrhythmogenic substrate.

Table 2. **Drug Therapy for Supraventricular Tachycardia in Children**

Drug	Dosage	Product Availability
Adenosine	IV rapid push 0.1–0.2 mg/kg followed by immediate flush; if no response; double dose and repeat in 1–2 minutes Adult: 6 mg, then 12 mg IV bolus if no response	Solution: 3 mg/ml
Digoxin	Digitalization (load): give 1/2 initially and 1/4 every 8h × 2 doses Premature or newborn: total dose 20–30 μg/kg/24 hr 1 month to 2 years: 30–50 μg/kg/24 hr 2–10 years: 30–40 μg/kg/24 hr >10 years: 10–15 μg/kg/24 hr Maintenance: infants: 8–10 μg/kg/day <2 years: 10–12 μg/kg/day 2–10 years: 8–10 μg/kg/day >10 years 2.5–5 mcg/kg/day	Tablets: 0.125, 0.25, 0.5 mg Liquid: 50 μg/ml PO
Propranolol	2–4 mg/kg/day PO divided every 6-8h	Liquid: 4 mg/ml Tablets: 10, 20, 40, 60, 80 mg SR capsules: 60, 80, 120, 160 mg
Verapamil	Children: PO 4–8 mg/kg/day divided tid Adults: 240–480 mg/day divided tid to qid	Tablets: 40, 80, 120 mg SR tablets: 120, 180 mg

IV, intravenous; *PO*, orally; *SR*, sustained release.

References

Chun TUH, Van Hare GF. Advances in the approach to treatment of supraventricular tachycardia in the pediatric population. Curr Cardiol Rep 2004;6:322–6.

Doniger, SJ, Sharieff GQ. Pediatric dysrhythmias. Pediatr Clin N Am 2006;53:85–105.

Erickson LC, Cocalis MW. The acute management of paroxysmal supraventricular tachycardia in children. Pediatr Rev 1993;14:273–4.

Etheridge SP, Judd VE. Supraventricular tachycardia in infancy: evaluation, management, and follow-up. Arch Pediatr Adolesc Med 1999;153:267–71.

Garson A Jr, Gillette PC, McNamara DG. Supraventricular tachycardia in children: clinical features, response to treatment, and long-term follow-up in 217 patients. J Pediatr 1981;98:875–82.

Ko JK, Deal BJ, Strasburger JF, Benson DW Jr. Supraventricular tachycardia mechanisms and their age distribution in pediatric patients. Am J Cardiol 1992;69:1028–1032.

Losek JD, Endom E, Dietrich A, et al. Adenosine and pediatric supraventricular tachycardia in the emergency department: multicenter study and review. Ann Emerg Med 1999;33:185–91.

Perry JC, Garson A Jr. Supraventricular tachycardia due to Wolff-Parkinson-White syndrome in children: early disappearance and late recurrence. J Am Coll Cardiol 1990;16:1215–20.

Weindling SN, Saul JP, Walsh EP. Efficacy and risks of medical therapy for supraventricular tachycardia in neonates and infants. Am Heart J 1996;131:66–72.

DENTAL

Facial Swelling and Odontogenic Infections

Ulrich Klein, DMD, DDS, MS

Facial swelling in pediatric patients is a common clinical problem with diverse causative factors and can be grouped according to its acuity and clinical presentation.

An *acute facial swelling* with inflammation may have odontogenic causes, such as dental caries or trauma, or nonodontogenic origins such as lymphadenitis, sinusitis, skin infections, insect/animal bites, or other puncture wounds. Less frequent reasons are viral and bacterial salivary gland infections, angioedema, and side effects of long-term steroid therapy. Although *nonprogressive swelling* is more indicative of a congenital anomaly, neoplasms are often the basis of *slowly* or *rapidly progressive swellings*. In one retrospective study on pediatric patients, odontogenic facial cellulitis accounted for almost 50% of emergency department visits with a diagnosis of facial infection. In another study, decayed primary maxillary anterior and posterior teeth were found as the most frequent source for upper face infections and primary mandibular posterior teeth for the lower face. From 362 patients reporting to the emergency department of a large children's hospital for dental caries-related emergencies, facial cellulitis accounted for 9% and 12% of the diagnoses pertaining to primary and permanent teeth, respectively. Unusual dental abscesses can also arise from developmental abnormalities of the dental hard tissues in the absence of caries.

This chapter describes causative factors, characteristics and clinical features, as well as pathology and management of facial swelling caused by odontogenic infections (Table 1).

CAUSATIVE FACTORS AND PATHOLOGY

Dental caries, an infectious disease caused mainly by *Streptococcus mutans* and *Lactobacilli,* begins as an enamel defect that can progress within a few months into dentin from where it moves toward the pulp tissue. The ensuing pulpal hyperemia causes minor intermittent pain that is provoked by hot, cold, and sweet. If caries that progressed through enamel into dentin is not excauated and filled with a dental restoration, acute pulpitis will eventually develop. The pain associated with this stage is more intense, lingers longer or does not subside at all, and presents often with a nocturnal exacerbation. Dental treatment now requires removal of the infected coronal pulp (pulpotomy) or both the coronal and radicular pulp (pulpectomy) and subsequent replacement with a root canal filling material or extraction of the tooth.

If not treated, the infected pulp tissue eventually becomes necrotic and bacteria will exit through the apical foramen, resulting in acute periapical periodontitis. As more inflammatory cells such as granulocytes accumulate to isolate the infection from the surrounding tissues, a localized periapical abscess will form at the tooth apex. This stage is generally characterized by significant pain. If the host is unable to resolve the infection, the purulent material will extravasate through medullary spaces and eventually perforate through the cortical plate and spread diffusely along the path of least resistance the fascial planes

Table 1. **Comparison of Simple vs. Complex Odontogenic Infections**

Category	Simple	Complex
Medical history	WNL	Complicated medical history, uncontrolled metabolic disease, immunodeficiency, malignancy
Appearance of patient	Stable, "well"	Unstable, ill, lethargic, malaise
Signs and symptoms	Nutritional status WNL, mandibular range of motion WNL	Dehydration, dysphagia, trismus, lymphadenopathy
Vital signs	WNL	↑ HR, ↑ RR, ↑ temperature > 101° F (39° C), weight loss
Laboratory and other tests	WNL, panoramic and intraoral radiographs	↑ ESR, ↑ leukocytes, ↑ CRP, CT, MRI, sensitivity culture
Clinical examination	Localized soft cellulitis or fluctuant swelling, sinus tract with parulis	Diffuse, boardlike cellulitis, involvement of several fascial spaces
Treatment options	Root canal therapy or extraction of offending tooth, I&D; may require oral antibiotics	Hospitalization, I&D under IV sedation or general anesthesia; extraction of offending tooth; IV antibiotics and fluids
Social factors	Intact, caring social structure	Noncompliant patient, suspicion of unreliable home care
Treatment facility and care providers	Dental office; general or pediatric dentist	Hospital, acute-care facility, emergency department, dental and medical specialists

CT, computed tomography; *ESR,* erythrocyte sedimentation rate; *HR,* heart rate; *I&D,* incision and drainage; *IV,* intravenous; *MRI,* magnetic resonance imaging; *RR,* respiratory rate; *WNL,* within normal limits.

of the overlying soft tissues. This acute inflammatory process is called *cellulitis* and represents the acute initial phase of the infection. It can progress rapidly or become chronic and form an abscess if local host mechanisms are able to wall off and consolidate the purulent material. In its early stage, cellulitis feels soft and doughy to palpation, whereas its advanced and serious form is indurated ("boardlike") and painful because of tissue distension. The site of perforation relative to muscle attachments determines the fascial space involved and the location of the soft tissue swelling. The more fascial spaces are involved, the more serious the facial cellulitis will be. One such potentially life-threatening complication is Ludwig angina, a diffuse infection of the submandibular and sublingual spaces that causes airway compromise. As another pathway, purulent material from a periapical abscess may penetrate the surface epithelium near the apex of the tooth and form a fistula. At its intraoral opening, inflamed granulation tissue appears as parulis ("gumboil") from which drainage occurs. In this case, the periapical abscess becomes asymptomatic because purulent material can no longer accumulate. The abscess may also drain extraorally via a cutaneous sinus tract.

This periapical route of inoculating bacteria into the soft tissue is typical in children, whereas in adults the cause may also be a deep periodontal pocket. It is important to note that primary teeth cause infections of the same severity and system toxicity compared with permanent teeth. Rare but severe systemic complications of odontogenic origin are bacterial endocarditis, meningitis, cavernous sinus thrombosis, abscesses of the orbit or brain, and infections of the mediastinum or the lungs.

MICROBIOLOGY OF ODONTOGENIC INFECTIONS

Odontogenic infections are generally polymicrobial and from endogenous oral flora. They are mixed aerobic/anaerobic with 60% caused by anaerobic and aerobic bacteria, 35% by aerobic bacteria, and 5% by anaerobic bacteria only. Of the aerobic group, *Streptococci* comprise about 90% and *Staphylococci* about 5%. In the anaerobic group, gram-positive cocci and gram-negative rods can be isolated most frequently among many others. *Streptococcus viridans* was found in 54% of the aerobic/facultative anaerobic group, whereas *Prevotella* spp. were found in 53% of the anaerobes. Initially, more virulent bacteria such as the aerobic *Streptococcus* spp. dominate the infection, but after local conditions deteriorate for them, anaerobic bacteria take over. An increased prevalence of β-lactamase–producing bacteria among gram-negative anaerobes has been noted. Before the advent of *Haemophilus influenzae* type B (Hib) vaccine, *H. influenzae* was mainly responsible for facial cellulitis of unknown origin, whereas thereafter it has been supplanted by *Streptococcus pneumoniae* and *Staphylococcus aureus*. A blood culture should be obtained in such cases.

PATIENT ASSESSMENT AND PHYSICAL EXAMINATION

A. History/Physical Examination: The patient is initially questioned about the onset, duration, rapidity, and pattern of the progress of the facial infection, and if any trauma or treatment has occurred earlier. The patient's medical history must be evaluated for conditions that affect host defenses (e.g., uncontrolled metabolic diseases such as diabetes and renal disease), malignancies, or use of immunosuppressive drugs. In these individuals, treatment of the infection may require more aggressive surgery or parenteral antibiotics. The patient should then be evaluated for symptoms of pain, swelling, hot skin areas, redness, as well as reduced function such as limited opening (trismus) and difficulty in swallowing, breathing, or chewing. Patients with moderate to severe infections will feel ill and lethargic (malaise), and generally show an increased heart and respiratory rate and a temperature greater than 101°F. The patient's recent fluid intake and voiding must be assessed. The *extraoral examination* should identify any asymmetry in the neck and face, assess the mandibular range of motion, the temporomandibular joint, and include palpation of the bony margins of the facial bones to assure their continuity. Lymphadenopathy is a sign of an infection that has spread. *Intraorally,* the mouth must be checked for carious teeth, unusual tooth mobility, gingival or vestibular mucosal swellings, ulcers, and fistulas to determine a specific cause for the infection. Findings from these previous assessments will determine the type of special test required to make the final diagnosis.

B. Further evaluation: Tooth vitality tests, bacterial cultures, fine-needle aspiration cytology, and biopsy may be ordered as necessary. Radiographic examination may include intraoral and/or extraoral (panoramic) radiographs, a computed tomography (CT) scan, or a magnetic resonance image if intracranial spread is suspected. Abnormal complete blood cell count (CBC) values such as generalized leukocytosis, neutrophilia, monocytosis, eosinopenia, and basopenia can only be detected when the infection has reached the stage of acute cellulitis. A white blood cell shift to the left and an absolute band count greater than 500 cells/mm^3 should be suspicious of a nondental origin. In addition, mean erythrocyte sedimentation rate (ESR) values of 30 ± 4.5 mm/hr were observed in a group of 60 children with facial cellulitis.

C. Treatment: The primary treatment of odontogenic infections consists of removal of the cause of the infection and establishing local surgical drainage. Therapeutic modalities include root canal treatment for necrotic teeth, removal of the offending tooth, and incision and drainage (I&D) of an existing abscess or indurated soft tissues to release pressure from the area and to provide oxygen to an anaerobic environment. In situations with severe, extensive, or systemic infections, compromised host defenses, and particularly virulent pathogens, antibiotics may be a necessary adjunctive therapy to support the host. Treatment failures can occur if the surgical and/or antibiotic therapy or the host's defenses are inadequate. Hospitalization for surgical treatment and parenteral antibiotic therapy may be necessary for the noncompliant patient or when unreliable home care is suspected. Medical indications include the more severe infections that are characterized by difficulty breathing or swallowing, poor oral intake, dehydration, fever greater than 101° F (39° C), tachycardia and hypotension, and/or involvement of multiple fascial spaces.

D. Antibiotic therapy: Antibiotic therapy should be reserved for patients with compromised host defenses and serious infections that are persistent or systemic in nature or spreading rapidly. These are generally characterized by fever greater than 101°F, malaise, trismus, lymphadenopathy, and increased ESR and leukocyte count. Culturing is advised in immunocompromised patients or those with a history of bacterial endocarditis and if empiric therapy has failed. It is also appropriate in cases of recurrent postoperative infection, when dental treatment has been completed and the patient is not responding to the first antibiotic given within 48 hours, or when the infection progresses rapidly or to other fascial planes. Sampling of anaerobic bacteria is difficult because they are killed quickly when exposed to oxygen; therefore, needle aspiration and transfer with an inert gas is preferred. Empiric therapy can be used routinely because odontogenic infections are usually predictable and outcomes favorable. Penicillin is bactericidal and still considered the gold standard, but incidence of penicillin resistance is increased. When patients are allergic to or unresponsive to penicillin alone, clindamycin or β-lactamase inhibitors such as amoxicillin clavulanate (Augmentin) or ampicillin/sulbactam (Unasyn) should be given. Clindamycin and Unasyn were rated equally effective for treatment for complicated facial cellulitis of dental origin in children. Clindamycin was recommended for the more mature anaerobic infections, for serious intraosseous infections, and as a first-line antibiotic for all dental infections because of its unique antimicrobial properties, which include bacteriostatic activity, achievement of high tissue and bone concentrations, intracellular penetration, increased phagocytosis, and inhibition of toxin production. Although antibiotic-associated diarrhea is common in children, especially after administration of amoxicillin clavulanate, the incidence of pseudomembranous colitis in outpatient use is not greater for clindamycin as it is for ampicillin, amoxicillin, and the second- and third-generation cephalosporins. In a large, nested, case–control study, cephalexin and cefixime demonstrated an increased association with *Clostridium difficile* diarrhea compared with other antibiotics. When gram-positive organisms are suspected, first-generation cephalosporins may be used for their broader spectrum activity. Antibiotics should be prescribed for 5 to 7 days with an additional initial loading dose and the patient reassessed within 48 hours to ascertain effectiveness of treatment. Cost-effective generic drugs should be preferred over newer drugs. Patient compliance is usually greater if the drug can be taken with food and requires only three daily doses instead of four.

(Continued on page 98)

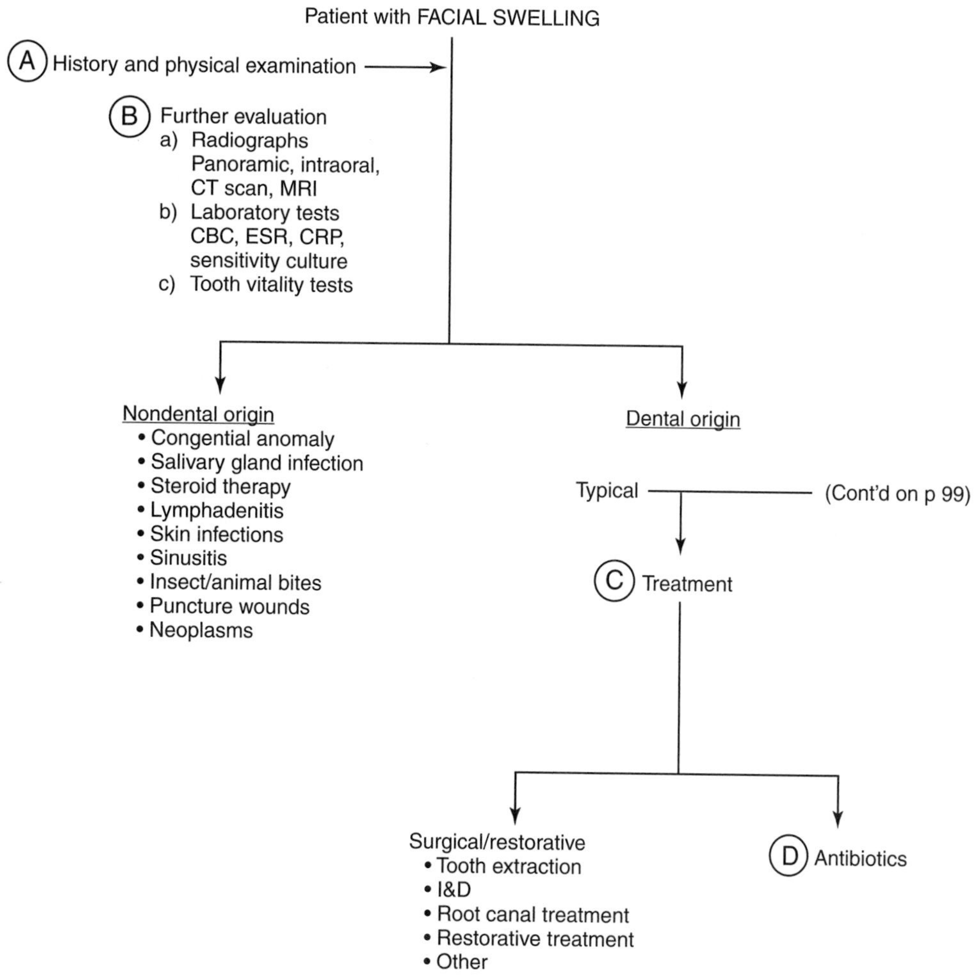
Patient with FACIAL SWELLING
A History and physical examination
B Further evaluation
a) Radiographs
Panoramic, intraoral,
CT scan, MRI
b) Laboratory tests
CBC, ESR, CRP,
sensitivity culture
c) Tooth vitality tests
Nondental origin
• Congential anomaly
• Salivary gland infection
• Steroid therapy
• Lymphadenitis
• Skin infections
• Sinusitis
• Insect/animal bites
• Puncture wounds
• Neoplasms
Dental origin
Typical
(Cont'd on p 99)
C Treatment
Surgical/restorative
• Tooth extraction
• I&D
• Root canal treatment
• Restorative treatment
• Other
D Antibiotics

E. Dental Abscesses of Unusual Dental Origin: In the absence of dental caries, unusual dental abscesses occur in individuals with developmental anomalies of the teeth caused by a local aberration of tooth development, a general manifestation of systemic conditions, or by acquired conditions. Dens invaginatus (dens-in-dente) is found in approximately 1% to 2% of the population and most frequently affects the maxillary permanent lateral incisor. Oral bacteria can enter the pulp through a deep palatal pit and cause an infection. In a similar fashion, the pulp becomes exposed and infected if the fragile tubercle of a dens evaginatus (incidence rate about 2% mainly in Asiatic races) fractures off. Both are local conditions and generally can be treated by root canal treatment. Systemic conditions include dentin dysplasias, dentinogenesis imperfecta, regional odontodysplasia ("ghost teeth"), and X-linked hypophosphatemia (X-H). All are characterized by abnormal formation of the dental hard tissues resulting in obliterated pulps (dentin dysplasias, dentinogenesis imperfecta), abnormally large pulp chambers (regional odontodysplasia, X-H), and dysplastic and poorly mineralized dentin (X-H). In these patients, enamel and dentin wear or fracture off easily, leading to exposed dentinal tubuli through which oral bacteria can ingress the pulp without difficulty particularly if the channels are abnormally large (X-H). In addition, limited vascular supply through pulp obliteration contributes to pulp necrosis. Treatment options other than extraction of the affected teeth are limited mainly because obliterated pulps make root canal treatment impossible. Prophylactic coverage of the affected teeth with metal or resin crowns is another therapeutic option to protect defective tooth structure from chipping off and oral microorganisms from entering the pulp. Dental abscesses are sometimes the first presenting clinical sign of X-linked hypophosphatemia when systemic manifestations are mild. Acquired conditions include pre-eruptive intracoronal resorption and mandibular infected buccal cyst. In pre-eruptive intracoronal resorption, resorptive cells stemming from undifferentiated cells of the developing dental follicle or from the surrounding bone enter the tooth through a break in the enamel surface and resorb its dentin after mineralization. When the tooth erupts into the oral cavity, caries forms in the resorbed cavity and eventually leads to pulp degeneration and subsequent abscess formation. However, early recognition of an intracoronal radiolucency presents the option of immediate restoration after tooth eruption. In mandibular infected buccal cyst, the infected operculum or pericoronitis around an erupting tooth, usually mandibular molars, causes its dental follicle to undergo cystic changes and displacement of adjacent teeth leading to deep periodontal pockets, pain, and swelling. The therapy of choice with a good success rate is curettage and removal of the cyst with concomitant antibiotic therapy. A tuberculoid granuloma can present as a solitary unilateral diffuse swelling with induration and extraoral sinus tract formation. In a panoramic radiograph, it generally presents as an ill-defined osteolytic lesion, whereas in an intraoral occlusal radiograph, it shows a typical "onion-peel" appearance. Differential diagnoses include osteomyelitis and Ewing sarcoma.

SUMMARY

Many acute facial swellings in children are due to odontogenic infection. Although most of these can be successfully treated with elimination of the source of the infection, a number of them require additional antibiotic therapy, as well as more extensive surgical treatment and hospitalization. Facial swellings of nonodontogenic origin require interdisciplinary evaluation by various medical specialties.

References

Batra P, Tejani Z, Mars M. X-linked hypophosphatemia: dental and histologic findings. J Can Dent Assoc 2006;72(1):69–72.

Brook I. Pseudomembranous colitis in children. J Gastroenterol Hepatol 2005;20(2):182–6.

Brook I, Lewis MA, Sandor GK, et al. Clindamycin in dentistry: more than just effective prophylaxis for endocarditis? Oral Surg Oral Med Oral Pathol Oral Radiol Endod 2005;100(5):550–8.

Dinkar AD, Prabhudessai V. Primary tuberculous osteomyelitis of the mandible: a case report. Dentomaxillofac Radiol 2008;37(7):415–20.

Dodson TB, Kaban LB. Infections of the maxillofacial region. In: Kaban LB, Troulis MJ, editors. Pediatric oral and maxillofacial surgery. Philadelphia: Saunders; 2004, p. 171–84.

Flynn TR. Principles of management and prevention of odontogenic infections. In: Happ JR, Ellis E, Tucker MR, editors. Contemporary oral and maxillofacial surgery. 5th ed. St. Louis: Mosby Elsevier; 2008, p. 291–315.

Khanna G, Sato Y, Smith RJ, et al. Causes of facial swelling in pediatric patients: correlation of clinical and radiologic findings. Radiographics 2006;26(1):157–71.

Levy DG, Stergachis A, McFarland LV, et al. Antibiotics and Clostridium difficile diarrhea in the ambulatory care setting. Clin Ther 2000;22(1):91–102.

Lin YT, Lu PW. Retrospective study of pediatric facial cellulitis of odontogenic origin. Pediatr Infect Dis J 2006;25(4):339–42.

Rush DE, Abdel-Haq N, Zhu JF, et al. Clindamycin versus Unasyn in the treatment of facial cellulitis of odontogenic origin in children. Clin Pediatr (Phila) 2007;46(2):154–9.

Seow WK. Diagnosis and management of unusual dental abscesses in children. Aust Dent J 2003;48(3):156–68.

Sheller B, Williams BJ, Lombardi SM. Diagnosis and treatment of dental caries-related emergencies in a children's hospital. Pediatr Dent 1997;19(8):470–5.

Sigal MJ, Levine N. Facial swelling and asymmetry in children: systematic diagnosis and review. J Can Dent Assoc 1989;55(10):799–805.

Swift JQ, Gulden WS. Antibiotic therapy—managing odontogenic infections. Dent Clin North Am 2002;46(4):623–33, vii.

Tervonen SA, Stratmann U, Mokrys K, Reichart PA. Regional odontodysplasia: a review of the literature and report of four cases. Clin Oral Investig 2004;8(2):45–51.

Travis RT, Steinle CJ. The effects of odontogenic infection on the complete blood count in children and adolescents. Pediatr Dent 1984;6(4):214–219.

Turck D, Bernet JP, Marx J, et al. Incidence and risk factors of oral antibiotic-associated diarrhea in an outpatient pediatric population. J Pediatr Gastroenterol Nutr 2003;37(1):22–6.

Unkel JH, McKibben DH, Fenton SJ, et al. Comparison of odontogenic and nonodontogenic facial cellulitis in a pediatric hospital population. Pediatr Dent 1997;19(8):476–9.

Warnke PH, Becker ST, Springer IN, et al. Penicillin compared with other advanced broad spectrum antibiotics regarding antibacterial activity against oral pathogens isolated from odontogenic abscesses. J Craniomaxillofac Surg 2008;36(8):462–7.

Patient with FACIAL SWELLING

(Cont'd from p 97)

(E) Unusual

- Dens evaginatus/invaginatus
- Dentin dysplasia
- Dentinogenesis imperfecta
- Regional odontoplasia
- X-linked hypophosphatasia
- Pre-eruptive intracoronal resorption
- Mandibular infected buccal cyst
- Tuberculoid granuloma

Dental Caries and the Primary Care Provider

Mark G. Koch, DDS, MS

BACKGROUND

Dental caries is the most common chronic disease affecting children in the United States, and it is mostly preventable. It is five times more common than asthma and seven times more common than hay fever. Research indicates that, although general oral health has been improving over the past three decades, the prevalence of early childhood caries has increased in recent years. New epidemiologic studies indicate 2- to 5-year-old and 6- to 11-year-old children now have prevalence rates of 28% and 51%, respectively.

The consequences of childhood caries can be multifaceted and far ranging. Pain and infection, difficulty with eating, tooth loss with potential malocclusion, poor weight gain, expensive and difficult treatment, and predilection toward adult decay are all potential sequelae of dental caries. The complications associated with dental caries can lead to missed school, inability to concentrate, impaired speech, poor self-esteem, systemic illness, hospitalization for treatment of infection, and even death.

CARIES PROCESS

Dental caries is directly attributable to the demineralization and breakdown of the enamel surface of the tooth. It is biofilm (plaque)-induced, which, in concert with substrate (fermentable carbohydrate, sucrose) and time, may induce demineralization. Further progression results in cavitation and loss of tooth structure.

A child's oral cavity has little cariogenic potential until it becomes colonized with the appropriate bacteria. Caregivers can transmit cariogenic bacteria (principally mutans streptococci) to infants before the eruption of any teeth. Vertical transmission of dental caries occurs between the primary caregiver (usually the mother) and the child. Caries is also horizontally transmissible via family members, siblings, or between children in group childcare settings. The bacteria can be passed via saliva to the infant by blowing on, tasting, or chewing the infant's food, sharing of utensils, and even kissing. The infant is at greatest risk for transmission during the first 2 years of life. Consequently, reduction of mutans streptococci in mothers and family members can inhibit or delay transmission to their infants.

CARIES-RISK ASSESSMENT

The caries process is influenced by multiple factors, including diet, susceptibility of the host, and oral flora that interact with social, cultural, and behavioral influences. The American Academy of Pediatric Dentistry recognizes that caries-risk assessment is an integral element of current clinical pediatric care. Risk assessment enables a provider to recognize risk factors and to intervene in the disease process rather than the outcomes of the disease. A policy statement was adopted and a Caries-risk Assessment Tool (CAT) developed to assess the level of risk for caries development in infants, children, and adolescents based on a set of clinical, environmental, and general health factors. The included caries-risk assessment form (see Table 1) provides guidance for nondental healthcare providers in the clinical decision-making process as a predictor of patients' risk for future disease of young children.

COLLABORATIVE EFFORTS

In 2003, the Office of the Surgeon General released the *National Call to Action to Promote Oral Health*. This release was in response to the Surgeon General's 2000 wake-up call report *Oral Health in America*, which highlighted the "silent epidemic of oral diseases." As a result, collaborative efforts were initiated between medical and dental professionals, private industry, private and government agencies, foundations, and universities. All joined the effort to improve the nation's overall health through promoting oral health.

The American Academy of Pediatrics cultivates the concept of a medical home by "well-trained physicians who provide primary care and help to manage and facilitate essentially all aspects of pediatric care." Likewise, the American Academy of Pediatric Dentistry encourages physicians to promote the concept of a pediatric dental home with their patients to develop an ongoing relationship with a pediatric dentist and to initiate and maintain dental health habits and keep children free of oral disease.

ROLE OF THE PRIMARY HEALTHCARE PROVIDER

A. Medical providers have integral responsibilities in pediatric oral health. Complete health history, parental dental history, and social history should be taken. Risk assessment, oral screening, anticipatory guidance, fluoride varnish application, and referrals to dental professionals are appropriate services to be provided by healthcare providers. Children at high risk should be referred to pediatric dentists by 6 months of age. All children should receive dental evaluation by 1 year of age.

An oral health assessment can be easily incorporated into a well-child visit. It can be performed in approximately

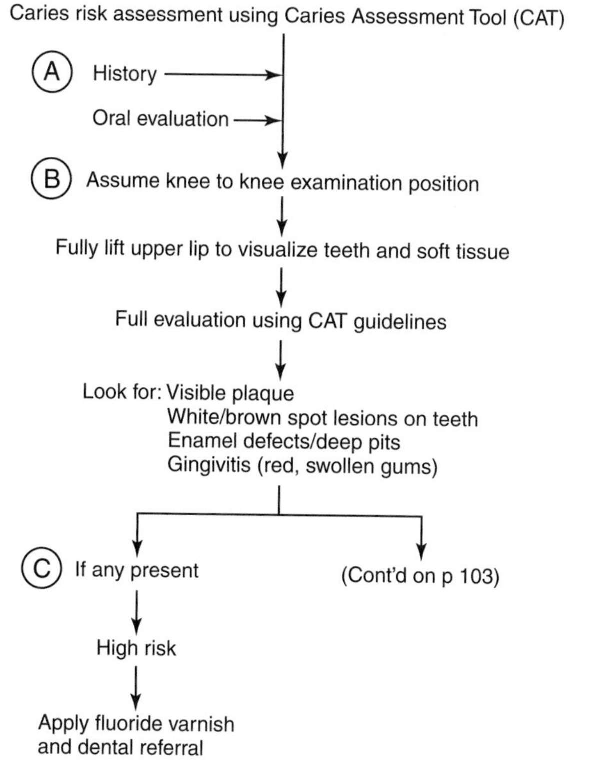
Caries risk assessment using Caries Assessment Tool (CAT)
A
History
Oral evaluation
B
Assume knee to knee examination position
Fully lift upper lip to visualize teeth and soft tissue
Full evaluation using CAT guidelines
Look for: Visible plaque
White/brown spot lesions on teeth
Enamel defects/deep pits
Gingivitis (red, swollen gums)
C
If any present
(Cont'd on p 103)
High risk
Apply fluoride varnish
and dental referral

1 minute and does not require a dental chair. An oral health assessment includes:

- Identification of existing or potential dental problems
- Caries risk assessment
- Anticipatory guidance to caregivers
- Application of fluoride varnish when indicated
- Referral to oral health professional as appropriate

EARLY CHILDHOOD ORAL ASSESSMENT

B. Children younger than 3 years can be examined in a knee-to-knee position. The child is placed in the caregiver's lap facing the caregiver. As the examiner, you and the caregiver should sit facing one another with knees touching. The child lays back with his or her legs around the caregiver's waist so that the child's head is in your lap and is secured against your abdomen. The child's hands should be held by the caregiver to prevent interfering with the examination process. It is quite common for the child to cry and struggle during the examination.

Initiate the evaluation by lifting the upper lip to fully expose the teeth and soft tissues. A dental mirror is recommended to facilitate examination of the lingual sides of the anterior teeth and to visualize the posterior molars. The provider should evaluate the teeth for white spot lesions, enamel defects, cavities, restorations, and plaque accumulation on the teeth, according to CAT guidelines.

Plaque will appear as a sticky film particularly noticeable on the smooth surfaces of the teeth. It is usually richly colonized with cariogenic bacteria, which promote demineralization of the enamel. Plaque is removed with effective oral hygiene (brushing and flossing). Primary teeth should be brushed at least twice per day, once in the morning and at bedtime. The examination is an ideal opportunity to demonstrate and reinforce proper toothbrushing with the caregiver.

White spot lesions can appear as a chalky white band along the gumline. This is indicative of initial demineralization of the enamel and is an early clinical sign of the caries process. Early intervention and possible remineralization may be possible through improved oral hygiene, diet modification, and fluoride therapy. As the primary care provider, you may apply fluoride varnish to facilitate the remineralization process. White spots can lead to frank decay if left untreated.

As the decay process advances, brown or black cavitations appear. This represents penetration of the demineralized enamel. Referral to a dentist, particularly a pediatric dentist, is indicated for evaluation and restoration.

Advanced decay can lead to total destruction of the crowns of the maxillary anterior teeth, leaving only a decayed stump of the root imbedded in the jaw. Advanced decay can also result in severe pain and infection secondary to the bacterial penetration into the pulp of the tooth. You may observe dental abscesses in such circumstances. These may appear as fluctuant swelling in the vestibular areas of the teeth or as a pointed area of draining pus (parulis). Immediate dental referral is indicated. If left untreated, abscessed teeth can progress into facial cellulitis with potential orbital involvement or submandibular swelling with airway compromise. Hospital-based care may be required for treatment.

C. Interventions: Physicians, nurses, and other healthcare professionals are more likely to see new mothers and infants at an early age than dentists. An understanding of the dental infectious process and the associated risk factors of early childhood caries is essential to make appropriate decisions regarding effective intervention and appropriate referrals. The ultimate goal is to help families find a dental home for their children.

Nondental healthcare professionals can also play a leading role in dental prevention. Primary care providers offering first-line assessment have the initial opportunity to educate caregivers about the relation between oral bacteria and cariogenic diet, nutrition, oral hygiene, and the vertical transmission of cariogenic bacteria from caregiver to infant.

Table 1. **Caries-Risk Assessment Form for 0–3 Year Olds (For Physicians and Other Nondental Healthcare Providers)**

Factors	High Risk	Moderate Risk	Protective
Biological			
Mother/primary caregiver has active cavities	Yes		
Parent/caregiver has low socioeconomic status	Yes		
Child has >3 between meal sugar-containing snacks or beverages per day	Yes		
Child is put to bed with a bottle containing natural or added sugar	Yes		
Child has special health care needs		Yes	
Child is a recent immigrant		Yes	
Protective			
Child receives optimally-fluoridated drinking water or fluoride supplements			Yes
Child has teeth brushed daily with fluoridated toothpaste			Yes
Child receives topical fluoride from health professional			Yes
Child has dental home/regular dental care			Yes
Clinical Findings			
Child has white spot lesions or enamel defects	Yes		
Child has visible cavities or fillings	Yes		
Child has plaque on teeth		Yes	

Circling those conditions that apply to a specific patient helps the health care worker and parent understand the factors that contribute to or protect from caries. Risk assessment categorization of low, moderate, or high based on preponderance of factors for the individual. However, clinical judgment may justify the use of one factor (e.g., frequent exposure to sugar-containing snacks or beverages, visible cavities) in determining overall risk.

Overall assessment of child's dental caries risk: High ☐ Moderate ☐ Low ☐

D. Fluoride Varnish: Fluoride renders the crystalline structure of tooth enamel less susceptible to the demineralizing effects of the acidic oral environment. It inhibits bacterial acid production and, in instances of early decalcification, it can even reverse some of the effects through remineralization. Adequate exposure to fluoride via drinking water, fluoride supplementation, or topical application is integral to caries reduction.

Fluoride varnish is easily applied to at-risk children by nondental professionals. The fluoride is available in individual prepackaged kits that include a small brush and the fluoride varnish. Position the child in the same knee-to-knee position as for the examination technique. Wipe the teeth dry with gauze and paint a thin layer of the varnish on the dry tooth surfaces. The varnish will solidify when contacted by the saliva. The solidified fluoride should be allowed to remain on the teeth for an extended period. Routine oral hygiene, to include brushing and flossing, may be delayed until the following day, if possible.

BARRIERS

Over the past five years various barriers to the implementation of preventive dental services for pediatric patients in primary medical practices have been reported. Among the chief barriers indicated has been lack of knowledge about dental preventive services, difficulty with the technique of applying fluoride varnish, integration of the procedures into the practice routine, staff resistance, and lack of dental referral sources. Many practices indicated that after initial concerns about the services, they were able to overcome obstacles through continuing education and staff training, increased familiarity with the procedures, and fostering of partnerships with local dental providers.

Caries risk assessment using Caries Assessment Tool (CAT)

(Cont'd from p 101)

↓

(D) If none present

↓

Low risk

↓

Encourage establishing a dental home

References

Alaluusua S, Renkonen OV. Streptococcus mutans establishment and dental caries experience in children from 2 to 4 years old. Scand J Dent Res 1983;91(6):453–7.

American Academy of Pediatric Dentistry, American Academy of Pediatrics. Policy on early childhood caries (ECC): classifications, consequences, and preventive strategies. Pediatr Dent 2008;30(7 Suppl):40–3.

American Academy on Pediatric Dentistry Council on Clinical Affairs. Policy on the dental home. Pediatr Dent 2008 30(7 Suppl):22–3.

American Academy on Pediatric Dentistry Council on Clinical Affairs. Guideline on caries-risk assessment and management for infants, children, and adolescents. Pediatr Dent 2010;32(special issue):101–8.

Beltran-Aguilar ED, Goldstein JW, Lockwood SA. Fluoride varnishes: a review of their clinical use, cariostatic mechanism, efficacy and safety. J Am Dent Assoc 2000;131(5):589–96.

Berkowitz RJ. Mutans streptococci: acquisition and transmission. Pediatr Dent 2006;28(2):106–9, discussion 92–8.

Carletto Korber FP, Cornejo LS, Gimenez MG. Early acquisition of Streptococcus mutans for children. Acta Odontol Latinoam 2005;18(2):69–74.

Caufield PW, Cutter GR, Dasanayake AP. Initial acquisition of mutans streptococci by infants: evidence for a discrete window of infectivity. J Dent Res 1993;72(1):37–45.

Close K, Rozier RG, Zeldin LP, et al. Barriers to the adoption and implementation of preventive dental services in primary medical care. Pediatrics 2010; 125(3): 509–17.

Dye BA, Tan S, Smith V, et al. Trends in oral health status: United States, 1988-1994 and 1999–2004. Vital Health Stat 2007;11(248):1–92.

Fontana M, Young DA, Wolff MS. Evidence-based caries, risk assessment, and treatment. Dent Clin North Am 2009;53(1): 149–61.

Gift HC, Reisine ST, Larach DC. The social impact of dental problems and visits. Am J Public Health 1992;82(12):1663–8.

Kohler B, Bratthall D, Krasse B. Preventive measures in mothers influence the establishment of the bacterium Streptococcus mutans in their infants. Arch Oral Biol 1983;28(3):225–31.

Lewis C, Lynch H, Richardson L. Fluoride varnish use in primary care: what do providers think? Pediatrics 2005; 115(1):e69–76.

Loesche W. Dental caries: a treatable infection. Grand Haven (MI): Automated Diagnostic Documentation, Inc., 1993.

Milgrom P, Riedy CA, Weinstein P, et al. Dental caries and its relationship to bacterial infection, hypoplasia, diet, and oral hygiene in 6- to 36-month-old children. Community Dent Oral Epidemiol 2000;28(4):295–306.

Mouradian WE. The face of a child: children's oral health and dental education. J Dent Educ 2001;65(9):821–31.

National call to action to promote oral health (NIH Publication No. 03-5303). Rockville (MD): U.S. Department of Health and Human Services, Public Health Service, National Institute of Health, National Institute of Dental and Craniofacial Research, 2003.

Oral Health in America: A Report of the Surgeon General (NIH Publication No. 00-4713). Rockville (MD): U.S. Department of Health and Human Services, National Institute of Dental and Craniofacial Research, National Institutes of Health, 2000.

Otto M. For want of a dentist. The Washington Post, February 28, 2007.

Weintraub JA, Ramos-Gomez F, Jue B, et al. Fluoride varnish efficacy in preventing early childhood caries. J Dent Res 2006;85(2):172–6.

Dermatology

Evaluation of Skin Lesions

Dermatitis

Reactive Erythemas and Erythematous Maculopapular Lesions

Nonblistering, Nonerythematous Skin Lesions

Papulosquamous Disorders

Vesiculobullous Disorders

Nail Disorders

Evaluation of Skin Lesions

Arelis Burgos-Zavoda, MD, and Joanna M. Burch, MD

A. In the history, determine the onset, progression, distribution, duration, and recurrence of the lesions. Note the presence of prodromal and associated symptoms, including pruritus, fever, cough, coryza, vomiting, diarrhea, jaundice, lymphadenopathy, altered mental status, arthritis, and failure to thrive. Identify any precipitating factor or agent, including infection, medications, trauma, sunburn, frostbite, water immersion, food, and agents contacting the skin in the area of involvement. Note predisposing conditions, such as atopic disease (atopic dermatitis, allergic rhinitis, asthma), malignant neoplasia, collagen vascular disease, liver disease, renal disease, and mucocutaneous diseases.

B. In the physical examination, recognize primary lesions, including macules, papules, plaques, nodules, wheals, vesicles, bullae, pustules, and cysts. According to accepted definitions, a macule is a color change in the skin that is flat to the surface and not palpable. A papule is a firm, raised lesion with distinct borders 1 cm or less in diameter. A plaque is a firm, raised, flat-topped lesion with distinct borders and an epidermal change larger than 1 cm in diameter. A nodule is a raised lesion with indistinct borders and a deep palpable portion. A wheal is an area of tense edema within the upper dermis producing a flat-topped, slightly raised lesion. A vesicle is a papule filled with clear fluid. A bulla is a lesion larger than 1 cm in diameter filled with clear fluid. A pustule is a papule filled with a fluid exudate, giving it a yellowish appearance. A cyst is a raised lesion containing a sac filled with liquid or semisolid material. Recognize secondary changes such as scale, oozing and crusting, erosions, atrophy, excoriations, and fissures. Note the specific location of the rash (generalized, truncal, flexural creases, extremities, hands, and feet). With any rash, determine its color, distribution, and arrangement. Lesions arranged in a straight line are called *linear;* those in a circular configuration are described as *annular.* Lesions may be discrete if alone, or in groups. Many congenital mosaic disorders of skin will be in curvilinear or whorled arrangements and located on one side of the body. Note associated signs of infection or systemic disease, such as lymphadenopathy, hepatomegaly, splenomegaly, arthritis, jaundice, and heart murmur.

C. Common laboratory procedures related to dermatologic conditions include potassium hydroxide (KOH) preparations to identify fungal infection, scabies oil preparation, exfoliative cytology, and skin biopsy. To perform a KOH preparation, scrape scale from the lesion onto a glass slide and add a drop of 10% KOH to dissolve the stratum corneum cells. Heat the slide gently to dissolve the cells more quickly. Cover the slide with a coverslip and examine for branching hyphae. A scabies preparation should be performed if scabies is suspected. Perform a scraping by placing a drop of mineral oil on a glass slide. Dip a 15 blade scalpel in the oil, then scrape several papules in a linear array and place the cells in the mineral oil on the slide. Look for mites, eggs, or scybala (feces) on low power. Perform exfoliative cytology by breaking the blister and scraping its base. Place the scrapings on a glass slide. After drying, stain the slide with Wright or Giemsa stain and examine for the presence of epidermal giant cells (herpes simplex or herpes zoster) or acantholytic cells (pemphigus).

D. In the neonatal period, pustular disorders include neonatal acne, erythema toxicum, transient neonatal pustular melanosis, miliaria profunda, and folliculitis. Suspect candidiasis when satellite papulopustular lesions are present around a central, deeply raised erythematous area. In infants and older children/adolescents, consider acne when pustules and white papules (closed comedones) are located on the face, upper back, and upper chest. Drug-induced acne can be produced by glucocorticosteroids, androgens, adrenocorticotropic hormone, diphenylhydantoin, or isoniazid. In drug-induced acne, bacterial or chemical folliculitis, all lesions are in the same stage at the same time. Scabies infestation, basic bacterial folliculitis, perioral dermatitis, and psoriasis can all present with pustules. Suspect bacteremia with gonococcus or meningococcus when the patient has fever, signs of toxicity, and an acral distribution of pustules.

Reference

Weston WL, Lane AT, Morelli JG. A color textbook of pediatric dermatology. 4th ed. St. Louis: Mosby-Elsevier; 2007.

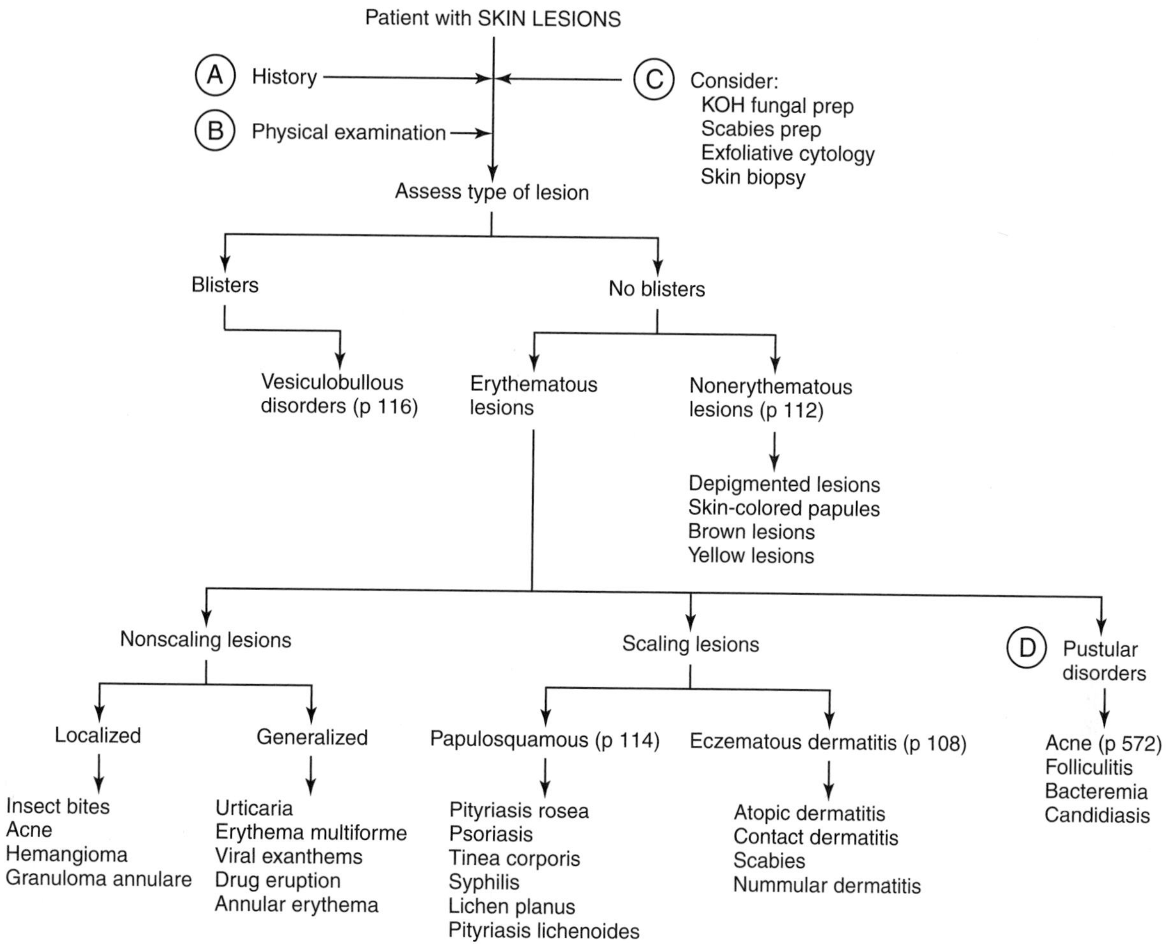
Patient with SKIN LESIONS
A History
B Physical examination
C Consider:
KOH fungal prep
Scabies prep
Exfoliative cytology
Skin biopsy
Assess type of lesion
Blisters
No blisters
Vesiculobullous disorders (p 116)
Erythematous lesions
Nonerythematous lesions (p 112)
Depigmented lesions
Skin-colored papules
Brown lesions
Yellow lesions
Nonscaling lesions
Scaling lesions
D Pustular disorders
Localized
Generalized
Papulosquamous (p 114)
Eczematous dermatitis (p 108)
Acne (p 572)
Folliculitis
Bacteremia
Candidiasis
Insect bites
Acne
Hemangioma
Granuloma annulare
Urticaria
Erythema multiforme
Viral exanthems
Drug eruption
Annular erythema
Pityriasis rosea
Psoriasis
Tinea corporis
Syphilis
Lichen planus
Pityriasis lichenoides
Atopic dermatitis
Contact dermatitis
Scabies
Nummular dermatitis

Dermatitis

Arelis Burgos-Zavoda, MD, and Joanna M. Burch, MD

Eczematous dermatitis, or inflammation of the epidermis and superficial dermis, causes erythema, pruritus, and secondary skin changes of marked dryness, oozing, crusting, erosions, vesiculations, and epidermal thickening.

A. Identify substances that cause contact dermatitis by direct irritation or an allergic mechanism. The most common form of irritant dermatitis is diaper rash, which is related to prolonged contact with urine and feces. Prolonged contact with water is central to the pathogenesis of the dermatitis. Diaper dermatitis present for longer than 3 days or with red satellite lesions or erosions suggests secondary infection with *Candida albicans*. Treat diaper rash with frequent diaper changes and minimal washing of the diaper area with a moistened soft cloth or fragrance-free diaper wipe. Diaper area cleansing is necessary only when stool is present. Zinc oxide and petrolatum-based formulations tend to be most effective in forming a barrier to further skin contact with urine and feces. Candidal infection requires the use of a topical antifungal agent, such as an imidazole or nystatin cream.

B. Suspect allergic contact dermatitis when the rash has a local distribution and geometric shape, especially on the hands or feet. Secondary changes of vesiculation, oozing, and excoriation are common. A linear arrangement on the arms or legs suggests contact with a plant, such as poison ivy or poison oak. Allergic contact dermatitis is related to cell-mediated immunity. Common allergens that act as haptens include pentadecacatechol, found in poison oak and poison ivy; nickel in jewelry and zippers; dichromates in tanned leather; and several chemicals in glues, rubber, dyes, cosmetics, shampoos, and topical medications. Once sensitization occurs, repeated exposure to the antigen may result in a widespread papulovesicular dermatitis, or so-called id reaction. This is particularly observed in nickel allergy. If a child presents with widespread, papular eczematous eruption, always check the periumbilical skin. A lichenified eczematous plaque near the umbilicus is nickel allergy until proved otherwise. When appropriate, consider patch testing to identify a specific allergen. Treatment consists of topical glucocorticosteroid ointments of moderate potency for 2 to 3 weeks. Use wet dressings for severe generalized pruritus. Wet dressings result in increased humidity at the skin that relieves the pruritus, causes vasoconstriction, and débrides crusting. Instruct the parent to place tight-fitting cotton or mostly cotton pajamas in warm water and thoroughly wring out the excess water. Have the child wear dry pajamas over the damp ones. Consider oral prednisone 1 mg/kg once daily for 14 to 21 days when allergic contact dermatitis is severe.

C. Suspect atopic dermatitis (AD) when its characteristic age-dependent distribution is seen. AD is a hereditary disorder characterized by dry skin, the presence of eczematous plaques, and onset under 2 years. The exact pathogenesis is unknown. Recent data have suggested that loss-of-function genetic variants in the filaggrin gene are associated with AD. Filaggrin is a protein in the skin involved in "sealing the skin" and preventing water loss. The distribution of the clinical findings in AD is primarily on the scalp, face, trunk, and extensor surfaces of the arms and legs in infancy. The flexor surfaces of the arms and legs are often involved in toddlers and small children. Involvement of the feet is especially common in school-age children and adolescents. Treat acute exacerbations with topical steroids of the appropriate strength depending on body area (Box 1) and antihistamines; avoid oral steroids. Recognize secondary infections with *Staphylococcus aureus* and *Streptococcus pyogenes*, and treat with systemic antibiotics. Secondary infection by herpes simplex virus results in fever and widespread vesicles that may become eroded, punched out pits with hemorrhagic crusts (eczema herpeticum). This should be treated with antiviral therapy. Consider wet dressings when oozing, excoriations, and crusting are marked. Maintain adequate skin hydration with routine use of lubricant creams and ointments (Box 2). Use antihistamines when necessary for pruritus, especially if it interferes with sleep. Avoid occlusive clothing, frequent soaping, wool clothes, and cleaning agents and chemicals (Box 3). The evidence suggests that avoidance of allergenic foods during pregnancy or the use of hydrolyzed or soy formula milks does not prevent eczema. Delayed introduction of solids may decrease eczema risk. Children who are not responding to treatment may be referred to a dermatologist for further treatment.

D. Suspect nummular eczema when coinlike lesions 1 to 10 cm in diameter are distributed symmetrically on the extremities or trunk. The lesions can be dry and scaly or wet and oozing. Patients usually describe severe pruritus. Dry lesions can be confused with tinea corporis and wet lesions with impetigo. The treatment is the same as for AD, although high-potency topical steroids are often required. Four to 6 weeks of therapy are required to reverse the thickening.

E. Greasy scale on the face and scalp of infants and also in the nasolabial folds of the face, posterior auricular areas, scalp, or chest of adolescents suggests seborrheic dermatitis. Treat these cases with a low-potency topical steroid two times daily for 1 to 2 weeks. Topical ketoconazole cream and shampoo has been shown to be effective for seborrheic dermatitis. "Cradle cap" in infants with widespread eczema should just be treated as if all of it is eczema.

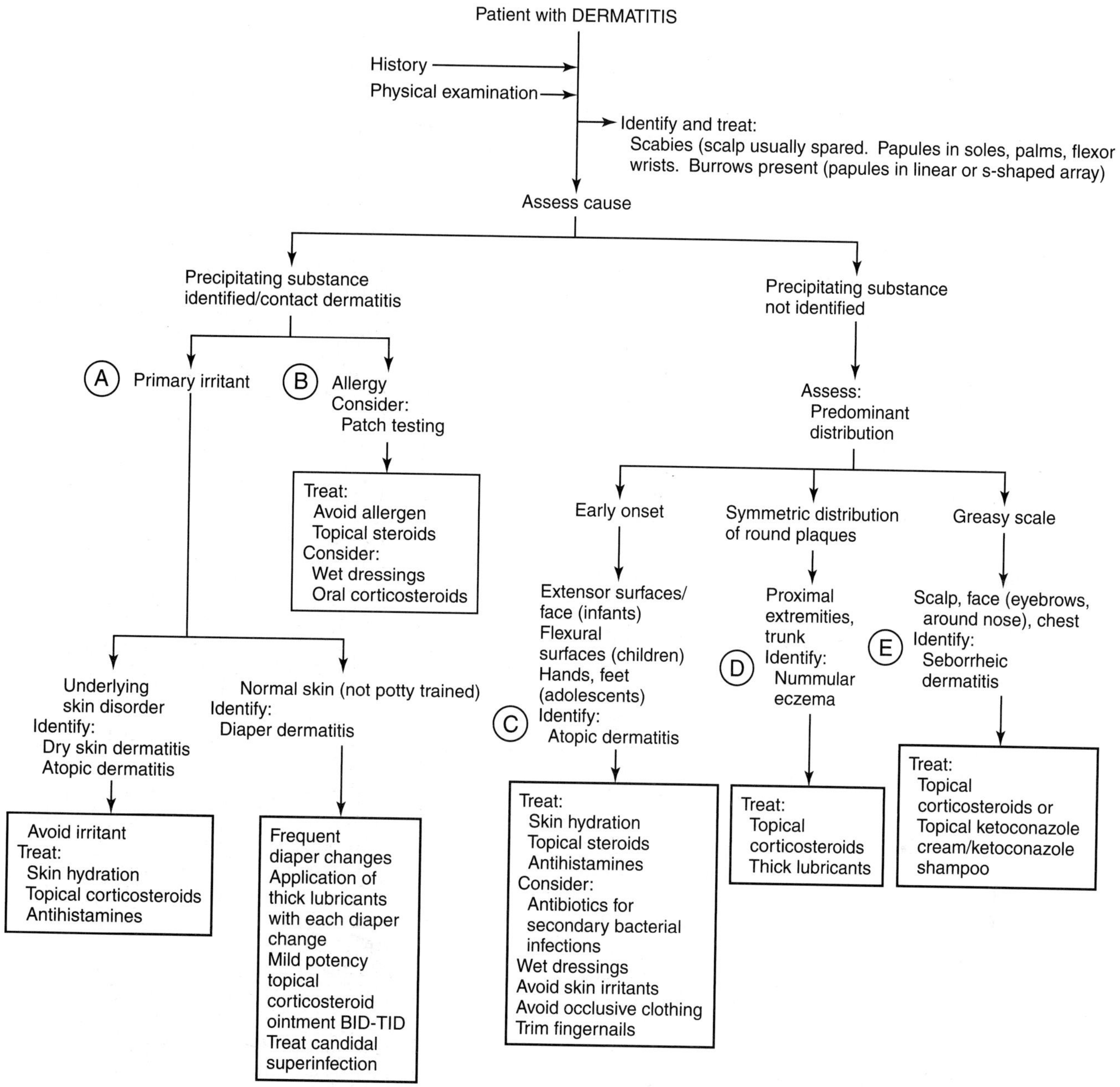
Patient with DERMATITIS
History
Physical examination
Identify and treat:
Scabies (scalp usually spared. Papules in soles, palms, flexor wrists. Burrows present (papules in linear or s-shaped array)
Assess cause
Precipitating substance identified/contact dermatitis
Precipitating substance not identified
A Primary irritant
B Allergy
Consider:
Patch testing
Treat:
Avoid allergen
Topical steroids
Consider:
Wet dressings
Oral corticosteroids
Underlying skin disorder
Identify:
Dry skin dermatitis
Atopic dermatitis
Avoid irritant
Treat:
Skin hydration
Topical corticosteroids
Antihistamines
Normal skin (not potty trained)
Identify:
Diaper dermatitis
Frequent diaper changes
Application of thick lubricants with each diaper change
Mild potency topical corticosteroid ointment BID-TID
Treat candidal superinfection
Assess:
Predominant distribution
Early onset
Extensor surfaces/ face (infants)
Flexural surfaces (children)
Hands, feet (adolescents)
C Identify:
Atopic dermatitis
Treat:
Skin hydration
Topical steroids
Antihistamines
Consider:
Antibiotics for secondary bacterial infections
Wet dressings
Avoid skin irritants
Avoid occlusive clothing
Trim fingernails
Symmetric distribution of round plaques
Proximal extremities, trunk
D Identify:
Nummular eczema
Treat:
Topical corticosteroids
Thick lubricants
Greasy scale
Scalp, face (eyebrows, around nose), chest
E Identify:
Seborrheic dermatitis
Treat:
Topical corticosteroids or
Topical ketoconazole cream/ketoconazole shampoo

Box 1. Topical Steroids for Use in Childhood Atopic Dermatitis

Low potency (face)
Hydrocortisone 2.5%
Desonide 0.05%
Moderate potency
Fluocinolone acetonide 0.025% (Fluonid, Synalar)
Mometasone furoate 0.1% (Elocon)
Triamcinolone 0.1% (Kenalog, Aristocort)

Box 2. General Instructions for Long-Term Management of Atopic Dermatitis

- Infrequent bathing
- Keep the skin lubricated
- Keep fingernails trimmed short
- Avoid overheating of skin
- Always use a soap substitute

Box 3. Lubricants Useful for Atopic Dermatitis

- Hydrophilic petrolatum (Vaseline)
- Aquaphor
- Cetyl alcohol cream (Cetaphil)
- Vanicream
- Eucerin
- Moisturel

References

Brenninkmeijer EE, Schram ME, Leeflang MM, et al. Diagnostic criteria for atopic dermatitis: a systematic review. Br J Dermatol 2008;158(4):754–65.

Hanifin JM. Evolving concepts of pathogenesis in atopic dermatitis and other eczemas. J Invest Dermatol 2009;129(2):320–2.

Sinyer LJ, Decroix J, Lagner A, et al. Ketoconazole gel 2% in the treatment of moderate to severe seborrheic dermatitis. Cutis 2007;79(6):475–82.

Weston WL, Lane AT, Morelli JG. A color textbook of pediatric dermatology. 4th ed. St. Louis: Mosby; 2007.

Williams HC, Grindlay DJ. What's new in atopic eczema? An analysis of the clinical significance of systematic reviews on atopic eczema published in 2006 and 2007. Clin Exp Dermatol 2008;33(6):685–8.

Reactive Erythemas and Erythematous Maculopapular Lesions

Arelis Burgos-Zavoda, MD, and Joanna M. Burch, MD

A. Insect bite reactions (papular urticaria) generally occur in crops and are usually few. Urticarial lesions are distinguished by their transient nature. Papular urticaria is characterized by a chronic or recurrent eruption of 2- to 5-mm papules with tiny central puncta. Vesicles and bullae may occasionally be seen. The eruption is caused by hypersensitivity to a variety of biting arthropods. It is often pruritic. Eruptions are most common in the summer and late spring, and can last 3 to 9 months. It is most common in children 18 months to 7 years. Treatment includes antihistamine therapy or topical corticosteroids for pruritus, or both. Apply a safe insect repellent to the affected areas. Have all pets around the child checked by a veterinarian for fleas and mites. If mites or fleas are in the home environment, call an extermination service.

B. Urticaria is characterized by sudden onset of erythematous raised wheals that can occur anywhere. The edematous skin lesions usually are flat topped and will change shape or disappear, usually within 20 minutes to several hours. They can be arcuate or annular, with a clear or sometimes a violaceous-appearing center, making them easily confused with erythema multiforme (EM). Up to half of children with urticaria can also have a deeper swelling (angioedema), most commonly on the face, hands, and feet. Urticaria is most commonly associated with infection but can be associated with foods, medications, stinging/biting insects, and rarely systemic disease (e.g., collagen vascular disease). Treat new-onset, uncomplicated urticaria with daily antihistamine therapy (use a nonsedating antihistamine in the morning and a sedating antihistamine before bed). After 2 to 4 weeks of suppression, try to wean the medication. Prednisone may be indicated for severe cases.

C. Lesions of EM have a symmetric distribution mostly on the extremities. Lesions begin as red papules and progress during 7 to 10 days to lesions with concentric color change with a dusky center and red border. They may form blisters or crusts centrally. Lesions are fixed and last 7 to 21 days. There is not a prodrome with this eruption and the child should look well. EM is an inflammatory response in the skin to herpes simplex virus DNA processing. EM lesions can be recurrent and may be preceded by a lesion of herpes labialis. Always inquire about cold sores in the child or family/caregivers. Treat symptomatically with wet compresses or oral antihistamines for symptomatic relief. If there is an obvious herpes lesion, treat with antivirals. In children with recurrent episodes of EM, prophylaxis with oral acyclovir at 20 mg/kg/day may be considered. Corticosteroids are not indicated for the treatment of EM. EM does not become Stevens–Johnson syndrome.

D. Many viral illnesses can have associated exanthems that are red and maculopapular. Often, they will last 2 weeks and resolve spontaneously without intervention. Reassurance and antihistamines for itching are all that is required. Several viral illnesses have exanthems with distinct features. Erythema infectiosum (fifth disease) presents in childhood on the face as a bright red erythema (slapped-cheek appearance), then evolves into an erythematous maculopapular rash distributed primarily over the extremities. As the rash fades, it develops a lacelike appearance. This lacelike eruption can reappear intermittently for weeks. The presence of high fever without associated symptoms for 3 to 4 consecutive days with abrupt defervescence, followed by the development of a light pink lacy rash is suggestive of roseola. The rash usually appears first on the trunk, then spreads to involve the neck, upper extremities, face, and lower extremities. The rash lasts 1 to 2 days. Roseola occurs most often in children 6 months to 3 years of age. Consider enterovirus in cases of a viral exanthem with associated aseptic meningitis.

E. Infectious mononucleosis presents with a rash in 10% to 15% of cases. The rash is most commonly an erythematous maculopapular eruption but can appear scarlatiniform, urticarial, or hemorrhagic. Associated findings may include pharyngitis, lymphadenopathy, splenomegaly, hepatitis, pneumonitis, and central nervous system involvement (meningitis, encephalitis, or Guillain–Barré syndrome). The acute phase with fever and sore throat lasts 2 to 3 weeks. Extreme fatigue and lethargy may persist for 3 months. The most distinctive rash associated with infectious mononucleosis is an abrupt onset of diffuse red papules over the entire trunk after the administration of amoxicillin, often given for the mistaken diagnosis of streptococcal pharyngitis. Prompt withdrawal of the amoxicillin is indicated.

F. Suspect scarlet fever when pharyngitis, fever, abdominal pain, and malaise are associated with an erythematous, punctiform (sandpaper) rash. This eruption is more impressive to palpation than to observation. Associated findings include circumoral pallor, flushed cheeks, a strawberry tongue, and Pastia's sign (transverse lines in antecubital fossae). The rash often desquamates. At least three types of erythrogenic toxin have been identified. Treat with penicillin VK, 125 to 250 mg two times daily for 10 days. Erythromycin is used in patients who are allergic to penicillin. If staphylococcal scarlet fever is suspected, dicloxacillin 15 to 50 mg/kg/day orally for 10 days is recommended.

G. Maculopapular (morbilliform) drug eruptions are the most common of all drug-induced eruptions in children. This eruption usually occurs 7 to 21 days after the onset of the offending medications. The eruption is usually symmetric, widely distributed, and may have

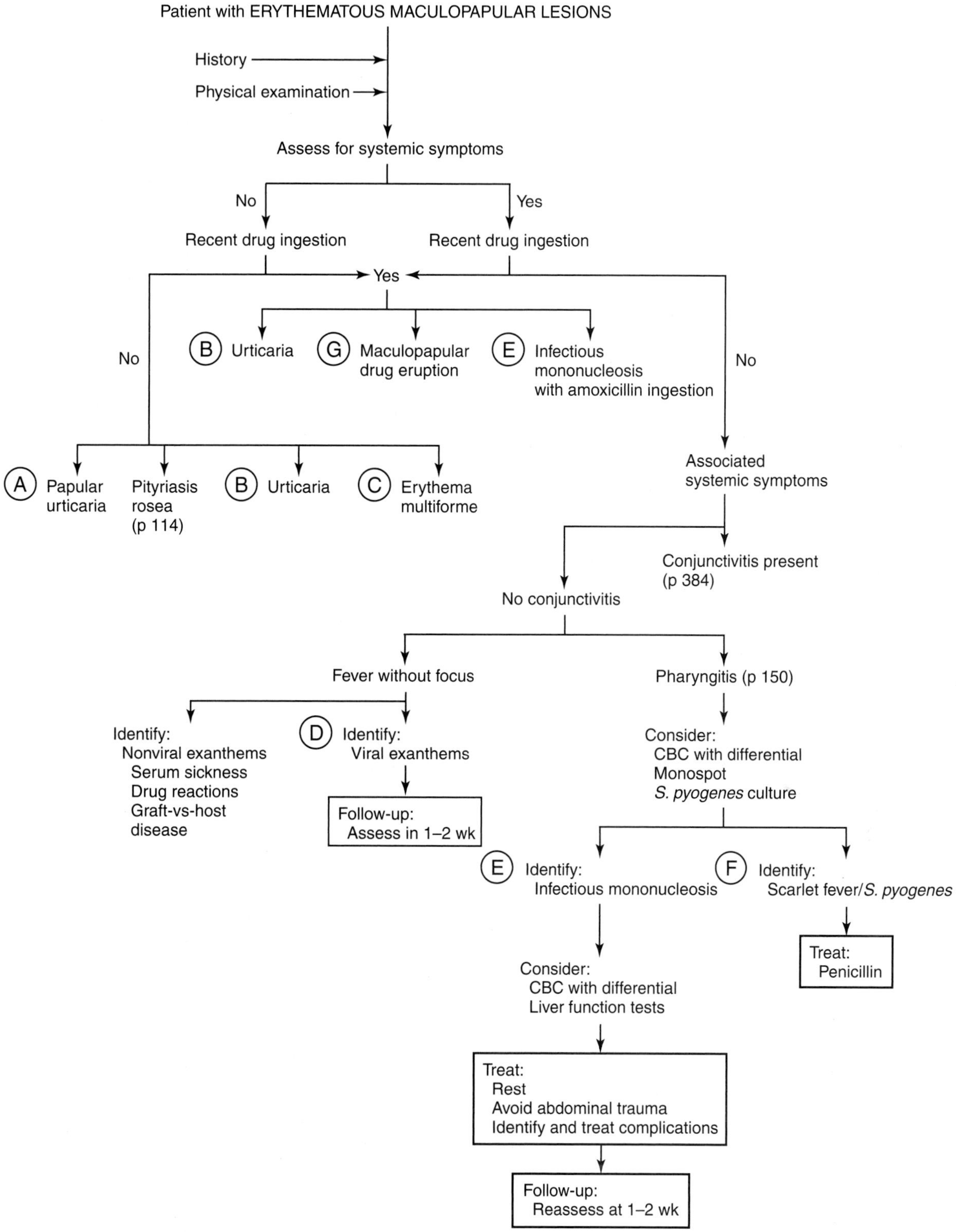
Patient with ERYTHEMATOUS MACULOPAPULAR LESIONS
History
Physical examination
Assess for systemic symptoms
No
Yes
Recent drug ingestion
Recent drug ingestion
Yes
No
B Urticaria
G Maculopapular drug eruption
E Infectious mononucleosis with amoxicillin ingestion
No
A Papular urticaria
Pityriasis rosea (p 114)
B Urticaria
C Erythema multiforme
Associated systemic symptoms
Conjunctivitis present (p 384)
No conjunctivitis
Fever without focus
Pharyngitis (p 150)
Identify: Nonviral exanthems Serum sickness Drug reactions Graft-vs-host disease
D Identify: Viral exanthems
Follow-up: Assess in 1–2 wk
Consider: CBC with differential Monospot S. pyogenes culture
E Identify: Infectious mononucleosis
F Identify: Scarlet fever/S. pyogenes
Treat: Penicillin
Consider: CBC with differential Liver function tests
Treat: Rest Avoid abdominal trauma Identify and treat complications
Follow-up: Reassess at 1–2 wk

areas of totally normal skin surrounded by erythematous macules and papules. The eruption typically lasts 7 to 14 days. Pruritus may be present. Associated fever, malaise, and arthralgias are sometimes present. Antibiotics, particularly penicillins, are common causes.

References

Carneiro SC, Cestari T, Allen SH, Ramos e-Silva M. Viral exanthems in the tropics. Clin Dermatol 2007;25(2):212–20.

Dyer JA. Childhood viral exanthems. Pediatr Ann 2007;36(1):21–9.

Paller AS, Mancini AJ. Hurwitz clinical pediatric dermatology. 3rd ed. New York: Elsevier; 2006.

Weston WL, Lane AT, Morelli JG. A color textbook of pediatric dermatology. 4th ed. St. Louis: Mosby; 2007.

Woo SB, Challacombe SJ. Management of recurrent oral herpes simplex infections. Oral Surg Oral Med Oral Pathol Oral Radiol Endod 2007;103(Suppl):S12.e1–e18.

Nonblistering, Nonerythematous Skin Lesions

Arelis Burgos-Zavoda, MD, and Joanna M. Burch, MD

A. Common warts (verruca vulgaris) usually appear on the extremities (especially hands and feet) as papules with an irregular scaly (verrucous) surface. These epithelial tumors are induced by human papillomavirus. There are more than 100 types of human papillomavirus, and different types cause different types and locations of warts. By age 11, 5% of children will have a wart. Filiform warts have a narrow stalk and longer, finger-like spiny projections on the surface. They are most common around the nose and eyes. Warts on the sole are called plantar warts (verruca plantaris), and are often painful and surrounded by thick callus because of their weight-bearing location. Warts in the genital area are called *condyloma acuminata.* Treatment options for warts are listed in Box 1. Epidermal nevi have a warty appearance and may be arranged in a linear pattern. They are usually present at birth, but occasionally new lesions can develop into adolescence. For localized lesions, surgical excision is the best treatment. Extensive lesions may be improved with the use of mild keratolytics or with bland lubricant therapy.

B. Flat warts are broad, flat-topped, skin-colored papules, usually grouped together and found on the face and extremities. Flat warts have a smooth surface that is flat or planar rather than dome shaped as seen in molluscum contagiosum (MC; see D). Flat-topped, skin-colored papules on the face that do not respond to wart therapy may be a benign adnexal tumor of the skin (e.g., trichoepithelioma). These should be referred to dermatology.

C. Keratosis pilaris is a follicular plug of scale within a body hair opening. Lesions usually develop on the extensor surfaces of the extremities and on the cheeks in children between 18 months and 3 years of age. The lesions are occasionally pink and rarely erythematous or pustular. Keratosis pilaris on facial skin is often accompanied by telangiectatic erythema (cheeks look rosy). The use of lubricants applied to wet skin may be sufficient to improve the condition. Other treatment options include lactic acid 12% cream (Lac-Hydrin), 20% urea cream (Carmol 20), or cream with both lactic acid and urea (Eucerin Plus). The 40% urea cream is available by prescription. Patients should be counseled that this is a lifelong disorder. Closed comedones of acne appear as discrete papules that are skin colored or slightly whitish. They first appear over the forehead and cheeks when the child is 8 to 10 years old. Treat with topical keratolytic agents (e.g., tretinoin, adapalene gel, or benzoyl peroxide gel).

D. MC lesions are dome-shaped, solitary papules with central umbilication. They may be grouped together anywhere on the skin surface but tend to like skin-fold areas. The lesions, which are produced by a pox virus (MCV-1, -2, and -3), may be passed from person to person by skin-to-skin contact and in water. Surrounding dermatitis around MC lesions ("molluscum dermatitis") is common. Spontaneous clearing of MC often occurs over 18 months to 3 years. Removal of a papule is curative. In-office treatment options are curettage of the papules, application of cantharidin, or podophyllum. Home treatments include daily application of imiquimod 5% cream, oral cimetidine, or benign neglect. Pustular molluscum lesions do not require antibiotics.

E. Pityriasis alba usually presents in childhood as multiple oval, scaly, flat, hypopigmented patches on the face, extensor surface of the arms, and upper trunk. The lesions have indistinct borders, do not itch, and are usually distributed symmetrically. Treat with mild topical corticosteroids or calcineurin inhibitors for a few weeks, followed by frequent application of lubricants and protection from sun exposure. Lesions of tinea versicolor, caused by *Malassezia* yeasts, are smaller and have distinct borders and a fine scale. They are distributed most often on the shoulders, upper chest, and back. Diagnose these cases with a potassium hydroxide examination of a lesion, which will show short, curved hyphae and numerous spores. Treatment with antifungal cream or shampoo is curative, although recurrences are common. Vitiligo is associated with complete depigmentation rather than the hypopigmentation of pityriasis alba or tinea versicolor. A Wood's lamp examination will reveal a dramatic porcelain-white change in vitiligo, but only subtle changes in color with pityriasis alba or tinea versicolor. Treatment options include potent topical steroid or topical calcineurin inhibitors. If large areas of skin are depigmented or patient has not responded successfully to topical therapy, phototherapy should be considered.

F. Café-au-lait spots are tan macules and are usually in sun-protected areas. They are larger than freckles and are not sun responsive. They usually appear in early life. Suspect neurofibromatosis when six café-au-lait

Box 1. **Treatment of Viral Warts**

Type of Warts	Treatment
Common	Cryotherapy/salicylic acid/laser
Periungual	Imiquimod cream/salicylic acid/cantharidin/laser
Flat	Imiquimod cream/tretinoin
Filiform	Cryotherapy with forceps/laser
Plantar	Salicylic acid plaster with duct tape/laser
Condyloma acuminata	Podophyllum/imiquimod cream/cryotherapy (older patients)

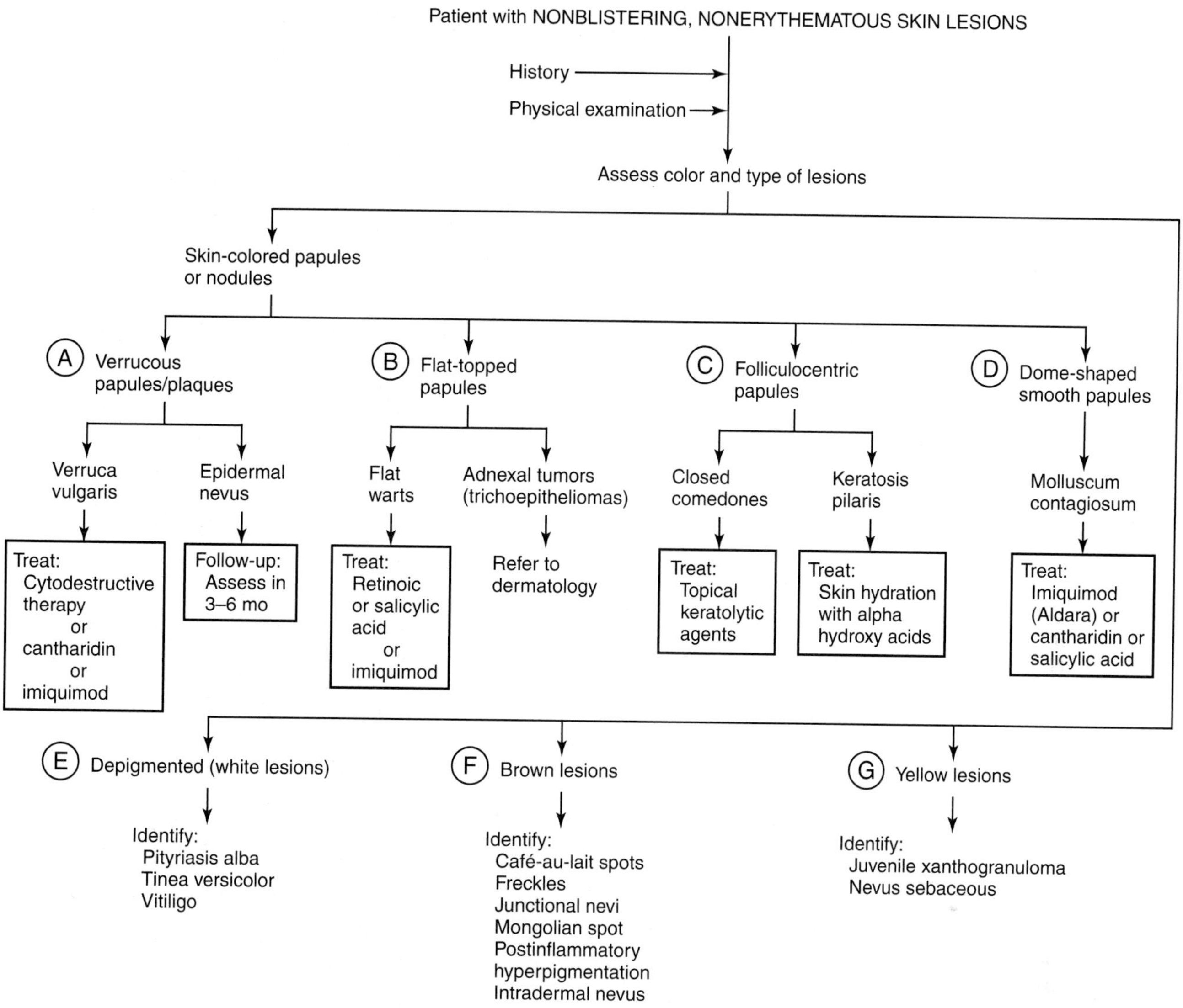
Patient with NONBLISTERING, NONERYTHEMATOUS SKIN LESIONS
History
Physical examination
Assess color and type of lesions
Skin-colored papules or nodules
A Verrucous papules/plaques
B Flat-topped papules
C Folliculocentric papules
D Dome-shaped smooth papules
Verruca vulgaris
Epidermal nevus
Flat warts
Adnexal tumors (trichoepitheliomas)
Closed comedones
Keratosis pilaris
Molluscum contagiosum
Treat: Cytodestructive therapy or cantharidin or imiquimod
Follow-up: Assess in 3–6 mo
Treat: Retinoic or salicylic acid or imiquimod
Refer to dermatology
Treat: Topical keratolytic agents
Treat: Skin hydration with alpha hydroxy acids
Treat: Imiquimod (Aldara) or cantharidin or salicylic acid
E Depigmented (white lesions)
F Brown lesions
G Yellow lesions
Identify: Pityriasis alba Tinea versicolor Vitiligo
Identify: Café-au-lait spots Freckles Junctional nevi Mongolian spot Postinflammatory hyperpigmentation Intradermal nevus
Identify: Juvenile xanthogranuloma Nevus sebaceous

spots are present or multiple café-au-lait spots are found in the axilla or groin area. Nevi can be brown, reddish brown, skin colored, dark brown, or blue. Some nevi are flat (junctional), whereas others are raised (dermal or compound). They can occur anywhere. Mongolian spots are present at birth and may fade with time. They are always flat and are blue or blue–black and have indistinct borders.

G. Juvenile xanthogranulomas commonly present as orange to yellow–brown soft papules or nodules most often on the head or neck. Multiple lesions in children younger than 2 years may have associated eye lesions that can be misdiagnosed as retinoblastoma. Ophthalmology examination is indicated for multiple juvenile xanthogranulomas. A nevus sebaceous (a hamartoma of the sebaceous glands) appears clinically from birth as a yellow linear plaque on the face or scalp. At puberty, the lesion develops a warty appearance and has a predisposition for benign tumor growth and growth of basal cell carcinoma.

References

Boulanger JM, Larbrisseau A. Neurofibromatosis type 1 in a pediatric population: Ste-Justine's experience. Can J Neurol Sci 2005;32(2):225–31.

Ferner RE, Huson SM, Thomas N, et al. Guidelines for the diagnosis and management of individuals with neurofibromatosis 1. J Med Genet 2007;44(2):81–8.

Gawkrodger DJ, Ormerod AD, Shaw L, et al. Therapy Guidelines and Audit Subcommittee, British Association of Dermatologists; Clinical Standards Department, Royal College of Physicians of London; Cochrane Skin Group; Vitiligo Society: Guideline for the diagnosis and management of vitiligo. Br J Dermatol 2008;159(5):1051–76.

Jena DK, Sengupta S, Dwari BC, Ram MK. Pityriasis versicolor in the pediatric age group. Indian J Dermatol Venereol Leprol 2005;71(4):259–61.

Lin RL, Janniger CK. Pityriasis alba. Cutis 2005;76(1):21–4.

Paller AS, Mancini AJ. Hurwitz clinical pediatric dermatology. 3rd ed. New York: Elsevier; 2006.

Prcic S, Djuran V, Mikov A, Mikov I. Vitiligo in children. Pediatr Dermatol 2007;24(6):666.

Weston WL, Lane AT, Morelli JG. A color textbook of pediatric dermatology. 4th ed. St. Louis: Mosby; 2007.

Papulosquamous Disorders

Arelis Burgos-Zavoda, MD, and Joanna M. Burch, MD

Papulosquamous disorders are skin lesions consisting of red or purple papules or plaques with scale.

A. Suspect pityriasis rosea when pink to red oval papules appear parallel to the lines of skin stress. A larger, erythematous, scaly plaque called the *herald patch* occurs in many cases. When present before the outbreak of other lesions, the herald patch is easily confused with tinea corporis. A viral-like prodrome with fever and malaise may occur but is uncommon. In adolescents, consider secondary syphilis when fever and adenopathy are associated with palmar lesions. The lesions of pityriasis rosea usually occur on the trunk, but in black children may be mostly in the inguinal and axillary areas and extremities. Lesions persist for 4 to 8 weeks, but pruritus usually resolves sooner. Treat with sun exposure or phototherapy (narrow-band ultraviolet B) to reduce the pruritus and quicken resolution.

B. Pityriasis lichenoides, a rarer skin disease, occurs in two forms: chronic and acute. Chronic pityriasis lichenoides resembles pityriasis rosea but can persist for 2 to 3 years. It is most common in a "swim trunk" distribution. Suspect chronic pityriasis lichenoides when pityriasis rosea fails to clear within 2 to 3 months. The acute form of pityriasis lichenoides, also called *Mucha–Habermann disease* or *PLEVA* (pityriasis lichenoides et varioliformis acuta), presents with red papules that have central petechiae and crusting. The rash, which can be confused initially with varicella, persists for more than 9 months. This diagnosis should be considered in children with "recurrent chicken pox." When the diagnosis is uncertain, consider skin biopsy. Treatment with oral erythromycin, 40 mg/kg/day for 1 to 2 months, may benefit some children. Phototherapy for pityriasis lichenoides is the treatment of choice.

C. Suspect psoriasis when red plaques with silver scale involve the elbows, knees, or scalp. Other common sites are ears, eyebrows, superior gluteal crease, genitalia, and nails. Involvement of the scalp with nongreasy thick scale is not associated with hair loss. Nail changes include pitting, yellowing, thickening, and separation of the nail plate from the nail bed. The presence of multiple, discrete, droplike papules with scales suggests guttate psoriasis, which is seen in approximately one third of psoriasis cases. Guttate psoriasis flares are frequently associated with streptococcal pharyngitis. Skin biopsy in cases of psoriasis show signs of epidermal proliferation and rapid turnover. Treatment is dependent on the severity of the disease. Topical corticosteroids of moderate-to-high potency, often in combination with topical calcipotriene (Dovonex) twice a day for 1 to 3 months, may provide relief. Tazarotene is the best agent for psoriatic nails. For the scalp, salicylic acid 3% in mineral oil or tar shampoo is helpful to reduce scale. In resistant scalp lesions, add a topical corticosteroid in addition to scale-reducing therapies. Natural sunlight in the summer helps control outbreaks, and in indicated cases, phototherapy is effective. Systemic agents such as oral retinoids, methotrexate, and anti–tumor necrosis factor biologic agents should always be managed by an experienced dermatologist. Systemic corticosteroids are contraindicated because of the rebound effect on psoriasis once discontinued. Recognize and treat secondary staphylococcal infection of the lesions.

D. Suspect lichen planus when flat-topped, pruritic, purple, polygonal papules are present. The papules often have a shiny appearance. Oral, penile, and scalp lesions may occur. Scalp lesions may be associated with hair loss. Nail involvement is rare. Treat cases with topical steroids for 4 to 8 weeks. Consider oral prednisone, 1 to 2 mg/kg/day, for 1 to 2 weeks in severe generalized cases. Phototherapy is helpful with pruritus and at times will speed clearing. Skin biopsy shows epidermal basal cell injury of unknown cause.

References

Balasubramaniam P, Ogboli M, Moss C. Lichen planus in children: review of 26 cases. Clin Exp Dermatol 2008 33(4):457–9.

Benoit S, Hamm H. Childhood psoriasis. Clin Dermatol 2007;25(6): 555–62.

Chuh A, Lee A, Zawar V, et al. Pityriasis rosea—an update. Indian J Dermatol Venereol Leprol 2005;71(5):311–5.

Ersoy-Evans S, Greco MF, Mancini AJ, et al. Pityriasis lichenoides in childhood: a retrospective review of 124 patients. J Am Acad Dermatol 2007;56(2):205–10.

Ott H, Frank J, Poblete-Gutiérrez P. Eruptive lichen planus in a child. Pediatr Dermatol 2007 24(6):637–9.

Paller AS, Mancini AJ. Hurwitz clinical pediatric dermatology. 3rd ed. New York: Elsevier; 2006.

Wahie S, Hiscutt E, Natarajan S, Taylor A. Pityriasis lichenoides: the differences between children and adults. Br J Dermatol 2007;157(5): 941–5.

Weston WL, Lane AT, Morelli JG. A color textbook of pediatric dermatology. 4th ed. St. Louis: Mosby; 2007.

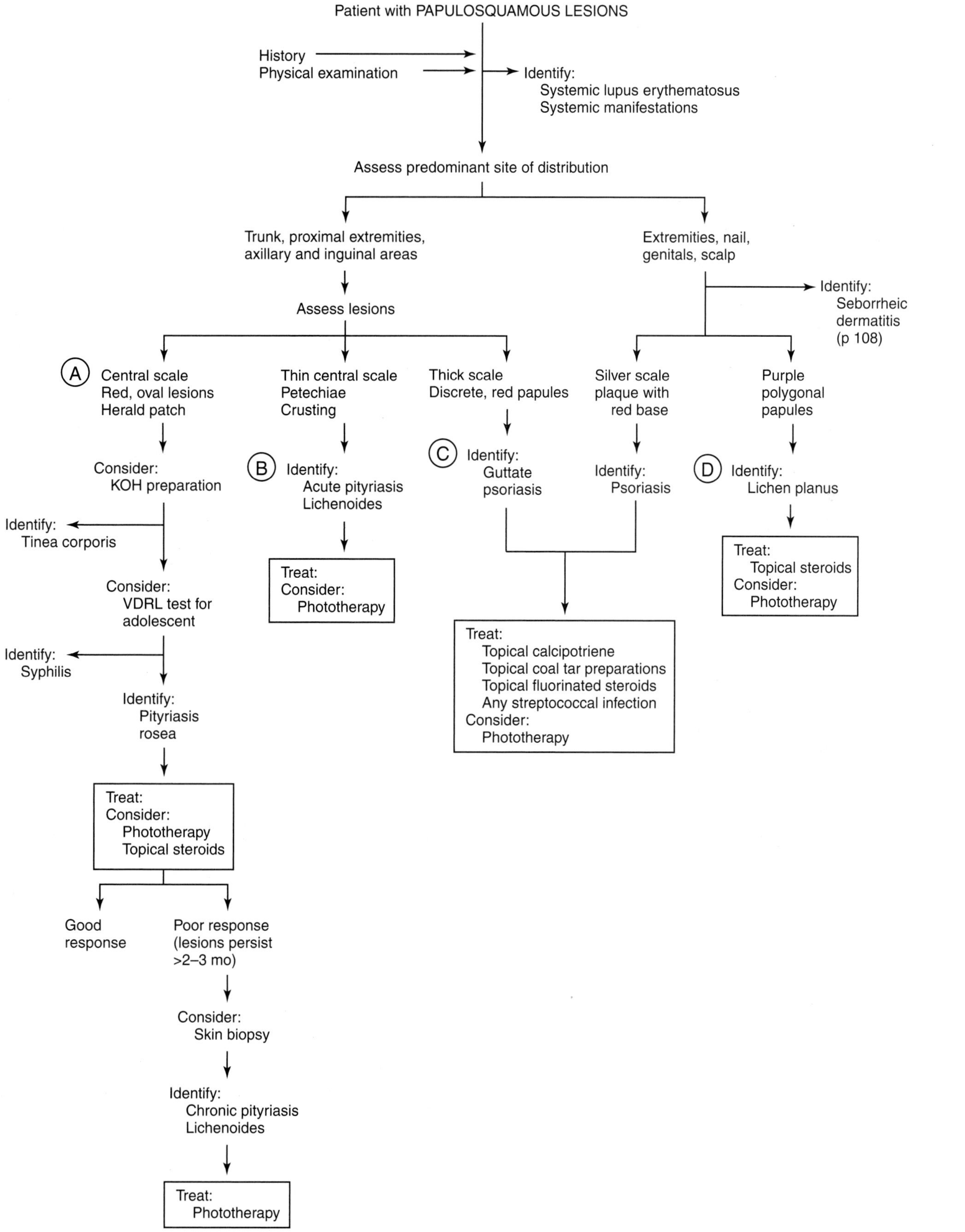
Patient with PAPULOSQUAMOUS LESIONS
History
Physical examination
Identify:
Systemic lupus erythematosus
Systemic manifestations
Assess predominant site of distribution
Trunk, proximal extremities, axillary and inguinal areas
Extremities, nail, genitals, scalp
Assess lesions
Identify:
Seborrheic dermatitis
(p 108)
A
Central scale
Red, oval lesions
Herald patch
Thin central scale
Petechiae
Crusting
Thick scale
Discrete, red papules
Silver scale plaque with red base
Purple polygonal papules
Consider:
KOH preparation
B
Identify:
Acute pityriasis
Lichenoides
C
Identify:
Guttate psoriasis
Identify:
Psoriasis
D
Identify:
Lichen planus
Identify:
Tinea corporis
Treat:
Consider:
Phototherapy
Treat:
Topical steroids
Consider:
Phototherapy
Consider:
VDRL test for adolescent
Treat:
Topical calcipotriene
Topical coal tar preparations
Topical fluorinated steroids
Any streptococcal infection
Consider:
Phototherapy
Identify:
Syphilis
Identify:
Pityriasis rosea
Treat:
Consider:
Phototherapy
Topical steroids
Good response
Poor response (lesions persist >2–3 mo)
Consider:
Skin biopsy
Identify:
Chronic pityriasis
Lichenoides
Treat:
Phototherapy

Vesiculobullous Disorders

Arelis Burgos-Zavoda, MD, and Joanna M. Burch, MD

A. Four forms of mastocytosis are observed in childhood. The most common forms are the solitary mastocytoma and urticaria pigmentosa (UP). The solitary mastocytoma presents at birth or shortly after as a reddish brown plaque that will urticate and sometimes blister on rubbing (Darier sign). UP is a disease characterized by brown maculars and papules that appear in the first year of life. Stroking of these lesions will also result in a positive Darier sign. Most patients with UP have the nonhereditary form that remits around age 7. Systemic symptoms, such as flushing, wheezing, diarrhea, and syncope, occur infrequently in UP. There seems to be a hereditary form in less than 2% of cases that has later onset and does not remit. Systemic symptoms develop with time. When necessary, treat patients with a long-acting, nonsedating antihistamine during the day and 0.6 to 1 mg/kg hydroxyzine hydrochloride about 1 hour before bedtime. If symptoms are not controlled by antihistamines, or if there is a family history of UP, refer the patient to a dermatologist. Telangiectasia eruptiva macularis perstans and diffuse cutaneous mastocytosis are rarer and more serious forms of the disease. Prompt referral for widespread blistering/urtication is warranted.

B. Incontinentia pigmenti usually occurs in girls and is characterized by linear patterns of red plaques with blisters on the extremities. The blisters evolve into wartlike lesions that persist for about 1 year and then resolve. Older children and adults often have swirls of brown pigmentation on the trunk and at the sites of previous lesions. Although mental retardation, microcephaly, and eye and skeletal anomalies occur in some individuals, many have no significant findings. Referral to an ophthalmologist for a baseline eye examination in the newborn period is indicated.

C. Epidermolysis bullosa (EB) is a congenital absence or dysfunction of a part of the complex that anchors the epidermis to the dermis. EB can be divided into three basic categories: simplex (epidermal), junctional (dermal-epidermal junction), and dystrophic (dermal). Scarring does not usually occur in the simplex types but is common in the junctional and dystrophic types. The inheritance of the simplex types is usually dominant, whereas that of the junctional types is recessive. The dystrophic forms may be dominant (less severe) or recessive (more severe). All three forms of EB can present in the newborn period, although the milder simplex and dominant dystrophic forms can present much later. Children with spontaneous blistering with mild trauma and newborns born with blisters or erosion should be referred to a regional EB center or a dermatologist for prompt diagnosis and appropriate intervention.

D. Epidermolytic hyperkeratosis, also known as congenital bullous ichthyosiform erythroderma, is a genetic disorder characterized by blistering, diffuse erythema, and thickened scaling of the skin. Bullae predominate early, but with time the skin becomes less fragile and more thickened and scaly. Inheritance is autosomal dominant. The disease is caused by mutations in type 1 and type 10 keratin genes that are expressed in the upper layers of the epidermis. Refer patients suspected of having epidermolytic hyperkeratosis to a dermatologist.

E. Superficial skin infection with bacteria, viruses, and fungi can produce vesicles or erosions (exposed bases of superficial vesicles). Bacterial impetigo produces red plaques with moist, honey-colored crusts on each lesion. Bullous impetigo results if the causative staphylococcal species produces an exfoliative toxin, a toxin that cleaves the desmoglein 1 attachments between keratinocytes in the superficial epidermis. Because the split is superficial, the blister roof is flaccid, and often ruptured, leaving a central crust over erosions with desquamation of the epidermis at the periphery. Early burns, contact dermatitis, or friction blisters are in the differential of early bullous impetigo. Viral infections that present with vesicular eruptions include varicella, herpes zoster, hand-foot-and-mouth disease (coxsackievirus), enteroviral infections, and herpes simplex. Grouped vesicles on an erythematous base suggest herpes simplex. Consider obtaining bacterial or viral cultures and staining a smear of the blister's contents with Wright stain (Tzanck preparation) to identify epidermal giant cells associated with viral infections. Infestations with the scabies mite can produce vesicles or pustules. Bullous lesions on the palms and soles suggest scabies infestation or possibly bullous papular urticaria (see F). Interdigital webs, palms, and soles with S-shaped burrows in infants and young children are suggestive of scabies. Do mineral oil scraping for definitive diagnosis (see Evaluation of Skin Lesions). If present, treat with 5% permethrin cream.

(Continued on page 118)

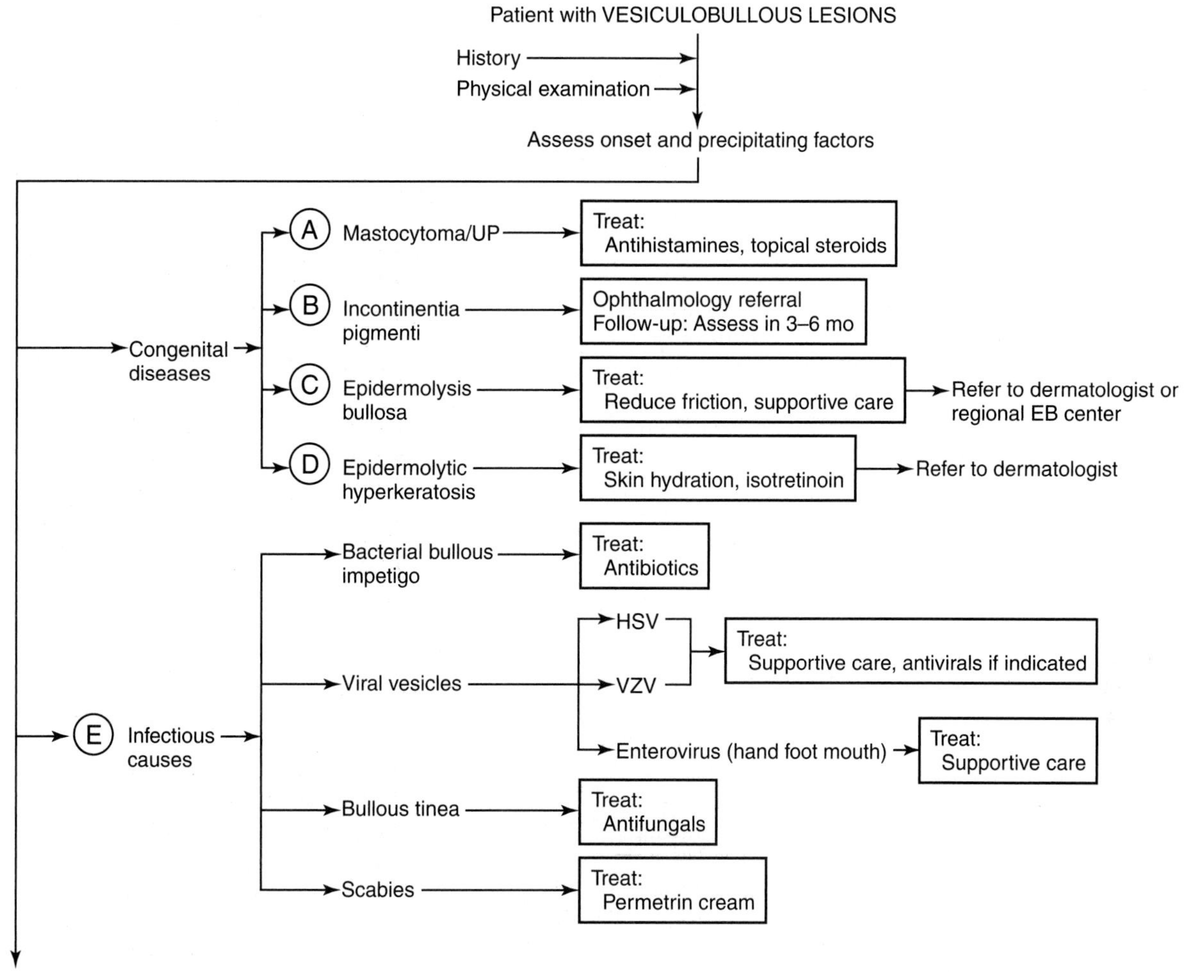
Patient with VESICULOBULLOUS LESIONS
History
Physical examination
Assess onset and precipitating factors
Congenital diseases
A Mastocytoma/UP
Treat: Antihistamines, topical steroids
B Incontinentia pigmenti
Ophthalmology referral
Follow-up: Assess in 3–6 mo
C Epidermolysis bullosa
Treat: Reduce friction, supportive care
Refer to dermatologist or regional EB center
D Epidermolytic hyperkeratosis
Treat: Skin hydration, isotretinoin
Refer to dermatologist
E Infectious causes
Bacterial bullous impetigo
Treat: Antibiotics
Viral vesicles
HSV
VZV
Treat: Supportive care, antivirals if indicated
Enterovirus (hand foot mouth)
Treat: Supportive care
Bullous tinea
Treat: Antifungals
Scabies
Treat: Permetrin cream

(Cont'd on p 119)

F. Vesicles or bullae on the skin have several noninfectious causes. Friction blisters are usually solitary, on areas of known rubbing or trauma, are not inflamed, and resolve spontaneously. A history of repetitive frictional forces should differentiate from infectious blisters. Less than 1% of healthy newborns will have a sucking blister, usually on the back of the hand, finger, or forearm, presumably from vigorous sucking of the skin in utero. These also are usually isolated, noninflammatory, and resolve rapidly and without sequelae. Blockage of the sweat ducts can lead to a vesiculopapular eruption called *miliaria.* The skin findings vary depending on the depth of the sweat duct obstruction. Miliaria crystallina occurs with plugging of the sweat duct within or just beneath the stratum corneum. Clinically, 1- to 2-mm, clear, thin-walled vesicles appear in crops most commonly on intertriginous areas or areas covered with clothing. The eruption is asymptomatic. Miliaria rubra, also called *prickly heat,* is the most common form. The obstruction is deeper than with miliaria crystallina. Nonfollicular, red papules or papulovesicles with a predilection for occluded areas of skin are present, especially on the upper trunk, back, volar aspects of arms, and body folds. Treatment includes cooling of the skin and the prevention of occlusion of the skin surface. Any dermatitis (atopic, irritant, nummular, or contact) that is acute and severe enough can cause sufficient swelling between the keratinocytes of the epidermis to result in vesiculation. This clinically presents as red, scaly plaque with much oozing/crusting and some vesicle formation. There is a type of hand/foot dermatitis called *pompholyx,* or dyshidrotic eczema, that presents with very pruritic vesicles along the lateral surface of the palms and digits, often with associated red plaques with scale and crust of the hands and feet. Attacks may occur several times a year and last for weeks. Treat with a topical corticosteroid of appropriate strength. Papular urticaria is an inflammatory reaction to biting arthropods. It presents as recurrent crops of pruritic, grouped red papules with a central pinpoint punctum. Often, it is only the toddler or small child in the house that is affected. On the hands and feet, if the inflammatory reaction is acute, bullae can form. The child is usually exposed to fleas, mites, or other small, biting arthropods in this environment. A skin biopsy of a bullous papular urticaria lesion will show acute inflammation with edema in the epidermis and a brisk inflammatory infiltrate in the dermis with many eosinophils. Treatment of papular urticaria involves removing the arthropods from the environment if they can be identified, the use of topical corticosteroids, and oral antihistamines as needed for symptomatic control. The use of a safe insect repellant daily on the arms and legs of the child may prevent bites. This is usually a phenomenon that resolves after 6 to 12 months (one biting season).

G. Bullous drug eruptions include Stevens–Johnson syndrome (SJS) and toxic epidermal necrolysis (TEN). Vancomycin is the most common cause of a drug-induced linear IgA bullous dermatosis, which is often a childhood autoimmune blistering disorder (see H) not associated with drug ingestion. SJS is more common in childhood than is TEN. It is most commonly associated with drugs and *Mycoplasma pneumoniae* infection. Drugs most frequently implicated are anti-infective sulfonamides, anticonvulsant agents, and nonsteroidal anti-inflammatory drugs. SJS usually has onset 7 to 21 days after starting a new medication, and almost always occurs within the first 8 weeks of beginning the causative drug. SJS is preceded by a 1- to 14-day prodrome of fever, headache, sore throat, and malaise. The eruption is characterized by widespread, maculopapular, targetoid lesions (they do not form the distinct three-zoned target lesions like in EM) that can progress to blisters. There may be areas of confluence with widespread epidermal sloughing. Mucosal involvement of two surfaces is required for diagnosis and is often florid. The oral mucosa (involved in most cases) and eyes are most commonly involved, but genitourinary involvement must be ruled out. Painful, hemorrhagic crusts on the lips often interfere with oral intake. Severe eye pain and photophobia are common with eye involvement, and early ophthalmology consultation with any eye signs or symptoms is indicated. TEN often has higher fever and more severe prodromal symptoms, less mucosal involvement, and more widespread cutaneous involvement. The mortality rate for SJS is around 5%, whereas that of TEN is 15% to 30%. The initial treatment is prompt removal of any drugs started in the last 8 weeks of onset of symptoms. Hospitalization with burn unit care, fluid replacement, enteral feeding, monitoring for infection, ophthalmologic consultation and treatment, and pain control is often required. Systemic steroids and intravenous immunoglobulin (IVIG) use has not been proved effective in randomized, controlled, double-blind studies. The most common long-term sequela is skin dyspigmentation.

H. Autoimmune-mediated blistering disorders are due to immunoglobulin deposition in the skin against a specific protein antigen that leads to separation of the epidermis or the epidermis from the dermis. These disorders often require systemic therapy including prednisone and other immunosuppressive agents. Children suspected of having an immunobullous disorder should be referred promptly to a dermatologist. These disorders include linear IgA bullous dermatosis, characterized by the spontaneous, widespread eruption of tense bullae and smaller blisters, often in an annular array with a crusted depressed center, like a "string of pearls." IgA is deposited in a thin line along the dermoepidermal junction. Dermatitis herpetiformis (DH) is characterized by very pruritic, small, crusted papules and vesicles, often on the extensor neck, arms, and low back. It is related to gluten intolerance. IgA is deposited in clumps at the top of the rete ridges in the dermis. Children with dermatitis herpetiformis should be worked up for Celiac disease. Bullous pemphigoid is rare in children but is characterized by tense bullae, pruritus, and IgG against a protein in the dermoepidermal junction. Pemphigus is characterized by more superficial blistering, often with just blister bases and erosions noted on skin examination and involvement of the oral mucosa. This is caused by immunoglobulin directed against proteins in the keratinocyte desmosomes. When acquired blistering lesions

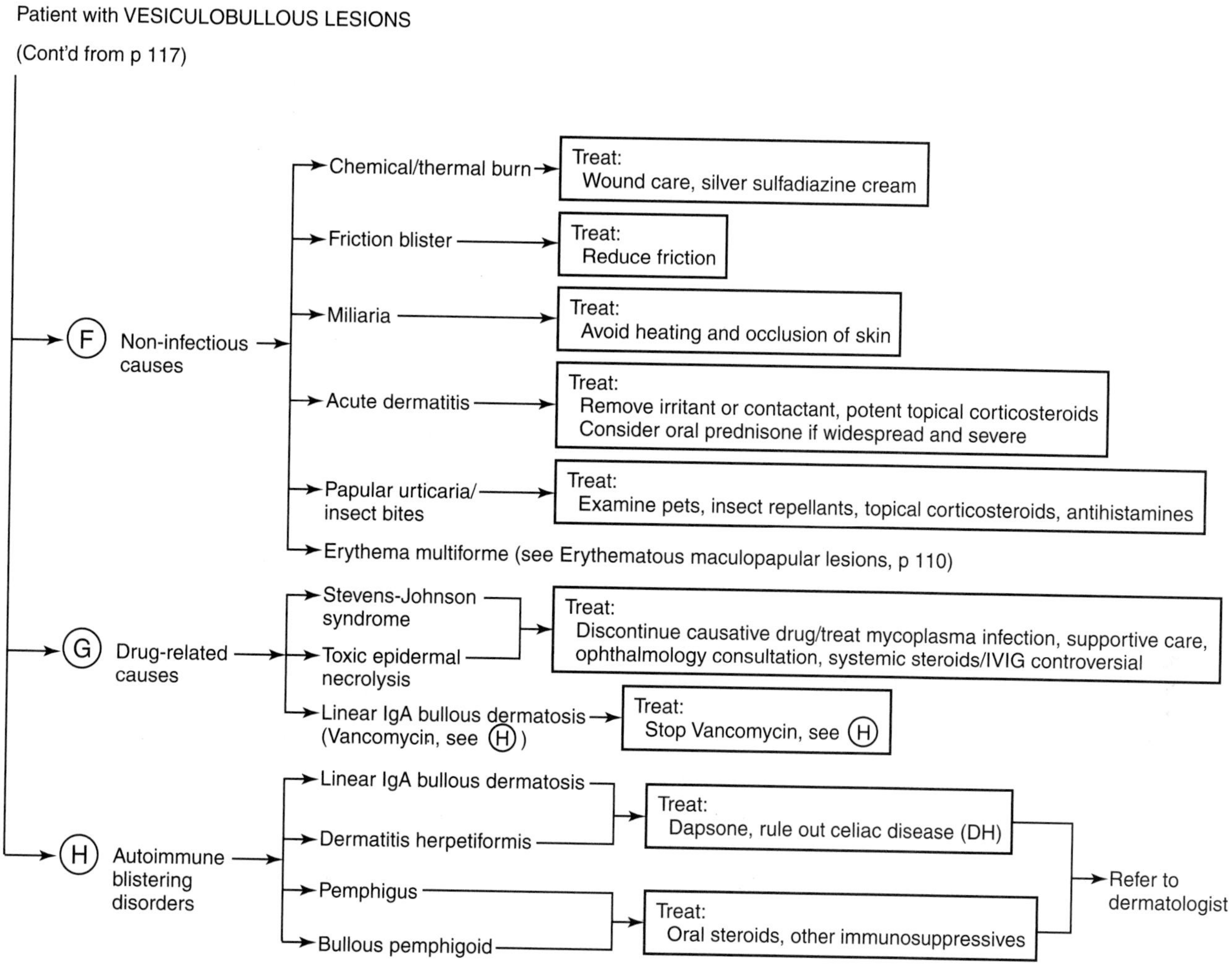
Patient with VESICULOBULLOUS LESIONS
(Cont'd from p 117)
F Non-infectious causes
Chemical/thermal burn
Treat: Wound care, silver sulfadiazine cream
Friction blister
Treat: Reduce friction
Miliaria
Treat: Avoid heating and occlusion of skin
Acute dermatitis
Treat: Remove irritant or contactant, potent topical corticosteroids Consider oral prednisone if widespread and severe
Papular urticaria/insect bites
Treat: Examine pets, insect repellants, topical corticosteroids, antihistamines
Erythema multiforme (see Erythematous maculopapular lesions, p 110)
G Drug-related causes
Stevens-Johnson syndrome
Toxic epidermal necrolysis
Treat: Discontinue causative drug/treat mycoplasma infection, supportive care, ophthalmology consultation, systemic steroids/IVIG controversial
Linear IgA bullous dermatosis (Vancomycin, see H)
Treat: Stop Vancomycin, see H
H Autoimmune blistering disorders
Linear IgA bullous dermatosis
Dermatitis herpetiformis
Treat: Dapsone, rule out celiac disease (DH)
Pemphigus
Bullous pemphigoid
Treat: Oral steroids, other immunosuppressives
Refer to dermatologist

persist for longer than 1 month, obtain a skin biopsy for routine histopathology and immunofluorescence to look for these immunobullous disorders. Treat linear IgA bullous dermatosis or dermatitis herpetiformis with sulfapyridine or dapsone; treat bullous pemphigoid with systemic corticosteroids. Pemphigus often requires other immunosuppressive agents.

References

Darmstadt GL. A guide to superficial strep and staph infections. Contemp Pediatr 1997;14:95.

Levi N, Bastuji-Garin S, Mockenhaupt M, et al. Medications as risk factors of Stevens-Johnson syndrome and toxic epidermal necrolysis in children: a pooled analysis. Pediatrics 2009;123(2):e297–e304.

Mann JA, Siegel DH. Common genodermatoses: what the pediatrician needs to know. Pediatr Ann 2009;38(2):91–8.

Nishifuji K, Sugai M, Amagai M. Staphylococcal exfoliative toxins: "molecular scissors" of bacteria that attack the cutaneous defense barrier in mammals. J Dermatol Sci 2008;49(1):21–31.

Paller AS, Mancini AJ. Hurwitz clinical pediatric dermatology: a textbook of skin disorders of childhood and adolescence. 3rd ed. New York: Elsevier-Saunders; 2006.

Rzany B, Correia O, Kelly JP, et al. Risk of Stevens-Johnson syndrome and toxic epidermal necrolysis during first weeks of antiepileptic therapy: a case-control study. Study Group of the International Case Control Study on Severe Cutaneous Adverse Reactions. Lancet 1999;353(9171):2190–4.

Wagner A. Distinguishing vesicular and pustular disorders in the neonate. Curr Opin Pediatr 1997;9:396–405.

Weston WL, Huff JC, Morelli JG. Misdiagnosis, treatments and outcomes in the immunobullous diseases of children. Pediatr Dermatol 1997;14:264–72.

Weston WL, Lane AT, Morelli JG. A color textbook of pediatric dermatology. 4th ed. St. Louis: Mosby-Elsevier; 2007.

Nail Disorders

Arelis Burgos-Zavoda, MD, and Joanna M. Burch, MD

When a patient presents with a nail disorder, the clinician must determine whether the disorder is congenital or acquired. Is this purely a nail disorder, or a sign of a widerspread skin disorder, a sign of a systemic disorder, or nutritional deficiency? Nail thickness and color change can be clues to the diagnosis. It is also important to be aware of normal changes in the nails. Concave nail plates are normal in the first 3 years of life. A rare pit in the nail plate can be normal. Scattered white spots are normal and are usually the result of minor trauma. Longitudinal ridging of the nail plates that worsens with age is common.

A. The history should ascertain the onset of the nail disorder (congenital or acquired). Does the patient wear tight shoes or tight stockings? How are the nails cut? Is there evidence that the patient bites and/or picks the nails, or sucks the thumb/finger with the nail changes? Is there any erythema, tenderness, or discharge? Are there other changes in the skin, mucous membranes, or hair?

B. Examine all 20 nails (have patient remove any polish) and the associated nail folds, as well as the skin in general and oral mucous membranes. Look for congenital malalignment, overcurvature of the nail plate, involvement of more than one nail, erythema, tenderness, exudate, granulation tissue, and other skin and joint involvement.

C. The main diagnostic tests used in the workup of nail disorders include a potassium hydroxide (KOH) preparation of nail scrapings, culture of any discharge from the periungual areas for bacteria and fungus, and culture of nail plate that can be obtained by using a spoon-shaped curette to obtain cells from the thickened distal nail plate and placed on Sabouraud dextrose agar or dermatophyte test media. A positive KOH preparation or culture should be obtained and documented before starting oral antifungal medication for onychomycosis. Nail clippings can be sent on saline gauze in a sterile urine cup to be processed by surgical pathology with hematoxylin and eosin and stained with periodic acid-Schiff (PAS), which will mark the walls of any hyphae in the nail plate. This is a more sensitive method to detect dermatophyte infection than KOH or culture. A nail biopsy may be indicated if there is concern of an associated disease and the nail plate, as well as the matrix or nail bed, must be evaluated. This should be referred to a dermatologist or a practitioner experienced in nail biopsy techniques. The patient may have permanent nail-plate deformities after a biopsy of the matrix.

D. Nail surface changes include pitting, scaling, ridging (longitudinal or horizontal), or splitting. Generalized roughness of the nail plate surface is called *trachyonychia* and can be idiopathic or may signal psoriasis, alopecia areata, lichen planus, dermatitis, and sometimes inherited ectodermal dysplasias. Long-term follow-up is often required to determine whether the nail changes resolve over time, as is common for idiopathic trachyonychia, or whether the patient shows signs of other more widespread skin diseases involving the nails. Pitting of the nails is most commonly seen in psoriasis and alopecia areata. Transverse ridges called *Beau's lines* occur in one to two nails after a severe illness or after a toxic or traumatic event (e.g., surgery). Self-induced trauma, such as thumb sucking, nail biting, and nail picking, can cause roughness, ridging, and inflammation of the nail folds (see F). This should be avoided. Habit-tic dystrophy of the nail is self-induced and usually involves the thumbnail. It is characterized by a central depression of the nail plate with several irregularly spaced horizontal ridges extending from the depression. Onychomycosis, in which disruption of the nail plate is often accompanied by distal thickening (see E) is becoming more common in children.

E. Many disorders that cause thickening of the nails also cause roughness of the surface. Psoriasis, lichen planus, and idiopathic trachyonychia (20-nail dystrophy) are the most common cause of widespread thickening of the nails. Infections of the nail (onychomycosis) make the nail yellowed, crumbly, and thickened. In both psoriasis and onychomycosis, thickening begins distally. In onychomycosis, usually only a few nails are involved. Pachyonychia congenita is an autosomal dominantly inherited disorder in which there is a mutation in nail keratin proteins that is associated with congenital or early onset of thickening of the nails, in addition to other associated findings. Poorly developed or absent nails are often associated with a variety of congenital syndromes. Hidrotic ectodermal dysplasia is an inherited disorder associated with nail atrophy/dystrophy. Children with epidermolysis bullosa often have dystrophic or nails that shed. Periodic shedding of one or two nails can be inherited as an autosomal dominant trait. Acquired causes of thin or absent nails include trauma, bullous drug eruptions, erythema multiforme, or poor acral circulation (as in Raynaud disease). Koilonychia, or spoon nails, can be normal in early life, associated with other nail disorders (lichen planus), and have been reported in patients with severe iron deficiency.

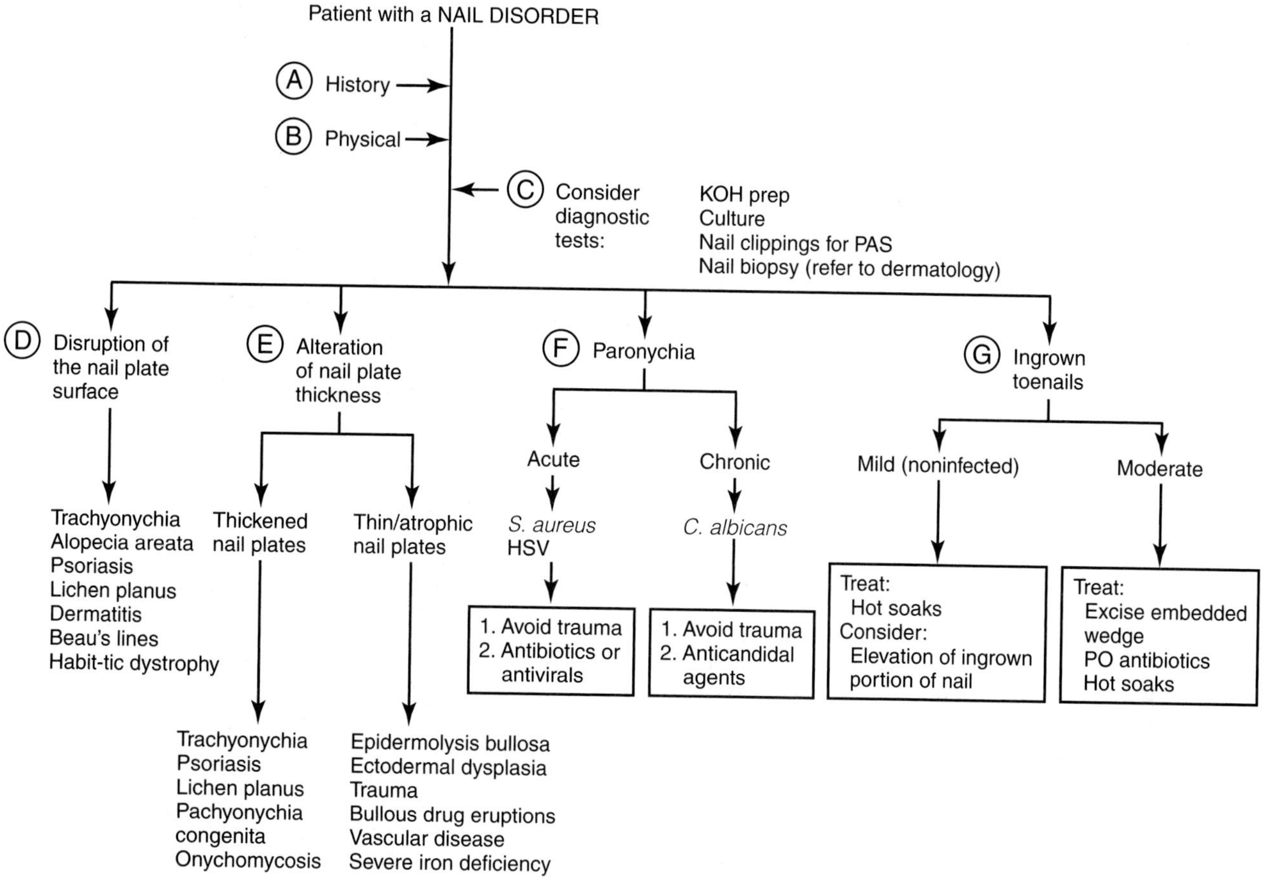

Patient with a NAIL DISORDER
A History
B Physical
C Consider diagnostic tests:
KOH prep
Culture
Nail clippings for PAS
Nail biopsy (refer to dermatology)
D Disruption of the nail plate surface
E Alteration of nail plate thickness
F Paronychia
G Ingrown toenails
Trachyonychia
Alopecia areata
Psoriasis
Lichen planus
Dermatitis
Beau's lines
Habit-tic dystrophy
Thickened nail plates
Thin/atrophic nail plates
Trachyonychia
Psoriasis
Lichen planus
Pachyonychia congenita
Onychomycosis
Epidermolysis bullosa
Ectodermal dysplasia
Trauma
Bullous drug eruptions
Vascular disease
Severe iron deficiency
Acute
S. aureus
HSV
1. Avoid trauma
2. Antibiotics or antivirals
Chronic
C. albicans
1. Avoid trauma
2. Anticandidal agents
Mild (noninfected)
Treat: Hot soaks
Consider: Elevation of ingrown portion of nail
Moderate
Treat: Excise embedded wedge
PO antibiotics
Hot soaks

F. Paronychia is inflammation of the tissues surrounding the nail caused by infection. Acute paronychia is most often caused by *Staphylococcus aureus*. The tissue surrounding the nail is painful, red, and edematous. There may be associated purulent drainage. The periungual areas may also be infected with herpes simplex virus (HSV; herpetic whitlow). This infection is very inflammatory, and grouped vesicles on an erythematous base should be visible. Chronic paronychia is characterized by a more violaceous color without exudates or tenderness. It is most commonly caused by *Candida albicans*. Thumb suckers, nail biters and pickers, and patients with type I diabetes mellitus are most commonly affected. Cultures should be taken, and antibiotics, antivirals, or anticandidal agents should be used as indicated. Habits or hobbies that cause recurrent trauma to the nail folds should be avoided.

G. An ingrown nail occurs when the lateral or free edge of the nail penetrates the epidermis and becomes embedded in the adjacent soft tissue either laterally or anteriorly. Ingrown nails are the result of one or more of the following: (1) faulty footwear, (2) improper nail care, (3) injury, (4) congenital malalignment, and (5) overcurvature of the nail plate. In mild cases, the ingrowing nail has penetrated the soft tissues of the nail groove and there is inflammation but no sign of infection. Hot soaks three times a day may be adequate therapy. Elevation of the embedded area of the nail with placement of cotton between the nail and the adjacent soft tissue is sometimes required. In more severe or frequently infected cases, the embedded nail should be excised and a small cotton wad placed to keep the nail plate separate from the inflamed area. Continue hot soaks. Infection is most often due to *Staphylococcus aureus*, and less frequently to *Candida*, *Pseudomonas*, or *Proteus*. Antibiotic coverage should be chosen accordingly. Prophylaxis includes avoidance of tight-fitting shoes and socks, trimming the nails straight across rather than in an arc, and cutting the nail only when it is beyond the distal end of the lateral nail fold.

References

Lawry MA, Haneke E, Strobeck K, et al. Methods for diagnosing onychomycosis: a comparative study and review of the literature. Arch Dermatol 2000;136(9):1112–6.

Paller AS, Mancini AJ. Hurwitz clinical pediatric dermatology: a textbook of skin disorders of childhood and adolescence. 3rd ed. New York: Elsevier-Saunders; 2006.

Weston WL, Lane AT, Morelli JG. A color textbook of pediatric dermatology. 4th ed. St. Louis: Mosby-Elsevier; 2007.

Ear/Nose/Throat

Acute Otitis Media

David M. Spiro, MD, MPH, and Donald H. Arnold, MD, MPH

DEFINITIONS

Acute otitis media (AOM) is the most common infection diagnosed in the outpatient setting, with U.S. healthcare costs greater than $5 billion annually. AOM is defined as an infection of the middle-ear space with rapid onset of signs and symptoms (<48 hours) of inflammation, such as otalgia, fever, irritability, anorexia, vomiting, and otorrhea. Otoscopic findings include a yellow–red exudate behind the tympanic membrane (TM). The TM is often bulging, with loss of ossicular landmarks and decreased mobility of the TM. Unresponsive AOM is characterized by clinical signs and symptoms associated with otoscopic findings of inflammation that continue beyond 48 to 72 hours of therapy with an appropriate antimicrobial. Unresponsive AOM suggests continued active infection with persistence of the bacterial pathogen in the middle-ear space. However, prolonged symptoms associated with a concomitant viral infection may be misdiagnosed as an unresponsive infection when the AOM is actually resolving. Clinical judgment is required, with attention to the patient's overall clinical status, if antibiotic use is to be limited appropriately.

PATHOGENESIS

The pathogenesis of AOM involves interactions among host characteristics, infectious agents, and environmental factors. Colonization of *Streptococcus pneumoniae*, nontypeable *Haemophilus influenzae*, or *Moraxella catarrhalis* of the middle-ear space associated with eustachian tube dysfunction likely causes AOM. Viral upper respiratory infections may increase bacterial adherence to mucosa, promote bacterial overgrowth, and increase colonization of the nasopharynx with bacterial pathogens. Aspiration of infected secretions may then occur into the middle-ear space. Factors that increase the frequency of viral respiratory infections include child-care attendance, and absence of breast-feeding also predisposes children to AOM. Sidestream smoking also increases the risk for AOM by impairing normal mucociliary function and promoting the attachment of the pathogen to respiratory epithelium in the middle-ear space. AOM is more common during the first 2 years of life because of an immature immune response against bacterial polysaccharides, in addition to the anatomic orientation and structure of the eustachian tube.

CAUSATIVE FACTORS

Respiratory viral infection may predispose to bacterial infection if these infections cause eustachian tube dysfunction. However, it remains unclear whether purulent effusions associated with AOM can result from viral infection alone or require bacterial coinfection. Bacterial pathogens can be isolated in about 80% of AOM middle ear aspirates. The most common bacterial pathogens in AOM are *S. pneumoniae* and nontypeable *H. influenzae,* the same bacterial pathogens most frequently associated with sinusitis. With initial treatment failure, *H. influenza* is more commonly isolated and *S. pneumonia* is likely to be penicillin nonsusceptible. Less frequent bacterial pathogens include *M. catarrhalis, Streptococcus pyogenes, Staphylococcus aureus,* gram-negative enteric organisms, and anaerobic organisms. AOM resolves spontaneously in the majority of cases. Often a wait-and-see, observational approach can be used as a primary management scheme to prevent unnecessary use of antibiotics. Prevention of AOM burden is possible through the use of pneumococcal vaccine that includes protection from seven serotypes of *S. pneumoniae.*

CLINICAL APPROACH

A. In the patient history, ask about earache and discharge, fever, respiratory symptoms, conjunctivitis, irritability, crying, decreased feeding, difficulty sleeping, vomiting, and ataxia. Inquire about the timing and treatment of the most recent AOM episode and frequency of episodes during the past 6 and 12 months. Ear tugging and other nonspecific symptoms are not reliable predictors of AOM. Identify children with immune disorders, acquired immunodeficiency syndrome, cystic fibrosis, or Kartagener syndrome (immotile cilia).

B. Examine the TM with pneumatic otoscopy. Use a pneumatic otoscope head and remove sufficient cerumen to have an adequate view of the membrane. It is important to create an adequate seal with an appropriately sized speculum, to have adequate light intensity with a halogen light source. Signs of AOM are bulging contour with exudate (bulging pus), and diminished or absent eardrum mobility. On occasion, bullae form between the outer and middle layers of the TM (bullous myringitis). Look for signs of middle-ear damage, such as tympanosclerosis (chalky white deposits in the eardrum), retraction pocket, perforation, or cholesteatoma (yellow greasy mass). Examine the mastoid area behind the ear for tenderness, swelling, protrusion of the ear, or erythema.

C. The most important step is to establish the proper diagnosis of AOM. Antibiotic therapy is not recommended for otitis media with effusion or for upper respiratory infections. The American Academy of Pediatrics developed a clinical guideline that establishes a diagnosis of AOM based on three components:

1. Acute onset (<48 hours) of signs and symptoms,
2. Middle-ear effusion, and
3. Signs and symptoms of middle-ear inflammation

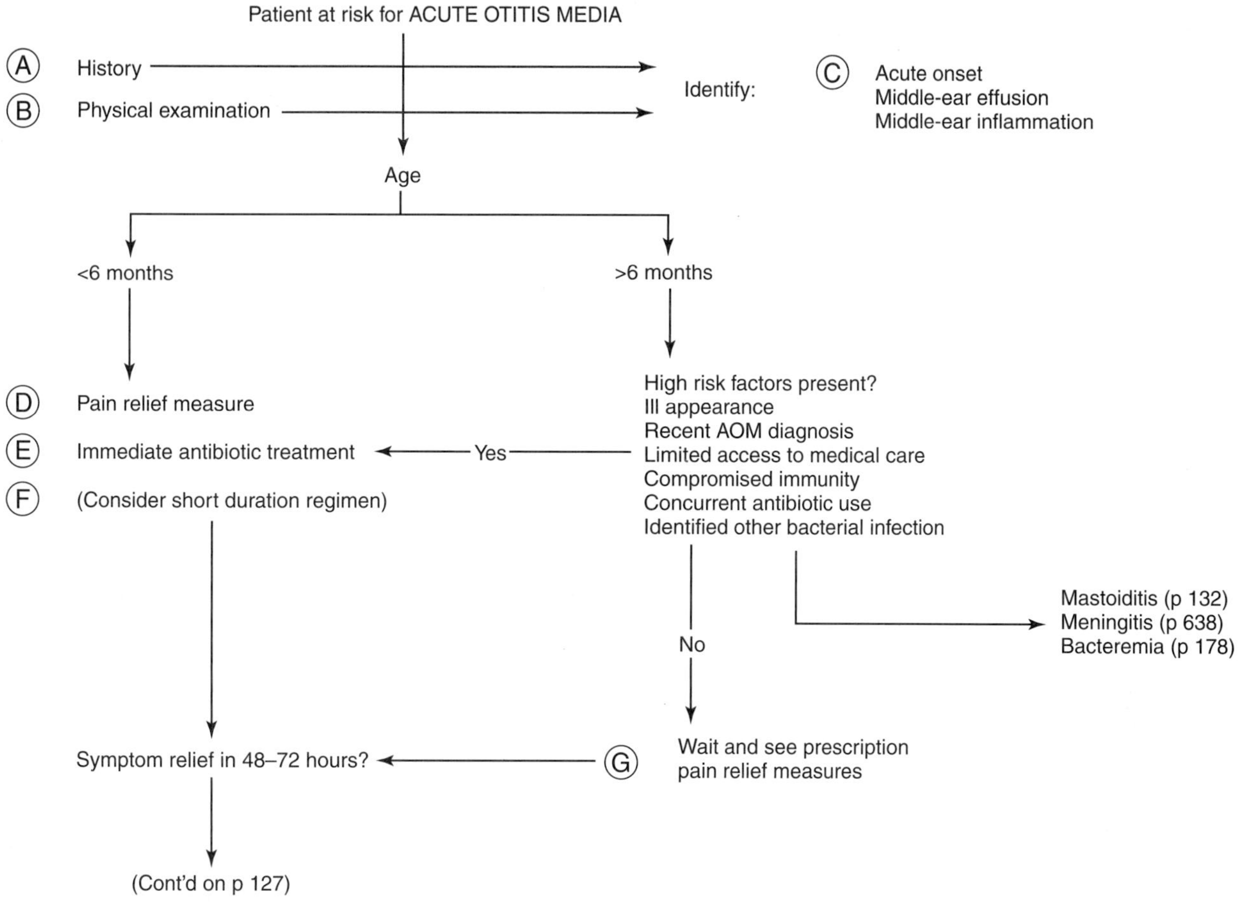
Patient at risk for ACUTE OTITIS MEDIA
A History
B Physical examination
Identify:
C Acute onset
Middle-ear effusion
Middle-ear inflammation
Age
<6 months
>6 months
D Pain relief measure
E Immediate antibiotic treatment
F (Consider short duration regimen)
Yes
High risk factors present?
Ill appearance
Recent AOM diagnosis
Limited access to medical care
Compromised immunity
Concurrent antibiotic use
Identified other bacterial infection
Mastoiditis (p 132)
Meningitis (p 638)
Bacteremia (p 178)
No
Symptom relief in 48–72 hours?
G Wait and see prescription
pain relief measures
(Cont'd on p 127)

D. *The pain associated with AOM should be uniformly treated. Antibiotics have no analgesic properties.* A small number of trials have demonstrated the short-term effectiveness of topical analgesic drops such as benzocaine-antipyrine and lignocaine. Systemic analgesics such as ibuprofen have been shown to improve symptom relief and may improve clinical outcomes. When pain is severe, tympanocentesis results in prompt relief.

E. Immediate treatment of AOM with antibiotics is controversial because of questions about efficacy and concerns about increasing the prevalence of drug-resistant microbes. A meta-analysis of the results of 33 randomized clinical trials found that treatment with antibiotics increased the resolution rate by only 13.7%. First-line therapy in a nonallergic child is high-dose amoxicillin (Table 1). High-dose amoxicillin will usually eradicate the most invasive pathogen, *S. pneumoniae,* and if no improvement occurs, a second-line antibiotic may be chosen to cover *M. catarrhalis* and β-lactamase–producing *H. influenzae.* Consider an initial single intramuscular dose of ceftriaxone when the patient is unable to take oral antibiotics because of vomiting. If the patient is allergic to penicillin or amoxicillin, treat with azithromycin when there is a history of a serious type I hypersensitivity reaction (severe urticaria, respiratory distress, anaphylaxis), or with cefdinir, cefuroxime, or cefpodoxime when there is a history of a less severe reaction. *Antihistamines, decongestants, and steroids are of no benefit in treatment of AOM.*

F. The optimal duration of amoxicillin therapy is controversial. According to Dagan and colleagues (2001), using a shorter duration regimen of 5 to 7 days appears to decrease drug-resistant pneumococcal carriage after therapy. This is important because nasopharyngeal flora determines the pathogen of the next AOM.

G. Most clinicians in the United States routinely treat AOM with antibiotics. Some European countries frequently use a wait-and-see, observational approach to avoid unnecessary use of antibiotics, with similar rates of mastoiditis compared with the United States. Counsel parents of untreated children who do not improve within 48 to 72 hours of diagnosis to fill the prescription or return to be reassessed and treated with antibiotics if the AOM is immediately treated with an antibiotic. Approximately two of every three families will fill the wait-and-see prescription. Observational therapy should be considered when children do not meet high-risk criteria: ill appearance, recent AOM diagnosis, limited access to medical care, compromised immunity, concurrent antibiotic use, or an identified bacterial infection other than AOM.

Table 1. **Antibiotic Therapy for Acute Otitis Media in Children**

Antibiotic	Dosage	Product Availability
Amoxicillin	High-dose: 80–90 mg/kg/24 hr bid	80–90 mg/kg/24 hr bid (200, 400 mg/5 ml) Chewables: 200, 400 mg
Amoxicillin-clavulanate (Augmentin ES)	High dose: 90 mg/kg/24 hr bid (maximum dose: 875 mg bid)	200 mg/5 ml, 400 mg/5 ml Chewables: 200, 400 mg
Azithromycin (Zithromax)	10 mg/kg/24 hr, one dose day 1 (maximum dose: 500 mg), followed by 5 mg/kg daily on days 2–5 (maximum dose: 250 mg)	Suspension: 100, 200 mg/5 ml Capsules: 250 mg
Cefdinir (Omnicef)	14 mg/kg/24 hr qd (maximum dose: 600 mg)	Suspension: 125 mg/5 ml Capsules: 300 mg
Cefpodoxime proxetil (Vantin)	10 mg/kg bid	Liquid: 50, 100 mg/5 ml Tablets: 100, 200 mg
Ceftriaxone (Rocephin)	50 mg/kg/24 IM/IV for 3 days (1 g maximum)	Vials: 250, 500 mg, 1 g
Cefuroxime (Ceftin, Zinacef)	30 mg/kg/24 hr bid	Suspension: 125, 250 mg/5 ml Tablets: 250, 500 mg
Clindamycin	10–30 mg/kg/24 hr tid (maximum dose: 450 mg)	Granules: 75 mg/5 ml Capsules: 75, 150, 300 mg

IM, intramuscularly; *IV*, intravenously.

H. A scheduled re-examination of the ear is usually not necessary for the previously healthy child.

I. Risk factors for unresponsive infections include age younger than 18 months, a history of recurrent AOM in the child or a sibling, and a history of antibiotic treatment of AOM within the preceding month. Parents of children older than 15 months usually know when their child's infection has resolved. Consider treating unresponsive AOM with amoxicillin-clavulanate, cefdinir, cefuroxime, or cefpodoxime to cover both *S. pneumoniae* and β-lactamase–producing pathogens. This type of second-line agent is also indicated when a child experiences another symptomatic infection within 4 weeks of stopping amoxicillin; however, repeated use of amoxicillin is indicated if more than 4 weeks have passed without symptoms because a new pathogen is usually present.

J. If a child remains symptomatic longer than 3 days while taking a second-line agent, consider performing a tympanocentesis or treating with oral clindamycin (effective against resistant pneumococci but not β-lactamase–producing organisms) or intramuscular ceftriaxone (one dose a day for 3 days; effective against both resistant pneumococci and β-lactamase–producing organisms). Tympanocentesis is performed by placing a needle through the TM and aspirating the middle-ear fluid. Indications for a tympanocentesis or myringotomy are: (1) AOM in an infant younger than 6 weeks with a past neonatal intensive care hospitalization, because the pathogens may be gram-negative; (2) AOM in a patient with compromised host resistance, because the organism may be unusual; (3) unresponsive AOM despite courses of two to four different antibiotics; (4) acute mastoiditis or suppurative labyrinthitis; and (5) severe pain.

References

Appelman CL, Claessen JQ, Touw-Otten FW, et al. Co-amoxiclav in recurrent acute otitis media: placebo controlled study. BMJ 1991;303:1450–2.

Arola M, Ziegler T, Ruuskanen O. Respiratory virus infection as a cause of prolonged symptoms in acute otitis media. J Pediatr 1990;116:697.

Berman S. Current concepts: otitis media in children. N Engl J Med 1995;332:1560–5.

Berman S, Roark R. Factors influencing outcome in children treated with antibiotics for acute otitis media. Pediatr Infect Dis J 1993;12:20–4.

Bertin L, Pons G, d'Athis P, et al. A randomized, double-blind, multicentre controlled trial of ibuprofen versus acetaminophen and placebo for symptoms of acute otitis media in children. Fundam Clin Pharmacol 1996;10(4):387–92.

Block SL, Hedrick JA, Tyler RD, et al. Microbiology of acute otitis media recently treated with aminopenicillins. Pediatr Infect Dis J 2001;20:1017–21.

Bluestone CD, Klein JO. Otitis media in infants and children. 2nd ed. Philadelphia: WB Saunders; 1995.

Carlin SA, Marchant CD, Shurin PA, et al. Host factors and early therapeutic response in acute otitis media. J Pediatr 1991;118:178.

Dagan R, Hoberman A, Johnson C, et al. Bacteriologic and clinical efficacy of high dose amoxicillin/clavulanate in children with acute otitis media. Pediatr Infect Dis J 2001;20:829–37.

Dagan R, Leibovitz E, Cheletz G, et al. Antibiotic treatment in acute otitis media promotes superinfection with resistant *Streptococcus pneumoniae* carried before initiation of treatment. J Infect Dis 2001;183:880–6.

Dagan R, Leibovitz E, Leiberman A, Yagupsky P. Clinical significance of antibiotic resistance in acute otitis media and implication of antibiotic treatment on carriage and spread of resistant organisms. Pediatr Infect Dis J 2000;19:S57–S65.

Dagan R, McCracken Jr GH. Flaws in design and conduct of clinical trials in acute otitis media. Pediatr Infect Dis J 2002;21:894–902.

Damoiseaux RA, van Balen FA, Hoes AW, et al. Primary care based randomised, double blind trial of amoxicillin versus placebo for acute otitis media in children aged under 2 years. BMJ 2000;320:350–4.

del Prado G, Martinez-Marin C, Huelves, L et al. Soriano impact of ibuprofen therapy in the outcome of experimental pneumococcal acute otitis media treated with amoxicillin or erythromycin. Pediatr Res 2006;60(5):555–9.

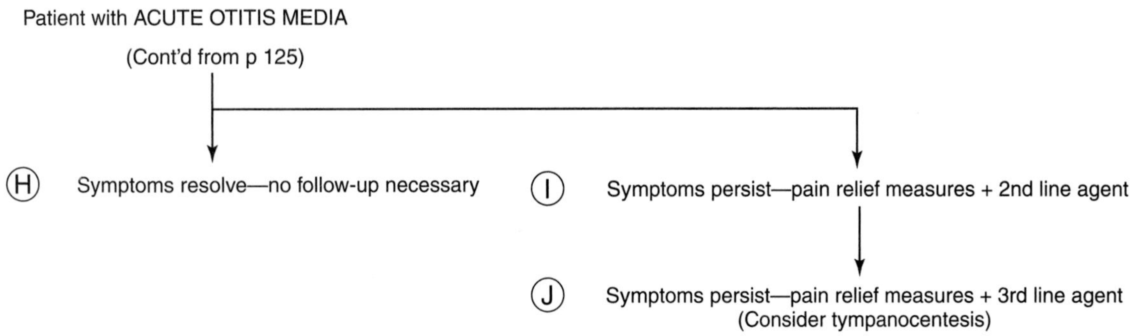
Patient with ACUTE OTITIS MEDIA
(Cont'd from p 125)
H
Symptoms resolve—no follow-up necessary
I
Symptoms persist—pain relief measures + 2nd line agent
J
Symptoms persist—pain relief measures + 3rd line agent
(Consider tympanocentesis)

Dowell SF, Butler JC, Giebink SG, et al. Acute otitis media: Management and surveillance in an era of pneumococcal resistance—a report from the Drug-Resistant Streptococcus pneumoniae Therapeutic Working Group. Pediatr Infect Dis J 1999;18:1–9.

Englehard D, Strauss N, Jorczak-Sarni L, et al. Randomised study of myringotomy, amoxycillin/clavulanate, or both for acute otitis media. Lancet 1989;2:141–3.

Hathaway TJ, Katz HP, Dershewitz RA, Marx TJ. Acute otitis media: who needs posttreatment follow-up? Pediatrics 1994;94:143–7.

Heikkinen T, Ruuskanen O. Signs and symptoms predicting acute otitis media. Arch Pediatr Adolesc Med 1995;149:26–9.

Heikkinen T, Thint M, Chonmaitree T. Prevalence of various respiratory viruses in the middle ear during acute otitis media. N Engl J Med 1999;340:260.

Hoberman A, Paradise JL, Reynolds E, Urkin J. Efficacy of Auralgan for ear pain in children with acute otitis media. Arch Pediatr Adolesc Med 1997;151:675–8.

Leibovitz E, Raiz S, Piglansky L, et al. Resistance pattern of middle ear fluid isolates in acute otitis media recently treated with antibiotics. Pediatr Infect Dis J 1998;17:463–9.

Marchant C. Acute otitis media, antibiotics, children and clinical trial design. Pediatr Infect Dis J 2002;21:891–3.

Pichichero ME, Casey JR, Hoberman A, Schwartz R. Pathogens causing recurrent and difficult-to-treat acute otitis media, 2003–2006. Clin Pediatr 2008;47(9):901–6.

Rosenfeld RM. Natural history of untreated otitis media. Laryngoscope 2003;113(10):1645–57.

Rosenfeld RM, Vertrees JE, Carr J, et al. Clinical efficacy of antimicrobial drugs for acute otitis media: metaanalysis of 5400 children from 33 randomized trials. J Pediatr 1994;124:355–67.

Schrag SJ, Phil D, Pena C, et al. Effect of short-course, high-dose amoxicillin therapy on resistant pneumococcal carriage: a randomized trial. JAMA 2001;286:49–56.

Spiro DM, Tay K-Y, Arnold DH, et al. Wait-and-see prescription for the treatment of acute otitis media: a randomized controlled trial. JAMA 2006;296(10):1235–41.

Subcommittee on Management of Acute Otitis Media. Diagnosis and management of acute otitis media. Pediatrics 2004;113(5):1451–65.

Van Zuijlen DA, Schilder AG, Van Balen FA, Hoes AW. National differences in incidence of acute mastoiditis: relationship to prescribing patterns of antibiotics for acute otitis media? Pediatr Infect Dis J 2001;20(2):140–4.

Otitis Media with Effusion

Donald H. Arnold, MD, MPH, and David M. Spiro, MD, MPH

DEFINITIONS AND EPIDEMIOLOGY

Otitis media with effusion (OME) and other disorders of the middle ear commonly encountered in infants and children have been described by various and inconsistent terms. We refer to otitis media (OM) as an umbrella term including acute otitis media (AOM) and OME. This is biologically plausible terminology, because OME is frequently a result of AOM, and the two disorders generally have the common causative pathway of eustachian tube dysfunction.

OME is defined as the presence of fluid in the middle ear not accompanied by signs or symptoms of acute infection or inflammation. Previously, OME was subcategorized as residual (≤4 months) or persistent (>4 months). However, this categorization has no clinical relevance because in the absence of risk factors (see later), surgical interventions based on duration-based criteria have been demonstrated to not improve developmental outcomes. Duration and laterality should nonetheless be documented, with duration defined as the time since the AOM episode or from the time the effusion was noted.

OME is common, occurring in 90% of children before school age, and is most prevalent between 6 months and 4 years of age. As duration of OME increases, the likelihood of spontaneous resolution decreases. However, most episodes resolve spontaneously within 3 months.

PATHOGENESIS

Eustachian tube dysfunction is the common pathway to AOM and OME. Frequent causes of eustachian tube dysfunction include upper respiratory viral infections, secondhand smoke or other environmental insults, craniofacial anomalies, and concurrent AOM. The result is a middle-ear effusion that, in the presence of negative middle-ear pressure, becomes more viscous and thick over time.

Risk factors have been identified that may increase the likelihood of developmental delay or dysfunction as a result of OME. These include permanent hearing loss unrelated to OME, craniofacial abnormalities (e.g., Robin sequence, CHARGE association, cleft palate), syndromes with cognitive or language delay (e.g., trisomy 21 syndrome), underlying speech or language disorder, visual dysfunction (because these children depend more on the sense of hearing), or established developmental delays.

CLINICAL MANIFESTATIONS AND DIAGNOSIS

Signs and symptoms of OME in children include mild otalgia, a sensation of fullness in the ear, a popping sound, decline in school performance, and mild ataxia manifesting as clumsiness or delayed motor development. Infants and younger children may have more nonspecific signs including irritability and disrupted sleep. The manifestation most frequently of concern is conductive hearing loss with potential speech and language delay. Nonetheless, up to 50% of patients with OME have no signs or symptoms.

The tympanic membrane (TM) may be cloudy with confluent fluid, an air–fluid level, or bubbles. The most important distinction during the examination is between AOM and OME, and it must be emphasized that the former requires evidence of middle-ear inflammation.

This is of great importance to the child, because OME should not be treated with antibiotics. In this regard, it is important to obtain an atraumatic examination; when an infant or child cries, the TM turns red almost immediately. Indeed, this examination is the high art of pediatric care.

The primary diagnostic tool for OME should be pneumatic otoscopy. This is a cost-effective, sensitive, and specific bedside tool, particularly in the hands of an experienced examiner. The examination can be performed painlessly if the speculum is gently inserted only into the cartilaginous portion (outer third) of the ear canal.

Tympanometry is a valuable adjunct, allowing reliable documentation of middle-ear status in patients 4 months and older. Although acoustic reflectometry is an alternative method that does not require an airtight seal, pneumatic otoscopy remains the criterion standard.

OVERALL CLINICAL APPROACH

Practice primary prevention: Eliminate or decrease secondhand smoke, move the infant or child to a day-care setting with fewer than four to six children or out of day-care altogether, encourage breast-feeding, and avoid bottle propping and other at-risk practices.

"Watchful waiting" is the key management principle. Resist the urge to intervene for this self-limited condition ("just don't do something, stand there") while monitoring for hearing deficits, language or other developmental delay, coordination or other motor problems, behavioral dysfunction and complications such as cholesteatoma, retraction pockets, and other TM and middle-ear abnormalities. Antibiotics do not prevent any of these complications.

Refer to an otolaryngologist if any of the events in item E occur. Advocate for the patient, particularly for appropriate and prudent use of pneumatic equalization tube (PET) placement and other surgical interventions. The risk associated with anesthesia and the procedures is low, but it is not zero.

COMPLICATIONS

OME may predispose to retraction pockets or atelectasis of the TM, ossicular damage, and cholesteatoma. As noted earlier, the most important element of management is watchful waiting, with emphasis on "watchful" to recognize these complications early and to provide appropriate otolaryngologic referral.

MANAGEMENT

A. Because OME is self-limited in most instances, with effusion resolving within 3 months, management consists primarily of watchful waiting. Children without risk factors should be monitored for 3 months, the specific interval based on physician and parental preference and individual patient characteristics. Evaluations at these visits should include pneumatic otoscopy, tympanometry, or both.

B. Patients without risk factors who have OME for more than 3 months should have their hearing tested and should have retesting at 3- to 6-month intervals. Initial testing for children older than 4 years may be performed by the primary care physician. Patients who cannot be tested in the primary care setting and those who are younger than 4 years should be tested by an audiologist. Patients with moderate hearing loss *in the better hearing ear* (≥40 dB) are surgical candidates. Those with mild deficits (21–39 dB) should be managed based on duration of effusion, language development, severity of hearing deficit, and parental preference. Those with normal hearing (<20 dB deficit) should have repeat testing at 3- to 6-month intervals. Language testing by a speech-language pathologist should be considered for patients with hearing deficits.

C. For infants and children with risk factors, the earlier recommendations for monitoring and testing should be accelerated. Other interventions (e.g., hearing aids) may be necessary, and surgical intervention (e.g., PET scans) may be applied earlier.

D. Medications have no role in management of OME. Antibiotics may have minimal short-term (2–8 weeks) benefit but have statistically and clinically nonsignificant benefit overall. Treating OME with antibiotics only results in exposing the child to the risks of these medications (e.g., allergy, bacterial resistance). Antihistamines and decongestants are similarly ineffective, and decongestant preparations are not safe in young children and infants. Corticosteroids have no benefit over placebo and also expose the patient to undue risk. Intranasal steroids are safer but of no benefit.

E. Surgery is indicated in three settings:

1. Patients with OME for 4 months or longer with persistent signs and symptoms or hearing loss
2. Patients with risk factors who have recurrent or persistent OME
3. Patients with OME and structural damage to the middle ear or TM

F. PET placement is the initial recommended procedure. For patients who have PET extrusion and who continue to meet one of the three earlier criteria, one of the following is appropriate:

1. Adenoidectomy with PET placement (for age <4 years)
2. Adenoidectomy with myringotomy or PET placement (for children >4 years of age)

Adenoidectomy may be contraindicated in the patient with cleft palate.

References

American Academy of Family Physicians, American Academy of Otolaryngology-Head and Neck Surgery, American Academy of Pediatrics Subcommittee on Otitis Media with Effusion. Otitis media with effusion. Pediatrics 2004;113:1412–29.

Burke P, Bain J, Robinson D, Dunleavey J. Acute red ear in children: controlled trial of non-antibiotic treatment in general practice. BMJ 1991;303:558–62.

Butler CC, Van Der Voort JH. Oral or topical nasal steroids for hearing loss associated with otitis media with effusion in children. Cochrane Database Syst Rev 2002;(4):CD001935.

Marchant CD, Shurin PA, Turczyk VA, et al. Course and outcome of otitis media in early infancy: a prospective study. J Pediatr 1984;104:826–31.

Paradise JL, Feldman HM, Campbell TF, et al. Effect of early or delayed insertion of tympanostomy tubes for persistent otitis media on developmental outcomes at the age of three years. N Engl J Med 2001;344:1179–87.

Paradise JL, Feldman HM, Campbell, TF, et al. Early versus delayed insertion of tympanostomy tubes for persistent otitis media: developmental outcomes at the age of three years in relation to prerandomization illness patterns and hearing levels. Pediatr Infect Dis J 2003;22:309–314.

Paradise JL, Rockette HE, Colborn DK, et al. Otitis media in 2253 Pittsburgh-area infants: prevalence and risk factors during the first two years of life. Pediatrics 1997;99:318–33.

Rosenfeld RM, Goldsmith AJ, Tetlus L, Balzano A. Quality of life for children with otitis media. Arch Otolaryngol Head Neck Surg 1997;123:1049-54.

Rovers MM, Krabbe PF, Straatman H, et al. Randomised controlled trial of the effect of ventilation tubes (grommets) on quality of life at age 1-2 years. Arch Dis Child 2001;84:45-9.

Rovers MM, Schilder AG, Zielhuis GA, Rosenfeld RM. Otitis media. Lancet 2004;363:465-73.

Rovers MM, Straatman H, Ingels K, et al. The effect of ventilation tubes on language development in infants with otitis media with effusion: a randomized trial. Pediatrics 2000;106:E42.

Shekelle P, Takata G, Chan LS, et al. Diagnosis, natural history, and late effects of otitis media with effusion. Evid Rep Technol Assess (Summ) 2002;(55):1-5.

Stool SE, Berg AO, Berman S, Carney CJ. Otitis media with effusion in young children (Clinical practice guideline, no. 12; AHCPR Publication No. 94-0622). Washington, DC: Agency for Health Care Policy and Research, Public Health Service, U.S. Department of Health and Human Services; 1994.

Teele DW, Klein JO, Rosner BA. Epidemiology of otitis media in children. Ann Otol Rhinol Laryngol Suppl 1980;89:5-6.

Tos M. Epidemiology and natural history of secretory otitis. Am J Otol 1984;5:459-62.

Tracy JM, Demain JG, Hoffman KM, Goetz DW. Intranasal beclomethasone as an adjunct to treatment of chronic middle ear effusion. Ann Allergy Asthma Immunol 1998;80:198-206.

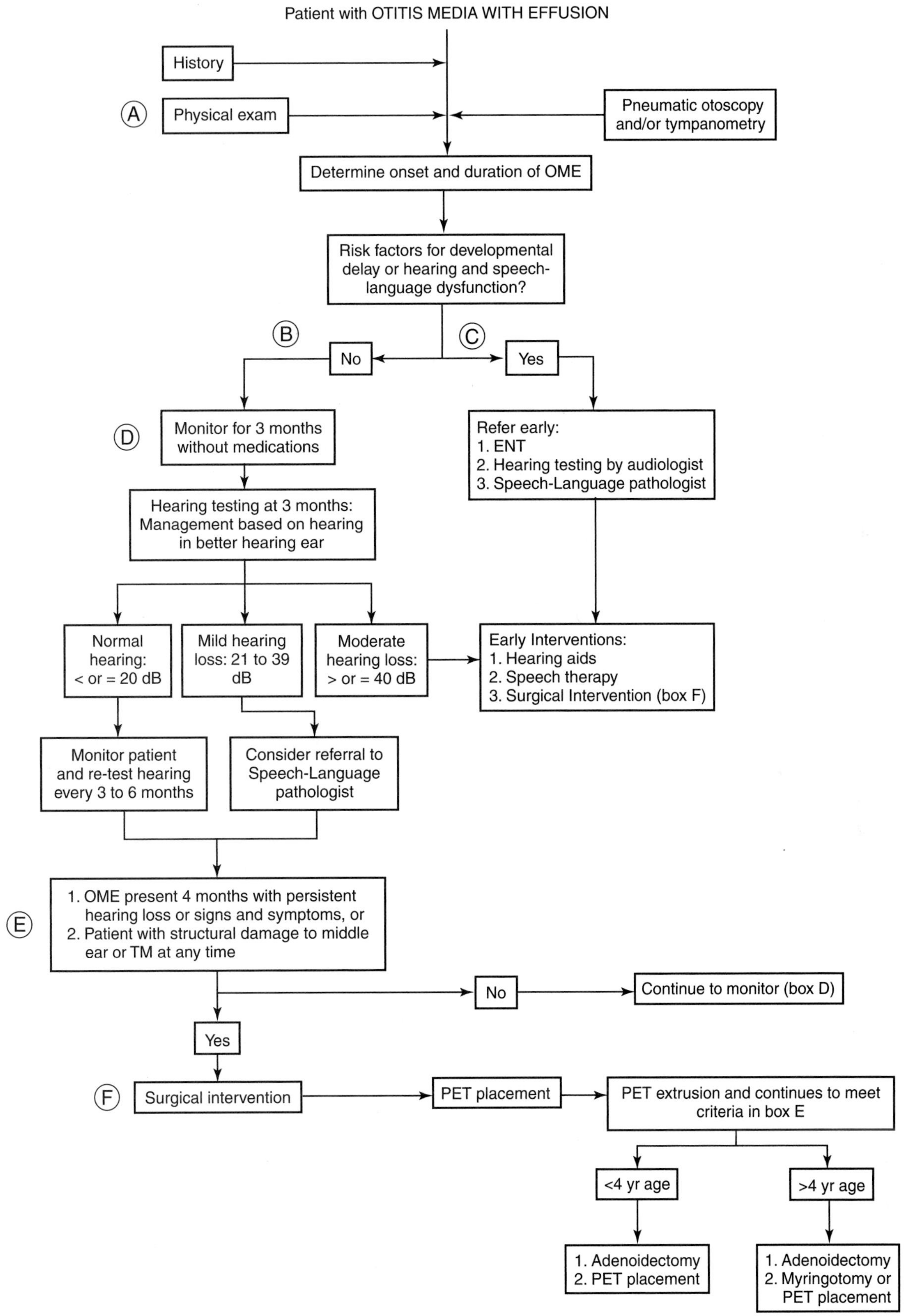

Patient with OTITIS MEDIA WITH EFFUSION
History
A
Physical exam
Pneumatic otoscopy and/or tympanometry
Determine onset and duration of OME
Risk factors for developmental delay or hearing and speech-language dysfunction?
B
No
C
Yes
D
Monitor for 3 months without medications
Refer early:
1. ENT
2. Hearing testing by audiologist
3. Speech-Language pathologist
Hearing testing at 3 months: Management based on hearing in better hearing ear
Normal hearing: < or = 20 dB
Mild hearing loss: 21 to 39 dB
Moderate hearing loss: > or = 40 dB
Early Interventions:
1. Hearing aids
2. Speech therapy
3. Surgical Intervention (box F)
Monitor patient and re-test hearing every 3 to 6 months
Consider referral to Speech-Language pathologist
E
1. OME present 4 months with persistent hearing loss or signs and symptoms, or
2. Patient with structural damage to middle ear or TM at any time
No
Continue to monitor (box D)
Yes
F
Surgical intervention
PET placement
PET extrusion and continues to meet criteria in box E
<4 yr age
>4 yr age
1. Adenoidectomy
2. PET placement
1. Adenoidectomy
2. Myringotomy or PET placement

Mastoiditis

Donald H. Arnold, MD, MPH, and David M. Spiro, MD, MPH

DEFINITIONS

The mastoid air cells are a mucous membrane–lined, diploic portion of the temporal bone. At birth, this structure consists of the one-cell antrum, and by 3 years of age, most children have experienced development of multiple mastoid air cells. This structure communicates with the distal end of the middle-ear cavity via a small canal, the *aditus ad antrum.*

PATHOGENESIS

Because of this direct communication with the middle ear, inflammation of the mastoid accompanies episodes of acute otitis media (AOM). Mastoiditis is defined as clinically significant inflammation and/or infection of the mastoid that leads to purulent material within the air cells and obstruction to drainage of this material. It remains the most frequent extracranial complication of AOM. The infection may spread to form a subperiosteal abscess. This might be suspected when the patient does not improve within 48 hours of initiating antibiotic treatment and may require incision and drainage.

Acute mastoiditis was a common complication of AOM before effective antibiotics were available for this infection. It is generally categorized as acute or chronic, and this chapter pertains to acute mastoiditis. Acute mastoiditis remains a potentially serious complication of AOM.

CAUSATIVE FACTORS

The bacterial organisms causing acute mastoiditis do not entirely parallel those causing AOM. The most common are *Streptococcus pneumoniae* and *Pseudomonas aeruginosa,* as well as *Staphylococcus aureus* and nontypeable *Haemophilus influenzae.* Anaerobic organisms may also cause mastoiditis. However, the prevalence of bacterial organisms may be dependent on age and location. A recent comprehensive review of published cases noted a mean age of 32 months, and *S. pneumoniae* as the most frequently isolated bacterium. Reports note equal prevalence of *S. pneumoniae* and *P. aeruginosa* (20%–25% each) and group A Streptococcus (15%). In contrast, studies from the United States have demonstrated a younger median age (12 months) in children with mastoiditis caused by *S. pneumoniae.*

Risk factors for mastoiditis are those for AOM and include underlying congenital or acquired immune deficiencies and anatomic abnormalities such as cholesteatoma. However, the most frequent predisposing factors include sidestream smoke, day-care attendance, and supine feeding position.

CLINICAL MANIFESTATIONS AND DIAGNOSIS

The classic clinical manifestation of acute mastoiditis is protrusion of the auricle and anterior bowing of the external auditory canal. Although mastoiditis may occur in the absence of these findings, most often the diagnosis can be established at the bedside based on these clinical features. Additional physical findings may include postauricular pain, erythema and swelling, tenderness of the mastoid process, and the nonspecific findings of sleep disruption, irritability, and decreased oral intake. In patients pretreated with antibiotics, physical findings may be modified and subtle, and the course of illness more indolent.

Plain radiographs are of limited utility because they may be normal in the presence of mastoiditis and, conversely, abnormal in the absence of the infection. Noncontrast computed tomography (CT) scan of the temporal bone is the imaging modality most often used. However, this diagnosis can generally be made clinically without exposing the child to CT radiation. Consultation with a pediatric otolaryngologist is recommended once mastoiditis is suspected clinically.

TREATMENT

Gram stain may provide valuable information for initial antibiotic selection, and culture results are the most definitive source for antibiotic choice. In most cases, a third-generation cephalosporin (e.g., ceftriaxone, cefotaxime) in combination with clindamycin (for anaerobe and staph coverage) is an appropriate antibiotic regimen. In patients with concern for *P. aeruginosa* (e.g., a child with a history of chronic AOM), an aminoglycoside (e.g., gentamicin, tobramycin), meropen em, or semisynthetic penicillin with antipseudomonal coverage (e.g., ticarcillin-clavulanate, piperacillin-tazobactam) should be added to the regimen. Recommended duration of treatment has ranged from 10 to 21 days, and the portion of this composed of parenteral treatment must be based on clinical response.

Surgical intervention is indicated in the presence of intracranial complications and may include simple mastoidectomy with or without tympanoplasty or pneumatic equalization tube placement. Indications for mastoidectomy are not uniform but may include the presence of cholesteatoma or extratemporal bone suppurative complications. Patients treated surgically appear to respond after surgery to oral antibiotics.

COMPLICATIONS

Extracranial complications include CN6 (abducens) or CN7 palsy, jugular venous thrombosis, internal carotid artery inflammation, and erosion. Intracranial complications include meningoencephalitis, venous sinus thrombosis, epidural or subdural abscess, and brain abscess. Changes in mental status or neurologic examination mandate immediate imaging to evaluate for these complications.

CLINICAL APPROACH

A. In the patient's history, ask about pain in the retroauricular area, as well as concerning central nervous system signs such as headache, emesis, neck pain, and mental status changes. Identify predisposing conditions such as recurrent or chronic otitis media and acquired or inherited immunodeficiency.

B. During the physical examination, observe and note any swelling, erythema, or tenderness of the retroauricular area. Examine the external auditory canal for anterior bowing or edema. Evaluate the child for meningeal signs, facial or abducens nerve palsies, and evidence of increased intracranial pressure.

C. Consider immediate ear, nose, and throat (ENT) consultation, particularly for the child who appears significantly ill. Mastoidectomy may be necessary to facilitate treatment of the abscess and to avoid intracranial or extracranial complications.

D. As noted earlier, CT imaging is not always necessary, and mild cases of mastoiditis may be diagnosed clinically and treated without imaging. However, if the child appears ill, has significant swelling or tenderness of the mastoid area, or notable pouting of the auricle, CT may be indicated to evaluate for subperiosteal abscess.

E. Gram stain and culture (anaerobic and aerobic) are essential to choosing appropriate antibiotic therapy. Initial antibiotics generally include a third-generation cephalosporin (e.g., ceftriaxone, cefotaxime) in combination with clindamycin (for anaerobe and staph coverage). In patients with concern for *P. aeruginosa* (e.g., a child with a history of chronic AOM), an aminoglycoside (e.g., gentamicin, tobramycin), meropenem, or semisynthetic penicillin with antipseudomonal coverage (e.g., ticarcillin-clavulanate, piperacillin-tazobactam) should be added to the regimen.

References

Brook I. Current management of upper respiratory tract and head and neck infections. Eur Arch Otorhinolaryngol 2009;266:315–23.

Butbul-Aviel Y, Miron D, Halevy R, et al. Acute mastoiditis in children: Pseudomonas aeruginosa as a leading pathogen. Int J Pediatr Otorhinolaryngol 2003;67:277–81.

Grant JCB. Grant's atlas of anatomy. 6th ed. Baltimore, MD: Williams & Wilkins; 1972.

Kaplan SL, Mason EO Jr, Wald ER, et al. Pneumococcal mastoiditis in children. Pediatrics 2000;106:695–9.

Moore JA, Wei JL, Smith HJ, Mayo MS. Treatment of pediatric suppurative mastoiditis: is peripherally inserted central catheter (PICC) antibiotic therapy necessary? Otolaryngol Head Neck Surg 2006;135:106–10.

Mostafa BE, El Fiky LM, El Sharnouby MM. Complications of suppurative otitis media: still a problem in the 21st century. ORL J Otorhinolaryngol Relat Spec 2009;71:87–92.

Nelson's pocket book of pediatric antimicrobial therapy. 16th ed. Buenos Aires: Alliance for World Wide Editing; 2006.

Oestreicher-Kedem Y, Raveh E, Kornreich L, et al. Complications of mastoiditis in children at the onset of a new millennium. Ann Otol Rhinol Laryngol 2005;114:147–52.

Taylor MF, Berkowitz RG. Indications for mastoidectomy in acute mastoiditis in children. Ann Otol Rhinol Laryngol 2004;113:69–72.

van den Aardweg MT, Rovers MM, de Ru JA, et al. A systematic review of diagnostic criteria for acute mastoiditis in children. Otol Neurotol 2008;29:751–7.

Zanetti D, Nassif N. Indications for surgery in acute mastoiditis and their complications in children. Int J Pediatr Otorhinolaryngol 2006;70:1175–82.

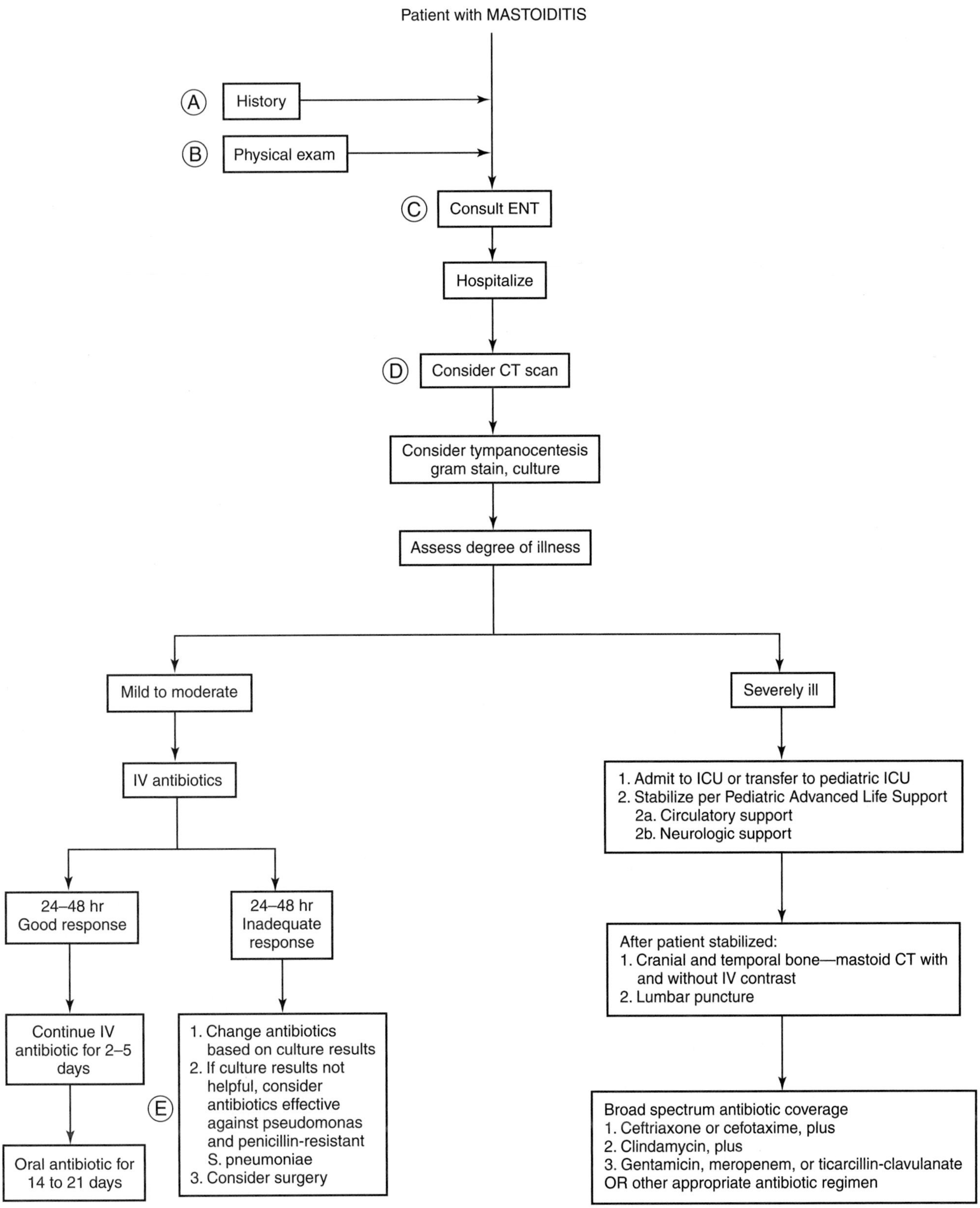
Patient with MASTOIDITIS
A
History
B
Physical exam
C
Consult ENT
Hospitalize
D
Consider CT scan
Consider tympanocentesis gram stain, culture
Assess degree of illness
Mild to moderate
IV antibiotics
24–48 hr Good response
Continue IV antibiotic for 2–5 days
Oral antibiotic for 14 to 21 days
24–48 hr Inadequate response
E
1. Change antibiotics based on culture results
2. If culture results not helpful, consider antibiotics effective against pseudomonas and penicillin-resistant S. pneumoniae
3. Consider surgery
Severely ill
1. Admit to ICU or transfer to pediatric ICU
2. Stabilize per Pediatric Advanced Life Support
2a. Circulatory support
2b. Neurologic support
After patient stabilized:
1. Cranial and temporal bone—mastoid CT with and without IV contrast
2. Lumbar puncture
Broad spectrum antibiotic coverage
1. Ceftriaxone or cefotaxime, plus
2. Clindamycin, plus
3. Gentamicin, meropenem, or ticarcillin-clavulanate
OR other appropriate antibiotic regimen

Epistaxis

Patricia J. Yoon, MD

The nose has a rich vascular supply, receiving blood flow from both the internal and external carotid arteries. These two systems meet in an area of the anterior septum known as Little's area or the Kiesselbach plexus. This area accounts for most pediatric epistaxis. Epistaxis is relatively uncommon before age 2 years and is most frequent between the ages of 3 and 8 years.

A. In the patient's history, note the frequency, duration, and volume of the bleeding. It is important to note laterality: Does the bleeding predominantly occur from one side, both sides separately but equally, or out of both sides simultaneously? Identify any precipitating factors such as trauma (e.g., nose picking). Inquire about nasal allergies and whether the epistaxis is worse during certain seasons. Allergies may exacerbate epistaxis, as may dry winter air. Has the patient had problems with easy bruising or excessive bleeding from procedures such as dental work or circumcision? Is there a family history of bleeding disorders? Medications such as NSAIDs and nasal corticosteroid sprays may worsen epistaxis. Note any other medical conditions that may contribute to bleeding such as hypertension (e.g., renal disease) or chronic liver disease. Inquire about nasal obstruction; neoplastic lesions may present with bleeding and nasal obstruction.

B. Perform a complete physical examination. Examination of the nose will usually reveal a dry or excoriated anterior septum with fresh clots or old crusts. Prominent blood vessels are often seen in this area. Look for signs of nasal trauma. Note the appearance of the turbinates; boggy, pale turbinates are indicative of allergic rhinitis. Look for signs of infection/sinusitis, such as purulent nasal drainage. Septal deviation can cause turbulent airflow and resultant dryness and epistaxis. Are there any nasal masses such as polyps or other obstructing tumors? Are telangiectasias, hemangiomas, varicosities, or petechiae present in the nose or elsewhere?

C. Blood tests are not routinely obtained for most patients who initially present with recurrent epistaxis. However, they are indicated if the patient has had copious prolonged bleeding, recurrent bleeding despite preventive measures, or a personal or family history of easy bleeding or a bleeding disorder. A complete blood cell count (CBC; including hematocrit and platelet count), prothrombin time (PT), and activated partial thromboplastin time (aPTT) should be obtained. Further testing such as bleeding time, platelet function assay, and other coagulation assays may be ordered if warranted. A computed tomography (CT) scan may be ordered if neoplasm is suspected.

D. The differential diagnosis of epistaxis is extensive (Table 1). Most commonly, recurrent epistaxis is due to inflammation or trauma. Hematologic conditions may cause epistaxis, as may vascular abnormalities. Epistaxis is the most common manifestation of hereditary hemorrhagic telangiectasia (HHT). Neoplastic lesions (benign or malignant) may present with bleeding, nasal obstruction, or both. Juvenile nasopharyngeal angiofibroma is a highly vascular tumor that presents in adolescent boys with nasal obstruction and usually severe, recurrent epistaxis. CT scan should be obtained if this is suspected.

E. For patients who have a history of recurrent epistaxis, without current active bleeding and without otherwise concerning history or examination, the first line of preventive management is improved nasal moisture. This may be accomplished by use of a room humidifier (particularly in cold, dry climates), nasal saline spray, and once or twice daily application of a water-based lubricant (such as a nasal saline gel), antibiotic ointment, or petroleum jelly (Vaseline) to the anterior septum. Digital trauma or nose rubbing should be discouraged. If allergies seem to be exacerbating the nosebleeds, treatment with antihistamines may decrease the frequency. If a patient is using nasal corticosteroid sprays, proper technique must be used that directs the spray superolaterally, and away from the anterior septum. If bleeding persists, the spray may need to be discontinued. If a patient has persistent recurrent epistaxis despite these measures, cautery with silver nitrate may be elected. The laterality of the bleeding is important to note: Only one side of the septum should be cauterized at a time, because simultaneous bilateral cauterization carries a risk for septal perforation. In children aged 10 and older, this can often be accomplished in the clinic; younger children usually require a general anesthetic.

F. In the setting of active bleeding, the patient should gently blow out any clots, sit upright, and lean forward so that blood is not swallowed. A topical vasoconstrictor, such as oxymetazoline, may be sprayed into the nose. Firm, constant pressure should then be applied to the anterior septum by pinching the nose shut for 5 minutes by the clock. This will control most cases of epistaxis. If a bleeding source can be identified, it may be cauterized with silver nitrate. If the bleeding persists, anterior nasal packing may be necessary. CBC, PT, and PTT should also be ordered. In children, oxidized cellulose or microfibrillar collagen have typically been used for anterior packing, because these dissolve and usually do not need to be removed. Because of the risk for toxic shock syndrome, the packing material should be coated with antibiotic ointment before insertion, and the patient should be placed on oral antibiotic therapy for the duration. If bilateral packs are necessary, the airway must also be monitored. In recent years, topical hemostatic agents have been developed for epistaxis control, such as collagen-derived particles and topical bovine-derived thrombin applied as a viscous gel. These also obviate the need for pack removal.

(Continued on page 138)

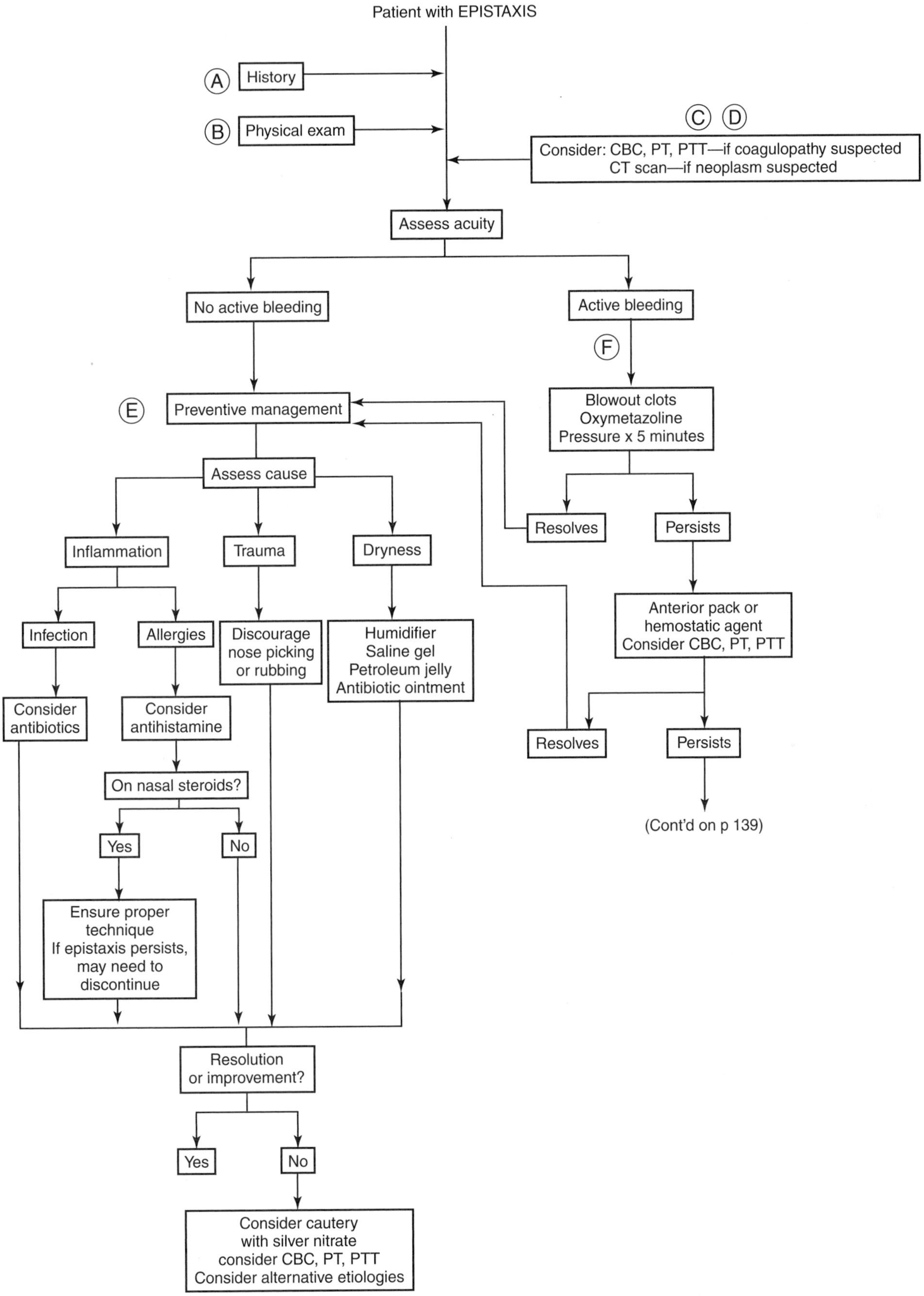
Patient with EPISTAXIS
A History
B Physical exam
C D
Consider: CBC, PT, PTT—if coagulopathy suspected
CT scan—if neoplasm suspected
Assess acuity
No active bleeding
Active bleeding
F
Blowout clots
Oxymetazoline
Pressure x 5 minutes
E Preventive management
Assess cause
Resolves
Persists
Inflammation
Trauma
Dryness
Anterior pack or
hemostatic agent
Consider CBC, PT, PTT
Infection
Allergies
Discourage
nose picking
or rubbing
Humidifier
Saline gel
Petroleum jelly
Antibiotic ointment
Consider
antibiotics
Consider
antihistamine
Resolves
Persists
On nasal steroids?
(Cont'd on p 139)
Yes
No
Ensure proper
technique
If epistaxis persists,
may need to
discontinue
Resolution
or improvement?
Yes
No
Consider cautery
with silver nitrate
consider CBC, PT, PTT
Consider alternative etiologies

Table 1. **Causes of Epistaxis in Children**

Common Causes

Inflammation

Upper respiratory infections
- Viral
- Bacterial

Allergic rhinitis
Childhood exanthems
Vestibulitis (furunculosis)
Nonallergic rhinitis with eosinophilia
Foreign body

Trauma

Dry air
Outdoor and indoor air pollution
Patient-induced (nose picking)
Facial fracture or blunt trauma
Sudden barometric pressure changes

Uncommon Causes

Anatomic

- Severe septal deviation
- Postsurgical adhesions or atrophic rhinitis

Hematologic

- Platelet abnormalities
  - Primary (idiopathic thrombocytopenic purpura)
  - Acquired (aspirin, leukemia)
- Coagulation defects
  - Primary (von Willebrand, hemophilia)
  - Acquired (warfarin, liver disease)

Neoplasms

- Benign
  - Nasopharyngeal angiofibroma
  - Pyogenic granuloma
  - Papillomas
- Malignant
  - Rhabdomyosarcoma
  - Lymphoma

Vascular Abnormalities

- Hereditary hemorrhagic telangiectasia
- Internal carotid pseudoaneurysm
- Hemangioma

Trauma

- Nasogastric or nasotracheal tube placement
- Postsurgical
- Chemical and caustic agents

From: Manning SC, Culbertson MC. Epistaxis. In: Bluestone CD, Stool SE, Alper CM, et al, editors. Pediatric otolaryngology. 4th ed. Philadelphia: Saunders; 2003. p. 925–30.

G. In the rare instances where these measures fail to control bleeding, a superior or posterior source of bleeding must be suspected. In a stable patient, nasal endoscopy should be performed in an effort to visualize the source. If a posterior/superior source can be identified, cautery may be performed under a general anesthetic. Alternatively, in the emergent setting, a posterior pack may be placed in conjunction with the anterior pack. This may consist of gauze or a saline-filled balloon that sits in the nasopharynx. Patients with posterior packing must be admitted for airway observation.

H. For uncontrolled bleeding, angiography and arterial ligation or embolization may be required. The anterior and posterior ethmoidal arteries and the internal maxillary artery may be ligated.

I. HHT may be treated with laser coagulation or septodermoplasty. There are reports that hormone therapy may decrease epistaxis in HHT, but this has yet to be proved.

References

Burton MJ, Doree CJ. Interventions for recurrent idiopathic epistaxis (nosebleeds) in children. Cochrane Database Syst Rev 2004;(1):CD004461.

Douglas R, Wormald PJ. Update on epistaxis. Curr Opin Otolaryngol Head Neck Surg 2007;15:180–3.

Manning SC, Culbertson MC. Epistaxis. In: Bluestone CD, Stool SE, Alper CM, et al, editors. Pediatric otolaryngology. 4th ed. Philadelphia: Saunders; 2003. p. 925–30.

Sharathkumar AA, Shapiro A. Hereditary haemorrhagic telangiectasia. Haemophilia 2008;14:1269–80.

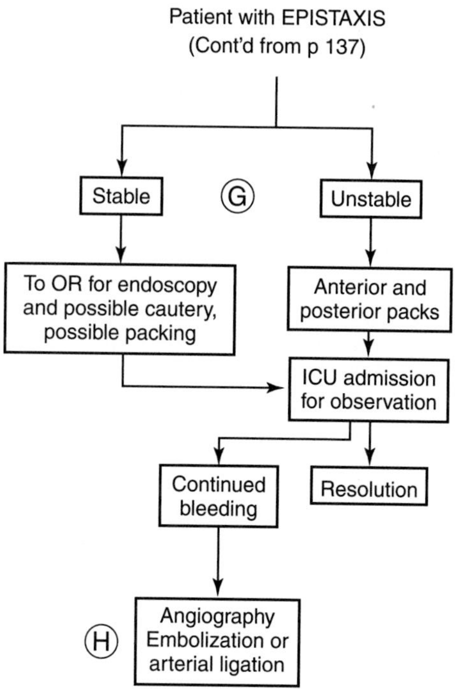
Patient with EPISTAXIS
(Cont'd from p 137)
Stable
G
Unstable
To OR for endoscopy and possible cautery, possible packing
Anterior and posterior packs
ICU admission for observation
Continued bleeding
Resolution
H
Angiography Embolization or arterial ligation

Nasal Congestion

Megan G. Henderson, MD, FAAP

Nasal congestion (rhinitis) is inflammation of the nasal passages with subsequent production of rhinorrhea. The most common cause is viral rhinosinusitis, otherwise known as the common cold. The exact incidence is estimated to average 6 to 12 upper respiratory infections each year in the pediatric population. Usually these will spontaneously resolve within 7 to 10 days. However, about 6% to 13% of children with viral rhinosinusitis go on to acquire acute bacterial sinusitis (ABS). Another principle cause of chronic rhinitis is allergic rhinitis of the seasonal or perennial type. All other causes are less frequent (Table 1). A directed history and examination of the patient should help clarify the diagnosis and subsequent treatment plan.

A. History: In the patient's history, generalized malaise and decrease appetite is quite common. Fever early in the course may occur in rhinosinusitis but is clearly not necessary for a diagnosis. Inflammation of the nasal-pharyngeal epithelium can cause sneezing, pharyngitis, cough, postnasal drip, and throat clearing. Headache and facial pain, with or without intermittent periorbital swelling, may be present in sinusitis. Inquire about symptom onset, duration, and severity, as well as other contributing factors. Seasonal variations of watery rhinorrhea and pruritic eyes or nose are indicative of allergic processes. Ask about exposure to allergens, irritants, climate changes, and current medications. Note a history of other atopic conditions in the family such as eczema, asthma, or allergies. Clear or purulent nasal discharge of less than 10 days, or improvement of symptoms by the tenth day, is an important factor to help discern between viral rhinosinusitis and bacterial processes, thus eliminating unnecessary use of antibiotics. ABS is defined as bacterial infection of the paranasal sinuses lasting longer than 10 days, but less than 30 days. Infection persisting between 30 to 90 days is called *subacute bacterial sinusitis.* Conditions persisting longer than 90 days are termed *chronic sinusitis.* Individuals with a history of allergic rhinitis, structural anomalies that obstruct the sinus cavity drainage (deviated nasal septum, nasal polyps), and gastroesophageal reflux disease are all more susceptible to ABS or recurrent bouts of ABS.

Disorders can be superimposed on each other or contribute to other disease states. Viral rhinosinusitis is the most common antecedent to bacterial sinusitis. Allergic rhinitis can predispose patients to sinus infections and contribute to poorly controlled asthma. Seasonal allergic rhinitis can be superimposed on perennial rhinitis. Overuse of nasal decongestants can exacerbate the symptoms as well.

B. Physical Examination: A good history is important because it may be impossible to discern between viral rhinovsinusitis and ABS by physical examination alone. Older patients may have facial tenderness to palpation with ABS. Any swelling of the area overlying the sinuses should be investigated to rule out Pott puffy tumor. Examination for dental abscesses and caries may reveal another cause of facial pain. The periorbital area should be examined for signs of vascular congestion: periorbital edema, infraorbital bluish discoloration (allergic shiners), Morgan–Dennie lines (skin folds under the lower eyelid), and ocular conjunctivitis—all of which are consistent with allergic processes. The nasal passages should be investigated for foreign bodies, anatomical obstruction, swollen pale blue turbinates (vascular congestion from allergies), or friable dry nasal membranes (rhinitis medicamentosa). An allergic crease may be visible across the nasal bridge from the allergic salute—a repetitive upward wiping of the nose in allergic rhinitis. The pharynx may have a cobblestoning pattern from postnasal drip. The lungs should be auscultated to assess for wheezing. With any mental status changes, focal neurologic deficits, or severe headache, severe sinusitis or cavernous venous thrombosis should be suspected.

C. Diagnostic Tests and Imaging: Laboratory and imaging tests are rarely indicated and are not helpful in the workup of a patient with rhinitis. Screening for an immunodeficiency, cystic fibrosis, or ciliary dyskinesias may be indicated with recurrent or persistent infections, the finding of nasal polyps, concomitant poor growth of a child, or a significant family history. Imaging studies of the sinuses to differentiate between viral and bacterial processes is not recommended for the diagnosis of uncomplicated ABS. Computed tomography (CT) may be indicated in the evaluation of individuals with recurrent or complicated ABS, who may be considered for surgery. Therefore, patients with severe pain, periorbital cellulitis, facial swelling, or suspected central nervous system involvement should have CT sinus studies performed and blood collected to rule out sepsis. Occasionally, sinus aspiration or lavage to obtain cultures will be indicated in the more severe cases.

Although an IgE-mediated process, serum RAST or skin prick testing is also rarely indicated in allergic rhinitis. Avoidance measures, antihistamines, and topical steroidal measures are certainly first-line therapies. However, serum RAST or skin-prick testing can help guide avoidance measures and/or immunotherapy when necessary for persistent severe allergic symptoms or worsening asthma with poorly controlled allergies.

D. Treatment: Most uncomplicated episodes of viral rhinosinusitis resolve within 5 to 7 days. One can consider analgesics, mechanical nasal clearance, and decongestants in older children. ABS is defined as inflammation of the normally sterile paranasal sinuses caused by a bacterial infection. Clinically, ABS has a persistence that differentiates it from viral rhinosinusitis. Most

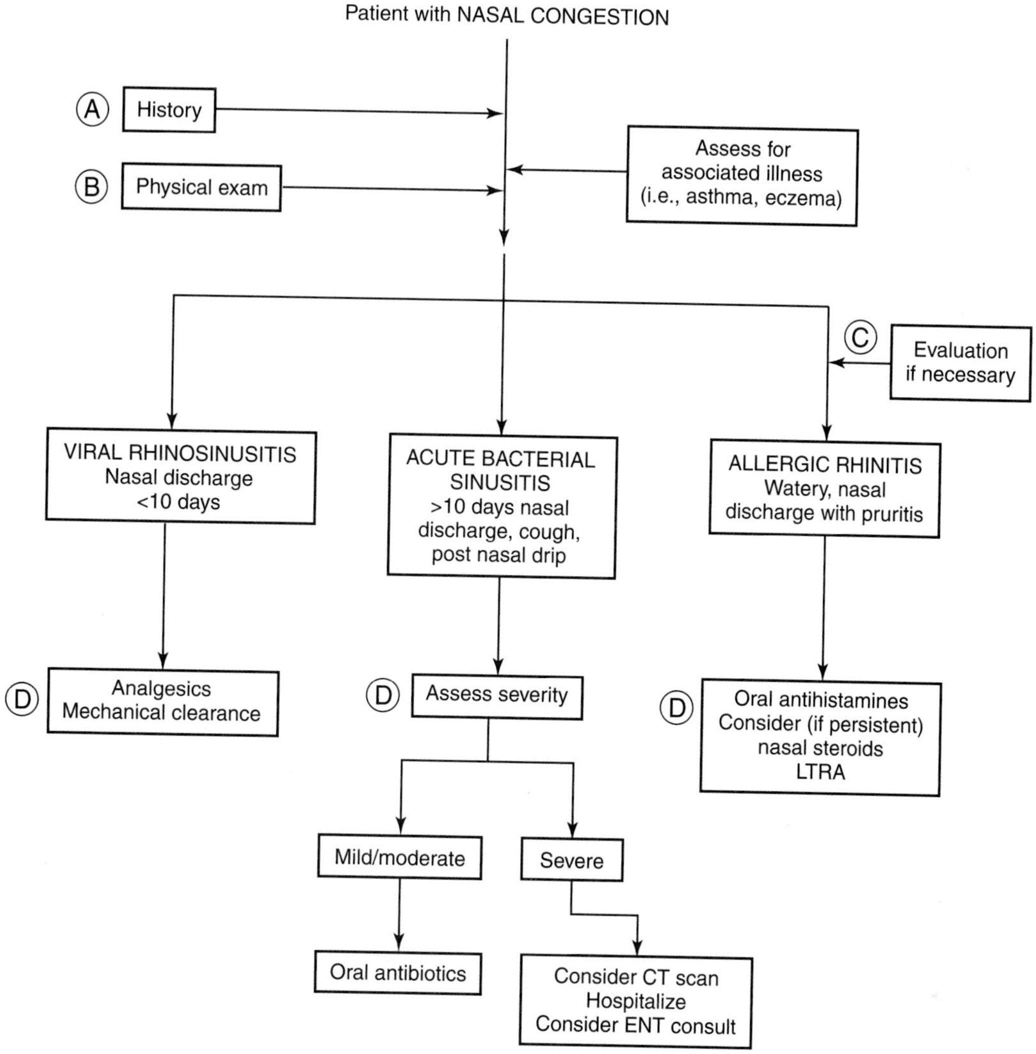
Patient with NASAL CONGESTION
A
History
B
Physical exam
Assess for associated illness (i.e., asthma, eczema)
C
Evaluation if necessary
VIRAL RHINOSINUSITIS
Nasal discharge
<10 days
ACUTE BACTERIAL SINUSITIS
>10 days nasal discharge, cough, post nasal drip
ALLERGIC RHINITIS
Watery, nasal discharge with pruritis
D
Analgesics
Mechanical clearance
D
Assess severity
D
Oral antihistamines
Consider (if persistent) nasal steroids
LTRA
Mild/moderate
Severe
Oral antibiotics
Consider CT scan
Hospitalize
Consider ENT consult

commonly, the complaint is nasal discharge of any quality (thin or thick; clear or purulent) or daytime cough, with worsening at night, for greater than 10 days without improvement. The child may not appear very ill but will complain of the persistence of the symptoms. Low-grade fever, headache, facial pain, and/or malodorous breath may also be reported.

The most common pathogens responsible for ABS are *Streptococcus pneumoniae,* nontypeable *Haemophilus influenzae,* and *Moraxella catarrhalis.* Less frequently, *Staphylococcus aureus* and anaerobic organisms are implicated in chronic bacterial sinusitis. Amoxicillin is the first-line drug for treatment of ABS, with high dosages of 80 to 90 mg/kg/day for children younger than 2 years and other risk factors for bacterial resistance—that is, day-care attendance or antibiotic exposure within the last 30 days. Patients with a penicillin allergy can be treated with an oral second- or third-generation cephalosporin. Patients with both penicillin and cephalosporin allergies can be treated with a macrolide, such as azithromycin. If oral therapy is not an option because of vomiting, a single dose of parenteral ceftriaxone, followed by a course of oral antibiotic is another option. Evidence is not clear on the optimal duration of therapy, including 10-, 14-, or 21-day courses. However, the treatment for 7 days after resolution of symptoms is well accepted.

Adjuvant therapies such as antihistamines, decongestants, and anti-inflammatory agents for the treatment of ABS have not been validated. Investigations into antihistamine and decongestant use are the most equivocal with results showing as much harm as benefit. Further study of topical nasal steroids would be helpful. Nasal irrigation with saline has shown to have some positive effect and is inexpensive. Certainly patients with severe ABS, with orbital or possible central nervous system involvement, should be hospitalized for receipt of intravenous antibiotics, subspecialty consult, and surgical drainage, if indicated.

First-line treatment of allergic rhinitis is an intranasal corticosteroid spray. Options include beclomethasone, flunisolide, fluticasone, and mometasone; they can also improve eye symptoms. Antihistamines can be a useful adjunct. The nonsedating antihistamines (loratadine, cetirizine, and fexofenadine) are available in pediatric liquid preparations. Oral decongestants (i.e., pseudoephedrine) are useful to decrease nasal congestion but are not indicated in younger children (<6 years of age), and topical decongestants (i.e., oxymetazoline) can be helpful but should not be used for more than 3 days secondary to the risk for rebound vasocongestion. Leukotriene receptor antagonists (i.e., montelukast) are approved for use in allergic rhinitis and asthma.

Table 1. **Differential Diagnosis of Rhinitis**

Disorder	Clinical Features
Viral rhinosinusitis	Clear or purulent rhinorrhea and cough with resolving symptoms by 7–10 days
Acute bacterial sinusitis	Nasal or postnasal discharge for longer than 10–14 days with sinus pressure, malodorous breath, headache
Allergic rhinitis	Watery rhinorrhea with pruritus of the nose, eyes, ears, or throat, sneezing, and allergic stigmata (allergic salute, swollen nasal turbinates)
Rhinitis medicamentosa	Rhinitis with dry, sore nasal mucosa and overuse of nasal decongestants
Chronic (recurrent) bacterial sinusitis	Greater than 90 days of acute bacterial sinusitis symptoms (see earlier)
Anatomic Abnormalities	
Foreign body	Unilateral nasal drainage with foreign matter visualized in the nares
Obstructing masses	Unilateral nasal drainage with deviating septum, nasal polyps
Ciliary dyskinesia	Situs inversus, recurrent otitis media, family history of ciliary dysfunction
Cystic fibrosis	Poor growth, diarrhea, clubbing of digits, recurrent pneumonias
Immunodeficiency	Poor growth, notable lack of tonsillar tissue or lymph nodes, recurrent or severe infections

Table 2. **Antibiotic Therapy for Paranasal Sinusitis in Children**

Antibiotics	Dosage	Product
Availability		
Oral Antibiotics		
Amoxicillin	45 mg/kg/day ÷ bid (usual dosage) or 90 mg/kg/day ÷ bid (high dosage)	Liquid: 125, 250, 400 mg/5 ml Capsules: 250, 500 mg Chewables: 125, 250 mg
Amoxicillin-clavulanate (Augmentin ES)	80–90 mg/kg/day with 6.4 mg/kg/day clavulanate ÷ bid	Liquid: 600 mg/5 ml Tablets: 2 g
Azithromycin	10 mg/kg/day on day 1, then 5 mg/kg/day for 4 days	Suspension: 100, 200 mg/5 ml Capsules: 250 mg, 600 mg
Cefdinir	14 mg/kg/day in 1 or 2 doses	Suspension: 125 mg/5 ml Capsules: 300 mg
Clindamycin	30–40 mg/kg/day ÷ tid	Suspension: 75 mg/5 ml Capsules: 75, 150, 300 mg
Intravenous Antibiotics for Hospitalized Patients		
Cefotaxime (Claforan)	50 mg/kg/dose IV every 8h	
Ceftriaxone (Rocephin)	75 mg/kg/dose IV every 24h	
Clindamycin (Cleocin)	10 mg/kg/dose every 6–8h	
Nafcillin	25 mg/kg/dose IV every 6h	
Vancomycin	40 mg/kg/24 hr divided every 6–8h	

Table 3. **Medications to Treat Rhinitis**

Drug Name	Age-Appropriate Dosage
Intranasal Corticosteroid	
Flunisolide	6–14 years: 1 spray/nostril tid, or 2 sprays bid >14 years: 1–2 sprays/nostril 2–4 times per day
Fluticasone propionate	≥4 years: 1 spray/nostril daily Adults: 2 sprays/nostril daily or 1 spray bid
Triamcinolone acetonide	6–12 years: 1–2 sprays/nostril daily >12 years: 2 sprays/nostril daily
Intranasal Antihistamine	
Azelastine	5–11 years: 1 spray per nostril bid ≥12 years: 2 sprays/nostril bid
Olopatadine	≥5 years: 2 sprays/nostril bid to tid
Intranasal Decongestant	
Oxymetazoline	≥6 years: per pediatric drug dosing
Oral Antihistamine—Nonsedating/Less Sedating	
Cetirizine	5 mg/5 ml syrup, 5-mg chew tablet, 10-mg chew tablet: 6–12 months: 2.5 mg once a day 1–5 years: 2.5 mg once or twice a day ≥6 years: 5 or 10 mg once a day
Desloratadine	2.5 mg/5 ml syrup, 2.5 mg RediTab, 5 mg RediTab/ tablet: 6–11 months: 2 ml = 1.0 mg daily 12 months to 11 years: 2.5 mg daily ≥12 years: 5 mg daily
Fexofenadine	30 mg/5 ml syrup, 30-/60-/180-mg tablets 6–11 years: 30 mg bid ≥12 years: 60 mg bid or 180 mg daily
Levocetirizine	2.5 mg/5 ml syrup, 5-mg tablet 6–11 years: 2.5 mg each evening ≥12 years: 5 mg each evening
Loratadine	5 mg/5 ml syrup, 5 mg RediTab, 10-mg tablet 2–5 years: 5 mg daily ≥6 years: 10 mg daily
Oral Antihistamine—Sedating	
Diphenhydramine	12.5 mg/5 ml syrup, 25-mg tablets 6 months to 2 years: per pediatric drug dosing ≥2 years: 5 mg/kg/day ÷ every 6h
Hydroxyzine HCL	10 mg/5 ml syrup; 10-/25-/50-mg tablets
Hydroxyzine pamoate	25 mg/5 ml; 10-/25-/50-mg tablets 2 mg/kg/day ÷ every 6-8h
Leukotriene antagonist	
Montelukast	4-mg granules; 4-mg chewable, 5-mg chewable; 10-mg tablet 6–23 months: 4-mg granules daily 2–5 years: 4 mg daily 6–14 years: 5 mg daily ≥15 years: 10 mg daily

References

Kelly LF. Pediatric cough and cold preparations. Pediatr Rev 2004;25: 115–23.

Krouse JH. Allergic rhinitis—current pharmacotherapy. Otolaryngol Clin North Am 2008;41(2):xi–ii.

Leung RS, Katail R. The diagnosis and management of acute and chronic sinusitis. Prim Care 2008;35(1):11–24, v–vi.

Mahr TA, Sheth. Update on allergic rhinitis. Pediatr Rev 2005; 26:284–8.

Nash D, Wald E. Sinusitis. Pediatr Rev 2001;22:111–6.

Taylor A, Adam HM. Sinusitis. Pediatr Rev 2006;27:395–7.

Cervical Lymphadenitis/ Adenopathy

Patricia J. Yoon, MD, and Stephen Berman, MD

Lymphadenopathy, enlargement of lymph nodes, typically results from either inflammation (lymphadenitis) or neoplastic infiltration of the lymph nodes. The cervical nodes filter lymphatics from the head and neck, and may enlarge with a variety of infections ranging from viral upper respiratory to dental to soft tissue infections of the scalp or face. Cervical nodes that are tender, with or without erythema, suggest lymphadenitis. Unilateral acute cervical lymphadenitis is caused by *Staphylococcus aureus* or *Streptococcus pyogenes* in 80% of cases.

A. In the patient's history, note the duration for which the mass has been present, determine whether it has been changing in size or character, and whether it has been painful. If painful, determine whether salivation exacerbates the pain (sialadenitis). Record any treatment already undertaken (i.e., antibiotics), and its effect on the size and character of the mass. Ask about the history of dental problems. If the mass is thought to be a lymph node, inquire specifically about previous local infections in the area drained by the node. Reactive lymph nodes are the most common cause of adenopathy in children. Children with acute cervical lymphadenitis often have a history of preceding illness, such as an upper respiratory infection, tonsillitis, or otitis media. Note exposure to animals (cat-scratch disease [CSD], tularemia, brucellosis, anthrax, plague). If there has been exposure to cats, inquire about scratches, papules, or pustules in the area drained by the node (CSD). Inquire about ill contacts (tuberculosis). Determine the residence and type of travel (African trypanosomiasis, cutaneous leishmaniasis, scrub typhus). Note any systemic symptoms, such as fever, unexplained weight loss, night sweats, irritability, skeletal pain, cough, and wheezing.

B. Perform a complete physical examination. Laterality may offer clues: bilateral cervical adenitis is most commonly viral in nature (e.g., Epstein–Barr virus (EBV), adenovirus, cytomegalovirus (CMV), enterovirus, herpes simplex virus (HSV), whereas acute unilateral swelling is more often bacterial. Lymph node enlargement in more than two noncontiguous lymph node regions or hepatosplenomegaly suggests generalized lymphadenopathy (see p. 22). Characterize the mass: Note location, mobility (movable or fixed), consistency (solid or fluctuant, smooth or nodular), warmth, erythema, and tenderness. Note neck range of motion. Record accurate measurements of the mass in two dimensions. Parotid gland enlargement characteristically obscures the angle of the mandible, with at least half of the mass palpable above the angle. Note periodontal disease/dentition status. Examine the scalp (fungal lesions), face, ears, nose, and oropharynx for evidence of local infection (vesicles, ulcers, exudate) or neoplastic masses. Conjunctival involvement (injection or discharge) suggests adenoviral infection, CSD, Kawasaki disease (see p. 628), or tularemia. Note the presence of a rash (scarlet fever) or bruises or petechiae that suggest an oncologic condition. Look for sinus tract openings in the skin if the mass is midline (thyroglossal duct cyst) or anterior to the sternocleidomastoid muscle (branchial cleft cyst). Consider transillumination of any mass suspected of being cystic, particularly if it is lobulated and lies in the supraclavicular fossa of a young child (lymphatic malformation). Lymphatic malformations are usually soft masses but rarely are firm. Signs of acute inflammation suggest acute bacterial lymphadenitis or an infected congenital cyst. On occasion, non-Hodgkin lymphoma may present with persistent tonsillar enlargement and cervical adenopathy.

C. Complete blood cell count (CBC), erythrocyte sedimentation rate (ESR), C-reactive protein (CRP), purified protein derivative (PPD), Bartonella titers, lactate dehydrogenase (LDH), monospot test, and EBV titers may help identify the cause of lymph node enlargement, with laboratory test choice dictated by presentation. Computed tomography (CT) scan with contrast is the imaging modality of choice to help differentiate between cellulitis, phlegmon, and abscess. CT is not routinely indicated for children who present with cervical adenitis. However, it should be considered if there is a lack of response to antibiotic therapy, if abscess is suspected, or if airway concerns are present, because these may influence decision for surgical management. Ultrasonography may also help identify an abscess. In cases of a midline mass that moves with tongue protrusion, it is most likely a thyroglossal duct cyst, the most common congenital mass. In these cases, obtain a thyroid ultrasound to characterize the mass and to determine whether the child has a normal thyroid gland.

(Continued on page 146)

Patient with CERVICAL LYMPHADENITIS/ADENOPATHY

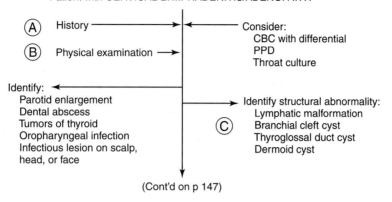

(A) History

(B) Physical examination

Consider:
- CBC with differential
- PPD
- Throat culture

Identify:
- Parotid enlargement
- Dental abscess
- Tumors of thyroid
- Oropharyngeal infection
- Infectious lesion on scalp, head, or face

Identify structural abnormality:
(C)
- Lymphatic malformation
- Branchial cleft cyst
- Thyroglossal duct cyst
- Dermoid cyst

(Cont'd on p 147)

Table 1. **Differential Diagnosis of Lymphadenopathy in the Pediatric Patient**
Infections
Bacterial
Localized:
Staphylococcus aureus, group A Streptococcus (e.g., pharyngitis), anaerobes (periodontal disease), cat-scratch disease, tularemia, bubonic plague, diphtheria, chancroid
Generalized:
Brucellosis, leptospirosis, lymphogranuloma venereum, typhoid fever
Viral
Epstein–Barr virus, cytomegalovirus, herpes simplex virus, human immunodeficiency virus, hepatitis B, mumps, measles, rubella, dengue fever
Mycobacterial
Tuberculosis, atypical mycobacteria
Fungal
Coccidiomycosis, cryptococcosis, histoplasmosis
Protozoal
Toxoplasmosis, leishmaniasis
Spirochetal
Lyme disease, syphilis
Malignancy
Leukemia, lymphoma, metastasis from solid tumor
Immunologic
Angioimmunoblastic lymphadenopathy with dysproteinemia, autoimmune lymphoproliferative disease, chronic granulomatous disease, dermatomyositis, drug reaction, rheumatoid arthritis, hemophagocytic lymphohistiocytosis, Langerhans cell histiocytosis, serum sickness, systemic lupus erythematosus
Endocrine
Addison disease, hypothyroidism
Miscellaneous
Amyloidosis, Castleman disease, Churg–Strauss syndrome, inflammatory pseudotumor, Kawasaki disease, Kikuchi disease, lipid storage diseases, sarcoidosis

From Friedmann AM. Evaluation and management of lymphadenopathy in children. Pediatr Rev 2008;29:56.

D. The differential diagnosis of cervical lymphadenitis/adenopathy is extensive. Therefore, the diagnostic approach should consider whether the process is acute or chronic, whether it is inflammatory, whether the lymphadenitis/adenopathy is localized or general, and whether there are signs of systemic disease. Lymphadenopathy may be caused by infections, malignancy, immunologic disorders, or various other miscellaneous disorders (Table 1). Worrisome features include supraclavicular or scalene lymphadenopathy; unexplained constitutional symptoms such as weight loss or night sweats; size greater than 2 cm; a hard, firm or matted consistency, lack of associated infection; onset during the neonatal period; history of rapid or progressive growth, particularly in the absence of any inflammation. Patients exhibiting these characteristics should be referred for biopsy. Adjunctive studies that may be helpful include CBC, ESR, and chest radiograph. Corticosteroids should not be given to patients in whom lymphoma or leukemia are suspected, because these can mask the diagnosis and affect prognosis.

(Continued on page 148)

Patient with CERVICAL LYMPHADENITIS/ADENOPATHY

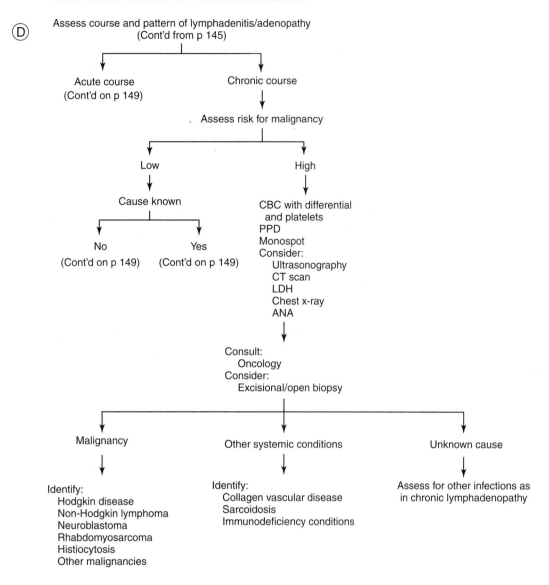

(D) Assess course and pattern of lymphadenitis/adenopathy
(Cont'd from p 145)

- Acute course
  (Cont'd on p 149)
- Chronic course
  - Assess risk for malignancy
    - Low
      - Cause known
        - No
          (Cont'd on p 149)
        - Yes
          (Cont'd on p 149)
    - High
      - CBC with differential and platelets
        PPD
        Monospot
        Consider:
        - Ultrasonography
        - CT scan
        - LDH
        - Chest x-ray
        - ANA
      - Consult:
        - Oncology

        Consider:
        - Excisional/open biopsy
        - Malignancy
          - Identify:
            - Hodgkin disease
            - Non-Hodgkin lymphoma
            - Neuroblastoma
            - Rhabdomyosarcoma
            - Histiocytosis
            - Other malignancies
        - Other systemic conditions
          - Identify:
            - Collagen vascular disease
            - Sarcoidosis
            - Immunodeficiency conditions
        - Unknown cause
          - Assess for other infections as in chronic lymphadenopathy

E. In the absence of severe caries or dental infections (anaerobes), acute unilateral cervical adenitis is most often caused by *S. aureus* or *S. pyogenes.* Consider dicloxacillin, a cephalosporin or amoxicillin with clavulanate for empiric therapy. Penicillin-allergic patients may be treated with clindamycin or a macrolide (Table 2). Failure to respond to outpatient oral therapy suggests the need for admission for intravenous antibiotic therapy (ampicillin-sulbactam, nafcillin, oxacillin, or clindamycin) and possible needle aspiration or surgical drainage. Consider obtaining blood cultures in patients with fever. Early antibiotic therapy is often successful in preventing suppuration; however, once fluctuant, the abscess will likely require surgical drainage for resolution. The possibility of methicillin-resistant *S. aureus* (MRSA) must be considered in all patients, particularly those who do not respond successfully to treatment, and cultures should be obtained at the time of surgical drainage to facilitate culture-directed therapy. Patients with signs of airway compromise warrant immediate otolaryngology consultation.

F. Chronic cervical lymphadenitis can be caused by nontuberculous or atypical mycobacteria. The most common pathogen has changed from *Mycobacterium scrofulaceum* to *Mycobacterium avium.* The adenitis is often indolent, developing over a long period, but the node may also grow rapidly over 4 to 8 weeks. There are typically no systemic signs or much local pain. The overlying skin often becomes erythematous, and over time, the node may suppurate and drain chronically through the skin. Atypical mycobacterial infections are often associated with PPD skin reactions less than 10 mm. A positive PPD test may raise concern about the possibility of tuberculosis. Obtain a chest radiograph and consider a referral to a regional tuberculosis clinic for patients older than 12 years because of the greater risk for *Mycobacterium tuberculosis* infection in these patients. Fluctuant cervical nodes should be aspirated for Gram stain and culture. Surgical excision is considered optimal treatment. When surgery is not feasible or jeopardizes the facial nerve, antimicrobial therapy is indicated with a combination of two to four medications (e.g., clarithromycin, ethambutol, Isoniazid, rifampin). Susceptibility testing is needed to optimize therapy.

G. CSD produces a chronic cervical lymphadenitis. It is caused by a pleomorphic gram-negative bacillus, *Bartonella henselae,* transmitted by kittens through scratches and bites or by flea bites. However, cat exposure is not always documented. The presentation begins with the development of a papule at the contact site with subsequent involvement of regional lymph nodes. Adenopathy is tender and can progress to suppuration. Conjunctivitis, together with mild malaise and fever, may accompany the adenitis. Serologic testing is available to support the diagnosis. PCR assays are also available. CSD is self-limited, with resolution of symptoms in about 3 months. Treatment with azithromycin may speed resolution. Surgical resection is generally not indicated.

H. Patients with localized cervical adenopathy, without features concerning for malignancy, may reasonably be observed for 3 to 4 weeks. A 7- to 10-day course of oral antibiotics may also be given to evaluate for response. A patient should be referred for biopsy if the adenopathy progresses or does not improve within 4 to 6 weeks. Although longstanding, stable lymph nodes have a low likelihood of being malignant, Hodgkin lymphoma is an exception, because it may remain quite indolent. This diagnosis should be considered, particularly in adolescents, teenagers, and young adults. An open/excisional biopsy is preferred over needle biopsy for diagnosis of hematopathologic disorders.

Table 2. **Antibiotic Coverage for Children with Cervical Adenitis**

Antibiotic	Dosage
Staphylococcus Aureus, Streptococcus Pyogenes	
Erythromycin	10 mg/kg/dose qid (maximum: 2 g/day)
Amoxicillin-clavulanate	10–15 mg/kg/dose tid (maximum: 2 g/day)
Dicloxacillin	7.5–10 mg/kg/dose qid (maximum: 2 g/day)
Cephalexin	10–25 mg/kg/dose qid (maximum: 4 g/day)
Atypical Mycobacteria	
Clarithromycin	7.5 mg/kg/dose bid (maximum: 1 g/day)
Cat-Scratch Disease	
Azithromycin	12 mg/kg/day for 5 days (maximum: 500 mg/day)

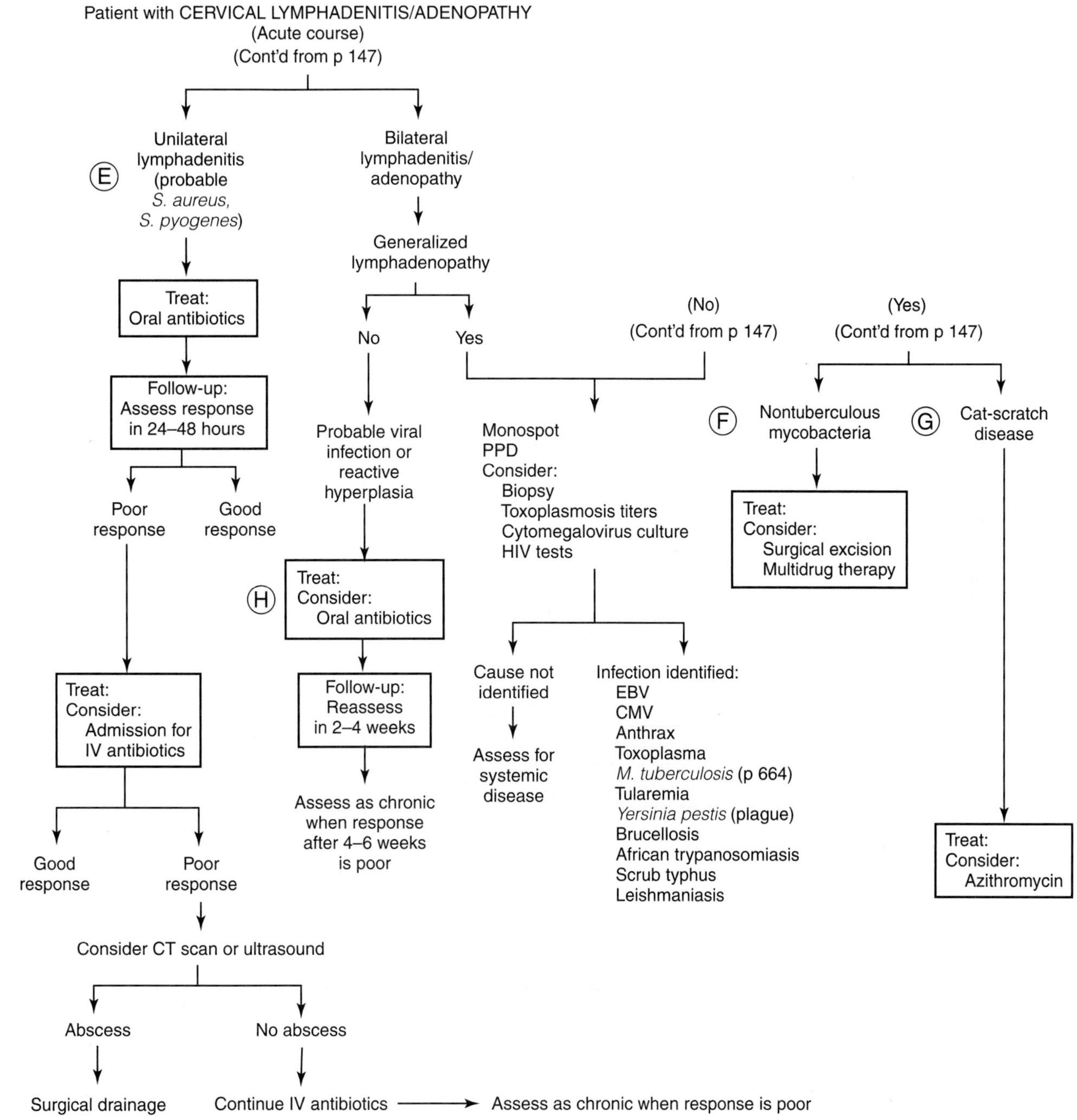
Patient with CERVICAL LYMPHADENITIS/ADENOPATHY
(Acute course)
(Cont'd from p 147)
E
Unilateral lymphadenitis (probable *S. aureus*, *S. pyogenes*)
Bilateral lymphadenitis/ adenopathy
Generalized lymphadenopathy
Treat: Oral antibiotics
No
Yes
(No) (Cont'd from p 147)
(Yes) (Cont'd from p 147)
Follow-up: Assess response in 24–48 hours
Probable viral infection or reactive hyperplasia
Monospot
PPD
Consider:
Biopsy
Toxoplasmosis titers
Cytomegalovirus culture
HIV tests
F
Nontuberculous mycobacteria
G
Cat-scratch disease
Poor response
Good response
Treat: Consider: Surgical excision Multidrug therapy
H
Treat: Consider: Oral antibiotics
Cause not identified
Infection identified:
EBV
CMV
Anthrax
Toxoplasma
M. tuberculosis (p 664)
Tularemia
Yersinia pestis (plague)
Brucellosis
African trypanosomiasis
Scrub typhus
Leishmaniasis
Treat: Consider: Admission for IV antibiotics
Follow-up: Reassess in 2–4 weeks
Assess for systemic disease
Assess as chronic when response after 4–6 weeks is poor
Treat: Consider: Azithromycin
Good response
Poor response
Consider CT scan or ultrasound
Abscess
No abscess
Surgical drainage
Continue IV antibiotics
Assess as chronic when response is poor

References

Brook I. Microbiology and antimicrobial management of head and neck infections in children. Adv Pediatr 2008;55:305–25.

Elliott DJ, Zaoutis TE, Troxel AB, et al. Empiric antimicrobial therapy for pediatric skin and soft-tissue infections in the era of methicillin-resistant staphylococcus aureus. Pediatrics 2009;123:e959–66.

Friedmann AM. Evaluation and management of lymphadenopathy in children. Pediatr Rev 2008;29:53–60.

Inman JC, Rowe MR, Ghostine M, et al. Pediatric neck abscesses—changing organisms and empiric therapies. Laryngoscope 2008;118:2111–4.

Meyer AC, Kimbrough TG, Finkelstein M, et al. Symptom duration and CT findings in pediatric deep neck infection. Otolaryngol Head Neck Surg 2009;140:183–6.

Peters TR, Edwards KM. Cervical lymphadenopathy and adenitis. Pediatr Rev 2000;21:399–405.

Timmerman MK, Morley AD, Buwalda J. Treatment of non-tuberculous mycobacterial cervicofacial lymphadenitis in children: critical appraisal of the literature. Clin Otolaryngol 2008;33:546–52.

Acute Pharyngitis in Children

Jody Ann Maes, MD

CAUSATIVE AGENTS

Acute pharyngitis is one of the most common illnesses for which children visit a healthcare facility. Many viruses and bacteria can cause acute pharyngitis in children and adolescents. A partial list of the most common microorganisms that cause pharyngitis in children and adolescent is provided in Table 1. Group A Streptococcus (GAS) is the most important of the bacterial causes of pharyngitis. It accounts for 15% to 30% of cases of acute pharyngitis. GAS pharyngitis is uncommon in children younger than 3 years and rare in children younger than 15 months.

Goals of Diagnosis and Treatment of Group A Streptococcus

1. Prevent acute rheumatic fever (ARF): Although the incidence of ARF is rare, significant sequelae are associated with ARF. Children younger than 4 years are not usually at risk for ARF. Treatment begun up to 9 days after GAS infection prevents ARF.
2. Prevent suppurative sequelae (peritonsillar, retropharyngeal abscess).
3. Shorten the duration of symptoms.
4. Interrupt transmission to family member or classmates.

Table 1. **Causative Agents of Acute Pharyngitis**

Causative Agent	Associated Disorder
Bacterial Agents	
Group A beta-hemolytic streptococci	Acute pharyngitis, Scarlet fever
Groups C, G beta-hemolytic streptococci	
Corynebacterium diphtheriae	Diphtheria
Neisseria gonorrhoeae	
Chlamydophila pneumoniae	
Chlamydia trachomatis	
Mycoplasma pneumoniae	
Mixed anaerobes	Vincent angina
Francisella tularensis	Tularemia
Viral Agents	
Rhinovirus	Common cold
Coronavirus	Common cold
Adenovirus	Pharyngoconjunctival fever
Herpes simplex virus	Gingivostomatitis
Parainfluenza	Common cold, croup
Influenza	Flu
Coxsackievirus	Herpangina; hand-foot-and-mouth disease
Epstein–Barr virus	Infectious mononucleosis

It is important to identify children with GAS pharyngitis not only for the reasons listed earlier, but to reduce antibiotic use for those children who have a viral cause of pharyngitis (Tables 2 and 3).

COMPLICATIONS OF GROUP A STREPTOCOCCUS

GAS is a self-limited illness, generally not lasting more than 3 to 5 days, even in the absence of treatment. The *main* reason to treat GAS pharyngitis is to prevent complications. Complications of GAS pharyngitis are:

1. Rheumatic fever
2. Peritonsillar abscess (see Table 4 for features)
3. Retropharyngeal abscess (abscess formation between the posterior pharyngeal wall and prevertebral fascia; see Table 5 for features)
4. Poststreptococcal glomerulonephritis: no evidence has been reported that treating GAS prevents the development of poststreptococcal glomerulonephritis

A. History and Physical Examination: Some typical features of viral pharyngitis include cough, rhinorrhea, nasal congestion, conjunctivitis, hoarseness, oral/pharyngeal vesicles or ulcers, viral exanthema, and age younger than 3 years. Some typical features of GAS pharyngitis include abrupt onset of fever, throat pain, headache, abdominal pain with or without vomiting, tender anterior cervical lymph nodes, exudative pharyngitis, palatal

Table 2. **Features of Group A Streptococcus Pharyngitis**

Abrupt onset of fever, throat pain
Headache
Abdominal pain with or without vomiting
Tender anterior cervical lymph nodes
Exudative pharyngitis
Palatal petechiae
Scarlet fever rash
Absence of cough, rhinorrhea, nasal congestion
Recent confirmed exposure (especially household)

Table 3. **Features of Viral Pharyngitis**

Cough, rhinorrhea, nasal congestion
Conjunctivitis
Hoarseness
Oral/pharyngeal vesicles or ulcers
Viral exanthema
Age <3 years

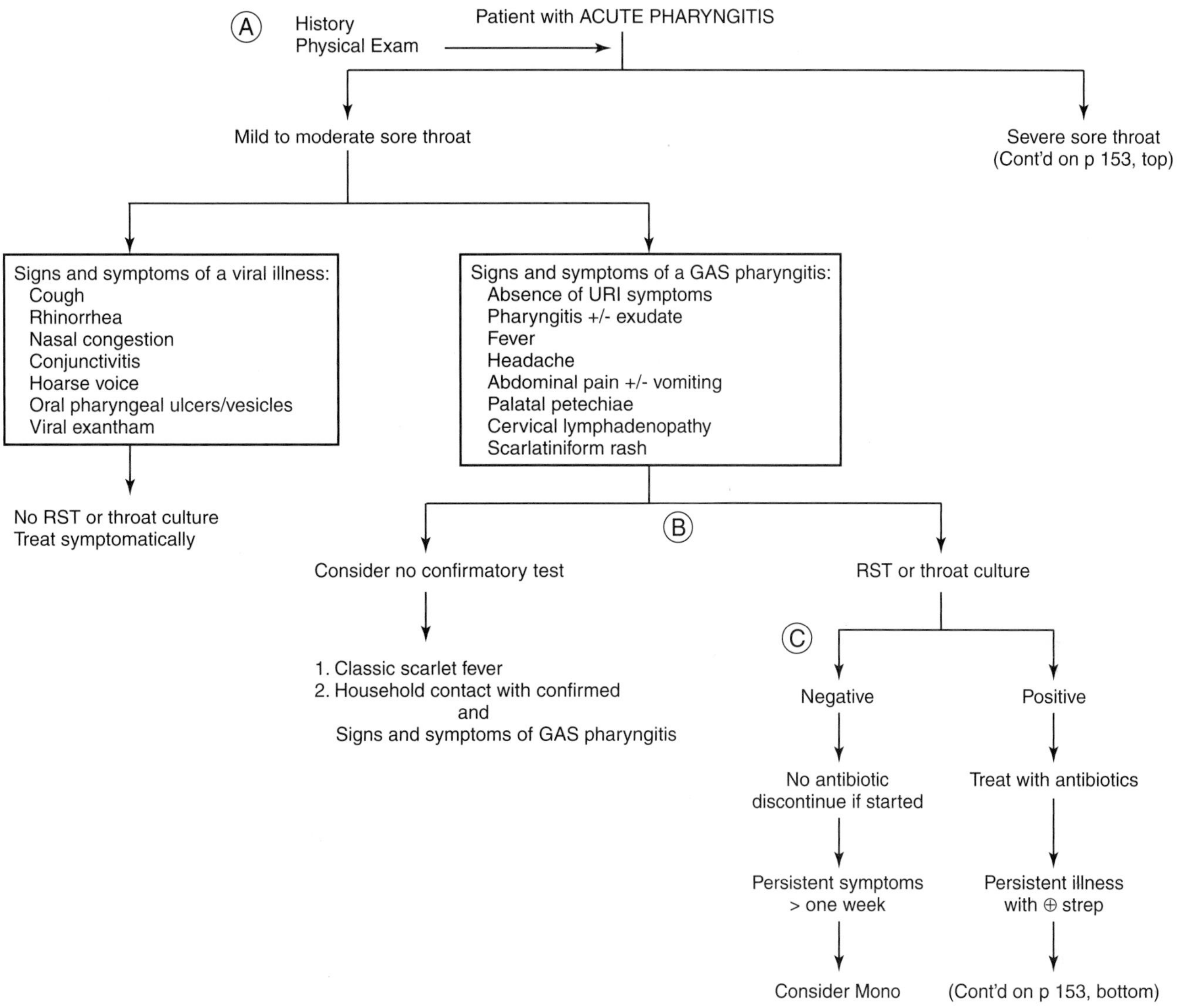
A
History
Physical Exam
Patient with ACUTE PHARYNGITIS
Mild to moderate sore throat
Severe sore throat
(Cont'd on p 153, top)
Signs and symptoms of a viral illness:
Cough
Rhinorrhea
Nasal congestion
Conjunctivitis
Hoarse voice
Oral pharyngeal ulcers/vesicles
Viral exantham
Signs and symptoms of a GAS pharyngitis:
Absence of URI symptoms
Pharyngitis +/- exudate
Fever
Headache
Abdominal pain +/- vomiting
Palatal petechiae
Cervical lymphadenopathy
Scarlatiniform rash
No RST or throat culture
Treat symptomatically
B
Consider no confirmatory test
RST or throat culture
1. Classic scarlet fever
2. Household contact with confirmed
and
Signs and symptoms of GAS pharyngitis
C
Negative
Positive
No antibiotic
discontinue if started
Treat with antibiotics
Persistent symptoms
> one week
Persistent illness
with ⊕ strep
Consider Mono
(Cont'd on p 153, bottom)

petechiae, scarlet fever rash, absence of cough, rhinorrhea, nasal congestion, and recent confirmed exposure (especially household). The features of a peritonsillar abscess are important to recognize because it is a frequent complication of pharyngitis. They include prolonged sore throat, severe sore throat, muffled voice, trismus, dysphagia, drooling, asymmetric bulge and enlarged tonsil on affected side, deviated uvula to the contralateral side, and adolescence (peritonsillar abscess is rare in young children). A retropharyngeal abscess is characterized by ill appearance, reluctance to move neck, and often neck swelling, and it usually occurs in younger children.

B. Evaluation: Although there are signs and symptoms more suggestive of GAS pharyngitis, several studies have demonstrated that the diagnosis of GAS pharyngitis based on clinical signs and symptoms alone even by experienced clinicians is unreliable. Based on these studies, many children who do not have GAS pharyngitis would be treated unnecessarily with antibiotics. Therefore, guidelines from the Infectious Disease Society of America, as well as from the American Academy of Pediatrics (AAP), indicate that microbiologic confirmation either with a throat culture or a Rapid Antigen Detection Test (RADT) is required for the diagnosis of GAS pharyngitis. A throat culture is the gold standard for diagnosis of GAS pharyngitis. If performed correctly, it has a sensitivity of 90% to 95%. The disadvantage of doing a throat culture only is that results may take up to 48 to 72 hours. In addition, many patients with viral pharyngitis are started on antibiotics pending throat culture results, some of which complete a 10-day course anyway. The majority of currently available RADTs have specificities of 95%. However, sensitivity is between 70% and 90%. Throat swabs should be obtained from the surface of both tonsils and the posterior pharyngeal wall. In the more severely ill patients or those you are concerned may have complications, a complete blood cell count and blood culture may be useful. A computed tomographic scan of the neck may also be indicated (Table 6).

Table 4. **Features of Peritonsillar Abscess**
• Prolonged sore throat
• Severe sore throat
• Muffled voice
• Trismus
• Dysphagia
• Drooling
• Asymmetric bulge and enlarged tonsil on affected side
• Deviated uvula to the contralateral side
• Adolescents (peritonsillar abscess is rare in young children)

Table 5. **Features of Retropharyngeal Abscess**
• Symptoms similar to acute pharyngitis
• Looks ill
• Reluctance to move neck
• Usually occurs in younger children
• Usually diagnosed by computed tomographic scan

Table 6. **Advantages and Disadvantages of Rapid Antigen Detection Tests**
Advantages
Increased patient satisfaction
Speed clinical improvement
Reduce the risk for spread of group A Streptococcus
Decrease treatment of viral pharyngitis
Disadvantages
Greater cost, especially if negative
Need for a backup culture if negative
Possible increased wait times (provider performed vs. laboratory performed)
Some evidence that suggest early treatment may compromise the antibody response

C. Treatment of GAS Pharyngitis: GAS remains universally sensitive to penicillin and is currently recommended by the AAP as first-line therapy for GAS pharyngitis secondary to its narrow spectrum and low cost. The disadvantage of oral penicillin is that it must be taken for 10 days. Amoxicillin is a low-cost alternative and is often preferred to penicillin because it tastes better than penicillin. In addition, several studies have demonstrated that amoxicillin given as a single daily dose is as effective as orally administered penicillin given for 10 days. A myriad of other drugs treat GAS pharyngitis, including cephalosporins, macrolides, erythromycin, and clindamycin. Erythromycin or azithromycin can be used for patients allergic to penicillin. Cephalosporins are also acceptable in penicillin-allergic patients, except for patients with an immediate or type 1 hypersensitivity to penicillin. A short-course regimen of 5 to 7 days with several cephalosporins has been shown by several studies to produce a bacteriologic eradication rate similar to a 10-day course of penicillin. However, only azithromycin and cefpodoxime have been approved by the U.S. Food and Drug Administration as a 5-day treatment course for GAS pharyngitis. Although a shorter course therapy is associated with increased compliance, most of these antibiotics are significantly more expensive than penicillin or amoxicillin. Penicillin-resistant strains of GAS have never been identified. Therefore, treatment failure is not likely secondary to penicillin resistance. The causes of treatment failure are unrecognized carrier state (with repeated episodes of viral pharyngitis), poor compliance with prescribed therapy, or reinfection. Another possible cause is suppression of immunity with prompt antibiotic treatment. Antibody suppression has been associated with relapse and recurrence of GAS pharyngitis.

D. An algorithm is included on the evaluation and treatment of a peritonsillar abscess.

References

Fleisher GR. Evaluation of sore throat in children. Up to Date; June 9, 2008.

Gerber MA. Pharyngitis. In: Long, SS, Pickering LK, Prober CG, Ed. Principles and practices of pediatric infectious diseases. 3rd ed. Philadelphia, PA: Saunders/Elsevier; 2009.

Jaggi J, Shulman S. Group A Streptococcal infections. Pediatr Rev 2006;27:99–105.

Pichichero ME. Group A beta-hemolytic Streptococcal Infections. Pediatr Rev 1998;19(9):291–302.

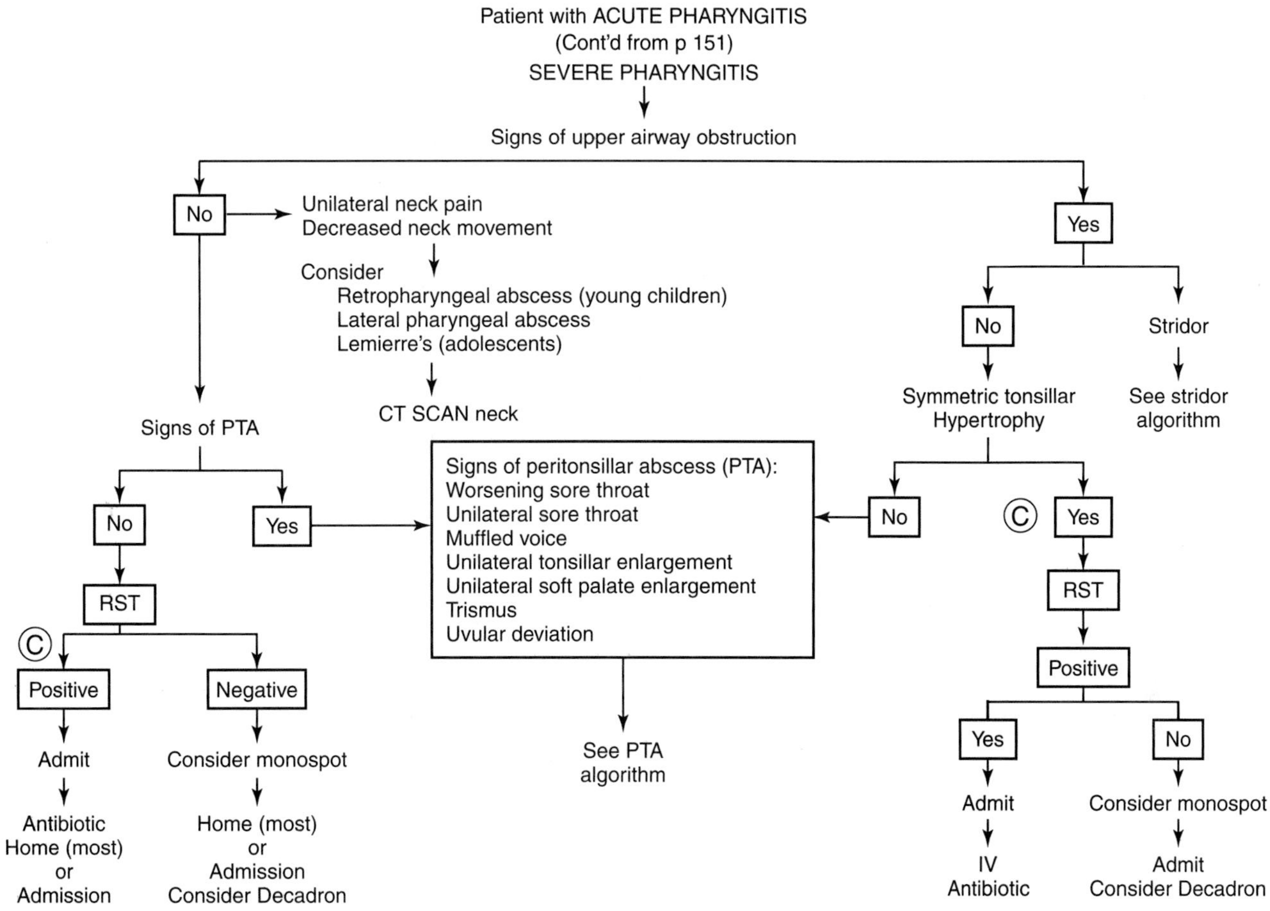
Patient with ACUTE PHARYNGITIS
(Cont'd from p 151)
SEVERE PHARYNGITIS
Signs of upper airway obstruction
No
Unilateral neck pain
Decreased neck movement
Consider
Retropharyngeal abscess (young children)
Lateral pharyngeal abscess
Lemierre's (adolescents)
CT SCAN neck
Yes
No
Stridor
Symmetric tonsillar Hypertrophy
See stridor algorithm
Signs of PTA
No
Yes
RST
C
Positive
Negative
Admit
Consider monospot
Antibiotic
Home (most)
or
Admission
Home (most)
or
Admission
Consider Decadron
Signs of peritonsillar abscess (PTA):
Worsening sore throat
Unilateral sore throat
Muffled voice
Unilateral tonsillar enlargement
Unilateral soft palate enlargement
Trismus
Uvular deviation
See PTA algorithm
No
C
Yes
RST
Positive
Yes
No
Admit
Consider monospot
IV
Antibiotic
Admit
Consider Decadron

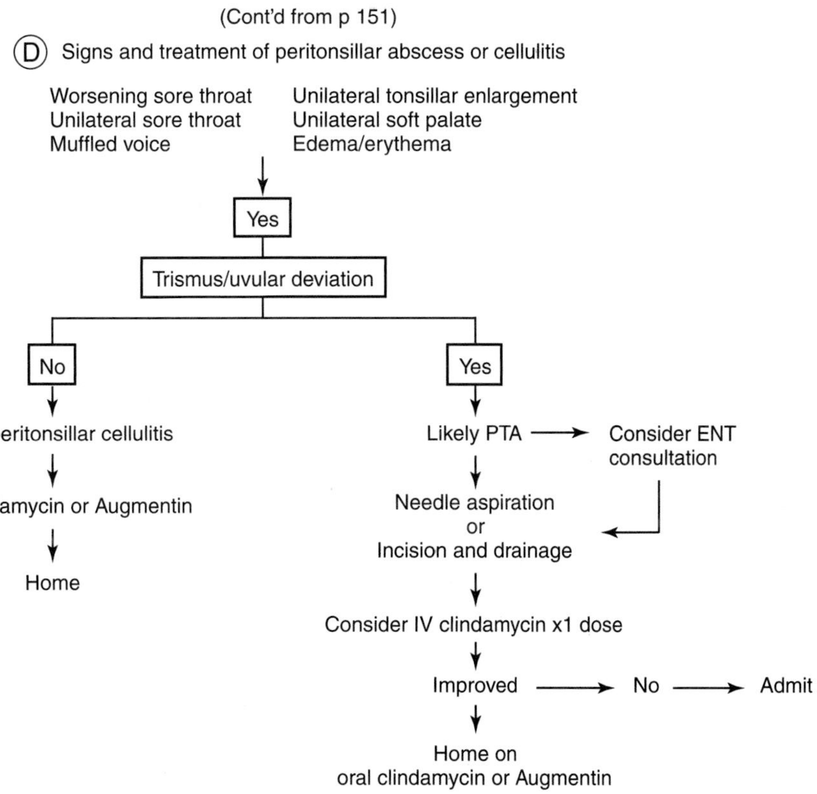
(Cont'd from p 151)
D Signs and treatment of peritonsillar abscess or cellulitis
Worsening sore throat
Unilateral sore throat
Muffled voice
Unilateral tonsillar enlargement
Unilateral soft palate
Edema/erythema
Yes
Trismus/uvular deviation
No
Yes
Likely peritonsillar cellulitis
Oral clindamycin or Augmentin
Home
Likely PTA
Consider ENT consultation
Needle aspiration
or
Incision and drainage
Consider IV clindamycin x1 dose
Improved
No
Admit
Home on
oral clindamycin or Augmentin

Endocrine

Ambiguous Genitalia

Megan Kelsey, MD, MS

A. In the patient's history, note predisposing factors and conditions, such as a family history of ambiguous genitalia, congenital adrenal hyperplasia, infant deaths, or maternal virilization.

B. In the physical examination, accurately describe the infant's phallus (stretched length and diameter), labioscrotal folds and degree of fusion, and the relation of the urethral opening to the glans and number of perineal openings. Presence of at least one palpable gonad (testis) suggests the Y chromosome in the karyotype. The absence of palpable testis in the scrotal, labial, or inguinal region implies that the child is a female with salt-losing congenital adrenal hyperplasia until proved otherwise. Associated abnormalities in the genitourinary system suggest a dysmorphic syndrome as opposed to an inherited metabolic-endocrine disorder.

C. Some of the causes of ambiguous genitalia involve enzymatic defects in steroid biosynthesis that may result in life-threatening, salt-losing crises. Early assessment and monitoring of serum electrolytes and plasma renin activity is crucial. Except when the patient presents with clearly defined 21-hydroxylase deficiency (e.g., through the newborn screen), definitive karyotyping should be done. The results of karyotyping separate cases into genetic males (XY) with incomplete virilization, genetic females (XX) with excessive virilization, and chromosomal aberrations fitting neither genotype.

D. A multidisciplinary team, including endocrinology, urology, genetics, and psychology or social work, should be involved as soon as possible. Gender assignment may be difficult and should be done using a team approach, including the parents in the decision-making process.

E. Much information can be gained about internal anatomy of the child with ambiguous genitalia with the use of pelvic ultrasonography, as well as a genitogram (i.e., a contrast study delineating the extent of the posterior vagina and presence of the cervix), to help identify the gonads and uterus if present.

F. The evaluation of incomplete virilization in a genetic male may be most readily accomplished by measuring serum luteinizing hormone (LH), testosterone (T), and dihydrotestosterone (DHT). This enables the physician to distinguish between defects of the hypothalamic-pituitary axis and those of the testes. In addition, it helps identify defects in the androgen receptor causing end-organ insensitivity to androgens. It is imperative that age-appropriate norms be used to interpret these results; the normal serum concentrations of LH, T, and DHT change considerably during the first 3 months of life. If these labs cannot be drawn within the first 48 hours of life, during the initial perinatal surge, it is best to wait until 2 months of life when the "mini-puberty" of infancy is at its peak. Alternatively, these tests can be performed after β-chorionic gonadotropin hormone (β-hCG) stimulation.

G. The combination of low levels of LH, T, and DHT suggests a hypothalamic-pituitary defect. These defects do not ordinarily cause ambiguity, but they do cause micropenis and can affect testicular descent. The degree of incompleteness of virilization is not nearly as severe as with either testicular or end-organ (receptor) defects. Assessment of hypothalamic-pituitary function should be done with the help of an endocrinologist, as described in Short Stature (see p. 162).

H. High LH and normal-to-high T and DHT levels usually suggest end-organ insensitivity to androgens. High T associated with low DHT suggests 5-α-reductase deficiency. In these patients, testes are present, but external and internal virilization is defective, resulting in ambiguous genitalia on physical examination and absent or severely compromised Wolffian duct development. This includes the epididymis, vas deferens, seminal vesicles, and ejaculatory ducts. Müllerian derivatives (cervix, uterus, and oviducts) are absent because the testes produce normal amounts of müllerian inhibitory factor in utero.

I. A high level of LH with low T and DHT levels suggests an inborn error of androgen or T biosynthesis (Figure 1). Because errors of androgen biosynthesis may also involve enzymes necessary for the production of cortisol and aldosterone (namely, 17-hydroxylase and 3-β-ol-dehydrogenase), these infants should have an assessment of adrenocortical metabolism by an adrenocorticotropic hormone (ACTH; Cortrosyn) stimulation test. Infants with a more "distal" metabolic defect (e.g., 17-ketosteroid reductase or 5-α-reductase) do not have other clinically significant adrenal metabolic defects. A deficiency of 5-α-reductase is characterized by normal plasma T but low plasma DHT levels.

(Continued on page 158)

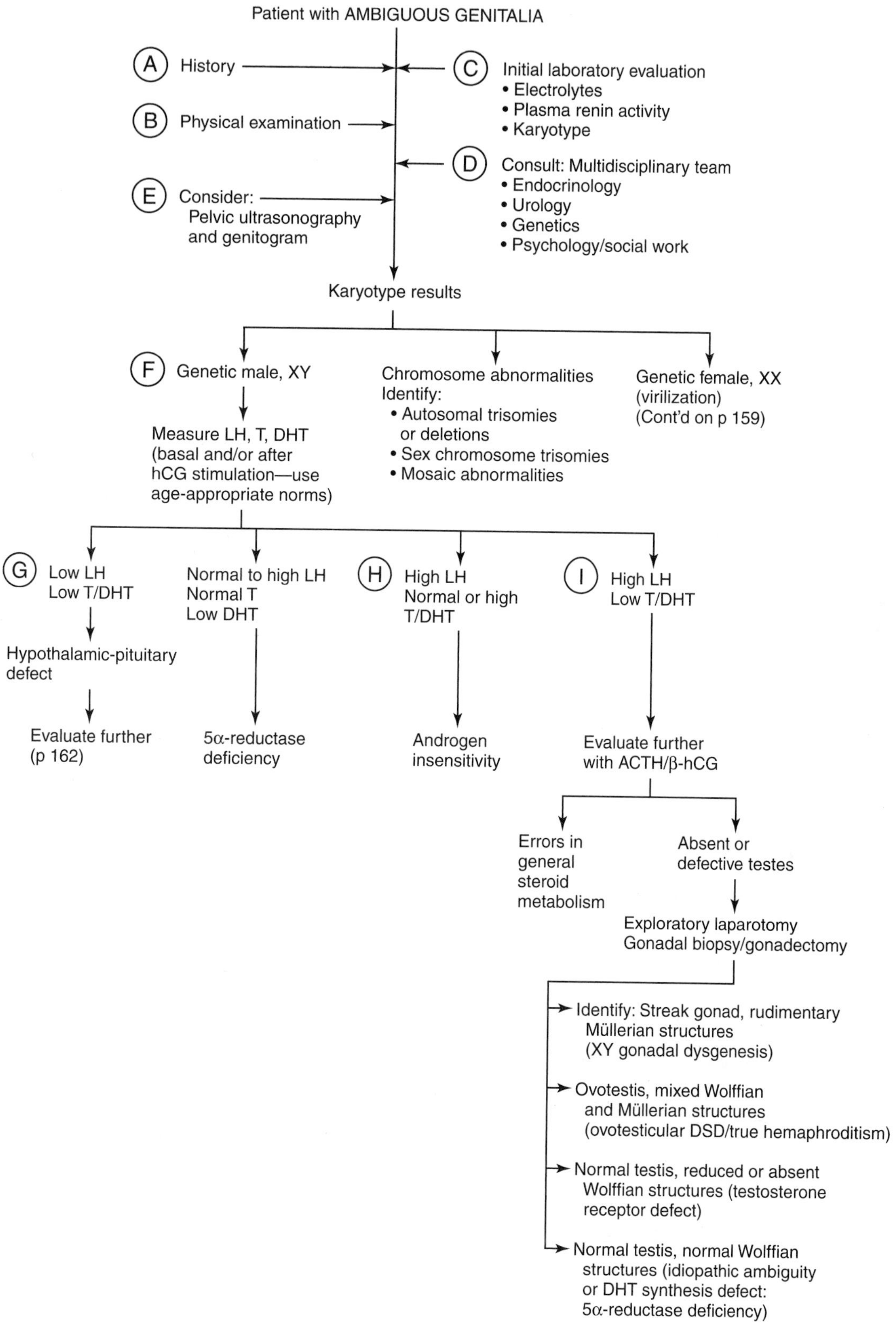
Patient with AMBIGUOUS GENITALIA
A History
B Physical examination
C Initial laboratory evaluation
• Electrolytes
• Plasma renin activity
• Karyotype
D Consult: Multidisciplinary team
• Endocrinology
• Urology
• Genetics
• Psychology/social work
E Consider:
Pelvic ultrasonography and genitogram
Karyotype results
F Genetic male, XY
Measure LH, T, DHT (basal and/or after hCG stimulation—use age-appropriate norms)
Chromosome abnormalities
Identify:
• Autosomal trisomies or deletions
• Sex chromosome trisomies
• Mosaic abnormalities
Genetic female, XX (virilization) (Cont'd on p 159)
G Low LH Low T/DHT
Hypothalamic-pituitary defect
Evaluate further (p 162)
Normal to high LH Normal T Low DHT
5α-reductase deficiency
H High LH Normal or high T/DHT
Androgen insensitivity
I High LH Low T/DHT
Evaluate further with ACTH/β-hCG
Errors in general steroid metabolism
Absent or defective testes
Exploratory laparotomy
Gonadal biopsy/gonadectomy
Identify: Streak gonad, rudimentary Müllerian structures (XY gonadal dysgenesis)
Ovotestis, mixed Wolffian and Müllerian structures (ovotesticular DSD/true hemaphroditism)
Normal testis, reduced or absent Wolffian structures (testosterone receptor defect)
Normal testis, normal Wolffian structures (idiopathic ambiguity or DHT synthesis defect: 5α-reductase deficiency)

J. The presence of maternal virilization is not always obvious and should be pursued (e.g., congenital adrenal hyperplasia [CAH], adrenal or ovarian tumor), particularly if the evaluation of a genetically female infant is unproductive.

K. The absence of maternal virilization or increased androgens suggests idiopathic ambiguity (dysmorphia) or ovotesticular disorder of sexual differentiation (ovotesticular DSD/true hermaphroditism). 17-hydroxyprogesterone may be falsely low on the first test. Thus, "normal" findings for these hormones in the presence of a virilized girl should not be considered conclusive. Alternatively, normal infants may have false increases of 17-hydroxyprogesterone or androstenedione compared with reference levels for age, especially if they are studied in the first day or two of life when plasma 17-hydroxyprogesterone levels are high, particularly in premature or stressed newborns. All 50 states in the United States and many countries include a 17-hydroxyprogesterone in the newborn screening program. Some states send a second newborn screen, which can be helpful in these cases. Otherwise, a repeat 17-OH progesterone should be sent.

L. Monitoring electrolytes alone is not sufficient for the diagnosis of mineralocorticoid deficiency in cases of congenital adrenal hyperplasia because infants who are salt losers often maintain normal serum concentrations of electrolytes at the expense of increased plasma renin activity. Thus, a high plasma renin activity in the face of normal electrolytes is indicative of compensated salt losing and may be as common as overt salt loss manifested by hyponatremia and hyperkalemia. Both degrees of salt-losing tendency are generally treated with mineralocorticoid replacement as fludrocortisone acetate with or without NaCl supplementation (Table 1).

Table 1. **Drug Therapy for Congenital Adrenal Hyperplasia**

Glucocorticoid replacement: cortisol (hydrocortisone, Cortef) PO 10–25 mg/m²/day divided into 3 doses; administer morning dose as early as possible
Mineralocorticoid replacement: 9-fludrocortisone acetate (Florinef Acetate) PO 0.05–0.3 mg daily

References

Bin-Abbas B, Conte F, Grumbach MM, Kaplan SL. Congenital hypogonadotropic hypogonadism and micropenis: effect of testosterone treatment on adult size—why sex reversal is not indicated. J Pediatr 1999;134:579.

Lee PA, Houk CP, Ahmed SF, Hughes LA. Consensus statement on management of intersex disorders. Pediatrics 2006;118:e488–500.

Meyer-Bahlberg HFL. What causes low rates of child-bearing in congenital adrenal hyperplasia? J Clin Endocrinol Metab 1999;84:1844.

Migeon CJ, Berkovitz GD, Brown TR. Sexual differentiation and ambiguity. In: Kappy MS, Blizzard RM, Migeon CJ, editors. The diagnosis and treatment of endocrine disorders in childhood and adolescence. 4th ed. Springfield, IL: Charles C Thomas; 1994. p. 573.

Root AW. Genetic errors of sexual differentiation. Adv Pediatr 1999;46:67.

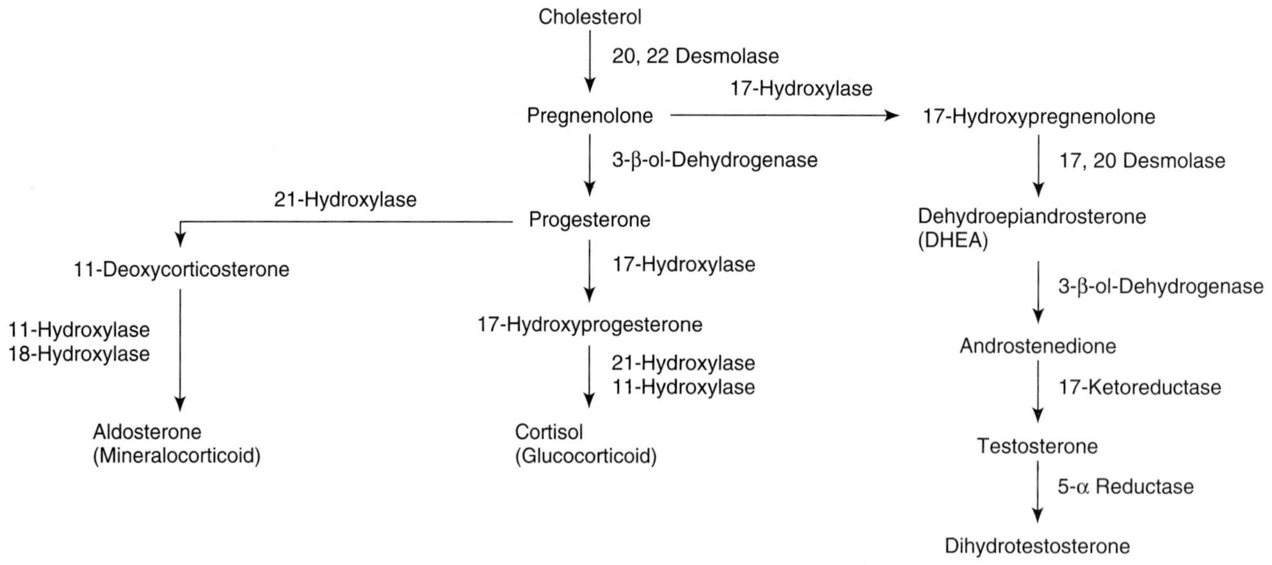

Cholesterol
20, 22 Desmolase
Pregnenolone
17-Hydroxylase
17-Hydroxypregnenolone
3-β-ol-Dehydrogenase
17, 20 Desmolase
21-Hydroxylase
Progesterone
Dehydroepiandrosterone (DHEA)
11-Deoxycorticosterone
17-Hydroxylase
3-β-ol-Dehydrogenase
11-Hydroxylase
18-Hydroxylase
17-Hydroxyprogesterone
Androstenedione
21-Hydroxylase
11-Hydroxylase
17-Ketoreductase
Aldosterone (Mineralocorticoid)
Cortisol (Glucocorticoid)
Testosterone
5-α Reductase
Dihydrotestosterone

Figure 1 Steroid hormone biosynthesis.

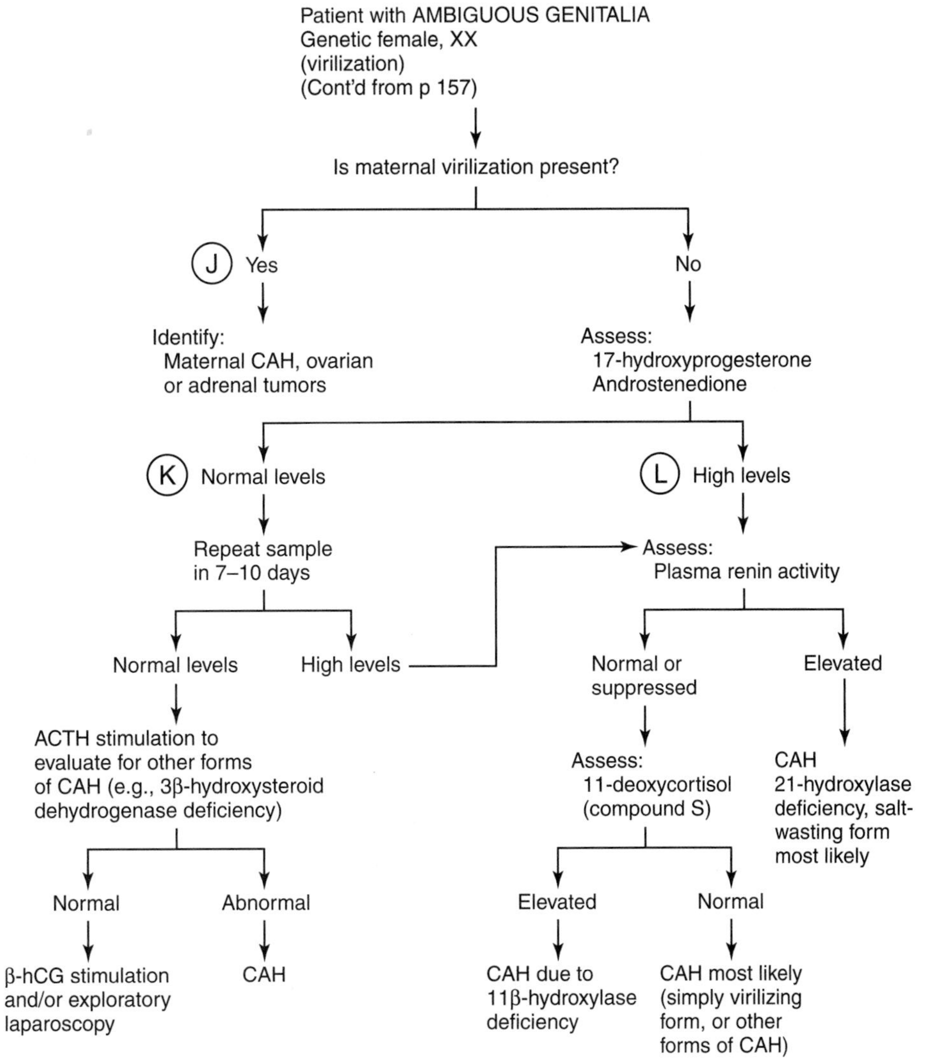

Patient with AMBIGUOUS GENITALIA
Genetic female, XX
(virilization)
(Cont'd from p 157)
Is maternal virilization present?
J Yes
No
Identify:
Maternal CAH, ovarian or adrenal tumors
Assess:
17-hydroxyprogesterone
Androstenedione
K Normal levels
L High levels
Repeat sample in 7–10 days
Assess:
Plasma renin activity
Normal levels
High levels
Normal or suppressed
Elevated
ACTH stimulation to evaluate for other forms of CAH (e.g., 3β-hydroxysteroid dehydrogenase deficiency)
Assess:
11-deoxycortisol (compound S)
CAH
21-hydroxylase deficiency, salt-wasting form most likely
Normal
Abnormal
Elevated
Normal
β-hCG stimulation and/or exploratory laparoscopy
CAH
CAH due to 11β-hydroxylase deficiency
CAH most likely (simply virilizing form, or other forms of CAH)

Delayed Puberty

R. Paul Wadwa, MD, and Michael S. Kappy, MD, PhD

An evaluation of delayed puberty in a child of either sex depends on the judgment of the physician, who is guided by the upper limits of ages for the development of normal pubertal events. For example, if there is no breast development in a girl by age 14 years, pubertal delay is significant. Likewise, if no testicular or penile enlargement occurs in a boy by age 14 years, puberty is significantly delayed and further evaluation is warranted. The condition most likely to be confused with pathologically delayed pubertal maturation is constitutional delay, and often it is not easy to differentiate the two at the first visit.

Constitutional delay is the most common form of delayed pubertal maturation. In this condition, the child's rate of physical maturation is slower than that of peers. The bone age is usually delayed for chronologic age but is equal to the height age. Pubertal maturation is correspondingly delayed, and often one or both parents give a similar history (i.e., delayed menarche in the mother or growth after high school in the father). There is considerable variation in the onset and development of secondary sexual characteristics in both boys and girls (Figures 1 and 2). Variation in the onset of puberty by race/ethnicity should also be considered. In boys with constitutional delay, short-term (4–6 months) treatment with testosterone (Depo-Testosterone), 50 to 80 mg intramuscularly monthly, may be beneficial.

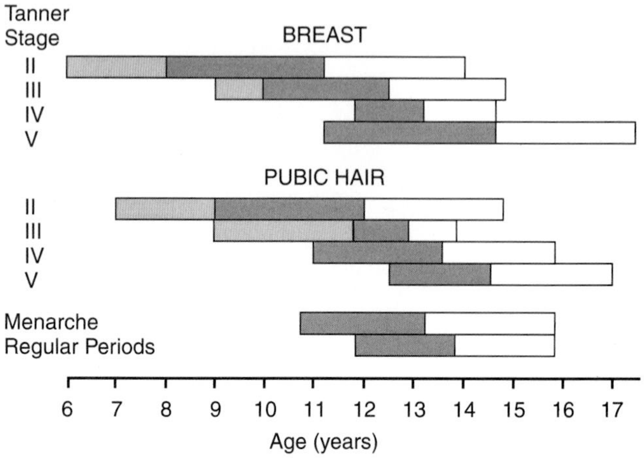
Tanner Stage
BREAST
II
III
IV
V
PUBIC HAIR
II
III
IV
V
Menarche
Regular Periods
6 7 8 9 10 11 12 13 14 15 16 17
Age (years)

Figure 1 Mean ages of pubertal development in girls. *(From Lee PA. Normal ages of pubertal events among American males and females. J Adolesc Health Care 1980;1:26; and Herman-Giddens ME, Macmillan JP. Prevalence of secondary sexual characteristics in a population of North Carolina girls ages 3 to 10. Adolesc Pediatr Gynecol 1991;4:21.)*

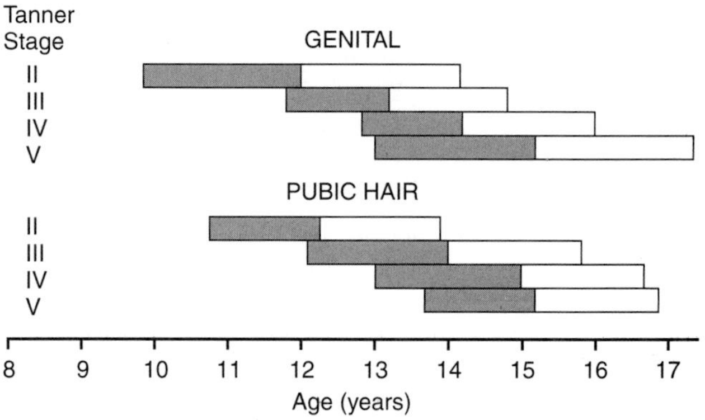
Tanner Stage
GENITAL
II
III
IV
V
PUBIC HAIR
II
III
IV
V
8 9 10 11 12 13 14 15 16 17
Age (years)

Figure 2 Mean ages of pubertal development in boys. *(Data derived from Lee PA. Normal ages of pubertal events among American males and females. J Adolesc Health Care 1980;1:26.)*

A. In the patient's history, ask about significant central nervous system disease, including surgery, chemotherapy, and cranial irradiation for tumor treatment; infection; and trauma. Similarly, gonadal trauma, infection, chemotherapy, or irradiation can delay puberty because of gonadal insufficiency. Obtain a history of excessive physical activity (e.g., gymnastics), general systemic chronic illness, anorexia, and stress.

B. A careful Tanner staging is necessary, as is a comparison with age-specific norms for the various aspects of secondary sexual development (see Figures 1 and 2). Only significant pubertal delay should be evaluated comprehensively. Exclude syndromes such as Turner, Noonan, Klinefelter, and Prader–Willi by formal karyotyping, and syndromes such as Laurence–Moon–Biedl, which may be diagnosed by the patient's obesity and associated findings.

C. If the diagnosis remains in question, measure luteinizing hormone (LH) and testosterone (T) in boys, and follicle-stimulating hormone (FSH) and estradiol (E_2) in girls. When basal measurements of LH and FSH are inconclusive, consider obtaining leuprolide-stimulated LH levels at 30 to 40 minutes. Persistence of prepubertal basal or stimulated LH and FSH levels accompanied by prepubertal T or E_2 suggests a hypothalamic-pituitary defect. Exclude panhypopituitarism with the help of an endocrinologist. In addition, cranial magnetic resonance imaging including the pituitary gland may help to rule out intracranial disease. Kallmann syndrome is accompanied by anosmia and occasionally by an abnormal cranial magnetic resonance imaging scan. True gonadotropin deficiency is treated in boys with full-replacement testosterone, 100 mg/m^2 or 100 to 200 mg monthly intramuscularly injections, and in girls with oral estrogen (Premarin), 0.3 to 0.625 mg/day in divided doses (for 20 days; off 10 days; repeat until menses occur) for 1 to 2 years followed by a combination of estrogen and progesterone, either separately or with combination

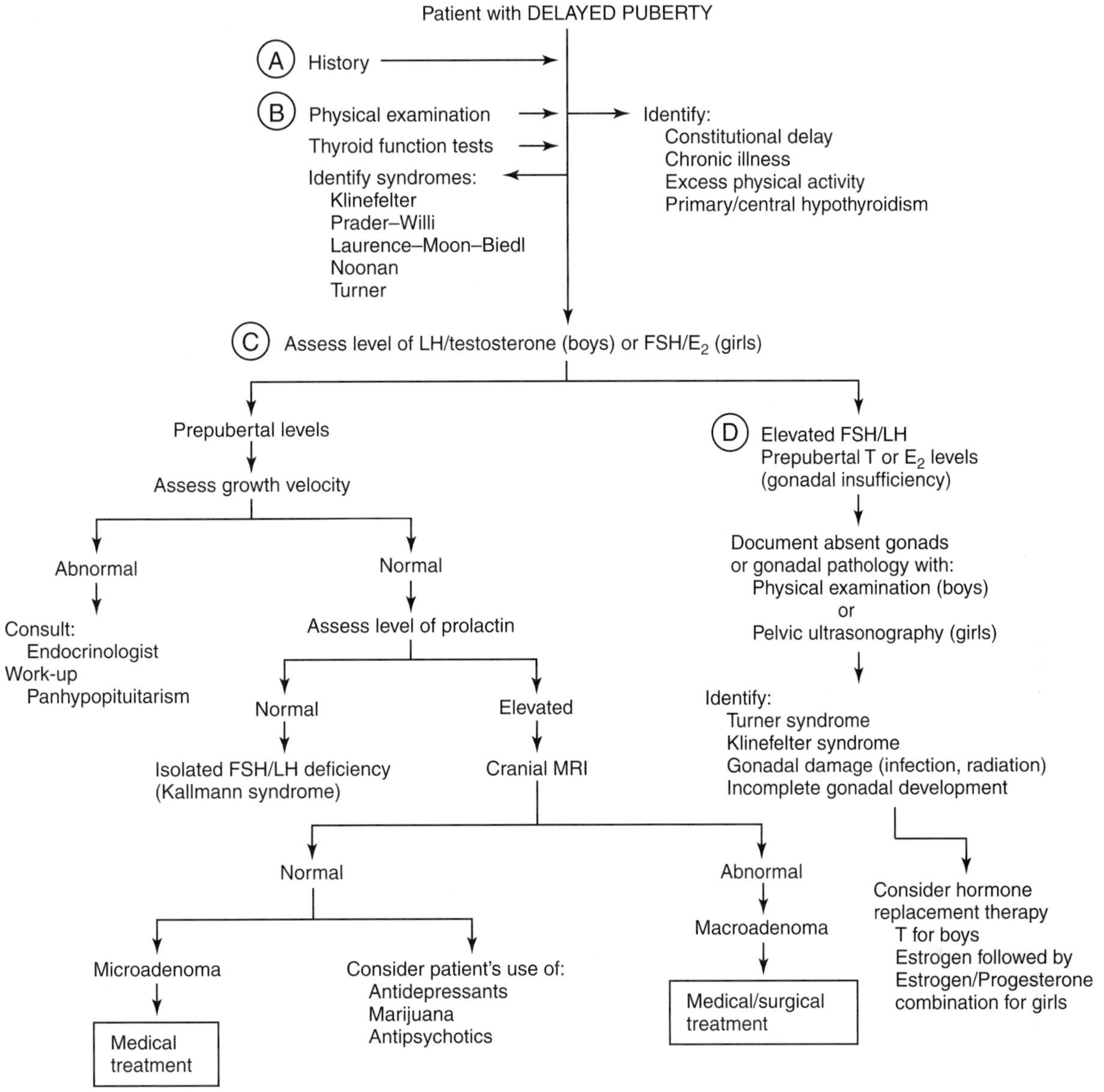
Patient with DELAYED PUBERTY
A History
B Physical examination
Thyroid function tests
Identify syndromes:
Klinefelter
Prader–Willi
Laurence–Moon–Biedl
Noonan
Turner
Identify:
Constitutional delay
Chronic illness
Excess physical activity
Primary/central hypothyroidism
C Assess level of LH/testosterone (boys) or FSH/E2 (girls)
Prepubertal levels
Assess growth velocity
Abnormal
Consult:
Endocrinologist
Work-up
Panhypopituitarism
Normal
Assess level of prolactin
Normal
Isolated FSH/LH deficiency
(Kallmann syndrome)
Elevated
Cranial MRI
Normal
Microadenoma
Medical treatment
Consider patient's use of:
Antidepressants
Marijuana
Antipsychotics
Abnormal
Macroadenoma
Medical/surgical treatment
D Elevated FSH/LH
Prepubertal T or E2 levels
(gonadal insufficiency)
Document absent gonads
or gonadal pathology with:
Physical examination (boys)
or
Pelvic ultrasonography (girls)
Identify:
Turner syndrome
Klinefelter syndrome
Gonadal damage (infection, radiation)
Incomplete gonadal development
Consider hormone
replacement therapy
T for boys
Estrogen followed by
Estrogen/Progesterone
combination for girls

pills. Daily application of topical testosterone gel for boys or weekly application of estrogen patches for girls are also options for hormone replacement if necessary.

D. Gonadal insufficiency may be related to a specific gonadal pathologic process. If Turner and Klinefelter syndromes have been eliminated by karyotyping, physical examination or pelvic ultrasonography may offer definitive information.

References

Gajdos ZK, Hirschhorn JN, Palmert MR. What controls the timing of puberty? An update on progress from genetic investigation. Curr Opin Endocrinol Diabetes Obes 2009;16(1):16–24.

Golden NH, Carlson JL. The pathophysiology of amenorrhea in the adolescent. Ann NY Acad Sci 2008;1135:163–78.

Herman-Giddens ME, Slora EJ, Wasserman RC, et al. Secondary sexual characteristics and menses in young girls seen in office practice. Pediatrics 1997;99:505.

Lee P. Stages of pubertal events among American males and females. J Adolesc Health Care 1980;1:26.

Rosenfield RL, Lipton RB, Drum ML. Thelarche, pubarche, and menarche attainment in children with normal and elevated body mass index. Pediatrics 2009;123(1):84–8.

Wu T, Mendola P, Buck GM. Ethnic differences in the presence of secondary sex characteristics and menarche among US girls: the Third National Health and Nutrition Examination Survey, 1988–1994. Pediatrics 2002;110(4):752–7.

Zeitler PS, Travers S, Kappy MS. Advances in the recognition and treatment of endocrine complications in children with chronic illness. Adv Pediatr 1999;46:101.

Short Stature

R. Paul Wadwa, MD, and Michael S. Kappy, MD, PhD

A. In the patient's history, ask about the heights of parents and siblings (familial short stature) and whether the mother had a history of delayed menarche or the father a delayed puberty ("late bloomer"), usually associated with continued growth after high school (constitutional delay with short stature as an adolescent). Calculate midparental height (for boys: [(mother's height + 13 cm) + father's height]/2; for girls: [mother's height + (father's height − 13 cm)]/2) and determine percentile at final adult height on Centers for Disease Control and Prevention (CDC) Growth Charts (www.cdc.gov/growthcharts). Obtain an appropriate nutritional and psychosocial database. Identify predisposing conditions, such as congenital infections; smallness for gestational age at birth (primordial short stature); congenital syndromes; chronic illness involving major organ systems, especially the gastrointestinal tract and cardiac, pulmonary, or renal systems; malnutrition; and medications, especially pharmacologic doses of oral or inhaled glucocorticoids (e.g., in asthma).

B. In the physical examination, accurately document the height of the child, preferably by use of a stadiometer or a ruler attached to the wall so that the child is reliably vertical. The metal bar attached to the scale in most physicians' offices is not accurate or reproducible enough for evaluation and monitoring of a child with short stature. Calculate body mass index (BMI) in kg/m^2, which may be graphed on CDC Growth Charts (www.cdc.gov/growthcharts). Body mass index is usually normal in endocrine and metabolic disorders, and reduced in malnutrition. "Weight age" and "height age" (the ages for which the patient's measurements are the 50th percentile) may also be helpful. Note the presence of congenital abnormalities or dysmorphic appearance and assess the gastrointestinal, cardiac, pulmonary, and renal systems. Note any goiter. Evaluate pubertal development and assess it according to age (see p. 160). Assess dentition and state of nutrition.

C. Consider Turner syndrome in girls, recognizing that 60% of such patients do not have marked stigmata of the syndrome (webbed neck, wide-spaced nipples, wide carrying angle to the arms), especially girls with Turner mosaicism. After 9 to 10 years of age, a random measurement of serum follicle-stimulating hormone and luteinizing hormone may signal ovarian failure (common in Turner syndrome); however, a karyotype is the definitive test.

D. Document the child's rate of growth during the longest period for which measurements are available. The lower limit of normal growth is approximately 4 cm/yr for children 5 to 10 years old, but it is greater in children younger than 5 years and during the pubertal growth spurt. Most standard pediatric texts have normal growth rate curves for comparison. A short child with a normal growth rate for age is unlikely to have significant illness or an endocrinopathy.

E. The bone age (single anteroposterior view of the left hand and wrist) is useful in correlating the degree of physical maturation with chronologic age. It is usually delayed for chronologic age but normal for height age in constitutional delay of puberty. Other causes of delayed bone age include emotional deprivation, chronic illness, malnutrition, growth hormone (GH) deficiency, and thyroid hormone deficiency.

F. Rule out thyroid and GH deficiency in children with a significantly delayed bone age who are growing at a rate abnormal for age (>2 standard deviations less than the mean for age). In primary hypothyroidism, a low free thyroxine (T_4) level or total T_4 is associated with increased levels of thyroid-stimulating hormone (TSH). Total or free T_4 level may be normal in compensated hypothyroidism, but TSH is increased. These children most likely have a disorder of the thyroid gland and should be treated with L-thyroxine: <12 years old 4 to 5 μg/kg/day (100–150 μg/day); ≥12 years old 2 to 3 μg/kg/day (≥150 μg/day).

G. Children with familial short stature have height at or near the percentile of the midparental height, normal findings on physical examination, normal (usually low-normal) growth rate for age, and bone age appropriate for chronologic age. Patients with primordial short stature were often small for gestational age at birth or may have (in addition) a congenital syndrome (e.g., Russell–Silver syndrome).

H. In constitutional delay, the child's tempo of physical maturation is slower than that of peers. The bone age is delayed for chronologic age but normal for height age. Pubertal maturation is appropriate for bone age. The ultimate height of these children is usually normal for their families because the pubertal growth spurt is not diminished but only delayed. In some boys for whom this delay causes undue psychological stress, a short course of low-dose, long-acting testosterone may be used. Testosterone depot, 50 to 80 mg intramuscularly monthly for 4 to 6 months, stimulates growth without unduly advancing the bone age. Although ultimate height is not increased by this treatment, the earlier growth spurt and appearance of secondary sexual characteristics make it a useful treatment option.

(Continued on page 164)

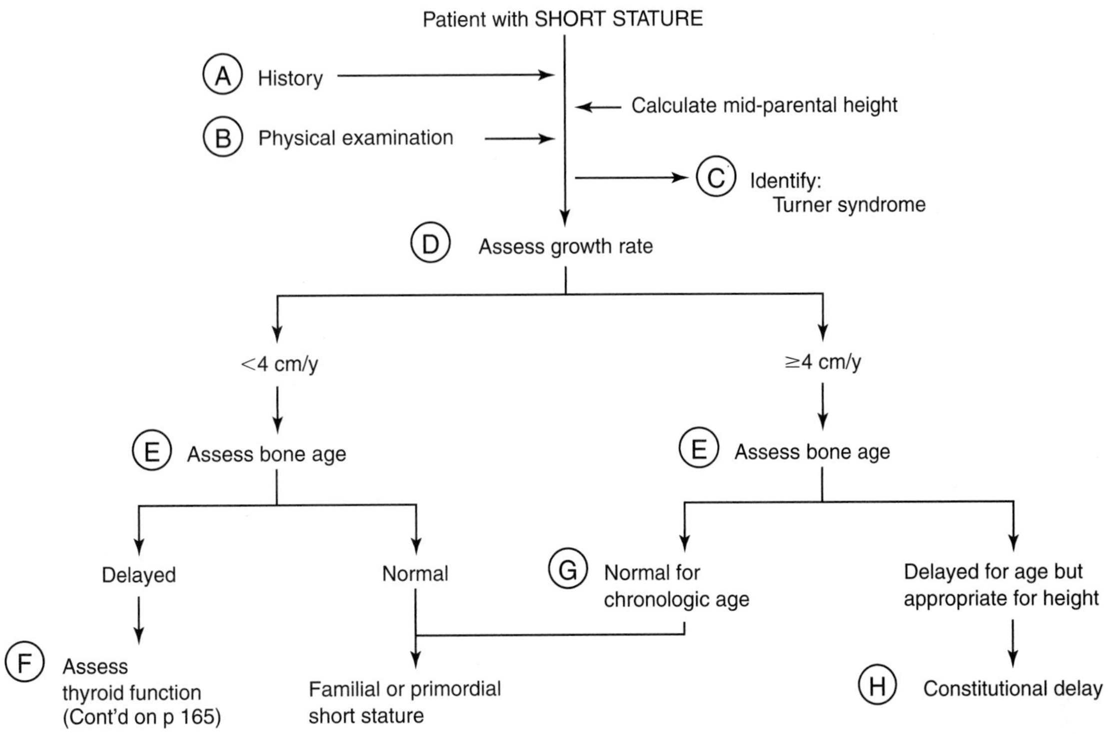
Patient with SHORT STATURE
A History
B Physical examination
Calculate mid-parental height
C Identify:
Turner syndrome
D Assess growth rate
<4 cm/y
≥4 cm/y
E Assess bone age
E Assess bone age
Delayed
Normal
G Normal for chronologic age
Delayed for age but appropriate for height
F Assess thyroid function (Cont'd on p 165)
Familial or primordial short stature
H Constitutional delay

I. Rule out GH deficiency in children with normal thyroid function, delayed bone age, and abnormal growth rate (usually <4 cm/yr).

J. Documentation of the extent of endogenous GH secretion is difficult. The standard provocative tests may yield normal results in children who are not growing well and who have low serum insulin-like growth factor 1 concentrations. Many of these children also respond well to a trial of GH therapy. Although such a trial has been advocated as a means of assessing or defining endogenous GH deficiency, many short children without true GH deficiency grow faster while receiving GH therapy. A concomitant increase in skeletal maturation also occurs; therefore, it is debatable whether this therapy actually adds inches to the child's ultimate height. GH treatment in children with idiopathic short stature is a complex issue with several potential caveats and pitfalls. Consultation with a pediatric endocrinologist should be considered in this scenario. Treatment of GH deficiency in children is recombinant human GH, 0.3 mg/kg/wk divided into daily subcutaneous injections doses.

K. A low T_4 level not accompanied by an increased TSH level suggests thyroxine-binding globulin deficiency, secondary (pituitary) disorders, or tertiary (hypothalamic) disorders. Refer patients with suspected pituitary or hypothalamic disorders for further evaluation.

References

Allen DB, Rose SR, Reiter EO. Normal growth and growth disorders. In: Kappy MS, Allen DB, Geffner ME, editors. Principles and practice of pediatric endocrinology. Springfield, IL: Charles C. Thomas; 2005. p. 77.

Rogol AD, Wit JM. Debate on the use of growth hormone in the treatment of children with idiopathic short stature (ISS) (Pro and Con). Pediatr Endocrinol Rev 2007;4(3):226–7.

Wajnrajch MP. Genetic disorders of human growth. J Pediatr Endocrinol Metab 2002;15(suppl 2):701–14.

Zeitler PS, Travers S, Kappy MS. Advances in the recognition and treatment of endocrine complications in children with chronic illness. Adv Pediatr 1999;46:101.

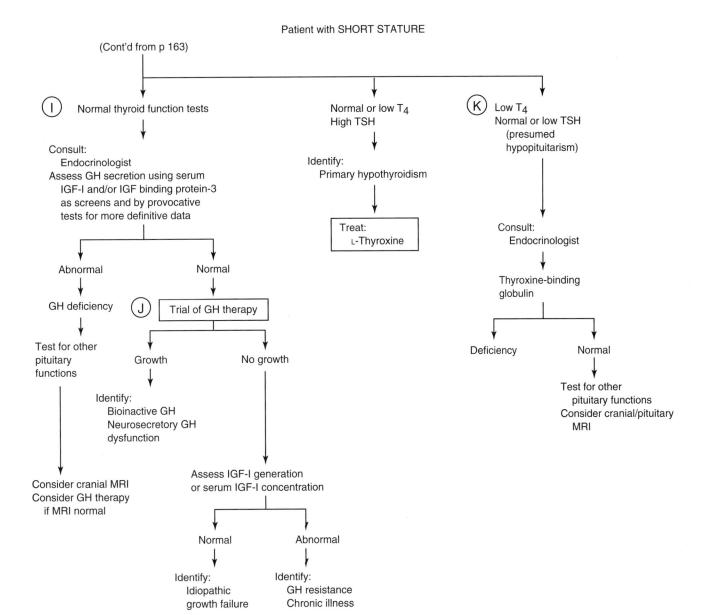

Patient with SHORT STATURE

(Cont'd from p 163)

- **(I)** Normal thyroid function tests
  - Consult:
    - Endocrinologist
  - Assess GH secretion using serum IGF-I and/or IGF binding protein-3 as screens and by provocative tests for more definitive data
    - Abnormal
      - GH deficiency
        - Test for other pituitary functions
          - Consider cranial MRI
          - Consider GH therapy if MRI normal
    - Normal
      - **(J)** Trial of GH therapy
        - Growth
          - Identify:
            - Bioinactive GH
            - Neurosecretory GH dysfunction
        - No growth
          - Assess IGF-I generation or serum IGF-I concentration
            - Normal
              - Identify:
                - Idiopathic growth failure
            - Abnormal
              - Identify:
                - GH resistance
                - Chronic illness
- Normal or low T_4, High TSH
  - Identify:
    - Primary hypothyroidism
      - Treat:
        - L-Thyroxine
- **(K)** Low T_4, Normal or low TSH (presumed hypopituitarism)
  - Consult:
    - Endocrinologist
      - Thyroxine-binding globulin
        - Deficiency
        - Normal
          - Test for other pituitary functions
          - Consider cranial/pituitary MRI

Precocious Puberty in Boys

Jennifer M. Barker, MD, and Michael S. Kappy, MD, PhD

DEFINITIONS

Pulsatile secretion of gonadotropic-releasing hormone (GnRH) from the hypothalamus initiates secretion of leuteinizing (LH) and follicle-stimulating hormones (FSH) resulting in estrogen release from the ovaries and the initiation of puberty. Testicular enlargement is usually the first sign of puberty in boys, followed by pubic and axillary hair development. Growth acceleration tends to occur during the later stages of puberty. Puberty is considered precocious when signs of puberty develop before 9 years of age in boys. Precocious puberty can be caused by release of LH and FSH from the pituitary, so-called central precocious puberty (GnRH dependent). When puberty is caused by unregulated estrogen release, it is referred to as peripheral precocious puberty (GnRH independent). Measurement of testicular size is important for the determination of central versus peripheral precocious puberty in boys with increased testicular size associated with central precocious puberty.

A. In the patient's history, note the age at onset of sexual development and recent increase in growth velocity. Identify predisposing central nervous system (CNS) conditions, such as head trauma, tumor, and meningitis. Obtain a family history of early male development that may be compatible with familial Leydig cell hyperplasia (testotoxicosis) and note parental heights. The normal mean age at onset of pubertal development (range in parentheses) in boys is as follows: testicular and penile enlargement, 11¾ years (9½ to 14 years); pubic hair, 12½ years (10¾ to 14 years); peak height growth velocity, 13¾ years (11¾ to 16 years); and axillary hair, 14 years (12 to 16 years).

B. In the physical examination, carefully plot height and weight, and note parental heights. Assess the genitalia (testicular volume and stretched penile length), and note any acne and pubic hair. In peripheral precocity, testosterone and other androgens are secreted without gonadotropin stimulation. Thus, the penis may be enlarged and pubic hair may be present, but the testes remain prepubertal in size (<4-ml volume with use of the Prader beads), unless a tumor is present (rare). In familial male limited precocious puberty or in congenital adrenal hyperplasia with adrenal rest tissue in the testes, the testes may be more than 4 ml in volume but are usually smaller than normal for the degree of observed virilization. In central precocity, early gonadotropin secretion stimulates the testes to grow and produce testosterone before the normal pubertal age. Thus, penile enlargement is accompanied by appropriate testicular enlargement. Note skeletal abnormalities (commonly in the lower extremities) and rough-bordered café-au-lait spots, which suggest McCune–Albright syndrome. Signs of androgen excess with moon face, central adiposity, and striae suggest Cushing syndrome. Evaluate growth chart for evidence of growth acceleration or growth deceleration.

C. Consider GnRH testing to determine the maturity of the hypothalamic-pituitary axis and if precocity is GnRH dependent (central) or independent (peripheral).

D. A plasma testosterone concentration less than 10 ng/dl and stimulated LH levels less than 10 IU/L suggests abnormal secretion of other androgens, usually from the adrenal glands. Measure these androgens (androstenedione, dehydroepiandrosterone) and 17-hydroxyprogesterone (17-OHP) directly in the blood. If necessary, remeasure these hormones after adrenocorticotropic hormone (ACTH) testing if basal results are equivocal.

E. In patients with congenital adrenal hyperplasia (CAH) or Cushing disease, low-dose dexamethasone will suppress endogenous production of cortisol by inhibiting ACTH secretion. In patients whose virilization results from autonomously functioning adrenal tissue (adrenal tumor or an ectopic ACTH-secreting tumor), dexamethasone will not suppress cortisol secretion.

F. CAH accounts for 70% to 80% of boys with peripheral precocity. An increased plasma 17-OPH concentration suggests this diagnosis.

G. Familial male limited precocious puberty (testotoxicosis) has been treated successfully with a combination of an antiandrogen (spironolactone) and an inhibitor of estrogen formation (testolactone) (Table 1).

H. The prevalence of CNS disease decreases as the patient's age at onset increases. Success in treatment of central precocity has been achieved with agonists of GnRH given intranasally or subcutaneously as a daily regimen or with a depot form of the agonist given monthly intramuscularly or subcutaneously (see Table 1).

Table 1. **Drug Therapy for Male Precocious Puberty**

Central (GnRH-Dependent) Precocity: GnRH Agonist
Leuprorelin (Lupron Depot-PED), 0.15–0.3 mg/kg/dose q4wk IM or SC (minimum dose: 7.5 mg)
Histrelin (Supprelin), 10 μg/kg qd SC
Nafarelin (Synarel), 1600–1800 μg/day, bid-tid
Peripheral (GnRH-Independent) Precocity, McCune–Albright Syndrome, or Familial Male Limited Precocious Puberty
Ketoconazole, 15–35 mg/kg/day divided into 2–3 doses PO
Spironolactone, 2–6 mg/kg/day divided into 2 doses PO
Testolactone, 20–40 mg/kg/day divided into 4 doses PO

GnRH, gonadotropic-releasing hormone; *IM*, intramuscularly; *PO*, orally; *SC*, subcutaneously.

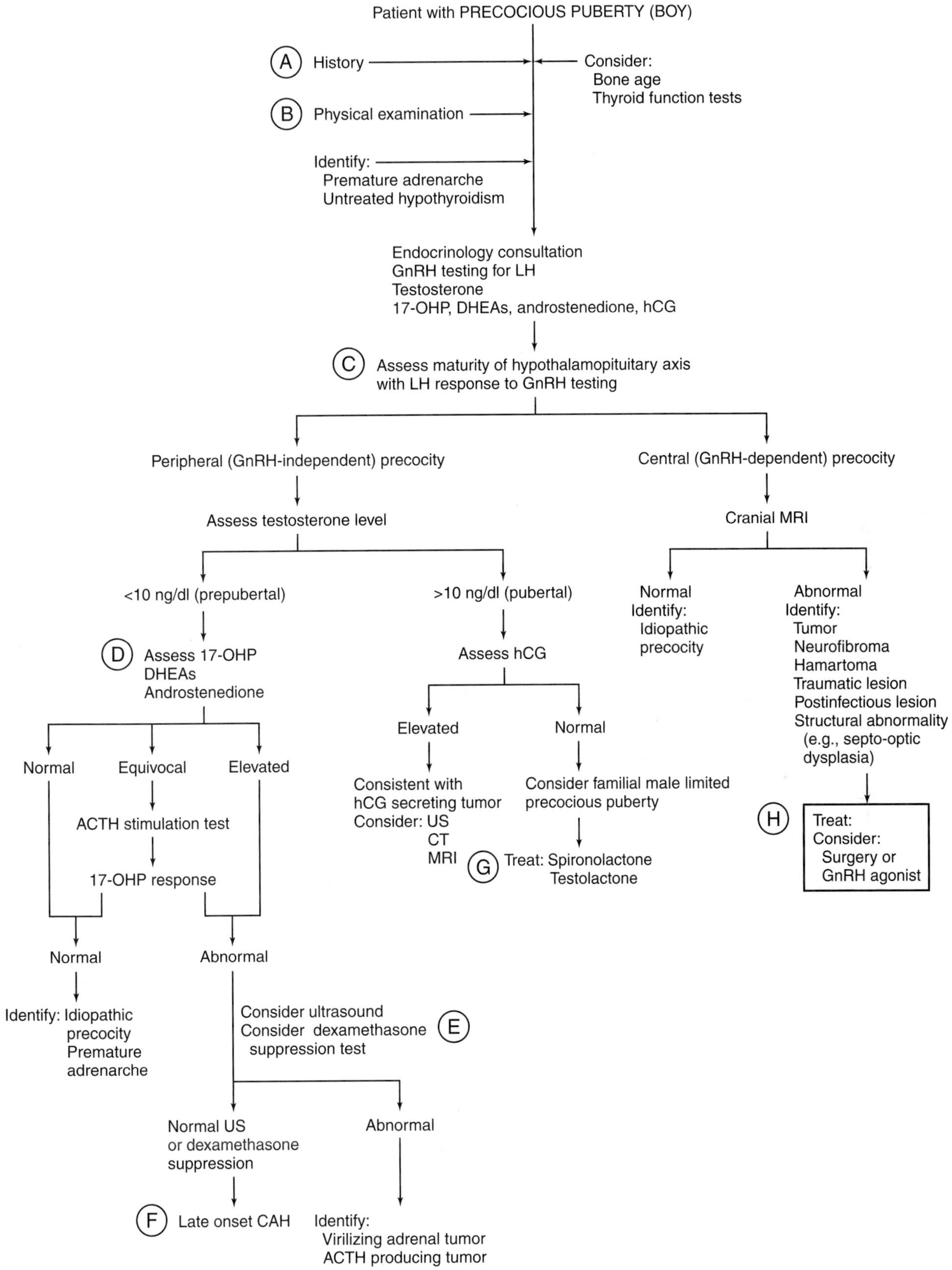
Patient with PRECOCIOUS PUBERTY (BOY)
A History
Consider:
Bone age
Thyroid function tests
B Physical examination
Identify:
Premature adrenarche
Untreated hypothyroidism
Endocrinology consultation
GnRH testing for LH
Testosterone
17-OHP, DHEAs, androstenedione, hCG
C Assess maturity of hypothalamopituitary axis
with LH response to GnRH testing
Peripheral (GnRH-independent) precocity
Central (GnRH-dependent) precocity
Assess testosterone level
Cranial MRI
<10 ng/dl (prepubertal)
>10 ng/dl (pubertal)
Normal
Identify:
Idiopathic
precocity
Abnormal
Identify:
Tumor
Neurofibroma
Hamartoma
Traumatic lesion
Postinfectious lesion
Structural abnormality
(e.g., septo-optic
dysplasia)
D Assess 17-OHP
DHEAs
Androstenedione
Assess hCG
Elevated
Normal
Normal
Equivocal
Elevated
Consistent with
hCG secreting tumor
Consider: US
CT
MRI
Consider familial male limited
precocious puberty
G Treat: Spironolactone
Testolactone
H Treat:
Consider:
Surgery or
GnRH agonist
ACTH stimulation test
17-OHP response
Normal
Abnormal
Identify: Idiopathic
precocity
Premature
adrenarche
Consider ultrasound
Consider dexamethasone
suppression test
E
Normal US
or dexamethasone
suppression
Abnormal
F Late onset CAH
Identify:
Virilizing adrenal tumor
ACTH producing tumor

References

Carel J-C, Leger J. Precocious puberty: clinical practice. N Engl J Med 2008;358:2366–77.

Dumitrescu CE, Collins MT. McCune-Albright syndrome. Orphanet J Rare Dis 2008;3:12.

Euling SY, Herman-Giddens ME, et al. Examination of US puberty-timing data from 1940–1994 for secular trends: panel findings. Pediatrics 2009;121:S182–91.

Reiter EO, Norjavaar E. Testotoxicosis: current viewpoint. Pediatr Endocrinol Rev 2005;3:77–86.

Precocious Puberty in Girls

Jennifer M. Barker, MD, and Michael S. Kappy, MD, PhD

DEFINITIONS

Pulsatile secretion of gonadotropic-releasing hormone (GnRH) from the hypothalamus initiates secretion of luteinizing (LH) and follicle-stimulating hormones resulting in estrogen release from the ovaries and the initiation of puberty. Breast development is usually the first sign of puberty in girls, followed by growth acceleration, pubic hair development, and menarche. Puberty is considered precocious when signs of puberty develop before 8 years of age in girls. Precocious puberty can be caused by release of LH and FSH from the pituitary, so-called central precocious puberty (GnRH dependent). When puberty is caused by unregulated estrogen release, it is referred to as peripheral precocious puberty (GnRH independent). Premature thelarche is early breast development in the absence of other signs of puberty. It is an innocent, nonpathologic finding and is not accompanied by rapid growth, advanced skeletal maturation, or pubertal plasma concentrations of estradiol or gonadotropins. Premature adrenarche is the early development of pubic hair without other signs of virilization. It is also a nonpathologic finding.

A. In the patient's history, ask about the age at onset of signs of puberty, what pubertal changes have been observed, and recent increase in growth velocity. The normal mean age at onset of pubertal development (range in parentheses) is as follows: breast development, 10 to 11 years (6 to 15 years); pubic hair, 10.5 to 11.5 years (7 to 15 years); menarche, 12.5 to 13 years (10½ to 16 years); peak height velocity at around the time of breast development. Identify any exogenous source of hormones (e.g., birth control pills or estrogen-containing creams). Note family history of early pubertal development and parental heights. Some studies suggest that normal breast development may begin in some girls as early as 6 years of age and pubic hair at 7 years.

B. In the physical examination, assess pattern and extent (use Tanner staging) of precocious development. Document any adrenal aspects of puberty (acne, pubic hair, axillary hair) and assess for clitoromegaly. Absence of adrenal aspects implies that estrogen excess produces the observed pubertal changes. Virilization without signs of estrogen effect (breast development or lightening of the color of the vaginal mucosa), suggests an excess of circulating androgens, usually from the adrenal glands. Perform a careful abdominal, rectoabdominal, or vaginoabdominal examination (depending on the age of the patient) to identify an adrenal or ovarian mass or uterine enlargement. Note signs of central nervous system abnormalities. Rough-bordered café-au-lait spots or skeletal abnormalities suggest McCune–Albright syndrome. Review growth chart for evidence of growth acceleration. Consider radiograph of left hand and wrist (anteroposterior view) to evaluate bone age to look for significant advancement. Consider thyroid function tests to rule out hypothyroidism. Consider endocrine consultation.

C. Assess pattern of precocious development. Use Tanner staging to document breast and pubic hair development. Evaluate growth chart for growth acceleration. If breast development is the only sign of puberty and bone age is not advanced, this could be consistent premature thelarche, which can be managed with conservative follow-up. Follow these girls for evidence of growth acceleration or other signs of puberty, which may require further evaluation. If virilization (pubic, axillary hair, and/or acne) is the only sign of puberty and the bone age is not advanced, careful follow-up for progression of puberty, growth acceleration, or advancement in bone age may be sufficient. All other patients require further evaluation.

D. Measure estradiol (E_2) and perform GnRH testing (see p. 166) in girls with breast development and advanced bone age. In peripheral precocity, estrogens are secreted without gonadotropin secretion, and GnRH testing shows a suppressed LH response. A pubertal response to GnRH testing is necessary for the diagnosis of central precocity. Increase of circulating estradiol without concomitant increase of gonadotropins (LH) suggests autonomous secretion of estrogens by a functional ovarian cyst, ovarian tumor, McCune–Albright syndrome, or adrenal tumor.

E. Studies have shown benefit in the treatment of central precocity from the use of a GnRH agonist given intranasally or subcutaneously daily or from a depot form of the agonist given once a month intramuscularly or subcutaneously (Table 1).

(Continued on page 170)

Table 1. **Treatment of Precocious Puberty in Girls**

Central GnRH-Dependent Precocity: GnRH Agonist	
Leuprorelin (Lupron Depot-PED), 7.5–15 mg q4wk IM; SC histrelin (Supprelin), 10 μg/kg qd; or SC nafarelin (Synarel), 1600–1800 μg/d bid to tid intranasally	
Peripheral GnRH-Independent Precocity	
Testolactone, 20–40 mg/kg/day divided into 4 doses PO	

GnRH, gonadotropic-releasing hormone; *IM*, intramuscularly; *PO*, orally; *SC*, subcutaneously.

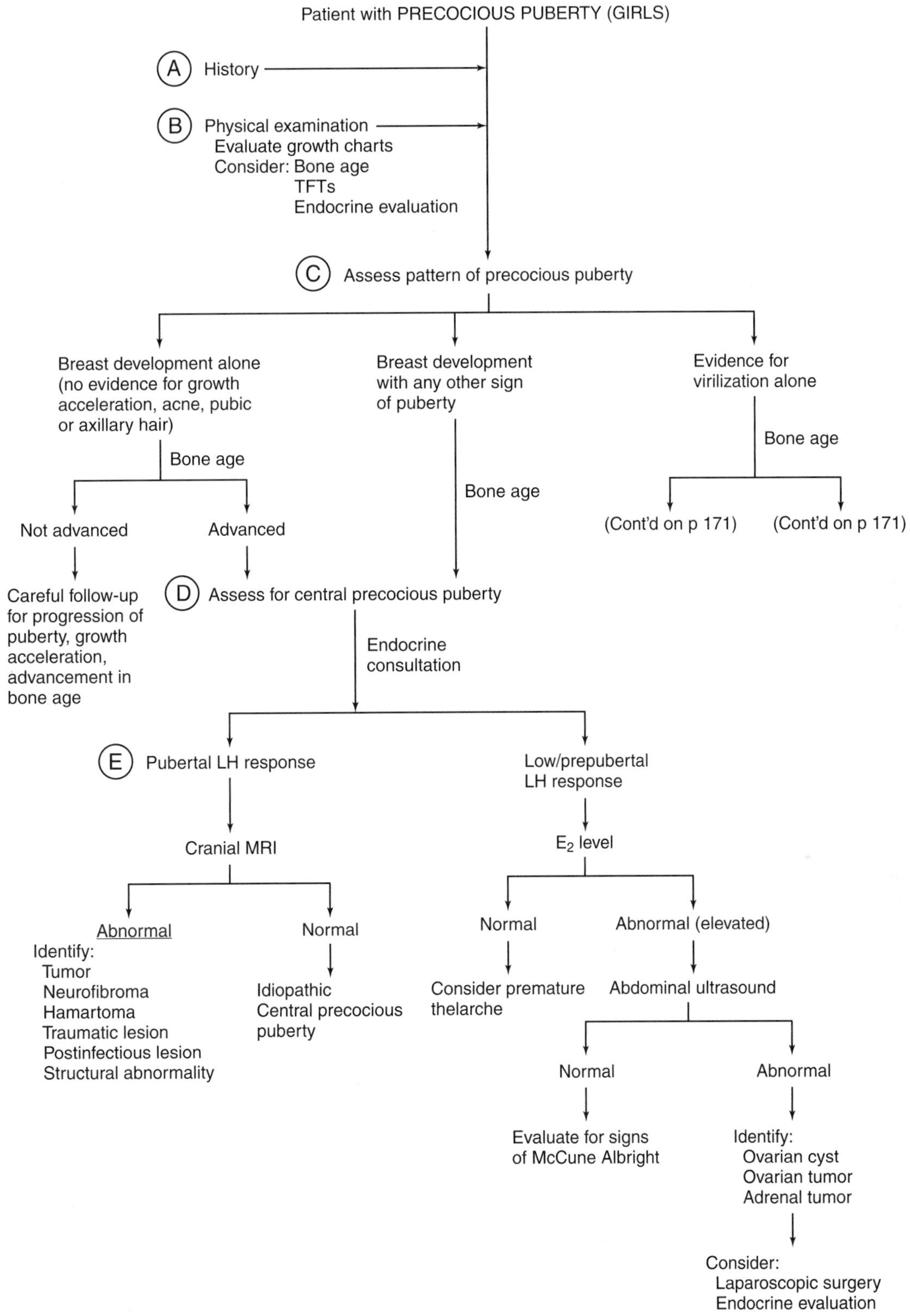
Patient with PRECOCIOUS PUBERTY (GIRLS)
(A) History
(B) Physical examination
Evaluate growth charts
Consider: Bone age
TFTs
Endocrine evaluation
(C) Assess pattern of precocious puberty
Breast development alone (no evidence for growth acceleration, acne, pubic or axillary hair)
Bone age
Not advanced
Careful follow-up for progression of puberty, growth acceleration, advancement in bone age
Advanced
Breast development with any other sign of puberty
Bone age
Evidence for virilization alone
Bone age
(Cont'd on p 171)
(Cont'd on p 171)
(D) Assess for central precocious puberty
Endocrine consultation
(E) Pubertal LH response
Cranial MRI
Abnormal
Identify:
Tumor
Neurofibroma
Hamartoma
Traumatic lesion
Postinfectious lesion
Structural abnormality
Normal
Idiopathic Central precocious puberty
Low/prepubertal LH response
E_2 level
Normal
Consider premature thelarche
Abnormal (elevated)
Abdominal ultrasound
Normal
Evaluate for signs of McCune Albright
Abnormal
Identify:
Ovarian cyst
Ovarian tumor
Adrenal tumor
Consider:
Laparoscopic surgery
Endocrine evaluation

F. Abnormal virilization in girls (pubic, axillary, or facial hair; acne; clitorimegaly) with evidence of bone age advancement warrants measurement of circulating androgens (testosterone, androstenedione, dehydroepiandrosterone [DHEA]) and 17-hydroxyprogesterone.

G. In a virilized girl who has increased 17-hydroxyoprogesterone levels, a diagnosis of late-onset congenital adrenal hyperplasia should be considered. In a virilized girl who has increased plasma testosterone, DHEA, or androstenedione concentrations, further evaluation with pelvic ultrasonography is indicated to rule out ovarian neoplasms. If findings on ultrasonography are abnormal, a laparoscopy or laparotomy is indicated for diagnostic and therapeutic purposes. With increase of DHEA or androstenedione alone, evaluation for late-onset congenital adrenal hyperplasia with ACTH stimulation testing is warranted.

H. Prepubertal concentrations of plasma testosterone in the absence of increased LH suggest the abnormal secretion of other androgens, most commonly from the adrenal glands. Measure the circulating androgens (see earlier) directly in the blood.

I. In patients with congenital adrenal hyperplasia or Cushing disease, low-dose dexamethasone will suppress endogenous secretion of cortisol by inhibiting adrenocorticotropic hormone (ACTH) secretion. Dexamethasone will not suppress cortisol secretion in patients whose virilization results from autonomously functioning adrenal tissue (tumor) or an ACTH-producing tumor.

References

Carel J-C, Leger J. Precocious puberty: clinical practice. N Engl J Med 2008;358:2366–77.

Dumitrescu CE, Collins MT. McCune-Albright syndrome. Orphanet J Rare Dis 2008;3:12.

Euling SJ, Herman-Giddens ME, Lee PA, et al. Examination of US puberty-timing data from 1940–1994 for secular trends: panel findings. Pediatrics 2008;121:S182–91.

Kaplowitz PB. Treatment of central precocious puberty. Curr Opin Endocrinol Diabetes Obes 2009;16:31–6.

Partsch C-J, Sippell WG. Pathogenesis and epidemiology of precocious puberty. Effects of exogenous oestrogens. Hum Reprod Update 2001;7:292–302.

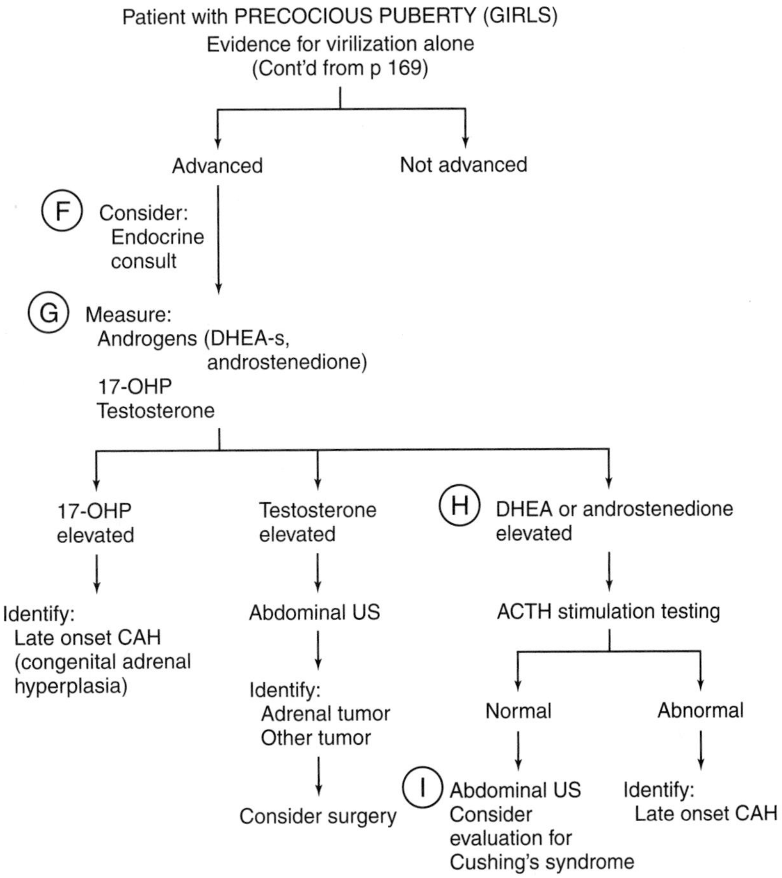
Patient with PRECOCIOUS PUBERTY (GIRLS)
Evidence for virilization alone
(Cont'd from p 169)
Advanced
Not advanced
F
Consider:
Endocrine consult
G
Measure:
Androgens (DHEA-s, androstenedione)
17-OHP
Testosterone
17-OHP elevated
Testosterone elevated
H
DHEA or androstenedione elevated
Identify:
Late onset CAH (congenital adrenal hyperplasia)
Abdominal US
ACTH stimulation testing
Identify:
Adrenal tumor
Other tumor
Normal
Abnormal
Consider surgery
I
Abdominal US
Consider evaluation for Cushing's syndrome
Identify:
Late onset CAH

Fever

Acute Fever in Infants Younger Than 3 Months

Acute Fever without a Source in Infants and Children 3 to 36 Months of Age

Fever, Rash, and Red Eyes

Frequent Infections

Fever of Unknown Origin

Acute Fever in Infants Younger Than 3 Months

John W. Ogle, MD

DEFINITIONS

Fever in early infancy is documented by a rectal temperature of 38° C (100.4° F) or greater in an infant 1 to 12 weeks of age. Fever without source is an acute febrile illness in which a probable cause cannot be identified with a careful history and physical examination. Serious bacterial infections include bacterial meningitis, bacteremia, bacterial pneumonia, urinary tract infections, bacterial enteritis, cellulitis, and bone and joint infections.

EPIDEMIOLOGY

Febrile illness during the first 3 months of life, although uncommon, can be serious. During the first 3 months of life, bacterial infections account for approximately 12% of febrile illnesses. Urinary tract infection is the most common serious bacterial infection (5.4%); bacteremia (1.8%), meningitis (0.5%), and pneumonia (3.3%) are also seen. Upper respiratory infection (25.6%), acute otitis media (12.2%), presumed viral (21.4%), bronchiolitis (7.8%), and gastroenteritis are also common.

RISK FACTORS

Age

Bacteremia is more than twice as frequent in the first month of life as in the second month and decreases further in the third month.

Temperature

For infants 4 to 12 weeks of age and appearing well or minimally ill, with temperature 38.6° C or greater, bacteremia or bacterial meningitis was present in 1.2% versus 0.4% if temperature is less than 38.6° C.

Prematurity

The frequency of late-onset group B streptococcus (GBS) infection is greater in premature infants than in full-term infants.

CAUSATIVE AGENTS

Bacterial pathogens responsible for meningitis and bacteremia are GBS, *Streptococcus pneumoniae, Escherichia coli,* other gram-negative rods, *Staphylococcus aureus,* group A streptococcus, *Enterococcus, Listeria monocytogenes, Salmonella,* and *Shigella.* During the first month, the most common pathogens are GBS and gram-negative enteric organisms; after the second month, *S. pneumoniae* is more common. Late-onset GBS infection can occur from 1 week to beyond 3 months of age. The most common viral pathogens are enteroviruses, respiratory syncytial virus, influenza, human herpes type 6, human metapneumovirus, adenovirus, and herpes simplex.

A. In the patient's history, ask about the following: onset, pattern, and degree of fever; perinatal risk factors (i.e., prematurity, maternal fever, herpes infection, premature rupture of membranes, prolonged nursery stay with antibiotic treatment); alterations in the mental status and normal level of activity (i.e., playfulness, irritability, feeding and sleeping patterns, responsiveness, seizures); respiratory symptoms (i.e., cough, congestion, coryza, fast or difficult breathing, chest indrawing [retractions]); and gastrointestinal symptoms (i.e., vomiting, diarrhea, abdominal distention, blood in stools).

B. On physical examination, look, listen, and feel for findings that suggest meningitis, such as a full fontanelle and being too weak to feed, difficult to arouse, or extremely irritable. It is more difficult to evaluate infants who have not developed a social smile (4–6 weeks) or the ability to make eye contact. An infant's smile is a useful negative predictor of meningitis. Note signs of perfusion, such as color and warmth of the extremities and capillary refill time (>2 seconds is abnormal). Findings of acute otitis media include tympanic membrane with decreased mobility, opaque rather than translucent, and bulging contour. Findings of pneumonia are tachypnea, retractions, grunting, and crackles. Soft tissue cellulitis or abscess (especially omphalitis) is suggested by swelling, erythema, induration, tenderness, and warmth of tissue. Bone or joint infection presents with limitation of motion, sometimes with pain or swelling; enteroviral infection presents with rash, erythematous macules, and hand, foot, and mouth lesions. *Neisseria meningitidis* bacteremia is often associated with petechiae or purpura.

C. The bacterial infections identified on physical examination and screening laboratory studies include acute otitis media, pneumonia, impetigo, adenitis, cellulitis, omphalitis, and bacterial enteritis (bloody diarrhea and septic arthritis-osteomyelitis). An associated bacteremia occurs in less than 10% of cases with bacterial enteritis and pneumonia. Some 10% of patients with urinary tract infection have bacteremia. Less than 5% of patients with acute otitis media have bacteremia or meningitis.

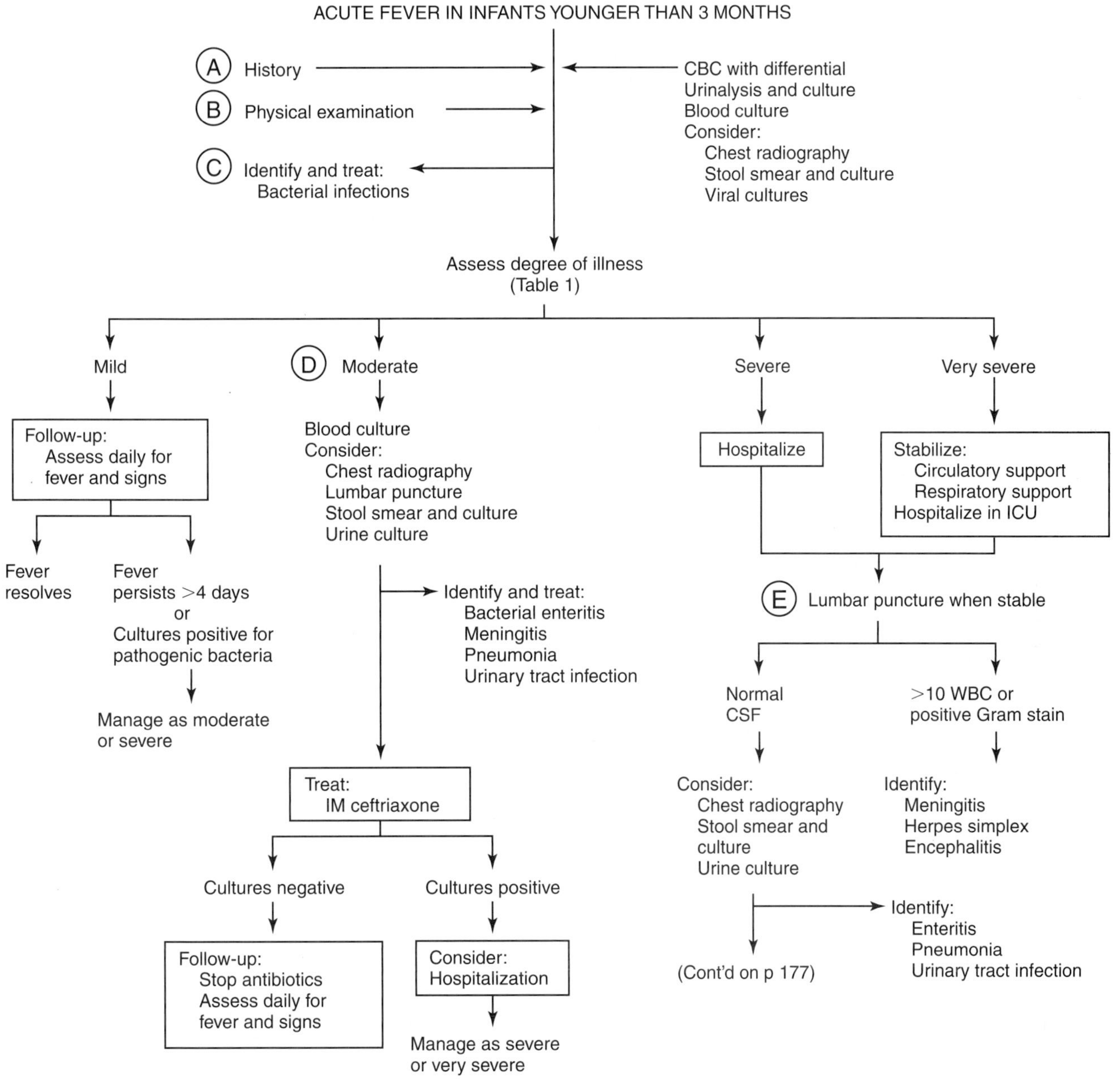
ACUTE FEVER IN INFANTS YOUNGER THAN 3 MONTHS
A History
B Physical examination
C Identify and treat: Bacterial infections
CBC with differential
Urinalysis and culture
Blood culture
Consider:
Chest radiography
Stool smear and culture
Viral cultures
Assess degree of illness (Table 1)
Mild
D Moderate
Severe
Very severe
Follow-up: Assess daily for fever and signs
Fever resolves
Fever persists >4 days or Cultures positive for pathogenic bacteria
Manage as moderate or severe
Blood culture
Consider:
Chest radiography
Lumbar puncture
Stool smear and culture
Urine culture
Identify and treat:
Bacterial enteritis
Meningitis
Pneumonia
Urinary tract infection
Treat: IM ceftriaxone
Cultures negative
Cultures positive
Follow-up: Stop antibiotics Assess daily for fever and signs
Consider: Hospitalization
Manage as severe or very severe
Hospitalize
Stabilize: Circulatory support Respiratory support Hospitalize in ICU
E Lumbar puncture when stable
Normal CSF
>10 WBC or positive Gram stain
Consider:
Chest radiography
Stool smear and culture
Urine culture
Identify:
Meningitis
Herpes simplex
Encephalitis
Identify:
Enteritis
Pneumonia
Urinary tract infection
(Cont'd on p 177)

D. An infant older than 4 weeks whose degree of illness is assessed as mild or moderate can be managed as an outpatient (Table 1). If blood and urine culture specimens have been obtained, there are two reasonable options: (1) Treat with intramuscular ceftriaxone, or (2) observe closely and follow up without antibiotic therapy. Follow-up should be daily until culture results are available and the child improves. If treatment with an antibiotic is planned, consider performing a lumbar puncture before treatment. When pathogens are isolated from blood, consider performing a lumbar puncture and admit to the hospital for parenteral antibiotic therapy. Infants with pathogens isolated from urine can be treated with outpatient oral antibiotics if they are afebrile, appear well, and are tolerating oral intake; if not, admit for parenteral antibiotics.

E. Perform a lumbar puncture as part of a workup to diagnose meningitis in infants who are admitted, regardless of appearance. Some will omit lumbar puncture if child is observed without antimicrobial therapy. Cerebrospinal fluid (CSF) pleocytosis is present when the total white blood cell count is greater than 10/ml. Most cases of meningitis are viral. Enteroviral meningitis is frequent in young febrile infants, particularly in summer. Herpes simplex infection also produces an abnormal spinal fluid. Herpes simplex virus polymerase chain reaction on spinal fluid and therapy with acyclovir should be considered in infants with a mononuclear CSF pleocytosis and/or an abnormal neurologic examination. The overall frequency of bacteremia or meningitis is 3% to 4% of infants with temperatures greater than 38.9° C.

F. Treat admitted patients with intravenous antibiotics (Table 2) pending culture results at 48 hours. Most positive blood and urine cultures will be recovered within 24 hours. In the first 4 weeks of age, consider ampicillin and gentamicin; from 4 to 8 weeks of age, consider ampicillin and cefotaxime or ceftriaxone. Ampicillin is recommended to cover *Listeria* and *Enterococcus*. Substitute nafcillin or another semisynthetic penicillin for ampicillin if an infection with *S. aureus* is suspected because of bullous skin lesions or a nursery outbreak. Enterococcus infections often require intravenous treatment with both ampicillin and gentamicin for 10 days. Intravenous antibiotics for GBS and *S. pneumoniae* bacteremia can be continued for 7 to 10 days. Consider acyclovir therapy when herpes simplex infection is suspected because of skin lesions, abnormal neurologic signs, or a CSF pleocytosis, and in any infant assessed as very severe. Ceftriaxone should be used with caution in infants with hyperbilirubinemia.

Table 1. **Degree of Illness**

Mild to Moderate	Severe	Very Severe
All infants aged ≥4 weeks with temperature <38.9°C without cardiopulmonary disease or a complicated nursery stay and who have a reliable caretaker	Infants aged <4 weeks* or infants with temperature >38.9°C or infants having cardiopulmonary disease or a complicated nursery stay regardless of degree of fever or who lack a reliable caretaker	
Mental status: smiles and not irritable, alerts quickly, feeds well	Mental status: irritable but consolable, poor eye contact (lethargic), feeds poorly	Mental status: irritable and not consolable, unresponsive, too weak to feed, or seizures
No signs of dehydration and good peripheral perfusion pink, warm extremities	Signs of dehydration or poor perfusion: mottled cool extremities	Shock, pale with thready pulse
No signs of respiratory distress	Respiratory rate >60, retractions, grunting	Apnea, cyanosis, respiratory failure
Absolute band count <1500/L, WBC 5000–15,000	Absolute band count ≥1500/L WBC <5000 or >15,000	
When diarrhea is present, <5 WBC/high-power field in stool and no blood in stool	When diarrhea is present, ≥5 WBC high-power field in stool or blood in stools	

Estimation of clinical usefulness of assessment criteria to identify cases with serious bacterial infection (SBI): sensitivity (proportion of SBI cases that will be classified as severe or very severe), 97%–99%; positive predictive value (proportion of cases classified as severe or very severe with SBI), 11.5% (range, 5.9%–24%); and negative predictive value (proportion of cases classified as mild to moderate with no SBI), 97.3% (range, 94.6%–100%).

*All febrile infants younger than 4 weeks should be hospitalized and treated pending culture results because of the lack of data correlating clinical assessment with outcome.

WBC, white blood cell count.

Table 2. **Therapy for Presumed Bacteremia or Herpes Simplex in Early Infancy**

Antibiotic	Dosage	Product Availability
Inpatient		
Acyclovir (Zovirax)	20 mg/kg/dose every 8h	500 mg/vial
Ampicillin sodium	50 mg/kg/dose IV every 6h	0.25, 0.5, 1, 2, 4 g
Cefotaxime (Claforan)	50 mg/kg/dose IV every 8h (bacteremia), every 6h (meningitis)	0.5, 1, 2 g
Ceftriaxone (Rocephin)	75 mg/kg/dose IV every 24h (bacteremia), 50 mg/kg/dose IV every 12h (meningitis)	0.25, 0.5, 1 g
Gentamicin	2.5 mg/kg/dose IV every 8h (neonates q12h)	20, 80 mg
Nafcillin	25–50 mg/kg/dose IV every 6h	250 mg
Outpatient		
Ceftriaxone (Rocephin)	50–75 mg/kg/dose IM every 24h	0.25, 0.5, 1 g

IM, intramuscularly; *IV*, intravenously.

ACUTE FEVER IN INFANTS YOUNGER THAN 3 MONTHS

(Cont'd from p 175)

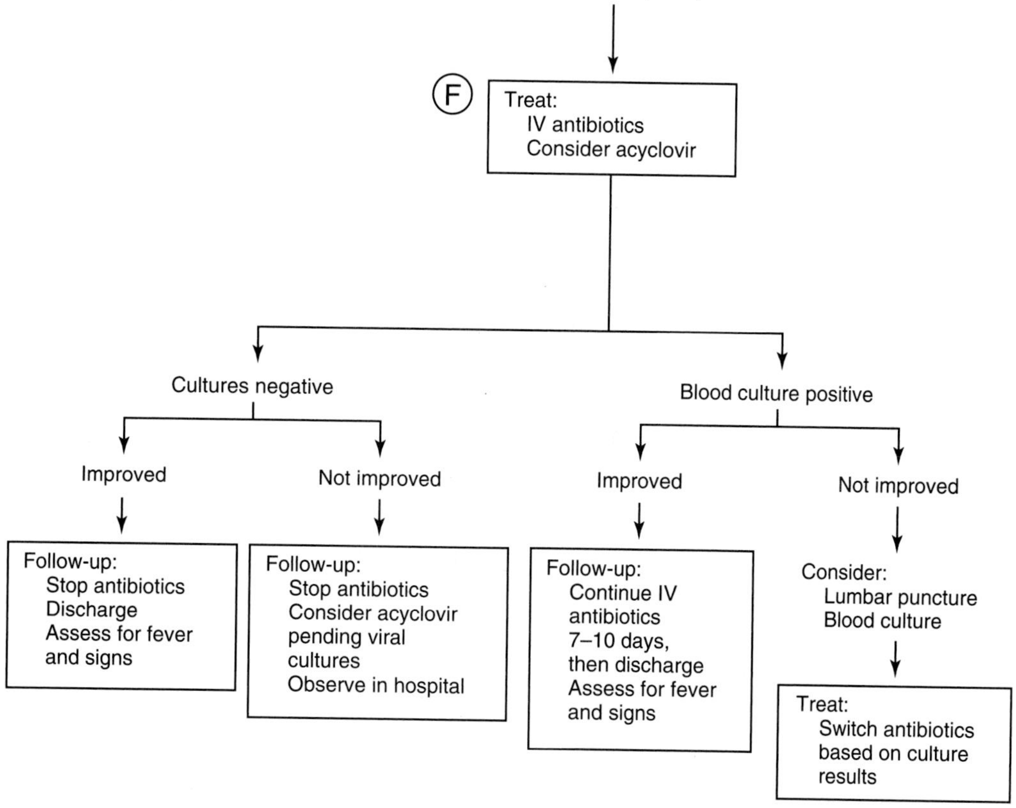
F
Treat:
IV antibiotics
Consider acyclovir
Cultures negative
Blood culture positive
Improved
Not improved
Improved
Not improved
Follow-up:
Stop antibiotics
Discharge
Assess for fever and signs
Follow-up:
Stop antibiotics
Consider acyclovir pending viral cultures
Observe in hospital
Follow-up:
Continue IV antibiotics 7–10 days, then discharge
Assess for fever and signs
Consider:
Lumbar puncture
Blood culture
Treat:
Switch antibiotics based on culture results

References

Albanyan EA, Bajer CJ. Is lumbar puncture necessary to exclude meningitis in neonates and young infants: lessons from the group B streptococcus cellulitis-adenitis syndrome. Pediatrics 1998;102:984–5.

Bachur RG, Harper MB. Predictive model for serious bacterial infections among infants younger than 3 months of age. Pediatrics 2001;108:311–6.

Baraff LJ, Bass JW, Fleisher GR, et al. Practice guideline for the management of infants and children 0 to 36 months of age with fever without source. Pediatrics 1993;92:1.

Baskin M, O'Rourke E, Fleisher G. Outpatient treatment of febrile infants 28 to 89 days of age with intramuscular administration of ceftriaxone. J Pediatr 1992;120:22.

Bonadio WA. Keeping febrile young infants out of the hospital. Contemp Pediatr 1994;11:73.

Bonadio WA, Smith D, Melzer M, et al. Reliability of observation variables in distinguishing infectious outcome of febrile young infants. Pediatr Infect Dis J 1993;12:111.

Bonadio WA, Webster H, Wolfe A, et al. Correlating infectious outcome with clinical parameters of 1130 consecutive febrile infants aged 0–8 weeks. Pediatr Emerg Care 1993;9:84.

Bramson RT, Meyer TL, Silbiger ML, et al. The futility of the chest radiograph in the febrile infant without respiratory symptoms. Pediatrics 1993;92:524.

Byington CL, Enriquez FR, Hoff C, et al. Serious bacterial infections in febrile infants 1 to 90 days old with and without viral infections. Pediatrics 2004;113:1662.

Caviness AC, Demmler GJ, Selwyn BJ. Clinical and laboratory features of neonatal herpes simplex virus infection: a case-control study. Pediatr Infect Dis J 2008;27:425.

Caviness AC Demmler GJ, Swint JM, Cantor SB. Cost-effectiveness analysis of herpes simplex virus testing and treatment strategies in febrile neonates. Arch Pediatr Adolesc Med 2008;162:665.

Hoberman A, Chao H-P, Keller DM, et al. Prevalence of urinary tract infection in febrile infants. J Pediatr 1993;123:17.

Jaskiewicz JA, McCarthy CA, Richardson AC, et al. Febrile infants at low risk for serious bacterial infection: an appraisal of the Rochester criteria and implications for management. Pediatrics 1994;94:390.

Kramer MS, Shapiro ED. Management of the young febrile child: a commentary on recent practice guidelines. Pediatrics 1997;100:128.

McCarthy J, Powell K, Jaskiewicz J, et al. Outpatient management of selected infants younger than 2 months of age evaluated for possible sepsis. Pediatr Infect Dis J 1990;9:385.

Pantell RH, Newman TB, Bernzweig J, et al. Management and outcomes of care of fever in early infancy. JAMA 2004;291:1203.

Yagupsky P, Menegus MA, Powell KR. The changing spectrum of group B streptococcal disease in infants: an 11-year experience in a tertiary care hospital. Pediatr Infect Dis J 1991;10:801.

Acute Fever without a Source in Infants and Children 3 to 36 Months of Age

John W. Ogle, MD

DEFINITIONS

Fever is documentation of a rectal temperature of at least 38° C (100.4° F) in an infant or child 3 to 36 months of age. Fever without source is an acute febrile illness in which no probable cause can be identified with a careful history and physical examination. Serious bacterial infections include bacterial meningitis, bacteremia, bacterial pneumonia, urinary tract infections, bacterial enteritis, cellulitis, and bone and joint infections.

COMPLICATIONS OF BACTEREMIA

Complications of occult bacteremia include delayed-onset meningitis, periorbital or buccal cellulitis, pneumonia, septic arthritis, osteomyelitis, epiglottitis, and pericarditis. Immunization with vaccines effective against *Haemophilus influenzae* and *Streptococcus pneumoniae* have substantially decreased bacteremia and subsequent complications. The 13-valent pneumococcal vaccine will further reduce the incidence of disease.

EPIDEMIOLOGY

Fever in early childhood (3–24 months) is common, accounting for 26% of sick visits to pediatricians and 55% of sick visits to hospital pediatric clinics. Approximately 25% of febrile sick visits are associated with temperatures of 39° C (102° F) or higher. The clinician cannot identify a focus of bacterial or viral infection (excluding a mild upper respiratory tract infection) in 15% to 30% of these cases. The incidence of occult bacteremia in patients without obvious focus of infection varies with age and degree of fever. Among immunized children with fever greater than 39° C, the incidence rate is about 0.5%. In many recent studies, the rate of contaminated blood cultures (2%–3%) is several-fold greater than recovery of true pathogens.

RISK FACTORS

The risk for bacteremia is low in this age, and age and height of fever are not predictive of serious bacterial infection.

CAUSATIVE FACTORS

Occult bacteremia is usually caused by *S. pneumoniae* or *Neisseria meningitidis*. *Salmonella*, *Staphylococcus aureus*, *Escherichia coli*, and *Streptococcus pyogenes* can also cause occult bacteremia. *Haemophilus influenzae* type B is rare in immunized populations. Invasive disease caused by *S. pneumoniae* is often caused by serotypes not covered by the current vaccine. Causes of bacterial enteritis include *Salmonella*, *Campylobacter*, *Shigella*, *Yersinia*, and invasive or toxigenic strains of *E. coli*.

A. In the history, ask about the onset, pattern, and degree of the fever. Evaluate the family's ability to care for the child at home, and their access to transportation and a telephone. Risk factors include immunization status; current medications; allergies; underlying conditions, such as cardiopulmonary, gastrointestinal, or renal disease; sickle cell disease; central venous catheter and other indwelling lines; and conditions and therapy that compromise immunity, especially human immunodeficiency virus infection. Assess alterations in the mental status and normal level of activity: playfulness, irritability, feeding and sleeping patterns, responsiveness, and seizures. Note any respiratory symptoms: cough, congestion, coryza, sore throat, earache, fast or difficult breathing, or chest indrawing (retractions). Check for gastrointestinal symptoms: vomiting, diarrhea, abdominal distention, abdominal pain, or blood in stools. Assess renal symptoms: pain with urination (dysuria), urinary frequency, flank pain, or lower abdominal pain.

B. On physical examination, look, listen, and feel for findings that suggest the following: meningitis (full fontanelle, too weak to feed, difficult to arouse, unresponsive, extreme or paradoxic irritability, nuchal rigidity, and Brudzinski and Kernig signs); an infant's smile is a useful negative predictor of meningitis; dehydration and poor perfusion (skin turgor, tears, moist mucous membranes, color and warmth of the extremities, and capillary refill time [>2 seconds is abnormal]); acute otitis media (tympanic membrane with decreased mobility, opaque with obscured landmarks, bulging contour); pneumonia (tachypnea,

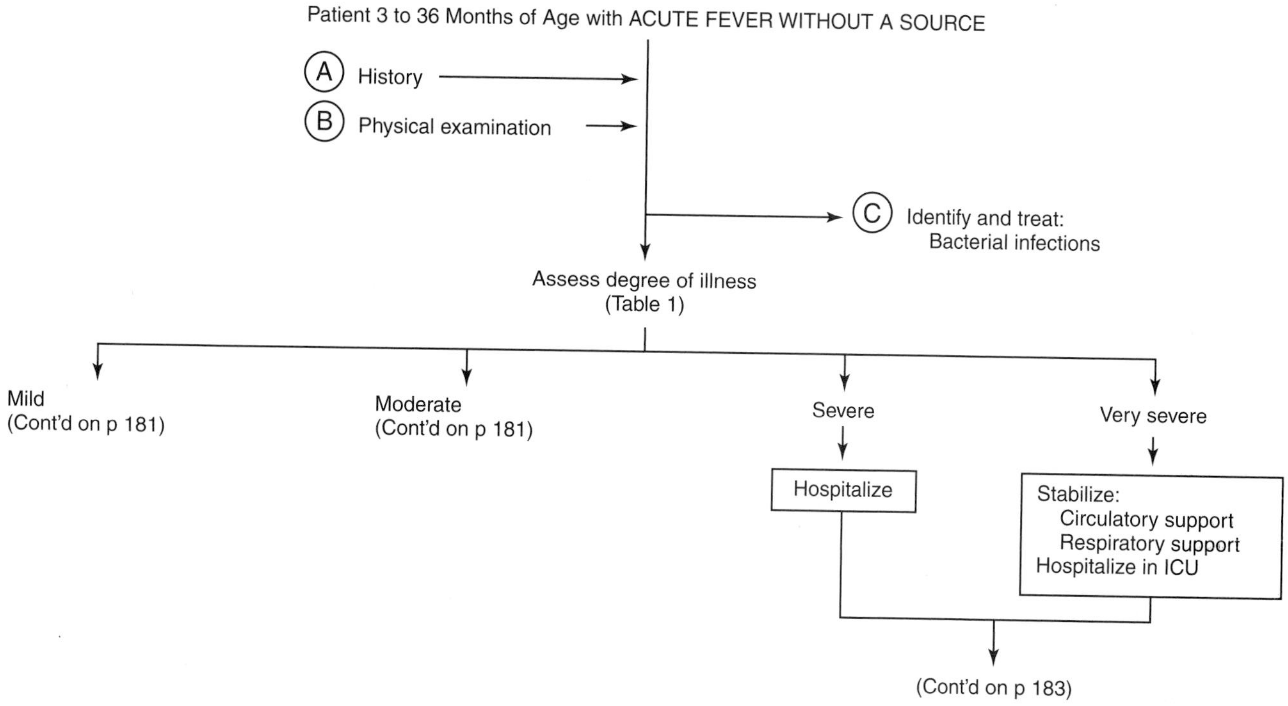
Patient 3 to 36 Months of Age with ACUTE FEVER WITHOUT A SOURCE
A History
B Physical examination
C Identify and treat:
Bacterial infections
Assess degree of illness
(Table 1)
Mild
(Cont'd on p 181)
Moderate
(Cont'd on p 181)
Severe
Very severe
Hospitalize
Stabilize:
Circulatory support
Respiratory support
Hospitalize in ICU
(Cont'd on p 183)

retractions, grunting, crackles); adenitis, soft tissue cellulitis, or abscess (swelling, erythema, induration, pain, warmth of tissue); bone or joint infection (painful swelling with limitation of motion); enteroviral infection (rash, erythematous exanthem, and hand, foot, and mouth lesions); *N. meningitidis* bacteremia (petechiae, purpura).

C. Bacterial infections identified or suspected on history and physical examination are acute otitis media, pneumonia, impetigo, adenitis, sinusitis, cellulitis, bacterial enteritis (bloody diarrhea), and septic arthritis or osteomyelitis. In most studies, the rate of bacteremia is the same in children diagnosed with acute otitis media compared with those with otitis media.

D. As the frequency of bacterial infection has decreased with immunization, clinicians frequently order complete blood cell count (CBC) with differential, urinalysis and urine cultures, and other diagnostic tests selectively rather than routinely. Age of the child, immunization status, degree of illness, and reliability of outpatient follow-up are factors used in determining whom to test. Urine specimens should be obtained by catheterization or suprapubic tap. A urine bag culture is only interpretable if negative. The CBC with differential can be used to screen moderately ill patients for occult bacteremia. Abnormal findings include an absolute band count greater than 500 and a white blood cell count greater than 15,000 or less than 5000. The risk of occult bacteremia is low in moderately ill patients with normal CBC. Increased C-reactive protein correlates better with bacteremia and other serious infections than either white blood count or band count.

E. Perform a lumbar puncture to diagnose meningitis in infants and children who are severely or very severely ill (Table 1). Consider it in selected moderately ill patients who will be treated with antibiotics. Cerebrospinal fluid pleocytosis is present when the total white blood cell count is greater than $10/mm^3$. The most sensitive indicator of bacterial meningitis is the cerebrospinal fluid Gram stain. The likelihood of isolating a bacterial pathogen from cerebrospinal fluid is very low if the Gram stain is negative and the cell count and chemistries are normal. Viral meningoencephalitis is much more common than bacterial meningitis. Do not routinely obtain chest radiographs of children who have no signs of respiratory illness. Obtain stool cultures when diarrhea is present with signs of invasive bacterial disease, such as blood or five white blood cells or more per high-power field. Most physicians recommend withholding empirical antibiotic treatment until the cause is confirmed by stool culture, for fear of worsening an *E. coli* O157 infection.

F. Selectively treat moderately ill patients without a source of infection with high-dose oral amoxicillin or intramuscular ceftriaxone. Although studies have suggested that parenteral antibiotics are more effective than oral antibiotics in preventing delayed-onset meningitis in bacteremic infants and children, the difference is attributed to infections with *H. influenzae*. Because immunization with *H. influenzae* type b vaccine has greatly reduced the frequency of these infections, oral antibiotics may adequately treat sensitive *S. pneumoniae* infections.

G. When a bacterial pathogen is isolated from the blood culture in a febrile patient managed as an outpatient, reassess the clinical status. All patients who remain febrile or who would continue to be assessed as moderately or severely ill without improvement should have a lumbar puncture, repeated blood culture, and consider admission for intravenous antibiotics. Children who are afebrile and appear well but who have bacteria isolated from blood can often be treated as outpatients. Treat afebrile patients assessed as mildly ill in whom sensitive *S. pneumoniae* has been isolated with 10 days of oral therapy with high-dose amoxicillin or parenterally with ceftriaxone. When a urine culture is positive and the patient is assessed as improved (well or mild illness), continue outpatient treatment with oral antibiotics. If the patient does not improve, consider admission for parenteral therapy.

(Continued on page 182)

Table 1. **Degree of Illness in Infants and Children 3 to 6 Months of Age with Acute Fever without a Source**

Mild	Moderate	Severe	Very Severe
All previously well infants and children with temperature <38.9°C and who have a reliable caretaker	All infants and children with chronic illness regardless of temperature and all patients with temperature >38.9°C or who lack a reliable caretaker	All infants and children with a condition that compromises immunity	All infants and children with petechiae, purpura
Mental status: smiles, playful, not irritable, alerts quickly, feeds well, cries strongly but is easily consoled by a caregiver	Mental status: brief smiles, irritable with crying and sobbing, still responsive to the caregiver and consolable, less playful and active than baseline	Mental status: irritable and not easily consolable, poor eye contact (lethargic), feeds poorly	Mental status: unresponsive, too weak to feed, seizures or signs of meningeal irritation
No signs of dehydration	Signs of mild or moderate dehydration	Signs of severe dehydration	
Good peripheral perfusion: pink, warm extremities	Good peripheral perfusion: pink, warm extremities	Poor perfusion: mottled, cool extremities	Shock, pale, with thready pulse
No signs of respiratory distress	No signs of respiratory distress	Respiratory rate >60, retractions, grunty	Apnea, cyanosis, respiratory failure

Estimation of clinical usefulness of assessment criteria to identify cases with serious bacterial infection (SBI): sensitivity (proportion of SBI cases that will be classified as severe or very severe), 44%–74%; positive predictive value (proportion of cases classified as severe or very severe that will have SBI), 33%; and negative predictive value (proportion of cases classified as mild or moderate that will not have SBI), 75%.

Patient 3 to 36 Months of Age with ACUTE FEVER WITHOUT A SOURCE

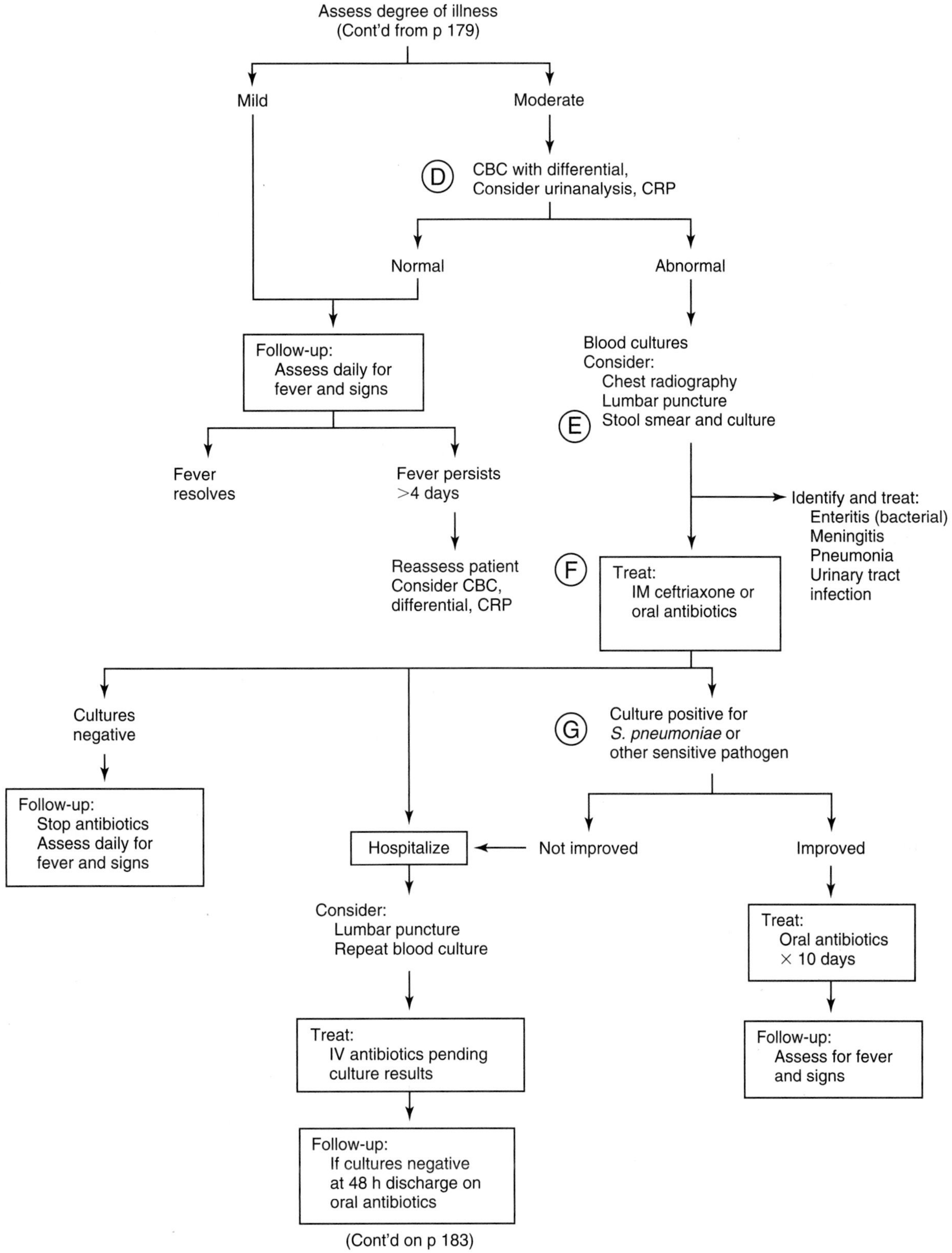

Assess degree of illness
(Cont'd from p 179)
Mild
Moderate
D
CBC with differential,
Consider urinanalysis, CRP
Normal
Abnormal
Follow-up:
Assess daily for
fever and signs
Fever
resolves
Fever persists
>4 days
Reassess patient
Consider CBC,
differential, CRP
Blood cultures
Consider:
Chest radiography
Lumbar puncture
E
Stool smear and culture
Identify and treat:
Enteritis (bacterial)
Meningitis
Pneumonia
Urinary tract
infection
F
Treat:
IM ceftriaxone or
oral antibiotics
Cultures
negative
Follow-up:
Stop antibiotics
Assess daily for
fever and signs
G
Culture positive for
S. pneumoniae or
other sensitive pathogen
Hospitalize
Not improved
Improved
Consider:
Lumbar puncture
Repeat blood culture
Treat:
IV antibiotics pending
culture results
Follow-up:
If cultures negative
at 48 h discharge on
oral antibiotics
(Cont'd on p 183)
Treat:
Oral antibiotics
× 10 days
Follow-up:
Assess for fever
and signs

Table 2. **Outpatient and Inpatient Antibiotics for the Treatment of Moderately to Severely Ill Children with Bacteremia**

Antibiotic	Dosage	Product Availability
Outpatient Antibiotics		
Cefuroxime (Ceftin)	75–150 mg/kg/day every 8h	Suspension: 125, 250 mg/5 ml Tablets: 125, 250, 500 mg
Amoxicillin-clavulanate (Augmentin)	80–90 mg/kg/24 hr bid (use 7:1 bid formulation)	Suspension: 200, 400 mg/5 ml Chewable: 200, 400 mg Tablets: 875 mg
Amoxicillin	80–90 mg/kg/24 hr bid	Suspension: 125, 250 mg/200, 400 mg/5 ml Chewable: 125, 200, 250, 400 mg Capsules: 250, 500 mg Tablets: 500–875 mg
Intramuscular Antibiotics		
Ceftriaxone (Rocephin)	50 mg/kg/dose every 12-24h	Vials: 0.25, 0.5, 1 g
Initial Intravenous Antibiotics		
Cefotaxime (Claforan)	50–75 mg/kg/dose every 6-8h	Vials: 0.5, 1, 2 g
Cefuroxime (Kefurox, Zinacef)	25–50 mg/kg/dose every 8h	Vials: 0.75, 2.5 g
Ceftriaxone (Rocephin)	75 mg/kg/dose every 24h	Vials: 0.25, 0.5, 1 g
Clindamycin (Cleocin)	8–13 mg/kg/dose every 8h	Vials: 2, 4, 6 ml (150 mg/ml)
Ampicillin sodium	50–75 mg/kg/dose every 6h	Vials: 0.25, 0.5, 1, 2, 4 g
Vancomycin (Vancocin)	10–15 mg/kg/dose every 8h	Vials: 500, 1000 mg Capsules: 125, 250 mg

H. Treat admitted patients assessed as severely ill with intravenous antibiotics (Table 2) pending culture results at 48 hours. The combination of antibiotics chosen depends on the severity of the illness. Treat patients assessed as very severely ill with vancomycin and a cephalosporin such as cefotaxime to provide additional coverage for resistant *S. aureus* and *S. pneumoniae*. Clindamycin should be considered if anaerobes or *S. aureus* is suspected.

References

Alpern ER, Alessandrini EA, Bell LM, et al. Occult bacteremia from a pediatric emergency department: current prevalence, time to detection, and outcome. Pediatrics 2000;106:505–11.

Bachur R, Harper MB. Reevaluation of outpatients with Streptococcus pneumoniae bacteremia. Pediatrics 2000;105:502–9.

Baraff LJ, Bass JW, Fleisher GR, et al. Practice guideline for the management of infants and children 0 to 36 months of age with fever without source. Pediatrics 1993;92:1.

Baraff LJ, Oslund S, Prather M. Effect of antibiotic therapy and etiologic microorganism on the risk of bacterial meningitis in children with occult bacteremia. Pediatrics 1993;92:140.

Black S, Shinefield H, Hansen J, et al. Post-licensure evaluation of the effectiveness of seven valent pneumococcal conjugate vaccine. Pediatr Infect Dis J 2001;20:1105.

Finkelstein JA, Christiansen CL, Platt R. Fever in pediatric primary care: occurrence, management, and outcomes. Pediatrics 2000;105:260–6.

Harper MB, Bachur R, Fleisher GR. Effect of antibiotic therapy on the outcome of outpatients with unsuspected bacteremia. Pediatr Infect Dis J 1995;14:760.

Herz AM, Greenhow TL, Alcantara J, et al. Changing epidemiology of outpatient bacteremia in 3- to 36-month-old children after the introduction of the heptavalent-conjugated pneumococcal vaccine. Pediatr Infect Dis J 2006;25:293.

Kramer MS, Shapiro ED. Management of the young febrile child: a commentary on recent practice guidelines. Pediatrics 1997;100:128.

Kyaw MH, Lynfield R, Schaffner W, et al. Effect of introduction of the pneumococcal conjugate vaccine on drug-resistant Streptococcus pneumoniae. N Engl J Med 2006;354:1455.

Lee GM, Fleisher GR, Harper MB. Management of febrile children in the age of the conjugate pneumococcal vaccine: a cost-effectiveness analysis. Pediatrics 2001;108:835–44.

Newman TB, Bernzweig JA, Takayama JI, et al. Urine testing and urinary tract infections in febrile infants seen in office settings. Arch Pediatr Adolesc Med 2002;156:44.

Pena BMG, Harper MB, Fleisher GR. Occult bacteremia with group B streptococci in an outpatient setting. Pediatrics 1998;102:67–72.

Pulliam PN, Attia MW, Cronan KM. C-reactive protein in febrile children 1 to 36 months of age with clinically undetectable serious bacterial infection. Pediatrics 2001;108:1275–9.

Rothrock SG, Harper MB, Green SM, et al. Do oral antibiotics prevent meningitis and serious bacterial infections in children with Streptococcus pneumoniae occult bacteremia? A meta-analysis. Pediatrics 1997;99:438–44.

Patient 3 to 36 Months of Age with ACUTE FEVER WITHOUT A SOURCE

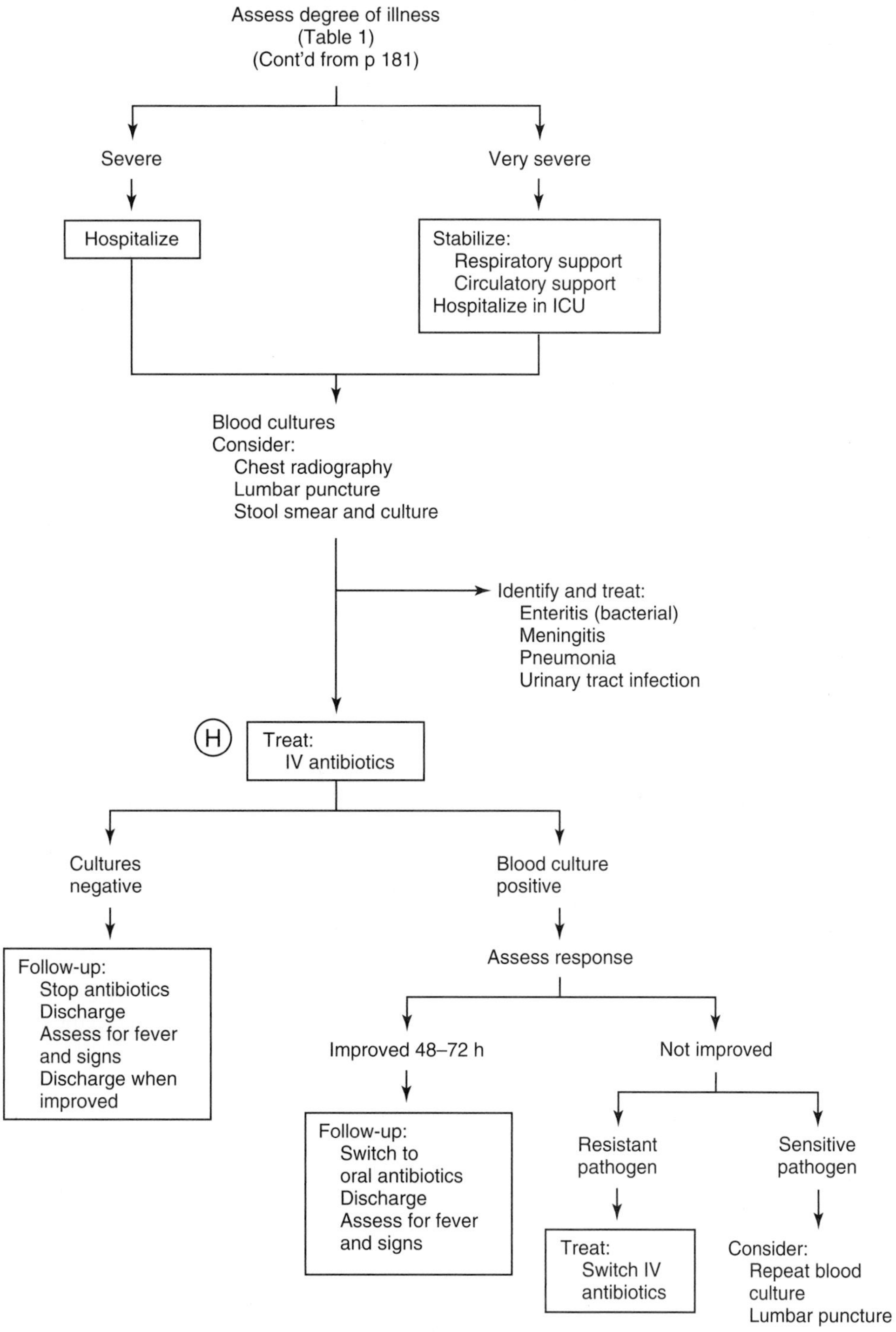
Assess degree of illness
(Table 1)
(Cont'd from p 181)
Severe
Very severe
Hospitalize
Stabilize:
Respiratory support
Circulatory support
Hospitalize in ICU
Blood cultures
Consider:
Chest radiography
Lumbar puncture
Stool smear and culture
Identify and treat:
Enteritis (bacterial)
Meningitis
Pneumonia
Urinary tract infection
H
Treat:
IV antibiotics
Cultures negative
Blood culture positive
Follow-up:
Stop antibiotics
Discharge
Assess for fever and signs
Discharge when improved
Assess response
Improved 48–72 h
Not improved
Follow-up:
Switch to oral antibiotics
Discharge
Assess for fever and signs
Resistant pathogen
Sensitive pathogen
Treat:
Switch IV antibiotics
Consider:
Repeat blood culture
Lumbar puncture

Fever, Rash, and Red Eyes

Samuel R. Dominguez, MD, PhD

A. In the patient's history, ask about the onset and duration of fever, rash, conjunctivitis, and other associated symptoms, such as sore throat, headache, photophobia, mouth lesions, coryza, cough, swelling of hands and feet, arthralgias or arthritis, diarrhea, vomiting, and abdominal pain. Ask about the distribution and progression of the rash and any temporal relationships between the onset of the fever and rash. Inquire about the use of current and past medications. Take a thorough exposure history, including history of recent travel (national and international), history of recent camping/hiking or tick exposure, exposure to animals, presence of sick contacts, and sexual history. Inquire about the patient's vaccination status and immune status. Note the season of the year.

B. On physical examination, note whether the conjunctivitis is purulent or hyperemic. Characterize the type of rash (morbilliform, maculopapular, erythrodermal, vesicular, petechial), as well as its distribution. Press on the lateral edge of a blister; extension and enlargement constitute presence of a Nikolsky sign. Look for mouth lesions (fissuring and crusting of lips, Koplik spots on the buccal mucosa, strawberry or raspberry tongue, oropharyngeal lesions, injection, or exudate). Characterizing the rash and conjunctivitis is helpful diagnostically. A purulent conjunctivitis and a diffuse erythroderma with bullae, tender skin, and presence of a Nikolsky sign suggest Stevens–Johnson syndrome (SJS) or staphylococcal scalded skin syndrome (SSSS). SSSS is often associated with a purulent rhinitis. Adenovirus may produce a serous conjunctivitis. An erythroderma suggests toxic shock syndrome, Kawasaki disease (KD), scarlet fever syndromes, or leptospirosis. Epstein–Barr virus (EBV) and adenovirus infections are often associated with an exudative pharyngitis. A morbilliform rash with Koplik spots suggests measles (rubeola).

C. Measles (rubeola) is associated with a 3- or 4-day prodrome of cough, coryza, fever, and conjunctivitis. The rash, which starts on the head and face, moves downward to involve the trunk and extremities. Lesions on the face, neck, and upper trunk become confluent. Koplik spots are usually present on the buccal mucosa and are pathognomonic for the disease. The rash resolves in approximately 1 week. Consider the diagnosis of measles in patients who have not been immunized.

D. A common presentation of adenovirus infection is pharyngoconjunctival fever. These children present with high fevers, upper respiratory infection symptoms, tonsillitis, cervical lymph node enlargement, conjunctivitis, and/or rash. Symptoms can persist for 3 to 10 days. The incidence is increased slightly during late winter, spring, and early summer. Unlike many other respiratory viral infections, adenovirus can mimic severe bacterial infections, and in one study, approximately 25% of children had C-reactive protein (CRP) levels greater than 7 mg/dl.

E. In working up a child with a fever, rash, and red eyes syndrome, it is important to diagnose diseases that are treatable. In particular, one should try to distinguish viral disease from bacterial disease and KD. Obtaining inflammatory markers can be helpful in distinguishing between these diseases. Most viral illness will have low erythrocyte sedimentation rates (ESRs), CRP levels, and procalcitonins (PCTs). In contrast, most bacterial diseases and KD will have increased inflammatory markers. Several studies have demonstrated that often the ESR and CRP are discordant, and thus obtaining both is useful. Several studies now suggest that PCT may be a more sensitive and specific test for helping to distinguish between a viral and bacteria disease process.

(Continued on page 186)

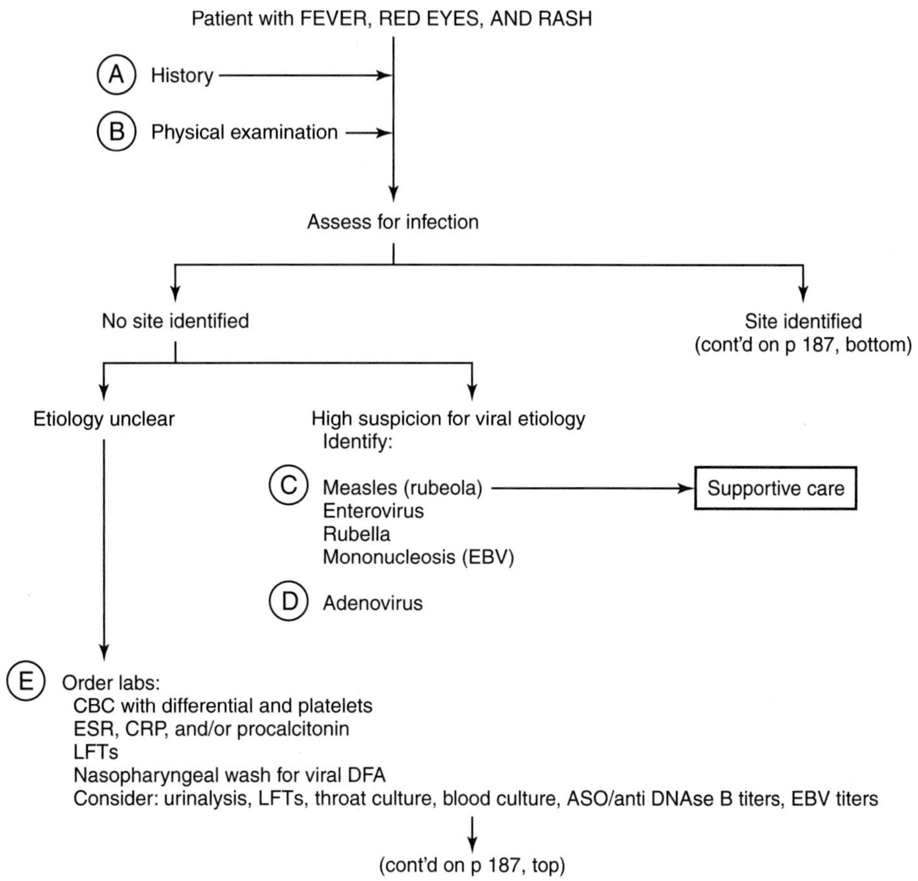
Patient with FEVER, RED EYES, AND RASH
A History
B Physical examination
Assess for infection
No site identified
Site identified
(cont'd on p 187, bottom)
Etiology unclear
High suspicion for viral etiology
Identify:
C Measles (rubeola)
Enterovirus
Rubella
Mononucleosis (EBV)
Supportive care
D Adenovirus
E Order labs:
CBC with differential and platelets
ESR, CRP, and/or procalcitonin
LFTs
Nasopharyngeal wash for viral DFA
Consider: urinalysis, LFTs, throat culture, blood culture, ASO/anti DNAse B titers, EBV titers
(cont'd on p 187, top)

F. SJS and toxic epidermal necrolysis represent a spectrum of the same illness associated with systemic signs, bullous lesions, a Nikolsky sign, and involvement of at least two mucous membranes (conjunctiva, oral cavity, genital mucosa, or esophagus). The rash of SJS often begins as poorly defined macules with purpuric centers (dusky red, morbilliform macules) that coalesce to form blisters and can progress to epidermal detachment. The lesions of SJS are often symmetrically distributed. The infectious agent most frequently associated with SJS in children is *Mycoplasma pneumoniae.* The most commonly associated drugs are antibiotics (sulfonamides, cephalosporins, quinolones, and aminopenicillins), anticonvulsants (carbamazepine, phenytoin, and phenobarbital), nonsteroidal anti-inflammatory drugs, corticosteroids, and allopurinol. In a patient with SJS caused by a medication, immediate discontinuation of the medication is required. Some experts advocate the use of intravenous immunoglobulin in the treatment of SJS. All patients with SJS require ophthalmology consultation to assess eye involvement and preserve vision with treatment.

G. Suspect SSSS when lateral pressure on the edge of the blister enlarges and extends the blister (Nikolsky sign) or bullous impetigo is present. The rash may be local or generalized. SSSS is often associated with a purulent rhinitis. Hospitalize and treat patients with antistaphylococcal antibiotics and for pain management.

H. Suspect KD when an erythematous rash and conjunctival hyperemia are associated with fever for more than 4 days, mouth lesions (red and/or cracked lips, strawberry tongue, or oropharyngeal injection), alterations of the hands or feet (erythema, edema, and induration followed by desquamation), and unilateral cervical lymphadenopathy. It is now recognized that many children with KD present without meeting full clinical criteria (see Kawasaki Disease, p. 628).

I. Lyme disease (causative agent: *Borrelia burgdorferi*) is the most common tick-borne (*Ixodes* ticks) disease in the United States and Europe. In the United States, Lyme disease is concentrated in three distinct geographical areas: in the Northeast from Maryland to Maine, in the Midwest primarily in Wisconsin and Minnesota, and in the West in Northern California and Oregon. More than 80% of patients with Lyme disease will present with the characteristic target-like rash erythema migrans. The skin lesions are frequently accompanied by influenza-like illness symptoms including fatigue, myalgias, arthralgias, headaches, and fever. Only about 10% of patients with Lyme disease have conjunctivitis. Lyme disease should be treated with doxycycline (first-line therapy) or amoxicillin (see Lyme Disease, p. 632).

J. Rocky Mountain spotted fever (RMSF) (causative agent: *Rickettsia rickettsii*) occurs most commonly in the Southeast United States and should be considered during the summer months when ticks are active (90% of cases occur from April to September). The rash of RMSF typically starts on the ankles and wrists, spreads to the palms and soles, and then spreads inward to the trunk. The rash will often begin as a maculopapular rash and can become petechial over time. Patients often have a classic triad of laboratory findings: hyponatremia, leukopenia, and thrombocytopenia. Diagnosis is made on clinical suspicion (can be confirmed only by convalescent serology) and is treated with doxycycline. Human monocytic ehrlichiosis and human granulocytic anaplasmosis are other tickborne rickettsial diseases that present similarly to RMSF but are associated less commonly with rash.

K. *Leptospira* organisms are secreted in the urine of animal; therefore, leptospirosis should be considered in patients with occupational exposure (i.e., farmers) or in association with swimming in freshwater. The most distinctive clinical findings of leptospirosis are conjunctival suffusion and myalgias of the calf and lumbar regions. Ten percent of patients have a life-threatening illness consisting of jaundice, renal failure, and hemorrhagic pneumonitis. Penicillin is the drug of choice.

L. Oral first-generation cephalosporins, dicloxacillin, and amoxicillin are comparable for treatment of superficial staphylococcal and streptococcal infections. However, because of the increase in community-acquired methicillin-resistant *Staphylococcus aureus* (MRSA) infections, treatment for suspected staphylococcal infections should include coverage for MRSA. Antibiotics should be chosen based on the susceptibility patterns of MRSA in the local community. Generally, clindamycin or trimethoprim-sulfamethoxazole (TMP-SMZ) is an acceptable choice. It is important to remember, however, that empiric coverage with TMP-SMZ does not provide adequate coverage for streptococcal infections.

M. Toxic shock syndrome is usually caused by a staphylococcal phage-related toxin. It can be caused by skin and wound infections, tampon use, vaginal infections, nasal packing, childbirth and abortion infections, and postinfluenza bacterial respiratory tract infections (tracheitis, pneumonia). Suspect toxic shock syndrome when erythroderma is associated with fever, hypotension, altered mental status, diarrhea, disseminated intravascular coagulation, and renal failure. Hospitalize these patients, stabilize their circulation, and begin intravenous antistaphylococcal antibiotic coverage. If a focus of infection is identified, efforts should be made to drain/remove it. Intravenous immunoglobulin (1 g/kg) should be considered in severely ill patients.

N. Group A streptococcus may also produce a toxin-mediated illness that is clinically similar to toxic shock syndrome. The diagnosis must be made by culture. Before culture results are available, use antibiotic coverage effective against both streptococcal and staphylococcal disease.

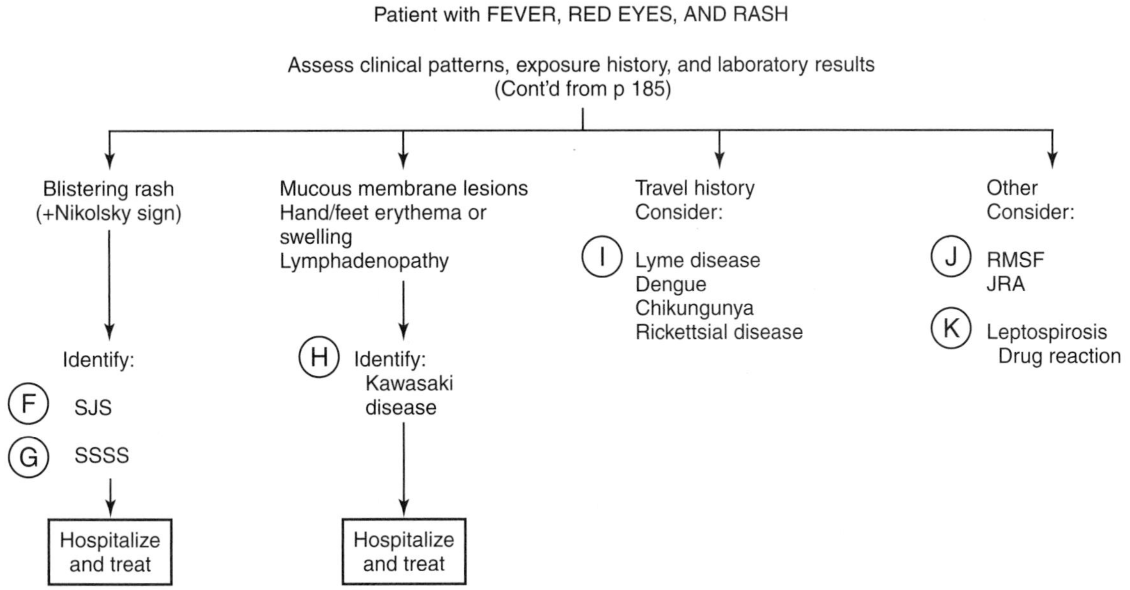
Patient with FEVER, RED EYES, AND RASH
Assess clinical patterns, exposure history, and laboratory results
(Cont'd from p 185)
Blistering rash
(+Nikolsky sign)
Identify:
F SJS
G SSSS
Hospitalize and treat
Mucous membrane lesions
Hand/feet erythema or swelling
Lymphadenopathy
H Identify:
Kawasaki disease
Hospitalize and treat
Travel history
Consider:
I Lyme disease
Dengue
Chikungunya
Rickettsial disease
Other
Consider:
J RMSF
JRA
K Leptospirosis
Drug reaction

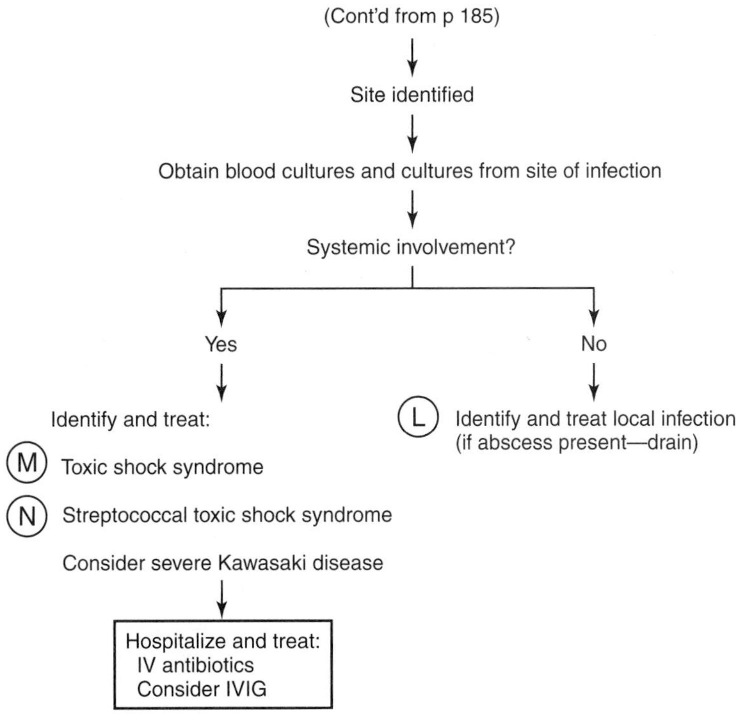
(Cont'd from p 185)
Site identified
Obtain blood cultures and cultures from site of infection
Systemic involvement?
Yes
Identify and treat:
M Toxic shock syndrome
N Streptococcal toxic shock syndrome
Consider severe Kawasaki disease
Hospitalize and treat:
IV antibiotics
Consider IVIG
No
L Identify and treat local infection
(if abscess present—drain)

References

Aber C, Alvarez Connelly E, Schachner LA. Fever and rash in a child: when to worry? Pediatr Ann 2007;36:30–8.

American Academy of Pediatrics (AAP). Red book: 2009 report of the Committee on Infectious Diseases. 28th ed. Elk Grove Village, IL: AAP; 2009.

Burns JC, Glode MP. Kawasaki syndrome. Lancet 2004;364:533–44.

Dantas-Torres F. Rocky Mountain spotted fever. Lancet Infect Dis 2007;7:724–32.

Daum RS. Clinical practice. Skin and soft-tissue infections caused by methicillin-resistant Staphylococcus aureus. N Engl J Med 2007;357:380–90.

Dominguez O, Rojo P, de Las Heras S, et al. Clinical presentation and characteristics of pharyngeal adenovirus infections. Pediatr Infect Dis J 2005;24:733–4.

Dyer JA. Childhood viral exanthems. Pediatr Ann 2007;36:21–9.

Roujeau JC, Kelly JP, Naldi L, et al. Medication use and the risk of Stevens-Johnson syndrome or toxic epidermal necrolysis. N Engl J Med 1995;333:1600–7.

Rzany B, Correia O, Kelly JP, et al. Stevens-Johnson syndrome and toxic epidermal necrolysis during first weeks of antiepileptic therapy: a case-control study. Study Group of the International Case Control Study on Severe Cutaneous Adverse Reactions. Lancet 1999;353:2190–4.

Wormser GP. Clinical practice. Early Lyme disease. N Engl J Med 2006;354:2794–2801.

Frequent Infections

Stephen Berman, MD, and Roberta L. DeBiasi, MD

Patients presenting for evaluation of frequent or recurrent infections are a heterogeneous group, including normal children, children with nonimmunologic causes of recurrent infection, or those with underlying immunodeficiency (primary or secondary). The likelihood of an underlying immunodeficiency disorder is closely related to the type, frequency, and severity of infections that the patient suffers. For example, patients with a history of frequent/recurrent minor childhood illnesses (such as viral upper respiratory infections) who are growing and developing normally are unlikely to have an underlying immunodeficiency predisposing them to frequent infections. In contrast, patients with a history of more than one episode of invasive bacterial infection, in which bacteria invade the bloodstream or other sterile body sites (such as bacteremia, bacterial pneumonia, septic arthritis, osteomyelitis, and meningitis), are statistically more likely to have an underlying immunologic defect that warrants evaluation.

Nonimmunologic causes of recurrent infection include increased exposure (day care), conditions that disrupt normal mucosal barriers (atopy: asthma, allergic rhinitis; passive smoke exposure, gastroesophageal reflux), anatomic abnormalities, cystic fibrosis, immotile cilia syndrome, malnutrition, and foreign bodies. An intact immune response includes components of innate, nonspecific immunity (such as physiologic barriers, spleen, phagocytes, complement and natural killer cells), as well as adaptive, specific immunity including cell-mediated (T lymphocyte) and humoral (antibody-mediated) immune responses. Defects within any of the arms of the immunologic system often lead to predictable types and patterns of recurrent infection that may provide clues to diagnosis. Furthermore, immunodeficiency disorders can be categorized as primary (inherited) or secondary to other illnesses, trauma, drugs, malnutrition, or protein loss.

EPIDEMIOLOGY

Overall, the incidence of primary immunodeficiency disorders is about 1 per 5000 to 10,000. Of these, approximately 50% are pure B-lymphocyte defects, 20% are T-lymphocyte defects, 10% combined B- and T-lymphocyte defects, and 15% are phagocyte defects; complement deficiency is rarer (2%–5%). The most common primary immune defect is selective IgA deficiency (usually asymptomatic), which occurs in 1 in 500 individuals. In contrast with the primary immunodeficiencies, acquired immunodeficiency is more common. For example, the incidence of human immunodeficiency virus (HIV) infection is as high as 1 in 1000 in some population groups within the United States, and thus should always be considered in the differential diagnosis of possible underlying immunodeficiency disorders. Other common causes of acquired immunodeficiency include immunoglobulin deficiency caused by nephrotic syndrome or protein-losing enteropathy, cell-mediated immunodeficiency caused by steroid therapy for asthma, asplenia caused by trauma or sickle cell disease, and impaired immune function caused by diabetes.

A. As a general rule of thumb, historical features that suggest underlying immunodeficiency include too many infections, infections that are of unusual severity or are difficult to treat, infections with unusual organisms (e.g., *Cryptococcus, Pseudomonas, Burkholderia, Pneumocystis*), or recurrent infections associated with growth or developmental delay. Ten warning signs that have been publicized for immunodeficiency include: eight or more ear infections within 1 year; two or more serious sinus infections within 1 year; 2 or more months on antibiotics with little or no effect; two or more pneumonias within 1 year; failure of an infant to gain weight or grow normally; recurrent, deep skin or organ abscesses; persistent thrush in mouth or elsewhere on skin, after age 1; need for intravenous antibiotics to clear infections; two or more deep seated infections; and family history of primary immune deficiency.

In the patient's history, ask about the types of infection and the pathogens isolated. Document the onset, severity, response to therapy, and pattern of infections. Onset of infections soon after birth suggests defects in cell-mediated immunity, neutrophil function, or complement because maternal antibody protects infants with B-cell disorders for 3 to 6 months. In the family history, note early unexplained infant deaths and other family members with frequent severe infections or known immunodeficiency diseases, especially HIV infection and malignant neoplasms. Risk factors include immunization status and adverse reactions to vaccines, current medications, allergies, underlying conditions (collagen vascular disease; cardiopulmonary, gastrointestinal, and renal disease; sickle cell disease), central venous catheter and other indwelling lines, and conditions or therapies that compromise immunity (especially HIV infection).

Review of systems should include:

Central nervous system symptoms, including alterations in the mental status and normal level of activity

Respiratory symptoms: cough recurrent sore throats, sinus and ear infections, pneumonia episodes

Gastrointestinal symptoms: chronic diarrhea, weight loss, malnutrition, failure to thrive

Renal symptoms: pain with urination (dysuria), urinary frequency, flank pain

Dermatologic symptoms: chronic *Candida* infection (involvement of skin, nails, and mucous membranes), severe eczema, delayed umbilical cord separation

B. On physical examination, look, listen, and feel for findings that suggest a current infection or sequelae of past infections. Note either abundance or absence of

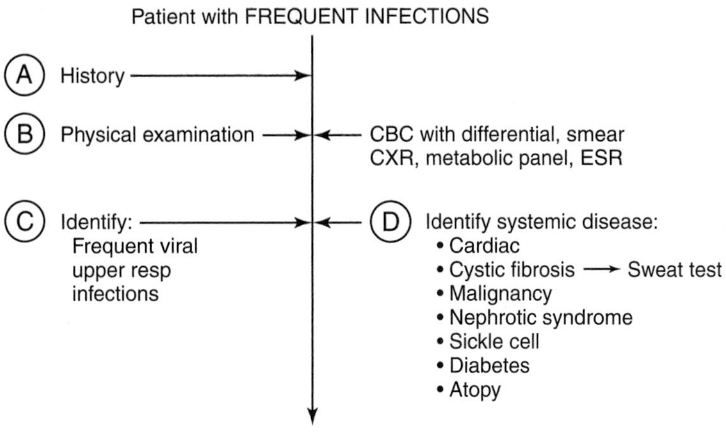

Patient with FREQUENT INFECTIONS
(A) History
(B) Physical examination
CBC with differential, smear
CXR, metabolic panel, ESR
(C) Identify:
Frequent viral
upper resp
infections
(D) Identify systemic disease:
• Cardiac
• Cystic fibrosis
Sweat test
• Malignancy
• Nephrotic syndrome
• Sickle cell
• Diabetes
• Atopy

(Cont'd on p 191)

lymphoid tissue (lymph nodes and tonsils); assess growth and development. Note petechiae (Wiskott–Aldrich syndrome), telangiectasia, and neurologic findings (ataxia-telangiectasia syndrome), scarring from adenitis (chronic granulomatous disease), hepatosplenomegaly, partial albinism (Chédiak–Higashi syndrome), periodontal disease (neutrophil defects), and nail/oral mucosal candidiasis (cell-mediated deficiency).

C. Children younger than 6 years may commonly have 6 to 12 viral infections per year. These episodes of upper respiratory infections and diarrhea are usually mild and self-limited. Children who attend nursery school or daycare centers are most likely to have frequent viral infections. Multiple episodes of otitis media are also not uncommon in infants/toddlers, and in isolation, do not necessarily warrant an immunologic evaluation. However, two or more otitis media per year in an adolescent or adult; two or more bacterial pneumonia, severe sinusitis, or bacterial gastroenteritis per year; or two or more life-threatening infections per lifetime warrant further evaluation.

D. A systemic disorder or malignant disease may predispose to frequent infections because of neutropenia, impaired mucociliary clearance (cystic fibrosis, atopy, ciliary dysfunction), or abnormal vascular perfusion (diabetes, nephrosis, congestive heart failure, infarction). Metabolic disorders and systemic diseases that predispose to frequent infection include diabetes mellitus, cystic fibrosis, severe malnutrition, allergic disorders (allergic rhinitis, eczema, reactive airway disease), central nervous system disorders (recurrent aspiration), and gastroesophageal reflux. Therapy with a corticosteroid or other immunosuppressive for renal disease, rheumatoid arthritis, or reactive airway disease alters immune defenses and may result in frequent infections.

E. Most patients fall into one of the following four patterns:

Pattern 1: recurrent bacterial infections involving one system only, such as recurrent meningitis, pneumonia, or osteomyelitis; consider nonimmunologic defects (such as anatomic-structural defects) and B-cell defects (Tables 1 and 3), as well as HIV infection

Pattern 2: recurrent bacterial infections involving multiple systems, especially respiratory (sinopulmonary disease) and gastrointestinal; consider B-cell defects (Tables 1 and 3), as well as HIV infection

Pattern 3: severe infections with opportunistic or intracellular pathogens, including viruses (herpesviruses, respiratory syncytial virus), fungi, protozoa (*Pneumocystis*), and intracellular bacteria (tuberculosis); consider T-cell defects (Tables 2 and 3), as well as HIV infection

Pattern 4: recurrent abscesses, soft tissue infections, and skin infections; consider neutropenia or neutrophil function defects (Table 4)

F. Suspect a defect in nonimmunologic defenses when two or more serious bacterial infections occur in the same anatomic site without infections in other sites. Nonimmunologic defects that allow frequent infections include anatomic alterations (ureteral stenosis, vesicoureteral reflux, eustachian tube dysfunction, tracheoesophageal fistula, skull defects or fractures, sinus tracts), impaired barriers (atopy, including asthma and eczema, burns, gastroesophageal reflux), and foreign bodies (catheters, heart valves).

G. Neutrophil disorders include abnormalities of quantity and function. Quantitative alterations include problems with bone marrow production (congenital and cyclic neutropenia, reticular dysgenesis), storage (bone marrow necrosis), migration or sequestration (hypersplenism, burns, trauma), and destruction (antineutrophil antibodies, infection, inflammation). Qualitative alterations include abnormalities of adhesion (leukocyte adhesion disorder), migration-chemotaxis (hyperimmunoglobulin E syndrome; Chédiak–Higashi syndrome, actin dysfunction; and systemic conditions, such as diabetes mellitus and collagen vascular disorders), phagocytosis (actin dysfunction, opsonin deficiency caused by hypogammaglobulinemia or complement deficiency, asplenia, Wiskott–Aldrich syndrome), bactericidal activity and cytotoxicity (enzyme defects), and oxidative burst activities (chronic granulomatous disease). Patients with chronic granulomatous disease do not respond to phagocytosis with chemiluminescence (emission of energy as light). Specific tests are available to evaluate

Table 1. **Selected B-Cell Disorders**

Disorder	Genetics and Presentation	Defect	Treatment
Bruton agammaglobulinemia	XLR inheritance; Xq21.3-q22 prenatal diagnosis available Absent/low-level B lymphocytes Absent immunoglobulins	Arrest in differentiation of pre-B cells	Monthly IVIG
Agammaglobulinemia	AR and AD forms; 14q32.33, 9q34.13	See above	Monthly IVIG
Immunoglobulin deficiency with hyper-IgM	XLR (Xq26), AR Low IgG, IgA, normal or high IgM	CD40 ligand signaling defect Impaired isotype switching from IgM to IgG, IgA, and IgE	Monthly IVIG
Common variable immuno- or late-onset hypogammaglobulinemia	Unknown inheritance; heterogeneous group of disorders	B cells do not differentiate into plasma cells Low normal B lymphocyte levels, poor antibody responses, autoimmunity	Monthly IVIG
Transient hypogammaglobulinemia of infancy	Unknown inheritance; spontaneous recovery by 4 years of age	Delayed maturation; response of B cells to T-cell–dependent stimulation depressed	Usually none

AD, autosomal dominant; *AR*, autosomal recessive; *IVIG*, intravenous immunoglobulin; *XLR*, X-linked recessive.

Table 2. **Selected T-Cell Disorders**

Disorder	Genetics and Presentation	Defect	Treatment
Purine-nucleoside phosphorylase deficiency	AR inheritance; prenatal diagnosis available (14q13); may present with autoimmune hemolytic anemia	Enzyme deficiency causes increase in deoxyguanosine triphosphate, which kills dividing T cells	Consider BMT, irradiated blood cell transfusions to replace enzyme
Thymic hypoplasia (DiGeorge syndrome)	Intrinsic genetic factors (22q11.2; 10p14-p13)	Malformation of cardiac outflow tract; absent or hypoplastic thymus, congenital hypoparathyroidism, abnormal facies	Consider graft with fetal epithelial; neonatal cells or BMT
Nezelof syndrome	Intrinsic genetic factors (22q11.2) Absent or low T lymphocytes	Thymic dysplasia	See above

AR, autosomal recessive; *BMT*, bone marrow transplantation.

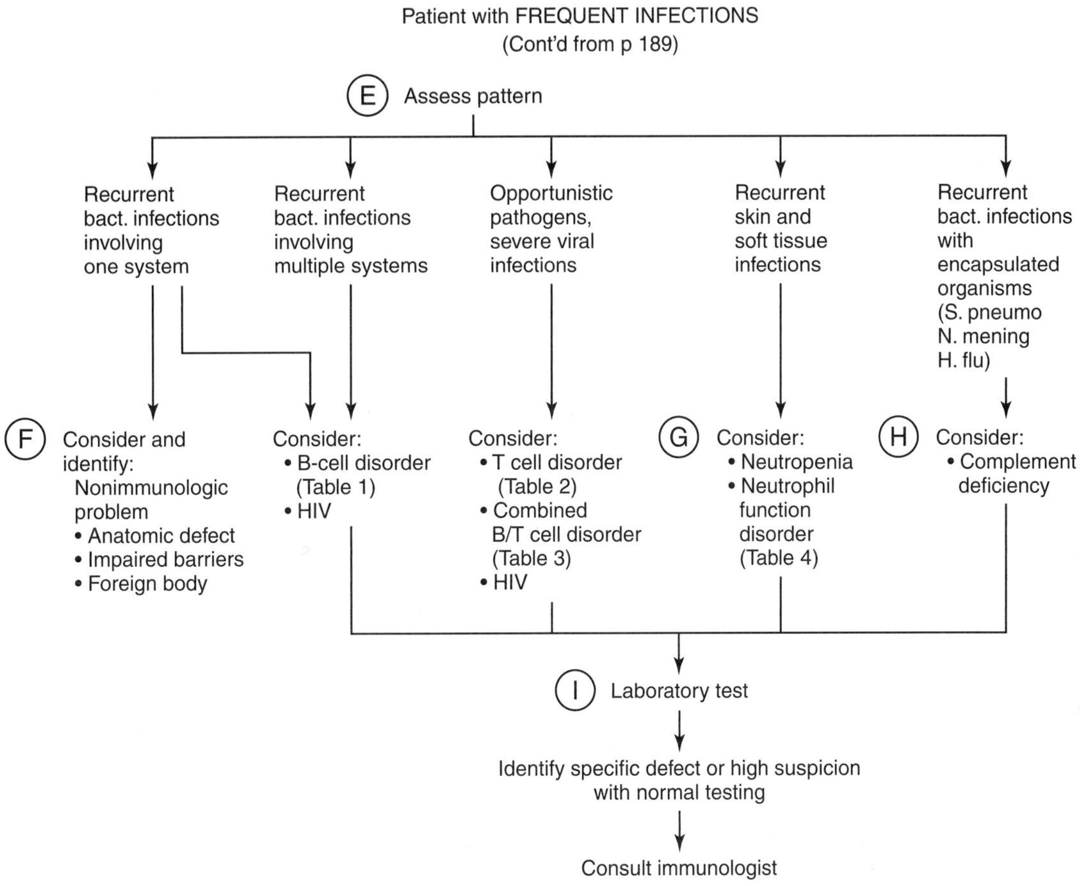
Patient with FREQUENT INFECTIONS
(Cont'd from p 189)
E Assess pattern
Recurrent bact. infections involving one system
Recurrent bact. infections involving multiple systems
Opportunistic pathogens, severe viral infections
Recurrent skin and soft tissue infections
Recurrent bact. infections with encapsulated organisms (S. pneumo N. mening H. flu)
F Consider and identify: Nonimmunologic problem • Anatomic defect • Impaired barriers • Foreign body
Consider: • B-cell disorder (Table 1) • HIV
Consider: • T cell disorder (Table 2) • Combined B/T cell disorder (Table 3) • HIV
G Consider: • Neutropenia • Neutrophil function disorder (Table 4)
H Consider: • Complement deficiency
I Laboratory test
Identify specific defect or high suspicion with normal testing
Consult immunologist

both quantitative and qualitative alterations. Neutrophil disorders are summarized in Table 4.

H. Disorders of complement have various clinical manifestations. Patients may be asymptomatic or have signs of autoimmune disease (systemic lupus erythematosus, angioedema, urticaria); failure to thrive; chronic diarrhea; seborrheic dermatitis; or recurrent severe infection, particularly with encapsulated bacteria *(Streptococcus pneumoniae, Haemophilus influenzae, Neisseria meningitidis).* Initial evaluation should include total complement (CH50, and in selected male patients, AH50). If abnormal, additional specific complement studies can be considered in conjunction with an immunologist. Terminal complement deficiency (C5-9) classically predisposes affected individuals to meningococcal disease; approximately 10% of individuals with their first episode of meningococcal disease have underlying complement deficiency.

I. First-tier laboratory evaluation should include the following: complete blood cell count (CBC) with manual differential and peripheral smear; note neutrophil quantity (high or low), cycling, granules, lymphocyte percentage and absolute number, thrombocytopenia, small platelets, Howell Jolly bodies (splenic dysfunction); quantitative immunoglobulins (IgG, IgA, IgM, IgE; IgG subclasses not recommended); quantitative B- and T-lymphocyte panel including T-lymphocyte subsets (CD4, CD8); HIV antibody or polymerase chain reaction (PCR) (age dependent); CH50 (and possibly AH50); oxidative burst testing; chest radiograph (CXR; bronchiectasis, pneumatoceles, thymic aplasia, cardiomegaly).

Second-tier laboratory evaluation to be considered to further assess cell-mediated immunity includes in vitro mitogen-stimulated responses (phytohaemagglutinin [PHA], ConA) and delayed-type hypersensitivity skin testing (candida, mumps, tetanus). Second-tier evaluation of humoral immunity includes functional assessment of antigen-specific antibody responses (isohemagglutinins, postvaccination titers for *Haemophilus influenzae* type B [HIB] and diphtheria, pertussis, tetanus [DPT] vaccines). Advanced testing for phagocyte dysfunction includes monitoring of weekly CBCs for cycling, CD11/18 markers (leukocyte adhesion deficiency), and specialized neutrophil function testing (chemotaxis, killing).

Table 3. **Selected Combination B- and T-Cell Disorders**

Disorder	Genetics and Presentation	Defect	Treatment
SCID	X-linked (Xq13) and AR inheritance; (multiple) prenatal diagnosis, carrier detection available for some	Absent T cells, B cells variable Adenosine deaminase deficiency in 50% of cases with AR SCID	BMT; consider enzyme replacement
Ataxia-telangiectasia syndrome	AR inheritance; carrier state detection (11q22.23); findings include increased serum AFP, telangiectasias, cerebellar ataxia (2–8 yr of age), high incidence of malignancy	Inability to repair DNA damage, interference with rearrangement of T- and B-cell genes	Supportive care, antibiotics for specific infections
Wiskott–Aldrich syndrome	XLR (rare AD); prenatal carrier detection (Xp11.23-p11.22) eczema, thrombocytopenia, bloody diarrhea, cerebral hemorrhage	Expression of a cell surface sialophorin	BMT; consider IVIG, prednisone, splenectomy
Chronic mucocutaneous candidiasis	Heterogeneous, unknown genetics Skin, nail, mucous membrane involvement association with endocrinopathies and autoimmune disorders	Unknown	Antifungal

AFP, alpha-fetoprotein; *AR,* autosomal recessive; *BMT,* bone marrow transplantation; *IVIG,* intravenous immunoglobulin; *SCID,* severe combined immunodeficiency; *XLR,* X-linked recessive.

Table 4. **Selected Neutrophil Function Disorders**

Disorder	Genetics and Presentation	Defect	Treatment
Chronic granulomatous gene disease	XLR, AD or AR inheritance; prenatal diagnosis available	Absent phagocyte superoxide production	γ-Interferon, BMT; therapy being studied
Leukocyte adhesion disorder	AR inheritance; prenatal diagnosis available; three types	Abnormal adhesion; leukocyte integrin deficiency with abnormal CD11/18 expression; selectin dysfunction	BMT; gene therapy being studied; oral fucose
Chédiak–Higashi syndrome	AR inheritance; prenatal diagnosis available, partial albinism, giant granules in neutrophils	Abnormal transport of granules including melanins and neurotransmitters	Vitamin C
Reticular dysgenesis	AR inheritance; no prenatal diagnosis, neutropenia	Uncertain	BMT
Cyclic neutropenia	AD, AR inheritance (19p13.3) *ELA-2* gene	Defect in neutrophil elastase	Granulocyte colony-stimulating factor
Hyper-IgE (Job) syndrome	Unknown inheritance (4q21); no prenatal diagnosis; severe eczema, recurrent sinopulmonary infections, increased IgE	Chemotaxis, T-cell function	Trials of γ-interferon, H_2 antagonists, vitamins C and E in progress

AD, autosomal dominant; *AR,* autosomal recessive; *BMT,* bone marrow transplantation; *XLR,* X-linked recessive.

References

Buescher ES. Evaluation of the child with suspected immunodeficiency. In: Long SS, Pickering LK, Prober CG, editors. Principles and practice of pediatric infectious diseases. 3rd ed. New York: Elsevier; 2008. p. 599–607.

Geha RS, Notarangelo LD, Casanova JL, et al. Primary immunodeficiency diseases: an update from the International Union of Immunological Societies Primary Immunodeficiency Diseases Classification Committee. J Allergy Clin Immunol 2007;120:776–94.

Johnson SL. Clinical immunology review series: an approach to the patient with recurrent superficial abscesses. Clin Exp Immunol 2008;152:397–405.

Sewell WA, Khan S, Dore PC. Early indicators of immunodeficiency in adults and children: protocols for screening for primary immunological defects. Clin Exp Immunol 2006;145:201–3.

Slattery MA, Gennery AR. Clinical immunodeficiency review series: an approach to the patient with recurrent infections in childhood. Clin Exp Immunol 2008;152:389–96.

Tedesco F. Inherited complement deficiencies and bacterial infections. Vaccine 2008;26(Suppl 8):13–8.

Wood P, Stanworth S, Burton J, et al. Recognition, clinical diagnosis and management of patients with primary antibody deficiencies: a systematic review. Clin Exp Immunol 2007;149:410–23.

Fever of Unknown Origin

Sean T. O'Leary, MD, and Mark J. Abzug, MD

DEFINITION

There are numerous definitions of fever of unknown origin (FUO), which generally include temperatures greater than 38° C to 38.3° C, but with durations ranging from longer than 1 week to longer than 3 weeks. We define FUO as daily temperature greater than 38.3°C lasting longer than 14 days with no diagnosis apparent after initial investigations, to distinguish children with FUO from those with common, generally benign, illnesses often associated with viral infections. Most patients with FUO may be initially evaluated as outpatients. In certain settings, however, inpatient evaluation may be more efficient.

CAUSATIVE FACTORS

Infectious causative agents are most common (20%–50%), followed by autoimmune disorders (6%–20%) and malignancies (2%–13%). Among infectious causative agents, occult presentations of common infectious agents are more likely than unusual infections. Many cases of FUO resolve with no diagnosis being made. The prognosis of pediatric FUO is generally favorable.

A. It is important to obtain a thorough history. Often, serial histories are crucial, as forgotten clues are recalled. The height and pattern of the fever are sometimes helpful, but most important is to document that there actually is a fever present. Nondiscriminating symptoms include anorexia, fatigue, weight loss, chills, and sweats. Symptoms that help narrow the focus of investigations include a history of rash, joint complaints, upper or lower respiratory complaints (even if mild), genitourinary complaints, and sometimes abdominal and central nervous system complaints.

An exposure history is critical and should include questions about ill contacts, place of residence and travel history (back to birth), pets and other possible contacts with animals (petting zoos, farms) and insects, medications, contacts with tuberculosis and HIV, and a dietary history (unpasteurized dairy, undercooked meat, and wild game).

B. A thorough physical examination is an essential part of the evaluation, and serial examinations are important because findings may develop over time. Nonspecific findings include adenopathy, hepatomegaly, and splenomegaly. More specific findings that may give a clue to a diagnosis include focal tenderness (bone or joint, abdomen, neck, etc.), rash, murmur, enanthema, or joint swelling. A normal physical examination generally portends a good prognosis.

C. A screening complete blood cell count (CBC) may identify cytopenias, blasts, atypical lymphocytes, or other clues that may point toward a specific diagnosis. Although increase of inflammatory markers such as erythrocyte sedimentation rate (ESR) and C-reactive protein (CRP) is nonspecific, their values (in addition to the clinical appearance of the patient) can guide the tempo of the workup. In addition, normal levels usually help eliminate certain diagnoses (systemic-onset juvenile rheumatoid arthritis [JRA], Kawasaki disease), and extremely high levels may help focus the differential diagnosis. A urinalysis (UA) and urine culture are important, although normal findings do not rule out urinary tract infections (UTIs) complicated by obstruction. A blood culture should be obtained and may lead to diagnoses such as occult osteomyelitis, endocarditis, or enteric fever caused by *Salmonella* infection. A posteroanterior and lateral chest radiograph may reveal an occult pneumonia, cardiomegaly, or a mediastinal mass.

D. If the history, physical, and screening laboratory evaluation give clues to a diagnosis, these should be pursued. For example, a history of recent travel to a developing country may prompt further evaluation, such as thick and thin smear evaluation for malaria, and blood and stool cultures for *Salmonella typhi*. A history of cat (particularly kitten) exposure would suggest sending serology for *Bartonella henselae*. Exudative pharyngitis with adenopathy or splenomegaly would warrant Epstein–Barr virus (EBV) serology. Persistent nasal discharge or congestion and headaches may suggest sinusitis and prompt imaging with plain films or computed tomography (CT) scan. Point tenderness of a bone, decrease in range of motion of a joint, or tenderness with pressure on the pelvis, is suggestive of osteomyelitis or arthritis, and a plain film of the affected area and/or additional imaging may be performed. Tenderness on abdominal examination may prompt evaluation by ultrasound or CT scan for evaluation of diagnoses such as missed appendicitis, biliary or urinary tract processes, or occult abscess. See Table 1 for clues to common and uncommon causes of FUO.

E. If fever persists and no diagnosis has become apparent after a thorough history and physical examination, screening laboratory studies, and focused investigations based on diagnostic clues, further evaluation may be pursued. A "shotgun" approach is not useful, because sending many undirected studies increases the likelihood of false-positive results. A thorough history and physical examination should be repeated. Initial screening studies should also be repeated, including CBC, ESR, CRP, urinalysis and urine culture, and blood culture. In addition, lactate dehydrogenase (LDH), uric acid, liver function tests, blood urea nitrogen (BUN), creatinine, and a stool heme test should be sent, and a tuberculin skin test (TST) for tuberculosis should be placed. Additional testing focused on any new clues from history, examination, and screening labs may be warranted. Other tests to consider with or after these "second-tier" investigations include EBV

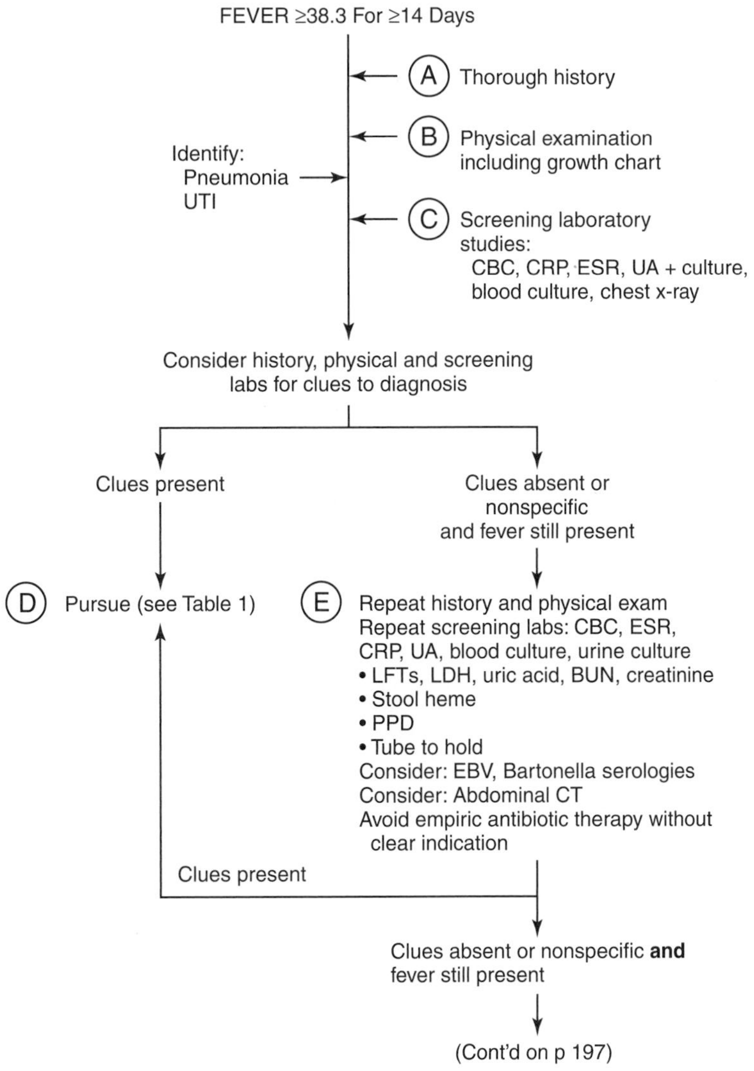
FEVER ≥38.3 For ≥14 Days
A Thorough history
B Physical examination including growth chart
Identify: Pneumonia UTI
C Screening laboratory studies: CBC, CRP, ESR, UA + culture, blood culture, chest x-ray
Consider history, physical and screening labs for clues to diagnosis
Clues present
Clues absent or nonspecific and fever still present
D Pursue (see Table 1)
E Repeat history and physical exam
Repeat screening labs: CBC, ESR, CRP, UA, blood culture, urine culture
• LFTs, LDH, uric acid, BUN, creatinine
• Stool heme
• PPD
• Tube to hold
Consider: EBV, Bartonella serologies
Consider: Abdominal CT
Avoid empiric antibiotic therapy without clear indication
Clues present
Clues absent or nonspecific **and** fever still present
(Cont'd on p 197)

and *Bartonella* serologies, if not previously obtained, and abdominal imaging by ultrasound or CT scan, because in series of pediatric patients with FUO, EBV and *Bartonella* infections and occult abdominal processes were among the most common, unsuspected diagnoses identified.

Trials of antibiotics should be avoided unless evaluations have identified a clear indication for treatment. Empiric antibiotics can mask the correct diagnosis, be a cause of drug fever, and ultimately prolong the period of illness and evaluation, rather than causing the FUO to resolve.

Table 1. **Clues and Diagnostic Studies for Common and Uncommon Causes of Fever of Unknown Origin**

Diagnoses	Clues	Diagnostic Studies
Epstein–Barr virus	Exudative pharyngitis, adenopathy, hepatosplenomegaly, increased LFTs, atypical lymphocytes	Serology
Cat-scratch disease	Cat (or dog) exposure, adenopathy, scratch	*Bartonella* serology and PCR
Vertebral or pelvic osteomyelitis	Decreased movement, refusal to walk (even with no point tenderness on examination)	Bone scan or MRI
Kawasaki disease	Infants may have incomplete presentations with prolonged fever predominating and without typical mucocutaneous findings; increased ESR and/or CRP generally present	CBC, ESR, CRP, LFTs, urinalysis, echocardiogram, pediatric infectious diseases and pediatric cardiology consultation
Cytomegalovirus	Leukopenia, hepatosplenomegaly	Serology
Enteric fever *(Salmonella)*	International travel, exposure to foods brought from other countries, reptile exposure; constipation may be present early in illness; leukopenia	Blood culture, stool culture
Infective endocarditis	Chest pain, murmur, anemia, red blood cells in urine, positive rheumatoid factor	Three large-volume blood cultures, echocardiogram
Lyme disease	Exposure to Lyme endemic region, season, erythema chronicum migrans rash, arthralgias/arthritis	Serology
Brucellosis	Exposure to unpasteurized dairy or farm animals, arthritis (particularly sacroiliac), hepatosplenomegaly	Blood culture, serology, PCR
Q fever *(Coxiella brunetti)*	Exposure to farm animals (particularly sheep) or unpasteurized dairy; culture-negative endocarditis, pneumonia, and/or hepatitis	Serology
Tularemia	Adenopathy, ulcerative lesion, tick bite, rabbit exposure, exposure to highly endemic region	Wound culture, blood culture, serology, PCR
Tuberculosis	High-risk group (born outside United States in highly endemic region), recent exposure, travel to endemic region	TST, chest radiograph
Histoplasmosis	History of travel to or living in endemic region, adenopathy, pancytopenia, hepatosplenomegaly	Serology, urine antigen, tissue biopsy
Malaria	Travel to endemic region (increased risk if failure to take prophylaxis), jaundice, pallor, splenomegaly	Three successive thick and thin blood smears
Sinusitis	Nasal congestion/discharge, halitosis, headaches	Sinus CT
Occult abdominal abscess	History of gastrointestinal illness in preceding weeks, history of trauma (even if minor)	Abdominal CT with contrast or ultrasound
Hemophagocytic syndrome	Hepatosplenomegaly, pancytopenia, hepatitis, multiorgan dysfunction, high LDH and ferritin	Ferritin level (extremely high), pediatric hematology consultation and bone marrow examination
Systemic-onset juvenile rheumatoid arthritis	Daily spiking fevers returning to normal or below normal, salmon pink rash present during fever, hepatosplenomegaly, very high ESR	Pediatric rheumatology consultation: no laboratory test is specific; normal ESR essentially rules out
Inflammatory bowel disease	Abdominal pain, diarrhea, anemia, short stature, high ESR	Endoscopy, upper GI contrast study

CBC, complete blood cell count; *CRP,* C-reactive protein; *CT,* computed tomography; *ESR,* erythrocyte sedimentation rate; *GI,* gastrointestinal; *LDH,* lactate dehydrogenase; *LFT,* liver function tests; *MRI,* magnetic resonance imaging; *PCR,* polymerase chain reaction; *TST,* tuberculin skin test.

F. Hospitalization should be considered if one or more of the following factors are present: (1) worrisome clinical appearance, (2) worrisome laboratory evaluations, (3) concern that fever may be factitious (or other social concerns), and (4) coordination of subspecialists and diagnostic testing. Hospitalization allows closer observation, serial physical examinations, and charting a detailed fever curve. Nuclear medicine scans such as gallium or white blood cell scans are of variable yield, and results are often of unclear significance. The role of newer imaging modalities such as positron emission tomography (PET) CT scan is yet to be determined. Bone marrow examinations have a low yield in the workup of FUOs in children, unless abnormalities are present in the CBC or there is concern for a disseminated infection involving the reticuloendothelial system, such as histoplasmosis or enteric fever caused by salmonella. Consultation with subspecialists, including pediatric infectious diseases, pediatric hematology/oncology, and pediatric rheumatology, should be considered as appropriate at this point. If the diagnosis remains unclear, the patient should be observed for development of clues to the correct diagnosis. The majority of FUOs that remain undiagnosed will ultimately self-resolve.

FEVER ≥38.3 For ≥14 Days

(Cont'd from p 195)

(F) Consider: hospitalization if:
- Clinically worrisome
- Labs worrisome
- Fever history suspect
- Need for evaluation by multiple subspecialists

Perform: serial physical exams

Consider as appropriate:
- Pediatric infectious diseases consult
- Hematology/oncology consult
- Rheumatology consult

References

Blockmans D, Knockaert D, Maes A, et al. Clinical value of [(18)F] fluoro-deoxyglucose positron emission tomography for patients with fever of unknown origin. Clin Infect Dis 2001;32:191–6.

Campbell JR. Fever of unknown origin in a previously healthy child. Semin Pediatr Infect Dis 2002;13:5, 64–6.

Jacobs RF, Schutze GE. Bartonella henselae as a cause of prolonged fever and fever of unknown origin in children. Clin Infect Dis 1998;26:80–4.

Kjaer A, Lebech AM, Eigtved A, Hojgaard L. Fever of unknown origin: prospective comparison of diagnostic value of 18F-FDG PET and 111In-granulocyte scintigraphy. Eur J Nucl Med Mol Imaging 2004;31:622–6.

Knockaert DC, Dujardin KS, Bobbaers HJ. Long-term follow-up of patients with undiagnosed fever of unknown origin. Arch Intern Med 1996;156:618–20.

Larson EB, Featherstone HJ, Petersdorf RG. Fever of undetermined origin: diagnosis and follow-up of 105 cases, 1970–1980. Medicine (Baltimore) 1982;61:269–92.

Long SS. Distinguishing among prolonged, recurrent, and periodic fever syndromes: approach of a pediatric infectious diseases subspecialist. Pediatr Clin North Am 2005;52:811–35, vii.

Massei F, Messina F, Talini I, et al. Widening of the clinical spectrum of Bartonella henselae infection as recognized through serodiagnostics. Eur J Pediatr 2000;159:416–9.

Miller LC, Sisson BA, Tucker LB, Schaller JG. Prolonged fevers of unknown origin in children: patterns of presentation and outcome. J Pediatr 1996;129:419–23.

Mourad O, Palda V, Detsky AS. A comprehensive evidence-based approach to fever of unknown origin. Arch Intern Med 2003;163: 545–51.

Murakami K, Tsukahara M, Tsuneoka H et al: Cat scratch disease: analysis of 130 seropositive cases, *J Infect Chemother* 8:349–352, 2002.

Noble JT, Mark EJ: Case records of the Massachusetts General Hospital. Weekly clinicopathological exercises. Case 22–2002. A 37-year-old man with unexplained fever after a long trip through South America, *N Engl J Med* 347:200–206, 2002.

Steele RW, Jones SM, Lowe BA, Glasier CM: Usefulness of scanning procedures for diagnosis of fever of unknown origin in children, *J Pediatr* 119:526–530, 1991.

Talano JA, Katz BZ: Long-term follow-up of children with fever of unknown origin, *Clin Pediatr (Phila)* 39:715–717, 2000.

Tsukahara M, Tsuneoka H, Iino H et al: Bartonella henselae infection as a cause of fever of unknown origin, *J Clin Microbiol* 38:1990–1991, 2000.

Ventura A, Massei F, Not T et al: Systemic Bartonella henselae infection with hepatosplenic involvement, *J Pediatr Gastroenterol Nutr* 29: 52–56, 1999.

Whiteford SF, Taylor JP, Dumler JS: Clinical, laboratory, and epidemiologic features of murine typhus in 97 Texas children, *Arch Pediatr Adolesc Med* 155:396–400, 2001.

Gastrointestinal

Acute Abdominal Pain

Judith A. O'Connor, MD

A. In the patient's history, focus on recent trauma, surgical and medical history, and the relationship of pain to fever, vomiting, diarrhea, dysuria, and menstruation. Determine the onset, frequency, pattern, nature, and location of the pain. Assess the severity of the pain (Table 1). Note associated symptoms of rectal bleeding, jaundice, weight loss, anorexia, and arthritis. Identify precipitating factors and predisposing conditions, including constipation, medications, spider/tick bite, sickle cell disease, pregnancy, prior abdominal surgery, and inflammatory bowel disease.

B. In the physical examination, assess the circulatory and hydration status. Note signs of peritoneal irritation, such as iliopsoas rigidity (psoas sign), pain with external thigh rotation (obturator test), pain with jarring movements, difficulty or inability to walk or jump, hyperesthesia, and referred pain to the neck or shoulder. Signs of intestinal obstruction include abdominal distention, decreased bowel sounds, and persistent vomiting. Gently palpate the abdomen with the patient's legs slightly raised to relax the abdominal rectus muscles. Signs of peritonitis include rigidity of the abdominal muscles, rebound tenderness, decreased bowel sounds, abdominal distention, and shock. Locate the sites of maximal pain and radiation of pain. With epigastric pain, consider peptic ulcer disease, hiatal hernia, gastroesophageal reflux, esophagitis, and pancreatitis. Right upper quadrant pain suggests hepatitis, liver abscess or tumor, Fitz–Hugh–Curtis syndrome, cholecystitis, or cholangitis. When mild abdominal pain is diffuse, periumbilical, or left-sided, consider constipation, mesenteric adenitis, food poisoning, pharyngitis, muscle strain, gastroenteritis, and psychogenic pain.

C. Abnormal radiographic findings include fecaliths (appendicitis), pneumatosis intestinalis (necrotizing enterocolitis), free air (perforation), obstructive patterns (mechanical and functional), air in an abscess, abdominal mass, and abdominal calcifications. Renal stones, pneumonia, or osteomyelitis may also be identified.

D. Nonaccidental abdominal trauma, suggested by a positive history or associated bruises or fractures, causes traumatic pancreatitis, intramural duodenal hematuria, and lacerations of the liver, spleen, or bladder.

E. Ultrasonography is a cost-effective diagnostic technique to identify many causes of acute abdominal pain, including appendicitis, intussusception, gallbladder disorders, biliary tract disease, pelvic masses, and renal disorders. It often fails to identify pelvic inflammatory disease, hepatitis, and pancreatitis. A negative sonogram does not exclude appendicitis or abscess. Abdominal computed tomographic (CT) scanning is the method of choice for blunt trauma.

(Continued on page 202)

Table 1. **Degree of Illness in Acute Abdominal Pain**

Mild	Moderate	Severe	Very Severe
Pain that interferes minimally with activity	Pain that interferes with activity	Signs of peritonitis or intestinal obstruction or intussusception	Signs of sepsis or septic shock with altered mental status
OR	OR	OR	OR
Pain associated with a known benign cause, such as viral gastroenteritis	Associated signs of bacterial infection (respiratory distress, urinary tract infection, *Streptococcus pyogenes*)	Alterations in mental status (delirium, confusion, lethargy)	Poor peripheral perfusion, hypotension Respiratory distress (adult respiratory distress syndrome)
	OR	OR	
	A history of abdominal surgery or necrotizing enterocolitis	Signs of moderate or severe dehydration	

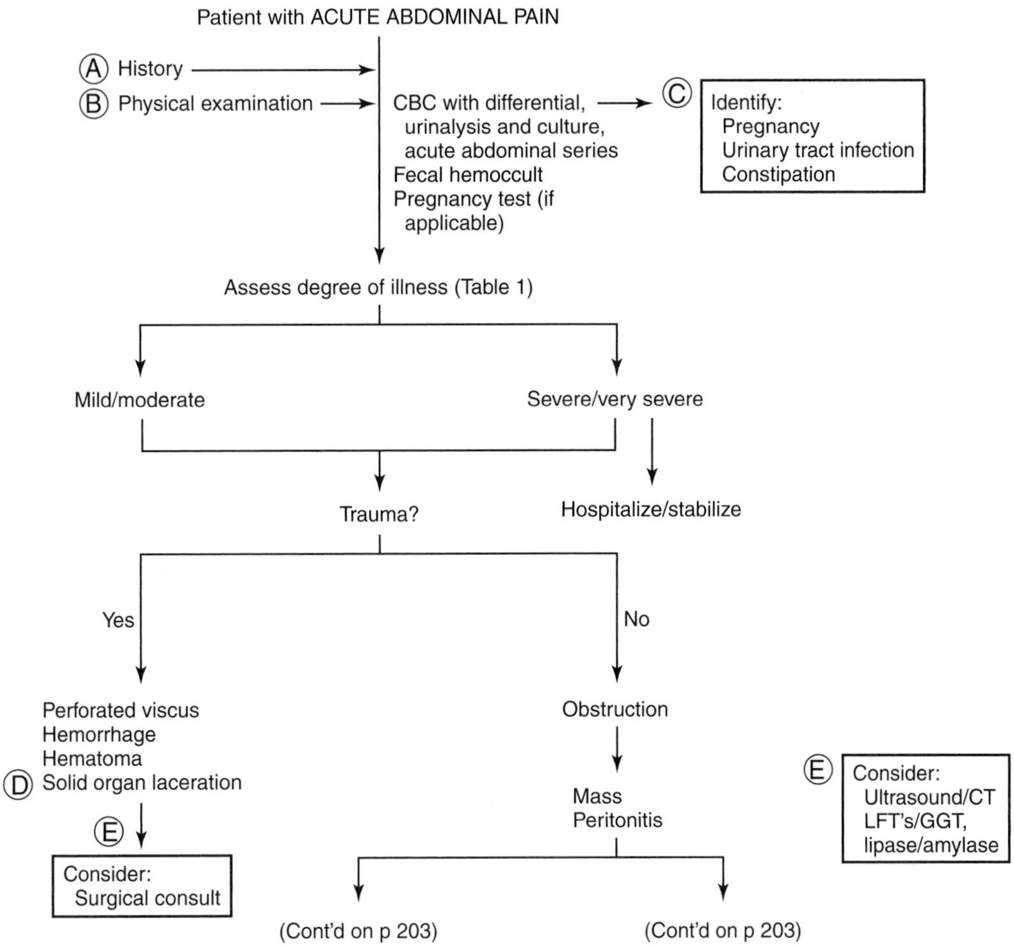
Patient with ACUTE ABDOMINAL PAIN
(A) History
(B) Physical examination
CBC with differential, urinalysis and culture, acute abdominal series
Fecal hemoccult
Pregnancy test (if applicable)
(C) Identify: Pregnancy Urinary tract infection Constipation
Assess degree of illness (Table 1)
Mild/moderate
Severe/very severe
Trauma?
Hospitalize/stabilize
Yes
No
Perforated viscus
Hemorrhage
Hematoma
(D) Solid organ laceration
(E) Consider: Surgical consult
Obstruction
Mass
Peritonitis
(E) Consider: Ultrasound/CT LFT's/GGT, lipase/amylase
(Cont'd on p 203)
(Cont'd on p 203)

F. Signs that suggest systemic disease or infection include jaundice (hepatitis); perianal lesions, weight loss, bloody stools (inflammatory bowel disease); bloody stools with antibiotic use (pseudomembranous colitis); bloody stools, hematuria, anemia, renal failure (hemolytic-uremic syndrome); bloody diarrhea, fever, no vomiting (bacterial enteritis); palpable purpura, arthritis, hematuria (Henoch–Schönlein purpura); prolonged fever, conjunctivitis, mucosal lesions, rash (Kawasaki disease); tick bite, erythema chronicum migrans (Lyme disease); vaginal discharge (pelvic inflammatory disease); fever, weight loss, lymphadenopathy, hepatosplenomegaly (malignant neoplasm); anemia (sickle cell disease); cough, rales, decreased breath sounds (lower lobe pneumonia); sore throat, exudate, adenitis (*Streptococcus pyogenes* pharyngitis); and bruises, fractures, abdominal distention (nonaccidental trauma) (Table 2).

G. Appendicitis presents classically with fever, vomiting, point tenderness over McBurney point, and signs of peritoneal irritation. The findings are variable, reflecting the location of the appendix (iliac, ascending, pelvic), the acuity of the inflammation, and after rupture, the size and site of the abscess. On rectal examination, a tender right lower quadrant mass may be palpated. Diarrhea or pyuria may occur. Leukocytosis is common but nonspecific. The absence of fever and vomiting suggests an alternative diagnosis (negative predictive value, 0.97). Appendicitis can be precipitated by fecaliths or parasitic infections. Perforation is most likely if treatment is delayed more than 36 hours or if the patient is younger than 8 years. CT can be performed quickly, does not require graded compression of the abdominal wall, and is less operator dependent. The examination should be performed with rectal contrast and be limited to below the liver edge. The sensitivity and specificity have been reported as 97% to 100% and 83% to 97%, respectively, with an overall accuracy rate of 97%. On CT, there is a fluid-filled appendix, often containing a fecalith, and periappendiceal fat "stranding" indicating inflammatory changes. Ultrasound (US) examination has a sensitivity of 80% to 94%, specificity of 86% to 98%, and an overall accuracy rate of 91%. The appendix will appear as a rigid, aperistaltic, noncompressible tubular mass in the appropriate location. A negative US does not exclude acute appendicitis.

H. Consider an intussusception when intermittent crampy abdominal pain is associated with vomiting, abdominal distention, or bloody stools and an epigastric sausage-shaped mass. Intussusception may cause an alteration in mental status that suggests central nervous system disease. Intussusception most commonly occurs in children 4 to 24 months of age. Plain abdominal radiography may be normal, show a paucity of gas on the right, or indicate small-bowel obstruction. Ultrasonography is the preferred method of confirming the diagnosis by demonstrating a sonolucent doughnut on cross section (edematous head of the intussusception). A cause such as a polyp, mass, Meckel diverticulum, anaphylactoid purpura, cystic fibrosis, celiac disease, foreign body, or infection (adenovirus or rotavirus) can be identified in about 15% of cases. Attempt an air–contrast or hydrostatic reduction with a barium enema before surgery only when the patient is stable without signs of shock, strangulated bowel, or perforation (free air, peritonitis). The use of analgesic premedication may increase the rate of successful hydrostatic reduction. Failure to reduce the intussusception with pneumatic or hydrostatic techniques requires a surgical intervention.

I. When an intestinal malrotation occurs, the mesentery is not fixed properly so that the midtransverse colon may twist around a narrow base and occlude the arterial blood supply, causing a volvulus. Neonates present with bilious vomiting and other signs of small-bowel obstruction. Assess for associated congenital anomalies including cardiac defects. Confirm an intestinal malrotation with an upper gastrointestinal series that documents the duodenojejunal junction on the right side of the spine or a barium enema study showing a mobile cecum. Refer patients with a volvulus to surgery immediately.

J. Acute ovarian torsion has signs of an acute abdomen. When the right ovary is involved, the presentation is similar to that of acute appendicitis. Perform ultrasonography to identify this condition. Early diagnosis and surgery are necessary to save the ovary and fallopian tube.

K. Suspect acute pancreatitis when acute abdominal pain radiates to the back or right upper quadrant and is associated with vomiting. Ascites, abdominal distention, and peritoneal signs may be present. Increase of serum amylase and lipase or a radioimmune assay of pancreatic trypsinogen suggests pancreatitis. Ultrasonography may show inflammation or a pseudocyst (5%–20% of cases). Consider performing a computed tomographic scan when an abscess (3%–5% of cases) is suspected. Causes of pancreatitis include acquired or congenital structural defects, trauma, metabolic disorders, infection, cystic fibrosis, autoimmune disorders, hemolytic-uremic syndrome, alcohol, and drug toxicity (valproic acid, thiazides, corticosteroids, sulfasalazine, antiretroviral, and many oncology medications). Assess for complications including fluid and electrolyte alterations leading to shock, respiratory distress and hypoxia, hypocalcemic tetany, severe anemia, acidosis, and hyperglycemia. Manage acute pancreatitis with gastric suction, intravenous fluids, bed rest, and adequate pain management. Consider blood transfusions, oxygen, and parenteral nutrition when indicated. Consult surgery when an obstructive lesion is identified, the gland has been ruptured by trauma, or an abscess or infected pseudocyst has not responded to antibiotic therapy.

L. Suspect ulcer disease when recurrent abdominal pain is associated with nausea, vomiting, hematemesis, or melena. The pain in older children is often epigastric, is relieved by food or antacids, and awakens the patient from sleep.

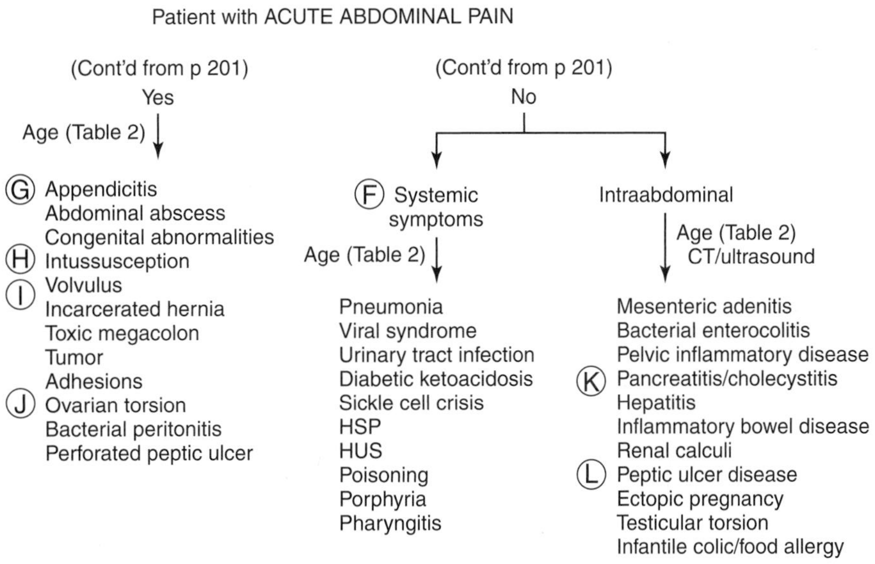

Patient with ACUTE ABDOMINAL PAIN
(Cont'd from p 201)
Yes
Age (Table 2)
G Appendicitis
Abdominal abscess
Congenital abnormalities
H Intussusception
I Volvulus
Incarcerated hernia
Toxic megacolon
Tumor
Adhesions
J Ovarian torsion
Bacterial peritonitis
Perforated peptic ulcer
(Cont'd from p 201)
No
F Systemic symptoms
Age (Table 2)
Pneumonia
Viral syndrome
Urinary tract infection
Diabetic ketoacidosis
Sickle cell crisis
HSP
HUS
Poisoning
Porphyria
Pharyngitis
Intraabdominal
Age (Table 2)
CT/ultrasound
Mesenteric adenitis
Bacterial enterocolitis
Pelvic inflammatory disease
K Pancreatitis/cholecystitis
Hepatitis
Inflammatory bowel disease
Renal calculi
L Peptic ulcer disease
Ectopic pregnancy
Testicular torsion
Infantile colic/food allergy

Table 2. **Differentiated Diagnosis for Acute Abdominal Pains by Age**

Neonate	Child <2 yr	School Age (2–13 yr)	Adolescent
Necrotizing enterocolitis	Colic (<3 months)	Acute gastroenteritis	Acute gastroenteritis
Hirschsprung disease	Acute gastroenteritis	Urinary tract infection	Urinary tract infection
Meconium ileus	Intussusception	Appendicitis	Appendicitis
Intestinal atresia/stenosis	Trauma	Trauma	Trauma
Incarcerated hernia	Incarcerated hernia	Constipation	Constipation
Volvulus	Volvulus	Pneumonia	Pelvic inflammatory disease
Trauma	Urinary tract infection	Inflammatory bowel disease	Inflammatory bowel disease
	Constipation	Testicular torsion	Ectopic pregnancy
	Esophageal reflux	Esophageal reflux	Esophageal reflux
	Hemolytic uremic syndrome	Pharyngitis	Ovarian torsion
	Henoch–Schönlein purpura		

References

Caty MG, Azizkhan RG. Acute surgical conditions of the abdomen. Pediatr Ann 1994;23:192.

Doria AS. Optimizing the role of imaging in appendicitis. Pediatr Radiol 2009;39:S144.

Eshel G, Barr J, Heyman E, et al. Intussusception: a nine year survey. J Pediatr Gastroenterol Nutr 1997;24:253.

Lowe LH, Penny MW, Scheker LE, et al. Appendolith revealed on CT in children with suspected appendicitis: how specific is it in the diagnosis of appendicitis? AJR Am J Roentgenol 2000;175:901.

Mason JD. The evaluation of acute abdominal pain in children. Emerg Med Clin North Am 1996;14:629.

Nance ML, Adamson WT, Hedrick NL. Appendicitis in the young child: a continuing diagnostic challenge. Pediatr Emerg Care 2000;16:160.

Reif S, Sloven DG, Lebenthal E. Gallstones in children. Am J Dis Child 1991;145:105.

Rothrock SG, Green SM, Harding M, et al. Plain abdominal radiography in the detection of acute medical and surgical disease in children: a retrospective analysis. Pediatr Emerg Care 1991;7:281.

Rothrock SG, Pagane J. Acute appendicitis in children: emergency department diagnosis and management. Ann Emerg Med 2000;36:39.

Scholer SJ, Pituch K, Orr DP, et al. Test ordering on children with acute abdominal pain. Clin Pediatr 1999;38:493.

Seashore JH, Touloukian RJ. Midgut volvulus: an ever-present threat. Arch Pediatr Adolesc Med 1994;148:43.

Sivit CJ. Abdominal trauma imaging: imaging choices and appropriateness. Pediatr Radiol 2009;39:S158.

Stevenson RJ, Ziegler MM. Abdominal pain unrelated to trauma. Pediatr Rev 1993;14:302.

Tenenbein M, Wiseman NE. Early coma in intussusception: endogenous opioid induced? Pediatr Emerg Care 1987;3:22.

Yeung CY, Lee HC, Huang FY, et al. Pancreatitis in children: experience with 43 cases. Eur J Pediatr 1996;155:458.

Persistent or Chronic Abdominal Pain

Edwin Liu, MD, and Edward J. Hoffenberg, MD

Abdominal pain is one of the most common childhood gastrointestinal (GI) complaints, and many are acute self-limited events. However, when the pain persists, physicians will be called on for an assessment. The majority of cases of abdominal pain are attributable to functional causes. Other causes broadly include psychogenic and organic. Multiple causes may interact to contribute to the pain with respect to personality and emotional characteristics, habits and lifestyle routines, critical events, and sources of stress. Functional abdominal pain syndromes are described in the Rome III diagnostic criteria for Functional GI Disorders (FGIDs), and in children, specifically under the category of Functional Abdominal Pain-Related FGIDs.

Childhood Functional Abdominal Pain is characterized by all of the following features present at least once per week for at least 2 months before diagnosis:

1. Episodic or continuous abdominal pain
2. Insufficient criteria for other FGIDs
3. No evidence of an inflammatory, anatomic, metabolic, or neoplastic process that explains the subject's symptoms

The addition of the two following criteria places the condition under the category of Childhood Functional Abdominal Pain Syndrome:

4. Some loss of daily functioning
5. Additional somatic symptoms such as headache, limb pain, or difficulty sleeping

Abdominal Pain-Related FGIDs include alternative diagnoses, primarily dependent on the location and specific features of pain, provided adequate exclusion of organic causes is ruled out. These include categories such as Functional Dyspepsia (pain located in the upper abdomen), Irritable Bowel Syndrome (discomfort associated with alterations in stool frequency and form—constipation, diarrhea, or both, relieved by defecation), and Abdominal Migraines.

Characteristics of paroxysmal episodes of intense, acute periumbilical pain include:

1. Pain lasts 1 hour or longer
2. Intervening periods of usual health last weeks to months
3. Pain interferes with normal activities
4. Pain is associated with two of the following: anorexia, nausea, vomiting, headache, photophobia, or pallor

It is important for a physician to recognize features of functional abdominal pain, to look out for atypical features that stand out as red flags, and to include FGIDs in the differential early on when counseling a family with a child with abdominal pain. Typical features associated with functional abdominal pain include (in general): poor localization of the pain (or periumbilical), a longer duration of symptoms, inconsistent pattern, the child losing function (missing school), and a pain response that is disruptive to the entire family dynamics. These children are typically high-achievers (type A personalities) but can also be seen in children with low self-esteem, a withdrawn personality, and few, if any, good friends—particularly when multiple somatic complaints are reported. Importantly, these children appear well, have a normal examination, and have a nonalarming history.

Although our understanding of FGIDs is incomplete, current thinking regarding abdominal pain involves intestinal hypersensitivity that can be exacerbated by psychologic and physiologic stimuli such as emotional stress, foods, and luminal distension. This has been demonstrated by studies involving gastric and rectal distension using an electronic barostat in children with functional pain versus control subjects; children with functional pain reported more pain on luminal distension compared with control subjects. Disturbances in intestinal motility are also being identified in functional pain syndromes and will play a larger role in the near future.

A. The initial visit should contain a history that notes the onset, frequency, pattern, and location of the pain. Is it associated with eating or defecating? What makes it better? What makes it worse? What has been tried for the pain? Look for any associated symptoms with the pain—for example, vomiting, diarrhea, rectal bleeding, headaches, weight loss, fever, rash, arthritis, and hematuria. Identify any possible precipitating factors such as medications (i.e., nonsteroidal anti-inflammatory drug use, pill esophagitis), menses, stress, and other concurrent conditions (i.e., sickle cell disease, cystic fibrosis). Look for a family history of other GI diseases, atopy (to suggest underlying food allergy or eosinophilic GI disease), and autoimmunity such as celiac disease, type 1 diabetes, and thyroid disease. In the presence of any red flag signs or symptoms, a focused workup is needed. This is a good time to explain that any testing performed is to "rule out" disease and not necessarily to diagnose a disease; this is particularly important when considering psychogenic disorders and FGIDs, because they will yield a normal workup.

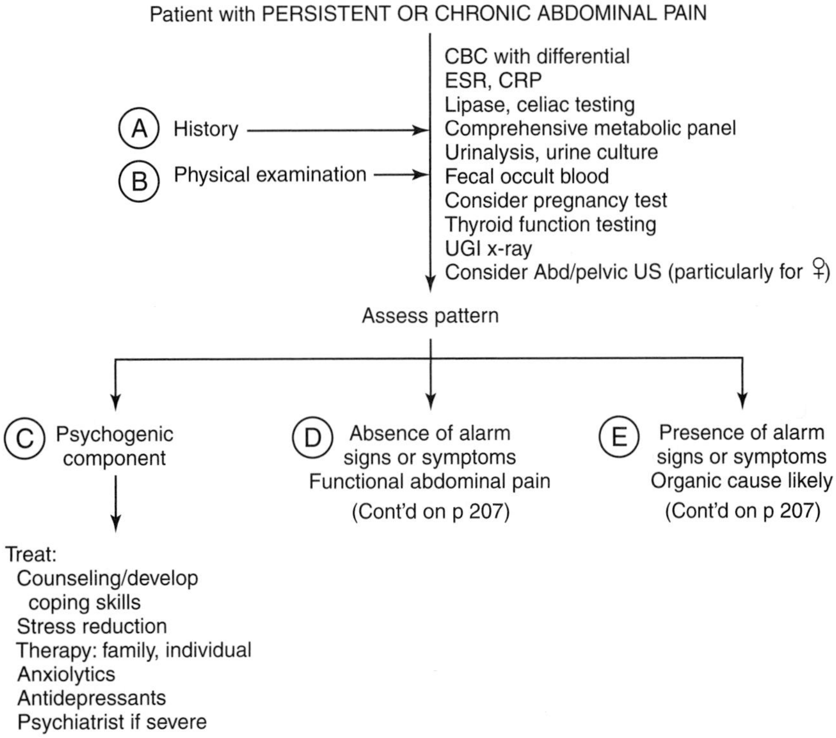
Patient with PERSISTENT OR CHRONIC ABDOMINAL PAIN
A History
B Physical examination
CBC with differential
ESR, CRP
Lipase, celiac testing
Comprehensive metabolic panel
Urinalysis, urine culture
Fecal occult blood
Consider pregnancy test
Thyroid function testing
UGI x-ray
Consider Abd/pelvic US (particularly for ♀)
Assess pattern
C Psychogenic component
D Absence of alarm signs or symptoms Functional abdominal pain
(Cont'd on p 207)
E Presence of alarm signs or symptoms Organic cause likely
(Cont'd on p 207)
Treat:
Counseling/develop coping skills
Stress reduction
Therapy: family, individual
Anxiolytics
Antidepressants
Psychiatrist if severe

B. The physical examination should note the general appearance of the child—abnormal growth velocity or percentiles to suggest chronic underlying disease, note skin for jaundice or rash, and digital clubbing to suggest inflammatory conditions. Note the site of the pain (in relation to the umbilicus is helpful). As a general rule of thumb, the farther away the abdominal pain is from the umbilicus, the less likely there will be organic disease. Is the abdomen focally tender and reproducible to suggest a possible surgical abdomen? Perform a rectal examination to look for occult blood, fecal impaction, anal fissures, anal tags, or mass.

C. In the absence of any alarm features and normal history, examination, and workup, consider psychogenic component. This may be associated with multiple somatic complaints including headaches, back pain, muscle or joint pain, and chest pain. There may be a focus on the complete relief of symptoms rather than adaptation to a chronic condition, or the patient may not take "ownership" of the symptoms, while placing high expectations on the physician to achieve symptom relief.

D. In the absence of any alarming features, symptoms could meet the criteria for FGIDs. Depending on the specific symptoms and presumed location of the pain (i.e., epigastric or left upper quadrant [LUQ] for gastric; lower abdomen, particularly lower left quadrant [LLQ] for colonic), a more tailored lifestyle and medical regimen can be recommended. Validate the child's pain as real, not imagined. Recognize and acknowledge that functional pain can cause children to cry, writhe in pain, turn pale and sweaty, and can occur even on stress-free days. Counseling is important at the onset to help relieve anxiety about symptoms and to help develop coping mechanisms. Focus on maintaining or re-establishing function (school attendance) and not pain resolution. If symptoms or loss of function is severe, then consider professional counseling. Treatment for functional pain also includes dietary management such as increasing daily fiber in foods or with a fiber supplement (goal for total daily intake should be "age + 5" g to a maximum of 35 g). Build up to the dose slowly because it may cause cramping and bloating. Try avoiding foods with sorbitol such as fruit juices, hard candy, gum, dried or rolled fruit snack foods, chocolate, as well as caffeine-containing and carbonated beverages. Families may identify triggering foods, particularly in irritable bowel syndrome, but less likely in Functional Abdominal Pain Syndrome. Consider lactose intolerance; give a trial of dairy and lactose elimination. In selected cases, there may be a role for antispasmodics (dicyclomine hydrochloride and hyoscyamine sulfate), or in teenagers, antidepressants. Amitriptyline in low doses (10–25 mg at night) can be particularly effective for chronic pain in teens, but can take weeks before there is an effect. An electrocardiogram is needed before starting this drug; also forewarn the parents that sedation during the first few weeks is common but typically resolves after prolonged use. In cases consistent with dyspepsia, an empiric trial of acid suppression (H2 blocker or proton pump inhibition) for at least 2 weeks is warranted, and if helpful, for a full 8-week course. Finally, although sufficient data are lacking, a trial of probiotics might be considered in refractory cases.

E. Target the workup for suspected organic disease. Consider the symptoms and examination, including location of pain. Is the disease more likely to be luminal or extraluminal, systemic or focal? In the case of acid peptic disease (LUQ/epigastric or substernal pain), Hemoccult-positive stools are supportive but rarely positive unless severe. Acid-induced injury can occur in the stomach or duodenum, and ulcers can even occur more distally in the small bowel. Older patients with acid reflux may be able to provide a reliable history of regurgitation or heartburn. However, be mindful that although acid reflux can be quite symptomatic, it is not necessarily a disease unless specific complications are present (esophagitis, stricture, weight loss, etc). For suspected inflammatory bowel disease (IBD; LLQ pain, hematochezia, and urgency for colitis vs. right lower quadrant [RLQ] pain, wasting, and anorexia for ileal disease), stool Hemoccult, complete blood cell count (CBC), and inflammatory markers are a good first step. Consider an abdominal computed tomography (CT) scan or Upper GI with small-bowel follow-through to assess the small bowel. The commercialized "IBD First Step" detecting antibodies against bacterial antigens is not recommended as a screen for IBD. In patients with a history of atopy (or strong family history), consider eosinophilic esophagitis, particularly in the presence of dysphagia. Allergy testing in this case can be useful. Celiac disease is more common in patients with type 1 diabetes (or a family history) and autoimmune thyroid disease, and should be considered. Screening is performed by measuring tissue transglutaminase IgA autoantibody and total IgA levels. When constipation is identified, treat appropriately, but avoid immediate presumption that constipation is the source of pain, and be sure to develop a broader differential. Extraluminal causes such as gallbladder disease (right upper quadrant [RUQ]), appendicitis (RLQ), and a numerous other causes will typically be seen by specific imaging such as ultrasound or CT scanning.

Finally, consider non-GI sources such as underlying neurologic disease, endocrine causes, collagen vascular disease (Henoch–Schönlein purpura), ischemia, drugs, and immunodeficiency, particularly in more atypical presentations of abdominal pain.

In all of these conditions, be aware that there can be overlap with psychogenic causes. It is also important to recognize that there is still incomplete understanding of functional pain syndromes. Standard testing (in non-GI motility centers) can readily identify structural or histologic abnormalities but are limited in assessing function (such as motility and nerve conduction). As we learn more about functional pain syndromes, we may have more success in getting families to accept such a diagnosis for which there is no specific and definitive test or treatment.

References

Clouse RE, Mayer EA, Aziz Q, et al. Functional abdominal pain syndrome. Gastroenterology 2006;130(5):1492–7.

Di Lorenzo C, Youssef NN, Sigurdsson L, et al. Visceral hyperalgesia in children with functional abdominal pain. J Pediatr 2001;139(6):838–43.

Rasquin A, Di Lorenzo C, Forbes D, et al. Childhood functional gastrointestinal disorders: child/adolescent. Gastroenterology 2006;130(5):1527–37.

Patient with PERSISTENT OR CHRONIC ABDOMINAL PAIN
(Cont'd from p 205)

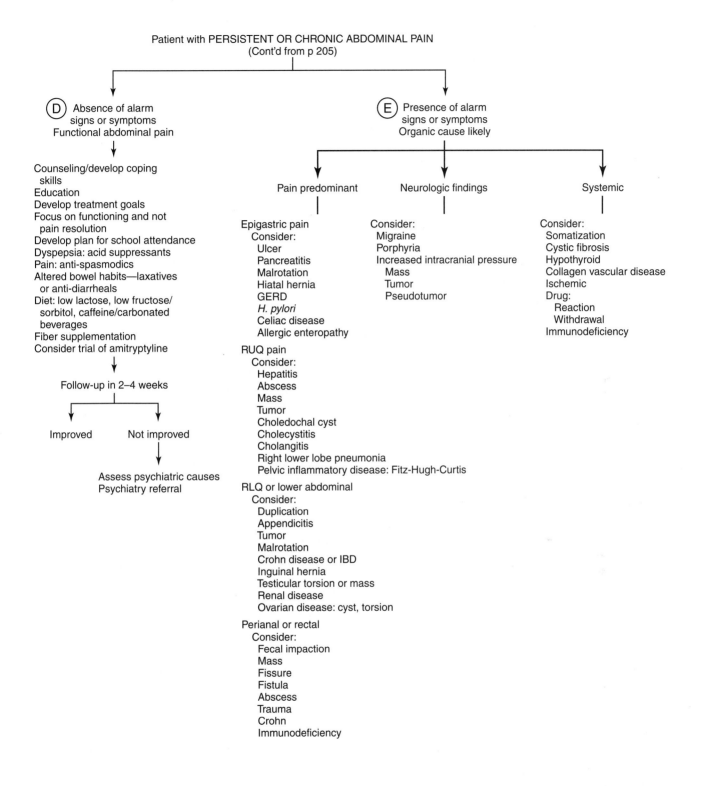

(D) Absence of alarm signs or symptoms
Functional abdominal pain

- Counseling/develop coping skills
- Education
- Develop treatment goals
- Focus on functioning and not pain resolution
- Develop plan for school attendance
- Dyspepsia: acid suppressants
- Pain: anti-spasmodics
- Altered bowel habits—laxatives or anti-diarrheals
- Diet: low lactose, low fructose/sorbitol, caffeine/carbonated beverages
- Fiber supplementation
- Consider trial of amitryptyline

→ Follow-up in 2–4 weeks

- Improved
- Not improved → Assess psychiatric causes; Psychiatry referral

(E) Presence of alarm signs or symptoms
Organic cause likely

Pain predominant

Epigastric pain
- Consider:
  - Ulcer
  - Pancreatitis
  - Malrotation
  - Hiatal hernia
  - GERD
  - *H. pylori*
  - Celiac disease
  - Allergic enteropathy

RUQ pain
- Consider:
  - Hepatitis
  - Abscess
  - Mass
  - Tumor
  - Choledochal cyst
  - Cholecystitis
  - Cholangitis
  - Right lower lobe pneumonia
  - Pelvic inflammatory disease: Fitz-Hugh-Curtis

RLQ or lower abdominal
- Consider:
  - Duplication
  - Appendicitis
  - Tumor
  - Malrotation
  - Crohn disease or IBD
  - Inguinal hernia
  - Testicular torsion or mass
  - Renal disease
  - Ovarian disease: cyst, torsion

Perianal or rectal
- Consider:
  - Fecal impaction
  - Mass
  - Fissure
  - Fistula
  - Abscess
  - Trauma
  - Crohn
  - Immunodeficiency

Neurologic findings

- Consider:
  - Migraine
  - Porphyria
  - Increased intracranial pressure
    - Mass
    - Tumor
    - Pseudotumor

Systemic

- Consider:
  - Somatization
  - Cystic fibrosis
  - Hypothyroid
  - Collagen vascular disease
  - Ischemic
  - Drug:
    - Reaction
    - Withdrawal
  - Immunodeficiency

Bloody Stools

Amethyst C. Kurbegov, MD, and Edward J. Hoffenberg, MD

Blood in the stools may be bright (hematochezia), dark black, tarry, shiny, and sticky (melena) or occult. Bright blood coating the stool is usually from the distal colon (sigmoid or rectum) or anus. A maroon color suggests a distal small-bowel source (such as a Meckel diverticulum); a currant-jelly appearance is characteristic of ischemic injury from intussusception. Upper gastrointestinal tract bleeding is usually melanotic, but if transit is rapid, it may be bright red. The most common causes of bloody stools differ according to age (Table 1).

A. In the patient's history, determine the onset, duration, frequency, and description of the bloody stools. Is the entire content blood? Does blood coat the stool? Is it mixed into the stool? Is the blood bright red or dark? Ask about associated symptoms, such as abdominal pain, tenesmus, diarrhea, vomiting, constipation, anorexia, and abdominal distention. Note extraintestinal symptoms, including fever, weight loss, delayed puberty, arthritis (each may suggest inflammatory bowel disease), purpura, easy bruising or bleeding, rash, and jaundice (consider chronic liver disease, Henoch–Schönlein purpura, or bleeding disorder). Exclude ingestion of substances that may be mistaken for melena or hematochezia, such as iron supplementation, bismuth, chocolate, grape juice, spinach, tomatoes, blueberries, food coloring, beets, gelatin, and red antibiotics. Identify possible precipitating factors or predisposing conditions, such as drug ingestions (maternal or child), use of salicylates or nonsteroidal anti-inflammatory agents, anticoagulant use, current antibiotic use, constipation, bleeding disorders, and milk or soy protein intolerance.

B. On physical examination, assess for active bleeding, hypovolemia, rash, edema, clubbing, ascites, jaundice, hepatosplenomegaly, hemorrhoids or anal fissures, and delayed puberty. Tags, perianal abscess, or fistulas suggest Crohn disease or immunodeficiency. In a preschool child with discoloration around an injured anus, suspect child abuse. Telangiectasias on mucous membranes, face, and hands suggest hereditary hemorrhagic telangiectasia.

C. Always test the stool material for occult blood even if it looks just like blood. False-positive results with a Hemoccult test may occur from foods that contain peroxidases such as broccoli, red meat, and radishes. Obtain a complete blood cell count (CBC) with differential and platelet count to document any anemia or thrombocytopenia. A low reticulocyte count may suggest an acute bleed. Identify hemolytic-uremic syndrome when thrombocytopenia and a microangiopathic hemolytic anemia are present. Thrombocytopenia may be an early sign of Wiskott–Aldrich syndrome or other systemic disease. Obtain a coagulation screen (prothrombin time/international normalized ratio [PT/INR], partial thromboplastin time [PTT]) when hemorrhagic disease of the newborn or other bleeding disorder is suspected. A low serum albumin concentration may suggest a protein-losing enteropathy. An increased sedimentation rate or C-reactive protein suggests infection, inflammatory bowel disease, or malignant disease. Serum amylase and lipase may reveal pancreatitis as cause of coagulopathy. Presence of fecal white blood cells indicates intestinal inflammation, likely infection, or inflammatory bowel disease. In the newborn period, the Apt–Downey or Kleihauer test distinguishes maternal blood from newborn blood. A positive nasogastric aspirate identifies bleeding proximal to the ligament of Treitz.

D. Consider placing a nasogastric tube. Blood in gastric aspirate identifies bleeding proximal to the ligament of Treitz (including oropharyngeal and nasal sources). Absence of blood, however, does not exclude an upper gastrointestinal tract source.

E. Assess the degree of illness and the need for resuscitation if a large volume of blood may have been lost (Table 2).

F. Anal fissures are a common cause of painless blood in the stool of a healthy infant. Fissures, usually associated with constipation and straining, may be infected with *Candida, Streptococcus,* or *Staphylococcus* and require antimicrobial therapy.

G. Nonspecific colitis related to milk, soy, or other protein intolerance presents in infants younger than 6 months with flecks or globs of blood mixed in the stool. Severe allergy may present with systemic signs, including vomiting, diarrhea, pain, distention, and weight loss. Obtain a stool culture for bacterial pathogens and a CBC with differential to assess for anemia, eosinophilia, and thrombocytopenia. When no other cause of bleeding is identified in a breast-fed baby, initiate a trial of excluding milk and soy from the maternal diet. When a child is not breast-fed, or when a dietary modification was not successful in a breast-fed baby, recommend a hydrolyzed formula (such as Nutramigen, Alimentum, or Pregestimil) or an amino acid formula (Neocate, EleCare, or Nutramigen AA). Visible blood usually resolves within 2 weeks. Gradual reintroduction of increasing amounts of soy or milk formula may begin after a few months. Anaphylaxis is a rare complication on repeated challenge. Remember that 30% to 40% of infants with allergy to cow milk protein also react to soy milk protein.

(Continued on page 210)

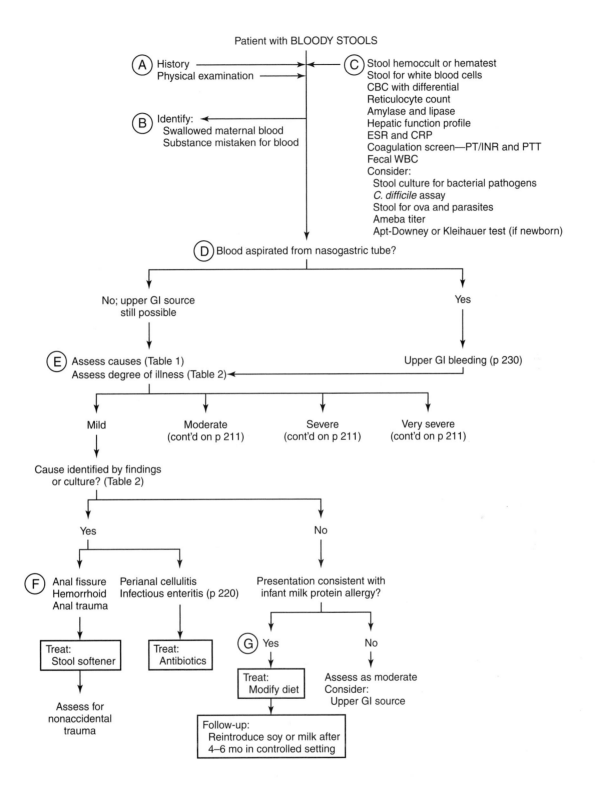

Patient with BLOODY STOOLS

(A) History
Physical examination

(B) Identify:
- Swallowed maternal blood
- Substance mistaken for blood

(C) Stool hemoccult or hematest
Stool for white blood cells
CBC with differential
Reticulocyte count
Amylase and lipase
Hepatic function profile
ESR and CRP
Coagulation screen—PT/INR and PTT
Fecal WBC
Consider:
- Stool culture for bacterial pathogens
- *C. difficile* assay
- Stool for ova and parasites
- Ameba titer
- Apt-Downey or Kleihauer test (if newborn)

(D) Blood aspirated from nasogastric tube?

- No; upper GI source still possible → (E)
- Yes → Upper GI bleeding (p 230) → (E)

(E) Assess causes (Table 1)
Assess degree of illness (Table 2)

- Mild
- Moderate (cont'd on p 211)
- Severe (cont'd on p 211)
- Very severe (cont'd on p 211)

Mild → Cause identified by findings or culture? (Table 2)

- Yes
  - (F) Anal fissure / Hemorrhoid / Anal trauma → **Treat:** Stool softener → Assess for nonaccidental trauma
  - Perianal cellulitis / Infectious enteritis (p 220) → **Treat:** Antibiotics
- No → Presentation consistent with infant milk protein allergy?
  - (G) Yes → **Treat:** Modify diet → **Follow-up:** Reintroduce soy or milk after 4–6 mo in controlled setting
  - No → Assess as moderate. Consider: Upper GI source

Table 1. **Causes of Bloody Stools by Age**

Type of Cause	AGE 0–1 yr	1–5 yr	>5 yr
Common	Allergic colitis (milk, soy) Intussusception Meckel diverticulum Volvulus Enterocolitis (necrotizing) Hirschsprung disease Infection* Fissure	Fissure Infection* Polyp Intussusception Lymphonodular hyperplasia Meckel diverticulum	Infection* IBD Polyp Fissure Upper GI source Hemorrhoid
Less common	Perianal cellulitis Vascular malformation Coagulopathy Swallowed blood	HUS IBD HSP Upper GI source (varices, ulcer)	HUS HSP Thrombocytopenia

*Infection: bacterial pathogens, *Clostridium difficile* and other toxins, virus, parasite.
GI, gastrointestinal; *HSP*, Henoch–Schönlein purpura; *HUS*, hemolytic-uremic syndrome; *IBD*, inflammatory bowel disease.

H. Hemolytic-uremic syndrome is a complication of *Escherichia coli* O157:H7 and other toxins, such as pneumococcal neuraminidase. Monitor for hemolysis and thrombocytopenia with a CBC and differential, and for proteinuria and renal failure. The petechial rash of Henoch–Schönlein purpura may develop before or after a gastrointestinal bleed; abdominal pain associated with this condition may be severe and indicate small-bowel intussusception. Causes of infectious enterocolitis include *Salmonella, Shigella, Campylobacter, Yersinia, E. coli,* and *Entamoeba histolytica* (see page 220 for infectious enteritis).

I. *Clostridium difficile* disease is mediated by toxins A and B. Toxin A is an enterotoxin; toxin B is a cytotoxin. Manifestations may include bleeding, watery diarrhea, crampy pain with fecal leukocytes, and a toxic appearance (pseudomembranous colitis). Infants in the first months of life frequently have toxins in the stool without disease because they lack the receptor necessary for toxin binding. Recent antibiotic use is the single largest risk factor for *C. difficile* disease. Stool testing may identify presence of toxin, whereas a flexible sigmoidoscopy can quickly reveal pseudomembranes and the extent of severe colitis. The course of the disease may be mild to severe with shock, bleeding, pain, or obstruction requiring hospitalization. Initial treatment is with oral or intravenous metronidazole or oral vancomycin, bowel rest, fluid resuscitation, correction of metabolic disturbances, and surgical consult. Recurrence is common and may require retreatment with antibiotics and probiotics.

J. Identify an intussusception when darkly bloody stools are associated with colicky abdominal pain, an abdominal mass, distention, or vomiting in the first 2 years of life. An air-contrast enema may be diagnostic, as well as lead to reduction of the intussusceptum. Ultrasonography or abdominal computed tomography (CT) scan may show a "donut" ring of intussuscepted bowel, as well as exclude an abscess or appendicitis. A full-term infant with necrotizing enterocolitis should be evaluated for Hirschsprung disease.

K. Suspect a vascular malformation when aortic stenosis, Turner syndrome, or a mucocutaneous disorder (Rendu–Osler–Weber syndrome or hereditary hemorrhagic telangiectasia) is present. Endoscopy and CT angiography may locate the source of the bleeding and the extent of the vascular involvement.

L. The most common polyp in children is the juvenile polyp. Juvenile polyps usually present with painless blood mixed in with the stool that persists despite achieving soft stools with laxatives. If a family history of polyposis, consider familial adenomatous polyposis/Gardner syndrome (associated with desmoid tumors, cysts, teeth malformations, and congenital hypertrophy of retinal pigment epithelium) or Peutz–Jeghers syndrome (small intestinal polyps, intussusception, mucocutaneous pigmentation). Both syndromes require periodic surveillance for malignancy.

M. Meckel diverticulum is usually located in the distal small bowel and contains gastric parietal cells. It most often causes symptoms in children younger than 2 years. Presentations include rapid, painless rectal bleeding (acid produced by the gastric tissue causes a bleeding ulcer), intussusception, and obstruction. A nuclear medicine scan identifies about 90% of bleeding Meckel diverticula. Enteric duplication can also contain ectopic gastric tissue and cause bleeding.

(Continued on page 212)

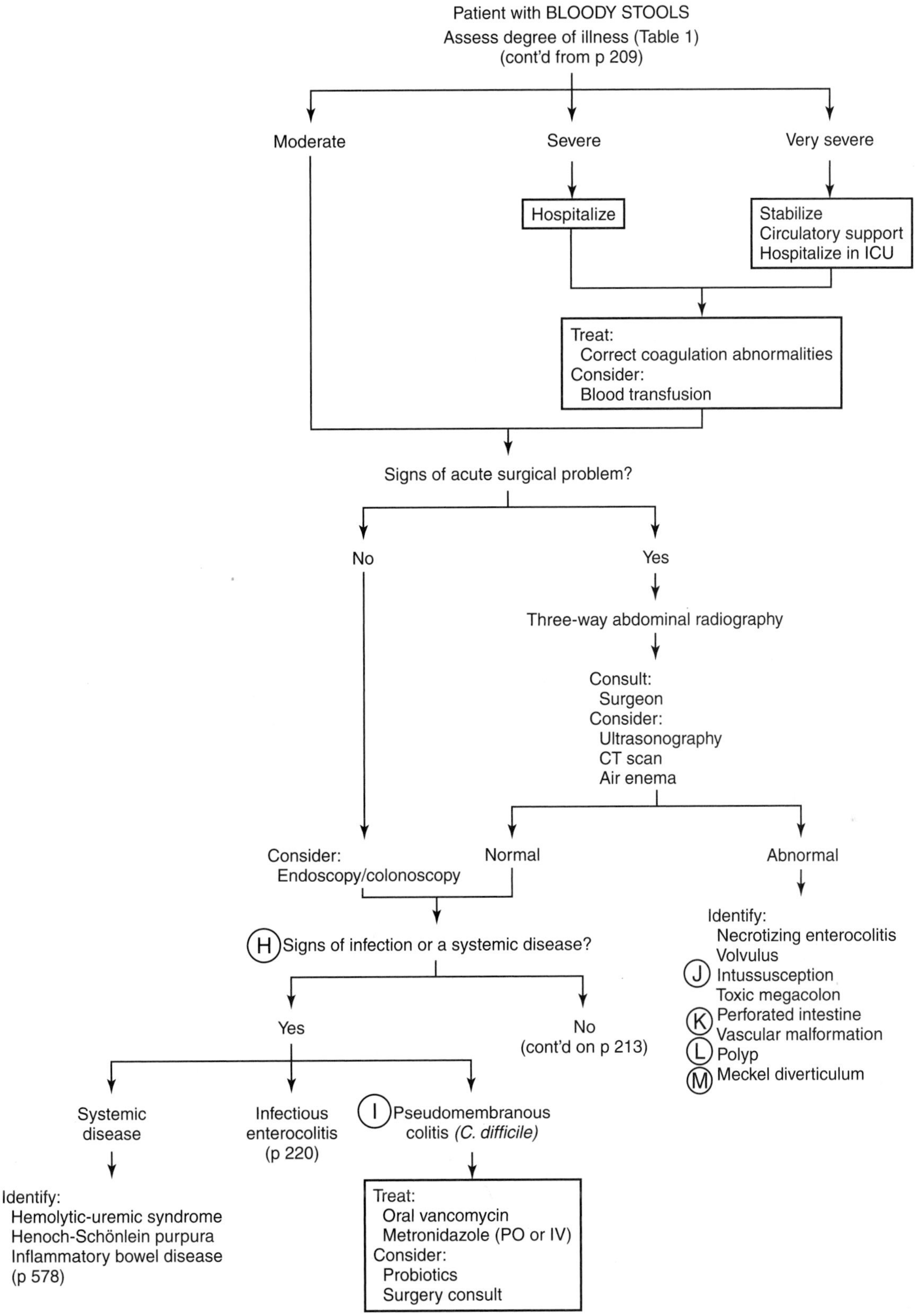

Patient with BLOODY STOOLS
Assess degree of illness (Table 1)
(cont'd from p 209)
Moderate
Severe
Very severe
Hospitalize
Stabilize
Circulatory support
Hospitalize in ICU
Treat:
Correct coagulation abnormalities
Consider:
Blood transfusion
Signs of acute surgical problem?
No
Yes
Three-way abdominal radiography
Consult:
Surgeon
Consider:
Ultrasonography
CT scan
Air enema
Consider:
Endoscopy/colonoscopy
Normal
Abnormal
Identify:
Necrotizing enterocolitis
Volvulus
J Intussusception
Toxic megacolon
K Perforated intestine
Vascular malformation
L Polyp
M Meckel diverticulum
H Signs of infection or a systemic disease?
Yes
No
(cont'd on p 213)
Systemic disease
Infectious enterocolitis
(p 220)
I Pseudomembranous colitis (C. difficile)
Identify:
Hemolytic-uremic syndrome
Henoch-Schönlein purpura
Inflammatory bowel disease
(p 578)
Treat:
Oral vancomycin
Metronidazole (PO or IV)
Consider:
Probiotics
Surgery consult

Table 2. **Degree of Illness in Patient with Bloody Stools**

Mild	Moderate	Severe	Critical
Minimal blood loss (no anemia) AND No systemic signs of illness	Signs of infection or systemic disease May have mild, chronic anemia OR Newborn, well appearing	Newborn, ill appearing OR Toxic appearance OR Dehydration OR Significant blood loss (acute anemia)	Shock or circulatory collapse OR Continued active hemorrhage OR Acute surgical abdomen (peritonitis, obstruction, ischemia)

References

Boyle JT. Gastrointestinal bleeding in infants and children. Pediatr Rev 2008;29(2):39–52.

Fox VL. Gastrointestinal bleeding in infancy and childhood. Gastroenterol Clin North Am 2000;29(1):37–66.

Xanthakos SA, Schwimmer JB, Melin-Aldana H, et al. Prevalence and outcome of allergic colitis in healthy infants with rectal bleeding: a prospective cohort study. J Pediatr Gastroenterol Nutr 2005;41(1):16–22.

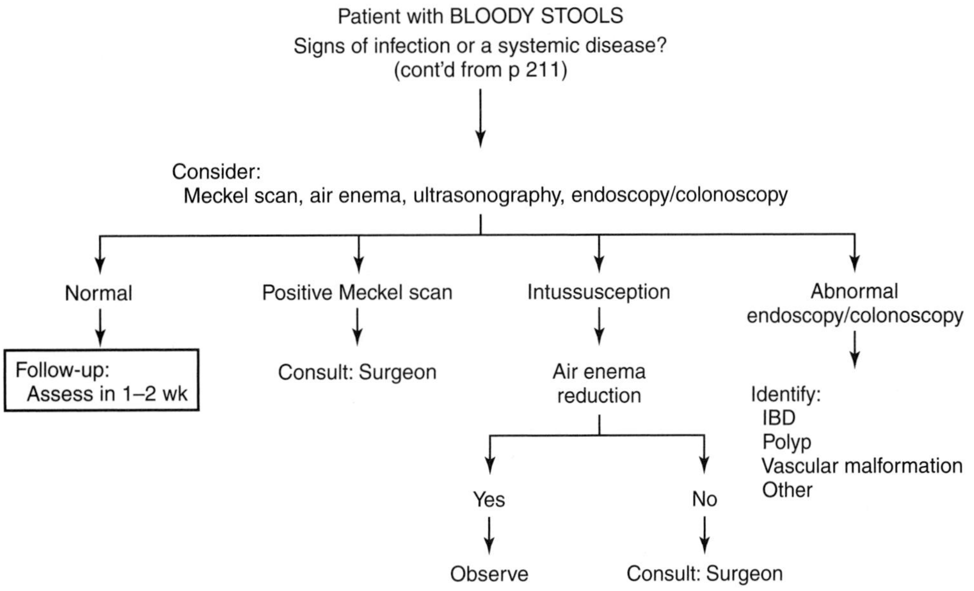
Patient with BLOODY STOOLS
Signs of infection or a systemic disease?
(cont'd from p 211)
Consider:
Meckel scan, air enema, ultrasonography, endoscopy/colonoscopy
Normal
Follow-up:
Assess in 1–2 wk
Positive Meckel scan
Consult: Surgeon
Intussusception
Air enema reduction
Yes
Observe
No
Consult: Surgeon
Abnormal endoscopy/colonoscopy
Identify:
IBD
Polyp
Vascular malformation
Other

Constipation

Christine Waasdorp Hurtado, MD, and Edward J. Hoffenberg, MD

Constipation accounts for 3% of all visits to general pediatricians and 25% of pediatric gastroenterology consultations. Changes in defecation patterns create anxiety and concern in parents, but thankfully, only small minorities of children have an organic causative factor. Constipation is defined as delay or difficulty with defecation lasting 2 or more weeks leading to distress in the patient (or parent). Parents pay significant attention to their children's bowel movements and will report when their child's stools are infrequent, hard, or large and painful to pass. Stooling patterns vary considerably between individuals and frequency decreases with age. The average newborn defecates four times per day (with some breast-fed babies stooling once every 5–7 days), decreasing to the adult pattern of one stool per day by the age of 4 years.

Functional constipation accounts for more than 90% of childhood constipation and is not associated with any pathologic condition. Stool retention is secondary to voluntary withholding, resulting in painful bowel movements and attempts to avoid future defecation, and thus setting up a cycle leading to worsening constipation. If enough stool is withheld in the rectum, the patient will experience overflow soiling, or encopresis. In addition to functional constipation, there are other less likely causes to be considered, including medical conditions and medications. In the child with constipation, specific medical conditions can be evaluated in a systematic fashion, with validation of the family's concerns.

A. A thorough history is important in investigating the cause of constipation. Timing of first bowel movement after birth and description of the typical stooling pattern and duration of the process should be obtained. Determine whether clear associations exist between stool pattern change and potty training or other stressful events. The provider should clarify what the family means by "constipation," duration of symptoms, frequency of bowel movements, consistency and size of the stool, presence of blood on or mixed in with the stool, in the toilet bowl, or on the toilet paper, and whether the child experiences pain with passage of stool. Stool-withholding behaviors, such as wriggling, leg crossing, or other posturing, reduce the concern for organic disease. A dietary history evaluating fluid intake, fiber intake, and general nutrition can be helpful. A complete medication list (medications, vitamins, and herbs) should be gathered as potential causes of constipation. A psychosocial history assesses family structure, interactions with other children, school performance, and any possibility of abuse. In addition, anxiety relating to restroom use at school and outside the home should be assessed. Acute retention increases suspicion for perianal strep or trauma.

Family history of Hirschsprung disease, other gastrointestinal disorders, as well as neurologic, endocrine, metabolic, cystic fibrosis, and developmental problems should be reviewed. The concern for organic causes increases with the report of fever, abdominal distension, anorexia, nausea, and poor weight gain.

B. A thorough physical examination is helpful in determining the severity of constipation. The patient should be examined for any evidence of neurologic, endocrine, metabolic, collagen vascular disease, or gastrointestinal disease. The back should be examined for presence of a sacral dimple or hair tuft. A neurologic examination including overall tone and deep tendon reflexes can suggest a neurologic cause. Close attention should be paid to physical findings suggestive of physical or sexual abuse. The abdomen should be evaluated for distension and masses, providing information about the severity of the constipation. Several anatomic abnormalities are associated with constipation including anal stenosis, anteriorly placed anus, and anorectal malformations. The rectal and perineal examinations are therefore central to the physical examination for constipation. Assess placement of the anus, presence of anal wink, evidence of fissures, hemorrhoids, perianal abscess, inflammation, or erythema; evaluate anal tone and rectal size; and document the presence of stool or stool impaction (firm ball of stool in an enlarged rectal vault) in the rectal vault. Explosive stool on withdrawal of finger in an infant is suggestive of an obstructive process such as Hirschsprung disease or anal stenosis.

C. An abdominal radiograph may be helpful when the rectal examination closely follows passage of a large bowel movement, or if because of psychosocial reasons the rectal examination is deferred. The radiograph has no role in the initial evaluation when the physical examination clearly shows evidence of constipation.

D. The differential diagnosis is extensive; however, most cases of constipation are functional and require minimal evaluation. The differential should be considered during the history and physical examination (see Table 1).

E. Hirschsprung disease is the most common cause of lower intestinal obstruction in neonates and rarely is the cause of constipation in toddlers and school-age children. In these children, the constipation is due to the absence of ganglion cells in the myenteric and submucous plexuses of the distal colon resulting in sustained contraction of the affected colon. The segment begins at the internal anal sphincter and extends in a continuous fashion. The disease is limited to the rectosigmoid area in 75% of cases. The incidence is 1 in 5000 live births, with the most common associated anomaly being trisomy 21. Early clues for diagnosis include the delayed passage of meconium with less than 10% of neonates with Hirschsprung disease passing meconium in the first 24 hours compared with 90% of normal neonates. Additional symptoms may include bilious vomiting,

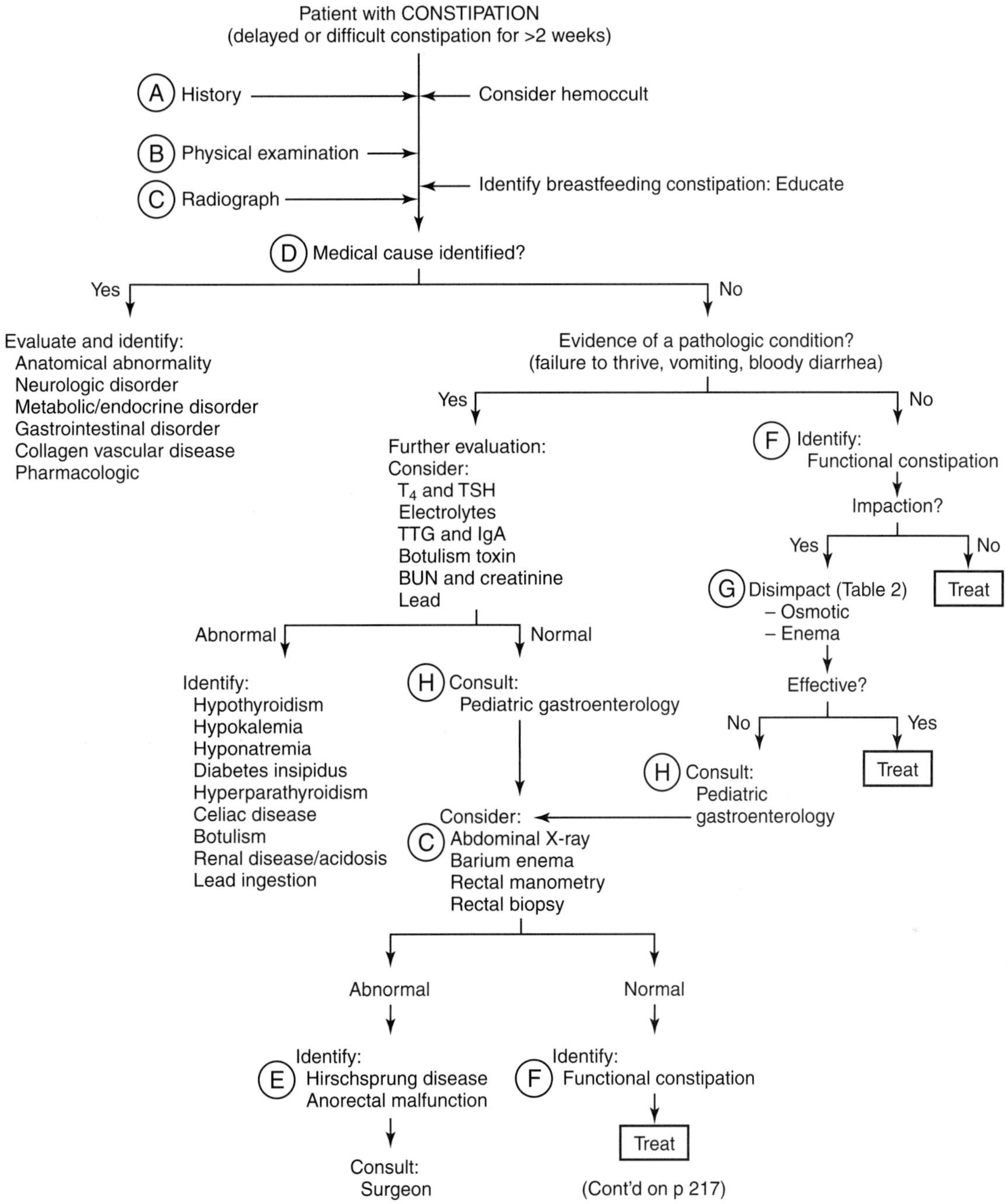
Patient with CONSTIPATION
(delayed or difficult constipation for >2 weeks)
A History
Consider hemoccult
B Physical examination
C Radiograph
Identify breastfeeding constipation: Educate
D Medical cause identified?
Yes
No
Evaluate and identify:
Anatomical abnormality
Neurologic disorder
Metabolic/endocrine disorder
Gastrointestinal disorder
Collagen vascular disease
Pharmacologic
Evidence of a pathologic condition?
(failure to thrive, vomiting, bloody diarrhea)
Yes
No
Further evaluation:
Consider:
T_4 and TSH
Electrolytes
TTG and IgA
Botulism toxin
BUN and creatinine
Lead
F Identify:
Functional constipation
Impaction?
Yes
No
G Disimpact (Table 2)
– Osmotic
– Enema
Treat
Abnormal
Normal
Identify:
Hypothyroidism
Hypokalemia
Hyponatremia
Diabetes insipidus
Hyperparathyroidism
Celiac disease
Botulism
Renal disease/acidosis
Lead ingestion
H Consult:
Pediatric gastroenterology
Effective?
No
Yes
H Consult:
Pediatric
gastroenterology
Treat
Consider:
C Abdominal X-ray
Barium enema
Rectal manometry
Rectal biopsy
Abnormal
Normal
Identify:
E Hirschsprung disease
Anorectal malfunction
Identify:
F Functional constipation
Treat
Consult:
Surgeon
(Cont'd on p 217)

abdominal distension, and refusal to feed. Enterocolitis is the most concerning complication, with a mortality rate of 20%; typically the presentation is sudden-onset fever, abdominal distention, and explosive bloody stools. Diagnosis of Hirschsprung disease is usually made by barium enema, rectal biopsy, or anorectal manometry.

F. Functional constipation is the most common cause of constipation in children in whom there are no other identified disorders. Onset is often associated with toilet training or following the passage of a large-caliber bowel movement resulting in pain. Children may withhold stool when they are busy playing or choose not to use bathrooms outside their comfort areas. Stool held in the rectum by the external sphincter (voluntary) often becomes dry, hard, and painful to pass. The negative experience often begins a challenging cycle of withholding increasingly dry, large-caliber stools and more pain with the urge to defecate. As the rectum stretches to accommodate the increased volume of stool, the decreased rectal sensation temporarily diminishes the urge to defecate. This cycle may be broken by disimpaction, a bowel regimen to support soft, small-caliber bowel movements, and positive reinforcement.

Table 1. **Differential Diagnosis of Chronic Constipation**

Gastrointestinal

Functional constipation
Hirschsprung disease
Anal stenosis
Anterior placement of anus
Celiac disease
Intestinal neuronal dysplasia

Neurologic

Spinal cord disorders (spina bifida, meningomyelocele, sacral teratoma, tethered cord)
Neurofibromatosis
Encephalopathy
Cerebral palsy

Metabolic/Endocrine

Hypothyroidism
Hypercalcemia
Hypokalemia
Diabetes mellitus
Hyponatremia

Connective Tissue Disorder

Scleroderma
Systemic lupus erythematosus
Ehlers–Danlos syndrome

Developmental

Mental retardation
Autism
Attention deficit disorder

Medications/Toxin

Anticholinergics
Phenobarbital
Antihypertensives
Sucralfate
Bismuth
Iron or lead
Opiates
Sympathomimetics
Antacids

Other

Botulism
Vitamin D intoxication
Cystic fibrosis
Perianal infection
Emotional disorder

G. Management consists of three main steps: disimpaction, maintenance, and finally weaning of medications. Disimpaction is necessary before starting a maintenance therapy and can be accomplished with either oral or rectal medications (see Table 2). The rectal approach is faster but more invasive. Soap suds, tap water, and magnesium enemas are not recommended because of toxicity risks. Maintenance therapy is started after successful disimpaction and is accomplished with dietary interventions, laxatives, and behavioral modification with the primary goal of preventing recurrence of constipation. The use of laxatives helps attain remission sooner. Daily treatment with laxatives (medication dosing titrated to effect) assists patients to meet the goal of one to two soft bowel movements daily. A stimulant laxative may be required to avoid recurrence of fecal impaction, with short-duration courses preferable over longer durations (>4 weeks). Behavioral modification with positive reinforcement is as important as medication for successful treatment of constipation. Scheduled toilet time 10 to 15 minutes after meals takes advantage of the gastrocolic reflex and can reduce soiling. A calendar or sticker chart provides positive reinforcement and charts success of bowel movements on the toilet. Dietary interventions are also important, with increasing fluids and fiber playing a role in maintenance therapy for constipation.

H. Children should be referred to a pediatric gastroenterologist when basic medical therapy has failed, if the concern for organic cause remains after initial evaluation and treatment or if management is complex. A consult will include re-evaluation for organic causative factors, specialized testing as indicated, change in frequency or dosing of medication, or a change in treatment regimen selection with close follow-up.

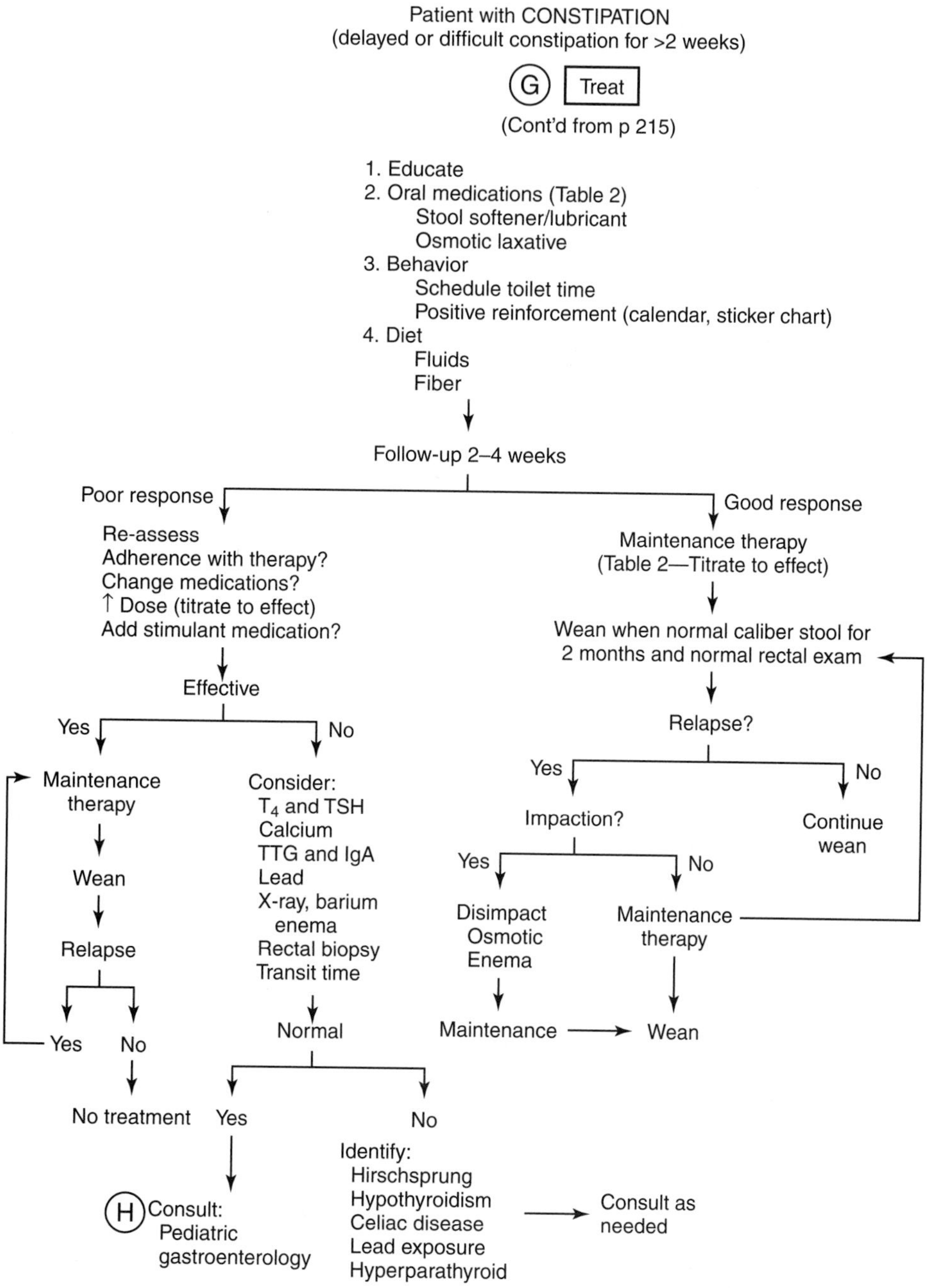
Patient with CONSTIPATION
(delayed or difficult constipation for >2 weeks)
G
Treat
(Cont'd from p 215)
1. Educate
2. Oral medications (Table 2)
Stool softener/lubricant
Osmotic laxative
3. Behavior
Schedule toilet time
Positive reinforcement (calendar, sticker chart)
4. Diet
Fluids
Fiber
Follow-up 2–4 weeks
Poor response
Good response
Re-assess
Adherence with therapy?
Change medications?
↑ Dose (titrate to effect)
Add stimulant medication?
Maintenance therapy
(Table 2—Titrate to effect)
Wean when normal caliber stool for
2 months and normal rectal exam
Effective
Yes
No
Relapse?
Yes
No
Maintenance
therapy
Consider:
T_4 and TSH
Calcium
TTG and IgA
Lead
X-ray, barium
enema
Rectal biopsy
Transit time
Impaction?
Continue
wean
Yes
No
Wean
Disimpact
Osmotic
Enema
Maintenance
therapy
Relapse
Yes
No
Normal
Maintenance
Wean
No treatment
Yes
No
Identify:
Hirschsprung
Hypothyroidism
Celiac disease
Lead exposure
Hyperparathyroid
H
Consult:
Pediatric
gastroenterology
Consult as
needed

Table 2. **Medications for Treatment of Chronic Constipation**

Medication	Dosage	Adverse Effects	Comments
Osmotic			
Lactulose	1–3 ml/kg/day in divided doses	Flatulence, abdominal cramps, hypernatremia if used in high dose for hepatic encephalopathy	Synthetic disaccharide. Well tolerated in long term
Sorbitol	1–3 ml/kg/day in divided doses	Same as lactulose	Less expensive than lactulose
Magnesium hydroxide	1–3 ml/kg/day of 400 mg/5 ml	Overdose can lead to hypermagnesemia, hypophosphatemia, and secondary hypocalcemia Infants are susceptible to magnesium toxicity	Releases cholecystokinin, which stimulates gastrointestinal secretion and motility Use with caution in renal impairment
Magnesium citrate	<6 years: 2–4 ml/kg/day 6–12 years: 100–150 ml/day >12 years: 150–300 ml/day Single or divided doses	Same as for magnesium hydroxide	
PEG 3350	Disimpaction: 1–1.5 g/kg/day for 3 days Maintenance: 1 g/kg/day	Flatulence, cramping, bloating, diarrhea	Superior palatability
Osmotic Enema			
Phosphate enema	>2 years: 6 ml/kg up to 135 ml	Risk for mechanical trauma, abdominal distention, and vomiting. May cause severe or lethal hyperphosphatemia, hypocalcemia with tetany	Most adverse effects in children with renal disease or Hirschsprung disease
Lavage			
Polyethylene glycol-electrolyte solution	Disimpaction: 25 ml/kg/hr to 1000 ml/hr via nasogastric tube until clear Maintenance: 1 mg/kg/day	Difficult to tolerate; nausea, bloating, cramps, vomiting; concerns for aspiration pneumonitis; long-term safety not well established	May require hospital admission and nasogastric tube placement
Lubricant			
Mineral oil	>1 year: Disimpaction: 15–30 ml per year of age up to 240 ml daily Maintenance: 1–3 ml/kg/day	Lipoid pneumonia if aspirated Minimal interference of fat-soluble vitamin absorption	Softens stools and decreases water absorption Anal leakage at high doses
Stimulants			
Senna	10–20 mg/kg/dose QHS Syrup: 8.8 mg/5 ml Also available as tablets or granules	Abdominal pain, cathartic colon Idiosyncratic hepatitis, melanosis coli, hypertrophic osteoarthropathy, analgesic nephropathy	Increased intestinal motility Melanosis coli resolves 4–12 months after discontinuation
Bisacodyl	≥2 years: 0.5–1 suppository, 0.3 mg/kg/day; max 30 mg	Abdominal pain, diarrhea, hypokalemia Case reports of urolithiasis	
Glycerin suppository		No adverse effects	

References

Clinical Practice Guideline: Evaluation and treatment of constipation in infants and children: recommendations of the North American Society for Pediatric Gastroenterology, Hepatology and Nutrition. J Pediatr Gastroenterol Nutr 2006;43:e1-e13.

Lewis NA, Levitt MA, Zallen GS, et al. Diagnosing Hirschsprung's disease: increasing the odds of a positive rectal biopsy result. J Pediatric Surg 2003;38:412–6.

Loenig-Baucke V. Constipation and encopresis. In: Wylie R, Hyams J, editors. Pediatric gastrointestinal and liver disease. 3rd ed. Philadelphia: Saunders-Elsevier; 2006. p. 177–91.

Loenig-Baucke V. Polyethylene glycol without electrolytes for children with constipation and encopresis. J Pediatr Gastroenterol Nutr 2002;34:372–7.

Pashankar DS, Loenig-Baucke V, Bishop WP. Safety of polyethylene glycol 3350 for the treatment of chronic constipation in children. Arch Pediatr Adolesc Med 2003;57:661–4.

Youssef NN, Peters JM, Henderson W, et al. Dose response of PEG 3350 for the treatment of childhood fecal impaction. J Pediatr 2002;141:410–4.

Acute Diarrhea

Steven Colson, MD, and Edward J. Hoffenberg, MD

Acute diarrhea is an abrupt but short-lived (<2 weeks) increase in the water content of stool and is usually associated with an increase in the frequency of stools. In children younger than 5, the frequency of yearly acute diarrhea episodes is one to two in the United States and three to eight in developing countries. Acute diarrhea is most commonly caused by an infection, including virus, bacteria, parasite, and toxin from food poisoning, as well as extraintestinal infections such as otitis media, pneumonia, and urinary tract infections. Noninfectious causes of acute diarrhea include drug effects, food allergy (most common in infants with milk or soy protein sensitivity), carbohydrate malabsorption from sucrase-isomaltase deficiency and hypolactasia (lactose intolerance), radiation- or chemotherapy-related enteritis, and anatomic conditions such as appendicitis or intussusception. Less common causes of acute diarrhea include niacin deficiency and toxicity from excess copper, tin, or zinc.

An infectious agent is detectable in about 70% of sporadic acute diarrhea cases, with viruses more common than other agents. These viruses include rotavirus, calicivirus (including Norwalk-like virus), astrovirus, and enteric adenovirus. Vaccination has reduced the frequency of severe acute diarrhea from rotavirus infection.

Diarrhea can be classified by the underlying pathogenic mechanism and location of disease. Secretory diarrhea, often infectious in nature, is accompanied by a high stool chloride content and normal stool osmotic gap. Osmotic gap equals the measured stool osmolality $-(2 [Na + K])$, and normal is less than 50 mOsm. The stool osmolality can be estimated at 290 mOsm when accurate measurement is not possible. Secretory diarrhea does not resolve in a fasting state. Osmotic diarrhea, often not infectious in nature, will have an increased stool anion gap (>100 mOsm/kg) and does improve during fasting. Diarrhea originating in the small bowel is marked by high stool sodium content, whereas diarrhea originating in the colon has low stool sodium content. Inflammation can be used to further classify secretory diarrhea. Noninflammatory secretory diarrhea results when the infection (or enterotoxin) promotes secretion of fluid and electrolytes or reduces absorption in the small bowel. The main pathogens causing noninflammatory diarrhea are the viruses listed earlier, the parasites *Giardia* and *Cryptosporidia,* enterotoxigenic and enteropathogenic *Escherichia coli, Vibrio cholerae,* and *Vibrio parahaemolyticus.* Food poisoning results from ingestion of preformed toxin. Bacteria forming these toxins include *Staphylococcus aureus* (improperly cooked or stored food), *Clostridium perfringens* (contaminated meat, vegetables, or poultry), and *Bacillus cereus* (fried rice and vegetable sprouts). Inflammatory secretory diarrhea, caused by invasion of the bowel mucosa, often presents with blood, mucus, and pus in the stool and tenesmus, severe cramps, and fever. The most common community-acquired pathogens include *Campylobacter, Escherichia coli* O157:H7 and other Shiga toxin-producing *E. coli, Salmonella, Shigella, Yersinia, Clostridium difficile, Entamoeba histolytica,* and possibly *Aeromonas.* Systemic bacteremic infections related to intracellular multiplication and penetration occur with *Salmonella typhi* (typhoid fever), *Yersinia,* and *Campylobacter.* The presence of bloody diarrhea and seizures suggest infection with *Shigella.* Acute bloody diarrhea is a medical emergency. A randomized, controlled intervention trial by Albano and colleagues recently showed that adherence to guidelines for management of acute gastroenteritis results in improved outcome, with excellent efficacy and good applicability. These guidelines can be applied to the child with acute diarrhea.

The following seven basic principles should guide treatment of acute diarrhea and dehydration:

1. Oral rehydration solutions (ORSs) should be used when possible.
2. Oral rehydration should be used rapidly (within 3–4 hours).
3. An age-appropriate, unrestricted diet is recommended after dehydration is corrected, to aid in rapid re-alimentation.
4. Continue nursing in breastfed infants.
5. Diluted formula is not recommended; special formula is usually not necessary.
6. Replace ongoing losses with additional ORSs.
7. Minimize unnecessary laboratory tests or medications.

A. In the history, ask about the onset, duration, frequency, pattern, and severity of the diarrhea. Ask if the stools contain blood or mucus and whether fasting (if done) decreases stooling amount. Document type and amount of oral intake, including breast milk, other fluids and food, and symptoms of dehydration including decreased frequency of urination, decreased activity level, irritability, weight loss and decreased tearing. Note associated gastrointestinal symptoms such as vomiting, abdominal pain (including location and intensity), and anorexia. Note systemic symptoms, such as fever, cough, coryza, arthralgias/arthritis and rash. Identify any potential precipitating factors including ingestions. Ask if other family members or contacts have recently had diarrhea. Past medical history should focus on underlying medical problems, recent infections, medications used, and human immunodeficiency (HIV) status.

B. In the physical examination, assess hydration (see Table 1) and circulatory status by documenting blood pressure, pulse, respiratory rate, skin color and turgor, capillary refill, tears, presence of sunken eyes, moistness of lips and mouth, fullness of

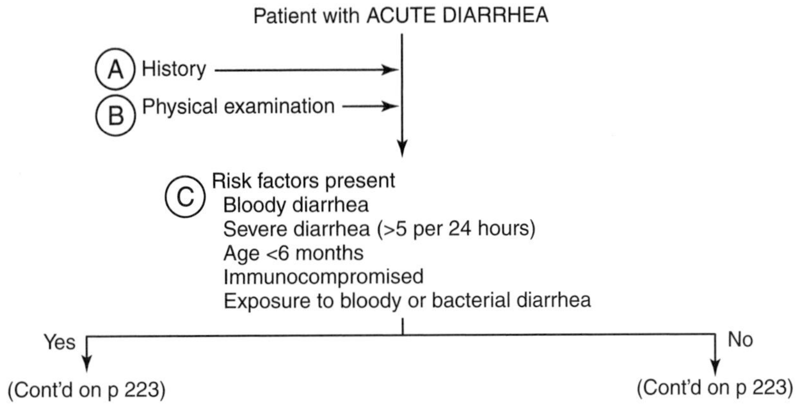
Patient with ACUTE DIARRHEA
A History
B Physical examination
C Risk factors present
Bloody diarrhea
Severe diarrhea (>5 per 24 hours)
Age <6 months
Immunocompromised
Exposure to bloody or bacterial diarrhea
Yes
No
(Cont'd on p 223)
(Cont'd on p 223)

the fontanel, and urine output. The anterior fontanel, though helpful at times, can be misleading as a dehydration marker. Increased heart rate and decreased peripheral perfusion are more sensitive signs than hypotension (a late sign) for dehydration. Decreased urination is also sensitive, though lacks specificity because it can be difficult to measure when mixed with diarrhea. A careful abdominal examination should be done assessing for location and severity of pain, masses (right lower quadrant may suggest intussusception), as well as for any peritoneal signs. Perianal inspection can also be helpful, looking for evidence of rash, ulceration, or active bleeding. Stool, if present, can be examined for blood or mucus. Assess mental status, noting any irritability, lethargy, seizures, or focal neurologic signs. Watch the child drink and note whether the child drinks normally, eagerly, or poorly. Note extraintestinal signs, such as rash, hepatomegaly, splenomegaly, lymphadenopathy, and arthritis.

C. Risk factors for bacterial acute diarrhea include age younger than 6 months, weight less than 8 kg, history of prematurity, immunosuppression, chronic illness, concurrent illness, fever, visible blood in the stool, fecal white blood cells present, ongoing losses including high-output diarrhea or frequent emesis, moderate-to-severe dehydration, change in mental status, and failed oral rehydration.

Table 1. **Degree of Dehydration**

Symptom	Mild	Moderate	Severe
Mental status	Alert, active	Restless, irritable	Lethargic, unresponsive
Thirst	Drinks normally	Drinks eagerly	Unable to drink or drinks poorly
Heart rate	Normal	Normal to increased	Tachycardia, bradycardia when most severe
Quality of pulses	Normal	Normal to decreased	Weak or impalpable
Breathing	Normal	Normal; fast	Deep
Eyes	Normal	Slightly sunken	Deeply sunken
Tears	Present	Decreased	Absent
Mouth and tongue	Moist	Dry	Parched
Skin fold	Instant recoil	Recoil in <2 seconds	Recoil >2 seconds
Capillary refill	Normal	Prolonged	Prolonged, minimal
Extremities	Warm	Cool	Cold, mottled, cyanotic
Urine output	Normal to decreased	Decreased	Minimal

Adapted from King CK, Glass R, Bresee JS, Duggan C; Centers for Disease Control and Prevention. Managing acute gastroenteritis among children: oral rehydration, maintenance, and nutritional therapy. MMWR Recomm Rep 2003;52(RR-16):1–16.

D. Acute Bloody Diarrhea: Of special concern is infection with *E. coli* O157:H7 because of the potential complication of hemolytic-uremic syndrome (HUS). Approximately 15% of children infected with *E. coli* O157:H7 will go on to experience development of HUS. Warning signs at time of presentation for *E. coli* O157:H7 infection include persistent bloody diarrhea that was initially nonbloody for 1 to 3 days, absence of fever, abdominal tenderness, greater than five stools in the past 24 hours, pain with defecation, and absence of bandemia in the white cell count differential. Other risk factors for a bacterial cause of bloody diarrhea are listed in Table 2. Send for a bacterial stool culture, making sure that *E. coli* O157:H7 is included or other testing for O157:H7 is done. If *E. coli* O157:H7 is detected, refer the patient to a center where dialysis can be done. Obtain a complete blood cell count (CBC) and pay special attention to the hemoglobin and platelet levels. Monitor electrolytes and serum creatinine when suspicious for *E. coli* O157:H7. Also obtain a blood culture in infants and immunocompromised patients when a bacterial cause is suspected, or when there is evidence of septicemia. It is unlikely that a computed tomographic (CT) scan will significantly change the diagnosis or management of a patient with acute bloody diarrhea. If signs of obstruction exist or dark currant jelly stool per rectum, consider intussusception. Obtain abdominal radiograph, air–contrast enema, and/or CT scan, and obtain surgical consult for intussusception. Avoid narcotics and antimotility agents. If significant pain exists, consider intravenous boluses of normal saline for pain relief. Avoid antibiotic therapy unless a treatable pathogen is found. *Shigella* and enteroinvasive *E. coli* should be treated once diagnosed. Patients with significant acute bloody diarrhea should be hospitalized to provide adequate hydration; to monitor for hypertension, volume overload, and signs and symptoms of HUS including oliguria and platelet, electrolyte, and creatinine abnormalities; and to help prevent secondary transmission of the infectious agent. Consideration should be made for an abdominal radiograph for pneumatosis or thumb printing. Once clinically improved, if the infectious agent is found not to be O157:H7 and the platelet count, if low, has increased or stabilized, the patient may be discharged. An important emerging pathogen is *C. difficile.* Though some patients may be asymptomatic carriers, clinical infection is typified by diarrhea that is often bloody. Patients may also have fever, nausea, abdominal cramping, or pain, and may experience development of pseudomembranous colitis, bacteremia and shock, and rarely, toxic megacolon. First-line therapy is oral metronidazole or, alternatively, oral vancomycin (Table 3). Repeated courses are often required to eradicate the organism. Any severe colitis can cause hypoalbuminemia and potassium shifts.

Table 2. **Risk Factors for Bacterial Cause of Acute Bloody Diarrhea**

Diarrhea turns from nonbloody to bloody within 5 days of onset
Abdominal pain and tenderness
Pain worse with defecation, especially with *Escherichia coli* O157:H7
Rectal prolapse: shigellosis and *E. coli* O157:H7
Absence of fever at time of initial evaluation: *E. coli* O157:H7
High fever (>39°C): shigellosis
Minimal vomiting
Greater than five stools 24 hours before evaluation
Contacts with bloody diarrhea or a culture-confirmed pathogen
Recent antibiotic usage

Adapted from Holtz LR, Neill MA, Tarr PI. Acute bloody diarrhea: a medical emergency for patients of all ages. Gastroenterology 2009;136(6):1887-98.

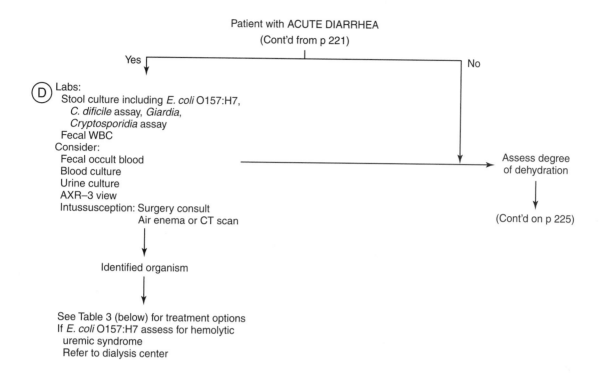

Patient with ACUTE DIARRHEA

(Cont'd from p 221)

Yes

(D) Labs:
- Stool culture including *E. coli* O157:H7, *C. dificile* assay, *Giardia*, *Cryptosporidia* assay
- Fecal WBC

Consider:
- Fecal occult blood
- Blood culture
- Urine culture
- AXR–3 view
- Intussusception: Surgery consult; Air enema or CT scan

→ Identified organism

→ See Table 3 (below) for treatment options

If *E. coli* O157:H7 assess for hemolytic uremic syndrome

Refer to dialysis center

No → Assess degree of dehydration

(Cont'd on p 225)

Table 3. **Treatment**

Infectious Agent	Treatment in Children
Clostridium difficile	Metronidazole, 7.5 mg/kg (maximum, 500 mg) tid; or Vancomycin, 10 mg/kg (maximum, 125 mg) qid for 10–14 days
Shigella	Azithromycin, 10 mg/kg/day once a day for 3 days; or Ceftriaxone, 50 mg/kg/day once a day for 3 days
Nontyphoid salmonellosis	None; or Ceftriaxone, 100 mg/kg/day divided bid for 7–10 days; or Azithromycin, 20 mg/kg/day once a day for 7 days
Salmonella typhi	Ceftriaxone, 100 mg/kg/day divided bid; or Azithromycin, 20 mg/kg/day once a day for 7 days
Campylobacter jejuni	None; or Azithromycin, 10 mg/kg/day once a day for 3–5 days; or Erythromycin, 30 mg/kg/day divided bid to qid for 3–5 days
Aeromonas	Treat as *Shigella*
Vibrio cholerae	Erythromycin, 30 mg/kg/day divided tid for 3 days; or Azithromycin, 10 mg/kg/day once a day for 3 days
Noncholeraic vibrios	None or treat as *Shigella*
Enterotoxigenic *E. coli*, enteroaggregative *E. coli*, or traveler's diarrhea	Azithromycin, 10 mg/kg/day once a day for 3 days; or Ceftriaxone, 50 mg/kg/day once a day for 3 days
E. coli O157:H7 and other *Shiga* toxin–producing *E. coli*	None
Enteroinvasive *E. coli*	Treat as *Shigella*
Giardia	Metronidazole, 15 mg/kg/day divided tid for 5–7 days; or Tinidazole, 50 mg/kg PO once (maximum: 2 g); or Nitazoxanide: 1–3 yr: 100 mg every 12 hours for 3 days 4–11 yr: 200 mg every 12 hours for 3 days >12 yr: 500 mg every 12 hours for 3 days
Cryptosporidium	Nitazoxanide: 1–3 yr: 100 mg bid for 3 days 4–11 yr: 200 mg bid for 3 days >12 yr: 500 mg every 12 hour for 3 days

Adapted from DuPont HL. Clinical practice. Bacterial diarrhea. N Engl J Med 2009;361(16):1560-9; and Pickering LK, editor. The Redbook: Report of the Committee on Infectious Diseases. 28th ed. American Academy of Pediatrics. <http://aapredbook.aappublications.org>; 2011.

E. For children with minimal or no dehydration, ORS should be used (see Table 4). A solution with glucose and electrolyte content similar to the World Health Organization formulation should be chosen. If diapers can be weighed, give 1 ml fluid per gram output. Otherwise, give 10 ml additional fluid per kilogram body weight for each watery stool and 2 ml/kg body weight for each episode of emesis. For simplicity, children less than 10 kg can be given 60 to 120 ml ORS for each episode of vomiting or diarrhea, and those greater than 10 kg given 120 to 240 ml. Nutrition need not be restricted.

F. For children with mild-to-moderate dehydration, give 50 to 100 ml ORS per kilogram body weight over 2 to 4 hours to replace the estimated fluid deficit (see Table 4). If losses are ongoing, additional ORS will also need to be given. This can be given in limited volumes using a teaspoon, syringe, or medicine dropper at first, increasing the amount as tolerated. For those refusing oral feeding, with continued vomiting, or oral ulcerations, nasogastric ORS feeding is an acceptable alternative. Rapid nasogastric rehydration has the benefits of being more cost-effective, is associated with fewer complications, has improved parental satisfaction, and often is well tolerated. To determine whether children in this category will respond to oral rehydration, observe them until dehydration signs subside. Also, those with unusually high output merit observation with regular assessment of hydration status. If attempts at correcting dehydration enterally have failed, intravenous fluid administration is indicated. Considerations for laboratory work include a stool culture in the case of bloody diarrhea, severe diarrhea (>5 per 24 hours), immunocompromised state, age younger than 6 months, or exposure to bloody or known bacterial diarrhea, and a CBC, and urine and blood culture when urinary tract infection and sepsis are of concern. Home management can be implemented once dehydration is corrected and after capable caregivers have been informed of potential complications, with a plan for close follow-up.

G. Severe dehydration constitutes a medical emergency and requires rapid intervention with isotonic intravenous fluids. Normal saline (NS) or lactated Ringer solution is given repeatedly, 20 ml/kg, with frequent assessment of hydration status until pulse, blood pressure, and mental status return to normal. Smaller volumes (5–10 ml/kg) should be used in those with impaired cardiac status, including malnourished infants. Obtain serum electrolytes, bicarbonate, blood urea nitrogen (BUN), creatinine (Cr), and serum glucose levels, as well as other labs clinically indicated (consider CBC, blood and urine culture, and stool culture). Lack of response to intravenous fluid resuscitation suggests other diagnoses including septic shock, metabolic disorders, cardiogenic shock, or a neurologic insult. NS and lactated Ringer solution are appropriate for initial management of both hyponatremic and hypernatremic dehydration. Once the patient stabilizes and dehydration has been improved to the point of normal cognition, ORS should be instituted and used to further correct for losses.

H. Consideration for admission should be made in the following circumstances:

1. Inadequate ability to care for child at home and/or inability to return if necessary
2. Intractable vomiting
3. Inadequate ORS intake because of refusal or inability to take (i.e., vomiting)
4. Lack of improvement despite adequate intake of ORS
5. Concern for complicating comorbid illnesses
6. Severe dehydration (>9% of body weight)
7. Young age, unusual irritability or drowsiness, progressive course of symptoms, or uncertainty of diagnosis
8. Other risk factors for worse outcome that should also be considered include prematurity, young maternal age, black race, and rural residence

I. Management of hospitalized patients with moderate or severe dehydration requires the correction of fluid deficit and electrolyte abnormalities. Rehydration during the 24-hour period is accomplished in three phases: circulatory stabilization (1–2 hours), deficit replacement (next 8 hours), and maintenance replacement (16 hours). After the patient has been stabilized, administer fluids to replace the deficit during 8 hours without providing maintenance fluid. During the following 16 hours of maintenance replacement, administer the amount of maintenance fluid needed for 24 hours for patients with isotonic or hypotonic dehydration. For patients with hypernatremic (sodium >150 mmol/L) dehydration, oral/nasogastric rehydration is safest. If intravenous fluids must be used, correction of the deficit should be done carefully to avoid complications of cerebral edema and convulsions. Replace the calculated fluid deficit over 8 hours with 0.45% normal saline with 5% dextrose, while carefully monitoring the plasma sodium level until normal.

Table 4. **Composition of Some Commercially Available Oral Rehydration Solutions**

	Carbohydrate (g/L)	Sodium (mmol/L)	Potassium (mmol/L)	Chloride (mmol/L)	Base (mmol/L)	Osmolarity (mOsm/L)
World Health Organization (2002)	13.5	75	20	65	30	245
Enfalyte	30	50	25	45	34	200
Pedialyte	25	45	20	35	30	250
Rehydralyte	25	75	20	65	30	305
CeraLyte	40	50–90	20	NA	30	220

NA, not applicable.

From King CK, Glass R, Bresee JS, Duggan C; Centers for Disease Control and Prevention. Managing acute gastroenteritis among children: oral rehydration, maintenance, and nutritional therapy. MMWR Recomm Rep 2003;52(RR-16):1–16.

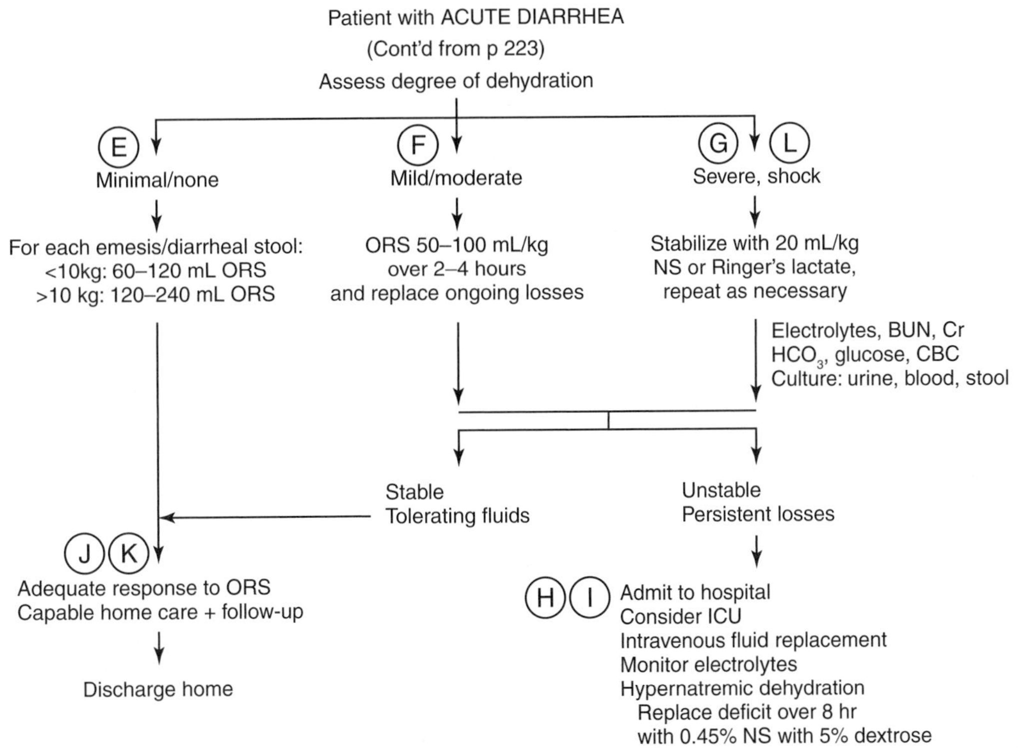
Patient with ACUTE DIARRHEA
(Cont'd from p 223)
Assess degree of dehydration
E
Minimal/none
For each emesis/diarrheal stool:
<10kg: 60–120 mL ORS
>10 kg: 120–240 mL ORS
F
Mild/moderate
ORS 50–100 mL/kg
over 2–4 hours
and replace ongoing losses
G
L
Severe, shock
Stabilize with 20 mL/kg
NS or Ringer's lactate,
repeat as necessary
Electrolytes, BUN, Cr
HCO3, glucose, CBC
Culture: urine, blood, stool
Stable
Tolerating fluids
Unstable
Persistent losses
J
K
Adequate response to ORS
Capable home care + follow-up
Discharge home
H
I
Admit to hospital
Consider ICU
Intravenous fluid replacement
Monitor electrolytes
Hypernatremic dehydration
Replace deficit over 8 hr
with 0.45% NS with 5% dextrose

J. Nutritional guidelines include avoiding foods with high amounts of simple sugars because of osmotic effects, including carbonated soft drinks, juice, and gelatin desserts. Early feeding helps with infection-induced intestinal permeability, reduces duration of illness, and improves nutritional outcomes. Highly specific diets such as the BRAT (bananas, rice, applesauce, and toast) diet are overly restrictive and can adversely effect nutritional recovery and gut healing. Instead, institute age-appropriate unrestricted diets, including complex carbohydrates, meats, yogurt, fruits, and vegetables.

K. Medical Therapy: Antidiarrheal agents, though commonly used, have only limited data supporting efficacy. Serious adverse effects include abdominal distension and bacterial overgrowth, and their use is generally not recommended. Zinc may be beneficial because numerous studies have shown the benefit of zinc supplementation in both treating and preventing diarrheal disease. A meta-analysis of probiotic use in children with acute diarrhea by Huang et al. showed a 1-day shortened duration, supporting their use in this setting. The majority of cases of bacterial diarrhea will not require antibiotic therapy, and empiric therapy while awaiting stool cultures is generally not recommended. Bacteria that should be treated are *Shigella,* enterotoxigenic and enteroinvasive *E. coli, Salmonella typhi,* and *Vibrio cholerae* (Table 3). Antibiotic use in uncomplicated nontyphoid *Salmonella* infection is contraindicated because it may prolong the carrier state. Decision on treatment of other bacteria depends on clinical factors including young infants (<3 months), immunocompromised state, and comorbid medical conditions.

L. Oral rehydration should be used with caution or avoided in cases of hemodynamic shock, abdominal ileus, concern for obstruction including intussusception, high-output diarrhea (>10 ml/kg/hr), and infants with evidence of carbohydrate malabsorption (diarrhea improves when not fed).

References

Albano F, Lo Vecchio A, Guarino A. The applicability and efficacy of guidelines for the management of acute gastroenteritis in outpatient children: a field-randomized trial on primary care pediatricians. J Pediatr 2010;156:226–30.

Ashkenazi S, Dinari G, Zevulunov A, Nitzan M. Convulsions in childhood shigellosis. Clinical and laboratory features in 153 children. Am J Dis Child 1987;141(2):208–10.

Bhupinder S, Devadason D. Management of diarrhea. In: Wylie R, Hyams JS, Kay M, editors. Pediatric gastrointestinal and liver disease. Cleveland, OH: Elsevier; 2006.

Centers for Disease Control and Prevention. Reduction in rotavirus after vaccine introduction—United States, 2000–2009. MMWR Morb Mortal Wkly Rep 2009;58(41):1146–9.

DuPont HL. Clinical practice. Bacterial diarrhea. N Engl J Med 2009;361(16):1560–9.

Guandalini S, Kahn SA: Acute diarrhea. In: Kleinman R, Goulet OJ, Mieli-Vergani G, Sanderson I, Sherman P, Shneider B, editors. Walker's pediatric gastrointestinal disease. 5th ed. Ontario, Canada: BC Decker; 2008.

Harris C, Wilkinson F, Mazza D, Turner T; Health for Kids Guideline Development Group. Evidence based guideline for the management of diarrhea with or without vomiting in children. Aust Fam Physician 2008;37(6 Spec No):22–9.

Holtz LR, Neill MA, Tarr PI. Acute bloody diarrhea: a medical emergency for patients of all ages. Gastroenterology 2009;136(6):1887–98.

Huang JS, Bousvaros A, Lee JW, et al. Efficacy of probiotic use in acute diarrhea in children: a meta-analysis. Dig Dis Sci 2002;47(11):2625–34.

King CK, Glass R, Bresee JS, Duggan C; Centers for Disease Control and Prevention. Managing acute gastroenteritis among children: oral rehydration, maintenance, and nutritional therapy. MMWR Recomm Rep 2003;52(RR-16):1–16.

McFarland LV. Renewed interest in a difficult disease: Clostridium difficile infections—epidemiology and current treatment strategies. Curr Opin Gastroenterol 2009;25(1):24–35.

Nager AL, Wang VJ. Comparison of nasogastric and intravenous methods of rehydration in pediatric patients with acute dehydration. Pediatrics 2002;109:566–72.

Shiau YF, Feldman GM, Resnick MA, Coff PM. Stool electrolyte and osmolality measurements in the evaluation of diarrheal disorders. Ann Intern Med 1985;102(6):773–5.

Persistent Diarrhea

Jason Soden, MD

Persistent diarrhea (PD) is defined as diarrhea lasting longer than 2 weeks. Persistent diarrhea is an important source of worldwide morbidity and mortality in infants and children, accounting for up to 2.2 million childhood deaths worldwide. In the developing world, where the burden of infectious diarrhea is most common, the spectrum of chronic diarrhea may represent consecutive acute infectious illnesses, persistent infections in human immunodeficiency virus/acquired immune deficiency syndrome (HIV/AIDS), or persistent malabsorption exacerbated by malnutrition or micronutrient deficiencies. In North America, persistent diarrhea is less likely to result from identifiable infectious agents.

In the evaluation of infants and children with diarrhea, consider causative factors of osmotic diarrhea (carbohydrate malabsorption), maldigestive diarrhea (pancreatic insufficiency), secretory diarrhea (infections, hormone-secreting tumors), motility disturbances, mucosal inflammatory conditions (allergy, celiac disease, inflammatory bowel disease), and structural abnormalities. In particular, special consideration should be made to the neonate with early-onset, persistent diarrhea. This population of neonates should be evaluated for rare, congenital structural, inflammatory, or transport defects of the enterocyte.

A. The first step in evaluating the clinical complaint of persistent diarrhea is to qualify the patient or caregivers' definition of diarrhea. Various changes in stool frequency or consistency, for instance, from breast-fed to formula-fed infants, may cause concern by a caregiver in nonpathologic settings. In practice, diarrhea is defined as increased stool frequency and decreased consistency (watery or loose). Objectively, stool volume >10 ml/kg (infant) or 200 ml/m^2 is abnormal.

B. The history should focus on relevant questions related to either a recent (or prolonged) infectious process, relevant medical/surgical history, recent medications (including antibiotics), diet history, travel history, and family history. Relevant descriptive features should be obtained, including time of onset, dietary patterns (including carbohydrate intake such as lactose or juice), relieving factors (including fasting/NPO), blood or mucus in the stool, concurrent abdominal pain, cramping, or tenesmus. Baseline stool patterns should be assessed, with specific questions of constipation and encopresis if relevant. Constitutional complaints including weight loss, fevers, oral ulcers, and perianal complaints should be addressed.

C. The most important aspects in the physical examination include nutritional status (weight and height percentiles), hydration, and general appearance. Abdominal examination should assess for peritoneal signs (perforation or abscess), distension, mass (including retained feces), and localized tenderness. Careful examination of the oral mucosa (aphthous ulcers) and perianal inspection (tags, fistulae) are relevant if Crohn disease is suspected. Digital rectal examination should be performed to evaluate for an anorectal anomaly, distal obstruction, or fecal impaction. Additional clues of systemic disease such as clubbing (cystic fibrosis [CF], inflammatory bowel disease, liver disease), bruising (fat-soluble vitamin deficiency), and rash (allergy or micronutrient deficiency) should be considered during the examination.

D. If available, examination of a stool sample in the office can help to validate the complaint and direct the diagnostic approach. If collected, watery (fresh) stool can be evaluated for reducing substances and stool pH (carbohydrate malabsorption). Hemoccult testing should be performed to evaluate for occult blood or confirm suspected visible blood. Microscopic evaluation of a water or saline stool prep may detect fecal leukocytes and (with or without a Sudan red stain) can visualize neutral (maldigested) fat, a sign of maldigestion (pancreatic insufficiency, including CF). Microscopic fat visualized after acid hydrolysis of the stool (split fat) suggests malabsorption (celiac disease or other disturbances of absorptive surface).

E. Stool laboratory examination should be performed. If office examination is not performed, laboratory assessment for fecal fat (spot check), occult blood, leukocytes, and, if indicated, reducing substances and stool pH may be performed on a watery, fresh sample. Although infectious sources are not frequently identified in persistent diarrhea, these should be considered and excluded. Routine evaluations for bacterial pathogens, relevant parasites (in North America, commonly *Giardia* and cryptosporidia), and *C. difficile* toxin should be considered. Although rotavirus rarely persists beyond 10 days, other viral pathogens (including adenovirus) may persist, and specific viral examinations (including culture or electron microscopic examination) may be considered. In certain settings (travel, developing countries, or immunocompromised patients), evaluation for other parasitic or viral pathogens should be performed.

F. Other laboratory examinations, when indicated, include complete blood cell count with differential, inflammatory markers, and electrolytes. To screen for celiac disease, consider measurement of IgA antibody to human recombinant tissue transglutaminase (TTG) early in the setting of persistent diarrhea and failure to thrive. Urine culture should be obtained if urinary tract infection is suspected, especially in an infant with diarrhea.

G. If possible, distinguish noninfectious causes of diarrhea as osmotic, secretory, or mixed. Osmotic diarrhea is more common, typically resolves when a patient is not fed (NPO), and typically results from excessive intake

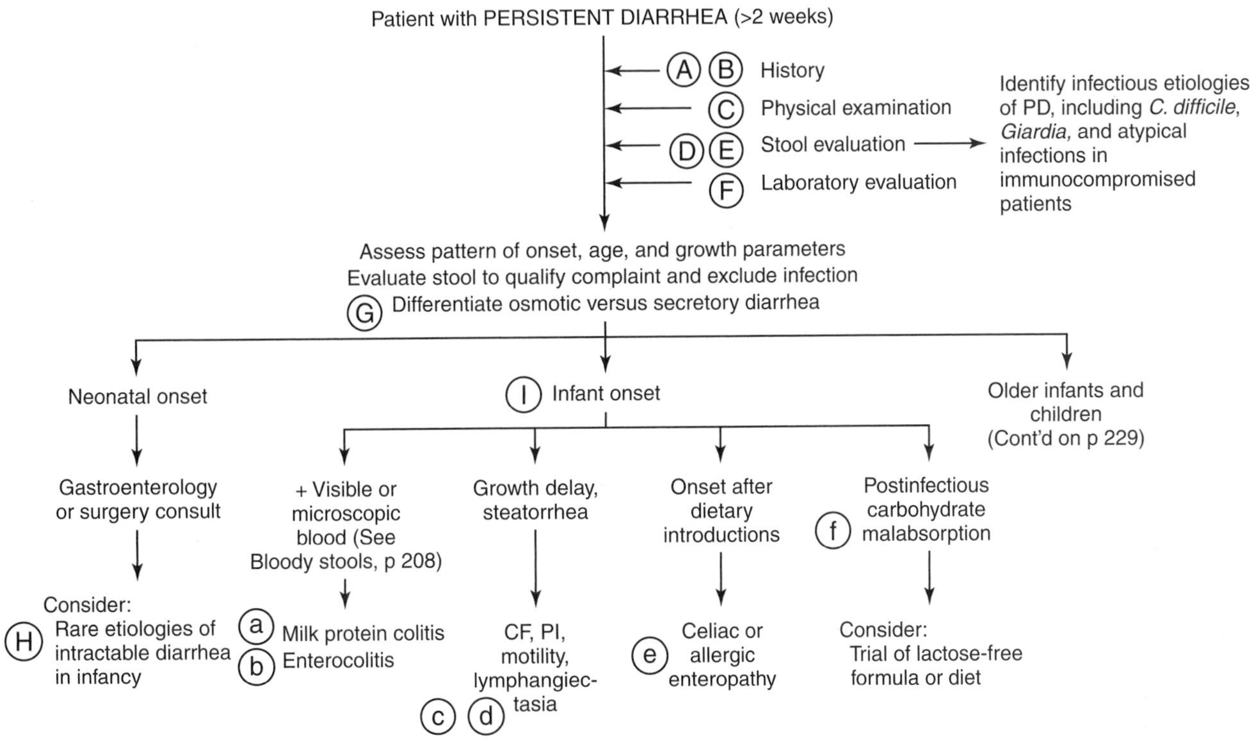

Patient with PERSISTENT DIARRHEA (>2 weeks)
A B History
C Physical examination
D E Stool evaluation
F Laboratory evaluation
Identify infectious etiologies of PD, including C. difficile, Giardia, and atypical infections in immunocompromised patients
Assess pattern of onset, age, and growth parameters
Evaluate stool to qualify complaint and exclude infection
G Differentiate osmotic versus secretory diarrhea
Neonatal onset
I Infant onset
Older infants and children (Cont'd on p 229)
Gastroenterology or surgery consult
H Consider: Rare etiologies of intractable diarrhea in infancy
+ Visible or microscopic blood (See Bloody stools, p 208)
a Milk protein colitis
b Enterocolitis
Growth delay, steatorrhea
CF, PI, motility, lymphangiectasia
c d
Onset after dietary introductions
e Celiac or allergic enteropathy
f Postinfectious carbohydrate malabsorption
Consider: Trial of lactose-free formula or diet

(carbohydrate), mucosal injury, or inherited (disaccharidase) deficiencies. Secretory diarrhea continues when the patient is not fed; causative factors include hormone-secreting tumors and rare, chronic enteropathies. Analysis of stool osmolality, anion gap, pH, and sodium can help in this differentiation.

H. The neonate with early-onset, persistent diarrhea should be evaluated for a subset of rare disorders that cause intractable (secretory) diarrhea in infancy. These include structural enterocyte disorders (microvillous inclusion disease), transport disorders (congenital chloride diarrhea), and congenital disaccharidase (lactase) deficiencies. Consultation with a gastroenterologist is beneficial in this setting.

I. In infants, common causes of persistent diarrhea include milk protein intolerance ("allergic colitis"), postinfectious carbohydrate malabsorption, CF, Hirschsprung disease, among others.

a. The onset of milk protein intolerance is typically around 2 months. Infants may present with visible bloody or mucoid, or Hemoccult-positive stools. Diagnostic and management strategies are typically conservative. Observation with no dietary change in a well-appearing, thriving infant without anemia is reasonable. Maternal dietary elimination of milk and soy in the breast-fed infant may be beneficial in some cases. Initiation of a protein hydrolysate formula or, in refractory cases, amino acid–based formulas are often beneficial. Expect 2 to 3 weeks to see improvement after a dietary intervention.

b. Enterocolitis may occur in the postneonatal period in infants with Hirschsprung disease, necrotizing enterocolitis/pneumatosis, or other potentially surgical diagnoses.

c. If maldigested (neutral) fat is visible in the stool, or if growth failure or other sequelae of CF or pancreatic insufficiency are found, consider a sweat test or pancreatic fecal elastase.

d. Fat malabsorption may also occur in structural or motility disorders (with or without small-bowel bacterial overgrowth) and protein-losing enteropathy states (including primary intestinal lymphangiectasia).

e. Persistent diarrhea that occurs later in infancy, after introduction of solids, should raise consideration for mucosal injury. More common conditions include allergy (with secondary enteropathy and malabsorption) and celiac disease. Dietary history, physical examination (eczema), stool examination for hydrolyzed fat, together with screening laboratory evaluations for IgE-mediated allergies, celiac disease, or allergy consultation should be considered.

f. In the setting of persistent diarrhea after an acute, diarrheal illness, consider changing to a lactose-free formula for a limited time to treat presumed postinfectious carbohydrate malabsorption.

J. In older infants or children with persistent diarrhea and no evidence of growth failure or systemic symptoms, consider several conditions.

a. Constipation with encopresis may present as "diarrhea" because of patient/parent complaint of abnormal stool frequency and consistency. Details of stooling history should be gathered in the history, and physical examination should include assessment for abdominal fecal mass, perianal inspection for soiling (common in encopresis), and digital rectal examination to assess for rectal fecal impaction.

b. Both infant overfeeding (>200 ml/kg/day) and chronic nonspecific diarrhea (toddler's diarrhea) may present with chronic diarrhea. Stools in toddler's diarrhea vary in consistency and frequency, and are often described in association with rapid transit (including undigested solids). Therapy should be aimed at reassurance and limitation of dietary juice intake.

c. Carbohydrate malabsorption may occur resulting in diarrhea and other symptoms (cramping, flatulence) that are most obvious after ingestion of the offending dietary carbohydrate. In the setting of a recent infectious gastroenteritis, postinfectious carbohydrate malabsorption may persist for several weeks. Older children may present with adult-type hypolactasia (primary lactose intolerance), which is more common in African American, Asian, and Latino populations. Congenital sucrase-isomaltase deficiency (CSID) may present with symptoms once dietary sucrose (including juices) have been introduced. Carbohydrate malabsorptive conditions may be suspected by history and confirmed by either hydrogen breath testing or disaccharidase activity measurement from duodenal biopsies. Treatment is aimed at dietary modification.

d. Irritable bowel syndrome may present with diarrhea predominant symptoms and in the absence of other underlying structural or metabolic abnormalities.

e. Antibiotic-associated diarrhea or other medication adverse effects should be considered.

f. Factitious diarrhea caused by laxative use (Münchausen syndrome) or poisoning (Münchausen by proxy) should be considered.

K. There is a broad differential diagnosis for older infants and children with chronic (noninfectious) diarrhea and growth failure or constitutional/systemic complaints. By assessing history, physical, and stool characteristics, one can direct the appropriate evaluation. Laboratory evaluation should include assessment of electrolytes and, if indicated, micronutrient status (including zinc). Involvement of pediatric gastroenterology specialists may be of benefit to obtain small-intestinal or colonic biopsies.

a. Fat malabsorption, failure to thrive, and sinopulmonary infections warrant evaluation for CF. Pancreatic insufficiency with fat malabsorption in other syndromes (e.g., Shwachman–Diamond) may be confirmed with fecal elastase.

b. Hypoalbuminemia and/or presence of fecal protein malabsorption raise concern for a protein-losing enteropathy, including lymphangiectasia.

c. Celiac disease should be considered if persistent diarrhea with FTT exists, or diarrhea and gastrointestinal (GI) symptoms in at-risk populations (dermatitis herpetiformis, dental enamel defects, type 1 diabetes, IgA deficiency, Down syndrome, Turner syndrome, Williams syndrome, and first-degree relatives of patients with celiac disease). Serologic evaluations should include antibody testing for celiac disease. The current standard evaluation is TTG IgA antibody, as well as a total serum IgA level (to screen for IgA deficiency, which would lead to a false-negative TTG). Serologic evaluations should be confirmed with duodenal biopsy.

d. Chronic diarrhea with blood, urgency, abdominal pain, growth failure, or other constitutional symptoms should raise concern for inflammatory bowel disease. Laboratory evaluations should include complete blood cell count and inflammatory markers. Upper GI with small-bowel follow-through or other small-bowel imaging studies may offer a clue toward small-bowel inflammatory changes, but endoscopy and colonoscopy with ileoscopy should be performed.

e. Several immunodeficiency syndromes may present with chronic diarrhea (with or without infectious organisms identified) and growth failure.

f. The distinction of a chronic, secretory diarrhea outside of the newborn period warrants evaluation for rare, hormone-secreting tumors. VIPomas (vasoactive intestinal polypeptide–secreting tumor) classically present with watery diarrhea, hypokalemia, and metabolic alkalosis.

g. Micronutrient deficiencies and starvation states may lead to secondary diarrhea, contributing to a vicious cycle of diarrhea and malnutrition. Zinc deficiency, specifically, may be accompanied by a characteristic rash (acrodermatitis enteropathica) and may occur as a primary or secondary disorder.

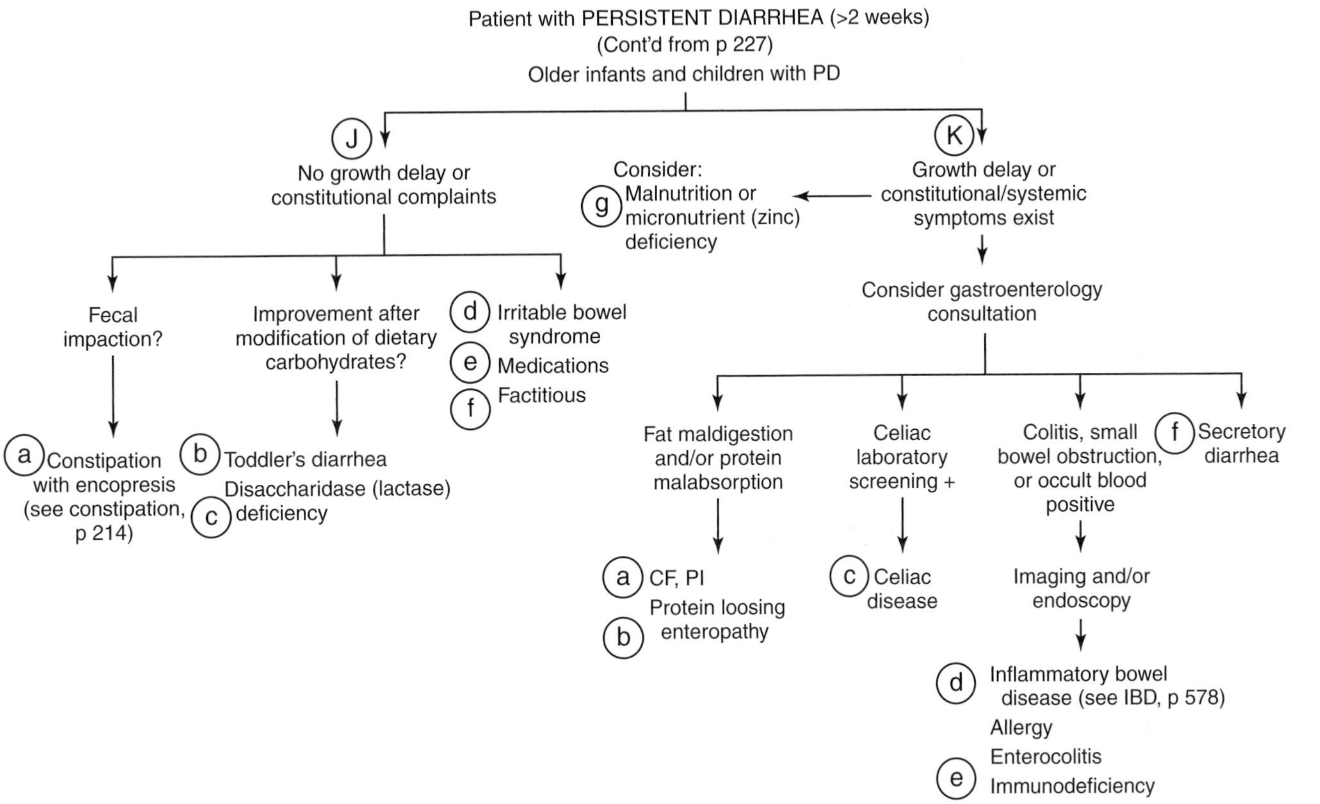

Patient with PERSISTENT DIARRHEA (>2 weeks)
(Cont'd from p 227)
Older infants and children with PD
J
No growth delay or constitutional complaints
K
Growth delay or constitutional/systemic symptoms exist
Consider:
g Malnutrition or micronutrient (zinc) deficiency
Fecal impaction?
Improvement after modification of dietary carbohydrates?
d Irritable bowel syndrome
e Medications
f Factitious
a Constipation with encopresis (see constipation, p 214)
b Toddler's diarrhea
c Disaccharidase (lactase) deficiency
Consider gastroenterology consultation
Fat maldigestion and/or protein malabsorption
Celiac laboratory screening +
Colitis, small bowel obstruction, or occult blood positive
f Secretory diarrhea
a CF, PI
b Protein loosing enteropathy
c Celiac disease
Imaging and/or endoscopy
d Inflammatory bowel disease (see IBD, p 578)
Allergy
e Enterocolitis
Immunodeficiency

References

Hill I, Dirks M, Liptak G, et al. Guideline for the diagnosis and treatment of Celiac disease in children: recommendations of the North American Society for Pediatric Gastroenterology, Hepatology, and Nutrition. J Pediatr Gastroenterol Nutr 2005;40:1–19.

Keating J. Chronic diarrhea. Pediatr Rev 2005;26:5–14.

Kneepkens CM, Meijer Y. Clinical practice: diagnosis and treatment of cow's milk allergy. Eur J Pediatr 2009;168:891–6.

Sondheimer JM. Office stool examination: a practical guide. Contemp Pediatr 1994; Supplement to Residents:5–14.

Vernacchio L, Vezina RM, Mitchell AA, et al. Characteristics of persistent diarrhea in a community-based cohort of young US children. J Pediatr Gastroenterol Nutr 2006;43:52–8.

Upper Gastrointestinal Bleeding

Robert E. Kramer, MD

Upper gastrointestinal (GI) hemorrhage is typically defined as a source of bleeding originating proximal to the ligament of Treitz. It may present with hematemesis, coffee-ground emesis, melena, occult heme-positive stools, or in the case of massive bleeding, hematochezia. The spectrum of potential causative factors resulting in upper GI hemorrhage in children is vast, ranging from mild, self-limited conditions to severe, life-threatening ones. The most likely causative factors vary significantly by age of the child (see Table 1). The clinical approach to the child with bleeding must be measured and methodical. Upper intestinal endoscopy is an important tool in the diagnosis and treatment of upper GI bleeding but may not always be necessary and rarely will be the initial step in management. Instead, initial steps should focus on careful assessment of hemodynamic status, stabilization, and supportive care.

A. Hemodynamic Status: The first step in the assessment of a child with upper GI hemorrhage is to determine whether they are hemodynamically stable. Accurate assessment of heart rate, blood pressure, and mental status are critical. Children have an impressive ability to maintain blood pressure until the late stages of shock; therefore, elevated heart rate may be the first clinical indicator of hemodynamic compromise. Orthostatic changes in the supine and upright positions should be assessed as well, with a decrease of 10 mm Hg in blood pressure or an increase of 20 beats/min in heart rate being defined as clinically significant. Evidence of instability should direct care toward providing acute stabilization, applying the principles of the ABCs of resuscitation (airway, breathing, circulation). This initial stabilization would typically take place in the emergency department, with transfer to an intensive care unit setting as soon as it is feasible. Good intravenous (IV) access is vital, and a central line or two large-bore peripheral IVs should be in place, followed by crystalloid boluses of at least 20 ml/kg for resuscitation. At least 2 units of packed red blood cells (RBCs) should be typed, crossmatched, and available at all times. An empiric dose of vitamin K should be strongly considered to optimize coagulation.

B. History and Physical Examination: In the stable patient, or the unstable patient after supportive care has been established, the history and physical examination provide the cornerstone for developing a differential diagnosis for the bleeding. Key elements in the history include the onset of bleeding (acute vs. chronic), the character of the blood (hematemesis, coffee-grounds, melena), the amount of blood observed, and associated symptoms (nausea/vomiting, epigastric pain, arthralgias, weight loss, dysphagia/odynophagia, skin rashes, diarrhea, epistaxis). Recurrent, forceful emesis without blood before the onset of hematemesis implies that a Mallory–Weiss tear of the esophagus may be responsible. Inquire about possible foreign body or caustic ingestions, as well as ingestion of red dyes or other substances that may be mistaken for blood (see section D). In breast-feeding infants, be alert to the possibility of swallowed maternal blood from cracked, bleeding nipples. It is important that review of the medical history include any personal or family history of liver disease, medication use (especially nonsteroidal anti-inflammatory drugs), history of prematurity (with umbilical venous catheter placement), and potential causes of nasopharyngeal bleeding, which may mimic GI hemorrhage.

Physical examination should, therefore, begin with a careful assessment of the nasopharynx, looking for evidence of a bleeding source in the nose or mouth. Abdominal examination should focus on any areas of tenderness, as well as the presence of hepatosplenomegaly or ascites, indicative of portal hypertension. Other findings associated with portal hypertension include spider angiomas, jaundice, and caput medusae. Skin examination should assess for petechiae or purpura, which might suggest a coagulation disorder or acute systemic illness, such as Henoch–Schönlein purpura. Cutaneous vascular lesions should also raise suspicion of a possible internal lesion within the GI tract as a cause of bleeding.

C. Laboratory Tests: The value of the complete blood cell count (CBC) is obvious in cases of GI bleeding, to help assess the severity of the illness, to establish a baseline at presentation, to evaluate the chronicity of bleeding, and to measure ongoing losses. In acute GI bleeding, however, the hematocrit may underestimate the true amount of bleeding because of the delay in hemodilution with rapid blood loss. Low mean corpuscular volume, consistent with a microcytic anemia, suggests chronic losses, systemic illness, or both. For hospitalized patients, serial hematocrits should be measured to determine the presence and severity of ongoing bleeding. The frequency of these hematocrits best is determined by the initial severity of the bleeding event and may range from every 6 to every 24 hours. A liver profile, including fractionated bilirubin and albumin, is helpful in assessing for occult chronic liver disease, which may present with acute variceal bleeding. Increased transaminases or direct bilirubin should then prompt further liver workup, as well as a Doppler ultrasound of the abdomen, looking for evidence of hepatosplenomegaly, varices, and ascites. Coagulation should be assessed with a prothrombin (PT) and partial thromboplastin time (PTT), and any coagulopathy should be corrected. Initial treatment with parenteral vitamin K should be given and then values reassessed. Blood urea nitrogen (BUN) and creatinine (Cr) provide a screen for underlying renal disease.

D. Assess for Fictitious Causes of Bleeding: A wide variety of substances other than blood may mimic GI bleeding. All emesis and stool suspected to contain blood should be

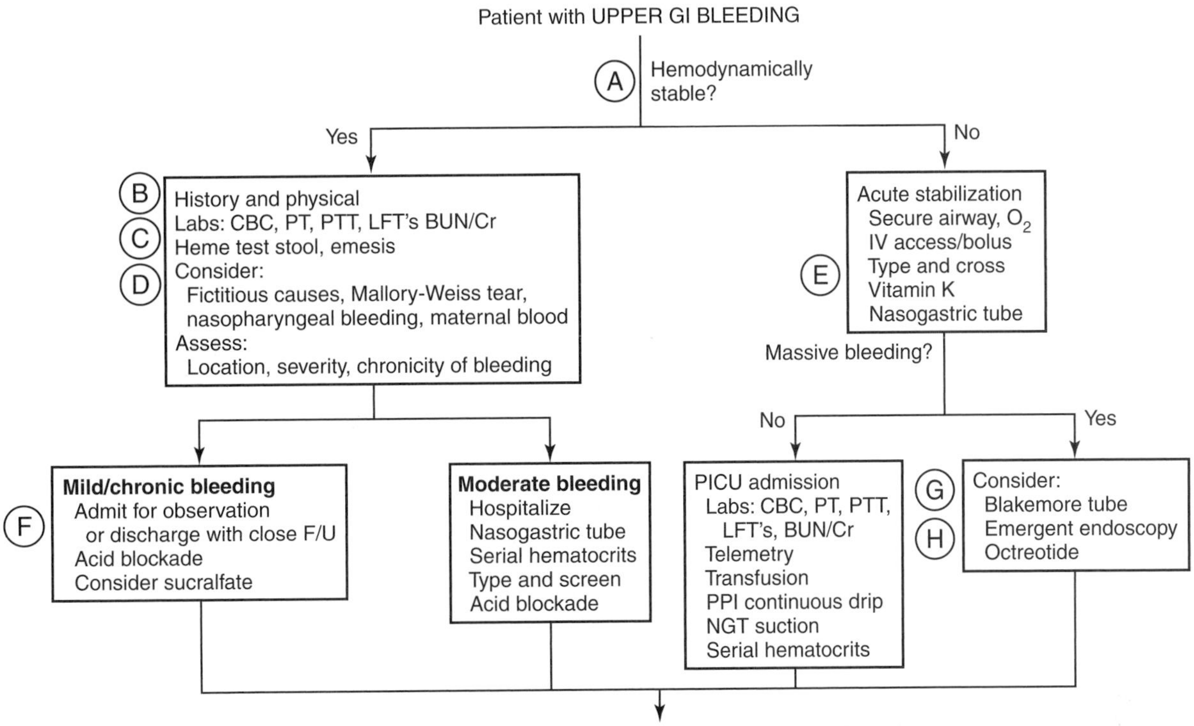
Patient with UPPER GI BLEEDING
A
Hemodynamically stable?
Yes
No
B
C
D
History and physical
Labs: CBC, PT, PTT, LFT's BUN/Cr
Heme test stool, emesis
Consider:
Fictitious causes, Mallory-Weiss tear, nasopharyngeal bleeding, maternal blood
Assess:
Location, severity, chronicity of bleeding
E
Acute stabilization
Secure airway, O2
IV access/bolus
Type and cross
Vitamin K
Nasogastric tube
Massive bleeding?
No
Yes
F
Mild/chronic bleeding
Admit for observation or discharge with close F/U
Acid blockade
Consider sucralfate
Moderate bleeding
Hospitalize
Nasogastric tube
Serial hematocrits
Type and screen
Acid blockade
PICU admission
Labs: CBC, PT, PTT, LFT's, BUN/Cr
Telemetry
Transfusion
PPI continuous drip
NGT suction
Serial hematocrits
G
H
Consider:
Blakemore tube
Emergent endoscopy
Octreotide
(Cont'd on p 233)

confirmed with Gastroccult or Hemoccult testing, regardless of how convincing they appear. Red blood may be simulated by food coloring, red candy, antibiotic syrups, beets, tomato skins, red gelatins, and juices. Dark stools from iron preparations, blueberries, spinach, grapes, licorice, or bismuth may be mistaken for melena. Swallowed maternal blood in the infant, either in the neonate as a consequence of vaginal delivery or in the older infant because of cracked or bleeding nipples, may result in hematemesis or coffee-ground emesis. The Apt–Downey test for fetal hemoglobin can be used to differentiate bleeding originating from the infant.

E. Nasogastric Tube: Placement of a nasogastric tube (NGT) and gastric lavage in the setting of upper GI bleeding has been somewhat of a controversial topic. Aspiration of frank blood from an NGT is diagnostic of upper GI bleeding and may be helpful for assessing ongoing losses through the course of treatment. Repeated lavage with room temperature normal saline may show clearing, suggestive of stabilization of bleeding. A negative aspirate, however, does not exclude upper GI bleeding, because blood may rapidly exit the stomach. From the therapeutic standpoint, there is no evidence that lavage is helpful in controlling bleeding and may, in fact, interfere with the development of clots at the bleeding site. Risk for exacerbating variceal bleeding is not a contraindication to placement to NGT placement.

F. Acid blockade: Many of the potential causes of upper GI bleeding in children are mucosal lesions, such as reflux esophagitis, reactive gastritis, duodenitis, nonsteroidal anti-inflammatory drug–induced injury, and stress ulcer that may resolve spontaneously. Protection from additional injury from acid exposure, however, may hasten healing and resolution of ongoing bleeding. Acid blockade may be achieved with a histamine-2 receptor antagonist or a proton-pump inhibitor (PPI) drug. Either class may be administered orally, intravenously by bolus, or with a continuous IV infusion. For mild or moderate cases, histamine-2 receptor antagonists are reasonable, but proton-pump inhibitors have demonstrated improved efficacy and are preferred for more severe cases. Adequacy of acid blockade can be assessed by measuring a trough pH of a gastric aspirate, with titration of dose to maintain the pH greater than 4.0.

G. Sengstaken–Blakemore Tube: Massive bleeding from the esophagus or fundus, typically as a result of variceal hemorrhage, may be stabilized by use of a Sengstaken–Blakemore tube. This device consists of an NGT with an inflatable balloon along the esophageal portion and an intragastric balloon at the tip, to be seated in the fundus. Pediatric sizes are available. A manometer is used to inflate the esophageal balloon to the desired pressure, and a defined volume of air is insufflated into the gastric portion. Traction is applied once the balloons are in place and used to provide direct pressure to tamponade bleeding lesions. If the site of bleeding is known to be solely esophageal or gastric, either balloon may be used independently. Pressure is maintained for a variable amount of time, not to exceed 24 hours.

H. Octreotide: Severe upper GI hemorrhage that has not responded to supportive measures may be treated with octreotide, a longer-acting analog of the GI inhibitory hormone somatostatin. Octreotide decreases portal pressure by reducing splanchnic blood flow. Typically it is bolused at a dose of 1 μg/kg, followed by a continuous drip at 1 to 4 μg/kg/hr. Blood sugars should be carefully monitored, because hyperglycemia and hypoglycemia are common adverse effects.

Table 1. **Causes of Upper Gastrointestinal Bleeding in Children**

Newborn	3 mo to 2 yr	>2 yr
Common		
Swallowed blood	Peptic	Peptic
Gastritis, esophagitis	Allergic	Mallory–Weiss
Ulcer	Mallory–Weiss	Nasopharyngeal
Vitamin K deficiency	Esophagitis	Varices
Uncommon		
Varices	Epistaxis	Salicylates
Coagulopathy	Varices	Thrombocytopenia
Vascular malformation	Vascular malformation	
Leiomyoma	Foreign body	

I. Upper Intestinal Endoscopy: Upper intestinal endoscopy/esophagogastroduodenoscopy is an important tool in the management of upper GI bleeding, offering the opportunity for both diagnostic and therapeutic benefit. Determining the optimal timing for endoscopy is critical to maximize this potential benefit. Except in cases of massive hemorrhage with little other therapeutic option, endoscopy is best reserved until the patient can be acutely stabilized, the airway secured, and rate of bleeding minimized as much as possible. This provides better visualization of the mucosal surface and a better chance that the site of bleeding can be properly identified and treated endoscopically. The endoscopist should be comfortable with the use of a wide variety of possible therapeutic maneuvers, including band ligation, sclerotherapy, injection therapy, clipping devices, and the various forms of electrocautery (monopolar, bipolar, argon plasma coagulation, etc). Proper supplies and equipment should be secured and set up before endoscopy.

J. Foreign Body: Foreign bodies rarely present with upper GI bleeding, even with ingestion of sharp, pointed objects. Typically, sharp objects such as straight pins, nails, and tacks proceed through the GI tract with the heavier, blunted end leading. In addition, the intestinal wall reflexively relaxes and withdraws away from sharp objects. The risk for bleeding is greatest for larger, irregularly shaped objects that are too large to pass through the narrower portions of the bowel, such as the lower esophageal sphincter, the pylorus, and possibly the duodenal sweep. Ingested button batteries, adherent to the mucosa, may result in severe GI bleeding and even death, either at the time of initial presentation or up to several weeks after removal. If a foreign body is identified at the time of endoscopy for upper GI bleeding, removal is obviously indicated. Objects imbedded in the mucosa, however, should be removed with care, because this may precipitate even greater amounts of bleeding. Alerting the surgical team of this potential and having them ready to intervene is prudent in these scenarios. Safe removal of large, sharp objects may be difficult without incurring greater mucosal damage on withdrawal of the endoscope. The use of hooding devices and overtubes should be used to minimize this risk.

K. Variceal Bleeding: Acute onset of severe upper GI bleeding is not an uncommon presentation in pediatric patients with both known and unknown portal hypertension or liver disease. As noted earlier, a careful history and physical examination, coupled with screening labs, may increase the level of suspicion for variceal hemorrhage as the cause of bleeding. Portal vein thrombosis, from either an umbilical venous catheter in the newborn period or an underlying coagulation disorder, may present years later with upper GI bleeding and no evidence of intrinsic liver disease. Esophageal varices may be treated endoscopically with either injection sclerotherapy or band ligation. Band ligation has become the favored approach in children old enough to pass the banding device, because of the relative technical ease of the procedure and decreased risk for ulceration and stricture of the esophagus. Persistent bleeding from gastric varices may require consideration of portosystemic shunts to reduce portal pressure.

L. Ulcer/Erosion: Ulcers, erosions, and other mucosal lesions are the most commonly identified sources of upper GI bleeding in children. Causative factors for mucosal inflammation include caustic, peptic, immune, allergic, and infectious causes. Treatment for these is largely pharmacologic, primarily focused on providing adequate acid blockade and, perhaps, adding a mucosal protective agent such as sucralfate. The endoscopic and/or histologic appearance, however, may suggest a causative factor that would require alternative medical therapy. Examples would include the characteristic nodular gastritis of *Helicobacter pylori* infection or ulcerations/lesions consistent with upper tract Crohn disease. Endoscopic therapy is generally reserved for discreet, actively bleeding lesions, such as an ulcer eroding into a visible vessel. Again, therapeutic options include injection of epinephrine, application of endoscopic clipping devices, or electrothermal coagulation of various types.

M. Unidentified Source of Bleeding: Even in the face of continued active bleeding, a normal-appearing mucosa at the time of endoscopy is not unusual. This implies that the bleeding has either resolved, is not coming from the upper GI tract, or is occurring intermittently via a lesion that is easily missed on endoscopy. Dieulafoy lesions, submucosal dilated arterioles, usually located in the upper portion of the stomach along the lesser curve, may present in this fashion, although they are a rare source of bleeding in children. Mallory–Weiss tears from forceful or repeated vomiting may also be easily missed in the distal esophagus if they are not actively bleeding at the time of endoscopy. Poor visualization of the mucosa, because of copious blood and clot formation, is another potential cause for unsuccessful identification of a bleeding source and underscores the importance of proper timing of endoscopy. Hemobilia and bleeding beyond the ligament of Treitz should also be considered when upper endoscopy yields no obvious source or site of bleeding. Further diagnostic studies to consider in these cases include angiography, tagged RBC scan, Meckel's scan, and capsule endoscopy, depending on the clinical context.

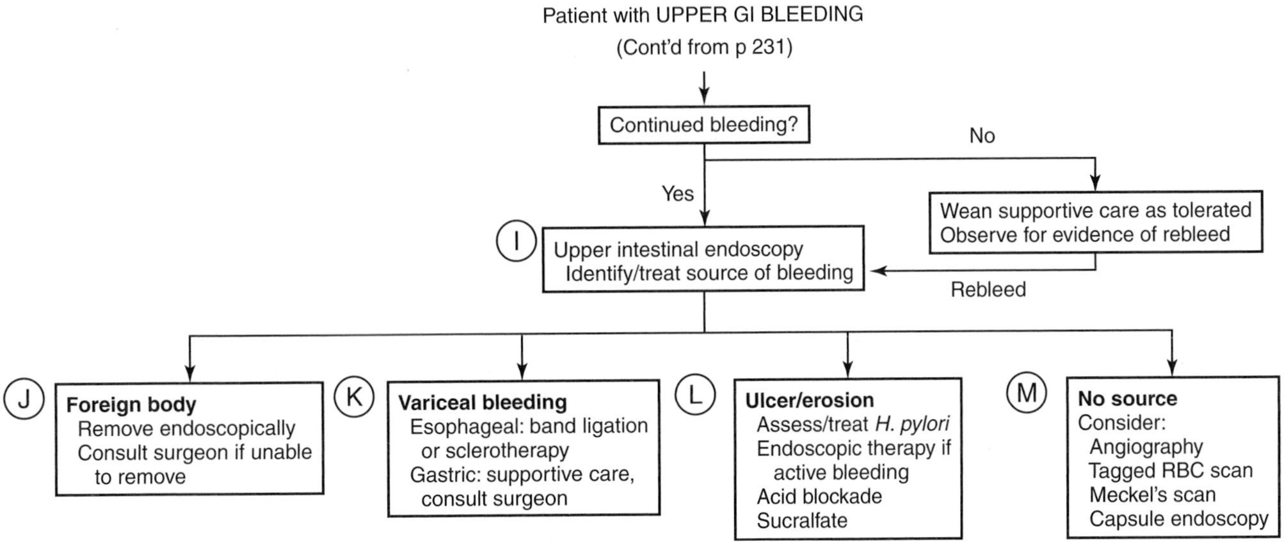

Patient with UPPER GI BLEEDING
(Cont'd from p 231)
Continued bleeding?
No
Yes
Wean supportive care as tolerated
Observe for evidence of rebleed
I
Upper intestinal endoscopy
Identify/treat source of bleeding
Rebleed
J
Foreign body
Remove endoscopically
Consult surgeon if unable to remove
K
Variceal bleeding
Esophageal: band ligation or sclerotherapy
Gastric: supportive care, consult surgeon
L
Ulcer/erosion
Assess/treat H. pylori
Endoscopic therapy if active bleeding
Acid blockade
Sucralfate
M
No source
Consider:
Angiography
Tagged RBC scan
Meckel's scan
Capsule endoscopy

References

Boyle JT. Gastrointestinal bleeding in infants and children. Pediatr Rev 2008;29(2):39–51.

Chawla S, Seth D, Mahajan P, Kamat D. Upper gastrointestinal bleeding in children. Clin Pediatr 2007;46(1):16–21.

Eisen GM, Dominitz JA, Faigel DO, et al. An annotated algorithmic approach to upper gastrointestinal bleeding. Gastrointest Endosc 2001;53(7):853–8.

Elevated Liver Tests after 6 Months of Age

Brandy Lu, MD, and Cara L. Mack, MD

A. In the patient's history, inquire about persistent or recurrent fevers; malaise/anorexia; emesis (bilious or bloody); jaundice or dark-colored urine; the stool color, frequency, consistency, presence of blood or mucous, and foul-smelling nature; abdominal pain; and pruritus. Document exposure to a hepatitis carrier, person with acute hepatitis, blood products, medications, or illicit drugs. Note whether the child attends a large child-care or residential facility, and whether there has been recent travel outside the United States. Identify hematologic abnormalities, such as hemolytic anemia, sickle cell disease, or thalassemia.

B. In the physical examination, note any right upper quadrant abdominal mass or tender hepatomegaly. Determine the firmness and size of the liver and the presence of splenomegaly. Signs of chronic liver disease include a firm and/or nodular liver, splenomegaly, ascites, cushingoid facies, digital clubbing, palmer erythema, asterixis, spider angiomata, caput medusae, and gynecomastia.

C. Abnormal liver tests include isolated increases in bilirubin only or variable increases in all liver tests. If the increased bilirubin is indirect in nature in the otherwise healthy-appearing child, the most likely cause is Gilbert syndrome. Gilbert syndrome is due to a partial deficiency of glucuronyl transferase and is benign. Isolated direct hyperbilirubinemia (with all other liver tests being normal) is rare in children and may be caused by Rotor or Dubin–Johnson syndromes.

Hepatitis is due to hepatocyte membrane disruption and is defined as two times the upper limit of normal of levels of the serum transaminases (alanine transaminase [ALT] and aspartate transaminase [AST]). If the AST is significantly more elevated than the ALT, consider nonhepatic sources of AST such as muscle (check creatine phosphokinase) or hemolysis (check lactate dehydrogenase, hematocrit). With extensive hepatocyte damage, serum albumin is depressed, the prothrombin time (PT)/international normalized ratio (INR) is prolonged, and the ammonia level may increase. Anemia associated with burr cells or severe thrombocytopenia suggests severe, chronic liver disease.

Pediatric acute liver failure is defined as: (1) children with no known evidence of chronic liver disease, (2) biochemical evidence of acute liver injury, and (3) hepatic-based coagulopathy defined as an INR of 1.5 or more not corrected by vitamin K in the presence of clinical hepatic encephalopathy or an INR of 2.0 or more regardless of the presence or absence of encephalopathy. Patients with liver failure should be transferred to a pediatric tertiary care center with consultation from a pediatric gastroenterology specialist.

D. In the patient with elevated liver tests, an abdominal ultrasound should be performed early in the evaluation and can identify structural problems such as a tumor, choledochal cyst, gallstones, or sludge and hydrops of the gallbladder.

(Continued on page 236)

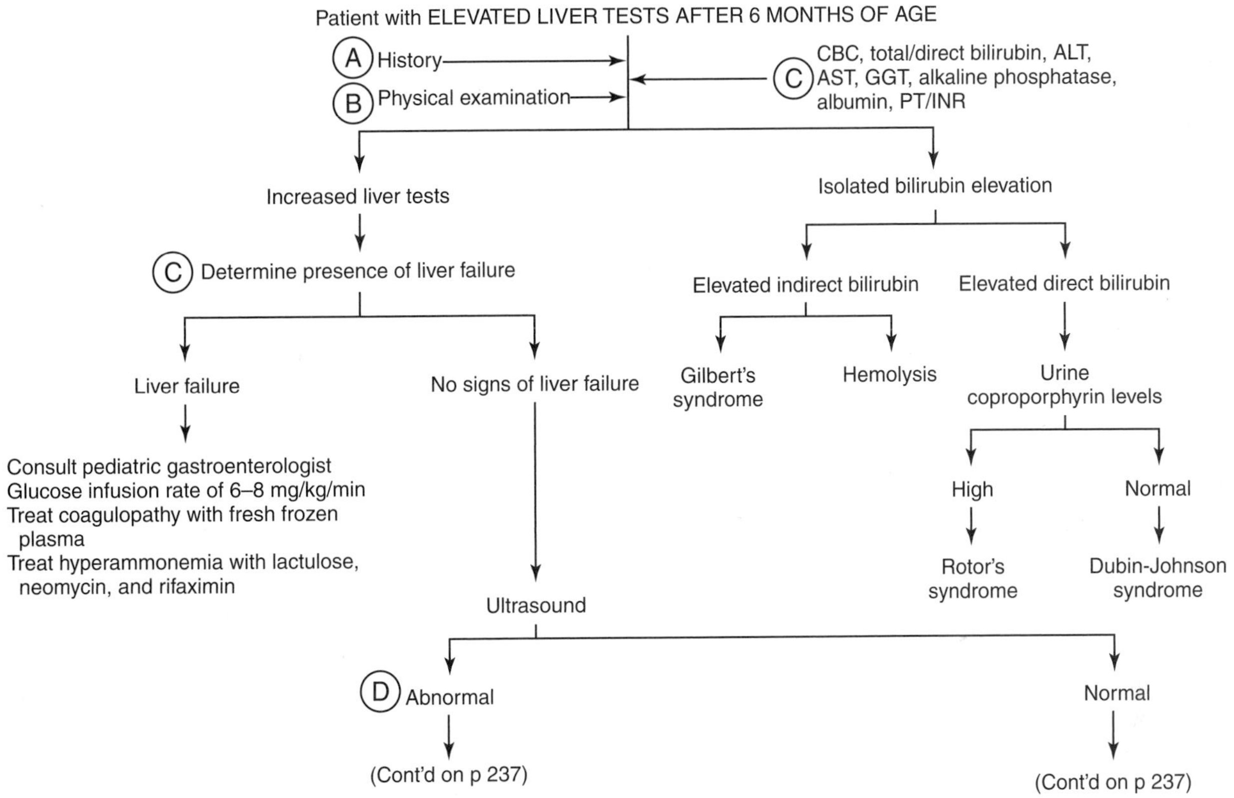

Patient with ELEVATED LIVER TESTS AFTER 6 MONTHS OF AGE
A History
B Physical examination
C CBC, total/direct bilirubin, ALT, AST, GGT, alkaline phosphatase, albumin, PT/INR
Increased liver tests
C Determine presence of liver failure
Liver failure
Consult pediatric gastroenterologist
Glucose infusion rate of 6–8 mg/kg/min
Treat coagulopathy with fresh frozen plasma
Treat hyperammonemia with lactulose, neomycin, and rifaximin
No signs of liver failure
Ultrasound
D Abnormal
(Cont'd on p 237)
Normal
(Cont'd on p 237)
Isolated bilirubin elevation
Elevated indirect bilirubin
Gilbert's syndrome
Hemolysis
Elevated direct bilirubin
Urine coproporphyrin levels
High
Rotor's syndrome
Normal
Dubin-Johnson syndrome

E. A homogeneous increase in echogenicity of the liver is compatible with nonalcoholic fatty liver disease (NAFLD) and should be considered in the overweight or obese patient. Ten to 20% of children will have NAFLD. Additional findings include acanthosis nigricans in up to 50% of children with NAFLD. ALT is often twofold elevated when compared with AST. However, because children with other chronic liver diseases can also be obese, it is important to screen for the other liver diseases discussed in Table 1 before giving the diagnosis of NAFLD.

F. Choledochal cysts are congenital anomalies consisting of dilation of various segments of the extrahepatic biliary tract and can also involve the large intrahepatic bile ducts. Choledochal cysts can lead to recurrent cholangitis and cholangiocarcinoma; therefore, surgical correction is necessary. Cholelithiasis, or gallstones, may be related to prolonged total parenteral nutrition, disease of the terminal ileum, hemolytic disease, hepatobiliary disease, abdominal surgery, cystic fibrosis, or obesity. The stones consist of calcium or cholesterol crystals, and ultrasonography usually identifies dilation of the intrahepatic and extrahepatic bile ducts, even if stones in the common duct are not visualized. Endoscopic retrograde cholangiopancreatography can be diagnostic, as well as therapeutic, with the removal of gallstones or sludge. Cholecystectomy is indicated for symptomatic patients.

G. Suspect acute hydrops of the gallbladder in children with Kawasaki disease and when ultrasonography demonstrates distention of the gallbladder without calculi and with normal extrahepatic bile ducts. Other conditions to consider include streptococcal or staphylococcal infection. Attempt treatment with supportive care (intravenous fluids) followed by a low-fat diet before considering surgery.

H. The most common cause of cholecystitis is due to cholelithiasis. Cholecystitis can also be caused by a postoperative state, burns, and infections with *Salmonella enterica, Escherichia coli, Streptococcus viridans, Leptospira, Rickettsia rickettsii, Cryptosporidium, Giardia, Cytomegalovirus, Candida,* and *Aspergillus.*

I. A number of potential underlying causative factors apply to the patient with elevated liver tests and a normal abdominal ultrasound. One of the most common causes of a transient, mild elevation in liver tests is an intercurrent viral illness. Other viral causes of hepatitis are discussed in the chapter "Infectious Hepatitis". Persistent elevation in liver tests may be caused by a variety of underlying chronic liver diseases. These include autoimmune diseases (autoimmune hepatitis, primary sclerosing cholangitis, lupus), genetic diseases (Wilson's copper storage disease, α_1-antitrypsin deficiency, cystic fibrosis, hemochromatosis, Alagille syndrome), metabolic diseases (tyrosinemia, other inborn errors of metabolism, mitochondropathies, fatty acid oxidation defects), and storage diseases (glycogen storage disease, Niemann–Pick disease, hemophagocytic lymphohistiocytosis). The workup for these conditions is outlined in Table 1. A liver biopsy is often needed to confirm many of these diagnoses. Furthermore, liver histology can aid in the diagnosis of nonalcoholic steatohepatitis, congenital hepatic fibrosis, and primary familial intrahepatic cholestasis. Finally, drug hepatotoxicity has been found with various antibiotics (amoxicillin/clavulanate, isoniazid, erythromycin, sulfonamides, sulfamethoxazole/trimethoprim, nitrofurantoin, minocycline), immunosuppressive drugs (methotrexate, azathioprine), and antiepileptic drugs (valproic acid, Dilantin, carbamazepine). Extrahepatic causes of liver disease include vascular lesions such as Budd–Chiari syndrome and right-sided heart disease.

Table 1. **Chronic Liver Disease Diagnostic Workup**

Disease	Workup (abnormality detected in disease)
Autoimmune hepatitis	ANA, anti-smooth muscle antibody, liver-kidney microsomal antibody (all elevated)
Primary sclerosing cholangitis	MRCP or ERCP (biliary strictures)
Wilson's disease	Ceruloplasmin (low), 24-hour urine copper (high), eye examination (Kayser–Fleischer rings)
α_1-Antitrypsin deficiency	α_1-Antitrypsin level (low) and phenotype (ZZ, SZ)
Cystic fibrosis	Sweat chloride test (high chloride)
Hemochromatosis	Transferrin saturation (high), ferritin (high)
Alagille syndrome	Echocardiogram (PPS, other), spine radiograph (butterfly vertebrae), eye examination (posterior embryotoxon)
Tyrosinemia	Urine succinylacetone (high)
Inborn errors of metabolism	Serum amino acids and urine organic acids (abnormal)
Mitochondropathy	Serum lactate/pyruvate ratio (high)
Fatty acid oxidation defect	Acylcarnitine profile (abnormal)
Glycogen storage disease	Triglycerides/cholesterol (high), lactate (high), uric acid (high)
Hemophagocytic lymphohistiocytosis	CBC (2 of 3 lineages low), triglycerides (high), fibrinogen (low)

ANA, antinuclear antigen; *CBC,* complete blood cell count. *ERCP,* endoscopic retrograde cholangiopancreaticogram; *MRCP,* magnetic resonance cholangiopancreaticogram; *PPS,* peripheral pulmonic stenosis.

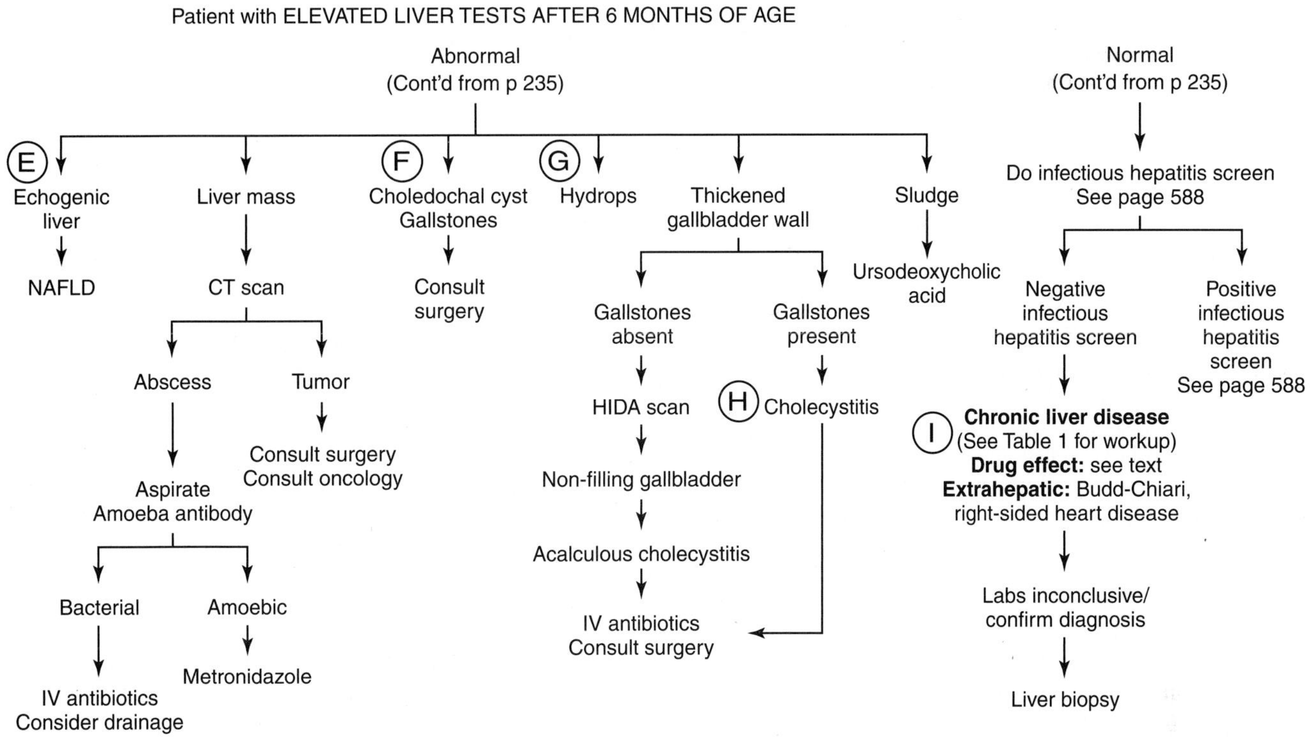
Patient with ELEVATED LIVER TESTS AFTER 6 MONTHS OF AGE
Abnormal
(Cont'd from p 235)
Normal
(Cont'd from p 235)
E
Echogenic liver
NAFLD
Liver mass
CT scan
Abscess
Tumor
Aspirate
Amoeba antibody
Consult surgery
Consult oncology
Bacterial
Amoebic
IV antibiotics
Consider drainage
Metronidazole
F
Choledochal cyst
Gallstones
Consult surgery
G
Hydrops
Thickened gallbladder wall
Gallstones absent
Gallstones present
HIDA scan
H
Cholecystitis
Non-filling gallbladder
Acalculous cholecystitis
IV antibiotics
Consult surgery
Sludge
Ursodeoxycholic acid
Do infectious hepatitis screen
See page 588
Negative infectious hepatitis screen
Positive infectious hepatitis screen
See page 588
I
Chronic liver disease
(See Table 1 for workup)
Drug effect: see text
Extrahepatic: Budd-Chiari, right-sided heart disease
Labs inconclusive/ confirm diagnosis
Liver biopsy

Reference

Suchy FJ, Sokol RJ, Balistreri WF, editors. Liver diseases in children. 3rd ed. Cambridge, NY: Cambridge University Press; 2007.

Vomiting during Infancy

Vincent Mukkada, MD, and Robert E. Kramer, MD

Vomiting is one of the most common signs of illness in infancy. In assessing symptoms, it is important to distinguish between true vomiting (the forceful expulsion of stomach/intestinal contents through the oral cavity) from the more common infant regurgitation ("spitting up"), which is effortless reflux of gastric contents into the esophagus or mouth. Vomiting typically occurs in three stages: (1) a prodrome with nausea or other autonomic signs; (2) a period of retching; and (3) vomiting with expulsion of emesis.

The first priority in the vomiting infant is to quickly assess hemodynamic stability, because small infants can rapidly become dehydrated. Second, the symptoms should be defined as either acute or chronic, with acute attacks occurring in an otherwise healthy infant raising suspicion of new or emergent issues such as infection, anatomic or surgical causes, trauma, or metabolic derangements. In addition, the character of the emesis (bilious vs. nonbilious) is important to ascertain quickly, because bilious emesis suggests intestinal obstruction, which may require urgent intervention. Obstruction may still present with nonbilious emesis if the site is proximal to the ampulla of Vater, as can be seen with hypertrophic pyloric stenosis, but these types of obstruction are less likely to be surgical emergencies.

A. In terms of history, a comprehensive description of the vomiting events is important (how often, how much volume, time of onset, single events vs. occurring in clusters, degree of forcefulness, presence of bile or blood). Feeding details are critical, including timing in relation to vomiting (during feeds, associated with choking, immediately after feedings, or hours later), protein source, volume, frequency, concentration of formula, other foods ingested, and whether any foods seem to make the vomiting worse. In addition, information about associated signs and symptoms such as pain, cough, respiratory distress, fever, rash, or nasal congestion can help to identify extraintestinal causes of vomiting. Questions regarding the infants overall status (dry mouth, urine output, activity level in the preceding hours, mental status changes) help to determine hydration status and the risk for shock. Infants who have a history of abdominal surgery or necrotizing enterocolitis (even if in the case of "medical necrotizing enterocolitis" not requiring resection) should be considered to be at greater risk for obstruction from adhesions or intestinal stenosis. A careful family history specifically directed toward perinatal deaths (suggesting inborn errors of metabolism or adrenal insufficiency) or surgical disorders such as pyloric stenosis may help direct the workup.

B. In the physical examination, the immediate concern is assessment of shock; therefore, careful examination for pulse, blood pressure, respiratory rate, capillary refill, skin color/turgor, status of mucous membranes, presence of tears, sunken or bulging fontanelle, and urine output is crucial. Plotting growth parameters (including head circumference, as rapidly expanding head circumference should raise suspicion for intracranial processes leading to vomiting) will help assess for chronicity of symptoms or presence of underlying organic disorders. Rapid decreases in weight compared with recent values should be used to help calculate the fluid deficit and assess the degree of dehydration. Examination should focus on other potential causes of vomiting, such as acute otitis, upper respiratory infections, or signs of neurologic diseases (irritability/lethargy, seizure activity, other focal neurologic abnormalities, nuchal rigidity). Abdominal examination should assess for signs of obstruction, including firm, distended abdomen, high-pitched or absent bowel sounds, or visible peristalsis, as well as signs of abdominal tenderness or palpable abdominal masses (such as the "olive" classically associated with pyloric stenosis). If the exam does not raise suspicion for an acute surgical abdomen, then observation of a feed may be instructive.

C. Initial nonspecific screening tests should include a complete blood cell count to gauge index of suspicion for an infectious causative agent, a basic metabolic panel to assess electrolyte abnormalities/dehydration, and a urinalysis to evaluate for dehydration or infection. In cases of prolonged vomiting, there can be hypochloremic alkalosis, which can be worsened by excretion of acidic urine as the kidney attempts to maintain adequate potassium stores in the face of intracellular potassium deficits. Fluid replacement with normal saline and gentle replacement of the potassium deficit is needed to correct this. Alkalinization of the urine indicates that potassium replacement is sufficient.

(Continued on page 240)

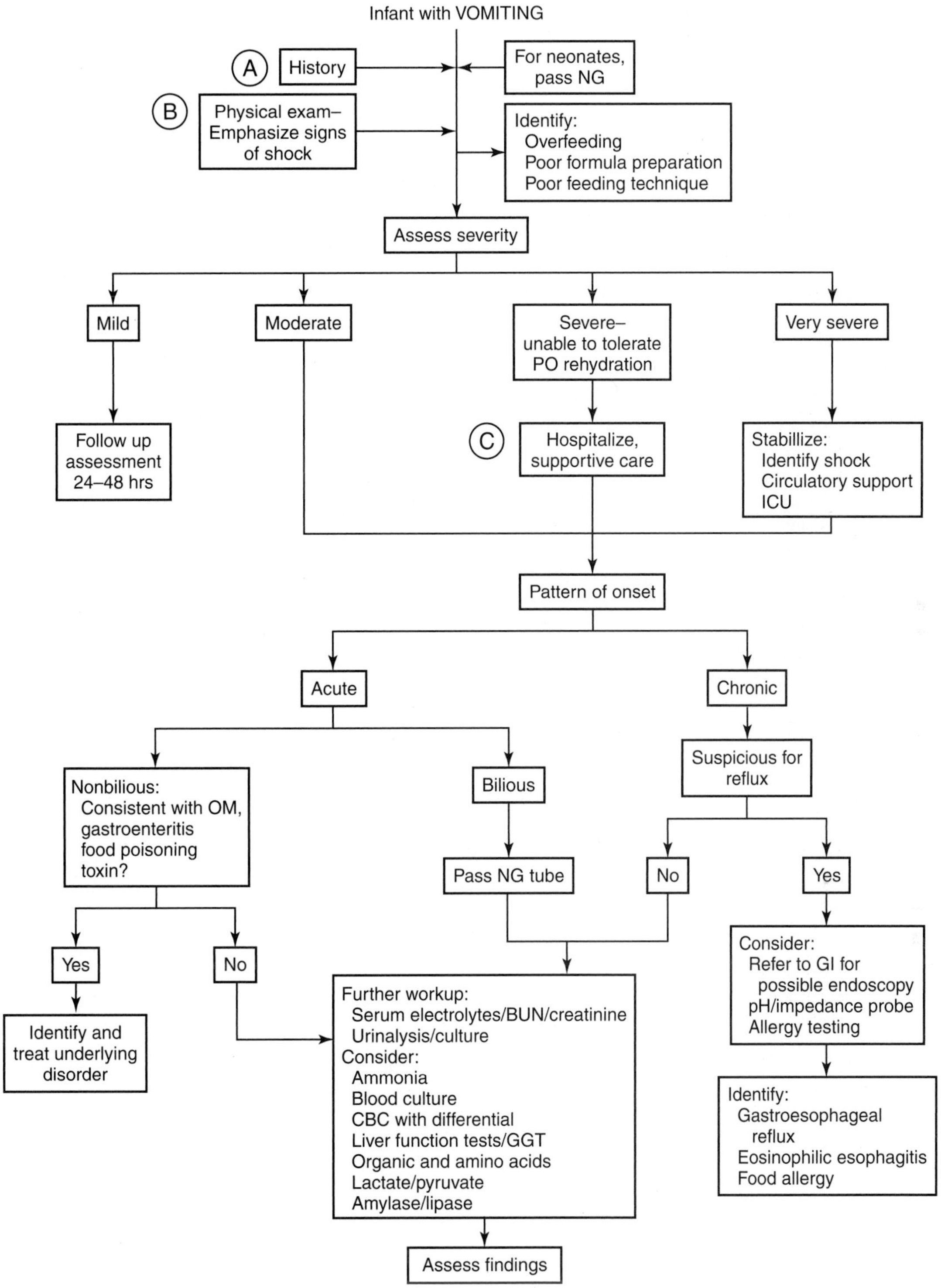

Infant with VOMITING
A
History
B
Physical exam–Emphasize signs of shock
For neonates, pass NG
Identify: Overfeeding Poor formula preparation Poor feeding technique
Assess severity
Mild
Moderate
Severe–unable to tolerate PO rehydration
Very severe
Follow up assessment 24–48 hrs
C
Hospitalize, supportive care
Stabillize: Identify shock Circulatory support ICU
Pattern of onset
Acute
Chronic
Nonbilious: Consistent with OM, gastroenteritis food poisoning toxin?
Bilious
Suspicious for reflux
Pass NG tube
No
Yes
Yes
No
Identify and treat underlying disorder
Further workup: Serum electrolytes/BUN/creatinine Urinalysis/culture Consider: Ammonia Blood culture CBC with differential Liver function tests/GGT Organic and amino acids Lactate/pyruvate Amylase/lipase
Consider: Refer to GI for possible endoscopy pH/impedance probe Allergy testing
Identify: Gastroesophageal reflux Eosinophilic esophagitis Food allergy
Assess findings

(Cont'd on p 241)

D. In considering the next steps in workup, it is important to remember that vomiting can be a symptom of a large variety of illnesses. Infectious causes for vomiting include bacterial or viral gastroenteritis, urinary tract infections, otitis media, meningitis, upper respiratory infections, pneumonia, and sepsis. Neurologic diseases causing increased intracranial pressure, including seizures, hemorrhage, intracranial masses, or Arnold–Chiari malformations, can present with vomiting. Similarly, a wide variety of endocrine/metabolic disorders, including adrenal insufficiency, diabetic ketoacidosis, and inborn errors of metabolism such as aminoaciduria, galactosemia, and fructosemia, urea cycle defects, and disorders of fatty acid metabolism (among many others) may also present with infantile emesis. Suspicion for metabolic disorders should be increased with severe acidosis, hyperammonemia, lethargy, or hypoglycemia/hyperglycemia. A variety of surgical/anatomic diseases, such as intussusception, hypertrophic pyloric stenosis, antral or duodenal webs, anatomic duplications, malrotation with volvulus, inguinal hernia, cholecystitis, annular pancreas, or vascular rings, can present with profuse vomiting. Intractable vomiting can also occur after trauma, either to the abdomen or to the head, and abuse needs to be considered in the absence of other identified causes. Allergic disease can present with emesis and should be considered especially if there is evidence of worsening with particular food. At its most severe, diseases such as food protein–induced enterocolitis can manifest with a shock/sepsis-like presentation, with profuse vomiting generally following reintroduction of a food after a period without exposure. A variety of gastrointestinal disorders such as gastroesophageal reflux, pancreatitis, eosinophilic gastrointestinal disease, gastritis, peptic ulcer disease, inflammatory bowel disease, or celiac disease can present as vomiting in infancy. A variety of toxins, both accidental exposures and therapeutic misadventures, can lead to vomiting; therefore, a careful history of all possible exposures is crucial.

References

Allen K. The vomiting child—what to do and when to consult. Aust Fam Physician 2007;30(9):684–7.

Kwon KT, Tsai VW. Metabolic emergencies. Emerg Med Clin North Am 2007;25:1041–60.

Li BK, Sunku BK. Vomiting and nausea. In: Wyllie R, Hyams J, editors. Pediatric gastrointestinal and liver disease: pathophysiology/diagnosis/management. 3rd ed. New York: Saunders Elsevier; 2006 [p. 127-50].

Morley CJ, Cole TJ. Bile stained vomiting in neonates. Arch Dis Child 2009;94(2):171.

Waseem M, Rosenberg HK. Intussusception. Pediatr Emerg Care 2008;24(11):793–800.

Infant with VOMITING

(Cont'd from p 239)

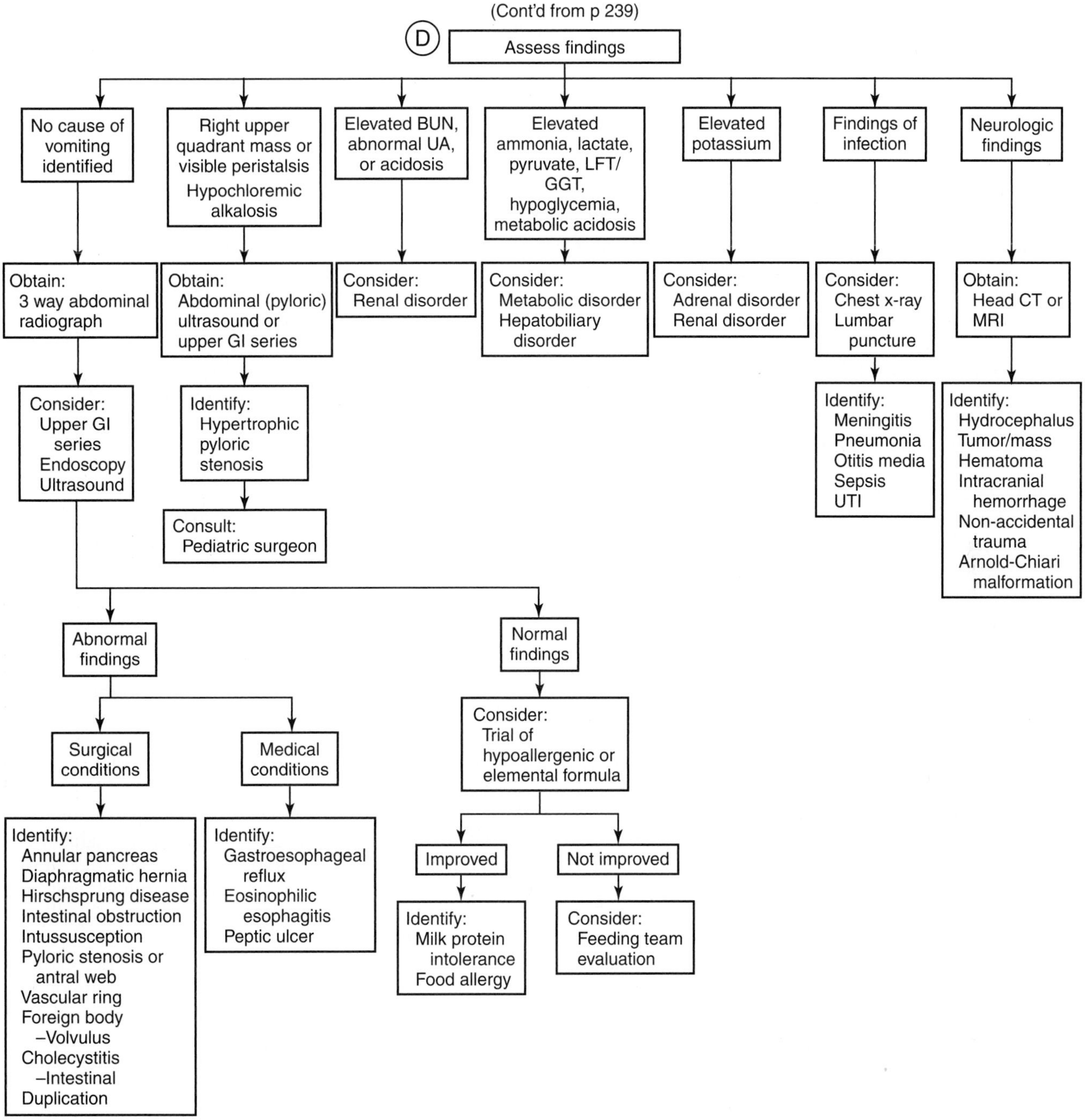
D
Assess findings
No cause of vomiting identified
Right upper quadrant mass or visible peristalsis
Hypochloremic alkalosis
Elevated BUN, abnormal UA, or acidosis
Elevated ammonia, lactate, pyruvate, LFT/GGT, hypoglycemia, metabolic acidosis
Elevated potassium
Findings of infection
Neurologic findings
Obtain: 3 way abdominal radiograph
Obtain: Abdominal (pyloric) ultrasound or upper GI series
Consider: Renal disorder
Consider: Metabolic disorder Hepatobiliary disorder
Consider: Adrenal disorder Renal disorder
Consider: Chest x-ray Lumbar puncture
Obtain: Head CT or MRI
Consider: Upper GI series Endoscopy Ultrasound
Identify: Hypertrophic pyloric stenosis
Consult: Pediatric surgeon
Identify: Meningitis Pneumonia Otitis media Sepsis UTI
Identify: Hydrocephalus Tumor/mass Hematoma Intracranial hemorrhage Non-accidental trauma Arnold-Chiari malformation
Abnormal findings
Normal findings
Surgical conditions
Medical conditions
Consider: Trial of hypoallergenic or elemental formula
Identify: Annular pancreas Diaphragmatic hernia Hirschsprung disease Intestinal obstruction Intussusception Pyloric stenosis or antral web Vascular ring Foreign body –Volvulus Cholecystitis –Intestinal Duplication
Identify: Gastroesophageal reflux Eosinophilic esophagitis Peptic ulcer
Improved
Not improved
Identify: Milk protein intolerance Food allergy
Consider: Feeding team evaluation

Vomiting after Infancy

Barrett H. Barnes, MD, and Edward J. Hoffenberg, MD

Vomiting involves the expulsion of stomach contents through the mouth. Retrograde gastric contractions are triggered by the central nervous system (CNS) vomiting centers. These centers can be stimulated through multiple pathways, such as gastrointestinal irritation and distention, the vestibular system, central nervous system abnormalities, and stress. Vomiting can be characterized as bilious or nonbilious (Table 1). Bilious vomiting occurs when green or yellow bile is present in the vomitus. Bilious vomiting usually indicates a process distal to the ligament of Treitz. In nonbilious vomiting, anatomic causes occur proximally to the ampulla of Vater, the point of bilious drainage into the intestine. Vomiting can also be characterized as bloody or nonbloody (bright red, maroon, or coffee-ground appearance).

A. In the patient's history, ask about the onset, frequency, severity (quantity and forcefulness), and timing of vomiting. Identify precipitating factors, such as feeding, cough, or activity. Note associated symptoms, such as abdominal pain, abdominal distention, alterations in mental status, bloody stools, coryza, constipation, cough, diarrhea, dysuria, failure to thrive, fever, headache, jaundice, polydipsia, and urinary frequency. Consider Reye syndrome with a recent history of chickenpox or influenza syndrome. Vomiting associated with bloody stools and intermittent abdominal pain suggests intussusception. Nighttime vomiting suggests a central nervous system disorder or possible exposure to a toxin (carbon monoxide poisoning). Identify predisposing conditions, such as hepatitis, inflammatory bowel disease, necrotizing enterocolitis, pregnancy, prior abdominal surgery, and sickle cell disease. Precipitating factors include current medications, ingestions (acetaminophen, salicylate), and toxins (lead). In adolescence, suspect bulimia or superior mesenteric artery syndrome when vomiting is associated with marked weight loss.

B. In the physical examination, assess the circulatory and hydration status (Table 2) by ascertaining blood pressure, pulse, respiratory rate, capillary refill, skin color and turgor, tears, fullness of the fontanelle, and urine output. Plot the child's height, weight, and head circumference on a growth grid to identify cases with failure to thrive or rapid head growth. Assess the mental status and note any irritability, lethargy, seizures, papilledema, retinal hemorrhage, ataxia, and focal neurologic signs. Assess the abdomen for any peritoneal signs such as distension, discoloration, or marked tenderness. Perform a rectal examination and note the quantity of stool and whether it contains blood (Hemoccult positive). Document extraintestinal manifestations, such as rash, arthritis, lymphadenopathy, hepatosplenomegaly, and infections.

C. Consider a diagnostic workup for infection, systemic disorders, and central nervous system disorders. Infections that can result in persistent vomiting include acute otitis media, urinary tract infection, pneumonia, sepsis, and meningitis. Systemic disorders with persistent vomiting include hepatobiliary disorders (hepatitis, cholangitis, choledochal cyst, cholecystitis), cystic fibrosis (meconium ileus equivalent), inborn errors of metabolism, and central nervous system abnormalities (hydrocephalus, tumors, cerebral edema, increased intracranial pressure). Consider also cyclic vomiting syndrome.

D. Suspect acute pancreatitis when acute abdominal pain radiates deep to the back, is epigastric or right upper quadrant, and is associated with vomiting after meals. Ascites, abdominal distention, and peritoneal signs may be present. Increase of serum amylase and/or lipase levels in the setting of normal kidney function suggests pancreatitis with possible biliary tract disease. Ultrasonography may show inflammation, dilated common bile duct or retained stone, or a pseudocyst. Causes of pancreatitis include gallstones, acquired or congenital structural defects, trauma, metabolic disorders, infection, vasculitis, hemolytic-uremic syndrome, and drug toxicity.

(Continued on page 244)

Table 1. **General Causes of Vomiting**

Nonbilious
Infectious-inflammatory
Metabolic-endocrinologic
Neurologic
Psychologic
Obstructive lesion
Bilious
Obstructive lesion distal to stomach

From Murray KF, Christie DL. Vomiting. Pediatr Rev 1998;19:337.

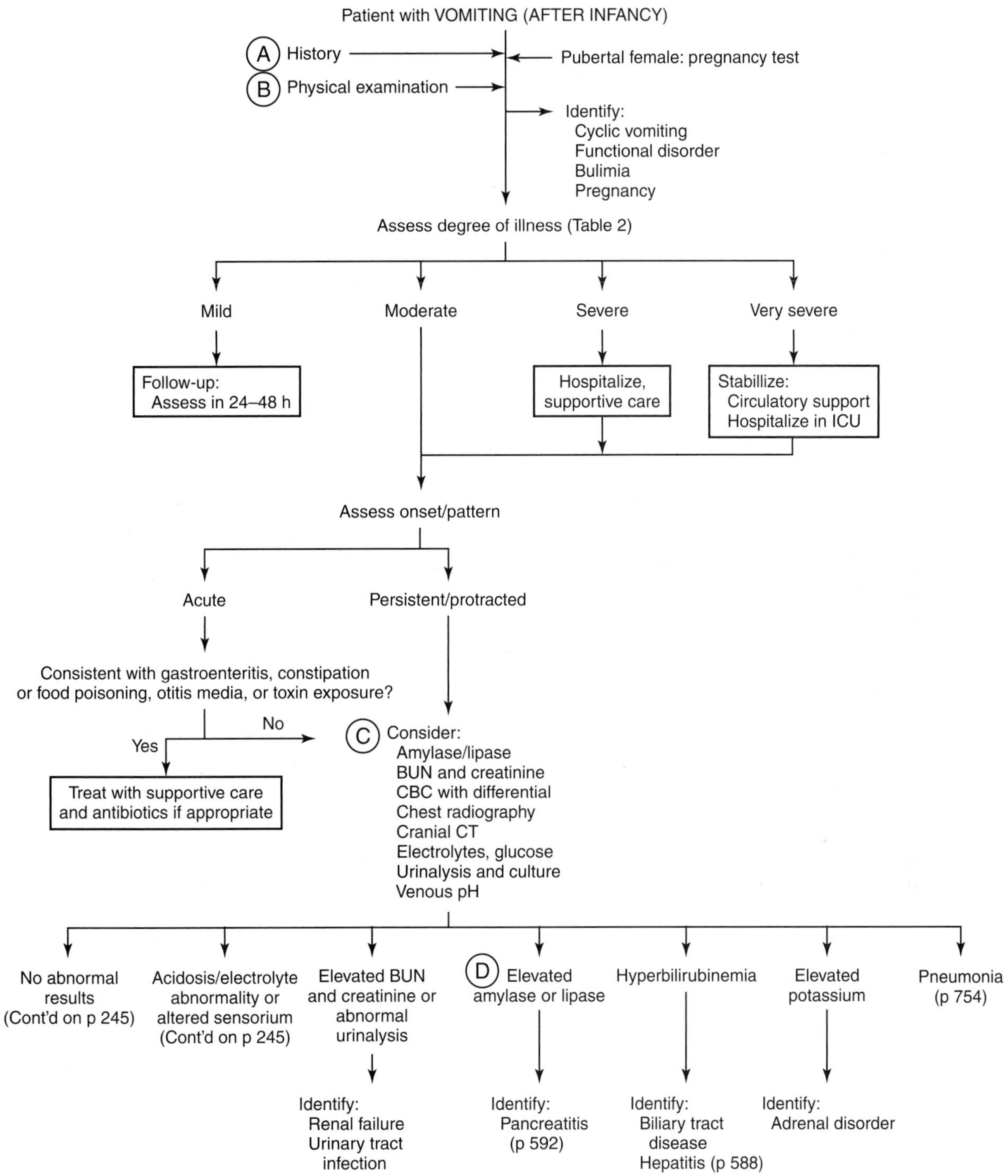
Patient with VOMITING (AFTER INFANCY)
A History
B Physical examination
Pubertal female: pregnancy test
Identify:
Cyclic vomiting
Functional disorder
Bulimia
Pregnancy
Assess degree of illness (Table 2)
Mild
Moderate
Severe
Very severe
Follow-up:
Assess in 24–48 h
Hospitalize,
supportive care
Stabillize:
Circulatory support
Hospitalize in ICU
Assess onset/pattern
Acute
Persistent/protracted
Consistent with gastroenteritis, constipation
or food poisoning, otitis media, or toxin exposure?
Yes
No
Treat with supportive care
and antibiotics if appropriate
C Consider:
Amylase/lipase
BUN and creatinine
CBC with differential
Chest radiography
Cranial CT
Electrolytes, glucose
Urinalysis and culture
Venous pH
No abnormal
results
(Cont'd on p 245)
Acidosis/electrolyte
abnormality or
altered sensorium
(Cont'd on p 245)
Elevated BUN
and creatinine or
abnormal
urinalysis
D Elevated
amylase or lipase
Hyperbilirubinemia
Elevated
potassium
Pneumonia
(p 754)
Identify:
Renal failure
Urinary tract
infection
Identify:
Pancreatitis
(p 592)
Identify:
Biliary tract
disease
Hepatitis (p 588)
Identify:
Adrenal disorder

Table 2. **Degree of Illness in Vomiting after Infancy**

Mild	Moderate	Severe	Very Severe
Previously healthy child with no signs of bacterial infection, systemic disorder, or dehydration	Signs of bacterial infection OR Systemic disorder OR Vomiting longer than 1 week OR Growth failure/ weight loss	Signs of dehydration OR Intestinal obstruction OR Acidosis OR Electrolyte abnormalities OR Altered mental status: lethargy, confusion, disorientation	Signs of shock OR Altered mental status: unresponsive, too weak to feed, seizures, signs of meningeal irritation

E. Constipation can present with abdominal pain and vomiting. Suspect pediatric constipation if irregular, hard, or very large bowel movements or physical examination suggests fecal impaction.

F. Suspect Reye-like syndrome or metabolic disease when the patient has persistent vomiting, hyperventilation, and altered mental status (confusion, combativeness, disorientation, stupor, coma) in association with hepatic dysfunction (increased serum transaminases, protime, and ammonia), acidosis, hypoglycemia, and lack of ketones despite dehydration and fasting.

References

Borowitz S, Sutphen J. Recurrent vomiting and persistent gastroesophageal reflux caused by unrecognized constipation. Clin Pediatr 2004;43:461–6.

Fuchs S, Jaffe D. Vomiting. Pediatr Emerg Care 1990;6:164–70.

Hall J, Driscoll P. 10 nausea, vomiting and fever. Emerg Med J 2005;22:200–4.

Li BU, Lefevre F, Chelimsky GG, et al. North American Society for Pediatric Gastroenterology, Hepatology, and Nutrition consensus statement on the diagnosis and management of cyclic vomiting syndrome. J Pediatr Gastroenterol Nutr 2008;47(3):379–93.

Murray KF, Christie DL. Vomiting. Pediatr Rev 1998;19:337–41.

Ramos AG, Tuchman DN. Persistent vomiting. Pediatr Rev 1994;15:24–31.

Sondheimer JM. Vomiting. In: Walker WA Durie PR, Hamilton JR et al, editors. Pathophysiology, diagnosis, management. Pediatric gastrointestinal disease, vol 1. Hamilton, (Ontario, Canada): BC Decker; 2004 p. 203–9.

Patient with VOMITING (AFTER INFANCY)

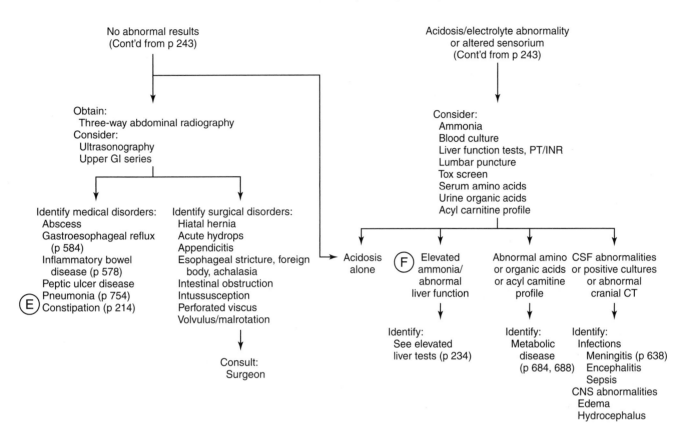

No abnormal results (Cont'd from p 243)

→ Obtain:
- Three-way abdominal radiography

Consider:
- Ultrasonography
- Upper GI series

→ Identify medical disorders:
- Abscess
- Gastroesophageal reflux (p 584)
- Inflammatory bowel disease (p 578)
- Peptic ulcer disease
- Pneumonia (p 754)
- (E) Constipation (p 214)

→ Identify surgical disorders:
- Hiatal hernia
- Acute hydrops
- Appendicitis
- Esophageal stricture, foreign body, achalasia
- Intestinal obstruction
- Intussusception
- Perforated viscus
- Volvulus/malrotation

→ Consult:
- Surgeon

→ Acidosis alone

Acidosis/electrolyte abnormality or altered sensorium (Cont'd from p 243)

→ Consider:
- Ammonia
- Blood culture
- Liver function tests, PT/INR
- Lumbar puncture
- Tox screen
- Serum amino acids
- Urine organic acids
- Acyl carnitine profile

→ Acidosis alone

→ (F) Elevated ammonia/abnormal liver function
- → Identify:
  - See elevated liver tests (p 234)

→ Abnormal amino or organic acids or acyl camitine profile
- → Identify:
  - Metabolic disease (p 684, 688)

→ CSF abnormalities or positive cultures or abnormal cranial CT
- → Identify:
  - Infections
    - Meningitis (p 638)
    - Encephalitis
    - Sepsis
  - CNS abnormalities
    - Edema
    - Hydrocephalus

Genitourinary

Vaginitis
Dysuria
Hematuria
Penile Complaints
Scrotal Swelling/Pain

Vaginitis

Stephen M. Scott, MD, FACOG

Vulvovaginitis is the most common genital complaint among prepubertal girls seen in an ambulatory setting. By far the most common cause is due to infection, coupled with a lack of estrogen, leading to thin atrophic mucosa that is prone to recurrent flares. Misdiagnosis and improper treatment can lead to persistence of symptoms and frustration for the child and parents. It is important to distinguish the common forms of vulvovaginitis from rarer, but more serious causative factors.

A. A thorough history and external genital examination in the office will often lead to the diagnosis of prepubertal vulvovaginitis. Symptoms include intermittent genital itching or pain. Dysuria from skin contact with acidic urine may lead to hesitancy and retention. Erythema of the vulva and vaginal mucosa may come and go, and yellow–green discharge may be seen coming from the vagina or on the underwear. Fever is uncommon unless the vaginitis is accompanied by genitourinary infections from the same bacteria. If in an acute cycle, the physical examination should reveal inflamed mucosa. Excoriations are possible if the child is scratching excessively. A gentle collection of discharge may reveal basal epithelial cells and numerous white blood cells indicating prepubertal estrogen levels and inflammation, respectively. Yeast is almost never a cause of vaginitis before puberty. Immunocompromised states such as diabetes or leukemia should be ruled out if yeast is found on a wet prep.

B. Because the gastrointestinal flora is the bacterial origin for these infections, the genital area will always be colonized. Therefore, treatment with antibiotics should be reserved only for acute stages of inflammation and is not the long-term solution. A broad-spectrum antibiotic, such as amoxicillin/clavulanic acid or clindamycin, is most effective if needed. The primary treatment of vaginitis is aggressive skin care to reduce bacterial contact with the mucosa. Initially, multiple daily sitz baths will dilute bacterial concentration in the genital area. After every immersion soak, application with any skin emollient will provide a barrier to prevent remaining bacterial contact with the mucosal layer. Adding baking soda or oatmeal to the baths may provide some initial symptomatic relief, but plain water is more than adequate treatment. Parents need to understand that the low estrogen environment will persist until puberty, and sitz baths and emollient application will need to continue (with lesser frequency eventually) until ovarian estrogen production begins. If discharge and symptoms persist, then other causes should be ruled out.

C. Estrogen stimulation of the genital area can lead to cervical mucus and vaginal transudate production, and may be mistaken for infectious vulvovaginitis. The acidification of the vaginal environment may lead to irritation of the mucosa and vaginitis symptoms until the mucosal layer has matured. The presence of estrogen may be physiologic in the first 2 months of life under the influence of maternal estrogen, and vaginal mucous production may be an early sign of puberty in young adolescents. Clues to distinguish pubertal discharge from prepubertal vulvovaginitis include secondary sexual signs such as breast tissue stimulation and/or the presence of superficial epithelial cells and lactobacilli on a vaginal wet prep. Any child between 3 months and 8 years of age should not have estrogen present. If seen, they need a workup for precocious puberty.

D. Careful history should include discussion of sexual contact to rule out sexually transmitted infections as a source of infection. Disruption of the hymen or perineal trauma should prompt the collection of gonorrhea and chlamydia samples, and a serum human immunodeficiency virus (HIV) screening. Sexually transmitted infection workup should also be performed if a wet prep reveals trichomoniasis.

E. Foreign bodies should be suspected if symptoms persist despite aggressive skin care for vaginitis. It may be suspected at the outset if severe odor and copious discharge is noted on examination. Patients may be reluctant to reveal placement, so sexual contact must be broached in this setting as well. Office evaluation may note the foreign body at the introitus and be removed easily. If the initial examination is negative, but a foreign body is still suspected, a vaginal flush with warm saline through a pediatric feeding tube connected to a large syringe may dislodge the object to the outside. If this does not achieve the goal, then a complete visualization of the vagina is necessary to rule out a foreign body. Although pediatric speculums, otoscopes, or laryngoscopes may provide visualization in the office, a vaginoscopy under sedation will allow for the best visualization of the upper vagina and cervix.

F. Lichen sclerosis can resemble vaginitis in its early stages. In later stages, the physical findings will evolve to show the typical leathery, parchment-like appearance of the skin located in an "hour glass" shape around the vulva and rectum. If left untreated, the vaginal entrance may become stenotic and create future problems, so early recognition and treatment is important. A moderate potency steroid cream, such as Temovate 0.05%, can be initiated with nightly applications for a few weeks. After that, a low-potency steroid cream, such hydrocortisone or betamethasone, should be used and tapered to the lowest frequency possible.

G. Labial adhesions are often present in the face of chronic irritation. Thus, they are frequently associated with vulvovaginitis. Oftentimes the adhesions are asymptomatic; therefore, the urge to separate should be resisted. Skin care with sitz baths and emollients should be the first line of treatment to address the underlying vulvovaginitis.

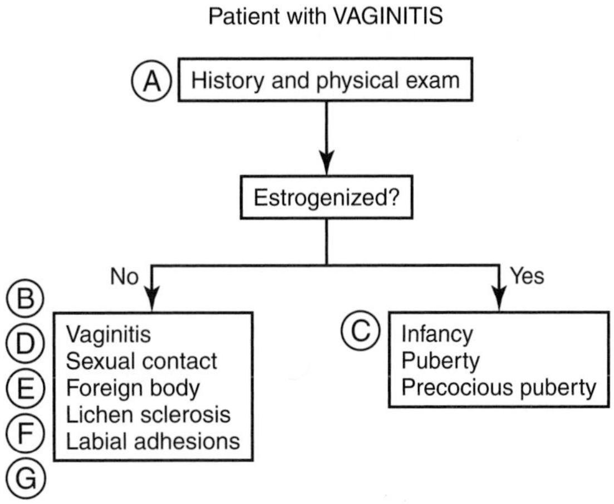

Patient with VAGINITIS
A
History and physical exam
Estrogenized?
No
Yes
B
D
E
F
G
Vaginitis
Sexual contact
Foreign body
Lichen sclerosis
Labial adhesions
C
Infancy
Puberty
Precocious puberty

Skin care should result in no further advancement in the adhesions if not in resolution. If symptoms are present such as pain with activity, recurrent urinary tract infections, or dribbling "accidents" after urination, then additional treatment may be used on top of baseline treatment. Topical estrogens and low-potency steroid creams may be substituted for one of the emollient applications to mature mucosa and reduce inflammation, respectively. Once symptoms have resolved, the emollient should be reintroduced. Blunt separation should be avoided because it leaves large areas of desquamated mucosa that rescar a majority of the time. Sharp dissection after estrogen and steroid cream priming will provide the least mucosal disruption and best chance for healing without adhesion reformation.

References

Jasper JM. Vulvovaginitis in the prepubertal child. Clin Ped Emerg Med 2009;10:10–3.

Koumantakis EE, Hassan EA, Deligeoroglou EK, Creatsas GK. Vulvovaginitis during childhood and adolescence. J Pediatr Adolesc Gynecol 1997;10:39–43.

Mayoglou L, Dulabon L, Martin-Alguacil N, et al. Success of treatment modalities for labial fusion: a retrospective evaluation of topical and surgical treatments. J Pediatr Adolesc Gynecol 2009;22:247–50.

Meffert J, Davis BM, Grimwood RE. Lichen sclerosis. J Am Acad Dermatol 1995;32:393–416.

Smith YR. Premenarchal vaginal discharge: findings of procedures to rule out foreign bodies. J Pediatr Adolesc Gynecol 2002;15:227–30.

Dysuria

Alison Brent, MD, and Meegan Leve, MD

Dysuria is defined as discomfort with urination often described as pain, burning, or stinging. Internal dysuria is the feeling of pain inside the body, and it occurs before or at the initiation of voiding. External dysuria is the feeling of pain after the initiation of voiding and may be felt as urine passes over inflamed external genitalia. Internal dysuria usually localizes to disorders of the bladder or urethra. External dysuria may be more suggestive of vaginitis, balanitis, or external genital lesions. Practically speaking, it may be difficult for children to distinguish internal from external dysuria.

Parents of preverbal children interpret nonspecific signs or symptoms such as crying with passage of urine as being reflective of dysuria. Verbal children who report pain with urination may have dysuria or pruritus. Adolescents most accurately report dysuria and more often than not have conditions related to the genitourinary (GU) tract.

CAUSES OF DYSURIA

Dysuria can be caused by myriad conditions in children, related to both infectious and noninfectious conditions, as referenced in Table 1. Most causes of dysuria are related to the GU tract and usually are benign, self-limited, or easily treatable. Systemic disease associated with dysuria or infectious causes extending beyond the GU tract can be serious and potentially life-threatening.

Localized Causes

Irritant

Topical or systemic exposure to a wide variety of agents has been reported to cause localized irritation in the GU area and may present as dysuria. Potential chemical irritants include bubble bath, scented soaps, and detergents, as well as systemically absorbed medications. Mechanical irritants include douching, prolonged exposure to wet diapers or undergarments such as with swimming, enuresis, and wearing tight clothing or nylon.

In infants and younger children who are not yet toilet trained, irritants can cause diaper dermatitis. Physical examination (PE) demonstrates erythema of the areas of skin that come into contact with the diaper, such as the perineal area, buttocks, lower abdomen, and thighs. Irritant diaper dermatitis generally spares the inguinal skin folds, which do not directly contact the diaper. In severe cases, superficial areas of breakdown or erosions may be noted. In older children, irritants can lead to redness of the vulva or vagina (vulvovaginitis) in girls, and inflammation of the glans penis or foreskin (balanitis or balanoposthitis) in boys. In both boys and girls, irritants may cause redness at the urethral entrance (urethritis). PE reveals few clues with the exception of localized minor erythema.

Infectious

Infection is the most common cause of dysuria. Urinary tract infection (UTI) is described as lower tract disease (cystitis) or upper tract disease (pyelonephritis). Risk factors for UTI include uncircumcised boys younger than 6 months, girls younger than 2 years, white, fever greater than 39° C, and urologic abnormalities. Cystitis, infection localized to the bladder or lower urinary tract disease, usually presents with dysuria, suprapubic pain, and low-grade fever. Hemorrhagic cystitis can be seen with bacteria, as well as with adenovirus infection. This affects boys more often than girls and causes dysuria, frequency, and gross hematuria, which will resolve spontaneously in 3 days. Schistosomiasis can cause a secondary UTI.

Diaper dermatitis can be related to streptococcal or *Candida albicans* infection. Candidal diaper infections present as erythematous plaques with satellite lesions. In contrast with irritant diaper dermatitis, *Candida* generally involves the skin folds. *Candida* infections may be associated with oral thrush or recent antibiotic use. Streptococcal diaper infections present with a sharply demarcated area of erythema and may be associated with perirectal fissures. Group A streptococcus is a cause of vulvovaginitis and perianal infection in preschool and early school-age children. The perineal area is described as "beefy" red. Other common symptoms are pruritus, perianal fissures, pain with bowel movements, and in girls, dysuria and discharge. Balanoposthitis refers to inflammation of the glans penis and foreskin. It can be caused by irritants or infection. In streptococcal balanoposthitis, the skin is usually "beefy" red and may be associated with discharge under the foreskin. Candidal balanoposthitis also causes erythema of the skin, often with satellite lesions and white discharge.

Enterobius vermicularis is a roundworm commonly known as pinworms or seatworms. Pinworms live in the large intestines, but at night, female pinworms lay eggs in the perineal, perianal, and vaginal areas. This can lead to vaginal irritation, dysuria, significant pruritus, and subsequently, sleep disturbance.

Minor Trauma

Minor urethral trauma is a relatively common cause of dysuria. Masturbation, sexual intercourse, and sexual abuse may result in trauma to the urethra. PE reveals minimal findings with the exception of localized erythema or a superficial abrasion or laceration. Foreign bodies can cause nonspecific vaginitis. There may be

ALGORITHM 1: EVALUATION OF DYSURIA

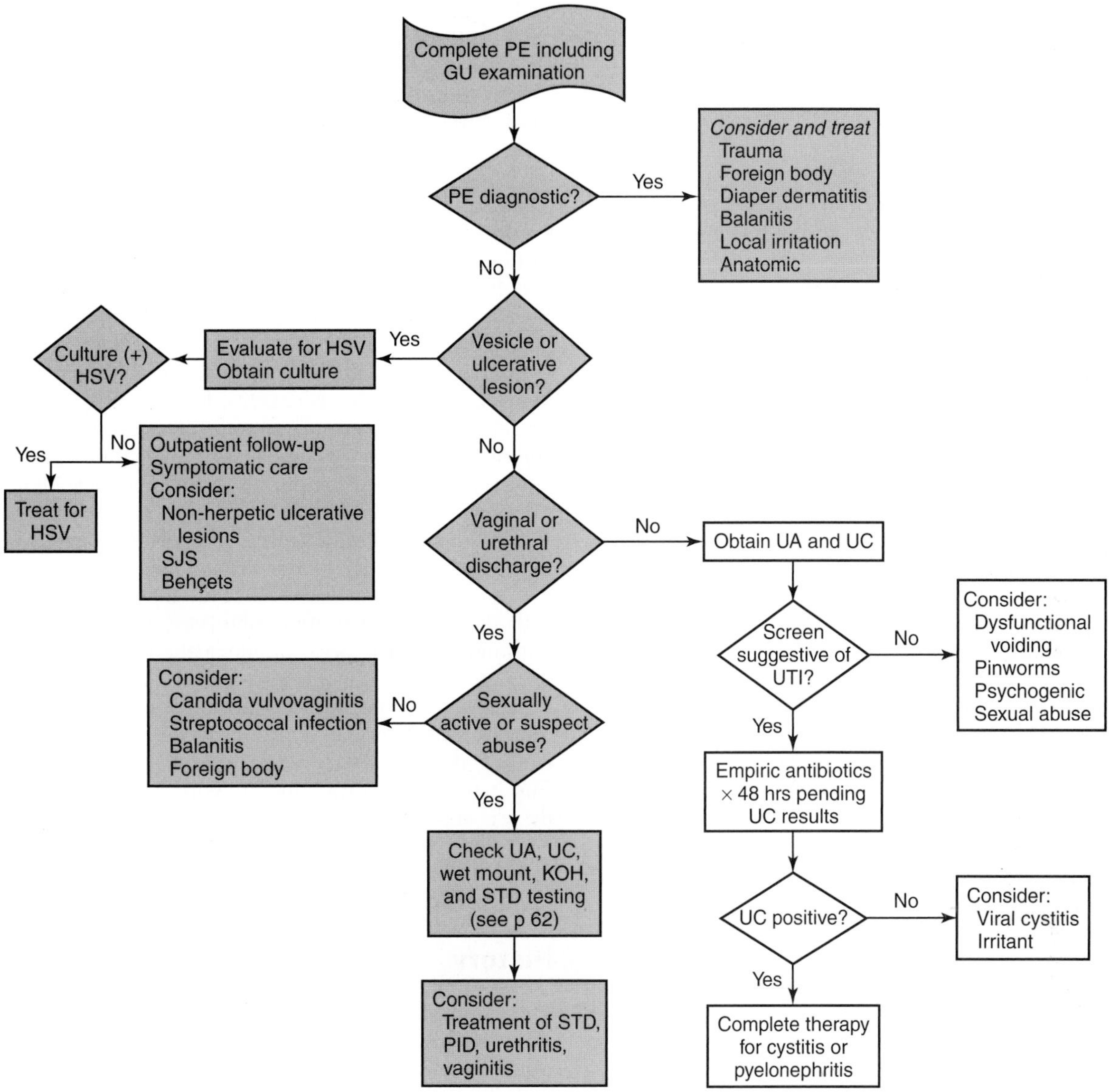
Complete PE including GU examination
PE diagnostic?
Yes
Consider and treat
Trauma
Foreign body
Diaper dermatitis
Balanitis
Local irritation
Anatomic
No
Vesicle or ulcerative lesion?
Yes
Evaluate for HSV
Obtain culture
Culture (+) HSV?
Yes
Treat for HSV
No
Outpatient follow-up
Symptomatic care
Consider:
Non-herpetic ulcerative lesions
SJS
Behçets
No
Vaginal or urethral discharge?
No
Obtain UA and UC
Screen suggestive of UTI?
No
Consider:
Dysfunctional voiding
Pinworms
Psychogenic
Sexual abuse
Yes
Empiric antibiotics × 48 hrs pending UC results
UC positive?
No
Consider:
Viral cystitis
Irritant
Yes
Complete therapy for cystitis or pyelonephritis
Yes
Sexually active or suspect abuse?
No
Consider:
Candida vulvovaginitis
Streptococcal infection
Balanitis
Foreign body
Yes
Check UA, UC, wet mount, KOH, and STD testing (see p 62)
Consider:
Treatment of STD, PID, urethritis, vaginitis

an associated bloody discharge. Common foreign bodies include retained toilet paper remnants, tampons, and condoms. Straddle injuries are common in children and occur when a child straddles an object during a fall such as a bike or monkey bars. This results in local trauma to the urogenital area. Straddle injuries can be penetrating or nonpenetrating. Nonpenetrating injuries are most common and result in superficial lacerations or abrasions to the labia in girls and scrotum or penis in boys. Penetrating injuries are more serious and extensive, and need to be differentiated from sexual assault.

Anatomic

Labial adhesions are common in young girls, with the greatest incidence being infants up to age 2 years. Adhesions frequently occur as a result of exposure to a wet diaper but can also occur after other minor trauma or irritation. Adhesions are usually asymptomatic but may result in dysuria if microtears are present. PE is diagnostic.

Meatal stenosis/urethral stricture is common in circumcised boys. It may occur as a result of chronic inflammation to the meatus, such as extended exposure to a wet diaper. Meatal stenosis/urethral stricture may not be detected until after toilet training. Boys may notice "difficult-to-aim stream," hesitancy, urgency, dysuria, or spots of blood on their underwear. It is not usually associated with significant obstruction or recurrent UTIs. Diagnosis is by evaluation of the meatal size, which may be difficult on examination, and observation of voiding.

Behavior/Functional

Voiding dysfunction is thought to be due to behavioral issues that occur during toilet training and affect the normal development of urinary control (see Enuresis, p. 70).

Table 1. **Causes of Dysuria**

Localized	Systemic
Irritants	
Diaper dermatitis, vulvovaginitis, urethritis, balanitis, and balanoposthitis can all be caused by irritants	Antidepressants Behçet syndrome
Chemical	
Bubble bath, scented soaps, detergents	Dysuria-hematuria syndrome Idiopathic hypercalcuria
Mechanical	
Douching, prolonged exposure to wet diaper or undergarments (swimming, enuresis), tight clothing or nylon	Malignancy Pelvic inflammatory disease
Infectious	
Balanitis/balanoposthitis Cervicitis Cystitis Diaper dermatitis Hemorrhagic cystitis Pinworms Schistosomiasis Urethritis Urinary tract infection Vulvovaginitis	Pyelonephritis Reactive arthritis Renal stones Stevens–Johnson syndrome Turpentine
Minor Trauma	
Abrasion/laceration Foreign body (tampon, toilet paper, condom, etc) Masturbation Sexual activity Straddle injury	
Anatomic	
Urethral stricture/meatal stenosis Posterior urethral valves Labial adhesions	
Behavioral/Functional	
Dysfunctional voiding Psychogenic	

Systemic Causes

Pyelonephritis or upper urinary tract disease usually presents with evidence of systemic illness including fever greater than 39° C. PE reveals flank pain and tenderness. Patients with Stevens–Johnson syndrome (SJS) may have erosive lesions of the GU mucosal surfaces and may complain of dysuria or the inability to void. Reactive arthritis (ReA), formerly known as Reiter syndrome, classically presents as the triad of arthritis, urethritis, and conjunctivitis, occurring several days or weeks after an enteric or urogenital infection. Bacteria that have been associated with ReA include *Shigella, Salmonella, Chlamydia trachomatis, Yersinia,* and *Clostridium difficile.* ReA is rare in the pediatric population and usually occurs after an enteric infection, until the adolescent age group when it more often follows a urogenital infection. The urethritis is culture negative because it is postinfectious in nature, and may cause dysuria or pelvic pain.

Behçet syndrome is a multisystem inflammatory disease characterized by recurrent aphthous ulcers, genital ulcers of varying size with yellow necrotic center and surrounding erythema, and uveitis. Genital lesions generally occur after oral lesions and are less painful. The lesions commonly occur in the scrotum in boys and the vulva in girls. Genital lesions often heal with scarring.

Any obstructive uropathy (renal calculi, posterior urethral valves, etc) can have ongoing illness with fever, dysuria, and ultimately renal failure. Posterior urethral valves are obstructing membranous folds within the lumen of the posterior urethra that are the most common causative factor of urinary tract obstruction in the male newborn. Renal stones present with dysuria, fever, flank pain, vomiting, and the child or adolescent will appear systemically ill. Rarely, patients with a malignancy (e.g., Wilms tumor) may present with dysuria and hematuria.

In dysuria-hematuria syndrome, the child complains of dysuria, but the urine is negative for infection but positive for microscopic or gross hematuria. This syndrome is most commonly seen in children of the toilet training age and may reflect hypercalciuria. The cause of this idiopathic hypercalciuria is not known. In children with hypercalciuria, microcrystallization of calcium with urinary anions may result in injury to the uroepithelium with resultant dysuria, incontinence, or UTI. There may be an association with skeletal diseases, nephrolithiasis, malignancy, human immunodeficiency virus, or medications (e.g., vitamin D supplements, furosemide loop diuretics).

Antidepressants, both cyclic and selective serotonin reuptake inhibitors, may produce GU adverse effects including dysuria, frequency, retention, and incontinence. The ingestion of turpentine, a hydrocarbon, can result in dysuria and hematuria.

EVALUATION

History

The child with dysuria requires a complete history and PE. The differential is broad, and historical clues and PE findings can help guide the workup.

It is important to ask about minor trauma, though it may not be recalled in young children or may be denied in the setting of sexual abuse or masturbation. A careful history must be obtained in children with straddle injuries and then the mechanism of injury correlated with the physical findings to rule out sexual assault.

First, ask about exposure to potential chemical and mechanical irritants. Obtain detailed information about other urinary symptoms in addition to the dysuria, such as frequency, urgency, hesitancy, and stream. In the toilet-trained child, ask about length of dryness after training, any day or nighttime wetting, and leakage. Elicit information about voiding patterns, such as holding behaviors, frequent voiding, and postponement of voiding. In girls, it is important to ask about symptoms of vaginitis such as itching, irritation, burning, and redness. In boys and girls, ask whether discharge is present, and if so, inquire about color, amount, and odor. Inquire about prior UTIs, known vesicoureteral reflux (VUR), neurogenic bladder, previously undiagnosed febrile illness, and constipation. Signs and symptoms of UTI vary by age and are listed in Table 2.

(Continued on page 254)

ALGORITHM 2: EVALUATION FOR UTI

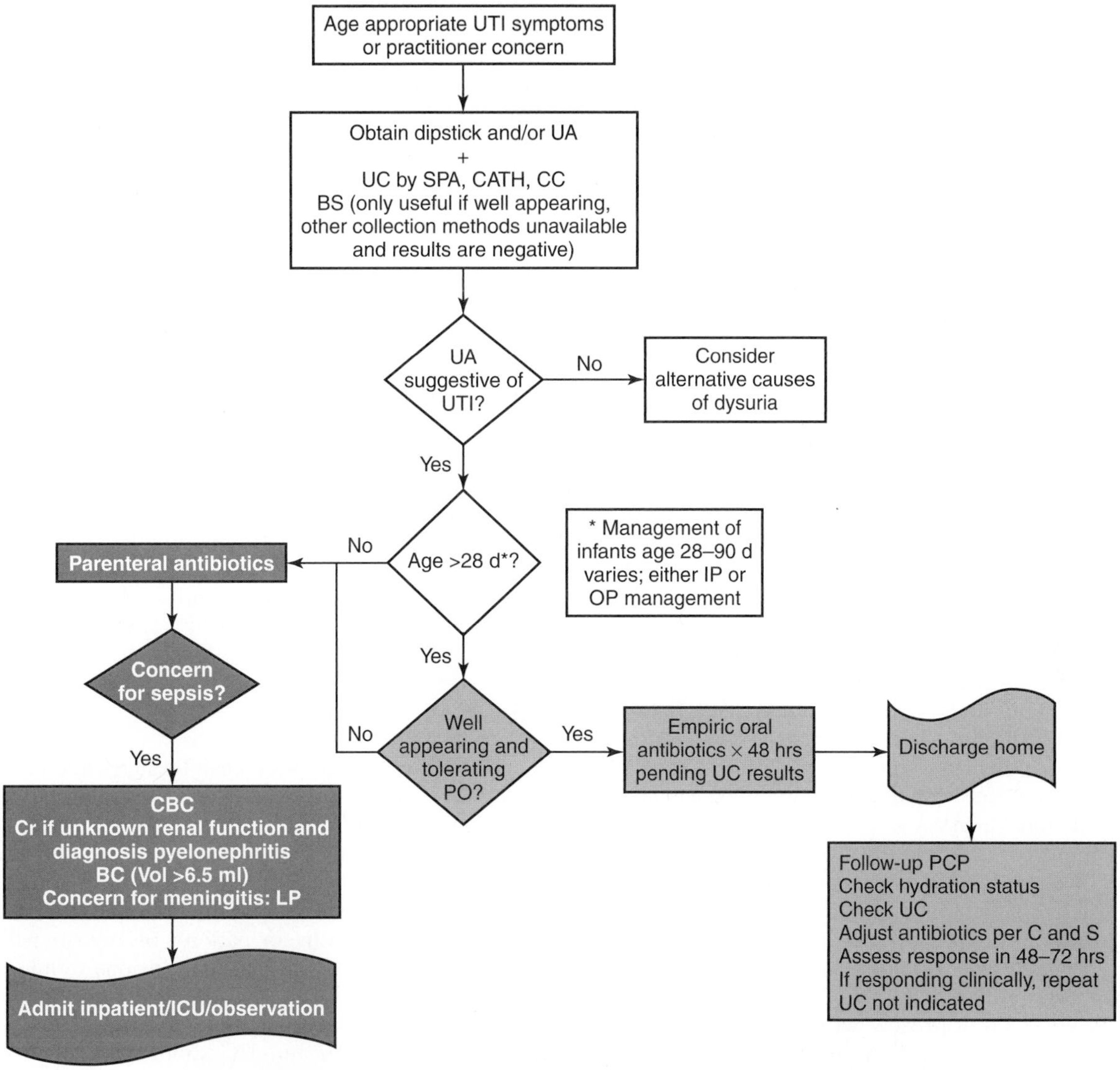

Age appropriate UTI symptoms or practitioner concern
Obtain dipstick and/or UA + UC by SPA, CATH, CC BS (only useful if well appearing, other collection methods unavailable and results are negative)
UA suggestive of UTI?
No
Consider alternative causes of dysuria
Yes
Age >28 d*?
* Management of infants age 28–90 d varies; either IP or OP management
No
Parenteral antibiotics
Concern for sepsis?
Yes
CBC
Cr if unknown renal function and diagnosis pyelonephritis
BC (Vol >6.5 ml)
Concern for meningitis: LP
Admit inpatient/ICU/observation
Yes
No
Well appearing and tolerating PO?
Yes
Empiric oral antibiotics × 48 hrs pending UC results
Discharge home
Follow-up PCP
Check hydration status
Check UC
Adjust antibiotics per C and S
Assess response in 48–72 hrs
If responding clinically, repeat UC not indicated

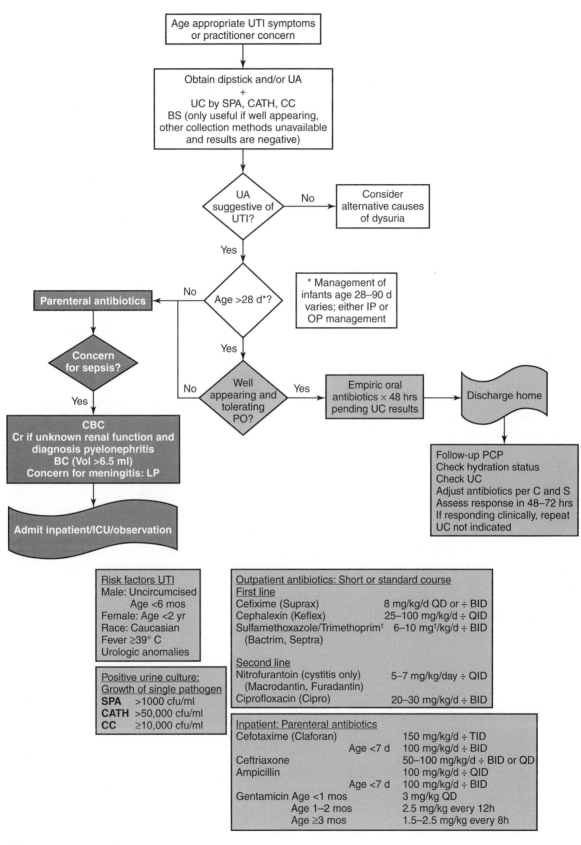

Risk factors UTI
- Male: Uncircumcised, Age <6 mos
- Female: Age <2 yr
- Race: Caucasian
- Fever ≥39° C
- Urologic anomalies

Positive urine culture: Growth of single pathogen

SPA	>1000 cfu/ml
CATH	>50,000 cfu/ml
CC	≥10,000 cfu/ml

Outpatient antibiotics: Short or standard course

First line	
Cefixime (Suprax)	8 mg/kg/d QD or ÷ BID
Cephalexin (Keflex)	25–100 mg/kg/d ÷ QID
Sulfamethoxazole/Trimethoprim[†] (Bactrim, Septra)	6–10 mg[†]/kg/d ÷ BID
Second line	
Nitrofurantoin (cystitis only) (Macrodantin, Furadantin)	5–7 mg/kg/day ÷ QID
Ciprofloxacin (Cipro)	20–30 mg/kg/d ÷ BID

Inpatient: Parenteral antibiotics

Cefotaxime (Claforan)		150 mg/kg/d ÷ TID
	Age <7 d	100 mg/kg/d ÷ BID
Ceftriaxone		50–100 mg/kg/d ÷ BID or QD
Ampicillin		100 mg/kg/d ÷ QID
	Age <7 d	100 mg/kg/d ÷ BID
Gentamicin	Age <1 mos	3 mg/kg QD
	Age 1–2 mos	2.5 mg/kg every 12h
	Age ≥3 mos	1.5–2.5 mg/kg every 8h

[†]Dosing is based on Trimethoprim component

Table 2. **Signs and Symptoms of Urinary Tract Infection by Age**

<3 mo	3 mo to 3 yr	3–10 yr
Fever	Fever	Fever/chills
FTT	FTT	Frequency
Loose stool	Diarrhea	Hematuria
Vomiting	Vomiting	Vomiting
Jaundice	Strong smell urine	Strong smell urine
Poor feeding	Abdominal/flank pain	Abdominal/flank pain
Irritability	Urinary incontinence	Urinary incontinence
	Dysuria	Dysuria
	Urgency	Urgency
	Suprapubic discomfort	Suprapubic discomfort
	CVA discomfort	CVA discomfort

CVA, costovertebral angle.

In adolescents, obtaining a sexual history is crucial to inquire about sexual activity, number of partners, history of prior sexually transmitted infections (STIs), condom use, and use of over-the-counter products, such as spermicidal agents, douches, and creams.

When a child has dysuria in addition to systemic symptoms, it is important to rule out significant systemic illness including SJS, ReA, Behçet syndrome, pelvic inflammatory disease (PID), and pyelonephritis. In this case, inquire for the presence of prodromal complaints (fever, sore throat, chills, headache, malaise, vomiting, and diarrhea) or systemic symptoms (rash, swollen joints, mucocutaneous lesions, abdominal pain).

The clinical presentation of posterior urethral valve is variable and often is diagnosed on prenatal ultrasound. In neonates, query anuria, poor or dribbling urine stream, abdominal distention, or failure to thrive. Severely affected male infants may present with urosepsis, dehydration, electrolyte abnormalities, or failure to thrive. Toddlers often present with voiding dysfunction or UTI, and school-age boys usually are identified because of urinary incontinence.

PHYSICAL EXAMINATION

The PE should target the abdominal and GU areas. It is also essential to evaluate skin, mucous membranes, joints, and spine for signs of systemic infection. The abdomen should be palpated for the presence of a mass or tenderness, including costovertebral angle (CVA) tenderness and suprapubic tenderness. GU examination can be diagnostic and direct the remainder of the evaluation. It is important to ensure patient comfort and maximum visualization. In girls, the GU examination is best performed in the lithotomy position for adolescents and in the frog leg position for younger children. Good lighting is essential. Palpate for inguinal lymphadenopathy. Examine the external genitalia of girls for erythema, edema, excoriations, abrasions, and bruising. In boys, inspect the penis for redness, lesions, discharge, and size of the urethral opening. Visualize the rectum in boy and girls, and the scrotum in boys. In girls, inspect the vaginal introitus for erythema, foreign body, lesions such as vesicles, and the presence of discharge. Remember that the vagina in prepubertal girls is normally more reddened, becoming lighter pink after puberty. Evaluate for the presence of discharge. Discharge can be normal in adolescent girls. This physiologic discharge is usually clear to white and does not stick to the vaginal walls, but rather accumulates in the posterior fornix. In sexually active adolescent girls, a speculum must be used to visualize the cervix. A bimanual examination, including evaluating for cervical motion tenderness, is also needed if evaluating for PID (see Sexually Transmitted Infections, p. 62).

Most straddle injuries are superficial, unilateral, and often involve the anterior portion of the genitalia in both girls and boys. Most straddle injuries in girls involve the mons, clitoral hood, and labia minora anterior or lateral to the hymen. Straddle injury to the hymen or posterior fourchette is rare and should raise the specter of sexual assault. Knowledge of normal hymenal variants is crucial for the distinction between normal and abnormal findings. Examination of straddle injuries can be hampered by pain and anxiety. Anxiolysis and local pain control (2% lidocaine jelly) may be needed for moderate injury, whereas procedural sedation and analgesia or general anesthesia may be necessary for complex injuries.

Clinical Evaluation

Many of the causes of dysuria can be suggested by history, in the case of irritant exposure, or PE in the case of trauma, foreign body, or anatomic disorders. However, in certain cases, further laboratory testing and evaluation will be needed to confirm the cause.

Febrile girls younger than 2 years, febrile boys younger than 6 months, or patients of any age with dysuria in the absence of discharge or lesions should have a urinalysis (UA) and urine culture (UC) obtained. Even in patients with historical findings suggestive of dysfunctional voiding, a UA and UC should be obtained, because patients may have a concomitant UTI. The presence of labial adhesions may present a quandary because these are usually asymptomatic; thus, a UA and UC should be obtained to rule out infection as a cause of the symptoms. Notably, there is considerable overlap in the patient's report of symptoms of vulvovaginitis and UTIs in girls. It is reasonable to start with a UA and UC, but keep in mind that pyuria is not specific for UTI. In sexually active girls with dysuria and abnormal discharge, testing for sexually transmitted diseases (STDs) and other vaginal infections should be strongly considered (see Vaginitis, p. 248).

Evaluation of balanitis or balanoposthitis in boys is usually clinical. If a history of irritants is elicited, no further testing may be needed. Gram stain and bacterial culture and potassium hydroxide (KOH) prep can be done to distinguish streptococcal and candidal infections. Sometimes it may be difficult to distinguish true urethral discharge from exudate or transudate of the foreskin associated with balanoposthitis. In sexually active adolescent boys with dysuria and abnormal discharge, a wet mount, Gram stain, and STI testing should be performed (see Sexually Transmitted Infections, p. 62).

Laboratory Evaluation

Diagnostic studies for potential UTI include a UA and UC. Indications for a UA are outlined in Table 3.

Appropriate mechanisms for collection are outlined in Table 4. In non–toilet-trained children, specimens ideally are obtained by suprapubic aspiration (SPA) or catheterization (CATH). In this group, bag specimens (BS) are useful only in well-appearing infants and children when other collection methods are unavailable and results are negative. If results are positive or sample is contaminated, a specimen obtained by SPA, CATH, or clean catch (CC) is necessary for accurate diagnosis. For toilet-trained patients, a CC specimen may be used with appropriate cleaning technique.

UA can be obtained by one of three methods: dipstick, standard, or enhanced as detailed in Table 5. A dipstick UA is easy and readily available. The presence of leukocyte esterase is suggestive of a UTI but not diagnostic. Nitrite is highly specific, but a negative test is not reliable. Always send a UC if dipstick negative but high clinical suspicion of a UTI. Remember that the presence of pyuria is nonspecific and can occur in conditions other than UTI, such as appendicitis, STI, trauma, foreign body, chemical irritation, or systemic illnesses associated with urethritis.

A UC is the gold standard for diagnosis of a UTI. A positive UC is defined as the growth of a single pathogen with colony counts meeting one of three criteria: >1000 colony-forming units (cfu)/ml from UC obtained by SPA, >50,000 cfu/ml from UC obtained by CATH, or >100,000 cfu/ml from high-quality midstream CC. Organisms associated with UTIs are detailed in Table 6.

The distinction between yeast and streptococcal diaper dermatitis is usually based on PE findings and a trial of empiric treatment. However, if the diagnosis is in question, a culture of the perineal area can be sent for streptococcal testing. The cellophane tape test can be used to diagnose pinworms. The tape is touched to the perineal area on awakening on three consecutive mornings. The tape is examined under the microscope for pinworm eggs.

Behçet syndrome may be suspected from the history and other systemic symptoms. However, it is reasonable to send samples from vesicular or ulcerative lesions to rule out herpes infection. ReA is generally suggested by constellation of clinical findings in the setting of a recent infection. It is prudent to ensure that patient has a "sterile" urethritis and to send appropriate testing for STDs. The diagnosis of SJS is usually clinical.

Dysuria-hematuria syndrome should be evaluated with a 24-hour urine, calcium, and creatinine excretion. In patients with an unrevealing PE and negative UA, possible causes include dysfunctional voiding, pinworms, or psychogenic.

Table 3. **Indications for a Urinalysis**

<2 mo	All febrile infants or if parental concern about crying with urination
2 mo to 2 yr	Fever ≥2 days without source with or without dysuria
>2 yr	Girls with dysuria and urinary symptoms

Table 4. **Mechanism of Urine Collection**

Suprapubic aspiration (SPA): most reliable
- Use for labial or penile adhesions
- Catheterized specimen inconclusive

Catheterization of bladder (CATH): alternative to SPA
Clean Catch (CC): toilet-trained and appropriate cleaning technique
Bag specimens (BS): useful only if well appearing, other collection methods unavailable, and results are negative; if results are positive or sample contaminated, need to obtain urine via SPA, CATH, or CC for diagnosis

TREATMENT

Treatment should be directed at the underlying cause. If an irritant cause is identified, it should be removed. If an infectious causative agent is found, antibiotics should be directed toward the underlying infection. If an anatomic defect or dysfunctional voiding is found, the patient should be referred to urology. Traumatic injuries usually require supportive care. Treatment of the systemic causes of dysuria such as SJS, Behçet syndrome, or ReA is beyond the scope of this chapter.

Table 5. **Urinalysis Methods**

Characteristics	Dipstick	Standard	Enhanced
Mechanism	Dipstick	Centrifuged urine, no Gram stain	Uncentrifuged urine + Gram stain + hemocytometer
Pyuria	Leukocyte esterase: suggestive but not diagnostic for urinary tract infection	≥5 white blood cells/high-power field (WBC/HPF)	≥10 WBC/mm^3
Bacteriuria	Nitrite: highly specific but negative test not reliable	Any bacteria/HPF (but correlates poorly with Gram stain and culture)	Any bacteria/10 oil immersion fields of Gram-stained urine
Sensitivity	Moderate 88% but not specific	Low <81%	Optimal sensitivity and specificity
Availability	Wide	Wide	Limited

If the UA and clinical evaluation are suggestive of infection, it is reasonable to start antibiotics pending culture results. Oral antibiotics are appropriate for simple cystitis as detailed in Table 7. In patients with pyelonephritis, the decision to start oral versus intravenous (IV) antibiotics depends on the age of the patient and the severity of illness. In general, infants younger than 28 days warrant hospitalization and IV therapy, whereas those age 28 to 90 days may be treated as outpatients or inpatients. Patients of any age with pyelonephritis who are vomiting, are dehydrated, have severe abdominal pain, or are otherwise ill appearing should be hospitalized. Initial antibiotics in the hospital are usually initiated IV and detailed in Table 8. Oral antibiotics can be considered in the hospital setting if there is no concern for sepsis or meningitis, patient has normal renal function, is not immunosuppressed, and can tolerate oral medication and fluids. Other supportive therapies should be given as needed, such as IV fluids or antipyretics.

Table 6. Organisms Associated with a Urinary Tract Infection

Gram-Negative Organisms

Escherichia coli (most common, >80% first UTI)
Klebsiella spp. (next most common organism)
Proteus spp.
Pseudomonas spp. (<2 %)
Enterobacter spp. (<2 %)

Gram-Positive Organisms

Enterococcus spp.
Coagulase-negative staphylococcus
Staphylococcus aureus
Group B streptococci

Fungal

Candida spp. (usually in premature infants)

Organisms Considered Contaminants

Lactobacillus spp.
Corynebacterium spp.
Coagulase-negative staphylococci
Micrococcus
Diphtheroids
Bacillus spp.

In patients in whom initial antibiotic therapy is IV, transition can be made to oral antibiotics after 3 to 5 days or once fever begins to defervesce. However, no randomized, controlled trials address the length of IV treatment in patients younger than 28 days. It appears safe to give IV antibiotics for 3 to 5 days if there is no meningitis and the patient is clinically improving.

A patient who is well appearing with pyelonephritis and can tolerate oral medications can be treated as an outpatient with oral antibiotics. Several studies have shown that oral antibiotics are equivalent to IV antibiotics in terms of time to symptom improvement, urine sterility, and renal scarring. In addition, an initial dose of intramuscular ceftriaxone in patients who will be treated on an outpatient basis does not hasten clinical improvement or prevent admission. Pyridium can be added in children older than 6 years to relieve symptoms of dysuria.

The choice of initial antibiotic therapy depends on the susceptibility patterns in your area. For options, see Tables 7 and 8. Antibiotic therapy may need to be adjusted based on the culture results and sensitivity testing. In patients with simple cystitis or lower UTI, a short course (2–4 days) of antibiotics has been shown to be as effective as the standard course (7–14 days). For pyelonephritis, the total duration of therapy should be 10 to 14 days. Repeat UC is not needed if responsive to therapy.

Irritant diaper dermatitis can be treated with topical zinc oxide or products that contain petrolatum. The treatment of candidal diaper rash or balanitis is topical antifungals. The first-line treatment of pinworms is mebendazole. Patients can be retreated in 2 weeks if symptoms persist. Household contacts must also be treated and bedding must be washed. The treatment of streptococcal infections of the GU area such as balanitis or perianal infection is amoxicillin/clavulanate because there may be other beta-lactam–resistant bacteria colonizing the perineal skin.

Because many cases of labial adhesions spontaneously resolve, they often can be managed with observation alone. However, if treatment is indicated, a topical estrogen cream may be used. If conservative management does not result in resolution of the adhesions, referral to a urologist may be considered. For treatment of STIs, PID, and vaginitis, see Sexually Transmitted Infections (p. 62).

Table 7. Outpatient Therapy: Oral Antibiotics for Urinary Tract Infection

First Line	
Cefixime (Suprax)	8 mg/kg/day once daily or divided bid
Cephalexin (Keflex)	25–100 mg/kg/day divided qid
Sulfamethoxazole/Trimethoprim* (Bactrim, Septra)	6–10 mg*/kg/day divided bid
Second Line	
Nitrofurantoin (cystitis only) (Macrodantin, Furadantin)	5–7 mg/kg/day divided qid
Ciprofloxacin (Cipro)	20–30 mg/kg/day divided bid

*Trimethoprim component

Table 8. Inpatient Therapy: Parenteral Antibiotics for Urinary Tract Infection

Cefotaxime (Claforan)	150 mg/kg/day divided tid
Age <7 days	100 mg/kg/day divided bid
Ceftriaxone	50–100 mg/kg/day divided bid or once daily
Ampicillin	100 mg/kg/day divided qid
Age <7 days	100 mg/kg/day divided bid
Gentamicin	
Age <1 month	3 mg/kg once daily
Age 1–2 months	2.5 mg/kg every 12h
Age ≥3 months	1.5–2.5 mg/kg every 8h

References

American Academy of Pediatrics. Practice parameter: the diagnosis, treatment, and evaluation of the initial urinary tract infection in febrile infants and young children. American Academy of Pediatrics, Committee on Quality Improvement, Subcommittee on Urinary Tract Infection. Pediatrics 1999;103:843-52 [erratum appears in 2000 Jan;105(1 Pt 1):141].

Baker PC, Nelson DS, Schunk JE. The addition of ceftriaxone to oral therapy does not improve outcome in febrile children with urinary tract infections. Arch Pediatr Adolesc Med 2001;155:135–9.

Bouissou F, Munzer C, Decramer S, et al. Prospective, randomized trial comparing short and long intravenous antibiotic treatment of acute pyelonephritis in children: dimercaptosuccinic acid scintigraphic evaluation at 9 months. Pediatrics 2008;121:e553–60.

Chang SL, Shortliffe LD. Pediatric urinary tract infections. Pediatr Clin North Am 2006;53:379–400.

Dore-Bergeron MJ, Gauthier M, Chevalier I, et al. Urinary tract infections in 1- to 3-month-old infants: ambulatory treatment with intravenous antibiotics. Pediatrics 2009;124:16–22.

Downs SM. Technical report: urinary tract infections in febrile infants and young children. The Urinary Tract Subcommittee of the American Academy of Pediatrics Committee on Quality Improvement. Pediatrics 1999;103:e54.

Gorelick MH, Shaw KN. Screening tests for urinary tract infection in children: a meta-analysis. Pediatrics 1999;104:e54.

Hoberman A, Wald ER. Treatment of urinary tract infections. Pediatr Infect Dis J 1999;18:1020–1.

Huicho L, Campos-Sanchez M, Alamo C. Metaanalysis of urine screening tests for determining the risk of urinary tract infection in children. Pediatr Infect Dis J 2002;21:1–11.

Magin EC, et al. Efficacy of short-term intravenous antibiotic in neonates with urinary tract infection. Pediatr Emerg Care 2007;23:83–6.

Newman TB, et al. Urine testing and urinary tract infections in febrile infants seen in office settings: the Pediatric Research in Office Settings' Febrile Infant Study. Arch Pediatr Adolesc Med 2002;156:44–54.

Pohl A. Modes of administration of antibiotics for symptomatic severe urinary tract infections. Cochrane Database Syst Rev 2007;CD003237.

Shaw KN, Gorelick MH. Urinary tract infection in the pediatric patient. Pediatr Clin North Am 1999;46:1111–24.

Hematuria

Nimisha Amin, MD, and Joshua J. Zaritsky, MD, PhD

Microscopic hematuria can be a common finding within a general pediatric practice and is generally benign in nature. Gross hematuria is much more distressing to the patient (and physician), but fortunately is not quite as common. The purpose of this chapter is to review the definition, common causes and evaluation of hematuria. This chapter also provides guidelines as to when a referral to a pediatric nephrologist is warranted.

DEFINITION

Hematuria refers to the presence of blood in the urine, as defined as more than 5 to 10 red blood cells per high-power field (RBC/hpf). A urine dipstick analysis is a highly sensitive measure for detection of blood, but it lacks specificity. This translates into a large number of false positives, in which case, the urine dipstick is positive, but microscopy reveals fewer than 5 to 10 RBC/hpf. This particular combination can be seen in the following benign or pathologic circumstances:

1. Ingestion of certain foods: beets, blackberries, food coloring
2. Ingestion of certain medications: chloroquine, ibuprofen, iron, sorbitol, nitrofurantoin, phenazopyridine, urates or rifampin (which often produces orange urine)
3. Hemoglobinuria: often in the setting of hemolytic anemia
4. Myoglobinuria: related to muscle damage (rhabdomyolysis), often after vigorous exercise or trauma
5. Urinary tract infection: secondary to the action of bacterial peroxidases on the dipstick
6. Delay in reading urine dipstick after submersion in urine

Given the large number of situations in which a positive dipstick may not represent true hematuria, all urine samples that test positive on dipstick analysis must be sent for microscopy to confirm hematuria. This applies in the setting of gross hematuria (where the urine may appear red, pink, amber, tea-colored, or brown) or with routine dipstick screening at well-child examinations.

CAUSES

The differential diagnosis for hematuria is extensive and is summarized in Table 1. The following discussion highlights some key features of the more common diagnoses. Overall, the most common causes for hematuria in children include urinary tract infection, benign familial hematuria, IgA nephropathy, and idiopathic hypercalciuria.

Table 1. **Causes of Hematuria in Children**

Benign Causes
Benign familial hematuria ("Thin basement membrane disease")
Transient conditions: exercise, dehydration, fever
Glomerulonephritis
With hypocomplementemia:
Postinfectious glomerulonephritis (PIGN)
Membranoproliferative glomerulonephritis (MPGN)
Systemic lupus erythematosus (SLE)
With normal complement levels:
IgA nephropathy
Alport syndrome
Henoch–Schönlein purpura (HSP)
Wegener granulomatosis
Goodpasture syndrome
Pauci-immune crescentic glomerulonephritis
Lower Urinary Tract Causes
Urinary tract infection/viral hemorrhagic cystitis
Nephrolithiasis
Trauma or foreign body
Hypercalciuria
Idiopathic
Drug induced (furosemide, corticosteroids)
Metabolic disorders
Dent's disease
Bartter syndrome
Wilson disease
Glycogen storage disease type 1a
Distal renal tubular acidosis (RTA)
Anatomic/Vascular Abnormalities
Hydronephrosis
Ureteropelvic junction obstruction
Arteriovenous malformation
Nutcracker syndrome
Renal vein thrombosis (neonates)
Hemolytic-uremic syndrome (HUS)
Cystic Kidney Disease
Autosomal recessive or dominant polycystic kidney disease
Multicystic dysplastic kidney
Others
Sickle cell trait, disease: papillary necrosis
Drugs/toxins (cyclophosphamide)
Wilms' tumor
Coagulopathy

Similar to proteinuria, benign and transient causes exist, and they should be considered early in the investigation. Examples of transient causes of hematuria include exercise, dehydration, and fever.

Hematuria associated with low complement levels is restricted to a few specific diagnoses, the most common of which are postinfectious glomerulonephritis, lupus nephritis, or membranoproliferative glomerulonephritis. In postinfectious glomerulonephritis, the patient classically develops tea-colored urine approximately 1 to 2 weeks after an episode of group A streptococcus pharyngitis or 3 to 4 weeks after streptococcal impetigo. C3 will initially be depressed, whereas C4 is usually normal. C3 will then normalize in the next 6 weeks after initial presentation with gross hematuria. Microscopic hematuria may be present for up to 2 years after initial presentation. Membranoproliferative glomerulonephritis and lupus nephritis will also cause hematuria and are associated with both low C3 and C4.

Among the remainder of normocomplementemic glomerulonephritides that cause hematuria, IgA nephropathy and benign familial hematuria are by far the most common. In contrast with the painless gross hematuria seen with postinfectious glomerulonephritis, IgA nephropathy will produce a "synpharyngitic" gross hematuria, which is occasionally painful.

Benign familial hematuria ("thin basement membrane disease") is an autosomal dominant condition often found in the setting of a well child (with normal growth, blood pressure, and laboratory workup) with family members who also have microscopic hematuria. When there is a negative family workup, it remains a diagnosis of exclusion. As the name implies, it is generally a benign condition; however, it does exist along a spectrum of disease related to Alport syndrome, given similar findings on renal biopsy and disruptions of the gene encoding collagen 4. A patient with Alport syndrome may present with gross or microscopic hematuria, in addition to a strong family history of renal disease, sensorineural hearing loss, or anterior lenticonus on ocular examination. Progression to end-stage renal disease ultimately occurs in nearly all affected males with Alport syndrome, while female carriers tend to have more mild disease.

Some glomerulonephritides causing hematuria will initially present with more pronounced systemic manifestations, such as hemoptysis (Wegener granulomatosis, Goodpasture disease), abdominal pain (Henoch–Schönlein purpura), or joint pains/rash (Henoch–Schönlein purpura, lupus).

Hematuria secondary to hypercalciuria is also quite common in the pediatric population and is defined as urinary calcium level of more than 4 mg/kg/day in a 24-hour urine sample or increase of the urinary calcium-to-creatinine ratio as follows: >0.8 in infants younger than 6 months, >0.6 in infants 6 to 12 months of age, or >0.2 in children age 2 and older. Idiopathic hypercalciuria likely develops secondary to a number of genetic and environmental factors, and can result in nephrocalcinosis or nephrolithiasis. Initial management is with sodium restriction and increased oral hydration.

Hematuria in association with a palpable mass on abdominal examination is a less frequently encountered condition but should not be overlooked. It may be reflective of Wilms' tumor, autosomal recessive polycystic kidney disease, multicystic dysplastic kidney, ureteropelvic junction obstruction, or severe hydronephrosis.

Rare vascular abnormalities, both structural and functional, may also cause hematuria. Structural anomalies include renal arteriovenous malformation or Nutcracker syndrome, in which the left renal vein is compressed between the abdominal aorta and superior mesenteric artery. Functional vascular abnormalities causing hematuria include hemolytic-uremic syndrome or renal vein thrombosis (typically seen in neonates).

Within the category of lower urinary tract conditions that can result in hematuria, viral hemorrhagic cystitis, trauma, or a urethral foreign body usually produce gross hematuria, whereas urinary tract infections and nephrolithiasis can result in either gross or microscopic hematuria.

EVALUATION

Two important principles relating to hematuria should be understood before the evaluation process is initiated:

1. In the asymptomatic well child with microscopic hematuria on a single urine specimen, repeat testing should be performed on at least 2 or more specimens, obtain ≥1 week apart. The rationale for this recommendation is based on studies of school-age children with hematuria on initial inspection, which disappears with subsequent testing.
2. When a child has gross hematuria, urinalysis may also help distinguish between glomerular and lower urinary tract bleeding. Hematuria secondary to glomerulonephritis often produces brown or tea-colored urine, with dysmorphic RBCs or RBC casts on microscopy. Conversely, lower urinary tract bleeding will result in red or pink urine, possibly with frank blood clots. Microscopy will reveal intact RBCs. If hematuria is noted only during a certain portion of the urinary stream (early or terminal), it is also more likely related to a lower urinary tract abnormality.

As noted earlier, it is unlikely that isolated microscopic hematuria in an otherwise well child is indicative of malignant renal disease, which would require immediate intervention. Hence the evaluation of hematuria is best performed in stepwise progression, beginning with simple and noninvasive investigations, followed by more aggressive interventions if positive results are obtained.

A. The first phase of investigation should include a thorough history and physical, and detailed urinary testing. Circumstances surrounding hematuria should be investigated, including history of strenuous exercise, fever, dehydration, recent ingestions as noted earlier, prior or concomitant infections, trauma, associated symptoms (abdominal, flank or urethral pain, dysuria, nausea, vomiting), frequency of hematuria and exact color of the urine. Constitutional and lupus-like symptoms should also be inquired about. Family history should include questioning about specific renal conditions (microscopic or gross hematuria, nephrolithiasis, lupus, end-stage renal disease, transplant, sickle cell disease, coagulopathies) and congenital hearing loss. If the family history is positive, consider obtaining urinalyses on family members.

B. Physical examination should be comprehensive, paying close attention to blood pressure, growth parameters, temperature, joint and skin examination (for arthritis or rash), abdominal examination for masses, and genital examination for evidence or trauma, discharge, or meatal stenosis. Accurate blood pressure assessment is critical in this phase of the workup because it may be the only sign of more significant renal disease.

C. From the patient's urine, initial evaluation should include urinalysis (with microscopic evaluation), urine culture, and urine calcium-to-creatinine ratio. If this entire portion of the evaluation is unremarkable, repeat urinalysis in 4 to 6 weeks is sufficient.

Should the history and physical be concerning for any reason (or if repeat urinalysis continues to show hematuria), the next level of investigation includes blood testing, but can also be tiered pending which portion of the history and physical is positive. Specific tests in this category include serum electrolytes, blood urea nitrogen/creatine (BUN/Cr), complete blood cell count, complement levels (C3 and C4), antinuclear antibody, anti–double-stranded DNA, and antistreptolysin titers. If concern exists about an abdominal mass or nephrolithiasis, a renal ultrasound should be obtained promptly. Also consider a hearing screen at this point, if the family history is suggestive of Alport syndrome.

If the earlier workup is entirely unremarkable, but the child continues with asymptomatic microscopic hematuria, re-evaluate the patient on a yearly basis. These visits should include a new history and physical examination, blood pressure, urinalysis (with microscopy), and serum BUN/Cr.

REFERRAL TO THE PEDIATRIC NEPHROLOGIST

Assistance from a pediatric nephrologist should be sought if certain positive findings during the evaluation are obtained, including strong family history, persistent painful and gross hematuria, concomitant hypertension or proteinuria, hypercalciuria, increased BUN/Cr, hypocomplementemia, positive serologies for lupus, or abnormal renal ultrasound.

References

Gubler MC, Heidt L, Antiganc C. Inherited glomerular disease. In: Avner ED, Harmon EH, Niaudet P, editors. Pediatric nephrology. Philadelphia: Lippincott William & Wilkins; 2004, p. 519–20.
Quigley R. Evaluation of hematuria and proteinuria: how should a pediatrician proceed? Curr Opin Pediatr 2008;20:140–4.
Vehaskari VM, Rapola J, Koskimies O, et al. Microscopic hematuria in school children: epidemiology and clinicopathologic evaluation. J Pediatr 1979;95:676-84.
Yadin O. Hematuria in children. Pediatr Annals 1994;23:475–85.

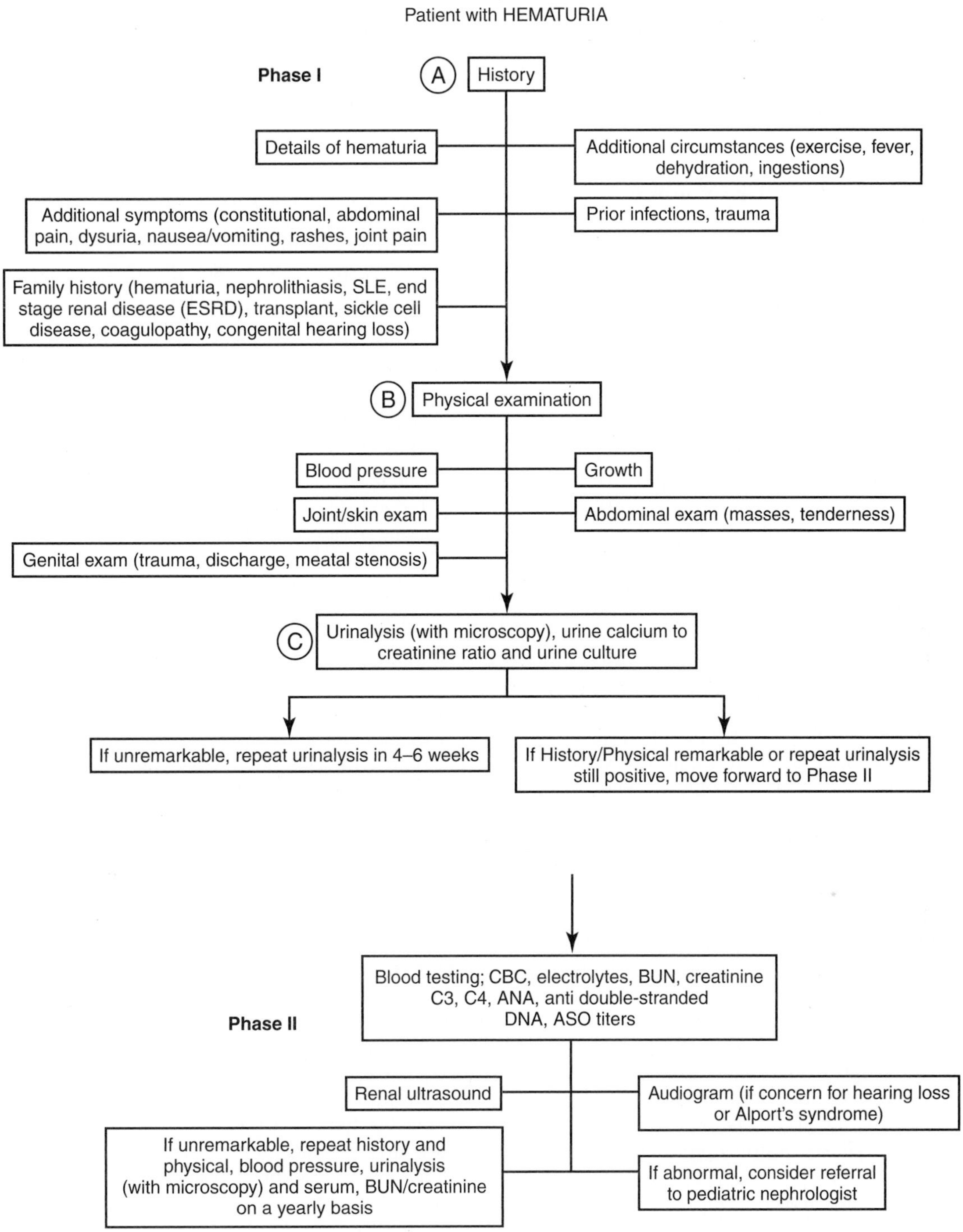

Patient with HEMATURIA
Phase I
A
History
Details of hematuria
Additional circumstances (exercise, fever, dehydration, ingestions)
Additional symptoms (constitutional, abdominal pain, dysuria, nausea/vomiting, rashes, joint pain
Prior infections, trauma
Family history (hematuria, nephrolithiasis, SLE, end stage renal disease (ESRD), transplant, sickle cell disease, coagulopathy, congenital hearing loss)
B
Physical examination
Blood pressure
Growth
Joint/skin exam
Abdominal exam (masses, tenderness)
Genital exam (trauma, discharge, meatal stenosis)
C
Urinalysis (with microscopy), urine calcium to creatinine ratio and urine culture
If unremarkable, repeat urinalysis in 4–6 weeks
If History/Physical remarkable or repeat urinalysis still positive, move forward to Phase II
Blood testing; CBC, electrolytes, BUN, creatinine C3, C4, ANA, anti double-stranded DNA, ASO titers
Phase II
Renal ultrasound
Audiogram (if concern for hearing loss or Alport's syndrome)
If unremarkable, repeat history and physical, blood pressure, urinalysis (with microscopy) and serum, BUN/creatinine on a yearly basis
If abnormal, consider referral to pediatric nephrologist

Penile Complaints

Kelly Casperson, MD, and Jeffrey B. Campbell, MD

ANOMALY OF PREPUCE/PENILE SHAFT SKIN

A. It is not unusual to encounter both *physiologic phimosis* and residual *preputial adhesions* in a male newborn, each precluding full retraction of the prepuce. Gentle, manual retraction of the prepuce with bathing and physiologic erections will stretch the phimotic ring, facilitating retraction of the prepuce. The natural process of separation of the inner preputial skin from the glans penis typically results in subpreputial accumulation of exfoliated epithelial cells, commonly referred to as *smegma*. The smegma is typically expressed over time as the preputial adhesions spontaneously lyse. The time required to achieve full retraction of the prepuce is variable. Should the patient remain asymptomatic, physiologic phimosis and residual preputial adhesions are of little concern. However, physiologic phimosis can be associated with a number of complications. It is not unusual for the tip of the prepuce to become erythematous on occasion, particularly in a child who is still in diapers. This usually resolves spontaneously. Ballooning of the foreskin with voiding can be a normal finding that typically resolves in time. However, should it be associated with discomfort or recurrent infection, treatment with a topical steroid (betamethasone cream BID × 6 weeks) or circumcision may be considered. Recurrent balanoposthitis (inflammation of the prepuce and glans) is another indication for treatment with either a topical steroid or circumcision. In these cases, referral to a pediatric urologist for evaluation and discussion of the management options is appropriate.

An *incomplete prepuce* is one in which the ventral aspect of the prepuce is incompletely fused. This is commonly seen in association with hypospadias but can be seen in isolation, or in association with ventral penile angulation. The altered anatomy precludes circumcision with the usual techniques used in the newborn period (i.e., Gomco clamp, Mogen clamp, Plastibell). In these cases, referral to a pediatric urologist for evaluation and discussion of the management options is appropriate. In most cases, a circumcision, with or without correction of penile angulation, is performed at 6 months of age, when the procedure can be safely performed as an outpatient procedure.

Examination of the phallus should also include evaluation of the penile raphe. *Deviation of the penile raphe* can be associated with hypospadias, penile angulation, and penile torsion, but can be seen in isolation. Gentle retraction of the prepuce will enable evaluation of the urethral meatus. Should the patient be found to have hypospadias, penile angulation, or more than 45 degrees penile torsion, consultation with a pediatric urologist should be obtained before proceeding with a newborn circumcision.

B. *Postcircumcision preputial adhesions* are commonly encountered after a newborn circumcision. This complication can be avoided by having the child's parents gently sweep the redundant inner preputial and penile shaft skin off the glans penis and apply an antibiotic ointment to the involved tissues with each diaper change for 2 weeks after the circumcision. Unlike physiologic preputial adhesions, postcircumcision preputial adhesions do not typically spontaneously lyse. Indeed, in some cases, the adhesions mature to become preputial skin bridges. Although not typically complicated by infection, the adhesions can result in tethering of the glans penis, particularly with an erection, and can be of some concern cosmetically. One may consider a trial of a steroid cream in an effort to soften the adhesions, enabling manual lysis. Alternatively, a topical anesthetic may be applied to the adhesions, followed by manual lysis in clinic. Successful lysis of the adhesions should be followed by gentle retraction of the redundant inner preputial and penile shaft skin off the glans penis and application of an antibiotic ointment to the involved tissues with each diaper change for 2 weeks. Should these measures fail, referral to a pediatric urologist for evaluation and further management is appropriate.

ANOMALY OF URETHRAL MEATUS

Anomalies of the urethral meatus include hypospadias and meatal stenosis. Although most commonly associated with an incomplete prepuce, *hypospadias* can also be seen in association with an intact prepuce. These cases are often identified at the time of a newborn circumcision. Most of these cases are mild and do not preclude completion of the circumcision. If in doubt, a consultation with a pediatric urologist may be obtained. In more severe cases, the preputial skin may be required for the urethroplasty and/or ventral skin coverage. It is for this reason that a circumcision is typically deferred in patients with more severe forms of hypospadias (i.e., hypospadias with an incomplete prepuce).

Meatal stenosis is a complication of circumcision, often presenting with upward deviation of a high-pressure, narrow-caliber urinary stream, with dysuria localized to the urethral meatus. It is the presence of symptoms, not the appearance of the urethral meatus, that determines the need for intervention, because the apparent caliber of the urethral meatus can often be quite misleading. In these cases, referral to a pediatric urologist for evaluation and discussion of the management options is appropriate.

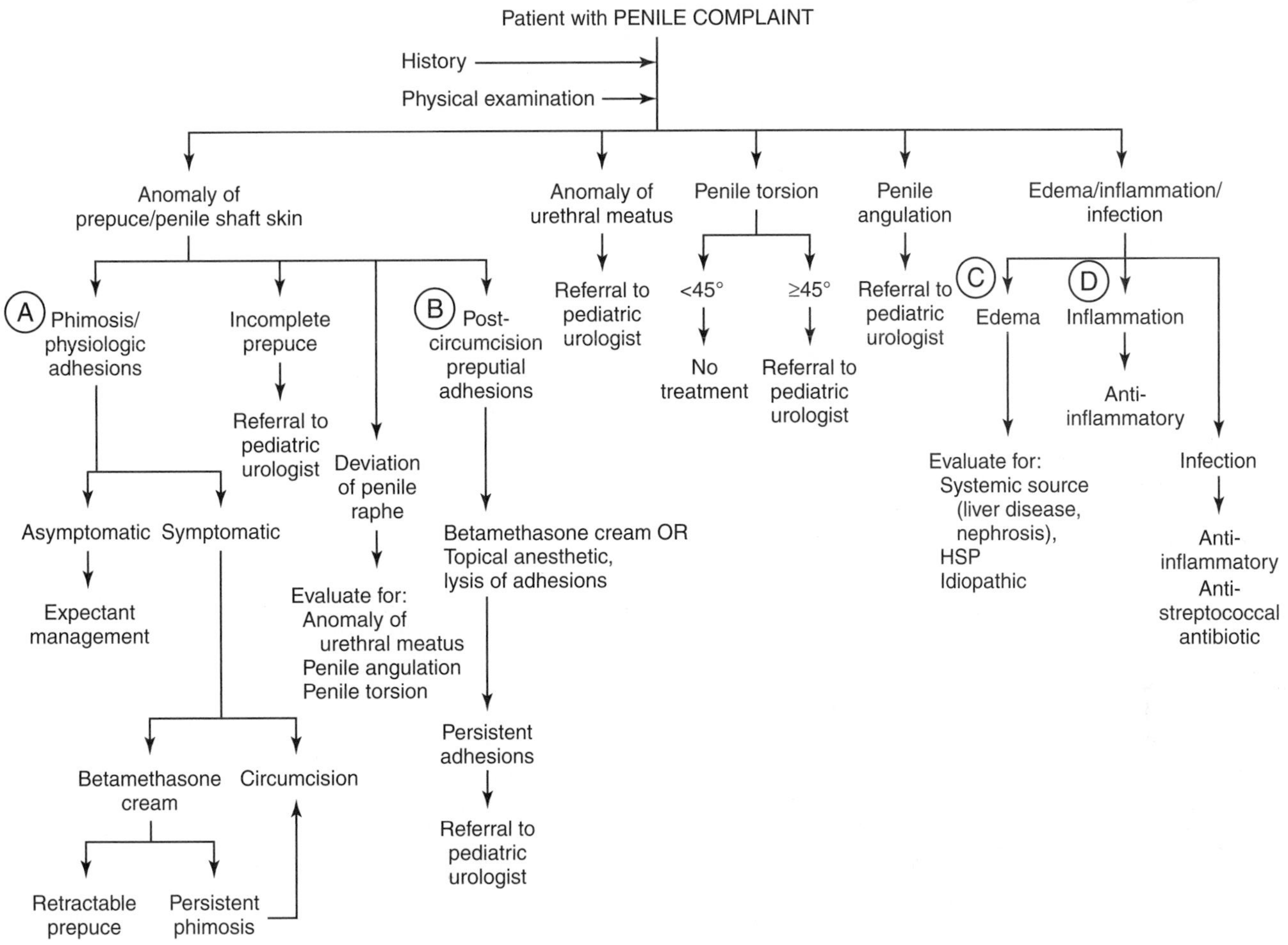
Patient with PENILE COMPLAINT
History
Physical examination
Anomaly of prepuce/penile shaft skin
Anomaly of urethral meatus
Penile torsion
Penile angulation
Edema/inflammation/infection
A Phimosis/physiologic adhesions
Incomplete prepuce
B Post-circumcision preputial adhesions
Referral to pediatric urologist
<45°
≥45°
No treatment
Referral to pediatric urologist
Referral to pediatric urologist
C Edema
D Inflammation
Anti-inflammatory
Referral to pediatric urologist
Deviation of penile raphe
Evaluate for: Systemic source (liver disease, nephrosis), HSP Idiopathic
Infection
Asymptomatic
Symptomatic
Betamethasone cream OR Topical anesthetic, lysis of adhesions
Anti-inflammatory Anti-streptococcal antibiotic
Expectant management
Evaluate for: Anomaly of urethral meatus Penile angulation Penile torsion
Persistent adhesions
Betamethasone cream
Circumcision
Referral to pediatric urologist
Retractable prepuce
Persistent phimosis

Penile Torsion

Penile torsion is best assessed by evaluating the orientation of the urethral meatus. Torsion greater than 45 degrees is thought to be of clinical significance and can be associated with penile angulation. In these cases, referral to a pediatric urologist for evaluation and discussion of the management options is appropriate.

Penile Angulation

Often seen in association with hypospadias, *penile angulation* can also occur in isolation. It is not uncommon, and in many cases, it is not clinically significant. The angulation is most commonly ventral but can be lateral or dorsal in orientation. Both the orientation and degree of angulation play a role in determining the need for surgical correction. The severity of the angulation is difficult to assess when the phallus is flaccid. Accordingly, the history obtained from the parent(s) plays a significant role in determining the need for further evaluation and possible correction of the penile angulation. In these cases, referral to a pediatric urologist for evaluation and discussion of the management options is appropriate.

EDEMA/INFLAMMATION/INFECTION

C. In a child who presents with *penile edema,* one should evaluate for a systemic source (e.g., hepatic, renal) or consider Henoch–Schönlein purpura or an insect bite as the cause. Idiopathic penile edema should be reserved as a diagnosis of exclusion. Management is dictated by the underlying diagnosis.

D. *Inflammation* (i.e., erythema and edema) of the preputial and penile shaft skin (balanoposthitis) can be seen in an uncircumcised phallus in response to local irritation, or secondary to *infection,* in which case purulent discharge may be expressed from beneath the prepuce. In the absence of infection, treatment includes the use of an anti-inflammatory for management of the pain and swelling. If an infection is suspected, the discharge is swabbed and sent for culture and sensitivities, and the infection is treated with an antibiotic that treats streptococcus. Recurrent balanoposthitis is an indication for treatment with either a topical steroid or circumcision. In such cases, referral to a pediatric urologist for evaluation and discussion of the management options is appropriate.

Scrotal Swelling/Pain

Jeffrey B. Campbell, MD

The differential diagnosis of scrotal pain/swelling is both vast and diverse. An approach to the more common causative factors is depicted in the accompanying algorithm. In addition to a thorough history and physical examination, an inguinoscrotal ultrasound (US) can be of some benefit in making a diagnosis. Although there may be some difficulty in differentiating a communicating hydrocele (or hernia) from a noncommunicating hydrocele, perhaps the greatest challenge is in differentiating epididymitis/epididymo-orchitis/orchitis from testicular torsion. Accordingly, the majority of this chapter focuses on these conditions and their management.

A. As the testis descends from the retroperitoneum into the scrotum, it associates with a finger-like projection of the peritoneum referred to as the processus vaginalis (PV). The PV usually obliterates along the course of the spermatic cord, trapping peritoneal fluid around the testis (noncommunicating hydrocele). In most cases, this fluid is gradually reabsorbed, with resolution of the noncommunicating hydrocele by 2 years of age. Should the hydrocele fail to resolve by this time, referral to a pediatric urologist (ped urol) is appropriate.

A noncommunicating hydrocele can also develop in association with trauma to the external genitalia, epididymo-orchitis, or a testicular tumor. In the setting of a *new-onset, noncommunicating* hydrocele, these diagnoses should be considered.

B. If the PV fails to obliterate (patent PV), communication remains between the peritoneal cavity and the scrotum. With increases in intra-abdominal pressure (e.g., crying, straining to have a bowel movement), peritoneal fluid may move into scrotum (communicating hydrocele). The patient's parents often relate a history of *intermittent* scrotal swelling or persistent scrotal swelling that appears to *fluctuate* in size. Given the intermittent nature of the scrotal swelling, a communicating hydrocele is not always appreciated on examination in the physician's office. In an effort to prevent the development of an indirect inguinal hernia and the complications thereof, surgical correction is usually recommended. In such cases, referral to a pediatric urologist is indicated.

C. An indirect inguinal hernia refers to the presence of omentum or bowel within the inguinal canal. The patient usually presents with mild inguinoscrotal discomfort and inguinoscrotal swelling. The hernia usually reduces spontaneously but may require manual reduction. In such cases, referral to a pediatric urologist is indicated. If the hernia cannot be reduced (incarcerated inguinal hernia), urgent consultation with a pediatric surgeon or a pediatric urologist is indicated.

The acute scrotum (acute scrotal pain with or without edema, erythema) should be considered an emergency requiring prompt evaluation and management. The key to successful management is in differentiating between testicular torsion and epididymitis/epididymo-orchitis/orchitis. A thorough history and physical examination are paramount in making this distinction. Although each condition has a classic presentation, there is considerable variation and many exceptions to the rule.

D. The classic presentation of testicular torsion is an acute onset of severe hemiscrotal pain, often associated with nausea and vomiting. On examination, the testis is high riding, with a horizontal lie. The cremasteric reflex is absent, and there is a negative Prehn sign (no symptomatic relief with manual elevation of the testis). With the onset of scrotal wall edema, the physical examination becomes more difficult and less informative. Testicular ultrasonography can be a helpful adjunct in making/confirming the diagnosis. Testicular torsion is a surgical emergency, with the best chance of testicular salvage within the first 6 hours after the onset of pain. In such cases, urgent consultation with a pediatric urologist is indicated.

E. Occasionally, testicular torsion resolves spontaneously (intermittent testicular torsion). These patients usually give a history consistent with testicular torsion, with resolution of the pain by the time they arrive to the emergency department. A testicular ultrasound is invariably found to be within normal limits. In such cases, referral to a pediatric urologist is indicated.

F. Epididymitis/epididymo-orchitis/orchitis can be associated with torsion of the appendix testis or appendix epididymis, or result from trauma to the external genitalia, viral or bacterial infection, or sterile reflux of urine. The classic presentation of torsion of the appendix testis or appendix epididymis is an acute onset of severe hemiscrotal pain. In some cases, the torsed appendage can be appreciated on examination as a blue dot visible through a thin, translucent hemiscrotal wall (blue dot sign). With the onset of scrotal wall edema, the physical examination becomes more difficult and less informative. Testicular ultrasonography can be a helpful adjunct in ruling out testicular torsion and making/confirming the diagnosis. In such cases, comfort measures (rest, anti-inflammatory) and follow-up with the patient's health care provider are appropriate.

G. The classic presentation of epididymitis/epididymo-orchitis/orchitis (epididymitis) is a gradual onset of increasing hemiscrotal pain, occasionally associated with irritative voiding symptoms (frequency, urgency, dysuria). On examination, the epididymis with or without the testis is enlarged and tender to palpation. The cremasteric reflex is present, and there is a positive Prehn sign (symptomatic relief with manual elevation of the testis). With the onset of scrotal wall edema, the physical examination becomes more difficult and less informative. Testicular ultrasonography can be a helpful adjunct in ruling out testicular torsion and making/confirming the diagnosis. A urinalysis (UA) is

(Continued on page 266)

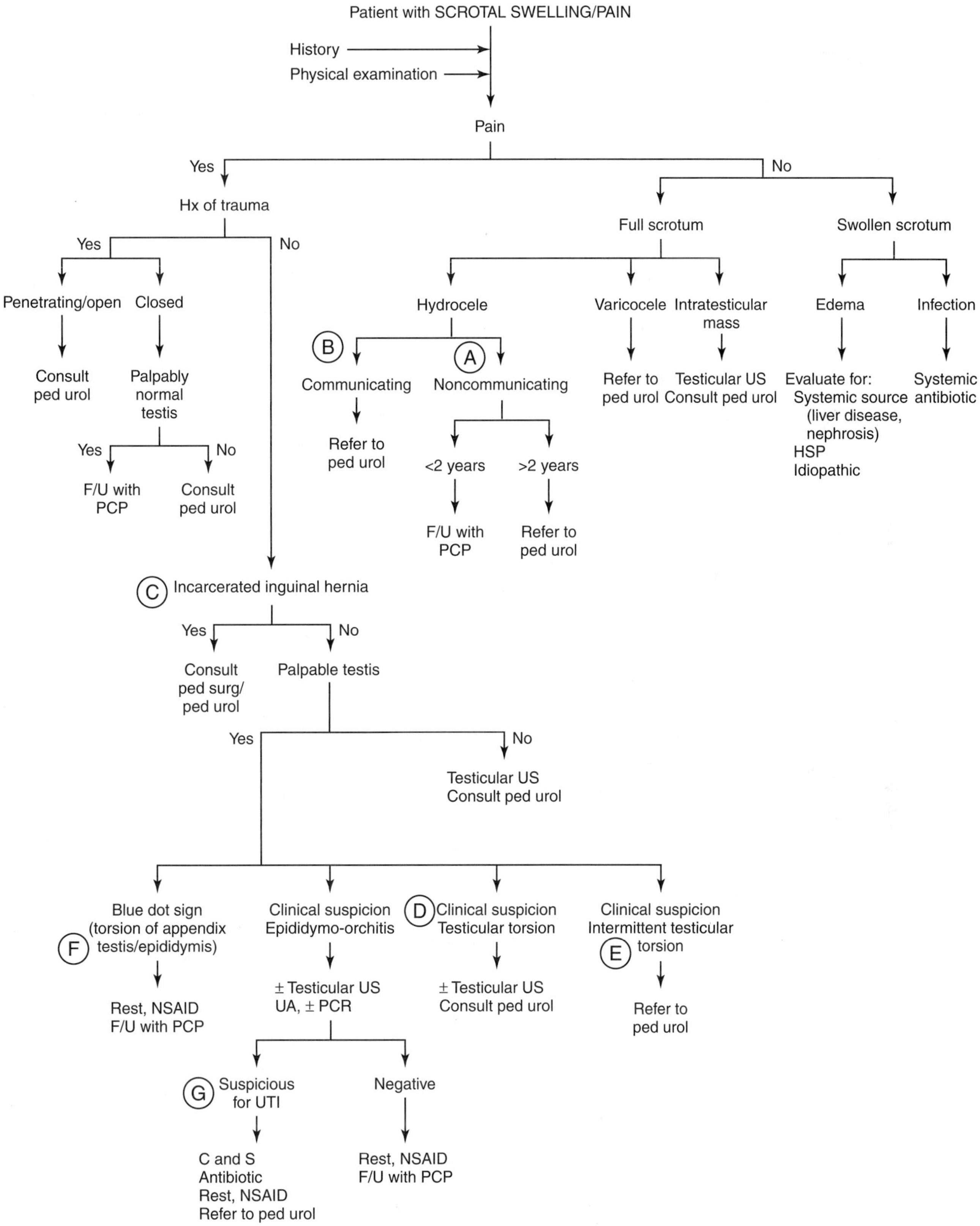
Patient with SCROTAL SWELLING/PAIN
History
Physical examination
Pain
Yes
No
Hx of trauma
Yes
No
Penetrating/open
Closed
Consult ped urol
Palpably normal testis
Yes
No
F/U with PCP
Consult ped urol
Full scrotum
Swollen scrotum
Hydrocele
Varicocele
Intratesticular mass
Edema
Infection
B
A
Communicating
Noncommunicating
Refer to ped urol
<2 years
>2 years
F/U with PCP
Refer to ped urol
Refer to ped urol
Testicular US
Consult ped urol
Evaluate for:
Systemic source (liver disease, nephrosis)
HSP
Idiopathic
Systemic antibiotic
C
Incarcerated inguinal hernia
Yes
No
Consult ped surg/ ped urol
Palpable testis
Yes
No
Testicular US
Consult ped urol
Blue dot sign (torsion of appendix testis/epididymis)
F
Rest, NSAID
F/U with PCP
Clinical suspicion Epididymo-orchitis
± Testicular US
UA, ± PCR
D
Clinical suspicion Testicular torsion
± Testicular US
Consult ped urol
Clinical suspicion Intermittent testicular torsion
E
Refer to ped urol
G
Suspicious for UTI
Negative
C and S
Antibiotic
Rest, NSAID
Refer to ped urol
Rest, NSAID
F/U with PCP

also obtained to assist in differentiating between bacterial and nonbacterial epididymitis. In sexually active patients, urine is sent for PCR (polymerase chain reaction) for *Neisseria gonorrhoeae* and *Chlamydia trachomatis*. Should the patient be found to have bacterial epididymitis, referral to a pediatric urologist is indicated. Otherwise, follow-up with the patient's health care provider is appropriate. Regardless of the cause, all patients are managed with comfort measures (rest, anti-inflammatory).

If the diagnosis is in doubt, always consider testicular torsion. If this cannot be ruled out on examination or with testicular ultrasonography, urgent consultation with a pediatric urologist is indicated.

Musculoskeletal

Chest Pain

Kristine Knuti, MD, and Simon J. Hambidge, MD, PhD

Chest pain, a common presenting complaint among children and adolescents, has many causative factors: idiopathic (12%–85%), musculoskeletal (15%–76%), pulmonary (12%–21%), psychogenic (4%–17%), gastrointestinal (GI; 4%–8%), cardiac (4%–6%), and miscellaneous (4%–25%). Chest pain is equally prevalent in boys and girls. Children younger than 12 years with chest pain are more likely to have a cardiopulmonary cause, whereas adolescents older than 12 years are more likely to have idiopathic or psychogenic causes. Though usually benign, chest pain results in missed school days and activity limitation in a significant portion of pediatric and adolescent patients. Thorough history and physical examination remain the cornerstones of accurate diagnosis and management of pediatric chest pain.

A. In the patient's history, ask about onset, duration, location, radiation, quality, and severity of the pain, as well as aggravating and alleviating factors. Pain that awakens the patient or is acute (duration less than 48 hours) is concerning for an organic cause. Note associated symptoms, such as fever, vomiting, cough, shortness of breath, palpitations, syncope, weight loss, hemoptysis, cyanosis, and fatigue. Ask about the effect of the pain on daily activities and school attendance. Note possible precipitating factors, especially trauma, exercise, eating, laying down, weight lifting, foreign body ingestion, caustic ingestion, acute respiratory infection, and stress. Assess history of and risk for underlying illnesses and conditions (especially Kawasaki disease, Marfan syndrome, cystic fibrosis, sickle cell disease, congenital and acquired heart disease, longstanding diabetes, pregnancy, neurofibromatosis, thrombophilia, hyperlipidemia, and migraines). Obtain a family history of cardiac disease and early sudden death, respiratory illnesses, gastroesophageal reflux and peptic ulcer disease, and rheumatologic disease. Assess the psychosocial situation, and identify sources of stress and anxiety. If appropriate, ask about cigarette and marijuana smoking, drug use (especially cocaine and amphetamines), recent or current pregnancy, and use of hormonal contraception.

B. Perform a complete physical examination with close attention paid to vital signs, specifically heart rate, respiratory rate, and blood pressure. Perform pulse oximetry. Assess respiratory rate, work of breathing, aeration, breath sounds (listening for wheezing, crackles, rales, and decreased breath sounds), and expiratory phase prolongation. Do a thorough cardiac examination, evaluating pulses in the four extremities, palpating chest for thrills, heaves, and the point of maximum intensity, and auscultating for murmurs, rubs, gallops, clicks, and pronounced or extra heart sounds. Palpate each rib cartilage with only one finger, because two or more fingers may splint the affected cartilage and not reproduce the pain. Note signs of arthritis, congestive heart failure, chronic respiratory disease, abdominal masses, and underlying conditions (such as Marfan syndrome and Kawasaki disease).

C. Cardiovascular causes of chest pain are less common than other causes, and include ischemia, infarction, arrhythmias, mitral valve prolapse, stenosis (pulmonic, aortic, subaortic, and supravalvular), coarctation of the aorta, myocarditis, pericarditis, pulmonary hypertension, and dissecting aortic aneurysm. Symptoms that point to a potential cardiac causes for chest pain include shortness of breath, syncope, pain associated with exercise, fever, palpitations, radiation of the pain to the jaw or left arm, nausea, sweating, dull pain or pressure, and substernal or precordial pain. Concerning family history includes early myocardial infarction, hyperlipidemia, early sudden death, arrhythmias, Marfan syndrome, and congenital and acquired heart disease (including hypertrophic cardiomyopathy). Personal history of Kawasaki disease, Marfan syndrome, hypertension, and congenital or acquired heart disease also warrants further investigation of cardiac causative factors. Physical findings that suggest cardiac causes include abnormal vital signs, murmurs, persistent tachycardia, increased intensity of the second heart sound, clicks, gallops, friction rubs, decreased femoral pulses, and signs of congestive heart failure. Chest radiography and electrocardiography (ECG)

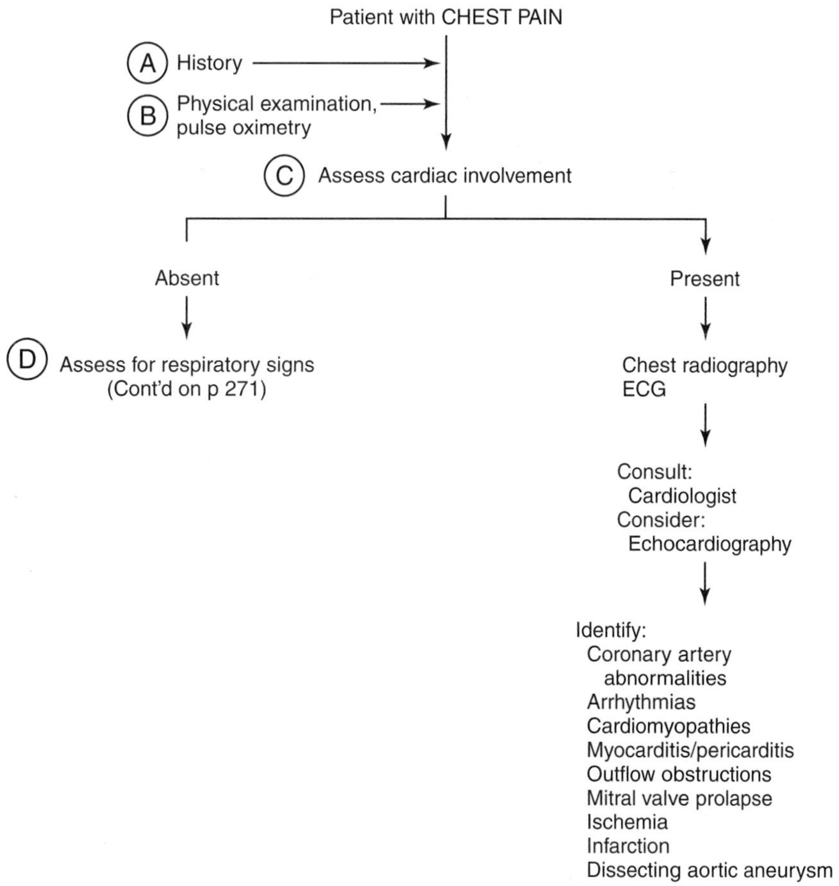
Patient with CHEST PAIN
A
History
B
Physical examination, pulse oximetry
C
Assess cardiac involvement
Absent
Present
D
Assess for respiratory signs
(Cont'd on p 271)
Chest radiography
ECG
Consult:
Cardiologist
Consider:
Echocardiography
Identify:
Coronary artery abnormalities
Arrhythmias
Cardiomyopathies
Myocarditis/pericarditis
Outflow obstructions
Mitral valve prolapse
Ischemia
Infarction
Dissecting aortic aneurysm

may also help to diagnose cardiac disease but are usually unnecessary in the diagnosis of pediatric chest pain. Pericarditis and myocarditis related to infection or vasculitis will often produce muffled heart sounds and show cardiomegaly on chest radiography and nonspecific ST abnormalities and/or low voltage on ECG. Aortic stenosis and idiopathic hypertrophic subaortic stenosis cause a systolic murmur and left ventricular hypertrophy. Primary pulmonary hypertension and pulmonary stenosis produce right ventricular hypertrophy and a pronounced second heart sound. Arrhythmias such as atrioventricular block, sick sinus syndrome, and supraventricular tachycardia are associated with abnormal conduction patterns on ECG. Acquired cardiac lesions include cardiomyopathy, myocarditis, pericarditis, endocarditis, rheumatic heart disease, valvular disease, and cardiac tumors. Coronary artery disease related to Kawasaki disease, hypercholesterolemia, aberrant left coronary artery, and lesions associated with decreased coronary artery blood flow (severe aortic stenosis, idiopathic hypertrophic subaortic stenosis) produce ischemic ST changes, abnormal T waves, and sometimes Q waves. Acute myocardial infarction, though exceedingly rare, has also been described in children and adolescents with otherwise normal coronary anatomy. Acute myocardial infarction during adolescence occurs more often in boys than girls. Other associated risk factors include hyperlipidemia, hypertension, smoking, drug use (specifically cocaine and amphetamines), and diabetes.

D. Pulmonary causes include asthma, pneumonia, pneumonitis, chronic cough, pleural effusion, pleurodynia, foreign body, congenital malformations, thoracic tumors, pneumothorax, and pulmonary embolism. Pulmonary disease can present as a variety of different types of chest pain, such as pleuritic pain, muscle strain related to cough, diaphragmatic irritation, tightness from asthma, and vague visceral pain from thoracic tumors. Signs and symptoms concerning for pulmonary causative factors include cough, fever, tachypnea, dyspnea, and hypoxia. Foreign body aspiration may be suspected from history, examination, or chest radiography. Mediastinal causes include pneumomediastinum, mediastinitis, and mediastinal tumors. Asthma remains a common and likely underreported cause of pediatric chest pain. Risk factors of pulmonary embolism include central venous catheter, pregnancy, trauma, malignancy, hormonal contraception, rheumatologic disease and vasculitis, nephrotic syndrome, recent surgery, history of previous venous thrombosis, obesity, sickle cell disease, immobilization, smoking, and familial thrombophilia.

E. Musculoskeletal pain is most often related to muscle overuse or trauma involving the pectoral, upper back, or shoulder muscles. Direct trauma may also fracture or bruise the ribs, and nonaccidental trauma needs to be considered. Costochondritis, inflammation of the costochondral junctures, produces anterior chest pain that may radiate. It is associated with tenderness to palpation of the costochondral junctions. Anterior chest wall syndromes cause chest wall pain that is exacerbated by trunk or shoulder movements. In Tietze syndrome, which is rare but has been described in children, there is isolated swelling of the upper costochondral area. In the slipping rib syndrome, the costal cartilages of the eighth, ninth, and tenth ribs are irritated and produce a slipping movement with pain. The pain is duplicated by pulling the lower rib cage anteriorly. In xiphoid process syndrome, inflammation of the xiphoid process produces anterior chest pain with chest movement. Precordial catch syndrome is related to irritation of the parietal pleura that produces a stabbing pain along the left sternal border. Osteomyelitis of the vertebrae or ribs, discitis, myositis, spondylolisthesis, and spondylolysis are rare causes of musculoskeletal chest pain.

F. GI disorders that cause chest pain include gastroesophageal reflux disease, peptic ulcer disease, esophagitis, esophageal spasm, gastritis, odynophagia, foreign bodies in the esophagus, caustic ingestions, and Mallory–Weiss tears. Pancreatitis, cholecystitis, Fitz–Hugh–Curtis syndrome, and subdiaphragmatic abscesses may also present with chest pain.

G. Psychogenic and psychiatric causative factors should also be considered, including stress, adjustment disorder, eating disorders (especially bulimia nervosa), panic attacks, anxiety, depression, hyperventilation, conversion disorder, and Münchausen syndrome. In one study, approximately a third of pediatric patients with chest pain reported a recent significantly stressful event. Hyperventilation produces reduction in carbon dioxide with subsequent alkalosis, decreased ionized calcium, and tetany. Hyperventilation syndrome is frequently associated with light-headedness, giddiness, dizziness, paresthesias, and chest pain.

H. Normal thelarche in a girl or gynecomastia in a boy may result in nipple tenderness or chest pain secondary to a high level of anxiety related to either appearance or concern about malignant neoplasia. Additional miscellaneous causes of chest pain include varicella zoster infection, nephrolithiasis, smoking, fibrocystic disease, mastitis, adenocarcinoma of the breast, illicit drug and medication ingestions, and acute chest syndrome in sickle cell disease.

References

Cava JR, Sayger PL. Chest pain in children and adolescents. Pediatr Clin North Am 2004;51:1553.

Evangelista JA, Parsons M, Renneburg AK. Chest pain in children: diagnosis through history and physical examination. J Pediatr Health Care 200;14:3.

Gokhale J, Selbst SM. Chest pain and chest wall deformity. Pediatr Clin North Am 2009;56:49.

Kanter RJ, Graham M, Fairbrother D, et al. Sudden cardiac death in young children with neurofibromatosis type 1. J Pediatr 2006; 149:718.

Kocis KC. Chest pain in pediatrics. Pediatr Clin North Am 1999;46:189.

Lane JR, Ben-Shachar G. Myocardial infarction in healthy adolescents. Pediatrics 2007;120:e938.

Mahle WT, Campbell RM, Favaloro-Sabatier J, et al. Myocardial infarction in adolescents. J Pediatr 2007;151:150.

Massin MM, Bourguignont A, Coreman C, et al: Chest pain in pediatric patients presenting to an emergency department or to a cardiac clinic. Clin Pediatr (Phila) 2004;43:863.

Mukamel M, Kornreich L, Horev G, et al: Tietze's syndrome in children and infants. J Pediatr 1997;131:774.

Ochsenschlager DW, Atabaki S, Holder MG, et al. Could it be cardiac? Clin Pediatr Emerg Med 2005;6:229.

Pantell RH, Goodman BW Jr. Adolescent chest pain: a prospective study. Pediatrics 1983;71:881.

Place RC. Pulmonary embolism in the pediatric emergency department. Clin Pediatr Emerg Med 2005;6:244.

Quinn CT, Buchanan GR. The acute chest syndrome of sickle cell disease. J Pediatr 1999;135:416.

Selbst SM, Ruddy RM, Clark BJ, et al. Pediatric chest pain: a prospective study. Pediatrics 1988;82:319.

Shirley KW, Adirim TA. Sudden cardiac death in young athletes. Clin Pediatr Emerg Med 2005;6:194.

Swenson JM, Fischer DR, Miller SA, et al. Are chest radiographs and electrocardiograms still valuable in evaluating new pediatric patients with heart murmurs and chest pain? Pediatrics 1997;99:1.

Wiens L, Sabath R, Ewing L, et al. Chest pain in otherwise healthy children and adolescents is frequently caused by exercise-induced asthma. Pediatrics 1992;90:350.

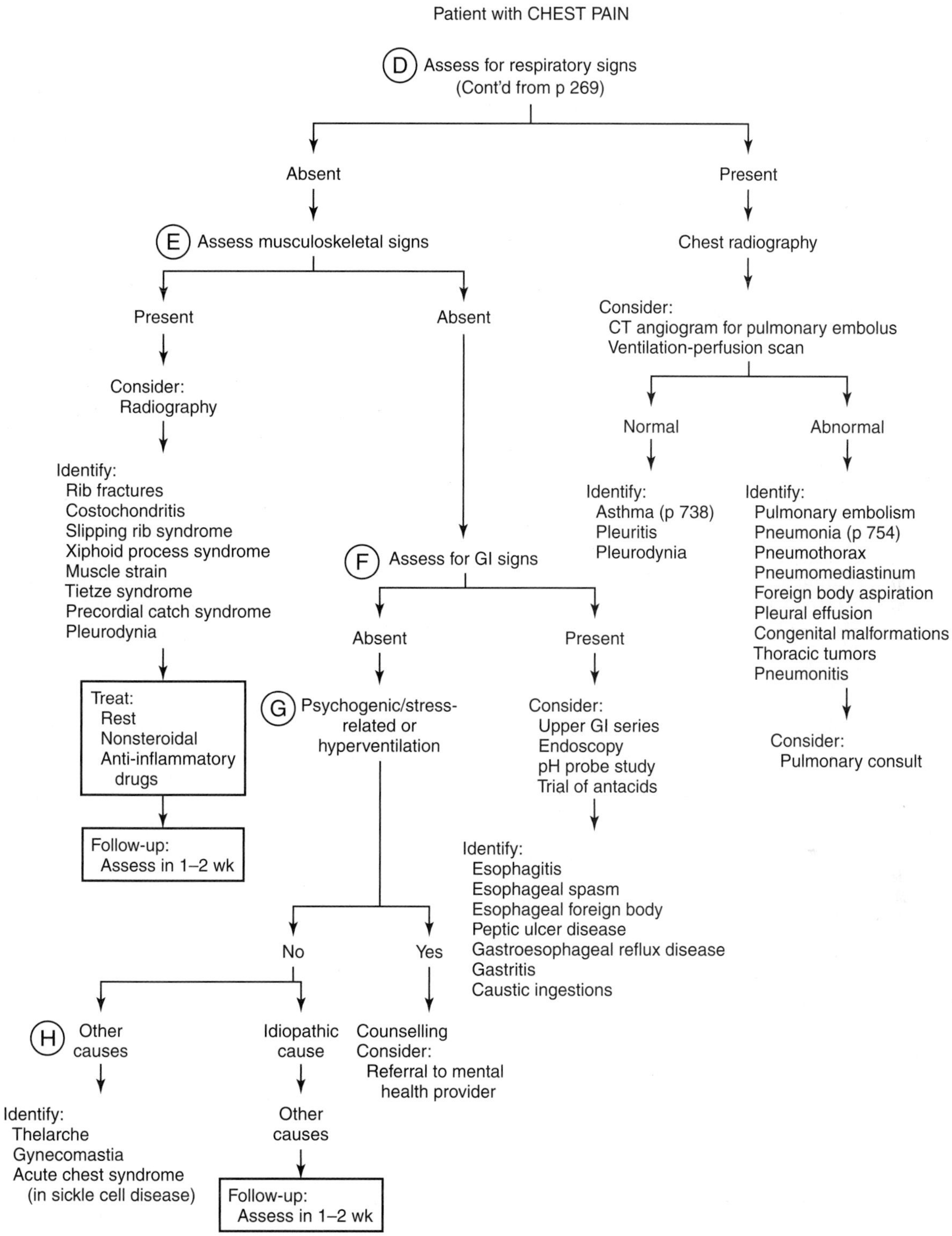
Patient with CHEST PAIN
D Assess for respiratory signs
(Cont'd from p 269)
Absent
Present
E Assess musculoskeletal signs
Chest radiography
Present
Absent
Consider:
CT angiogram for pulmonary embolus
Ventilation-perfusion scan
Consider:
Radiography
Normal
Abnormal
Identify:
Rib fractures
Costochondritis
Slipping rib syndrome
Xiphoid process syndrome
Muscle strain
Tietze syndrome
Precordial catch syndrome
Pleurodynia
Identify:
Asthma (p 738)
Pleuritis
Pleurodynia
Identify:
Pulmonary embolism
Pneumonia (p 754)
Pneumothorax
Pneumomediastinum
Foreign body aspiration
Pleural effusion
Congenital malformations
Thoracic tumors
Pneumonitis
F Assess for GI signs
Absent
Present
Treat:
Rest
Nonsteroidal
Anti-inflammatory
drugs
G Psychogenic/stress-related or hyperventilation
Consider:
Upper GI series
Endoscopy
pH probe study
Trial of antacids
Consider:
Pulmonary consult
Follow-up:
Assess in 1–2 wk
Identify:
Esophagitis
Esophageal spasm
Esophageal foreign body
Peptic ulcer disease
Gastroesophageal reflux disease
Gastritis
Caustic ingestions
No
Yes
H Other causes
Idiopathic cause
Counselling
Consider:
Referral to mental health provider
Identify:
Thelarche
Gynecomastia
Acute chest syndrome
(in sickle cell disease)
Other causes
Follow-up:
Assess in 1–2 wk

Foot Pain

K. Brooke Pengel, MD

A. In the patient's history, consider the age of the patient because certain injuries are more common during each stage of development. Determine whether the pain is acute or chronic because this historical fact can aid tremendously in narrowing the diagnosis. In the case of an acute trauma, clarify the specific mechanism of injury and the location of pain. Determine initial treatment and whether the child or adolescent was able to bear weight initially and shortly after the injury. More severe injuries tend to inhibit the ability to bear any weight on the foot. Elicit a history of swelling and bruising and whether these findings were focal or generalized. For chronic pain, ask about the schedule of repetitive motion activities and the recent ability to sustain the activity.

B. The physical examination of the foot, just like other joints, should proceed in a systematic fashion. The examination includes observation, palpation, range of motion/strength, and neurovascular status. In the physical examination, observe the foot with and without weight bearing, and the child's gait with and without shoes. Palpation of bone and soft tissue landmarks for specific areas of tenderness will aid in narrowing the differential diagnosis. Skeletally immature athletes have open growth plates (physes) that are particularly vulnerable to injury at certain stages of development. The foot may apear structurally normal or show obvious abnormality. In either case, if superficial causes for pain are excluded, radiography may provide further clarification as to the diagnosis.

A skin or soft tissue abnormality, such as plantar warts, paronychia, or subungual exostosis, may be the primary problem. Other abnormalities, including blisters and bursae, may be manifestations of underlying structural changes. Although rare, tumor and infection should be ruled out. A bunion may appear in the adolescent and is usually not symptomatic. The cause is not entirely clear, but theories include tight shoe wear, metatarsus primus varus, pronation, joint hyperlaxity, and hereditary. Pain, when present, arises over the first metatarsal head. When present at this age, the hallux valgus deformity (lateral deviation of the great toe) accompanies medial deviation of the first metatarsal. Standing radiographs are most helpful in evaluating this deformity. Bunionette (tailor's bunion) is a similar deformity of the fifth toe. Treatment consists of altering shoe wear, bunion pads, orthotics, and physical therapy. Surgery aims to realign the first metatarsal varus, but should be delayed as long as possible.

C. The most common fractures occur in the toes and metatarsals. The patient presents with an acute history of a crushing injury or axial force to the foot. Rapid swelling ensues and there is usually immediate difficulty bearing weight. Examination reveals swelling and, at times, deformity with the more severe injuries. With little or no displacement, toe and metatarsal fractures can be treated with a firm-soled shoe or a walking cast until the patient is no longer tender and healing bone is evident on radiographs. Intra-articular fractures, displaced fractures, or joint dislocations often need orthopedic referral. These injuries require prompt anatomic reduction, especially if the growth plate is involved. Fractures of the proximal fifth metatarsal can be more difficult to treat. The classic mechanism of injury is forceful inversion of the foot; the patient often presents with severe pain and difficulty walking. When this history is accompanied by focal swelling and tenderness at the base of the fifth metatarsal, a fracture is often present. Variations in the blood supply to the base of the fifth metatarsal explain the tendency toward delayed or incomplete healing depending on the location of the fracture. Fractures of the fifth metatarsal can be classified into three categories: tuberosity avulsion fractures, proximal diaphyseal fractures (Jones fracture), and stress fractures. Appropriate classification is important because the treatment and prognosis is quite different in the case of the Jones fracture and stress fracture compared with the avulsion fractures. Avulsion fractures are treated with immobilization with a hard-soled shoe, walking boot, or walking cast for 4 to 6 weeks. Prognosis is excellent. Treatment of the Jones fracture is more complicated because conservative treatment has a high failure rate. Referral to a specialist who can provide a balanced discussion with the family regarding the nonoperative and surgical options is warranted. Conservative care requires prolonged casting with a non–weight-bearing period of 6 to 8 weeks, a plan that poses a problem in terms of compliance. Stress fractures of the fifth metatarsal can also be problematic, with both conservative and surgical management as options for treatment.

D. Physiologic flatfeet, or pes planus, result from a fat pad in the arch of neonates, which disappears by 2 to 3 years of age. Flexible flatfeet, the most common variety, are often familial and may be accompanied by loose joints generally. Examination of the foot in a non–weight-bearing position and with toe walking yields a normal arch in a flexible flatfoot. Most commonly, flat feet are asymptomatic and do not require treatment. When symptoms arise, an arch support may be prescribed. In addition, running athletes with flat-feet and excessive pronation may benefit from orthotic treatment, because these athletes are at risk for overuse lower extremity injury. Rigid flatfeet can be distinguistred from physiologic flatfeet because they cannot be passively corrected. Physical examination reveals that the range of motion at the tarsal and subtalar joints is decreased, and the arch does not increase with toe raising.

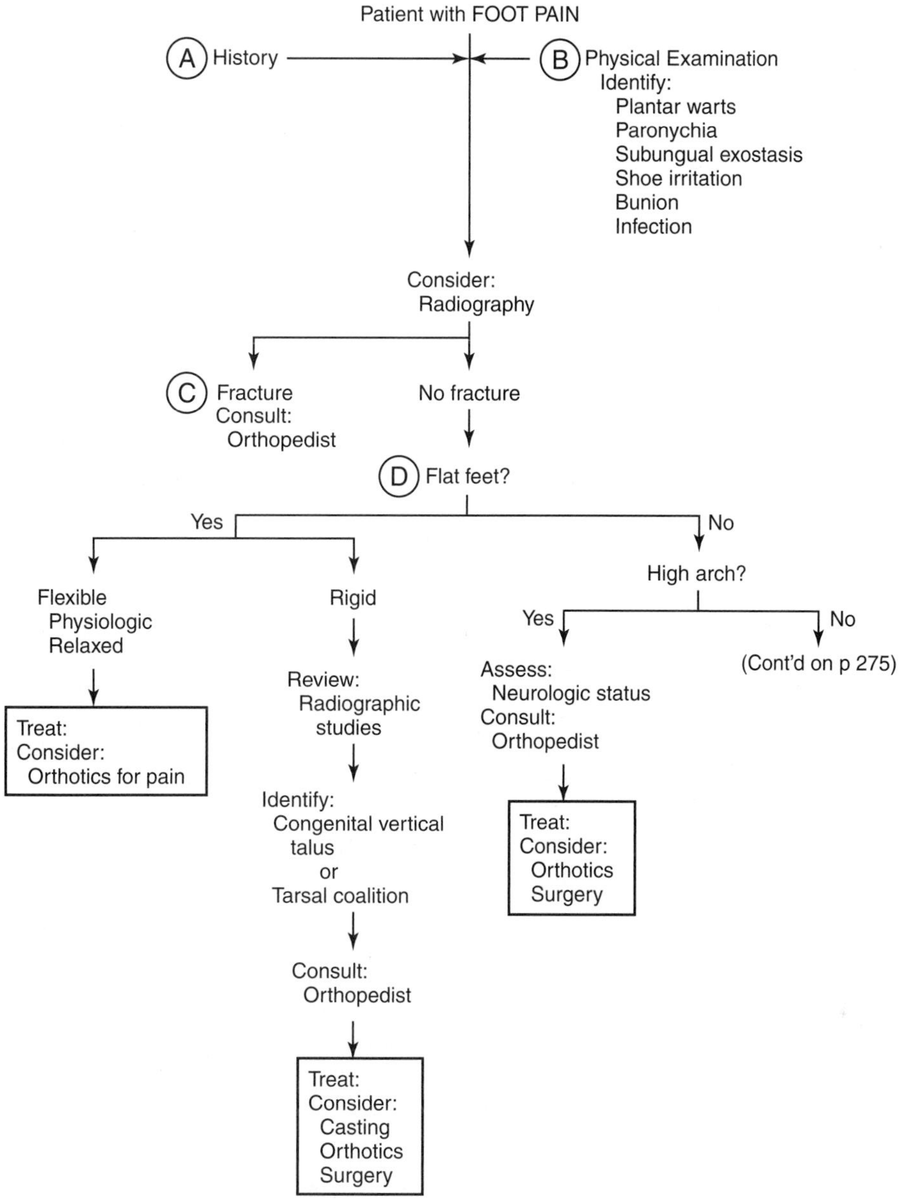
Patient with FOOT PAIN
A History
B Physical Examination
Identify:
Plantar warts
Paronychia
Subungual exostasis
Shoe irritation
Bunion
Infection
Consider:
Radiography
C Fracture
Consult:
Orthopedist
No fracture
D Flat feet?
Yes
No
Flexible
Physiologic
Relaxed
Treat:
Consider:
Orthotics for pain
Rigid
Review:
Radiographic
studies
Identify:
Congenital vertical
talus
or
Tarsal coalition
Consult:
Orthopedist
Treat:
Consider:
Casting
Orthotics
Surgery
High arch?
Yes
No
Assess:
Neurologic status
Consult:
Orthopedist
Treat:
Consider:
Orthotics
Surgery
(Cont'd on p 275)

Rigid flatfeet result from either a congenital vertical talus or a tarsal coalition. Vertical talus is usually associated with neuromuscular abnormalities, such as arthrogryposis and myelodysplasia. Treatment is surgical. Tarsal coalitions result from a cartilage and progressively developing bony bridge between tarsal bones. Most commonly, the calcaneal and navicular bones are involved, and an oblique radiograph may show the abnormality. A computed tomographic scan of the foot is often necessary to confirm the diagnosis. Initial treatment consists of a trial of casting or walking boot immobilization, supportive shoes, or activity modification. Surgery for resection of the bar or fusion may eventually be indicated for persistent symptoms. The high-arched (calcaneocavus) foot is abnormal and deserves a systematic work-up for underlying cause. This deformity can be progressive and is frequently the result of a central or peripheral neurologic abnormality. Imaging of the spine with magnetic resonance imaging (MRI) should be obtained to evaluate for a central neurologic cause. Other muscular and neurologic causes may be discerned by electromyography, muscle biopsy, or nerve conduction studies. Pes cavus deformity may also be a result of a residual clubfoot or may be post-traumatic or idiopathic in origin. The treatment of pes cavus depends on the cause of the deformity. Underlying neurologic problems should be addressed. Foot pain may respond initially to shoe alterations and orthotics. With progression, surgical correction will be necessary.

E. Köhler disease and Freiberg infraction are both considered to be osteochondroses, or diseases of the ossification centers characterized by osteonecrosis followed by recalcification. Köhler disease involves the tarsal navicular, affects children between 5 and 9 years of age, and presents with midfoot pain and limping. Examination reveals localized tenderness, and possibly swelling, over the navicular. Radiographs demonstrate sclerosis and tarsal navicular narrowing. Conservative treatment tends to be effective and consists of rest and if the pain warrants, immobilization. Freiberg infraction involves the metatarsal head and occurs most commonly in athletic adolescent girls. The history reveals the gradual onset of forefoot pain aggravated by activity. Examination is positive for focal tenderness over the affected metatarsal head (usually the second or third). Recalcification commonly occurs in a period of 2 to 3 years. Symptoms can be managed conservatively with activity modification, immobilization and orthotic treatment. Surgical intervention is reserved for patients who do not respond successfully to conservative treatment.

Osteochondritis dissecans (OCD) refers to a focal area of subchondral bone injury and progressive osteonecrosis. This process differs from osteochondroses because the latter usually is self-limiting, as opposed to OCD, which can be progressive and cause permanent impairment. Cause is poorly understood, yet trauma and overuse have been implicated. OCD of the talus commonly involves the medial or lateral corner of the talar dome and manifests as a gradual onset of pain, joint swelling, and occasionally locking if the fragment becomes mobile. Examination may reveal a joint effusion and tenderness about the anterior joint line. Radiographs are usually diagnostic, although MRI is often necessary for diagnosis and is also helpful in staging of the process. For early cases with a stable lesion, activity restriction and immobilization may be sufficient to allow the process to resolve. Younger, skeletally immature patients tend to have a better prognosis and higher chance of being managed successfully nonoperatively. If conservative measures of treatment fail, surgery is usually necessary.

F. Stress fractures are overuse injuries of bone that occur in the setting of chronic, repetitive activity that overwhelms the ability of the bone to recover. Stress fractures are characterized by an insidious onset of pain with activity that often progresses to pain at rest. The history usually reveals training errors, such as a recent increase in activity such as a sports camp. The metatarsals are a common site of stress injuries. Initial radiographs may be normal; the bone scan or MRI will be abnormal earlier. Treatment consists of bone rest, immobilization in a hard sole shoe or walking boot, physical therapy, and progressive return to activity. Certain stress fractures in the foot can be considered high risk, in that there is a considerable possibility for complications in healing such as the development of a nonunion. Stress fractures of the fifth metatarsal, as mentioned previously, are considered in this category. Tarsal navicular stress fractures are high risk and often require prolonged treatment. The young athlete presents with an insidious onset of medial foot pain aggravated by activity. Examination reveals focal tenderness over the navicular. Radiographs often fail to show the stress fracture and MRI is often needed to clarify the diagnosis. Treatment is initiated with a 6- to 8-week period of non-weight bearing in a cast, followed by further immobilization. Return to activity can take as long as 6 to 8 months. This treatment plan is understandably difficult for active children and motivated athletes. Despite appropriate conservative care, nonunion is still possible and requires operative fixation.

Overuse injury about the foot is common in youth especially with those who are involved in a high volume of activity without proper rest and recovery time. Overuse injury can affect the soft tissue or the bone (stress fracture). Soft tissue overuse manifests as a gradual onset of activity related pain with or without swelling. Examination typically reveals diffuse tenderness about the soft tissue of the foot. Imaging studies are negative for abnormality. Treatment is supportive with activity modification and physical therapy focusing on strength and proprioception.

Apophysitis refers to a condition in which pain is located around a developing ossification center and occurs characteristically in an age-dependent fashion in certain areas of the body during rapid growth spurts. In the foot, this traction apophysitis can occur around the age of 10 to 12 at the base of the fifth metatarsal, a condition referred to as *Iselin's disease.* The apophysis is often confused with a fracture but can easily be differentiated by the fact that the growth center always lies parallel to the long axis of the fifth metatarsal and usually has rounded, corticated edges. Sever's disease, or calcaneal apophysitis, occurs in active children beginning at age 9 through early adoleseence. The child has heel pain, particularly with running and jumping. Examination reveals tenderness of the calcaneal apophysis. The patient may also have tenderness over the Achilles tendon and its insertion into the os calcis apophysis, which likely results from a combination of a tight gastrocsoleus mechanism and overuse. Treatment is conservative and consists of activity modification based on pain, physical therapy, gel heel cups, and over-the-counter pain medication. Fortunately, apophysitis in the foot and heel tend to be self-limiting conditions.

Plantar fasciitis usually occurs in the adolescent athlete with closed physes. The history is one of a gradual onset of medial arch or heel pain aggravated by activity. Morning pain and stiffness are hallmark features. Examination reveals tenderness along the length of the plantar fascia, particularly medially. Radiographs do not contribute to the diagnosis, although they are reasonable to exclude other diagnoses. Treatment includes activity modification, ice, over-the-counter pain medication, orthotics, heel cups, and physical therapy. A mass over the medial aspect of the foot distal to the medial malleolus suggests an accessory navicular bone. The accessory bone most commonly occurs on the medial, planter border of the navicular, near the insertion of the tibialis posterior tendon.

Although the incidence rate of an accessory navicular is up to 15%, it is uncommon for the area to become

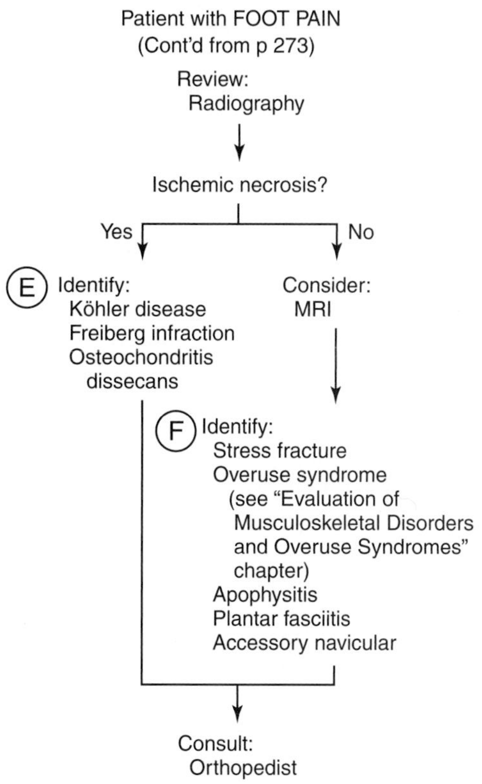
Patient with FOOT PAIN
(Cont'd from p 273)
Review:
Radiography
Ischemic necrosis?
Yes
No
E
Identify:
Köhler disease
Freiberg infraction
Osteochondritis dissecans
Consider:
MRI
F
Identify:
Stress fracture
Overuse syndrome
(see "Evaluation of Musculoskeletal Disorders and Overuse Syndromes" chapter)
Apophysitis
Plantar fasciitis
Accessory navicular
Consult:
Orthopedist

symptomatic. Adolescent athletes can experience symptoms around the accessory navicular, as a result from pressure over the bony prominence, irritation of the fibrous connection (synchondrosis), or inflammation or tendinopathy in the posterior tibialis tendon. Diagnosis is made from plain films, with an external oblique film the most helpful. Initial treatment includes activity modification, arch supports, and physical therapy. Recalcitrant symptoms may require cast or walking boot immobilization. Surgical excision might be necessary if symptoms persist despite conservative measures of care.

References

Evans AM, Rome K. A review of the evidence for non-surgical interventions for flexible pediatric flat feet. Eur J Phys Rehabil Med 2011;PMID:21304450
Lee MC, Sucato DJ. Pediatric issues with cavovarus foot deformities. Foot Ankle Clin 2008;13(2):199–219.
Malanga GA, Ramirez-Del Toro, JA. Common injuries of the foot and ankle in the child and adolescent athlete. Phys Med Rehabil Clin N Am 2008;19(2):347-71, ix.
Sullivan RJ. The pediatric foot and ankle. Foot Ankle Clin 2010;15(2):ix.
Zaw H, Calder JDF. Tarsal coalitions. Foot Ankle Clin 2010;15(2):349-64.

Gait Abnormalities

Susan D. Apkon, MD, and Jason T. Rhodes, MD

A. Observe the child walking toward and away from you. Observe the angle the thigh makes with the calf at the knee, the tibiofemoral angle. It varies with age and changes with growth (Figure 1). Varus is maximum at 18 months of age but may persist to age 3 years. This is followed by valgus angulation, which normally peaks by age 4 years. With further growth, it gradually declines to the adult value of about 6 degrees.

B. With the child standing or supine, measure varus angulation (bowlegs) along the major axis of the femur to the midpoint of the distal femur at the knee (which may be midpatella if there are no patellar alignment or dislocation issues) and distally to the center of the ankle joint. Until 2 years of age, 15 degrees of varus angulation is within the normal range. Significant varus angulation persisting beyond 2 years of age needs further evaluation and possibly surgical correction. Causes include Blount disease, rickets, skeletal dysplasia, and injury to the growth plate from infection or trauma. A second peak incidence of genu varum in the teens results from adolescent Blount disease. It is most common in African American children, is often unilateral, and usually requires surgical correction.

C. Valgus angulation (knock-knees) is measured the same way as varus angulation. However, it is best measured with the childbearing weight. In children younger than 6 years, values up to 15 degrees are normal. Progressive deformity beyond 6 years and unilateral deformity require further evaluation. The most likely causes of progressive valgus angulation include metabolic bone disease (renal disease), paralysis, and trauma to the proximal tibia.

D. Toe walking (equinus) can be considered habitual (idiopathic) or caused from a neurologic impairment. Signs of either an upper motor neuron process (spasticity, hyper-reflexia, or clonus) or lower motor neuron process (hypotonia, hyporeflexia, or weakness) should prompt an evaluation by a neurologist. Idiopathic toe walking should be considered in the absence of any of the above signs. Range of motion of the ankle may not be helpful in assisting in making the diagnosis.

E. Assess the angle of the foot with the straight line of progression, the foot progression angle (Figure 2). Define toeing-in as a negative angle and toeing-out as a positive angle. A normal foot progression angle is 0 to +30 degrees (Figure 3). Note the position of the patella. Medial deviation indicates the problem may be above the knee.

F. Signs of metatarsus adductus or medial deviation of the forefoot include convexity of the lateral border of the foot and a prominence at the base of the fifth metatarsal. An equinus contracture will not be present. A flexible deformity will resolve spontaneously or can be treated with physical therapy and/or home exercises. Inability to overcorrect the lateral convexity easily and a fixed crease suggest a fixed or rigid deformity. These children require serial casting followed by braces.

(Continued on page 278)

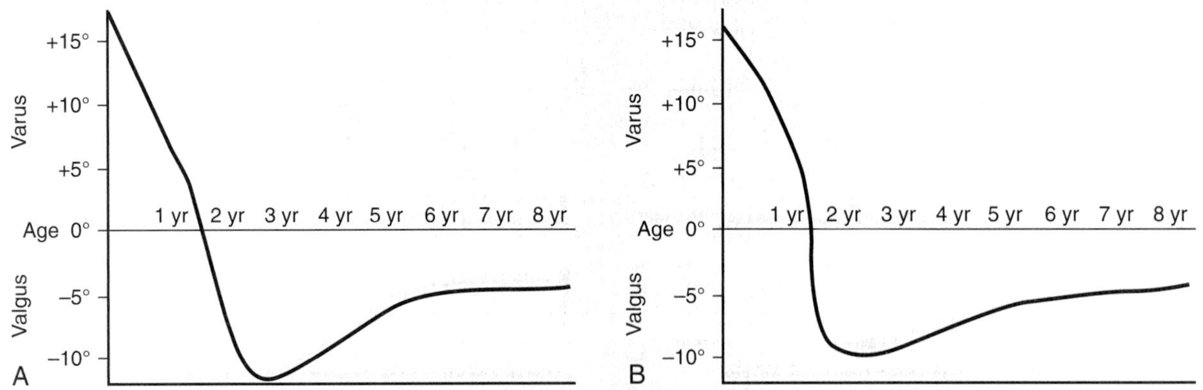
+15°
+10°
Varus
+5°
Age 0°
1 yr
2 yr
3 yr
4 yr
5 yr
6 yr
7 yr
8 yr
Valgus
−5°
−10°
A
B

Figure 1 Tibiofemoral angle in children. Mean values are shown for boys *(A)* and girls *(B)*. *(From Salenius P, Vanka E. The development of tibiofemoral angle in children. J Bone Joint Surg Am 1975;57:259-61.)*

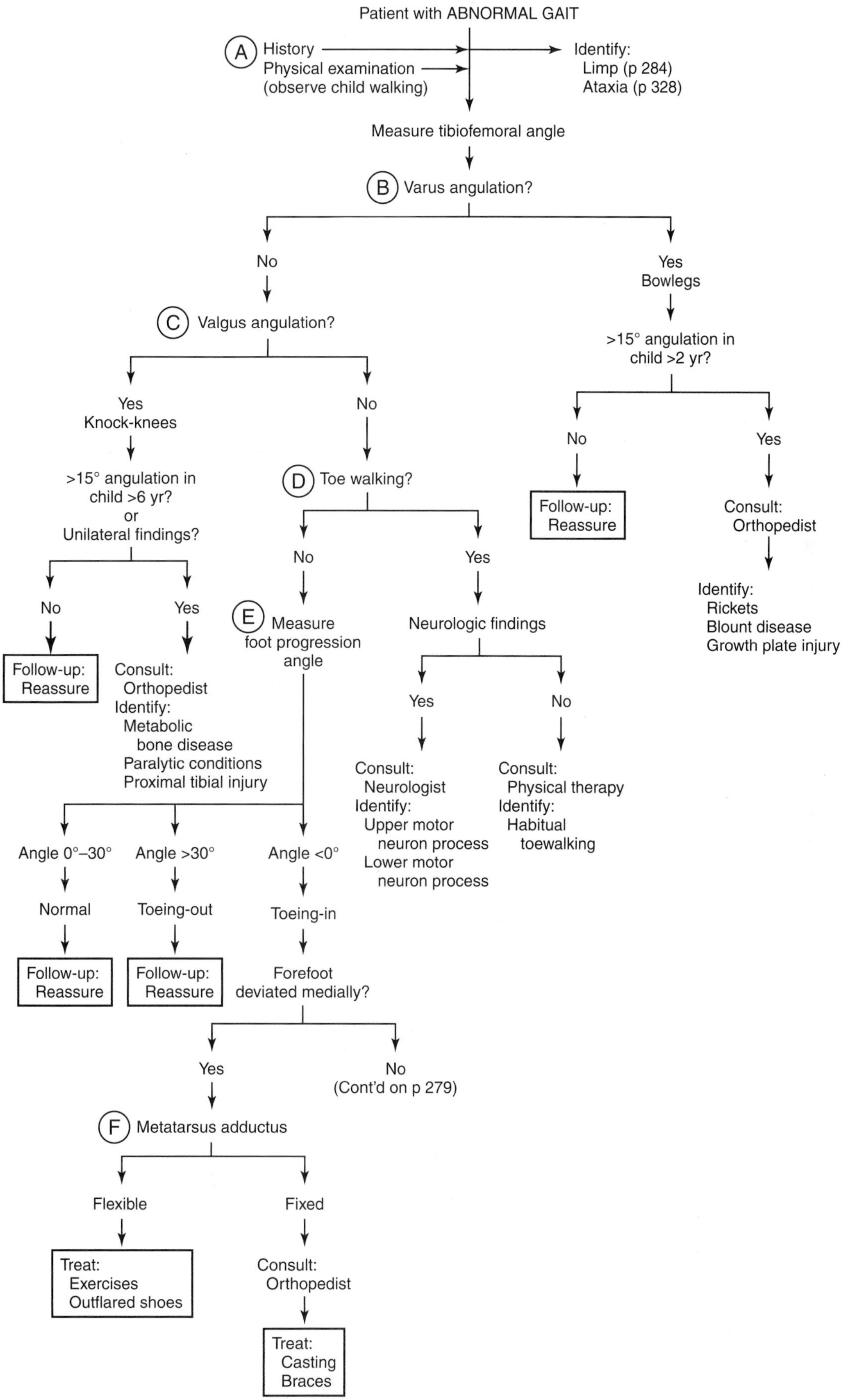
Patient with ABNORMAL GAIT
A History
Physical examination
(observe child walking)
Identify:
Limp (p 284)
Ataxia (p 328)
Measure tibiofemoral angle
B Varus angulation?
No
Yes
Bowlegs
C Valgus angulation?
>15° angulation in child >2 yr?
No
Yes
Follow-up: Reassure
Consult: Orthopedist
Identify:
Rickets
Blount disease
Growth plate injury
Yes
Knock-knees
No
>15° angulation in child >6 yr? or Unilateral findings?
D Toe walking?
No
Yes
Follow-up: Reassure
Consult: Orthopedist
Identify:
Metabolic bone disease
Paralytic conditions
Proximal tibial injury
No
Yes
E Measure foot progression angle
Neurologic findings
Yes
No
Consult: Neurologist
Identify:
Upper motor neuron process
Lower motor neuron process
Consult: Physical therapy
Identify:
Habitual toewalking
Angle 0°–30°
Angle >30°
Angle <0°
Normal
Toeing-out
Toeing-in
Follow-up: Reassure
Follow-up: Reassure
Forefoot deviated medially?
Yes
No
(Cont'd on p 279)
F Metatarsus adductus
Flexible
Fixed
Treat:
Exercises
Outflared shoes
Consult: Orthopedist
Treat:
Casting
Braces

G. Internal tibial torsion is common in children younger than 2 years, and it changes to external rotation with normal growth. The extent of internal tibial torsion can be estimated by measuring the angle formed by the axis of the thigh and the foot with the child prone and the knee flexed to 90 degrees. The normal range of this angle is between 0 and 30 degrees of external rotation, with the average being 10 degrees external by 8 years of age. The torsion of the tibia can also be measured by the transmalleolar axis, which looks only at the tibial rotation, thus removing the component of the foot from the measurements. Transmalleolar axis is measured by having the knee flexed to 90 degrees with the patient in the prone position. The axis is measured by comparing a line drawn across the medial and lateral malleoli to the long axis of the tibia. Average normal measurements are reported at 15 degrees. A severe degree of internal torsion produces an awkward gait and seems to cause affected children to trip over their toes, especially when they are tired. Mild deformities will correct spontaneously; correction may be hastened in young children by preventing them from sitting and sleeping with the feet turned out. Rarely, older children need corrective osteotomy, but this is usually not done until after 8 to 10 years of age because the rotation in the tibia continues to correct until 8 years of age.

H. Femoral anteversion produces toeing-in because of excessive internal rotation of the hip. Assess the degree of rotation of the hip with the child prone, the pelvis flat on the table, and the hips in a neutral position (Figure 4). Allow each leg to drop by gravity into full internal and external rotation. Internal rotation should not exceed 70 degrees; the sum of internal and external rotation should approximate 100 degrees. Femoral anteversion should correct spontaneously by 10 years of age. Parents can encourage the child to sit cross-legged, but this will not change the overall rotation. Exercises, braces, and orthopedic shoes are not indicated. Consider derotational osteotomy (major surgery) only in children older than 10 years with severe deformity.

References

Craig CL, Goldberg MJ. Foot and leg problems. Pediatr Rev 1993;14:395.
Morrissy RT, Weinstein SL. Lovell and Winter's pediatric orthopaedics. Philadelphia: Lippincott Williams & Wilkins; 2001.
Perry J. Gait analysis: normal and pathologic function. Thorofare, NJ: SLACK, 2010.
Staheli LT. Fundamentals of pediatric orthopedics. New York: Raven Press; 1992.
Staheli LT, Corbett M, Wyss C, King H. Lower extremity rotational problems in children: normal values to guide management. J Bone Joint Surg Am 1985;67:39–47.
Tolo VT, Wood B. Pediatric orthopaedics in primary care. Baltimore: Williams & Wilkins; 1993.

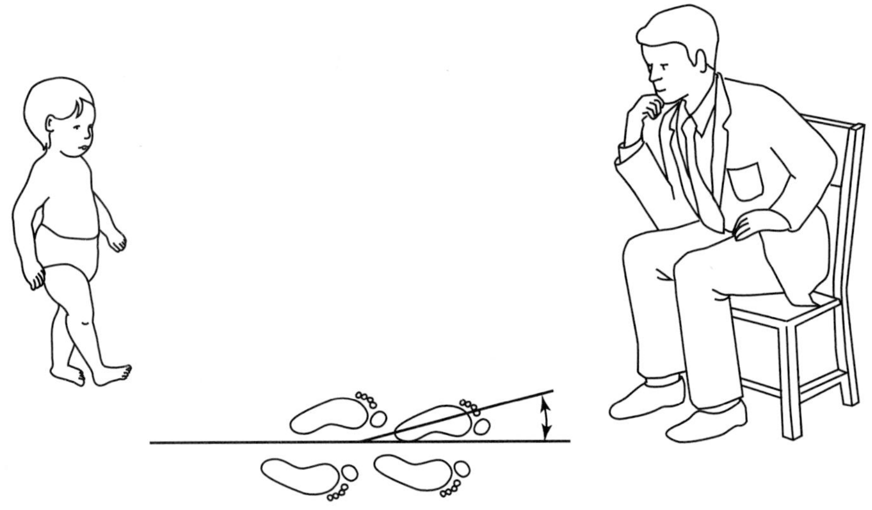

Figure 2 The foot progression angle is the average of the angles formed by the axis of the foot and the line of progression. *(From Staheli LT. Fundamentals of pediatric orthopedics. New York: Raven Press; 1992.)*

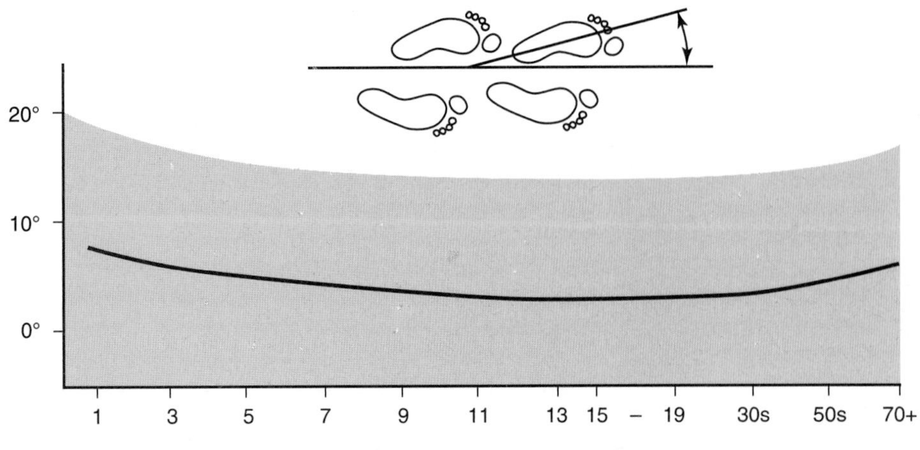

20°
10°
0°
1
3
5
7
9
11
13 15 – 19
30s
50s
70+

Figure 3 Normal range of foot progression angle *(shaded area). (From Staheli LT. Fundamentals of pediatric orthopedics. New York: Raven Press; 1992.)*

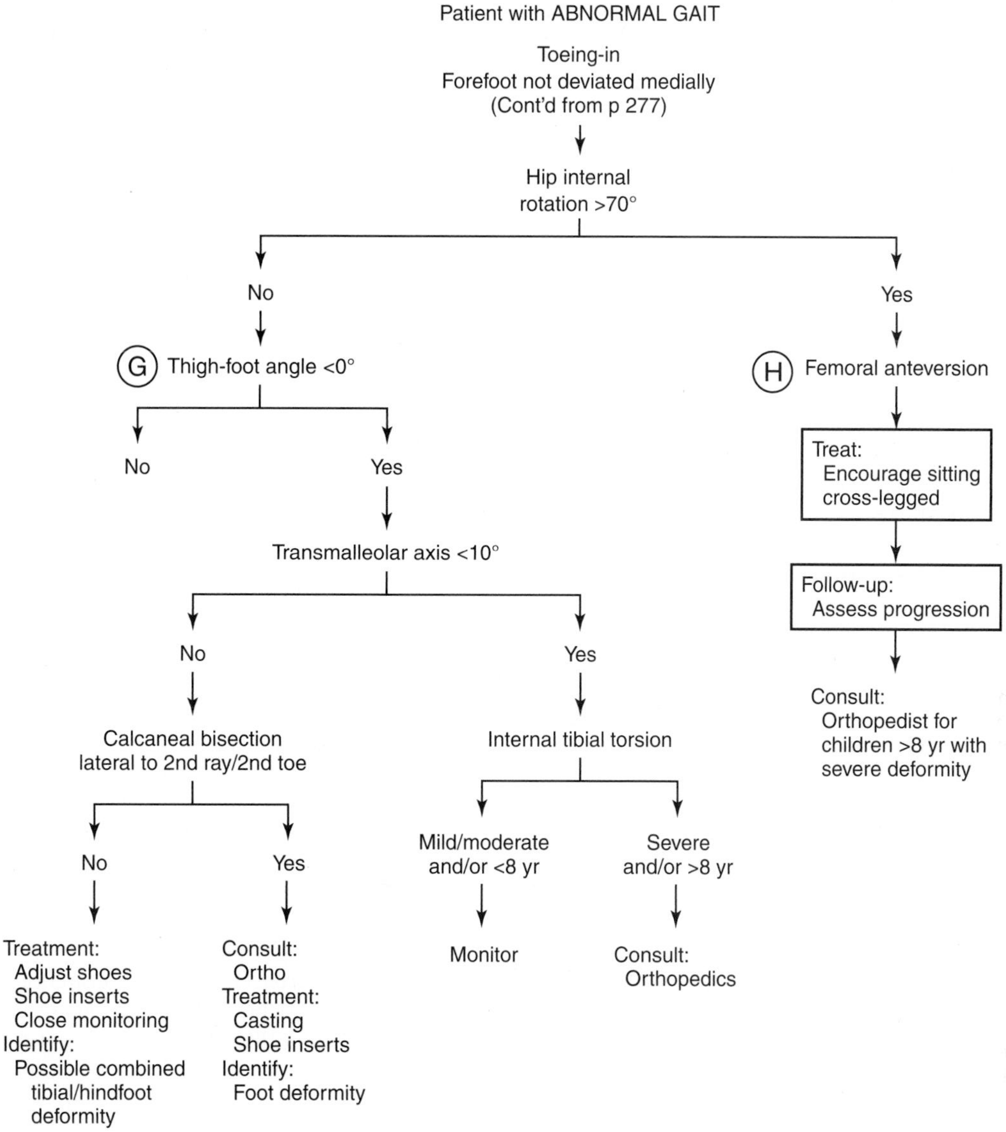

Patient with ABNORMAL GAIT
Toeing-in
Forefoot not deviated medially
(Cont'd from p 277)
Hip internal rotation >70°
No
G Thigh-foot angle <0°
No
Yes
Transmalleolar axis <10°
No
Calcaneal bisection lateral to 2nd ray/2nd toe
No
Treatment: Adjust shoes Shoe inserts Close monitoring Identify: Possible combined tibial/hindfoot deformity
Yes
Consult: Ortho Treatment: Casting Shoe inserts Identify: Foot deformity
Yes
Internal tibial torsion
Mild/moderate and/or <8 yr
Monitor
Severe and/or >8 yr
Consult: Orthopedics
Yes
H Femoral anteversion
Treat: Encourage sitting cross-legged
Follow-up: Assess progression
Consult: Orthopedist for children >8 yr with severe deformity

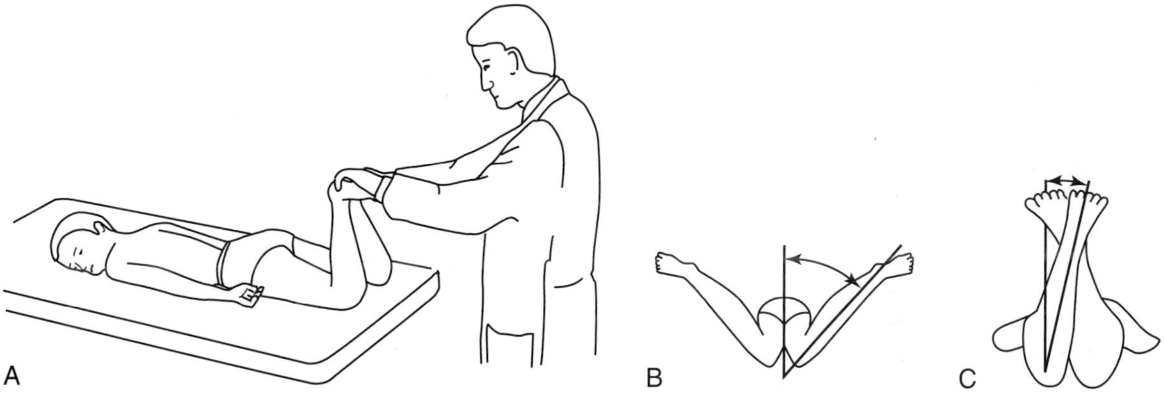

A
B
C

Figure 4 *A,* Assess hip rotation with the child prone and the knees flexed to a right angle. Allow the legs to fall into a comfortable maximum position in rotation. Level the pelvis and estimate or measure the degree of medial rotation *(B)* or lateral rotation *(C)*. *(From Staheli LT. Fundamentals of pediatric orthopedics. New York: Raven Press; 1992.)*

Knee Pain

K. Brooke Pengel, MD

A. In the patient's history, consider the age of the patient, as children of certain ages are vulnerable to specific knee injuries. Determine whether the pain is acute or chronic. In the absence of an acute injury, examine risk factors for the various overuse syndromes that affect the knee. In the presence of a known traumatic event, elicit the mechanism of injury and the specific location of pain because these facts can point to which structures may be injured. Determine initial treatment and whether the child or adolescent was able to bear weight initially and shortly after the injury. Complete inability to bear weight may signify a more severe injury such as a fracture. Elicit a history of swelling and, in the case of an acute injury, whether the swelling occurred rapidly, such as within an hour. A rapidly evolving hemarthrosis generally points toward a fracture, a high-grade ligamentous tear, or a patellar dislocation. Question the patient about the presence of mechanical symptoms such as locking, catching, or instability. Mechanical symptoms are worrisome for a loose body or a meniscal tear.

B. The physical examination of the knee, just like that of other joints, should proceed in a systematic fashion. The features of the examination include neurovascular status, inspection, range of motion, palpation, special testing, and screening of adjacent joints. The physical examination and approach to knee pain is firmly based in anatomy. Many structures in the knee can be directly palpated, which is quite helpful in arriving at the proper diagnosis. In the setting of acute injury and swelling, range of motion and examination can be limited secondary to patient discomfort and guarding. Skeletally immature athletes have open growth plates (physes) that are particularly vulnerable to injury at certain stages of development. Attention to the physis about the proximal tibia and distal femur is important in the assessment and treatment of a knee injury. Special testing about the knee is performed to narrow the diagnosis and largely refers to testing of stability.

C. Radiographs of the knee are obtained to further delineate the diagnosis and to confirm or deny the presence of current or underlying bone abnormality. General indications for knee radiographs include deformity, acute effusion, inability to bear weight, instability, and localized bone or physeal tenderness. Standard trauma views of the knee include anteroposterior, lateral, and oblique radiographs. Additional views used in the evaluation of acute or chronic knee pain include the sunrise view (useful to identify an avulsion fracture of the medial patella after an acute patellar dislocation) and the tunnel view (useful to identify osteochondal injury of femoral condyles). Magnetic resonance imaging (MRI) evaluation is warranted when plain radiographs fail to delineate the problem and there is a suspicion of a significant bone or soft-tissue injury (e.g., fracture, anterior cruciate ligament [ACL] tear, patellar dislocation, etc.). MRI evaluation is usually initiated after orthopaedic consultation.

D. Fractures about the knee can occur in the femur, tibia, fibula or patella. Younger patients are at greater risk for an injury to the physis, as opposed to the surrounding soft tissue, as the cartilaginous physeal plate is mechanically weaker than the adjacent ligament. In the history, there is often a significant mechanism of injury followed by rapid swelling and inability to bear weight. Physical examination is most commonly limited by pain and effusion. Radiographs, especially in skeletally immature patients, should be obtained before aggressive manipulation of the knee. Intra-articular fractures such as to the tibial spine may require surgery if there is any displacement affecting the joint surface. Injuries to the physis of the femur or tibia also need anatomic reduction if there is significant displacement or angulation. Immobilization in a fiberglass cast for approximately 4 weeks is followed by range of motion and progressive rehabilitation. Return to activity depends on the site of injury and the progression of healing radiographically and clinically. Families should be counseled about the risk for growth-related complication when the fracture involves the physis.

E. Knee contusions are common in children and adolescents given their activity level and their frequent participation in contact sports. The history consists of a fall onto the knee or a direct blow to the knee followed by swelling and bruising. When the fall or hit is significant, knee contusions can present similarly to more serious knee injuries. In addition to swelling and bruising, the knee examination often reveals limited range of motion and significant guarding that may even prevent the examiner from proceeding with stability testing. Radiographs are negative for fracture. Treatment consists of rest, protection, ice, and over-the-counter pain medication as needed. An MRI may be indicated in the setting of a large hemarthrosis to evaluate for radiographically occult fractures. MRI will show significant bone marrow edema and associated joint effusion. The use of a knee immobilizer should be limited to a few days and active range of motion should be encouraged. For patients who need a longer period of protection, a variety of knee braces can be used for comfort and support. In the case of severe contusions, the use of crutches for a short interval can aid in pain control and can facilitate healing. Return to activity is based on regaining normal range of motion, strength, and function, and usually occurs within a few weeks of the injury.

F. Ligament injuries about the knee, although possible in the skeletally immature patient, tend to occur in the adolescent once the physeal plates are more mature and less susceptible to trauma. Certain mechanisms are characteristic of serious ligament injury in the knee. Mild sprains in the knee may have minimal findings on examination and usually cause little disability.

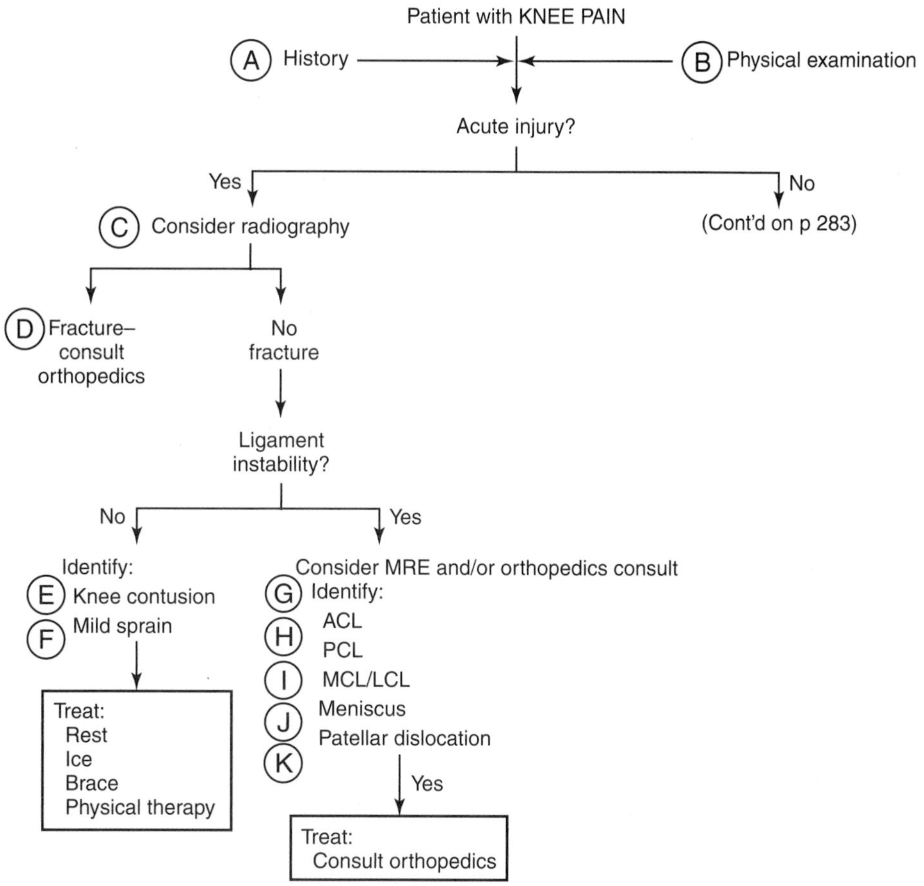
Patient with KNEE PAIN
A History
B Physical examination
Acute injury?
Yes
No
C Consider radiography
(Cont'd on p 283)
D Fracture– consult orthopedics
No fracture
Ligament instability?
No
Yes
Identify:
E Knee contusion
F Mild sprain
Treat:
Rest
Ice
Brace
Physical therapy
Consider MRE and/or orthopedics consult
G Identify:
H ACL
PCL
I MCL/LCL
J Meniscus
K Patellar dislocation
Yes
Treat:
Consult orthopedics

G. An ACL rupture can occur from either a contact or noncontact twisting injury, or by landing on a hyperextended knee. When one of these mechanisms is associated with a feeling of a "pop" and the presence of a rapidly evolving joint effusion, an ACL rupture should be suspected. The ACL injury can be isolated, but it is also quite possible that there is concomitant soft-tissue injury such as a collateral ligament injury or meniscal tear. The examination reveals a joint effusion and a positive Lachman test (both laxity and the absence of a solid end point noted when stressing the ligament in 20 degrees of flexion). Radiographs are usually negative but may show an avulsion of the lateral tibial plateau, also known as the Segond fracture. MRI is used to confirm and grade the injury, as well as to evaluate for other coexisting injuries. Initial treatment focuses on pain control and protection of the joint. Definitive treatment for a high-grade ACL sprain is largely surgical in children and adolescents to achieve joint stability and to allow safe return to the vigorous activity that is characteristic of this age group. Skeletally immature athletes with ACL injury represent a historically controversial population, although recent recommendations favor surgery in this age group as well. After ACL reconstruction, the patient is progressed through a comprehensive rehabilitation program. Return to sports can usually be achieved approximately 6 months after the surgery.

H. Posterior cruciate ligament (PCL) tears are far less common than ACL tears and may occur when there is a fall or a significant force to anterior aspect of the tibia when the knee is flexed. Examination shows a joint effusion, a positive sag sign, and increased laxity with the posterior drawer test. Radiographs are usually negative. MRI can characterize the injury and is done to evaluate for coexisting injury. Treatment is largely nonoperative because outcomes without surgery are quite good. Rehabilitation is prescribed and return to play is based on regaining motion, strength, and function. Bracing may be recommended upon return to play.

I. Medial collateral ligament (MCL) injuries usually occur when there is a blow to the lateral aspect of the knee, followed by immediate pain over the medial aspect of the knee. With high-grade injuries to the MCL, there can be a knee effusion; with less severe injury, the swelling is localized medially over the course of the MCL. Physical examination reveals tenderness over the MCL (and reproducible pain), as well as laxity, with valgus stress testing. Valgus stress testing is done at 0 and 30 degrees of knee flexion. If laxity is present at 0 degrees, a coexisting injury to the ACL should be suspected. Valgus stress testing in 30 degrees of flexion isolates the MCL and allows for grading of the injury in a cooperative patient. Radiographs are performed to evaluate for fracture, with special attention to the distal femoral physis, which is a structure more likely to mechanically fail with the same mechanism in the skeletally immature patient. MRI might be considered if an injury at the physis is suspected despite negative radiographs. MRI can also characterize the extent of the injury and assist in evaluating for other injuries. When the injury is isolated, rest, ice, protection, and pain medications are used to control pain.

Knee rehabilitation and progressive return to activity can usually be accomplished in 2 to 4 weeks. Knee bracing may be used for stability, as well as for return to activity. Lateral collateral ligament (LCL) injuries are less common than MCL injuries because sustaining a blow to the inside of the knee is an unusual injury. Assessment and treatment principles are similar to those for the MCL.

J. Meniscal cartilage tears can occur from a forceful twisting injuring when the knee is flexed. This injury is more common in the adolescent age group and rarely occurs younger children. The patient may describe an acute sensation of pain near the involved meniscus. Progressive symptoms may be mechanical in nature such as catching or locking. The physical examination may reveal a knee effusion. The most reliable physical examination finding is focal joint line tenderness. Other tests that load and twist the knee to elicit painful clicking on the joint line (such as in the McMurray's test) are not reliably helpful. MRI is obtained when the clinical suspicion is high. Surgery may be warranted for large tears, or for less severe tears if the patient is not responding successfully to conservative treatment of rest and physical therapy. When symptoms of meniscal pathology present in younger patients (swelling, catching, locking), a torn discoid meniscus should be suspected. The discoid meniscus is congenitally abnormal and prone to injury. MRI can detect a discoid meniscus. Surgery is usually recommended when a patient has significant symptoms.

K. Patellar dislocations occur from either direct contact to the knee or after a sudden change in direction. If the dislocation is transient or partial (termed a *subluxation*), the patient may not realize that the patella shifted position. Dislocations that require reduction in an emergency care facility are often accompanied by significant swelling, pain, and disability. Radiographs are used before and after reduction to confirm anatomic reduction and to evaluate for associated fracture. The sunrise view is particularly helpful to evaluate for fracture but is often not part of routine trauma series. MRI may be used by a specialist to evaluate for any associated cartilage injury or loose body that can result from a traumatic dislocation. Initial treatment consists of protection of the knee with bracing at 0 degrees for 3 to 4 weeks, rest, ice, and pain medication. If the MRI fails to show osteochondral or ligamentous injury that would warrant surgery, the patient is treated conservatively with protected bracing and progressive return to activities in approximately 10 to 12 weeks.

L. Sinding-Larsen-Johansson syndrome, or apophysitis of the inferior pole of the patella, refers to a condition that causes pain and localized swelling in the anterior knee in preadolescence. The patellar tendon creates traction over the cartilaginous component of the patellar apophysis, leading to a traction apophysitis. The condition usually occurs between the ages of 8 and 11, when the apophysis is rapidly developing and is susceptible to activity-related irritation. Together with the classic history, patients have focal swelling and exquisite tenderness over the inferior pole of the patella. Radiographs may show fragmentation of the inferior pole of the patella, although radiographs can also be normal. Treatment is conservative, consisting of activity modification, ice, over-the-counter pain medicine, stretching, and occasionally bracing. The condition tends to be self-limiting, and activity and sports are permitted based on pain tolerance.

M. Osgood-Schlatter disease, also known as tibial tubercle apophysitis, refers to a similar cause of anterior knee pain, although this condition occurs in a slightly older population closer to adolescence. Pain, swelling, and tenderness over the tibial tubercle apophysis between the ages of 10 and 14 are the hallmark features. Examination often shows dramatic swelling and significant tenderness over the tibial tuberosity. Radiographs may be obtained to evaluate the appearance of the apophysis, although significant variations in the appearance of the tibial tubercle apophysis exist. Most patients respond well to conservative treatment such as activity modification, ice, over-the-counter medicine, stretching, and occasionally bracing. As in Sindig, activity is allowed if the pain is not preclusive. Osgood Schlatter disease is largely self-limiting. However, in rare cases significant fragmentation at the apophysis can lead to painful malunion and require more aggressive treatment such as surgery.

N. Slipped capital femoral epiphysis (SCFE) can present as knee pain in the adolescent either with an acute or chronic history of pain. A screening examination of the hip in a young patient presenting with knee pain is essential to avoid missing this important diagnosis. The patient is usually between the ages of 10 and 16, and oftentimes overweight. Examination reveals pain with hip range of motion, loss of internal rotation of the hip, and obligatory external rotation of the femur (flexion of the hip results in involuntary external rotation of the leg). Radiographs of the bilateral pelvis including an anteroposterior and frog leg lateral are usually diagnostic. SCFE can be present bilaterally. SCFE is an orthopedic emergency, and treatment consists of strict non-weight bearing and orthopedic consultation for surgical management. Legg–Calvé–Perthe disease (Perthe disease, or LCP) can also present as knee pain in the younger patient and represents another diagnosis not to miss in the evaluation of the patient with knee pain. Perthe disease refers to avascular necrosis of the femoral head. Patients usually present between the ages of 2 and 12 with knee and/or hip pain and limping. Examination reveals limited range of motion of the hip with or without pain. Radiographs are useful in the diagnosis, and occasionally an MRI is needed. Orthopedic consultation is needed, and treatment depends on the stage and progression of the disease.

O. Patellofemoral pain syndrome (PFPS), occurring commonly in the adolescence, refers to an overuse injury causing anterior knee pain. Other terms that have been used to describe this condition are lateral patellar compression syndrome, runner's knee, and chondromalacia, although the latter term is falling out of favor. The symptoms are theorized to arise from dysfunction around the patellofemoral joint. The history reveals activity-related, chronic pain in the anterior knee that occurs without significant swelling or mechanical symptoms. Radiographs are obtained to screen for

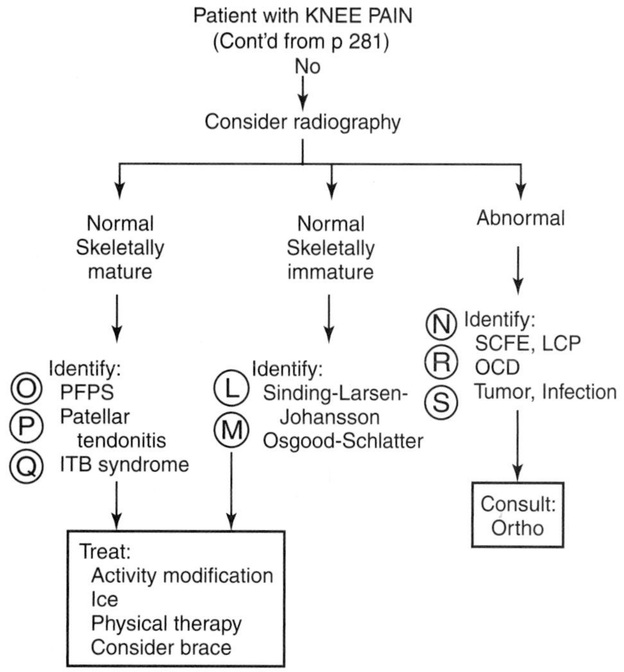
Patient with KNEE PAIN
(Cont'd from p 281)
No
Consider radiography
Normal
Skeletally
mature
Normal
Skeletally
immature
Abnormal
O
P
Q
Identify:
PFPS
Patellar
tendonitis
ITB syndrome
L
M
Identify:
Sinding-Larsen-
Johansson
Osgood-Schlatter
N
R
S
Identify:
SCFE, LCP
OCD
Tumor, Infection
Treat:
Activity modification
Ice
Physical therapy
Consider brace
Consult:
Ortho

other causes of knee pain, although radiographs are typically negative in this condition. MRI has little role in the initial evaluation of chronic, nontraumatic, anterior knee pain. Short-term treatment consists of activity modification, ice, and over-the-counter medications. Bracing of the knee may provide symptomatic relief especially during aggravating activity. Definitive management involves successful involvement in a systematic rehabilitation program focusing on lower extremity flexibility and strengthening, including pelvic and core strengthening to improve biomechanics. Return to activity is based on relief of symptoms and improved functioning of the knee. Failure to improve with conservative care may warrant more advanced consultation by an orthopaedic or sports medicine specialist.

P. Patellar tendonitis, also referred to as jumper's knee, is a type of overuse anterior knee pain. This condition commonly occurs in jumping athletes in adolescence. The history shows activity-related pain, and the examination shows focal tenderness over the course of the patellar tendon. Radiographs are commonly obtained and are usually normal. Treatment is supportive, focusing on controlling pain and regaining function. Bracing with a pateller tendon strap may be helpful for symptom relief. A progressive rehabilitation program is often helpful in returning athletes successfully to play.

Q. Iliotibial band (ITB) syndrome is an overuse injury that commonly occurs in running athletes. The history reveals lateral, nontraumatic knee pain that is aggravated by running. Examination reveals significant inflexibility of the ITB and focal tenderness over the lateral femoral condyle. Treatment is conservative and involves activity modification, identification of correctable biomechanical features, as well as active participation in a sound rehabilitation program focusing on correction of muscle imbalances, strengthening, and friction massage/stretching of the ITB. Recalcitrant cases may respond to a corticosteroid injection. For the rare cases that do not respond successfully to all conservative measures, surgical release of the ITB may be considered.

R. Osteochondritis dissecans (OCD) refers to an acquired injury to the subchondral bone and occurs most commonly in the medial femoral condyle. Most theories agree that the cause of this condition may be multifactorial, with repetitive overload or microtrauma a significant factor. The patient presents with a vague history of knee pain, occasional swelling, and at times mechanical symptoms of catching or locking. Radiographs tend to confirm the diagnosis, and MRI is useful in grading or clarifying the severity of the lesion. Progressive fragmentation and loose body formation is a complication of the disease. Management is largely conservative in skeletally immature patients. Surgical management may be required in adolescent patients or patients with more severe disease.

S. Although rare, tumor and infection are among the possibilities in the presentation of nontraumatic knee pain. Radiographs and MRI are excellent screening tools to evaluate for these conditions, and specialized testing is reserved depending on the clinical presentation.

References

Adirim TA, Cheng TL. Overview of injuries in the young athlete. Sports Med 2003;33:75–81.

Carry PM, et al. Adolescent patellofemoral pain: a review of evidence for the role of lower extremity biomechanics and core instability. Orthopedics 2010 Jul;33(7):498–507.

Frosch KH, et al. Outcomes and risks of operative treatment of rupture of the anterior cruciate ligament in children and adolescents. Arthroscopy 2010 Nov;26(11):1539–50. Review.

Gholve PA, Scher DM, Khakharia S, et al. Osgood-Schlatter syndrome. Curr Opin Pediatr 2007;19:44–50.

Polousky JD. Juvenile Osteochondritis Dissecans. Sports Med Arthrosc Rev 2011;19(1):56–63.

Siow HM, Cameron DB, Ganley TJ. Acute knee injuries in skeletally immature athletes. Phys Med Rehabil Clin N Am 2008;19:319–45.

Wijdicks CA, et al. Injuries to the medial collateral ligament and associated medial structures of the knee. J Bone Joint Surg Am 2010 May;92(5):1266–80.

Limp

Steven G. Federico, MD

A. Limp is defined as the deviation of one's standard ambulatory pattern. In pediatrics, this pattern is an evolution with age-dependent norms. The cause of a patient's limp can be categorized in one or more of the following: pain, weakness, and structural abnormality. The initial history taken on a patient who presents with a chief complaint of limp should include in its description several factors: duration, time of onset (night, day, with activity), age, sex, painful or nonpainful, location of pain (articular or nonarticular, monoarticular or polyarticular), history of trauma, presence of fever or other constitutional symptoms. Specific attention should be paid to the age of the patient. Although not completely absolute, many diagnoses of limp are more common in certain age ranges. For example, congenital hip abnormalities are more common in 1- to 3-year-olds, transient synovitis and Legg–Calve–Perthes syndrome are seen in 4- to 10-year-olds, and slipped capital femoral epiphyses and overuse injuries are more likely in 11- to 15-year-olds.

B. Careful attention should be placed on the physical examination of a child with a limp. This can be especially difficult in toddlers, but the determination of pain and/or anatomic location ultimately will dictate the evaluation, differential, and level of concern. Areas of focus should include a description of the gait highlighting the use of compensatory muscles/joints, limb lengths, point tenderness, site of pain (joint or soft tissue), areas of erythema, warmth, swelling, muscle strength, evidence of trauma, and presence of fever, rash, or other systemic findings.

C. Unequal leg length can be measured by having the patient stand barefoot on a smooth surface using a tape from the anterosuperior iliac spine to the medial malleolus or the sole of the heel. X-ray scanography can also be used. In toddlers, symmetry of the buttock and thigh creases and a Trendelenburg gait can point to asymmetric limb lengths. Congenital abnormalities of the proximal femur include bone malformations and dislocation of the hip.

D. Patients who lack trauma or systemic symptoms may require imaging studies, but laboratory analysis rarely is helpful. The anatomic location of pain should be delineated to maximize utility of imaging study. The assessment should specifically delineate between pain that is pinpoint versus diffuse, as well as the involvement of bone, soft tissue, and/or joints. Imaging usually consists of radiographs and should be targeted to area of pain with consideration of the joint(s) above and below.

E. Imaging is rarely helpful when cause of limp is not pinpoint or is migratory. Consider supportive management including anti-inflammatory medication, rest, ice, compression, and elevation. If limp persists, consider referral to orthopedics (chronic overuse or soft-tissue strain) or rheumatology (fibromyalgia, hypermobility, reflex sympathetic dystrophy, [RSD]).

F. Aseptic necrosis of the proximal femoral epiphysis (Legg–Calve–Perthes syndrome) and slipped capital femoral epiphysis (SCFE) both begin with a painless limp but usually have become symptomatic by the time of presentation. The pain may be mild and felt at the knee. Anteroposterior and lateral radiographs of both hips are important to the diagnosis. The treatment of aseptic necrosis is complex, requiring a period of no weight bearing and range-of-motion exercises, possibly followed by bracing or surgery. Slipping of the proximal femoral epiphysis is a surgical emergency.

G. Painful limp with systemic symptoms require prompt attention and evaluation. Prompt identification of infectious causative agents may significantly minimize morbidity and long-term sequelae. Radiographs of the involved area should be obtained, including consideration of the joint(s) above and below. It should be noted that radiographs can be negative in septic arthritis for up to 10 days. In addition, laboratory analysis should be obtained including complete blood cell count (CBC), erythrocyte sedimentation rate (ESR), C-reactive protein (CRP), and blood culture (in febrile, ill-appearing patient). Recent evidence suggests that a nonelevated CRP is the most accurate negative predictor of disease.

H. If either the radiographs or laboratory data are abnormal, further evaluation is urgently indicated. If arthritis is not present, further bone imaging such as bone scan or MRI may identify cause. Consider consultation with orthopedics and radiology to identify most useful imaging methodology. If monoarticular arthritis is present, ultrasound and arthrocentesis are indicated. Polyarticular disease usually requires additional analysis and rheumatology evaluation.

I. Transient or toxic synovitis is an inflammatory disease that affects the hip of unknown cause in children 3 to 10 years old, and is one of the most common causes of limp in young children. It is by definition self-limiting and benign. Patients may present with systemic symptoms, although they are rare. Laboratory values are generally normal but may be slightly elevated. The physical examination is significant for decreased active movement but good passive range of motion. It poses a diagnostic dilemma because its presentation can be difficult to differentiate from other inflammatory processes, most notably septic arthritis or fractures. These causative factors must be ruled out clinically, radiographically, or (especially if the child is febrile or has elevated inflammatory markers) microbiologically via aspiration.

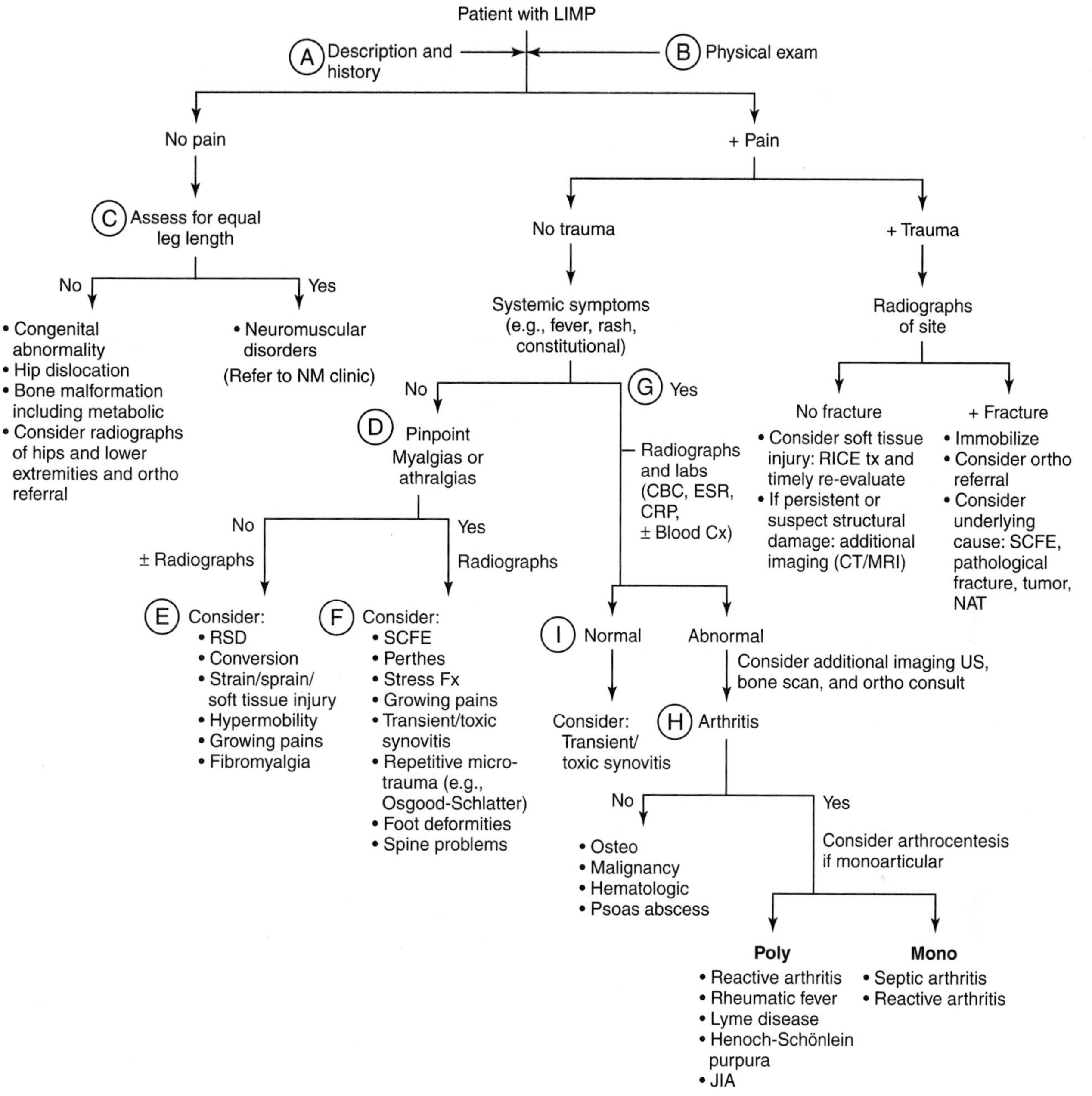
Patient with LIMP
A Description and history
B Physical exam
No pain
+ Pain
C Assess for equal leg length
No
Yes
• Congenital abnormality
• Hip dislocation
• Bone malformation including metabolic
• Consider radiographs of hips and lower extremities and ortho referral
• Neuromuscular disorders
(Refer to NM clinic)
No trauma
+ Trauma
Systemic symptoms (e.g., fever, rash, constitutional)
Radiographs of site
No
G Yes
D Pinpoint Myalgias or athralgias
Radiographs and labs (CBC, ESR, CRP, ± Blood Cx)
No fracture
• Consider soft tissue injury: RICE tx and timely re-evaluate
• If persistent or suspect structural damage: additional imaging (CT/MRI)
+ Fracture
• Immobilize
• Consider ortho referral
• Consider underlying cause: SCFE, pathological fracture, tumor, NAT
No
Yes
± Radiographs
Radiographs
E Consider:
• RSD
• Conversion
• Strain/sprain/ soft tissue injury
• Hypermobility
• Growing pains
• Fibromyalgia
F Consider:
• SCFE
• Perthes
• Stress Fx
• Growing pains
• Transient/toxic synovitis
• Repetitive micro-trauma (e.g., Osgood-Schlatter)
• Foot deformities
• Spine problems
I Normal
Abnormal
Consider additional imaging US, bone scan, and ortho consult
Consider: Transient/ toxic synovitis
H Arthritis
No
Yes
• Osteo
• Malignancy
• Hematologic
• Psoas abscess
Consider arthrocentesis if monoarticular
Poly
• Reactive arthritis
• Rheumatic fever
• Lyme disease
• Henoch-Schönlein purpura
• JIA
Mono
• Septic arthritis
• Reactive arthritis

References

Fleisher GR. Ludwig textbook of pediatric emergency medicine. 4th ed. Philadelphia: Lippincott Williams and Wilkins; 2000.

Onady G, Raslich MA. Evidence-based medicine for the pediatrician. Pediatr Rev 2002;23:318–22.

Renshaw TS. The child who has a limp. Pediatr Rev 1995;16:458–65.

Scherl SA. Common lower extremity problems in children. Pediatr Rev 2004;25:52–62.

Tse SML, Laxer RM. Approach to acute limb pain in childhood. Pediatr Rev 2006;27:170–80.

Zitelli BJ, Davis HW. Atlas of pediatric physical diagnosis. 5th ed. Philadelphia: Mosby; 2007.

Neonatal

Neonatal Hyperbilirubinemia

Betsey Chambers, MD, and Cara L. Mack, MD

Mild jaundice in the first few days of life is a normal part of the neonatal transition. Most jaundiced newborns do not require intervention. However, a small number of newborns will experience significant jaundice, which can lead to kernicterus if not properly treated. An even smaller number will have cholestatic jaundice, which requires prompt diagnosis and treatment. All newborns should be monitored clinically for jaundice to identify the subset of newborns who will require treatment.

A. History: A number of factors in the prenatal and postnatal history can put a newborn at risk for jaundice. They include:

1. Pregnancy complications such as intrauterine growth restriction (IUGR), gestational diabetes (GDM), and maternal use of certain medications
2. Family history of anemia, jaundice, or liver disease
3. African, Asian, or Mediterranean ethnicity
4. Delivery complications such as forceps or vacuum-assisted delivery, or delayed cord clamping
5. Poor feeding, exclusive breast-feeding, or poor voiding/stooling output

B. Physical Examination: A number of physical examination findings can put a newborn at risk for jaundice. They include:

1. Small or large for gestational age (SGA, LGA)
2. Preterm
3. Excessive weight loss since birth
4. Ruddiness
5. Bruising or cephalohematomas
6. Hepatosplenomegaly (as a sign of infection, hemolysis, or liver disease)
7. Abdominal distention (as a sign of obstruction)
8. Vital sign abnormalities (as a sign of infection)

C. Laboratory: All newborns with visible jaundice require a serum or transcutaneous total bilirubin level. In infants more than 35 weeks gestation, this level should be plotted on an age-specific nomogram to determine the risk level. The mother's blood type and antibody screen should also be reviewed in all cases, to determine risk for possible blood group incompatibility. If mother's blood type is O or Rh negative, or her antibody screen is positive, a blood type and Coombs test should be performed on the infant. Depending on history and examination findings, a subset of newborns will require additional laboratory testing. In cases of possible polycythemia (SGA, LGA, infants of diabetic mothers, ruddy complexion), a hematocrit should be checked. If concern exists for unexplained hemolysis, a complete blood cell count (CBC), reticulocyte count, and peripheral smear should be obtained. Lastly, in a small subset of cases in which the clinical course is atypical and other evaluations have not identified the cause of the jaundice, a direct bilirubin level, thyroid-stimulating hormone (TSH) level, and other testing may be indicated.

D. Physiologic Jaundice: The majority of jaundiced newborns will have jaundice that is likely to be explained simply by physiologic factors related to the newborn. The newborn has a greater rate of bilirubin production than an adult, because of relative polycythemia at birth, and a relatively shorter life span of fetal red blood cells. The newborn also excretes bilirubin much slower than an adult because of two factors: first, the conjugation mechanism is not fully functional at birth; and second, there is increased enterohepatic recirculation of bilirubin because of decreased stool output in the first few days of life and lack of normal gut flora in the neonatal intestines. The exact definition of "physiologic" jaundice is variable, depending on the source. However, newborns who are jaundiced in the first day of life, or who require phototherapy at any point, do not have simple physiologic jaundice.

E. Overproduction: Hyperbilirubinemia can result from overproduction, the causes of which can be divided into the following categories:

1. Hemolysis: ABO incompatibility is the most common cause of hemolysis in the neonate. Rh incompatibility is much rarer since the advent of RhoGAM. If untreated during pregnancy, Rh incompatibility can cause such severe hemolysis before birth that the presenting sign is fetal hydrops rather than neonatal jaundice. Other rare causes of hemolysis in the neonate include G6PD (glucose 6-phosphate dehydrogenase) deficiency (more common in persons of Asian, African, or Mediterranean descent) and red cell membrane defects such as elliptocytosis and spherocytosis. Sepsis can also present with hemolysis (among other symptoms).
2. Extravasated blood: Excessive bruising or cephalohematomas can lead to hyperbilirubinemia as the extravasated red blood cells are broken down and reabsorbed.
3. Polycythemia: Polycythemia causes hyperbilirubinemia because of increased red blood cell load. Infants born to diabetic mothers, or who are LGA, SGA, or ruddy in appearance are at particular risk for polycythemia. Delayed cord clamping is also a risk factor.

F. Underexcretion: Hyperbilirubinemia can result from underexcretion, the causes of which can be divided into the following categories:

1. Defective or delayed conjugation: Conjugation defects such as Crigler–Najjar or Gilbert syndrome

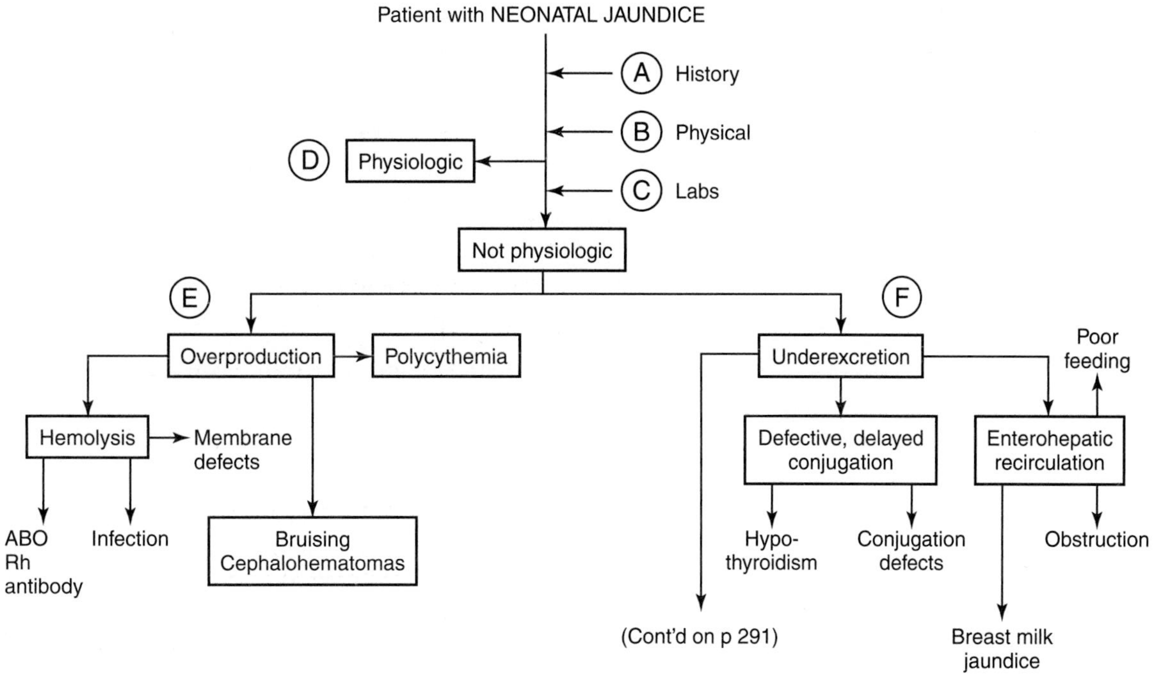

Patient with NEONATAL JAUNDICE
A History
B Physical
C Labs
D Physiologic
Not physiologic
E
F
Overproduction
Polycythemia
Underexcretion
Poor feeding
Hemolysis
Membrane defects
Defective, delayed conjugation
Enterohepatic recirculation
ABO Rh antibody
Infection
Bruising Cephalohematomas
Hypo-thyroidism
Conjugation defects
Obstruction
(Cont'd on p 291)
Breast milk jaundice

can cause hyperbilirubinemia. Crigler–Najjar type I causes severe early hyperbilirubinemia that will be difficult to control, even with treatment. Crigler–Najjar type II is less severe and can be controlled with medications. Hypothyroidism causes a delay in most metabolic processes, including conjugation of bilirubin. It should be considered in prolonged cases of hyperbilirubinemia in which a cause has not been identified. Asian infants are at greater risk for a DNA variant affecting the uridine diphosphate glucuronosyl-transferase protein, which also affects conjugation.

2. Increased enterohepatic recirculation: Conjugated bilirubin that remains in the intestines for prolonged periods is deconjugated by enzymes in the intestinal villi and reabsorbed. Poor feeding is the most common cause of increased enterohepatic recirculation. It is a contributing factor in breast-feeding jaundice, especially in preterm infants or infants experiencing breast-feeding problems. Breast-*feeding* jaundice should be distinguished from breast-*milk* jaundice. Breast-milk jaundice is a prolonged, unconjugated hyperbilirubinemia thought to be caused by enzymes in breast milk that deconjugate bilirubin, leading to enterohepatic recirculation. In rare cases, intestinal obstruction may be the cause of enterohepatic recirculation. Normal intestinal flora can decrease enterohepatic recirculation by further metabolizing bilirubin to a form that cannot be reabsorbed. However, neonates do not have the normal gut flora that adults have, which exacerbates enterohepatic recirculation.

3. Direct (conjugated) hyperbilirubinemia: See sections H and I and Table 1.

Table 1. **Neonatal Cholestatic Diseases**

Disease	Diagnostic Workup
Metabolic	
A1AT deficiency	A1AT level and phenotype
IEOM	Newborn screen (galactosemia) Urine succinylacetone (tyrosinemia) Serum amino acids, urine organic acids
BASD	Total serum bile acids; urine bile acid analysis
Infectious	
TORCH	Urine CMV culture; others as warranted
UTI	Urine culture for bacteria
Sepsis	Based on history, clinical picture, cultures
Hepatitis A	Hepatitis A IgM
Hepatitis B	Hepatitis B sAg
Genetic	
Cystic fibrosis	Newborn screen, sweat chloride test
Alagille syndrome	Echocardiogram, spine film, ophthalmologic examination
Endocrinopathy	
Hypothyroidism	Newborn screen, TSH, total and free T_4
Panhypopituitarism	TSH, total and free T_4, early morning cortisol
Toxin Induced	
TPN-related cholestasis (also known as intestinal failure-associated liver disease)	
Drug-induced hepatotoxicity	
Extrahepatic Biliary Obstruction	
Biliary atresia	See section H
Choledochal cyst	See section H

A1AT, alpha-1 antitrypsin; *BASD,* bile acid synthesis defects; *CMV,* cytomegalovirus; *IEOM,* inborn errors of metabolism; *IgM,* immunoglobulin M; *sAg,* surface antigen; T_4, thyroxine; *TORCH,* toxoplasmosis, other, rubella, cytomegalovirus, and herpes; *TPN,* total parenteral nutrition; *TSH,* thyroid-stimulating hormone; *UTI,* urinary tract infection.

G. Treatment of Unconjugated Hyperbilirubinemia:

1. Phototherapy: Initial treatment for hyperbilirubinemia is with phototherapy. Phototherapy causes a conversion of bilirubin into lumirubin, which is water soluble and more easily excreted from the body than bilirubin. Not all jaundiced newborns will need phototherapy. Guidelines for whom to start on phototherapy can be found in the American Academy of Pediatrics, Clinical Practice Guideline for the Management of Neonatal Hyperbilirubinemia.
2. Follow-up: Because most neonatal jaundice occurs in the first week of life, close follow-up in the first week of life is critical, even for infants who do not meet criteria for phototherapy at the time of discharge.
3. Other treatments: If phototherapy is unsuccessful in controlling the bilirubin level, other treatments may be considered. These include intravenous immunoglobulin (IVIG; which is helpful in cases of antibody-mediated hemolysis), albumin administration (which binds to bilirubin and prevents it from crossing the blood–brain barrier), and double-volume exchange transfusion. Infants who require these treatments need close monitoring in a neonatal intensive care unit.

H. Evaluation of Cholestatic Jaundice: Cholestatic jaundice in the neonatal period can be attributed to a variety of causative factors. All jaundiced infants older than 2 to 3 weeks require measurement of direct (or conjugated) bilirubin. Neonatal cholestasis is defined as a direct bilirubin of ≥2 mg/dL and ≥20% of the total bilirubin level. In assessing the jaundiced infant, make sure to visualize the stool color, as acholic stools are associated with biliary atresia, as well as other causes of biliary stasis. All patients with cholestasis should be worked up for the underlying cause as expediently as possible. The most important reason for this urgency is based on the fact that the success of the Kasai portoenterostomy surgical procedure for biliary atresia is dependent on an early age at diagnosis. It is generally regarded that effective bile drainage with resolution of jaundice can be achieved in up to 70% of patients with biliary atresia if the portoenterostomy is performed before 60 days of life as compared with 40% to 50% of patients if performed at 60 to 90 days of life, 25% of patients at 90 to 120 days, and only 10% to 20% of patients at 120 days.

Patients with neonatal cholestasis should have further liver evaluation including serum aspartate aminotransferase (AST), alanine aminotransferase (ALT), γ-glutamyl transferase (GGT), alkaline phosphatase, total protein, albumin, and prothrombin time (PT). Second, an abdominal ultrasound should be performed to rule out a choledochal cyst, biliary stones, sludge formation, or tumor compressing the extrahepatic bile duct. The size of the gallbladder and extrahepatic bile duct by ultrasound is variable in biliary atresia (from absent to normal caliber). Other abdominal abnormalities found in less than 20% of patients with biliary atresia include polysplenia, intestinal malrotation, discontinuous inferior vena cava, and preduodenal portal vein.

The majority of patients with neonatal cholestasis will require referral to a pediatric gastroenterologist to establish the underlying diagnosis. The causes of neonatal cholestasis include anatomic abnormalities (mentioned earlier), metabolic disorders, infectious agents, genetic syndromes, and endocrinopathies. Alert the surgeon for anatomic abnormalities including choledochal cyst, tumor, and spontaneous perforation of the bile duct. The stepwise approach to the diagnosis of biliary atresia entails a percutaneous liver biopsy and surgical intervention. If the liver histology is consistent with the diagnosis of biliary atresia, then the surgeon will perform an intraoperative cholangiogram. Intraoperative cholangiogram is considered the gold standard in the diagnosis of biliary atresia, and if the diagnosis is confirmed, the surgeon will proceed with the Kasai portoenterostomy.

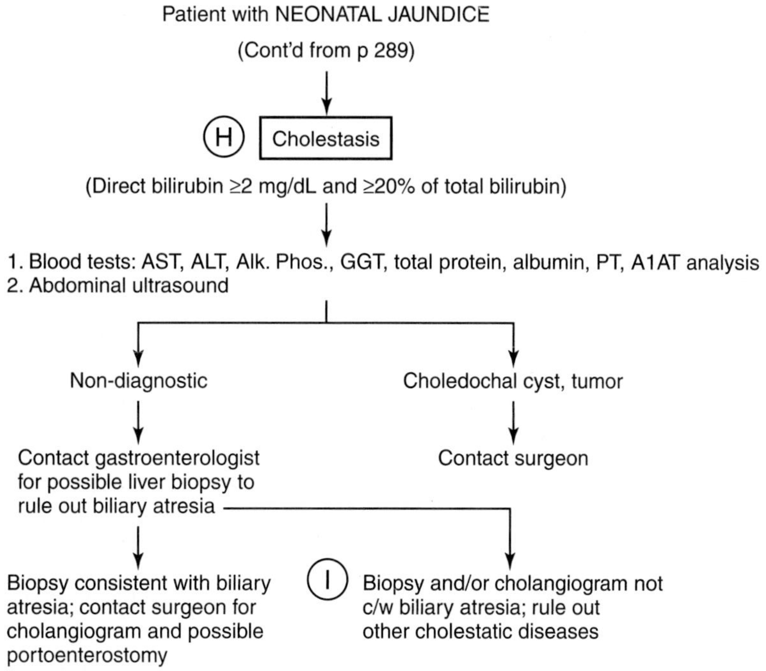
Patient with NEONATAL JAUNDICE
(Cont'd from p 289)
H
Cholestasis
(Direct bilirubin ≥2 mg/dL and ≥20% of total bilirubin)
1. Blood tests: AST, ALT, Alk. Phos., GGT, total protein, albumin, PT, A1AT analysis
2. Abdominal ultrasound
Non-diagnostic
Choledochal cyst, tumor
Contact gastroenterologist for possible liver biopsy to rule out biliary atresia
Contact surgeon
Biopsy consistent with biliary atresia; contact surgeon for cholangiogram and possible portoenterostomy
I
Biopsy and/or cholangiogram not c/w biliary atresia; rule out other cholestatic diseases

I. Uncommon Causes of Neonatal Cholestasis (see Table 1):

1. Metabolic disorders of neonatal cholestasis include alpha-1 antitrypsin (A1AT) deficiency, inborn errors of metabolism (IEOM), and bile acid synthesis defects (BASD). Approximately 10% to 15% of patients with A1AT deficiency have neonatal cholestasis, and it is diagnosed based on the serum A1AT level and phenotype. It is important to obtain this laboratory test early on in the evaluation of cholestasis because if A1AT deficiency is confirmed, then there is no need for further workup with a liver biopsy to rule out biliary atresia. IEOM that can present with cholestasis include, but are not limited to, galactosemia and tyrosinemia. Evaluation of galactosemia is part of the newborn screen and, if suspected, can be confirmed with the galactose-1-phosphate uridyl transferase serum level. Tyrosinemia can be diagnosed with the urine succinylacetone level. Other IEOM can be screened for with serum amino acid and urine organic acid studies. A primary test for BASD is measurement of total serum bile acids. Total bile acids in the serum will be below normal in BASD as compared with elevated in all other cholestatic diseases. If the total bile acids are low, then BASD is confirmed with measurement of individual bile acid levels by fast atom bombardment.
2. Infectious agents associated with neonatal cholestasis include the TORCH (toxoplasmosis, other, rubella, cytomegalovirus [CMV], and herpes) infections (particularly CMV), bacterial urinary tract infections (UTIs), and hepatitis A and B. Obtain a maternal history for TORCH infections and perform diagnostic workup if history or physical examination warrants. All infants with neonatal cholestasis should be screened for exposure to CMV with a urine CMV culture. Bacterial UTIs are associated with cholestasis, and cholestatic infants should have a catheter-obtained urine bacterial culture. Hepatitis A and B are uncommon causes of neonatal cholestasis and should be tested for with hepatitis A IgM and hepatitis B surface antigen only if the maternal or family history warrants.
3. Genetically associated causes of neonatal cholestasis include cystic fibrosis (CF), Alagille syndrome, and progressive familial intrahepatic cholestasis. If CF is suspected, then a sweat chloride test should be performed, even if the newborn screen result was negative. Alagille syndrome entails a constellation of physical findings including cholestasis caused by bile duct paucity, congenital heart disease such as peripheral pulmonic stenosis, abnormal facies, ophthalmologic abnormalities (posterior embryotoxon), and bony defects (butterfly vertebrae). Cholestatic neonates are screened for Alagille syndrome with an echocardiogram (if a murmur is detected), ophthalmologic examination, and spine film.
4. Endocrinopathies associated with neonatal cholestasis include isolated hypothyroidism and panhypopituitarism. Screening for these entities include TSH, total and free thyroxine (T_4), and early morning cortisol level.

References

American Academy of Pediatrics. Clinical Practice Guideline. Management of hyperbilirubinemia in the newborn infant 35 or more weeks of gestation. Pediatrics 2004;114(1):297–316.

Gourley GR, Arend RA. B-Glucuronidase and hyperbilirubinemia in breast-fed and formula-fed babies. Lancet 1986;1:644–6.

Suchy FJ. Neonatal cholestasis. Pediatr Rev 2004;25(11):388–96.

Wood AJ. Neonatal hyperbilirubinemia. N Engl J Med 2001;344(8):581–90.

Neonatal Seizures

Andrew White, MD, PhD, Lucy Zawadzki, MD, and Kelly Knupp, MD

Neonatal seizures can signify serious damage or malfunction of the immature brain and are considered a neurologic emergency requiring urgent diagnosis and treatment. The first month of life is the most vulnerable period for the development of seizures. The prevalence of neonatal seizures is greater in low-birth-weight and premature infants, and can be as high as 57 to 132 per 1000 live births. It is lower in term infants, ranging from 0.7 to 2.7 per 1000. The majority of seizures in neonatal period are classified as symptomatic (acute reactive) because of an underlying cause. Unprovoked seizures are usually classified into epileptic syndromes: two benign (benign neonatal convulsions and benign familial neonatal convulsions [BFNCs]) and two catastrophic (early myoclonic encephalopathy and early infantile epileptic encephalopathy).

CAUSATIVE FACTORS

The cause of provoked seizures can depend on the gestational age of the infant. Hypoxic ischemic encephalopathy (HIE) is the underlying cause in about 50% to 65% and is more common in term than premature infants. Seizures usually begin on first day of life and tend to be most severe in first 72 hours. In the majority of children with hypoxic ischemic encephalopathy, but not all, there is a clear history of fetal distress. Intracranial infections because of meningitis or sepsis are responsible for 5% to 10% of neonatal seizures. An additional 10% of seizures is provoked by intracranial hemorrhage. Subdural and subarachnoid bleeding are more commonly the result of trauma in term infants, and germinal matrix and intraventricular hemorrhages occur more frequently in premature infants. Aberrations in brain development, especially lissencephaly, pachygyria, and polymicrogyria, account for 5% to 10% of neonatal seizures. Metabolic causes include disturbances of glucose and calcium, and inborn errors of metabolism. Seizures secondary to intoxication or withdrawal because of intrauterine drug exposure can occur as early as 3 days of life or as late as 34 days of life.

A. History should include family history of seizures, history of infection, drug/alcohol/tobacco use during the pregnancy, details of maternal prenatal care and immunizations, birth history including mode of delivery and Apgar scores, as well as necessity for resuscitation at birth.

B. If possible, it is extremely helpful to visualize the episodes. Neonatal seizures are classified as follows:

1. Subtle: involving rocking, bicycling, swimming, eye deviation
2. Tonic: stiffening of arms, legs or trunk, upward eye deviation and apnea
3. Clonic: focal or multifocal nonsuppressible jerking movements of arms, legs, or face
4. Myoclonic: single or multiple jerks of an extremity

Notably, although not common, seizures can present as simple paroxysmal autonomic changes (tachycardia, hypertension) alone. Physical examination should include the measurement of head circumference, assessment of mental status (Is there tracking in a full term newborn?), identification of dysmorphic features and facial asymmetry, determination of neonatal tone and movement, evaluation of reflexes (tonic neck, suck, patellar, and Moro), presence of birthmarks or rashes, and evidence of accidental injection of anesthetic drug, trauma, or infection. Instability of temperature or blood pressure may indicate infection.

C. The electroencephalogram (EEG) can be valuable in the determining whether a particular behavior represents a seizure. Specific EEG patterns may correlate more closely with different pathologies. Background EEG rhythms (burst suppression as seen in Ohtahara) may allow for a more accurate prognosis. Either continuous (preferable) or repeat EEGs may be helpful in patient management.

D. Many mimics of neonatal seizures exist. These include jitteriness or tremulousness (noted in drug withdrawal, hypoxic-ischemic encephalopathy, or other metabolic conditions), benign neonatal sleep myoclonus (this occurs only during sleep), opisthotonus (possibly caused by meningeal irritation, associated with kernicterus or inborn errors of metabolism), and nonepileptic apnea (caused by cardiac, pulmonary, or gastrointestinal abnormalities). Methods that can be used to determine whether these are seizures include attempted suppression of movement (seizures are difficult to suppress), presence of eye deviation, nystagmus, and provocation using stimuli (seizures are not usually provoked).

E. Initial laboratory tests should include glucose, calcium, sodium, magnesium, phosphorous, liver function tests (LFTs), and a complete blood cell count. Infectious causative agents should always be ruled out. Maternal and neonatal drug screens can also be performed to check for drug withdrawal. If the child appears jaundiced, a bilirubin should be obtained. Tests that can be added if there is a suspicion of inborn error of metabolism include serum amino acids, urine organic acids, lactate, pyruvate, ammonia, and acylcarnitine profile. If no explanation is found for the seizure, cerebrospinal fluid should also be obtained and tested for amino

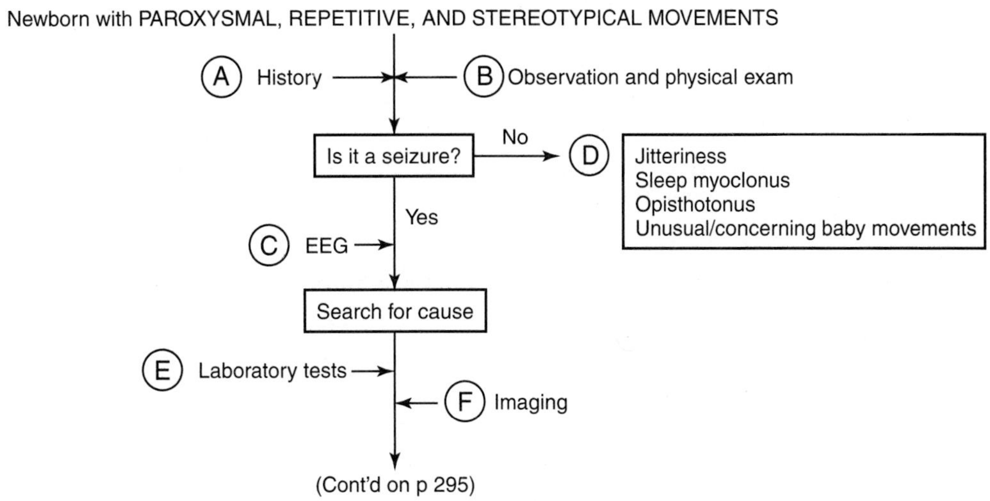
Newborn with PAROXYSMAL, REPETITIVE, AND STEREOTYPICAL MOVEMENTS
A History
B Observation and physical exam
Is it a seizure?
No
D
Jitteriness
Sleep myoclonus
Opisthotonus
Unusual/concerning baby movements
Yes
C EEG
Search for cause
E Laboratory tests
F Imaging

(Cont'd on p 295)

acids (specifically glycine), glucose, lactate, pyruvate, and to rule out meningoencephalitis.

F. Magnetic resonance imaging (MRI) with diffusion-weighted imaging is the most sensitive and therefore most preferred form of imaging. It is able to detect malformations of cortical development, strokes (even at a very early stage), changes from hypoxic-ischemic encephalopathy, meningeal enhancement associated with infection, and can often give clues to the type of inborn error of metabolism. It is not suited for a critically ill patient because it requires the patient to be brought to the machine and the study takes more time than other imaging modalities. It also is not very good at detecting blood unless specific sequencing is used. Computed tomography is able to detect more obvious parenchymal defects, bleeding, and when used with contrast, is excellent at detecting venous sinus thromboses. It takes much less time than an MRI but still requires patient transport. A more recent concern is that it also exposes the patient to radiation and increases the chance of subsequent malignancy. Ultrasound machines can be brought to the neonatal intensive care unit and hemorrhages can be identified. The technology, however, suffers from poor visualization of the cortex (specifically the convexities) and subarachnoid blood.

G. Infectious causes of meningitis in the neonate can be either bacterial (group B streptococcus, *Escherichia coli, Listeria monocytogenes*) or viral (herpes simplex virus [HSV] or cytomegalovirus [CMV]). Lumbar puncture is indicated in all infants suspected of having meningitis. Empiric treatment for neonatal meningitis usually consists of acyclovir, ampicillin, and cefotaxime. Treatment is refined when cultures and polymerase chain reaction (PCRs) are reported. MRI can be helpful in identifying stroke, hemorrhage, thrombosis, or abscess, and can be used to establish prognosis. MRI with diffusion-weighted imaging can also be useful in identifying seizure focality.

H. Vascular causes include both ischemic and hemorrhagic stroke, as well as arterial and venous thrombosis. All strokes should precipitate a hematologic workup. The timing of the workup is debatable. Typically, subarachnoid or subdural hemorrhages are seen in term infants, and germinal matrix bleeds (intraventricular hemorrhages) are seen in premature infants. Imaging and/or head circumference measurements can be used to follow resolution of hemorrhages.

I. There are many benign genetic causes of neonatal seizures, especially if there is a family history. BFNCs are focal or multifocal convulsions that occur within the first 2 weeks of life and are associated with a mutation in either the sodium or potassium ion channel. Benign infantile neonatal convulsions (BINCs or fifth-day fits) occur in otherwise healthy newborns and can be multifocal. They typically appear on the fourth or fifth day and continue for about 24 hours. They are refractory to drug treatment but resolve without sequelae. Other genetic causes that are associated with neonatal seizures include Smith–Lemli–Opitz, tuberous sclerosis, Aicardi syndrome, hypomelanosis of Ito, and incontinentia pigmenti. Chromosomal abnormalities can also lead to neonatal seizures.

J. Electrolyte abnormalities can also result in neonatal seizures. Hypoglycemia can be corrected with a dextrose 10% in water (D10W) bolus of 2 ml/kg, followed by an infusion of 6 to 8 mg/kg/min. Hypocalcemia is corrected using calcium gluconate (10%) 100 mg/kg intravenously (IV) over 1 to 3 minutes (monitor for bradycardia). A maintenance dose of 500 mg/kg/24 hour IV or PO should be instituted. Hypomagnesemia can be corrected using magnesium sulfate 25 to 250 mg/kg/dose IV or intramuscularly.

K. Many inborn errors of metabolism can result in seizures in the newborn period. Laboratory testing for these is described in section F. Two organic acidopathies that are strongly associated with neonatal seizures are propionic and methylmalonic academia. Other causes of neonatal seizures include nonketotic hyperglycinemia, urea cycle defects, amino acidopathies, and mitochondrial disorders. One other disorder that should be considered if the patient does not respond to standard antiepileptics is pyridoxine deficiency. This disorder is uniquely responsive to treatment with pyridoxine (vitamin B_6). It is recommended that this be done in an area with resuscitation equipment (because of the possibility of severe respiratory depression) using video-EEG.

L. Hypoxic-ischemic encephalopathy is the most common cause of neonatal seizures, and results from a lack of oxygen and blood flow to the newborn during the perinatal period. The injury and prognosis range from mild to severe and even fatal. MRI and EEG are both useful in establishing extent of injury and prognosis.

M. Malformations of cortical development are being identified more commonly as a cause of neonatal seizures. These stem from an abnormality in neuronal migration during development. Although the specific cause of the abnormality is usually not identified, it may be a result of drugs, infections (especially CMV), and genetics (e.g., LIS-1, ARX). Examples of malformations include focal cortical dysplasia, hemimegalencephaly, lissencephaly (smooth surface of the brain), pachygyria (thick cortex), and polymicrogyria (many small gyri).

N. The mainstays of treatment for neonatal seizures remain phenobarbital (20 mg/kg IV) or phenytoin (20 mg/kg). Levels of these drugs should be obtained 1 hour after the loading dose. Benzodiazepines (lorazepam, diazepam, or midazolam) may also be used if phenobarbital and phenytoin fail. Newer drugs including levetiracetam and topiramate are now commonly being used in tertiary care centers. Pyridoxine (50–100 mg IV) should always be tried for seizures that are resistant to treatment. A neonate should not be sent home on phenytoin because of its poor oral absorption.

O. There is a trend toward earlier withdrawal of medication (1–3 months). Although specific medication withdrawal techniques should be based on each individual patient, some general guidelines can be posed. The decision of whether to continue medication balances the likelihood of future seizures with the risks of the medication to the patient. If the seizures have stopped, the patient has a normal neurologic examination, and there is no identified cause that would make one suspect that seizures are likely, it is reasonable to discontinue medications at discharge. If the seizures have stopped and the neonate has an abnormal neurologic examination, but the follow-up EEG is normal, it is also reasonable to consider discontinuing antiepileptic medication. Follow-up with a neurologist should be scheduled for all neonates who have been discharged on antiepileptic medication. In addition, it is important to carefully monitor development of any child who has suffered seizures in the neonatal period. It is not uncommon for those individuals to suffer long-term sequelae, including the development of epilepsy, developmental delay, and behavioral disturbances.

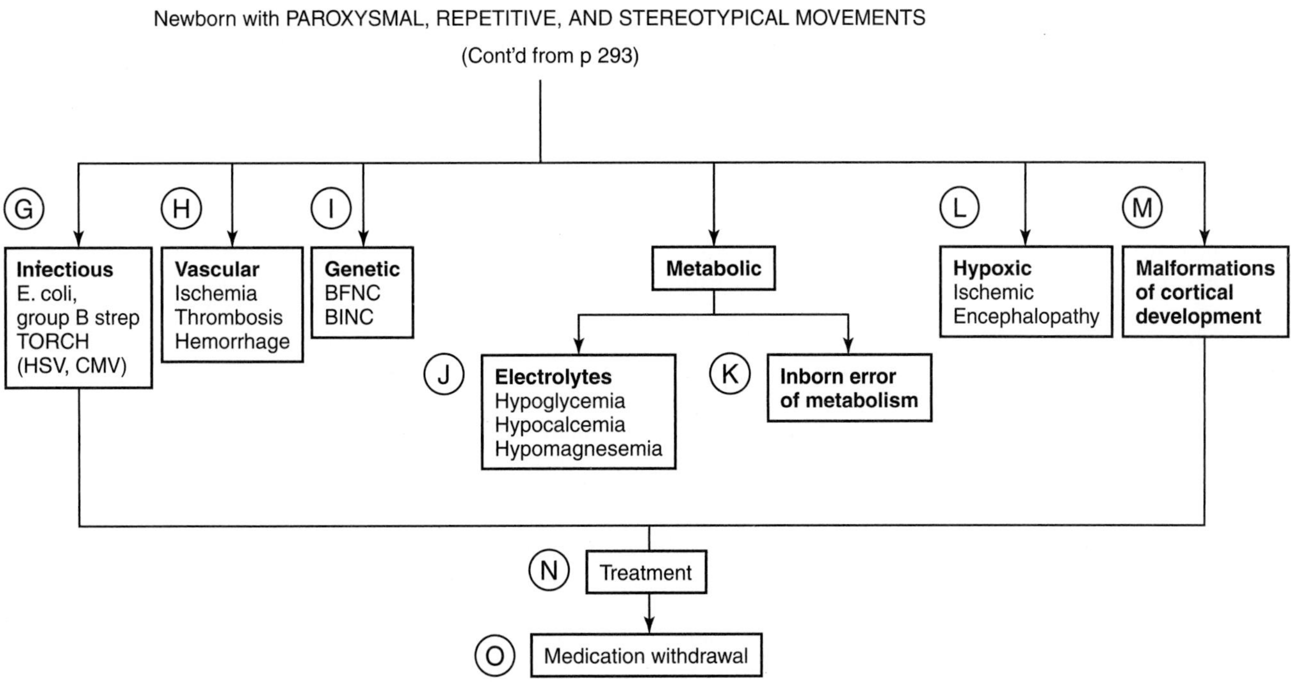
Newborn with PAROXYSMAL, REPETITIVE, AND STEREOTYPICAL MOVEMENTS
(Cont'd from p 293)
G
Infectious
E. coli,
group B strep
TORCH
(HSV, CMV)
H
Vascular
Ischemia
Thrombosis
Hemorrhage
I
Genetic
BFNC
BINC
Metabolic
J
Electrolytes
Hypoglycemia
Hypocalcemia
Hypomagnesemia
K
Inborn error
of metabolism
L
Hypoxic
Ischemic
Encephalopathy
M
Malformations
of cortical
development
N
Treatment
O
Medication withdrawal

References

Glass HC, Wu YW. Epidemiology of neonatal seizures. J Pediatr Neurol 2009;7(1):13–7.

Hauser WA, Kurland LT. The epidemiology of epilepsy in Rochester, Minnesota, 1935 through 1967. Epilepsia 1975;16:1–66.

Lanska MJ, Lanska DJ, Baumann RJ, Kryscio RJ. A population-based study of neonatal seizures in Fayette County, Kentucky. Neurology 1995;45:724–32.

Ronen GM, Penney S, Andrews W. The epidemiology of clinical neonatal seizures in Newfoundland: a population based study. J Pediatr 1999;134:71–5.

Sankar R, Painter MJ. Neonatal seizures: after all these years we still love what doesn't work. Neurology 2005;64:776–7.

Silverstein F, Jensen F, Inder T, et al. Improving the treatment of neonatal seizures: National Institute of Neurological Disorders and Stroke Workshop Report. J Pediatr 2008;153(1):12–5.

Volpe JJ. Neurology of the newborn. Philadelphia: WB Saunders; 2008.

Respiratory Distress Syndrome

Jason Gien, MD

Respiratory distress syndrome (RDS), once called *hyaline membrane disease,* results from surfactant deficiency, usually seen in premature infants, but can occur with decreased frequency in term infants. Incidence rates range from 86% at 24 weeks to less than 1% at 39 weeks. RDS should be anticipated in the setting of any preterm delivery, delivery where amniotic fluid indices indicate pulmonary immaturity, and in any infant born to a diabetic mother. Maternal corticosteroid therapy can prevent neonatal RDS when it is administered to the mother at least 24 to 28 hours before delivery.

A. In the physical examination, focus on the respiratory system; note the quality of respiratory effort (grunting, flaring, retractions, air entry, adventitial sounds), as well as respiratory rate. This assessment should include a decision about type of respiratory support needed. Search for evidence of congenital cardiorespiratory malformations (airway obstruction, congenital heart disease).

B. The chest radiograph in RDS is characterized by a diffuse reticulogranular or ground-glass pattern and hypoexpansion. Near-term infants may have a less specific hazy infiltrate. The radiographic appearance of RDS is often similar to that of group B streptococcal pneumonia, blood, or amniotic fluid aspiration, especially in term or near-term infants.

C. Included in the differential diagnoses are other systemic illnesses with pulmonary manifestations, such as congenital heart disease, hypoglycemia or cold stress, and polycythemia. Retained fetal lung fluid in near-term infants or aspiration syndromes (clear fluid, blood, or meconium) in term infants may lead to dilution or inactivation of surfactant, resulting in acquired surfactant deficiency and RDS.

D. Consider bacterial pneumonia (especially group B streptococcal disease) in patients with RDS. Risk factors for infection include maternal fever, chorioamnionitis, and premature or prolonged rupture of the membranes. Neutropenia (white blood cell count <2000 neutrophils/μl) or leukocytosis and a ratio of immature to total leukocytes greater than 0.2 are suggestive of infection. Draw blood culture specimens; consider tracheal aspirate samples in intubated infants. Initiate antibiotic therapy with ampicillin and an aminoglycoside (Table 1).

E. The natural history of RDS involves worsening of clinical symptoms, which occurs during the first 48 to 72 hours (Table 2). It is important to consider both the postnatal age of the patient and the severity of illness in choosing therapeutic interventions. Early initiation of continuous positive airway pressure (CPAP) by nasal prongs may stabilize alveoli and prevent atelectasis. A trial of CPAP in the first hours of life is useful if the patient is only mildly hypercapnic or ventilating normally and/or requiring a fractional inspired oxygen concentration (FiO_2) of less than 0.4 to maintain oxygenation. Extremely preterm infants and those with more severe disease often require intubation during delivery room resuscitation or shortly thereafter for mechanical ventilation and surfactant administration (see H). All neonates with RDS who have cardiac instability should have nothing by mouth and receive maintenance intravenous fluids and glucose (80 ml/kg fluids in the first 24 hours; 6–9 mg/kg per minute of glucose). Institution of total parenteral nutrition as soon as available is recommended, especially for preterm infants. In infants without cardiac instability, feeding via nasogastric tube is appropriate.

F. Monitor arterial oxygen saturation in every infant with RDS using pulse oximetry. Monitoring of preductal saturations and transcutaneous monitoring can provide information on PO_2 and PCO_2. Consider placement of an umbilical artery catheter or peripheral artery catheter in infants who require high oxygen, CPAP, or assisted ventilation. Connect arterial lines to pressure transducers for blood pressure monitoring and safety. Monitor glucose, electrolytes, and calcium and acid-base status.

G. Assisted ventilation is usually initiated with pressure-limited, time-cycled, synchronized intermittent mandatory ventilation. Synchronous intermittent mandatory ventilation delivers breaths that are synchronized to the onset of the patient's spontaneous breaths and allows spontaneous breaths between mechanical breaths. A peak inspiratory pressure that achieves some but not excessive chest rise is an appropriate starting point. Adjust peak inspiratory pressure and rate to normalize arterial blood gases. Positive end-expiratory pressure should be set initially at 5 cm water and adjusted accordingly for optimal inflation, being sure to avoid overinflation or underinflation. Synchronized pressure-limited volume ventilation when available may be preferable to pressure-limited ventilation. For extremely preterm infants, volumes of 4 to 6 ml/kg are appropriate; 6 to 8 ml/kg for near-term or term infants. High-frequency ventilation may be indicated under certain circumstances; consult a neonatologist.

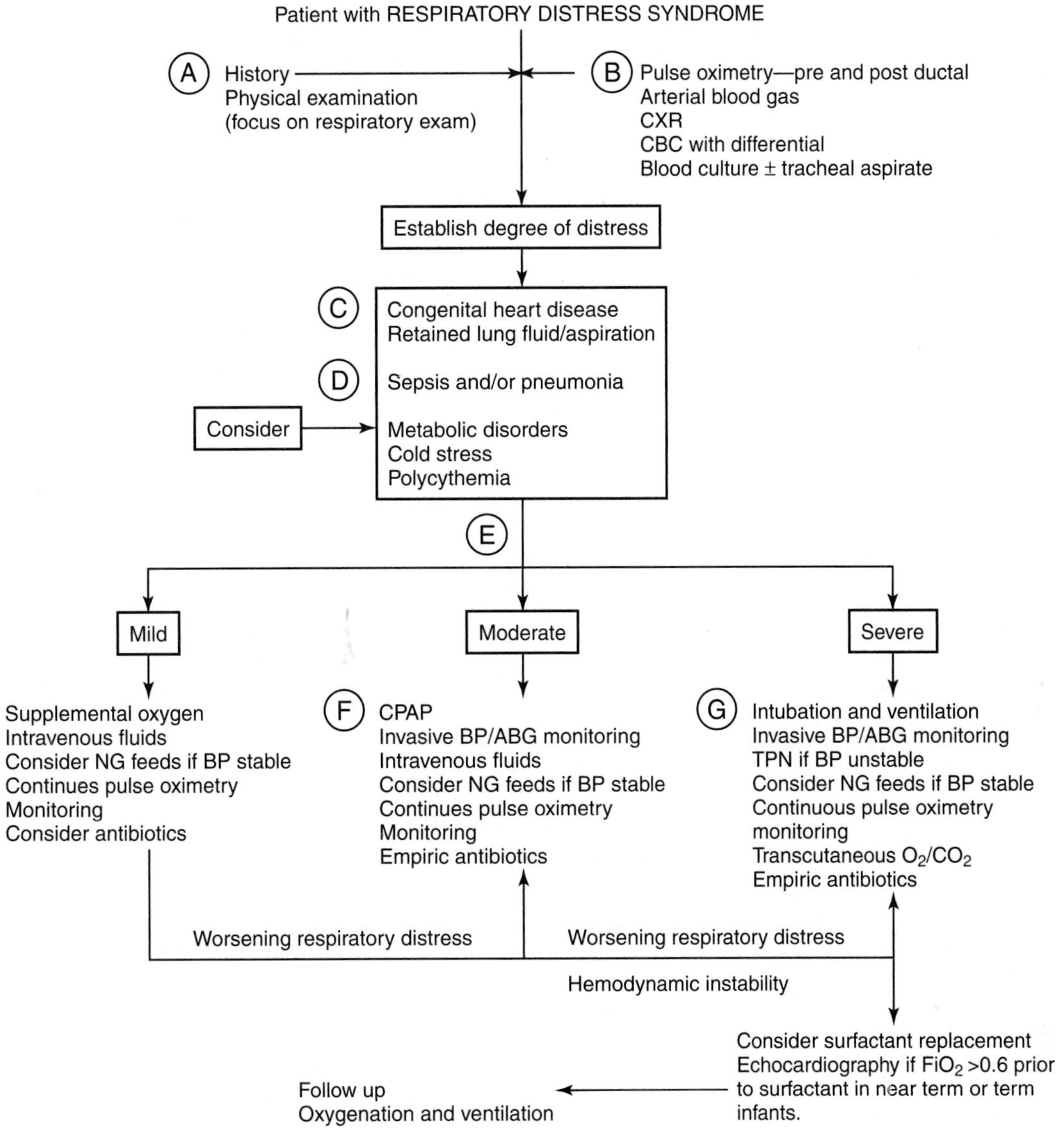

Patient with RESPIRATORY DISTRESS SYNDROME
(A) History
Physical examination
(focus on respiratory exam)
(B) Pulse oximetry—pre and post ductal
Arterial blood gas
CXR
CBC with differential
Blood culture ± tracheal aspirate
Establish degree of distress
(C) Congenital heart disease
Retained lung fluid/aspiration
(D) Sepsis and/or pneumonia
Consider
Metabolic disorders
Cold stress
Polycythemia
(E)
Mild
Moderate
Severe
Supplemental oxygen
Intravenous fluids
Consider NG feeds if BP stable
Continues pulse oximetry
Monitoring
Consider antibiotics
(F) CPAP
Invasive BP/ABG monitoring
Intravenous fluids
Consider NG feeds if BP stable
Continues pulse oximetry
Monitoring
Empiric antibiotics
(G) Intubation and ventilation
Invasive BP/ABG monitoring
TPN if BP unstable
Consider NG feeds if BP stable
Continuous pulse oximetry
monitoring
Transcutaneous O2/CO2
Empiric antibiotics
Worsening respiratory distress
Worsening respiratory distress
Hemodynamic instability
Consider surfactant replacement
Echocardiography if FiO2 >0.6 prior
to surfactant in near term or term
infants.
Follow up
Oxygenation and ventilation

Table 1. **Drugs Used to Treat Complications in Infants with Respiratory Distress Syndrome**

Drug	Dosage		
Ampicillin	Age <7 days	100 mg/kg/24 hr in 2 divided doses	Meningitis: 200 mg/kg/24 hr in 2 divided doses
	Age >7 days	<2000 g: 75 mg/kg/24 hr in 3 divided doses	Meningitis: 150 mg/kg/24 hr in 3 divided doses
Gentamicin	Premature newborn		
	Age <7 days	<1000 g and <28 wk GA: 2.5 mg/kg/dose every 24 hr <1500 g and <34 wk GA: 2.5 mg/kg/dose every 18 hr >1500 g and >34 wk GA: 2.5 mg/kg/dose every 12 hr	
	Age >7 days	<2000 g: 2.5 mg/kg/dose every 12 hr >2000 g: 2.5 mg/kg/dose every 8 hr	
Indomethacin	Initial dose:	0.2 mg/kg	
	Subsequent doses:		
	Age <48 hr at time of first dose	2 doses of 0.1–0.2 mg/kg at 12- to 24-hour intervals	
	Age 2–7 days at time of first dose	2 doses of 0.2 mg/kg at 12- to 24-hour intervals	

GA, gestational age.

Table 2. **Degree of Illness in Respiratory Distress**

	Moderate	Severe	Very Severe
FiO_2 to maintain adequate PaO_2	<0.4	>0.4	>0.6
PCO_2	<50 mm Hg	>50 mm Hg	>50 mm Hg
pH	Normal respiratory	Combined respiratory acidosis and metabolic acidosis	

H. Consider surfactant replacement therapy in patients with a diagnosis of RDS who require an FiO_2 greater than 0.4 with mechanical ventilation. Natural surfactants are preferable to synthetic surfactants. In term or near-term infants, screening echocardiogram for presence of pulmonary hypertension is advised before surfactant administration if FiO_2 in excess of 0.6.

I. Acute complications of RDS include pulmonary air leak (pneumothorax and pulmonary interstitial emphysema). Pulmonary hemorrhage can occur in the setting of patent ductus arteriosus (PDA). In term or near-term infants, persistent pulmonary hypertension may complicate RDS. RDS in premature infants is also associated with the chronic complications of retinopathy of prematurity, intracranial hemorrhage and its sequelae, necrotizing enterocolitis, hyperbilirubinemia, and anemia.

J. PDA is common in premature infants weighing less than 1500 g, including those who have received artificial surfactant for RDS. Suspect PDA with a continuous murmur, bounding pulses, diastolic blood pressure less than 26 mm Hg, and active precordium. The chest radiograph shows cardiomegaly with increased pulmonary blood flow or pulmonary edema. Color-Doppler echocardiography can confirm a left-to-right ductal shunt and demonstrate diastolic runoff from the aorta. Consider the use of indomethacin to promote ductal closure; indomethacin may be contraindicated for a patient with renal failure, thrombocytopenia or other coagulation disorders, or severe hyperbilirubinemia. Surgical ligation of the PDA may be necessary in urgent cases or if medical management is unsuccessful.

K. Persistent pulmonary hypertension in association with RDS most often occurs in near-term infants with congenital or acquired surfactant deficiency. Presentation may be immediately after birth or after several days of RDS. Right-to-left shunts through the ductus arteriosus or patent foramen ovale result in refractory hypoxemia. In the presence of a PDA, preductal saturations may be more than 15% to 20% greater than postductal PaO_2. Echocardiography can confirm right-to-left shunting through the ductus arteriosus and foramen ovale; the degree of pulmonary hypertension can be estimated by quantitation of a tricuspid regurgitation jet. Initial management includes adequate lung recruitment maintenance of adequate systolic blood pressure and circulating volume, correction of metabolic acidosis, and reversal of hypoxemia. High-frequency oscillatory ventilation (HFOV) and nitric oxide (NO) offer therapeutic alternatives followed by extracorporeal membrane oxygenation (ECMO) if the previous interventions fail.

References

Clark RH, Kueser TJ, Walker MW, et al. Low-dose nitric oxide therapy for persistent pulmonary hypertension of the newborn. Clinical Inhaled Nitric Oxide Research Group. N Engl J Med 2000;342:469–74.

Hein HA, Ely JW, Lofgren MA. Neonatal respiratory distress in the community hospital: when to transport, when to keep. J Fam Pract 1998;46:284–9.

Rodriguez RJ, Martin RJ. Exogenous surfactant therapy in newborns. Respir Care Clin North Am 1999;5:595–617.

Vyas J, Kotecha S. Effects of antenatal and postnatal corticosteroids on the preterm lung. Arch Dis Child 1997;77:F147–50.

Wright L. Effect of corticosteroids for fetal maturation on perinatal outcomes. Consensus Development Conference. Am J Obstet Gynecol 1995;173:253–62.

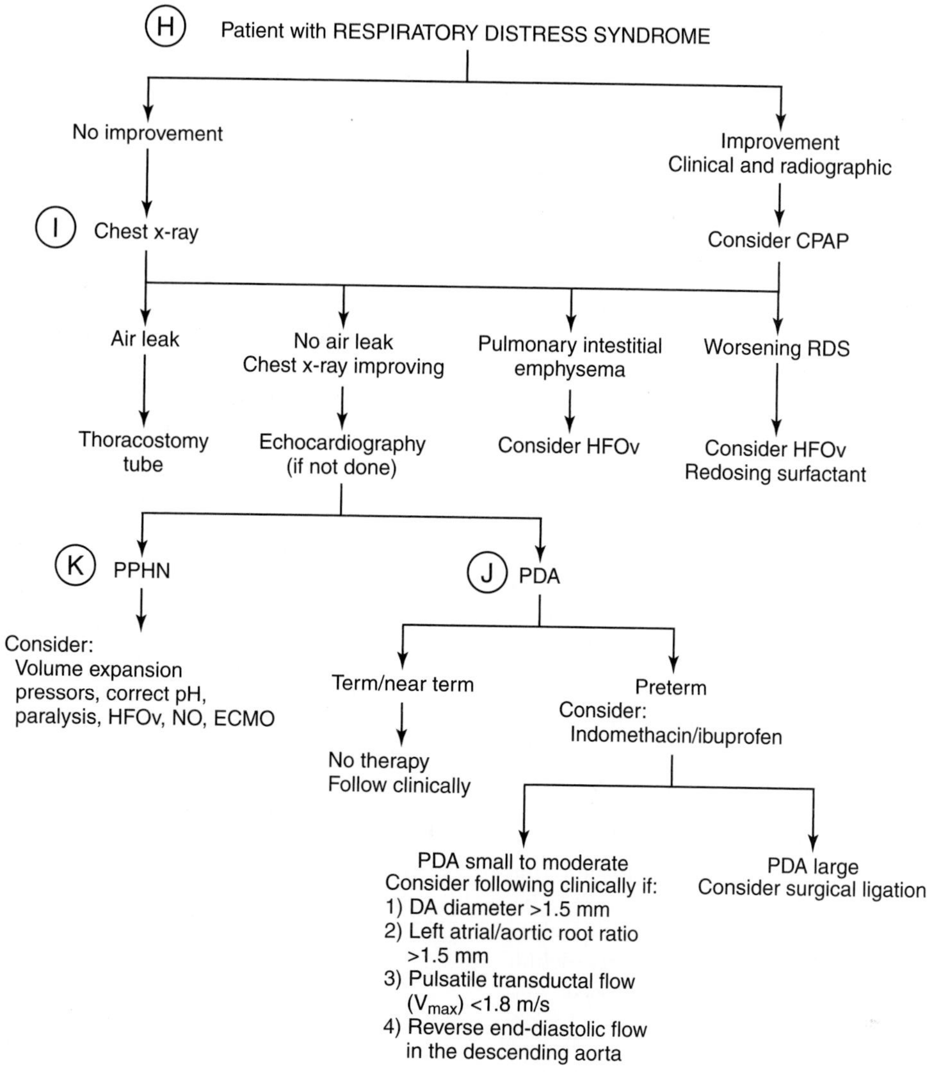
H Patient with RESPIRATORY DISTRESS SYNDROME
No improvement
Improvement
Clinical and radiographic
Consider CPAP
I Chest x-ray
Air leak
Thoracostomy tube
No air leak
Chest x-ray improving
Echocardiography
(if not done)
Pulmonary intestitial emphysema
Consider HFOv
Worsening RDS
Consider HFOv
Redosing surfactant
K PPHN
Consider:
Volume expansion
pressors, correct pH,
paralysis, HFOv, NO, ECMO
J PDA
Term/near term
No therapy
Follow clinically
Preterm
Consider:
Indomethacin/ibuprofen
PDA small to moderate
Consider following clinically if:
1) DA diameter >1.5 mm
2) Left atrial/aortic root ratio >1.5 mm
3) Pulsatile transductal flow (V_{max}) <1.8 m/s
4) Reverse end-diastolic flow in the descending aorta
PDA large
Consider surgical ligation

Neonatal Sepsis

Beena D. Kamath, MD, MPH

Perinatally acquired bacterial sepsis often presents with subtle or nonspecific signs but may progress rapidly to death. In such a condition with high mortality, low incidence, and relatively benign treatment, clinical practice dictates therapy for infants at risk on the basis of historical factors and diagnostic test results, as well as for those who are symptomatic.

CAUSATIVE FACTORS

Neonatal infection accounts for 29% of neonatal mortality around the world, or almost one million deaths per year. Epidemiology of neonatal infections depends on timing of the infection and whether the infected infant has risks because of ongoing hospitalization, prematurity, or central venous catheters. Early-onset infections occur within 48 hours of birth and represent infection acquired from vertical transmission in utero, either shortly before or during the process of birth. The most common causes of early-onset neonatal infection include group B streptococcus (GBS), *Escherichia coli,* and herpes (although symptoms may become apparent later). Late-onset sepsis occurs between 3 and 30 days after birth and is mostly hospital acquired. Common pathogens for late-onset sepsis include coagulase-negative *Staphylococcus, Staphylococcus aureus,* methicillin-resistant *Staphylococcus aureus,* gram-negative bacilli, and *Candida.* Finally, late late-onset sepsis occurs more than 30 days after birth and is particularly worrisome in a hospitalized patient for coagulase-negative *Staphylococcus,* resistant gram-negative organisms, or fungus. Infants who are admitted to the hospital after community exposure are at risk for respiratory viral pathogens, streptococcus, and methicillin-resistant *Staphylococcus aureus.*

Although the timing of neonatal infection affects the epidemiology of organisms seen, it is also important to know about the common pathogens and antibiotic resistance patterns of an individual hospital or locale. For example, in developing countries, the early versus late categories break down secondary to highly unclean environments, a large proportion of births that occur at home, and the lack of screening and prophylaxis for GBS infections. Increased use of screening and intrapartum antibiotic therapy to prevent neonatal GBS infections will continue to promote change in the cause of early-onset neonatal sepsis, with a marked decrease in the incidence of GBS infections, and an increase in ampicillin-resistant *Escherichia coli* and other gram-negative organisms.

This chapter focuses primarily on early-onset sepsis and, in particular, perinatally acquired bacterial infection. However, it is also important to consider congenital infection (bacterial and viral), perinatally acquired nonbacterial infection (e.g., herpes, enterovirus, mycoplasma, ureaplasma), and nosocomial infection (bacterial, viral, yeast) as other important causes of illness in the neonatal period.

A. The perinatal history provides important early information to assess the risk for sepsis in a newborn infant and should be complete to assess for risk factors (Table 1). Suspect chorioamnionitis with maternal temperature greater than 100.4° F (38° C), uterine tenderness, purulent or foul-smelling amniotic fluid, and maternal or fetal tachycardia. In the infant, hypothermia or temperature instability, hypoglycemia or hyperglycemia, and feeding intolerance can provide additional early signs of risk; however, such early signs may also be transient and nonspecific.

B. In the physical examination, note other nonspecific signs such as lethargy, hypotonia, fever or hypothermia, respiratory distress (tachypnea, cyanosis, grunting, apnea), tremulousness, irritability, weak suck, poor perfusion or shock, petechiae or purpura, and unexplained jaundice.

C. Obtain a blood culture specimen by sterile venipuncture or from a newly placed sterile umbilical catheter. Perform a lumbar puncture in neonates in whom sepsis is the primary diagnosis or who exhibit neurologic signs. Urine cultures have a low yield during the first 72 hours of life. Tracheal aspiration cultures are useful during the first 12 hours of life because the Gram stain may aid in early identification of bacterial causative agent. GBS antigen detection on serum likewise provides early, specific identification of an organism. Whereas neutropenia (white blood cell count $<5000/mm^3$) is a better predictor of sepsis than is neutrophilia (white blood cell count $>30{,}000/mm^3$), a ratio of immature to total neutrophils greater than 0.2 improves the predictive value. Toxic granulation or vacuolization of neutrophils and thrombocytopenia are useful but not definitive. The C-reactive protein (CRP) has low sensitivity, especially within the first 24 hours, but serial CRP determinations are more valuable in establishing a diagnosis of sepsis, because two negative CRP values have a high negative predictive value. No single laboratory test can accurately identify infected infants early in the disease course; therefore, various combinations of laboratory tests are used to identify neonatal sepsis. In addition, measures of cytokines, cell surface antigens, and bacterial genomes are currently under investigation to aid in the diagnosis of neonatal sepsis.

(Continued on page 302)

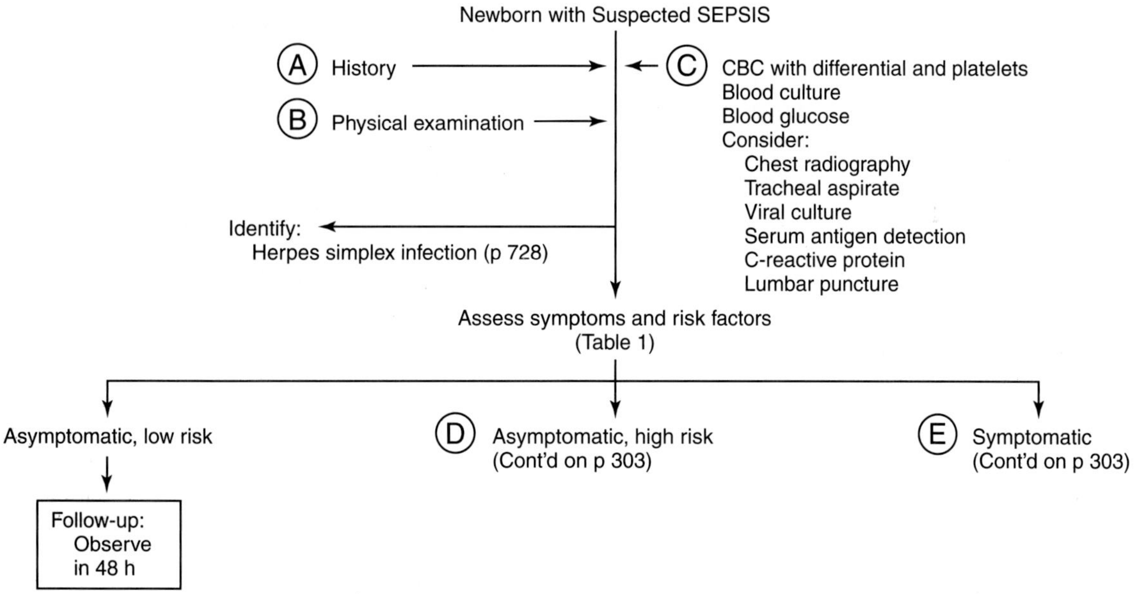
Newborn with Suspected SEPSIS
(A) History
(B) Physical examination
(C) CBC with differential and platelets
Blood culture
Blood glucose
Consider:
Chest radiography
Tracheal aspirate
Viral culture
Serum antigen detection
C-reactive protein
Lumbar puncture
Identify:
Herpes simplex infection (p 728)
Assess symptoms and risk factors
(Table 1)
Asymptomatic, low risk
Follow-up:
Observe
in 48 h
(D) Asymptomatic, high risk
(Cont'd on p 303)
(E) Symptomatic
(Cont'd on p 303)

Table 1. **Risk Factors for Neonatal Sepsis**

Condition	Incidence-Proven Sepsis	Incidence-Proven and Highly Suspected Sepsis*
PROM >18–24 hr	1%	1–2%
Maternal positive GBS	0.5–1%	1–2%
PROM and positive GBS	4–6%	7–11%
Positive GBS and maternal fever	3–5%	6–10%
PROM and chorioamnionitis	3–8%	6–10%
PROM or positive GBS and preterm	4–6%	7–11%
PROM and 5-min Apgar score <6	3–4%	6–10%
Male sex	Risk ↑ 4-fold	Risk ↑ 4-fold

*Highly suspected sepsis includes cases in which cultures were negative but the clinical presentation was highly consistent with bacterial infection, such as infants with pneumonia.

GBS, group B streptococcus; *PROM*, premature rupture of membranes.

Adapted from Gerdes JS. Clinicopathologic approach to the diagnosis of neonatal sepsis. Clin Perinatol 1991;18:361-81.

D. Treat the asymptomatic infant after evaluation of the risk factors. If maternal colonization with GBS is present but the infant is 35 weeks of gestation or more and the mother has received two or more doses of intrapartum antibiotic prophylaxis, the infant may be observed closely for 48 hours or longer. If one or two risk factors other than maternal colonization with GBS are present, perform laboratory screening and begin therapy as indicated. Consider treatment in the presence of three clinical risk factors, regardless of GBS status or results of screening.

E. Treat the symptomatic infant regardless of risk factors. Consider chest radiography in infants with respiratory symptoms. Monitor glucose concentration, oxygenation, blood pressure, renal function, electrolyte values, and coagulation. Consider viral cultures and serology if congenital infection or viral infection is possible.

F. Antibiotic therapy will vary according to whether neonatal sepsis is early- or late-onset sepsis. For early-onset sepsis, begin antibiotic therapy with intravenous or intramuscular ampicillin and an aminoglycoside (Table 2). For late-onset sepsis, intravenous or intramuscular ampicillin and an aminoglycoside can be started. A third-generation cephalosporin should also be considered if an infant has signs or symptoms for meningitis or community-acquired pneumonia. Otherwise, rapid emergence of cephalosporin-resistant, gram-negative organisms can occur if use is routine and has been documented as a problem in neonatal intensive care units that regularly use third-generation cephalosporins. For a hospitalized infant, or an infant with a central venous catheter, vancomycin can be given in place of ampicillin. Continue appropriate antibiotic treatment on the basis of culture results, with the goal to narrow antibiotic coverage as soon as identification and susceptibilities of the pathogen are known. Consider 7 to 10 days of therapy for positive GBS antigen. Treat positive blood culture for 7 to 14 days and meningitis for 14 to 21 days. Consider two antibiotics for coverage against gram negative bacteremia in extremely sick infants, or for treatment in infants with proven gram negative sepsis. If cultures are negative, discontinue antibiotics after 48 to 72 hours.

Table 2. **Medications Used in the Treatment of Neonatal Sepsis**

Drug	Dosage	Product Availability
Ampicillin	DOL 0–7 ≤2000 grams 25 mg/kg/dose every 12h Meningitis 50 mg/kg/dose every 12h DOL 0–7 >2000 grams 25 mg/kg/dose every 8h Meningitis 75 mg/kg/dose every 12h GBS meningitis: 66 mg/kg/dose every 8h DOL >7 <1200 grams 25 mg/kg/dose every 12h Meningitis 50 mg/kg/dose every 12h DOL >7 1200–2000 grams 25 mg/kg/dose every 8h Meningitis 50 mg/kg/dose every 8h DOL >7 > 2000 grams 25 mg/kg/dose every 6h Meningitis 50 mg/kg/dose every 6h GBS meningitis: 75 mg/kg/dose every 6h	Vials: 125, 250, 500 mg
Gentamicin	Postconceptional age ≤29 wk 0–7 days: 5 mg/kg/dose IV every 48h 8–28 days: 4 mg/kg/dose IV every 36h ≥29 days: 4 mg/kg/dose every 24h Postconceptional age 30–34 wk 0–7 days: 4.5 mg/kg/dose IV every 36h ≥8 days: 4 mg/kg/dose IV every 24h Postconceptional age >35 wk 4 mg/kg/dose IV every 24h	Intravenous solution: 10 mg/ml (2 ml)
Cefotaxime	≤7 days 50 mg/kg/dose IV every 12h >7 days 50 mg/kg/dose IV every 8h	Vials: 500 mg, 1 g, 2 g
Immunoglobulin, intravenous	Premature newborn: 500 mg/kg/dose Term newborn: 750 mg/kg/dose Reconstitute to 5% solution Graded, slow infusion	Vials: 2.5, 5 g

IV, intravenously.

G. Stabilize acutely ill infants with intubation, volume and pressor support, and coagulation factors as indicated. Treat seizures. Intravenous immunoglobulin may be useful in certain circumstances associated with neutropenia. Granulocyte transfusions and the use of cytokines continue to be under investigation.

(Continued on page 304)

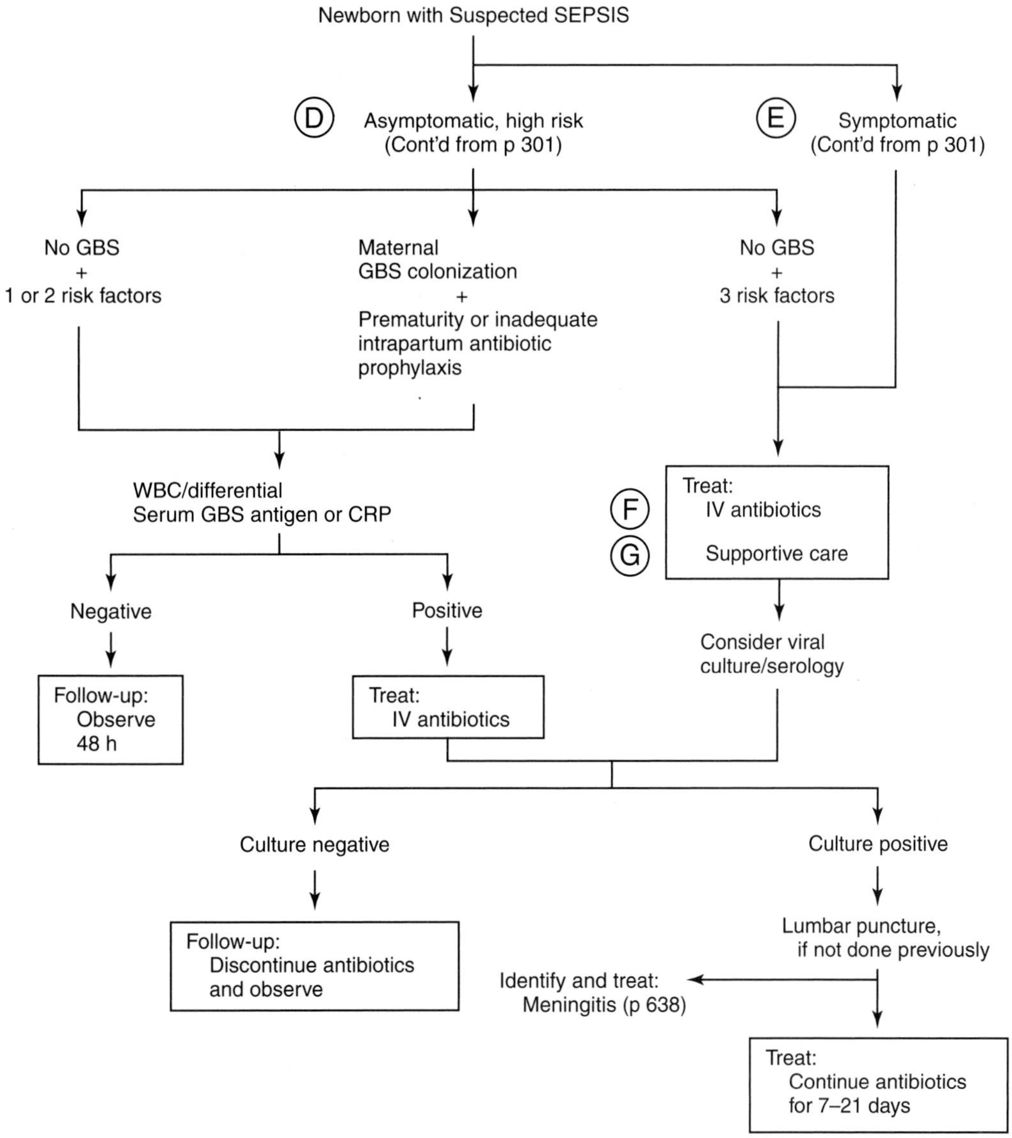
Newborn with Suspected SEPSIS
D
Asymptomatic, high risk
(Cont'd from p 301)
E
Symptomatic
(Cont'd from p 301)
No GBS
+
1 or 2 risk factors
Maternal
GBS colonization
+
Prematurity or inadequate intrapartum antibiotic prophylaxis
No GBS
+
3 risk factors
WBC/differential
Serum GBS antigen or CRP
Treat:
IV antibiotics
Supportive care
F
G
Negative
Positive
Consider viral culture/serology
Follow-up:
Observe
48 h
Treat:
IV antibiotics
Culture negative
Culture positive
Follow-up:
Discontinue antibiotics and observe
Lumbar puncture,
if not done previously
Identify and treat:
Meningitis (p 638)
Treat:
Continue antibiotics for 7–21 days

References

Allen SR. Management of asymptomatic term neonates whose mothers received intrapartum antibiotics—part 1: rationale for intrapartum antibiotic therapy. Clin Pediatr 1997;36:563–8.

Allen SR: Management of asymptomatic term neonates whose mothers received intrapartum antibiotics—part 2: diagnostic tests and management strategies. Clin Pediatr 1997;36:617–24.

Baltimore RS. Neonatal sepsis: epidemiology and management. Pediatr Drugs 2003;5(11):723–40.

Centers for Disease Control and Prevention. Revision of guidelines for the prevention of perinatal group B streptococcal disease. JAMA 2002;287:1106–7.

Garner AM, Hodgman JE. Can fullterm and nearterm infants at risk for sepsis be managed safely without antibiotics? J Perinatol 1999;19:589–92.

Gibbs RS, McDuffie RS Jr, McNabb F, et al. Neonatal group B streptococcal sepsis during 2 years of a universal screening program. Obstet Gynecol 1994;84:496–500.

Lawn JE, Kerber K, Enweronu-Laryea C, Cousens S. 3.6 million neonatal deaths—what is progressing and what is not? Sem Perinatol 2010;34:371–86.

Stoll BJ, Hansen N, Fanaroff AA, et al. Changes in pathogens causing early-onset sepsis in very-low-birth-weight infants. N Engl J Med 2002;347:240–7.

NEUROLOGIC DISORDERS

EVALUATION OF NEUROLOGIC DISORDERS

Evaluation of Neurologic Disorders

Timothy J. Bernard, MD, Paul Levisohn, MD,
and Stephen Berman, MD

Because it is increasingly possible to treat neurologic disorders, it is important to diagnose these conditions accurately. Keep in mind that many children will have disorders that cannot be cured, but that can be helped with palliative therapies. Case management aimed at addressing the physical, educational, and emotional needs of children with chronic neurologic disease, within the concept of a "medical home," is critically important for the child's well-being (see "Overview of Primary Care for the Child with Special Health Care Needs"). Presenting neurologic complaints can involve many areas; for example, weakness may be caused by disease throughout the nervous system, anywhere from the muscle to the cortex. The evaluation of neurologic disorders is based on the concept of localization, defining the areas of the involved nervous system associated with the patient's complaints and dysfunction to generate a differential diagnosis and to guide the subsequent diagnostic investigations.

A. In the patient's history, ask about the age at onset. Understand that parents may recognize a disorder only when a child reaches a certain developmental level. For example, parents may not recognize a congenital hemiparesis until the child begins to reach for objects at 4 months of age. Ask about the subsequent course of the illness to differentiate static from progressive disorders. Assess whether skills have been lost or whether there is a fixed deficit. Determining the age at which specific developmental landmarks were achieved can be useful in defining whether the difficulties reflect a delay in development or a loss of skills. It is important to recognize aspects of development that are never normal; for example, early hand preference (in infancy) is never normal, whereas some otherwise normal children will experience a delay, such as not walking until the middle of the second year of life. Consider obtaining family pictures and video recordings to document early developmental differences. School data may be helpful for both rate of progress and any loss of skills. Compare report cards, achievement test scores, and teacher evaluations. Most schools release these with proper authorization.

Clarify the words used by patients and parents. Patients may use dizziness to describe vertigo, lightheadedness, loss of balance and equilibrium, and even weakness. Numbness may mean loss of sensation, paresthesia, or loss of motor function in a limb, all suggesting a different localization. Ask about neck or back pain and injury (car accidents, slips, falls). Note episodes of significant head trauma. Mild closed-head injury, especially without loss of consciousness, is unlikely to lead to significant sequelae such as epilepsy or significant learning disabilities. Ask about vision, especially loss of vision. A mother can tell you about an infant who used to pick up small items and no longer does so. A child can often describe changes in the vision. This helps to diagnose an optic glioma or craniopharyngioma impinging on the optic pathways or visual compromise from increased intracranial pressure. Ask about head tilt and whether the child ever sees double. Ask about changes in hearing and any problems with swallowing, choking, sputtering, or aspirating food or liquid into the trachea. Ask about repetitive tasks (lifting smaller children, carrying a heavy backpack, helping with moving; sports such as gymnastics, wrestling, or football). Inquire about any sensory loss, as well as bowel and bladder control. When weakness is a concern, ask about the use of stairs and what time of day the child is weak (myasthenia often worsens during the day), and note trauma, pattern of weakness, sensory loss, and tingling. Ask about high-arched feet in the child and in the parents, as this may indicate peripheral nerve disease.

Evaluate the prenatal, perinatal, and neonatal history carefully, ideally with documentation of hospital records. Epilepsy and cerebral palsy are rarely related to perinatal events unless an acute neonatal encephalopathy is documented. Obtain a thorough family history, which can reveal genetic causes of neuromuscular disorders (Duchenne muscular dystrophy and myotonic dystrophy), epilepsy, migraine, tic disorders, and metabolic disorders that affect the central nervous system. Ask about family history of loss of walking ability or wheelchair use. Mitochondrial diseases may show evidence of maternal inheritance, as well as unexplained family history of hearing loss and diabetes.

B. Perform a careful neurologic examination with particular attention to the presence of findings that one might expect to occur together (neighborhood signs). When a formal neurologic examination is not possible in a young child, observe the child playing and interacting with parents. Note the mental status by observing speech and language.

Assess the cranial nerve function to the extent possible. Cranial nerve testing is reviewed in Table 1. With two or more dysfunctional cranial nerves, the brainstem is the most likely location. Examine the fundi. Ophthalmoscopic examination of infants and children can be particularly difficult if the child will not maintain fixation. This can often be achieved by the use of an appropriate target, such as a toy, and by maintaining sufficient ambient light to allow fixation. In addition to assessing the disk, observe the retinal vessels and the macula, noting chorioretinitis and retinal hemorrhages. In a child with headache, a careful ophthalmoscopic examination may reveal papilledema or absence of venous pulsations (although this finding can be normal). Consider performing visual field testing by presenting

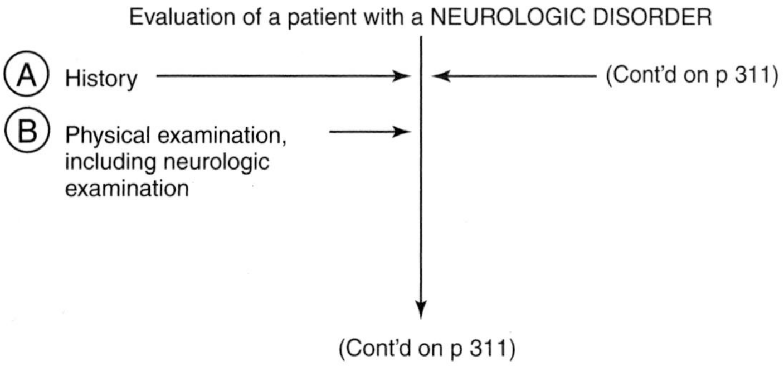
Evaluation of a patient with a NEUROLOGIC DISORDER
A History
B Physical examination, including neurologic examination
(Cont'd on p 311)
(Cont'd on p 311)

Table 1. **Cranial Nerve Testing**

Nerve	Testing Age	Comments
I (smell)	About 4 years	Head injury, coup-contrecoup Some frontal tumors
II (vision)	From birth	Optic nerve tumor in infancy Craniopharyngioma in childhood Increased ICP (hydrocephalus) Degenerative (neuronal ceroid-lipofuscinosis)
III, IV, VI	Some from birth	Eye does not move fully VI: ICP, tumor in brainstem III: herniation IV: often frontal trauma (e.g., fall off tricycle) Child reports double vision, may tilt head; try to determine field of diplopia Brainstem glioma; herpes or other brainstem infection
V	About 4 years	Touch three sensory divisions, palpate masseter while child bites
VII	From birth	Traumatic, facial nerve palsy Congenital, Moebius Acquired, Bell's palsy Brainstem glioma (requires others)
VIII	From birth	Audiologic testing, brainstem auditory-evoked response Early hearing test
IX	From birth	Acquired: document loss of gag Diagnosis of brainstem tumor requires other cranial nerve dysfunction
XI	From birth	Fasciculations, Werdnig–Hoffmann To one side, brainstem tumor (vs. infection)

ICP, intracranial pressure.

toys or objects of interest to the periphery, as well as by using an opticokinetic drum or tape. Pupillary response to light may indicate an afferent pupil (optic nerve dysfunction). A "swinging flashlight" assessment will reveal paradoxical pupillary dilatation to the light from the unaffected to the affected eye. A persistent head tilt may indicate abnormal ocular movements and lack of conjugate vision, and is often the first sign of a brain tumor. Asymmetric facies at rest or asymmetry of the nasolabial folds may indicate central facial weakness. Peripheral facial weakness and unilateral loss of taste support the diagnosis of Bell palsy. In infants, differentiate asymmetric facial movement (asymmetric crying facies caused by congenital absence of the depressor anguli oris) from mild Mobius sequence. Localization of a bell or rattle will help confirm grossly intact hearing, although this should not replace a more formal audiologic assessment in the young infant. Suck and swallow can be assessed by having the child suck on the examiner's finger.

Assess motor function. Note muscle bulk and tone; observe activity. Look for muscle fasciculations. Grade weakness as follows: 5, normal; 4, mild weakness against resistance; 3, antigravity strength only; 2, movement possible if gravity is eliminated (i.e., from side to side); 1, trace; 0, no muscle movement. Identify unilateral weakness by offering toys to a toddler to determine whether inappropriate hand preference is present. Assess gait in the young school-aged child by observing skipping, running, and hopping, and heel, toe, and side of foot walking. Test hand strength by asking the child to spread all fingers and not let you push them together. Then check the strength of index finger to thumb opposition, then little finger to thumb opposition, then all fingers flexed (slip your fingers under them and try to pull up). Then have the child extend the hand and you try to push it back. Throughout this, keep telling the child to be strong. Test upper body strength. Ask the child to flex arms and be strong while you try to pull against the arm (biceps). Ask the child to extend the arm; you push, trying to flex the arm (triceps). Ask the child to get up from a chair without using hands or arms, get up from the floor without using hands or arms (assessing for a Gower maneuver), and step up with each foot on a small step stool. Look at calves (gastrocnemius), especially of 3- to 5-year-old boys, for the enlargement of Duchenne disease. Test toe and heel walking; heel walking usually deteriorates first in patients with ataxia. Hemiparesis without sensory loss and with hyperreflexia suggests a long-standing deficit, usually at the level of the cortex or brainstem. Tap reflexes—biceps, triceps, brachioradialis, patella, and ankle—to identify alterations. Asymmetries are more significant than are mildly increased or decreased reflexes. Grade reflexes as follows: 0, no response; 1, trace or decreased response; 2, normal response for age; 3, increased but not pathologic; 4, pathologic with clonus/reduplication. Hypotonia with preserved reflexes suggests a central process; the absence of reflexes suggests a primary neuromuscular disorder, likely localized to the lower motor neuron. When appropriate, assess infantile reflexes, looking for asymmetries or failure to outgrow reflexes at an appropriate age (Table 2). Distinguish between delayed reflexes and abnormal reflexes (i.e., reflexes that never occur in a normal child or are asymmetric). In a child younger than 12 months, the plantar grasp reflex may obscure an extensor toe sign (Babinski). Persistent fisting, especially if it is unilateral, may represent a "cortical thumb," essentially the equivalent of a Babinski reflex.

Sensory function is often difficult to evaluate, particularly in the young child or infant. Assess sensory function if there is concern about a myelopathy (spinal cord dysfunction). Facial sensation can be assessed by eliciting the root reflex in an infant. Sensory loss contralateral to a motor deficit and weakness indicates the level of a spinal cord abnormality. Test the ulnar, median, and radial nerves by light touch to back of hand, little finger, thumb, and middle finger. Touch each hand and ask whether it can be felt on each hand and if it feels the same on both hands. If all have decreased sensation, use light touch from fingertips up the arm looking for the glove of glove-stocking distribution. Ask the child to tell you when he or she feels it better. Do three or four different routes. If you find glove-stocking on hands, be sure to do the feet and vice versa.

Assess coordination and cerebellar function. If the child is too young to do finger to nose, entice him or her to reach for an object, checking for ataxia. Children aged 4 years and older can do finger to nose, rapid alternating motion, and finger to thumb opposition. Active play with an infant may be sufficient to determine the presence of tremor or dysmetria. Distinguish limb ataxia (appendicular) from truncal ataxia. Note adventitious movements caused by tics (repetitive, monophasic movements), chorea, athetosis (dancelike), or tremor. Note myoclonus, a sudden rapid muscle contraction with slow recovery suggestive of a degenerative central nervous system disorder. Evaluate rapid alternating movements for both rhythmicity and asymmetry.

In the physical examination, note the presence of dysmorphic features that might aid in diagnosis of a specific inherited syndrome (see page 674). Measure the head circumference in all infants and in older children if there are concerns about megalencephaly caused by hydrocephalus or central nervous system storage diseases. Inspect the skin; neurocutaneous disorders are among the most common causes of brain problems. Look for adenoma sebaceum, shagreen patches, café-au-lait or depigmented spots, ecchymoses, and other evidence of trauma. Consider a Wood light examination to aid in diagnosis of tuberous sclerosis. The presence of organomegaly may help define an inherited storage disease. In the child with suspected myelopathy, carefully examine the spine for evidence of dysraphism (e.g., sacral dimple or tuft of hair) or disk space infection (localized tenderness to percussion). Assessment of the spine for scoliosis should be part of the routine examination in all school-aged children. Scoliosis and other abnormalities of the spine may indicate neuromuscular disorders.

(Continued on page 310)

Table 2. **Infantile Reflexes and Postural Reactions**

Postural Reflex	Age Reflex Appears	Age Reflex Disappears
Positive supporting action	Well developed in 50% of newborns	Indistinguishable from normal standing
Placing reaction	37 weeks	Covered up by voluntary action
Crossed extensor reflex	Newborn	7–12 months
Crossed adductor reflex to quadriceps jerk	3 months	8 months
Tonic neck reflex	Never complete and obligatory	
Grasp reflex		
Palmar	28 weeks	4–5 months
Plantar	Newborn	9–12 months
Moro reflex	28–32 weeks	4–5 months
Parachute reaction	4–9 months	Covered up by voluntary action
Postrotational nystagmus	Any age	

From Menkes JH. The neuromotor mechanism. In: Cooke RE, editor. The biologic basis of pediatric practice. New York: McGraw-Hill; 1968.

C. Diagnostic testing can confirm the localization and subsequently help define the pathophysiologic mechanism of the disorder. Obtain studies to assess a suspected underlying systemic disease, such as metabolic disorders (e.g., hypothyroidism, phenylketonuria) or bacterial infections (e.g., meningitis). Remember that early detection of inborn errors of metabolism may prevent long-term disability.

Structural central nervous system abnormalities can be defined by appropriate imaging techniques. With concerns about hydrocephalus or intracranial hemorrhage in the neonate, consider screening with a cranial ultrasound examination. Computed tomography, a more sensitive tool, is useful for early detection of calcifications from intrauterine infection, for assessment of ventricular size, and for determination of the presence of intracranial blood. Magnetic resonance imaging (MRI) can determine the presence of abnormalities of cerebral architecture (such as migrational disorders) and of white matter (leukoencephalopathy), as well as most tumors, brainstem disease, and myelopathy. MRI of very young patients may fail to reveal central nervous system dysplasia or heterotopia. Consider magnetic resonance angiography for suspected disorders of the major cranial vasculature. However, cerebral angiography may still be necessary for visualization of small vessels when a central nervous system vasculitis is present.

Electroencephalography remains important for the assessment of seizures. It also has a role in prognostication of neonatal encephalopathy, in monitoring of comatose patients, and in determining the depth of barbiturate coma in patients with acute increased intracranial pressure. The role of electroencephalography in determining irreversible coma ("brain death") is limited, particularly in the young infant. Evoked potentials have limited use in pediatrics except in the assessment of hearing in the young infant.

Lumbar puncture is primarily used for diagnosing central nervous system infection, but it is also important for defining increased intracranial pressure, as well as being part of the assessment for childhood central nervous system neoplasms. When there is a concern for increased intracranial pressure, a head image should precede the lumbar puncture to avoid herniation. Obtain measurements of cerebrospinal fluid lactate and pyruvate when mitochondrial disorders of intermediary metabolism are suspected.

Electromyography–nerve conduction velocity (EMG-NCV) testing is painful but may be useful in assessing weakness and neuropathies. Muscle biopsy is being replaced by specific molecular genetic testing in children with disorders of muscle (e.g., Duchenne muscular dystrophy) but remains useful in assessment of children with suspected mitochondrial disorders.

D. Assess the age at onset, pattern (acute, chronic, relapsing), progression (static or progressive), and localization. Neuromuscular disorders that occur in infancy have causes different from those of disorders that first occur in older children. Neurodegenerative disorders are best evaluated by defining the age at onset, as well as the rate of deterioration.

Assess the findings and symptoms as to whether the pattern is acute, chronic, or relapsing. It may initially be difficult to determine whether the disorder will become chronic or recurrent. Assess whether the condition is static versus progressive. Recognize that the determination of progressive deterioration in children can be difficult. The rate of developmental progress may be falling off even as the child continues to gain some new skills. In contrast, the child with mental retardation may appear to be losing skills relative to peers because a plateau has been reached on tests of cognitive skills and the child appears to have lost IQ "points."

E. Assess the patient for a systemic disorder (infection, toxin, metabolic disorder, neoplasia, hypoxia/ischemia, trauma, neurocutaneous disorders, degenerative disorder, and genetic disorder and syndromes). Altered mental status, for example, may be caused by a primary disorder of brain but may also reflect systemic illness. Headache may suggest increased intracranial pressure or may reflect disorders of intracranial vasculature (migraine), connective tissue (muscle tension headache), dental dysfunction (bruxism and temporomandibular joint dysfunction), sinusitis, or psychiatric disorders.

F. If you have obtained a careful history and physical examination and the signs, symptoms, and test results do not fit a well-recognized configuration, consider conversion hysteria. Psychogenic seizures, vision loss, and limb paralysis are all well-known to pediatric neurologists, but these diagnoses must be made with caution.

References

Berg BO. The clinical evaluation. In: Principles of child neurology. New York: McGraw-Hill; 1996. p. 5–22.

Blume WT, Kaibara M. Atlas of pediatric electroencephalography. Philadelphia: Lippincott-Raven; 1999.

Thompson RJ, Gustafson KE. Adaptation to chronic childhood illness. Washington, DC: American Psychological Association; 1996.

Evaluation of a patient with a NEUROLOGIC DISORDER

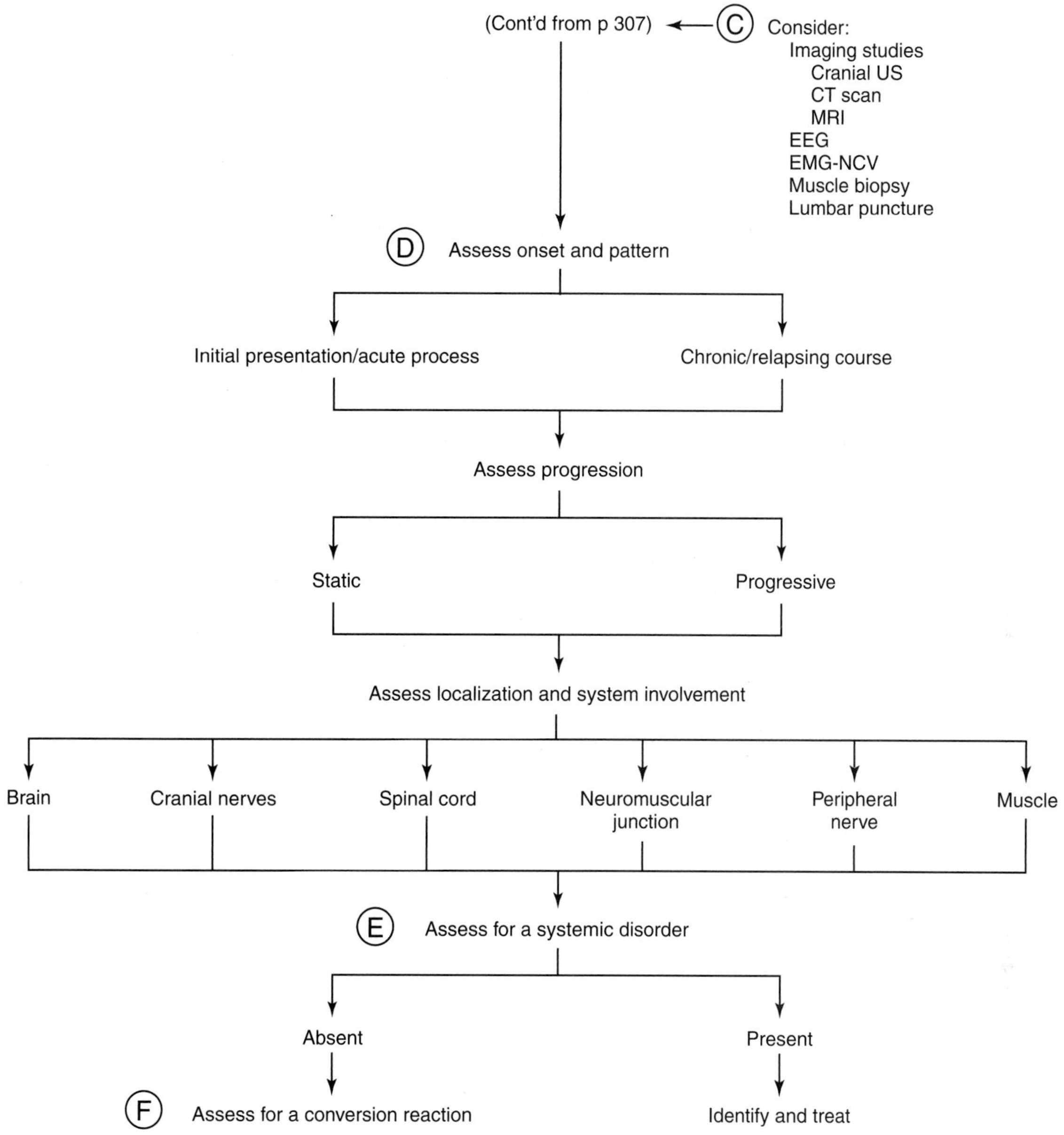
(Cont'd from p 307)
C
Consider:
Imaging studies
Cranial US
CT scan
MRI
EEG
EMG-NCV
Muscle biopsy
Lumbar puncture
D
Assess onset and pattern
Initial presentation/acute process
Chronic/relapsing course
Assess progression
Static
Progressive
Assess localization and system involvement
Brain
Cranial nerves
Spinal cord
Neuromuscular junction
Peripheral nerve
Muscle
E
Assess for a systemic disorder
Absent
Present
F
Assess for a conversion reaction
Identify and treat

NEUROLOGY*

*The editors and authors wish to express their appreciation to Dr. Tim Bernard for his work in coordinating the Neurology section of this book.

Abnormalities of Head Size and Shape

Ed Jernigan, MD, and Tonia Sabo, MD

HEAD SIZE

Macrocephaly

Macrocephaly is defined as a head size greater than two standard deviations above the mean for age, sex, and ethnicity. This criterion includes both benign anatomic variants of no clinical importance and a multitude of pathologic conditions. Diagnostic workup should be considered in any infant with documented macrocephaly or when serial measurements of head circumference cross percentile lines.

A. Clues to causative factors are usually found on history and examination. Medical history should focus on possible causes of hydrocephalus (e.g., prematurity, intraventricular hemorrhage, or meningitis). Family history may be significant for metabolic disease, neurocutaneous syndromes, or benign familial macrocephaly. Physical examination should focus on possible underlying causes. A bulging fontanelle, papilledema, or "sunsetting" of the eyes suggests hydrocephalus or increased intracranial pressure from a mass lesion. A bruit across the fontanelle or systemic signs of congestive heart failure indicate an intracranial vascular malformation. Hyperpigmented or hypopigmented macules may indicate a neurocutaneous syndrome. Dysmorphic features or organomegaly may be signs of a chromosomal or metabolic disease, respectively.

B. Diagnostic evaluation typically begins with head ultrasound to assess the size and shape of the ventricles. If unrevealing, the next step is usually magnetic resonance imaging (MRI) of the brain for identification of abnormalities such as tumors, congenital anatomic abnormalities, and vascular malformations.

C. If MRI shows only megalencephaly (i.e., proportionally large brain), then correct assessment of development becomes critical. If delayed—and especially if there has been a loss of milestones—then a neurodegenerative disorder should be suspected. Patients with family history of benign megalencephaly and with normal development may be observed over time without further intervention. Infants with megalencephaly and developmental delay may warrant neurologic consultation. If regression is present, a neurologic and probably metabolic evaluation is indicated.

Microcephaly

Microcephaly, a head size greater than two standard deviations below the mean for age, may be categorized as either primary or secondary. The primary type is caused by inherited conditions such as chromosomal abnormalities, migrational defects, or neurocutaneous syndromes. Secondary microcephaly is the result of an external injury, most commonly in the prenatal or perinatal period. Examples include hypoxic-ischemic encephalopathy, TORCH (toxoplasmosis, other, rubella, cytomegalovirus, and herpes) infection, and maternal malnutrition.

A. History should focus on pregnancy and perinatal complications, family history of microcephaly-associated syndromes, and early developmental milestones. Physical examination should focus on neurologic abnormalities (e.g., tone and reflexes), dysmorphic features, neurocutaneous stigmata, and abnormalities of cranial shape.

B. Brain MRI is relatively high yield in infants with microcephaly and developmental delay. Common findings include cerebral infarction and various structural abnormalities such as schizencephaly or polymicrogyria (among others). Laboratory testing may include chromosomes, microarray, amino or organic acids, or TORCH titers depending on associated features.

C. Microcephaly may be familial and benign, but also may indicate a severe central nervous system abnormality. Ultrasound or preferably MRI may show cerebral atrophy, dysgenesis, or old injury (e.g., in utero stroke). Computed tomographic (CT) scan is preferred to look for calcifications if TORCH infection is suspected.

(Continued on page 316)

Patient with ABNORMALITIES OF HEAD SIZE AND SHAPE

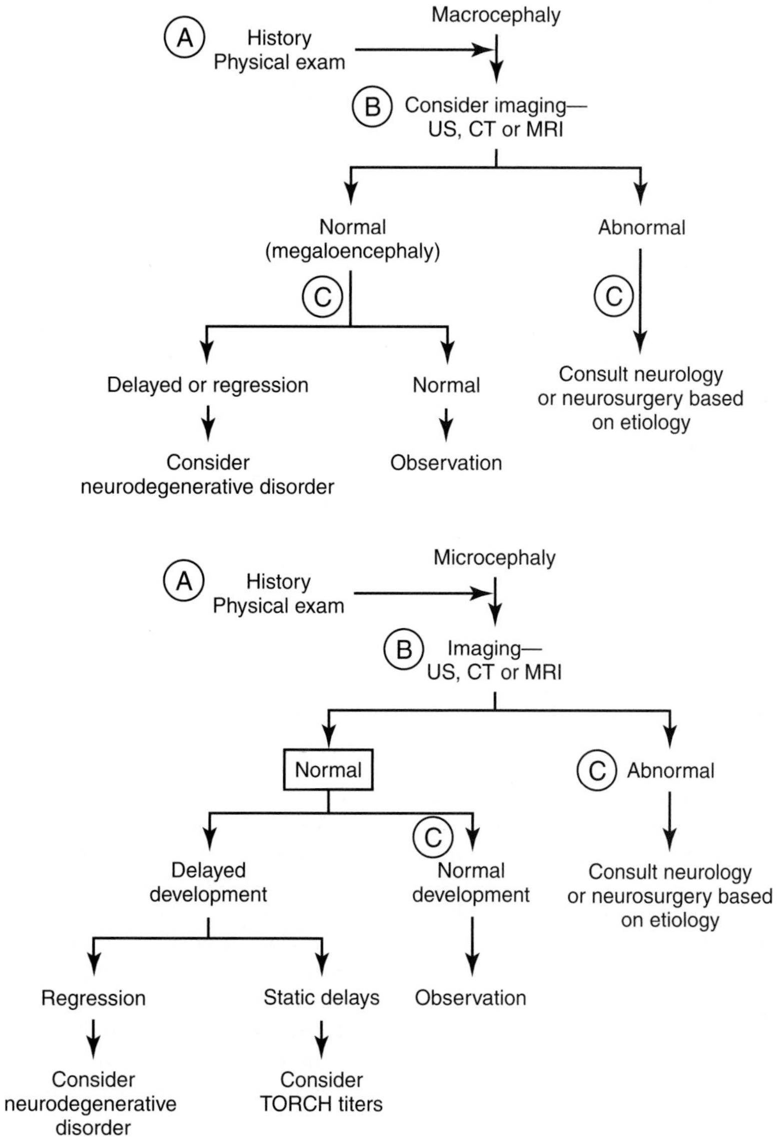
Macrocephaly
A
History
Physical exam
B
Consider imaging—
US, CT or MRI
Normal
(megaloencephaly)
Abnormal
C
C
Delayed or regression
Normal
Consult neurology
or neurosurgery based
on etiology
Consider
neurodegenerative disorder
Observation
Microcephaly
A
History
Physical exam
B
Imaging—
US, CT or MRI
Normal
C
Abnormal
C
Delayed
development
Normal
development
Consult neurology
or neurosurgery based
on etiology
Regression
Static delays
Observation
Consider
neurodegenerative
disorder
Consider
TORCH titers

HEAD SHAPE

A. Skull deformity in infants may be divided into three broad categories: positional deformity, isolated craniosynostosis, or craniosynostosis associated with an underlying metabolic syndrome.

B. The clinician's primary initial task is to distinguish between the relatively common positional deformity and the far less common—but more serious—*craniosynostoses*.

C. Craniosynostosis can also be associated with uncommon genetic syndromes, such as Apert syndrome, Crouzon syndrome, Jackson–Weiss syndrome, and Pfeiffer syndrome. Evidence of dysmorphology on physical examination, especially facial, dental, or hand/foot abnormalities, should warrant a genetics evaluation. A neurosurgical consult is warranted for consideration of surgical correction and proper timing of need of intervention. A true craniosynostosis may cause increased intracranial pressure and neuro-ophthalmologic complications in the medium term, and (if less severe) significant psychosocial distress later on.

Workup

Although the anterior fontanelle remains open, a head ultrasound is useful for evaluating the size and shape of ventricles. A noncontrast CT scan will show mass lesions, arteriovenous malformations, and subdural fluid collections. MRI is necessary when an underlying structural abnormality or neurodegenerative disease is suspected. Abnormalities on neuroimaging warrant further consultation based on causative factors. Common neurosurgical processes include hydrocephalus, space-occupying lesions, and subdural hematomas.

Abnormal head shape may be pathologic or benign. Severe deformity, any evidence of increased intracranial pressure, or evaluation of clinically or radiographically concerning anatomic variants warrants neurosurgical consultation. Any infant with other prominent or multiple dysmorphisms or prominent developmental delay without other explanation warrants genetics evaluation to identify possible syndromic craniosynostoses.

Standard descriptions of abnormal head shapes are as follows:

D. Dolichocephaly, or "long" head, is usually positional (especially with premature infants) and commonly benign. Dolichocephaly in premature infants is the result of lateral positioning of the head. It should resolve by 3 months of age in most cases. It should be distinguished from craniosynostosis in patients who do not have a history of prematurity.

E. Plagiocephaly, or "slanting" head, may be caused by a unilateral lambdoid synostosis, but more often is positional. Distinguishing positional plagiocephaly from unilateral lambdoid synostosis is based primarily on inspection. A positional plagiocephaly will typically show symmetric molding and a "parallelogram-shaped" head when viewed from above. In contrast, premature fusion of one lambdoid suture will produce a "trapezoid-shaped" head.

Trigonocephaly, or "three-angle" head, is caused by premature closure of the metopic suture. Severity differs greatly among individuals, and surgery is usually reserved for children with either severe deformity or evidence of increased intracranial pressure.

If an abnormal head shape is determined to be positional in nature, then the patient's sleep position should be modified and neck range-of-motion exercises initiated.

Positional skull deformity has no effect on brain function. Adjusting sleep position and stretching neck muscles should have positive effects in 1 to 2 months.

Failure to do so should warrant evaluation for poor head control, gross motor delay, and possibly visual function. If no improvement is noted at 1- to 2-month follow-up, then molded helmet therapy may also prove helpful.

Patient with ABNORMALITIES OF HEAD SIZE AND SHAPE

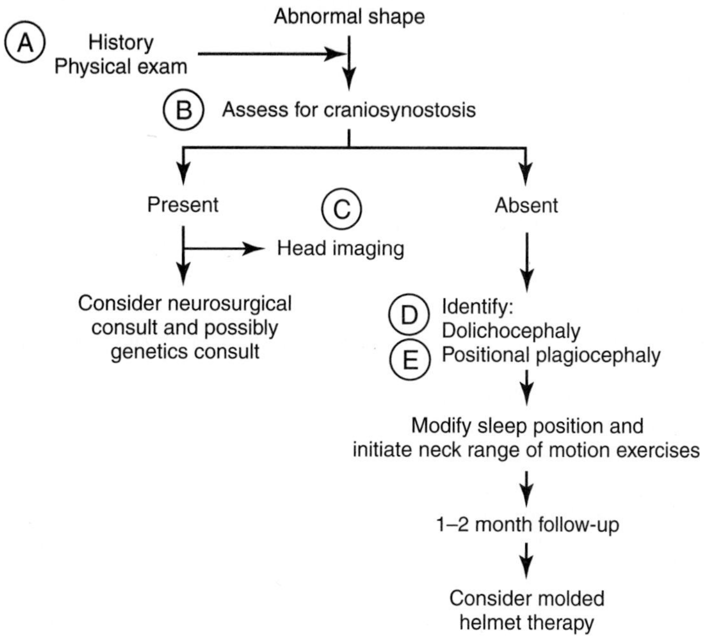
Abnormal shape
A
History
Physical exam
B
Assess for craniosynostosis
Present
C
Head imaging
Absent
Consider neurosurgical consult and possibly genetics consult
D
Identify:
Dolichocephaly
E
Positional plagiocephaly
Modify sleep position and initiate neck range of motion exercises
1–2 month follow-up
Consider molded helmet therapy

Abnormal Tone

Ed Jernigan, MD, and Julie Parsons, MD

Muscle tone refers to the involuntary continuous partial contraction of the muscles. Normal tone depends on the proper function of the central nervous system and various components of the motor unit. In infants, assessment of tone may reveal an increased, a decreased, or a mixed-type pattern.

A. History and Physical Examination: It is important to take a careful history and perform a careful clinical examination because it may not only identify tone abnormalities, but may provide clues to the cause.

B. Hypotonia: On initial evaluation of the infant with low tone, be careful to distinguish hypotonia from other possibly confounding processes. *Weakness* refers to the amount of active force the muscles can generate. Weak infants show poor tone, but hypotonic infants are not necessarily weak. *Fatigability* refers to the loss of force with repetitive contraction and indicates dysfunction of the motor unit. *Laxity* refers to increased range of motion in the joints. Essential clues to the cause of hypotonia are often found in the patient's history. Common examples include decreased fetal movement, polyhydramnios, traumatic delivery, or a family history of neuromuscular disease.

C. Once true hypotonia has been established by examination, identifying the site of pathology (e.g., brain, nerve, muscle) aids in narrowing the differential diagnosis. Abnormalities such as dysmorphism or hepatomegaly suggest a genetic or metabolic syndrome. On neurologic examination, determining the presence or absence of true muscle weakness is critical. Hypotonia without weakness suggests a central (i.e., brain or spinal cord) insult, whereas the presence of muscle weakness implies dysfunction of some component of the motor unit. Increased deep tendon reflexes with hypotonia almost always indicate a central cause (e.g., hypoxic-ischemic encephalopathy), whereas decreased or absent reflexes may suggest a peripheral process. Excessive fatigability may be difficult to assess in infants, but poor feeding may be significant. Fatigability most often indicates dysfunction at the level of the neuromuscular junction, such as a congenital myasthenic syndrome.

D. Diagnostic Evaluation: Infants in whom a central hypotonia is suspected should be screened for inborn errors of metabolism and electrolyte disturbances, including serum electrolytes, calcium, renal function, thyroid function, lactate, pyruvate, ammonia, serum amino acids, and urine organic acids. Serum creatine kinase levels may be checked but are likely to be normal in the absence of true weakness. Neuroimaging should also be considered. Magnetic resonance imaging (MRI) is generally preferred over computerized tomography (CT). The clarity of MRI allows for better assessment of many neurologic conditions, such as congenital malformations, white matter abnormalities, and malformations of cortical development. Abnormalities on general physical examination (especially dysmorphology) should prompt genetic screening. Invasive studies such as muscle or nerve biopsy should be deferred in infants who are clearly achieving developmental milestones, albeit with some delays. Electromyography/nerve conduction study and muscle biopsies are infrequently performed on infants because of both invasiveness and inherent difficulties with correct interpretation. Muscle biopsies are generally reserved for infants with true weakness or significantly increased creatine phosphokinase levels.

E. Hypertonia and Mixed Tone: Hypertonia refers to abnormally increased resistance to externally imposed movement around a joint. Whereas hypotonia in an infant may represent either a central or a peripheral process, hypertonia (or mixed tone) nearly always indicates an insult to the central nervous system. In fact, the most common clinical course in an infant with cerebral injury is diffuse hypotonia initially, followed by slow and segmental development of hypertonia, progressing over several days or weeks to spasticity and hyperreflexia.

Where possible, a further distinction between findings of spasticity, rigidity, or dystonia should be made. Spasticity is resistance of muscle to stretch and depends on rate of movement. Rigidity does not depend on velocity, and an affected limb will not typically return to a fixed posture after movement. Dystonia is an abnormal alteration of muscle contraction with either maintenance of posture or voluntary movement and, like rigidity, does not depend on velocity. These three may coexist and can be generalized or segmental.

F. The most sensitive study for identifying the cause of infant hypertonia is brain neuroimaging. Again, MRI is generally preferred over CT. Although hypoxic-ischemic encephalopathy is the most common cause of hypertonia, other possibilities include various maternal illnesses, placental dysfunction, sepsis, or an underlying structural lesion. Together with a careful history and examination, the pattern of imaging abnormality is likely to suggest the probable cause of brain injury.

G. Regardless of cause, the mainstay of treatment for infant hypertonia is physical (PT) and occupational therapy (OT).

References

Bodensteiner J. The evaluation of the hypotonic infant. Semin Pediatr Neurol 2008;15(1):10–20.

Crawford T. Clinical evaluation of the floppy infant. Pediatr Ann 1992;21(6):348–54.

Scher M. Neonatal hypertonia: I. Classification and structural-functional correlates. Pediatr Neurol 2008;39:301–6.

Scher M. Neonatal hypertonia: II. Differential diagnosis and proposed neuroprotection. Pediatr Neurol 2008;39:373–80.

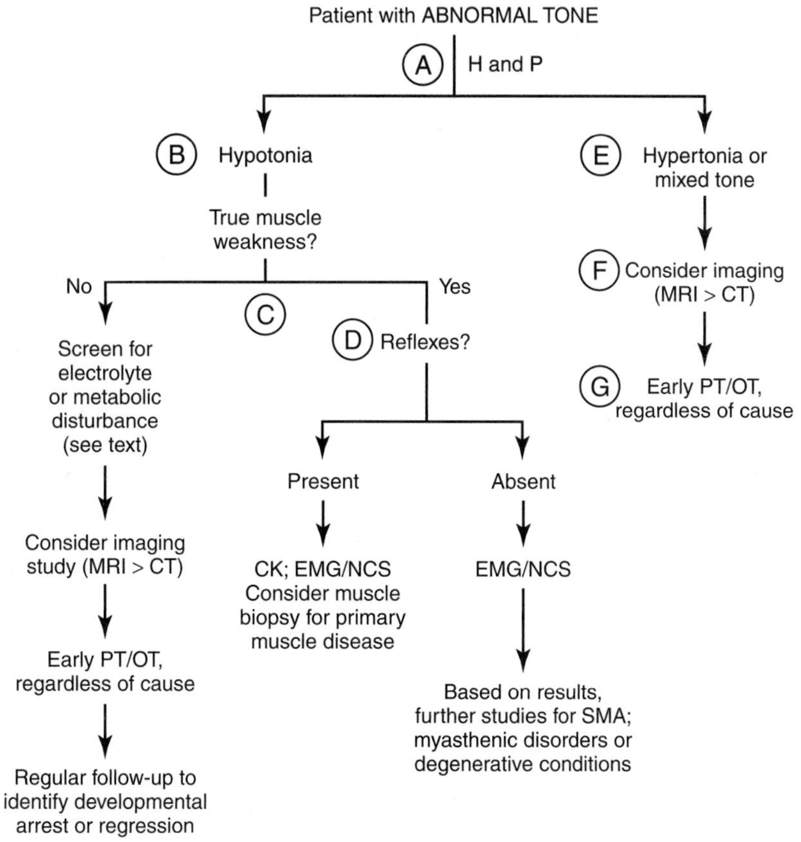
Patient with ABNORMAL TONE
A
H and P
B
Hypotonia
True muscle weakness?
No
Yes
C
Screen for electrolyte or metabolic disturbance (see text)
Consider imaging study (MRI > CT)
Early PT/OT, regardless of cause
Regular follow-up to identify developmental arrest or regression
D
Reflexes?
Present
Absent
CK; EMG/NCS Consider muscle biopsy for primary muscle disease
EMG/NCS
Based on results, further studies for SMA; myasthenic disorders or degenerative conditions
E
Hypertonia or mixed tone
F
Consider imaging (MRI > CT)
G
Early PT/OT, regardless of cause

Altered Mental Status/Coma

Jennifer Armstrong-Wells, MD, MPH, and Timothy J. Bernard, MD

Consciousness encompasses both wakefulness and awareness of self. Coma is defined as "a pathological state of deep and sustained unconsciousness (>1 hour) with the eyes closed, distinguishable from normal sleep by the inability to be aroused" (Plum and Posner, 2007). Coma results from global dysfunction of both cerebral hemispheres (awareness of self) or the disruption of the brainstem reticular activating system (wakefulness). It can arise from a variety of insults, ranging from widespread derangements (such as metabolic disturbances, drug/toxins, seizures, or infection) to direct brain injury, including anoxic brain injury, vascular events (stroke or hemorrhage) or trauma, or a combination of these factors. Thorough evaluation and examination for the underlying cause of unconsciousness is essential in determining the appropriate treatment and prognosis for the comatose child.

Brain death is the irreversible loss of brain/brainstem function with loss of consciousness, brainstem reflexes, motor response to noxious stimuli, and respiratory drive.

A. History and Physical Examination: Initially an assessment of airway, breathing, and circulation (ABCs) must always be performed. Level of alertness can be classified as either "difficult to arouse" or as "hyperalert, agitated, hallucinations (delirium)." It is important to avoid such terms as *somnolent, lethargic, obtundated,* and *stuporous,* because they are not uniformly used by practitioners. Vital signs can provide important clues to the cause. A heart rate assessment is key. If tachycardia is present, congenital heart defects, infection, shock, or drugs/intoxication can be suspected. If bradycardia is present, then Cushing triad of increased intracranial pressure (ICP; bradycardia, hypertension, irregular respirations), respiratory compromise, or shock is suspected. Blood pressure status should be assessed. Hypertension is seen with increased ICP (Cushing triad), drugs (cocaine, amphetamines), or hypertensive encephalopathy. Hypotension is seen in shock (septic, cardiogenic) and some toxins. As far as temperature is concerned, hyperthermia is seen in infection, seizures, and malignant hyperthermia, and hypothermia can be present in environmental hypothermia and shock. A careful assessment of respiratory pattern can also help elucidate causative factors. Cheyne–Stokes breathing is alternating increased respiration with apnea. It can be seen in bilateral hemisphere involvement, sleep apnea, congestive heart failure, and some pulmonary diseases. Ataxic breathing is irregular rate and volume. It points to the medulla in the brainstem and barbiturates and benzodiazepines as toxins. Apneustic breathing is a prolonged pause after inspiration and points to the pons. Hyperventilation points to the midbrain and pons, as well as systemic illness (i.e., shock, respiratory disease, infection, metabolic acidosis, nonorganic). Physical examination should look for evidence of trauma, infection (rash/purpura, meningismus), and drugs/toxins (i.e., anhidrosis, hyperhidrosis).

B. Neurological Evaluation (Brainstem Examination): Includes the assessment of level of consciousness. Cranial nerve examination details are essential. Pupils can be normal, which points to rostral and midbrain areas. Unilateral dilation points to ipsilateral uncal herniation; bilateral midposition and unreactive points to the midbrain; bilateral small, minimally reactive indicates pons or drugs (opioids, organophosphates/cholinergics); and bilateral dilated and unreactive points to drugs (amphetamines, anticholinergics, tetracyclic antidepressants), severe anoxic injury, central herniation, or brain death. Fundi examination can show optic disc swelling (increased ICP) or retinal hemorrhage (nonaccidental trauma). Gaze/doll's eyes/oculocephalics (should be deferred in cases of neck trauma) can show lateral deviation (i.e., seizure, structural [infarct, hemorrhage]). Gaze palsies can be seen in cranial nerve compression; upward deviation indicates bilateral cerebral hemisphere damage, and downward deviation indicates injury/compression of dorsal midbrain or thalamus (hydrocephalus, hemorrhage); and ocular bobbing points to the pons. Corneal reflex should be assessed, as well as a cough/gag. The patient can have a spinal reflex with deep suctioning, which is not a brainstem sign. Motor examination should assess for involuntary movements and reflexic movements. Involuntary movements such as myoclonus point to a metabolic or an anoxic injury. Generalized seizures can indicate a metabolic problem (i.e., glucose abnormalities, electrolyte disturbances, metabolic encephalopathy, drugs/toxins); focal seizures can indicate a structural abnormality (i.e., stroke, hemorrhage). Reflexic (stereotyped) responses are decorticate/flexor posturing (flexions of arms, extension of legs indicate bilateral hemispheric or thalamic injury; decerebrate/extensor posturing [extension of arms and legs] indicates brain or pons injury). Initial cursory evaluation can be summarized by the Glasgow Coma Scale (Table 1).

C. Workup: Standard components are serum blood glucose; arterial blood gases (ABG); complete blood cell count (CBC) with differential; electrolytes including calcium, blood urea nitrogen (BUN), and creatinine; liver function tests; ammonia, lactate; toxicology screen; thyroid function testing; and electrocardiogram (ECG). Further laboratory workup is determined by history and examination, that is, inborn errors of metabolism, expanded toxicology, blood/urine cultures, and lumbar puncture (head computed tomographic [CT] scan first). Imaging is also indicated. Head CT gives fast information about hemorrhage, severe cerebral edema, large tumor, hydrocephalus, and herniation. Causative factors such as early anoxic brain injury or infection may not appear on CT. Brain magnetic resonance imaging (MRI) is more sensitive but is usually limited by patient

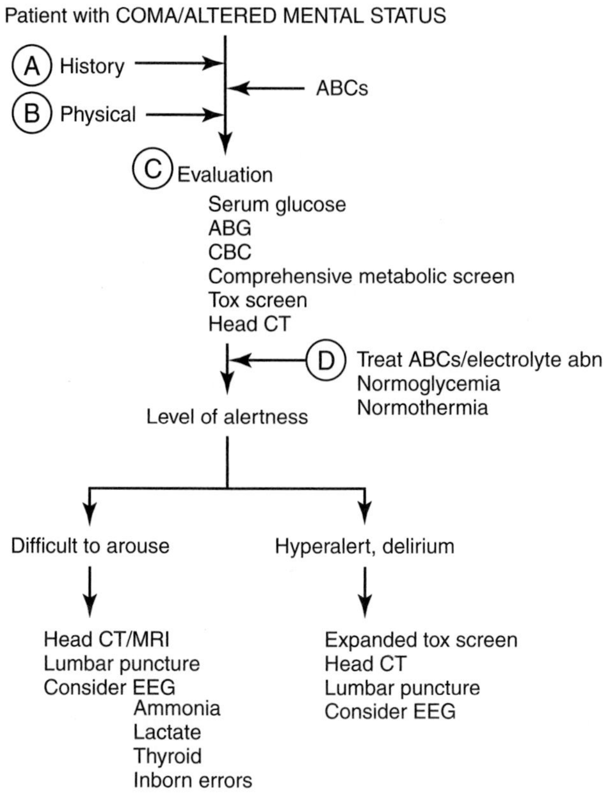
Patient with COMA/ALTERED MENTAL STATUS
A History
B Physical
ABCs
C Evaluation
Serum glucose
ABG
CBC
Comprehensive metabolic screen
Tox screen
Head CT
D Treat ABCs/electrolyte abn
Normoglycemia
Normothermia
Level of alertness
Difficult to arouse
Hyperalert, delirium
Head CT/MRI
Lumbar puncture
Consider EEG
Ammonia
Lactate
Thyroid
Inborn errors
Expanded tox screen
Head CT
Lumbar puncture
Consider EEG

acuity and stability. Should perform MRI if head CT scan is negative and coma is unexplained. Electroencephalogram (EEG) can be helpful to rule out nonconvulsive status epilepticus; it also may help in categorization (i.e., periodic lateralized epileptiform discharges in focal lesion—stroke, hemorrhage, herpes simplex virus encephalitis; triphasic waves—metabolic encephalopathy). "Alpha coma" resembles awake pattern and signifies extensive cerebral cortex or brainstem damage and generally poor prognosis. It is difficult to prognosticate based on EEG alone; entire clinical examination and information must be used.

D. Management includes ABCs, normoglycemia (avoid glucose-containing fluids unless hypoglycemic, as can cause hyperglycemia, hyperosmolarity, cerebral edema), normothermia, normal serum sodium, and treatment of underlying cause as indicated.

CONCLUSION

Prognosis is a combination of many factors (underlying cause, examination). Special attention should be made to conditions that can exacerbate coma, including hypothermia, drugs, and metabolic derangements. EEG can help if electrocerebral inactivity ("silence") lasting for a period of 6 to 12 hours. Patient cannot be hypothermic or have depressant drugs in system. Requires experienced electroencephalographers for interpretation. It can be difficult to interpret given interference of recording with equipment common in the intensive care unit. Rarely used for brain death evaluation. Cerebral flow study such as cerebral angiography can indicate brain death; that is, failure of intracerebral filling at the level of entry into the cranium by the carotid and vertebral arteries. Transcranial ultrasonography and cerebral scintigraphy (failure of uptake of radioisotope [technetium 99m hexametazime]) in brain can also be used.

Coma can mimic acute neuromuscular disease such as Guillain-Barré syndrome, botulism (pupils spared), myasthenic crisis, toxins (organophosphate poisoning), paralytics (iatrogenic or drugs/toxins), and critical illness neuropathy, as well as nonconvulsive status epilepticus and metabolic disease, together with locked-in syndrome (injury to the base of the pons). Injury involving the upper pons can be mistaken for coma; however, consciousness, voluntary eye movements, and blink are preserved. Psychogenic coma is a usually diagnosis of exclusion.

References

Michelson DJ, Ashwal S. Evaluation of coma and brain death. Semin Pediatr Neurol 2004;11(2):105–18.

Plum F, Posner JB. The diagnosis of stupor and coma. Philadelphia: FA Davis; 2007.

Wijdicks EF. The diagnosis of brain death. N Engl J Med 2001;344(16): 1215–21.

Table 1. **Glasgow Coma Scale with Modification for Children**

Sign	GCS	GCS for Children	Score
Eye opening	Spontaneous	Spontaneous	4
	To command	To sound	3
	To pain	To pain	2
	None	None	1
Verbal response	Oriented	Age-appropriate vocalization, smile, or orientation to sound	5
	Confused, disoriented	Irritable, consolable, uncooperative, aware of the environment	4
	Inappropriate words	Irritable, inconsistently consolable	3
	Incomprehensible sounds	Inconsolable, unaware of environment, restless, agitated	2
	None	None	1
Motor response	Obey commands	Obeys commands, spontaneous movements	6
	Localizes pain	Localizes pain	5
	Withdraws	Withdraws	4
	Abnormal flexion to pain	Abnormal flexion to pain	3
	Abnormal extension to pain	Abnormal extension to pain	2
	None	None	1
Best total score			**15**

GCS, Glasgow Coma Scale.
From Michelson DJ, Ashwal S. Evaluation of coma and brain death. Semin Pediatr Neurol 2004;11(2):105-18.

Headache

Sita Kedia, MD, and Tonia Sabo, MD

Headache is a common symptom in children and adolescents. Headaches can be grouped into two general categories: primary and secondary. Primary headaches include migraine, tension, and cluster headaches. Secondary headaches are those resulting from a variety of underlying conditions and include intracranial hypertension, infection, metabolic derangement, and vascular causative factors. The most important part of a patient evaluation is the history, followed by physical examination, and lastly, any supplemental imaging or laboratory testing. Headache expression is often affected by diet, sleep, stressors, and exercise habits, and it is important to get a clear understanding of the patient's typical routine. Migraine and tension headaches are the most common causes of recurrent headaches. Migraine headaches can be very debilitating, often interfering with school work and normal activities of daily living. Proper recognition, evaluation, and treatment strategies can be life changing for patients with frequent headaches.

A. A detailed history should be extensive and include the following: frequency, time of day, quality, location, severity, and radiation. Qualities of the headache may be throbbing/pounding, sharp, ice pick, dull, pressure, or bandlike. Migraine headaches are generally frontal; around the orbit can be bilateral or unilateral (in distinction to adults, which almost always is unilateral). Headaches that are new onset and progressive, described as the "worst headache of my life," occipital in location, associated with changes in the baseline neurologic function (ataxia, hemiparesis, etc.), accompanied by change in personality, or associated with new-onset seizures are more concerning for need for secondary headache, requiring imaging or other workup. Headaches that awaken a child in the middle of the night or in the morning are worrisome for increased intracranial pressure (ICP) syndromes or perhaps CO_2 retention in the setting of sleep apnea. Headaches that occur shortly after standing may be associated with low ICP syndromes, such as dural leak or overshunting. Common associated features immediately before, during, and/or after migraine headache include phonophobia and photophobia, association with physical activity, and visual changes. Focal neurologic deficit is less common and may include numbness, weakness, diplopia, ptosis, and pupil asymmetry. Less common general features to migraine include ringing in ears, dizziness, lacrimation, and rhinorrhea. Aggravating factors such as worsening of headache with Valsalva maneuvers (coughing, sneezing, bowel movements) and a sensation of a "swooshing" sound (pulsatile tinnitus) intermittently in the ears may be indicative of increased ICP.

Triggers and patterns such as dehydration, skipping meals, sleep deprivation, heat, bright light, changes in weather, physical exertion, computer use, hormonal cycle, caffeine intake, or changes in altitude should be established during the initial evaluation and are often easy for the patient to modify.

Medical history is important to review and useful to establish history of allergies, sinus infections, head injuries, concussions, seizures, and eye abnormalities.

Family history should focus on migraines, motion sickness, clotting disorders, mood disorders, cardiac, cancers, thyroid, and autoimmune disorders.

Social history should include review of psychosocial issues including ongoing/changing or new emotional stressors, sexual and drug use history, school work and grades, and changes in academic performance.

A full review of systems will help to classify headache and possibly lead to consideration of other systemic causes.

Patients may have tried many different forms of treatments for their headaches by the time they present for initial evaluation. They may be using abortive medications daily, thereby contributing to rebound effect. Determine whether any supplements such as vitamins or minerals are used. Alternative treatments are more widely used such as massage, chiropractic treatment, aromatherapy, physical therapy, or biofeedback. A full review of all medications used for all conditions for the patient is necessary.

B. Physical examination of the child must include both a general and thorough neurologic examination. Important points of the general examination include vital signs including evaluation of temperature, blood pressure, and pulse. Height, weight, and body mass index are important health indicators.

Head, ears, eyes, nose, and throat examination includes evaluation for sinus tenderness, postnasal drip, tonsillar enlargement, lymphadenopathy, dental examination, and temporomandibular joint tenderness. Cardiac and vascular examination should emphasize identification of murmurs or arrhythmias, and cranial, orbital, or carotid bruits. The skin evaluation is important to identify rashes and neurocutaneous stigmata. Neck stiffness may be associated with meningeal inflammation from central nervous system (CNS) structural, inflammatory, hemorrhagic, or infectious processes. Radiating pain down the neck may be associated with CNS foramen problem such as a Chiari 1 malformation or demyelinating condition. In children with tension headaches, physicians may find paraspinal or neck muscular spasm, trigger points, and/or tenderness.

The formal neurologic examination begins by general assessment of alertness, awareness, and affect. Excessive sleepiness may be indicative of a sleeping disorder, flat affect of depression, or altered mental status of more ominous causes such as infection or increased ICP.

Following is cranial nerve assessment starting with evaluation of the eyes. Visual examination includes funduscopic evaluation, which, although challenging, provides

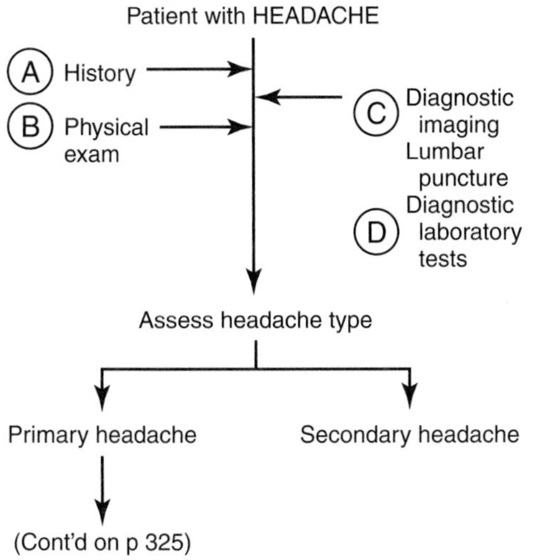
Patient with HEADACHE
A History
B Physical exam
C Diagnostic imaging
Lumbar puncture
D Diagnostic laboratory tests
Assess headache type
Primary headache
Secondary headache
(Cont'd on p 325)

valuable information for the presence of papilledema and of spontaneous venous pulsations, both markers of increased intracranial hypertension. Evaluation of the fundi is best done in the dark, causing the eyes to dilate and allowing for better visualization. Observe the color, as both hyperemic and pale fundi are abnormal. Focusing on the vessels is useful, often following the thinner edge of the vessels as they increase in diameter to the optic nerve head. Characteristics to note of the blood vessels are their appearance as they pass over the optic disk margins smoothly, increased tortuosity, hemorrhages, or pulsations. Reassuring findings are sharp optic disk margins and spontaneous venous pulsations; if these are present, the concern for increased ICP is very low. A good rule of thumb is any child with recurrent headaches should have a dilated eye examination by ophthalmologist. Visual fields, pupil symmetry and reactivity, and eye movements are all important. Loss of visual fields, asymmetric pupil, and ophthalmoplegia are all suggestive of possible structural anomaly such as mass, vascular malformation, or intracranial hypertension.

Remaining cranial nerves test primarily face, neck, and throat function. Motor (including tone, strength, and reflexes), sensory (including light touch and other modalities as indicated), and coordination (including truncal, extremities, and gait) tests are necessary to evaluate the CNS more fully.

If there is a new neurologic abnormality during the headache, migraine-associated symptomatology can be the cause; this is common if the symptoms are transitory (commonly before or at the apex of pain symptomatology). If a patient has a new neurologic deficit, consider very strongly the need for imaging, hypercoagulable workup, or possible manifestation of seizure.

C. Neuroimaging is not required for every patient with headache, and there is no consensus on its use in evaluating headache. After thorough history and examination, if there is clinical suspicion for intracranial hypertension or structural lesion (based on an abnormal examination or history), then proceed with imaging. Computed tomography (CT) should be used with careful consideration given radiation exposure risks in children and adolescents. CT of the head may be indicated for evaluation of acute headache after head trauma, for a patient with neurologic focality and altered mental status, or for immediate concerns of hydrocephalus or increased intracranial hypertension. As a general rule of thumb, if head imaging is emergent given clinical presentation, head CT should be obtained; if urgent or routine, try to obtain an MRI of the brain, which provides more detailed information without the radiation exposure. An advantage of MRI is the ability to evaluate structural components and vasculature of the brain. In addition, MRI evaluates superiorly the posterior fossa, cerebellum, and brainstem over CT. Sagittal views on MRI (not available on CT) help evaluate for Chiari 1 malformation and upper cervical spine. If there is a history of strokelike symptoms with headaches, obtain magnetic resonance angiography at the same time as cranial MRI. This provides a very detailed and three-dimensional reconstructive view of the neck and cranial vasculature, and is surpassed in detail only by formal invasive angiography. If intracranial hypertension is suspected, magnetic resonance venography can be useful in diagnosis of cranial venous thromboses.

Obtaining a lumbar puncture (LP) is important in the acute setting if there are any signs of CNS infection, with or without alteration of consciousness, concern for increased intracranial hypertension or hypotension, or concerning mental status changes (in most cases, this should be performed after head imaging to assess for increased ICP). If lateralizing features, associated trauma, or concern for increased ICP is present, obtain imaging before performing an LP. The LP should include an opening pressure (with patient lying on his or her side, and after manometer is in place, the patient should extend his or her legs from a fetal position). If opening pressure is elevated, then the patient should have enough fluid drained to have a closing pressure less than 18 to 20 cm H_2O. Opening pressures may vary depending on whether the LP is done in the sitting or lying position and may vary depending on the patient's weight (higher pressures can be seen with increased weight). Some patients may have "normal opening pressures" between 20 and 30 cm H_2O, but input of a neurosurgeon and evaluation with imaging would be recommended. Opening pressures less than 10 cm H_2O may be indicative of a low-pressure CSF headache syndrome and may indicate need for additional testing such as myelography or CT head with contrast, which may show diffuse meningeal enhancement. If signs or symptoms of infection are present, consideration and testing for appropriate infectious causative agents will be needed (viral, bacterial, fungal, etc.).

D. Laboratory testing and other ancillary testing is generally not needed for evaluation of headache unless systemic symptoms are present. Depending on clinical symptoms, consider complete blood cell count, metabolic panel including electrolytes and liver function, urinalysis, inflammatory markers such as C-reactive protein and erythrocyte sedimentation rate, antinuclear antibody, and thyroid function panel. Not routinely ordered but supported somewhat by the literature are consideration of serum testing of a coenzyme Q10 level, vitamin D analysis, and ionized magnesium/calcium ratio. Studies such as electroencephalogram, polysomnograph, and chest radiograph are not warranted unless there is a strong suspicion for seizures, sleep disorder, or lung pathology.

E. After history, physical examination, and any necessary diagnostic testing, headaches can generally be classified into primary or secondary. Secondary headache causative factors may warrant further testing and evaluation; these are not discussed here. Primary headaches are classified into migraine, tension, or cluster.

F. Estimates have found migraine prevalence rate in adolescents to be approximately 6%. The most widely used and accepted classification of migraines is that described by the International Headache Society. Migraines can present with or without aura. Migraine without aura is more common and generally lasts from 1 to 72 hours in children. These migraines are pulsating, moderate or severe in intensity, aggravated by routine physical activity, and associated with nausea and/or photophobia and phonophobia. In children, migraines are more commonly described as bilateral and emerge as unilateral in late adolescence or adulthood. Auras are reversible focal neurologic symptoms that generally develop gradually over 5 minutes and last for less than 60 minutes.

G. Tension-type headaches are generally described by the patient as bilateral, pressing/tightening quality, mild or moderate intensity, not aggravated by routine physical activity, and no associated symptoms of nausea, vomiting, photophobia, or phonophobia. These headaches generally last anywhere from 30 minutes to 7 days.

H. Cluster headaches are much less common than migraines and tension headaches. ICHD-II categorized cluster headaches amongst the trigeminal autonomic cephalgias. Cluster headaches are attacks of unilateral orbital, supraorbital, or temporal severe pain lasting from 15–180 minutes from once every other day to up to 8 per day. They are associated with ipsilateral conjunctival injection and/or lacrimation, nasal congestion and/or rhinorrhea, eyelid edema, forehead and facial sweating, miosis and/or ptosis, and/or sense of restlessness or agitation.

I. Treatments for headaches can be categorized as abortive or prophylactic. Abortive treatments for migraines and tension headaches are similar and overlap; therefore, they are discussed jointly here. Treatment options for a child suffering from a headache differ whether the child is at home or in the emergency department, where IV medication options can be given.

At home, parents should encourage fluid intake, in addition to rest, quiet surroundings, and a dark room. For some children and adolescents, simple over-the-counter medications have been successful in aborting the headache. These include acetaminophen, ibuprofen, naproxen (Naprosyn), or caffeine/aspirin/analgesic combinations, especially if they have been found useful previously with the patient. Overuse of aspirin-containing products or use during fever should be cautioned for concern of development of Reye syndrome. If typical "over-the-counter" medications have not been useful, then consider agents such as triptans (serotonin agonists), ergotamine-based medications (such as dihydroergotamine [DHE] nasal spray), and antinausea medications. Most of these medications are not U.S. Food and Drug Administration (FDA) indicated for adolescent migraine, but in general are well tolerated in children age 10 or older. Current clinical efficacy has been shown for rizatriptan, sumatriptan, and almotriptan. It probably will not be long until all triptans can be shown to have clinical significance in adolescents (as all have shown to be effective in studied adult migraineurs). Clinical studies to date have been challenging in proof of efficacy of triptan medications in the pediatric population because of the high placebo rate seen in trials to date. See Table 1 for considerations of abortive medications and associated class, dosage, formulations, and adverse effects.

In the emergency department, oral medications may be attempted but are often unsuccessful because the migraine headache is often prolonged and more resistant because of activated central pathways and altered enteric absorption. The patient will often need parenteral or rectal administration of medications. Most patients are able to abort their headache after an intravenous (IV) fluid bolus and the first abortive medication (commonly ketorolac [Toradol]). Many emergency department physicians and neurologists have favored giving several medications simultaneously as a "migraine cocktail" (such as perchlorperazine, diphenhydramine [Benadryl], and Toradol). Narcotic medication should be avoided because this class is often ineffective and may promote drug-seeking behavior.

J. Prophylactic medications are considered when migraines are debilitating and affecting one's quality of life. Typically, headaches occurring more than two times per week, several prolonged headache attacks per month, or debilitating but infrequent headaches with associated symptoms such as hemiparesis often are problematic enough to consider preventative pharmacologic treatment. Consideration of school attendance and inability to perform school activities or sports may warrant need for prophylactic medication. Migraine prophylactic medications are listed in Table 2. They can be generally classified into antidepressants, anticonvulsants, cardiac, and other. Patients generally younger than 10 to 12 years are initially tried on cyproheptadine, as opposed to amitriptyline in the older patient.

K. Many patients and parents prefer nonpharmacologic options in addition to medications such as vitamins and minerals. Petadolex, magnesium, feverfew, riboflavin, and coenzyme Q10 are promising micronutrients that may prove beneficial for patients with recurrent headaches. However, as with most complementary and alternative medicine choices, more randomized, double-blind, placebo–controlled efficacy studies need to be completed to document efficacy and dosing. Inconsistent preparation for Petadolex and feverfew warrant caution in use together with unclear safety profile. Coenzyme Q and magnesium dosages up to 10 mg/kg/day and riboflavin up to 100 mg/day have been used in previous adult studies and overall appear safe for use in the pediatric population; formal dietary analysis may reveal underlying nutritional deficit. Rarely is food allergy testing helpful, but dietary awareness of food triggers is often helpful.

L. Alternative treatments include biofeedback, massage, relaxation training, and acupuncture; parents and practitioners have used these approaches to help in preventing

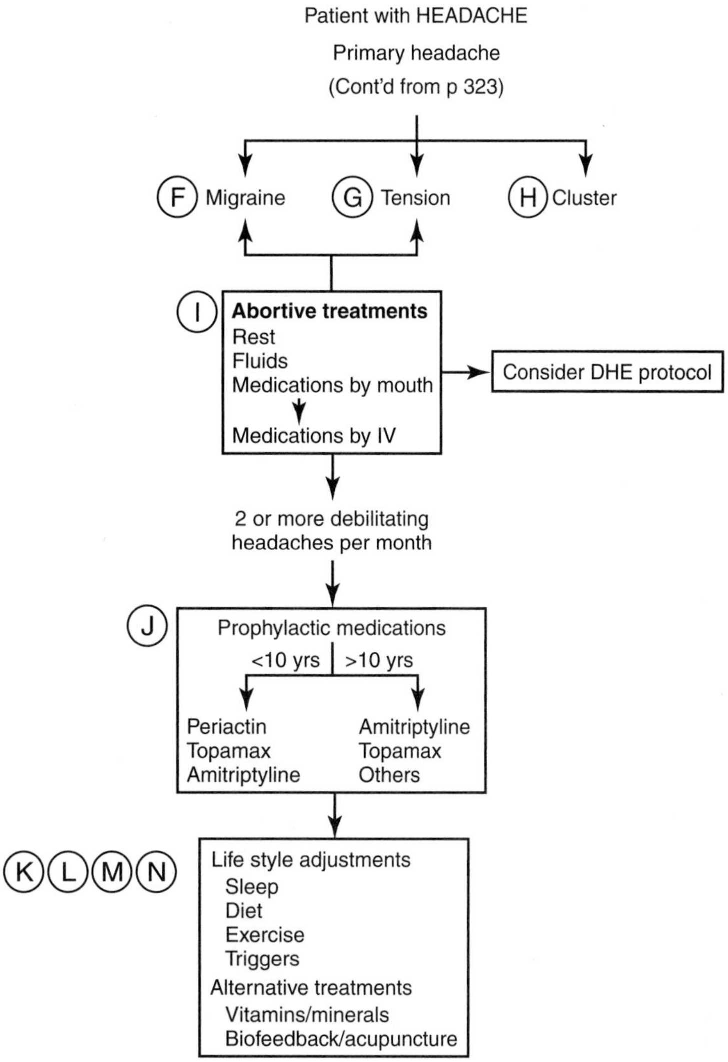
Patient with HEADACHE
Primary headache
(Cont'd from p 323)
F Migraine
G Tension
H Cluster
I
Abortive treatments
Rest
Fluids
Medications by mouth
Medications by IV
Consider DHE protocol
2 or more debilitating headaches per month
J
Prophylactic medications
<10 yrs
>10 yrs
Periactin
Topamax
Amitriptyline
Amitriptyline
Topamax
Others
K L M N
Life style adjustments
Sleep
Diet
Exercise
Triggers
Alternative treatments
Vitamins/minerals
Biofeedback/acupuncture

headaches. Given the nature of the treatment, randomized, double-blind, placebo-controlled trials are lacking. However, cohort studies show promising results as an adjunctive treatment. Psychological counseling may be important because many patients with recurrent headache have comorbid depression or anxiety.

M. Encouraging parents to keep a headache diary with a food, activity, and sleep log is very useful for parents to begin to recognize various triggers and make the medical encounter more productive.

N. Lifestyle interventions include sleep hygiene, improved diet, and exercise habits. Assessing body mass index and discussing goals for weight reduction and increased exercise is a known benefit for headache control. This is another area where a food diary is important, and the provider can help with strategies that are obtainable for the patient. These include reducing soda and high-sugar drinks and snacks, decreasing fat intake by suggesting a switch to 1% or skim milk, and reducing high-fat/calorie desserts. Develop an exercise plan where the patient works up to exercising 5 days a week for at least 30 minutes. Remember this may not be obtainable the first week; however, over several months, most children should be able to reach this goal.

(Continued on page 327)

Table 1. **Abortive Treatments for Acute Headache**

Medication	Forms	Dosage	Maximum Dose	Frequency	Adverse Effect Profile
NSAIDs					
Ibuprofen	PO	10 mg/kg/dose	600–800 mg	every 6–8h	GI bleed
Ketorolac	PO	>50 kg: 10 mg	10 mg	every 6–8h	GI bleed, deceased platelet function, drowsiness
	IV/IM	0.5 mg/kg/dose	30 mg	every 6–8h	
Naproxen	PO	5–7 mg/kg/dose	400 mg	every 8h	GI bleed, drowsiness, thrombocytopenia
Acetaminophen	PO/PR	15 mg/kg/dose	650–1000 mg	every 4–6h	Hepatic toxicity
Antiemetics					
Metoclopramide	PO/IV/IM	0.1–0.15 mg/kg/dose	10 mg	every 6h	Sedation, anxiety, leucopenia, diarrhea
Promethazine	PO/IM/IV/PR	0.25–1 mg/kg/dose	15–25 mg	every 4–6h	Sedation, blurred vision, dystonic reactions
Prochlorperazine	PO/PR	0.1 mg/kg/dose	10 mg	every 6–8h	
	IM	0.1 mg/kg/dose	10 mg	every 6–8h	
	IV	0.15 mg/kg/dose	10 mg	every 6–8h	
Diphenhydramine	PO/IV/IM	0.5 mg/kg/dose	50 mg/day	every 6h	Sedation, nausea, xerostomia, blurred vision
Triptans					
Almotriptan*	PO	6.25–12.5 mg/dose	12.5 mg	Can repeat in 2 hours	
Rizatriptan	PO	5–10 mg/dose			
Sumatriptan	PO	<50 kg 25 mg		Can repeat in 2 hours	Dizziness, chest pain and tightness, bad taste, paresthesias
	IN	>50 kg 50 mg	100 mg/dose		
	SC	<50 kg 5 mg			
		>50 kg 20 mg			
		>50 kg 6 mg	6 mg/dose		
Naratriptan	PO	1–2.5 mg/dose	2.5 mg/dose	Can repeat in 4 hours	
Zolmitriptan	PO	>50 kg give 2.5–5 mg/dose	5 mg/dose	Can repeat in 2 hours	
	IN	5 mg/dose			
Eletriptan	PO	>50 kg give 20–40 mg/dose	40 mg/dose	Can repeat in 2 hours	
Dihydroergotamine	IV	0.2–1 mg	1 mg	every 8h	Vasoconstrictor, flushing, nausea, diarrhea
	IN	0.5 mg/nostril	3 mg/day	every 15min × 2	
Caffeine (base)	IV	Up to 5–10 mg/kg		>30 minutes	Tachycardia, agitation, hyperactivity
Antiepileptics					
Valproate sodium	IV	10–20 mg/kg/dose	1500 mg/dose	Once	Sedation, tremor, transaminitis
Keppra	IV	20 mg/kg/dose	1000 mg	Once	Sedation
Magnesium	IV	30 mg/kg/dose	1000 mg/dose	Can repeat once in 4 h	

*Almotriptan is FDA approved for migraines in adolescents.
Some of these may not be U.S. Food and Drug Administration (FDA) indicated for use for headache in children and adolescents.
Fxn, platelet function; *GI*, gastrointestinal; *IM*, intramuscularly; *IN*, intranasally; *IV*, intravenously; *NSAID*, nonsteroidal anti-inflammatory drug; *PO*, orally; *SC*, subcutaneously.

Table 2. **Prophylactic Treatments for Recurrent Headache**

Medications	Initial Dose	Titration	Suggestions	Dosing	Adverse Effects
Antidepressants					
Amitriptyline	0.1 mg/kg/dose	Increase over 2–3 weeks to 0.5–2 mg/kg	Typical dose is 30–100 mg/dose	qhs-tid if needed	Constipation, dry mouth, arrhythmia, sedation
Nortriptyline	0.5–1 mg/kg	Increase over 2–3 weeks to 1–3 mg/kg	>11 years 25–35 mg	qhs	Constipation, dry mouth, arrhythmia, sedation
Anticonvulsants					
Topiramate	1–2 mg/kg/day	Increase in 1- to 2-week increments up to 10 mg/kg/day	Typical dose is up to 50 BID, which prevents side effects	bid	Weight loss, kidney stones, paresthesias, glaucoma
Valproic acid	20 mg/kg/day	Increase every 2 weeks to 40 mg/kg/day	Typical dose is 250–500 mg/dose	bid	Weight gain, bruising, hair loss, hepatotoxicity
Carbamazepine	5 mg/kg/day	Increase as tolerated to 15 mg/kg/day	Typical dose is 200 mg	bid	Sedation, rash, neutropenia, dizziness
Levetiracetam	20 mg/kg/day	Increase as tolerated to 60 mg/kg/day	Typical dose is 500–1000 mg/dose	bid	Sedation, behavioral disturbance
Cardiac					
Propranolol	≤35 kg 10 mg/dose >35 kg 20 mg/dose	Increase to 20 mg Increase to 40 mg		tid	Hypotension, vivid dreams depression
Metoprolol	2–6 mg/kg/day				same
Verapamil	4 mg/kg/day	Increase as tolerated to 8 mg/kg/day	Adolescents tolerate up to 240–480 mg	qd-tid	Hypotension, nausea, atrioventricular node block, weight gain
Antihistamine					
Cyproheptadine	0.25–1.5 mg/kg		Up to 12–14 mg tolerated	qhs	Sedation, weight gain
Other Treatments					
Magnesium	5 mg/kg/day	Increase as tolerated to 400 mg/day		qd-bid	Loose stools
Coenzyme Q10	5 mg/kg/day	Increase as tolerated to 200 mg/day		qd-bid	No reported significant side effects
Riboflavin (B_2)	25 mg/day	Increase as tolerated to 100 mg/day		qd-bid	Deep yellow urine

Some of these may not be U.S. Food and Drug Administration (FDA) indicated for use for headache in children and adolescents.
qhs, every hour of sleep

References

Bigal ME, Lipton RB, Winner P, et al. Migraine in adolescents: association with socioeconomic status and family history. Adolescent analysis of AMPP study. Neurology 2007;69:16–25.

Hershey AD. Current approaches to the diagnosis or management of paediatric migraine. Lancet Neurol 2010;9:190–204.

Lewis DW, Ashwal S, Dahl G, et al. Practice parameter: evaluation of children and adolescents with recurrent headaches: report of the Quality Standards Subcommittee of the American Academy of Neurology and the Practice Committee of the Child Neurology Society. Neurology 2002;59:490–8.

Movement Disorders

Ataxia, Chorea, Dystonia, Psychogenic Movements, Stereotypies, Infantile Self-Stimulation, and Tremor

Abigail Collins, MD, and Paul G. Moe, MD

Movement is one of the most important functions of the human body and is vital for our communication, artistic expression, reproduction, and survival. Movement can be categorized based on the degree of conscious control into automatic movements, which are learned behaviors performed without conscious effort (walking or running), voluntary movements, which are intentional (throwing a ball), semivoluntary movements, which are triggered by an inner stimulus or unwanted feeling (scratching an itch), and involuntary movements, which are not controlled but may be suppressible to some degree.

Abnormal movements are typically both unintentional and involuntary. They are grouped into broad categories of too much movement, including hyperkinesias (excessive movements) and dyskinesias (unnatural movements), and too little movement, including hypokinesia (decreased amplitude of movement), bradykinesia (decreased speed of movement), and akinesia (absence of movement). Given that disorders of too little movement are uncommon in pediatrics (when not caused by underlying weakness), this chapter focuses on hyperkinesias and dyskinesias (see Table 1). Tics were described in a separate chapter (see Tics and Tourette Syndrome chapter). Spasticity will not be discussed.

(Continued on page 330)

Table 1. **Categorization of Abnormal Movements**

Abnormal Movement	Description	Examination Features
Akathisia	Voluntary movements such as rubbing, rocking, and pacing caused by an intense inner restlessness and inability to remain still	Arrhythmical, nonsustained, *paroxysmal, at rest only,* nonpatterned, slow, suppressible
Ataxia	In-coordination of voluntary movements	Present with action only No abnormal movements at rest
Chorea	Random, brief, irregular, jerky movements that make the patient look like they are fidgeting and cannot sit still; large-amplitude, proximal chorea is ballismus	Arrhythmical, nonsustained, *continual, occur at rest and increase with action,* nonpatterned, intermediate speed, minimally suppressible
Dystonia	Abnormal twisting postures that are sustained for brief (milliseconds) to long (hours) periods	Arrhythmical, *sustained,* continual to continuous, at rest and with action, or with action only, *patterned,* mildly suppressible
Myoclonus	Sudden, brief, shocklike movements, typically in one direction	Arrhythmical or rhythmical, nonsustained, continual to continuous, at rest and with action, patterned or nonpatterned, *very fast, not suppressible*
Paroxysmal dyskinesias	Episodic abnormal movements that may be choreiform, dystonic, or a combination of movements	Arrhythmical, nonsustained, *paroxysmal, may be triggered by action,* nonpatterned, intermediate speed, minimally suppressible
Psychogenic movements	Any combination of abnormal movements that often are not consistent with any pattern by history or examination, may be distractible, vary in amplitude, direction, often with abrupt onset and atypical response to medications	*Any combination of features*
Restless leg syndrome	Abnormal sensations and discomfort in the legs typically at the end of the day when recumbent, which are relieved by voluntary movements of the legs and walking around	*Sensations occur at rest only*
Stereotypies	Highly stereotyped, repetitive, voluntary movements often involving the bilateral hands and arms, typically elicited by boredom or excitement and can be interrupted Child often stops what they are otherwise doing to engage in stereotypy	Arrhythmical, nonsustained, *paroxysmal, patterned,* intermediate speed, *highly suppressible* when attention called to behavior
Tardive dyskinesia	Repetitive movements often with tongue twisting, protrusion, lip pursing and chewing movements, and may involve the neck and trunk with extension, and extremities with rapid twisting postures	*Rhythmical,* nonsustained, continual, at rest more than with action, *patterned, combinations of movements,* intermediate speed, minimally suppressible
Tremor	Oscillatory, usually rhythmic and regular to and fro movements about an axis	*Rhythmical,* nonsustained, continuous, *may occur at rest, with action, or both, patterned,* intermediate speed, minimally suppressible

A. In general, the diagnosis of abnormal movements is clinical, made on history and physical examination alone. Categorizing the abnormal movement based on features of the patient's history and physical examination is crucial to determining a possible causative factor for the abnormal movements, and dictates the subsequent evaluation and treatment. Aspects of the history that must be explored for every patient with abnormal movements are outlined in Table 2. A general examination and thorough neurologic examination should be performed. The movement disorders examination includes additional maneuvers to specifically evaluate the abnormal movements (see Tables 3 and 4, and the following section).

When examining a patient with abnormal movements, first ask the patient to sit quietly without speaking or moving to determine whether the abnormal movements are present at rest. If they are, ask the patient to try to suppress them while you count the number of seconds that they are able to do so. Then have the patient do whatever seems to bring out the abnormal movements and go through the questions in Table 3 to help categorize the abnormal movement.

On cranial nerve testing, pay special attention to the eye movements, evaluating for nystagmus, breakdown of smooth pursuit on slow movements, and overshoot with large saccades. On speech examination, note the volume and speed of speech, modulation of pitch and intonation, and whether there is a clumsy quality to coordination of complicated sounds, such as the phrase "Presbyterian Episcopalian." Evaluate labial (p, b, m), lingual (l, t), and guttural (g, k) sounds separately. Have the patient hold the sound *eeeh* and *aaah* for about 10 seconds each to determine whether there is a vocal tremor, or strangulation or escape of air suggesting underlying laryngeal dystonia. Cerebellar speech is often described as "scanning," with slow- and clumsy-sounding speech that has abnormal pauses or intervals between syllables, a lack of normal inflection and intonation, variable volume but is typically loud, and difficulty with guttural sounds. Dysarthric speech is also slow but often affects both lingual and guttural sounds, and is typically more a problem of pronunciation when it involves the tongue and palate, and quality of sound when it involves the larynx. Have the patient protrude the tongue and assess the ease with which he can wiggle it from side to side. Uncoordinated and slow tongue movements may be caused by dystonia or cerebellar dysfunction. Inability to hold the tongue protruded for 10 seconds or longer represents motor impersistence and is often seen with chorea.

On motor examination, have the patient extend the arms in front of herself with the palms down, facing inward, upward, and completely rotated internally to face out for 5 seconds in each position to look for tremor or abnormal postures that emerge, noting in which position the tremor and/or postures are the most severe or absent (a null point that suggests dystonia). Have the patient squeeze your fingers to assess for a "milkmaid grip," with impersistence of pressure that results in a milking of the examiner's fingers and may be a manifestation of chorea.

Perform rapid alternating movements by having the patient rapidly open and close the hands as if flicking water off the fingers, tap the thumb and pointer finger repetitively, and rapidly pronate and supinate the hands at the wrist or held with elbows at 90 degrees (as if screwing in a light bulb) to assess for speed, amplitude, rhythmicity, abnormal postures, and coordination. Perform rapid alternating movements of the lower extremity with foot stomps and toe taps. For both the upper and lower extremities, determine whether volitional movement of one body part (the hands) causes abnormal postures to come out of that body part (dystonia) or other parts of the body (the feet, trunk, or neck) to suggest an overflow dystonia. Dystonia, chorea, and myoclonus are often worsened by purposeful movements, whereas tardive dyskinesia and tics are typically significantly decreased by purposeful movements of the involved body part.

On finger-to-nose testing, assess the accuracy of reaching the target (dysmetria), the path followed to arrive at the target (ataxia), and presence of tremor throughout the movement or only as the target is approached (intention tremor). Perform toe-to-finger and/or heel-knee-shin to assess for dysmetria and ataxia in the lower extremity. If a tremor is present, assess amplitude, frequency, and regularity, and whether the tremor is present at rest, with action or posture. To assess the handwriting, have the patient write a sentence, and do spiral and line drawing with both the dominant and nondominant hand with the hand and arm not resting on the table (unbraced) because this may dampen certain types of tremor.

Perform gait examination with bare feet and rolled-up pants to get a good look at the feet and ankles. Evaluate the position of the trunk and neck (flexed forward or arching back), how wide apart the feet are (base), stride length, heel-toe progression of each step, arm swing and posture, and whether the patient walks in a straight line or meanders. If abnormal postures are present, assess whether walking backward, sideways, or running eliminates them (which it often does for idiopathic dystonia). Determine whether walking increases abnormal movements (such as hand tremor or chorea) or whether there is a dancelike, irregular quality to the gait. Perform tandem gait and have the patient stand on one foot to assess for subtle balance impairment. If there is concern for a nonphysiologic gait abnormality, with wild swaying and embellishment, perform distracting maneuvers that require a great deal of concentration to determine whether the gait normalizes briefly, such as backward tandem gait.

Record your findings in writing and, if at all possible, on video. This is important for two reasons. First, it helps you assess the patient's course from visit to visit. Second, it allows you to send this information to a pediatric neurologist or movement disorder specialist to get advice about the categorization of abnormal movements, direction for further evaluation, and treatment if you need help and the patient does not have the means to travel for a second opinion. When the patient comes to clinic with a complaint of episodic abnormal movements that are not present on examination, asking the parents

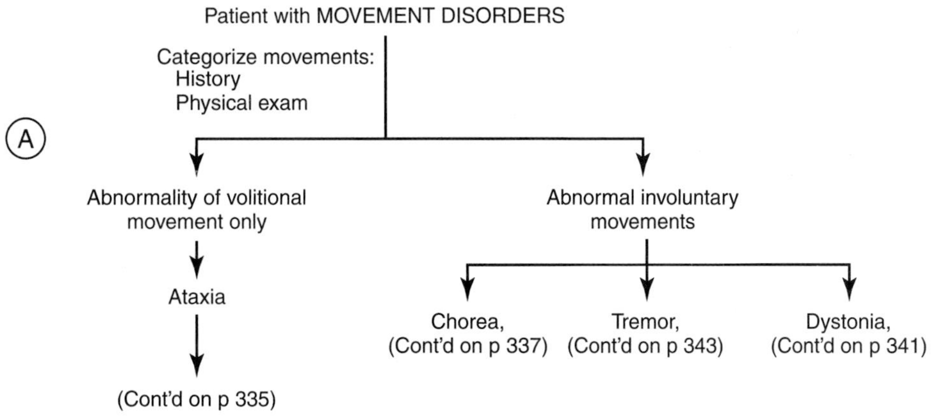
Patient with MOVEMENT DISORDERS
Categorize movements:
History
Physical exam
A
Abnormality of volitional movement only
Abnormal involuntary movements
Ataxia
(Cont'd on p 335)
Chorea, (Cont'd on p 337)
Tremor, (Cont'd on p 343)
Dystonia, (Cont'd on p 341)

Table 2. **Key Features of the Movement Disorder History**

Historical Feature	Details
Initial and subsequent manifestations	• Presence at rest • Presence with action, including examples of actions when it is noted • If present with both, determine whether more severe at rest or with action
Course	• Acute or gradual onset? • Slow or rapid progression? • Spontaneous remissions and recurrences?
Precipitating factors	• Medications • Exercise • Infection • Volitional movement
Aggravating factors	• Stress • Strong emotions including anger, anxiety, or excitement • Fever • Fatigue • Diurnal variation
Ameliorating factors	• Sleep • Medications • Distraction (concentration) • Alcohol • Touching another part of body (sensory trick)
Age at onset	
Family history of disorder or consanguinity	
Medical history including pregnancy, delivery, neonatal course	
Developmental history	
Comorbidities	

Table 3. **Questions to Help Categorize Abnormal Movements**

- Single abnormal movement or a combination of abnormal movements?
- Rhythmical or arrhythmical?
- Sustained posture (even briefly) or nonsustained?
- Patterned or random?
- Fast or slow?
- Large or small amplitude?
- More distal or proximal?
- Can you break it or inhibit it physically?
- Can the patient touch somewhere to help reduce or prevent it?
- Paroxysmal, continual (over and over), or continuous (without stopping)?
- Persist during sleep or occur only in sleep?
- Present with action, at rest, or both?
- How suppressible is it (completely, partially, or not at all)?
- What accompanies it (vocalizations, mutilation, sensory component)?

to make a video recording of the movements is often required to make an accurate diagnosis of the abnormal movements. See the video protocol (Table 5) for suggestions about making a useful video.

The most common abnormal movements in pediatric patients include tics, tremor, stereotypies, infantile self-stimulatory behavior (masturbation), psychogenic movement disorders, secondary dystonia from underlying brain injury, ataxia, chorea, and acute dystonic reactions. Rare movement disorders such as paroxysmal dyskinesias, myoclonus, akathisia, and tardive dyskinesia occur in children infrequently. The basic algorithms for evaluating the causative factors and treatment of abnormal movements are outlined in the algorithm.

When underlying conditions are causing abnormal movements, these should be addressed and managed appropriately. In contrast, abnormal movements should be treated *only* if they are causing a functional impairment to the child; the mere presence of abnormal movements that annoy or bother the parents or medical staff is not sufficient reason to expose the child to the potential side effects and toxicity of medications. This cannot be overstated. Abnormal movements should be treated only if they are or might cause an injury to the child, are functionally impairing the child, or are impeding their care. The general approach is to choose a medication that will be effective for the particular abnormal movement, with an acceptable side-effect profile for that patient. Start at a low dose and titrate up gradually over several weeks to months. If adverse effects emerge, lower or discontinue the medication over 1 to 2 weeks. Several medications may be required in combination to get adequate control of the abnormal movements.

(Continued on page 334)

Table 4. **Specific Components of the Neurologic Examination Helpful in Assessing Abnormal Movements and Ataxia**

Examination Component	Examination Maneuver	Examples of Abnormalities
General	Quiet sitting with and without suppression	Abnormal movements present at rest
Cranial nerves	Fixation of gaze	Square wave jerks
	Smooth pursuit	Breakdown with jerky saccades
	Large saccades	Overshoot or undershoot Blink to initiate saccade
	Speech	Abnormal movements elsewhere in body increase
	• Coordination of sounds	• Clumsy and ataxic
	• Quality of sound	• Soft, breathy, or strangulated
	• Pronunciation	• Dysarthric for labial, lingual, and/or guttural sounds
	• Modulation of pitch	• Abnormal
	• Inflection	• Abnormal
	• Holding *aah* and *eeh* sounds	• Tremor, strangulation, or breathy
	Tongue movements side to side	Slow Abnormal postures Abnormal movements (twisting or tremor)
Motor	Tone	Spastic Rigid Dystonia impairs assessment
	Arms extended with palms up, in, down, and out	Tremor Abnormal postures or movements
	Rapid alternating movements	Abnormal postures in part moving Abnormal postures in another part (not moving) Clumsy coordination Slow speed Low or diminishing amplitude Abnormal rhythm Superimposed abnormal movements
	Finger-to-nose and toe-to-finger	Ataxia Dysmetria Tremor throughout or as approach target Superimposed abnormal movements (chorea or myoclonus)
	Writing	Abnormal postures of hands Tremor Superimposed abnormal movements
Gait	Body posture	Trunk flexed Trunk extended
	Base	Wide Narrow (scissored)
	Stride length	Asymmetric Short
	Arm swing	Asymmetric
	Heel-toe progression	No heel strike
	Path	Meanders
	Tandem	Balance impairment
	Balance on one foot	Balance impairment
	Foot posture	Abnormal
	Reverse and sideways walking	Abnormal movements persist
	Assess whether any abnormal movements come out while walking	Increased abnormal movements

Table 5. **Movement Disorders Video Protocol**

Patient should be dressed in shorts and short sleeves with bare feet.

Film patient sitting quietly in a chair, not speaking with eyes open. Film the entire body first for 5 seconds, then zoom in on any part that has abnormal movements for 5 seconds (even if not present in that part at rest).

Patient speaking continuously for at least 10 seconds, film entire body for first ~5 seconds; then zoom in on part that has abnormal movements for additional 5 seconds.

Arms stretched straight out in front of body (as if you are a zombie):

- With palms facing upward (as if holding a pizza) for 5 seconds
- With palms facing inward (as if holding a ball between them) for 5 seconds
- With palms facing downward for 5 seconds
- With palms facing outward for 5 seconds
- Back to palms facing downward, make fists and open them up completely repeatedly, as fast as possible, 10 times
- Tap thumb and index finger together, as fast and as big as possible, 10 times

Stretch arms out to side, then touch your nose with one index finger, straighten it out, and touch with other index finger, straighten out. Repeat five times and focus in on finger as it approaches nose for the last few times.

Stomp right leg on floor 10 times, then left leg 10 times. Make it loud and big.

Keep the right heel on the ground and tap the toes of that foot 10 times. Tap the left toes 10 times.

Stand up and walk toward the camera at least 10 steps. Turn around and walk back. Walk toward the camera on your tip toes. Walk backward 10 steps. Then sit back down in chair.

If any particular activity is known to trigger the movement (e.g., writing, speaking, eating), then film that activity as well.

ATAXIA

B. Ataxia is an abnormality of voluntary movements and, therefore, is not present at rest. It is a perturbation of the coordination of movements including eye movements, speech, truncal and appendicular control, and balance. It may manifest with a number of different abnormalities on examination, depending on which part of the cerebellum or its outflow tracts is involved. Bifrontal lobe disease or a sensory ataxia from a peripheral neuropathy or posterior column disease of the spinal cord (with impaired joint position sense) may present with similar symptoms. The symptoms of acute-onset ataxia include feeling "dizzy" or unsteady, difficulty walking well, jumping eyes, and there may be associated headache, vomiting, or reduced awareness. Chronic ataxia typically presents with a longstanding history of clumsiness with frequent falls in ambulatory patients. Either acute-onset or chronic ataxia patients may appear drunk. Signs to look for on examination include nystagmus and jerky eye movements on smooth pursuit, dysarthria, head titubation, hypotonia, reduced reflexes, dysdiadochokinesis, an intention tremor, a rubral tremor, dysmetria and overshoot on finger-follow, wide-based stance and gait, ataxic gait, and difficulty with tandem gait and balancing on one foot.

The most common causes of acute-onset ataxia include drug toxicity or ingestion, postinfectious cerebellitis, basilar migraine, and psychogenic ataxia (Table 6). Ingestions are common in the toddler age group, whereas medication toxicity can occur at any age. It may present with nystagmus, encephalopathy, and/or seizures. Medications that may produce ataxia include antiepileptics such as phenytoin, carbamazepine, benzodiazepines, phenobarbital, and primidone, as well as antihistamines. Alcohol and lead may also cause acute-onset ataxia. The diagnosis is made by history, and drug and toxin levels in serum and/or urine. Postinfectious cerebellitis is common in the 2- to 7-year-old age group but can present up to 16 years of age. There is a history of a preceding viral syndrome in 50% of cases, and the male/female ratio is equal. The onset is typically explosive, with maximal ataxia within hours to a day or two from onset. It varies in severity from mild unsteadiness to complete inability to walk. There is always a clear sensorium without nausea or vomiting. Presence of these features should suggest increased intracranial pressure, prompting immediate head imaging. On examination, there may be normal or reduced reflexes and mild nystagmus. Absence of reflexes suggests the Miller Fisher variant of Guillain-Barré, whereas chaotic eye movements with extreme irritability and distal myoclonus should prompt a workup for opsoclonus-myoclonus ataxia syndrome. The course for postinfectious cerebellitis may be from days to months, and there is typically minimal waxing or waning of the symptoms. Imaging is usually normal and must be obtained to exclude other potentially dangerous causes of acute-onset ataxia, such as acute hydrocephalus, cerebellar hemorrhage, or edema. Opsoclonus-myoclonus-ataxia syndrome may initially present as postinfectious cerebellitis with ataxia, to be followed by the opsoclonus, myoclonus, and irritability 1 to 2 weeks later. The onset is from 1 month to 4 years old, with a mean age of 18 months. The ataxia characteristically waxes and wanes, as opposed to postinfectious cerebellitis. It is highly associated with an occult neuroblastoma, and a thorough workup must be undertaken to evaluate for this possibility. Treatment includes resection of the underlying tumor, adrenocorticotropic hormone (ACTH) or dexamethasone, intravenous immunoglobulin (IVIg), and rituximab. The outcome depends on how quickly treatment is initiated, with children who are treated earlier having a better motor and cognitive prognosis. Patients are prone to relapse with intercurrent infections or fever. Basilar migraines are recurrent attacks of brainstem or cerebellar dysfunction often followed by a severe, occipital throbbing headache and nausea and vomiting in a third of patients. The peak incidence is in adolescence, and it is more common in female than male individuals. Possible symptoms include gait ataxia in 50%, visual loss, tinnitus, alternating hemiparesis from one episode to the next, paresthesias, and decreased level of consciousness. Stroke and benign occipital epilepsy are other diagnostic considerations for this presentation. The workup includes an acute magnetic resonance imaging/magnetic resonance angiography (MRI/MRA) with diffusion-weighted imaging (DWI) to exclude stroke and consideration of an electroencephalogram (EEG). Treatment is the same as for other forms of migraine.

Chronic ataxias can be divided into nonprogressive ataxias, which are due to a congenital brain malformation or static brain injury, whereas progressive ataxias are due to a host of genetic and metabolic disorders, or slowly growing brain tumors (see Table 6). Patients with progressive ataxia should be referred to a pediatric neurologist for evaluation. The most common genetic causes include Friedreich ataxia and ataxia-telangiectasia. Friedreich ataxia is a recessively inherited disorder with an incidence of 1 to 2 per 50,000. It has no sex predilection but is most common in people of European descent and is rare in blacks or Asians. On examination, there is a progressive gait ataxia with early absent reflexes, upgoing toes, a peripheral neuropathy with vibration and joint position sense impairment, weakness and wasting of the lower extremities, and high arches, and is associated with scoliosis, cardiac arrhythmias and congestive heart failure, glucose intolerance and diabetes. It is diagnosed by gene testing. Ataxia telangiectasia has an incidence of 1 in 40,000 to 100,000. There is no sex or racial predilection, and it is an autosomal recessive condition with full penetrance. Patients have a slowly progressive ataxia with frequent sinopulmonary infections, telangiectasias in sun-exposed skin and conjunctivae, skin lesions, hypogonadism, and growth retardation. Neurologically, the first symptom is often hypotonia, followed by truncal ataxia, an oculomotor apraxia, chorea, and dystonia. Weakness and a peripheral neuropathy with loss of reflexes develop later. Mild mental retardation often is present in late childhood to adulthood. These patients are at high risk for development of tumors of the lymphoreticular system and are sensitive to radiation. At this time, there is no cure for either disorder.

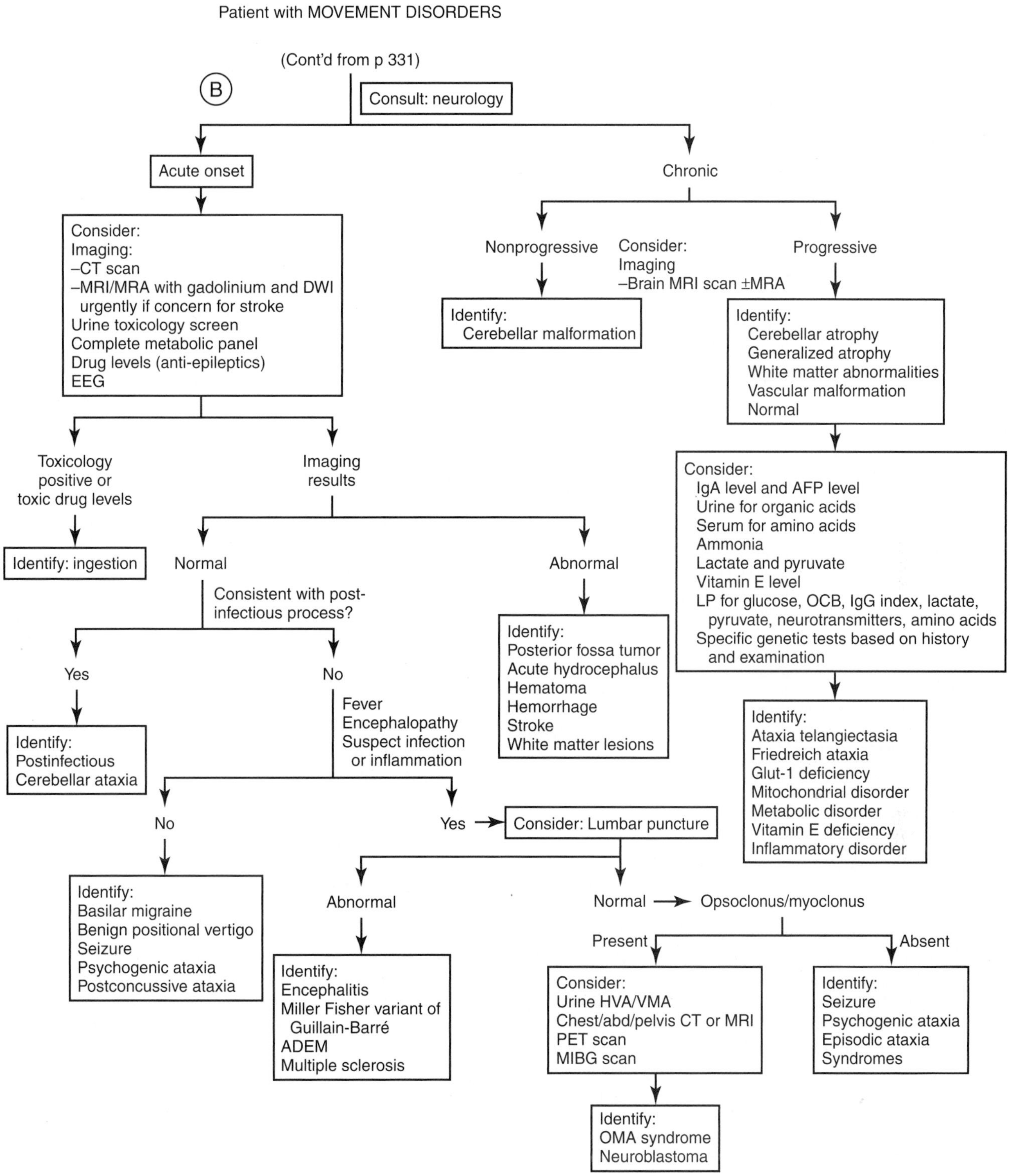
Patient with MOVEMENT DISORDERS
(Cont'd from p 331)
B
Consult: neurology
Acute onset
Consider:
Imaging:
–CT scan
–MRI/MRA with gadolinium and DWI urgently if concern for stroke
Urine toxicology screen
Complete metabolic panel
Drug levels (anti-epileptics)
EEG
Toxicology positive or toxic drug levels
Identify: ingestion
Imaging results
Normal
Consistent with post-infectious process?
Yes
Identify:
Postinfectious
Cerebellar ataxia
No
Fever
Encephalopathy
Suspect infection or inflammation
No
Identify:
Basilar migraine
Benign positional vertigo
Seizure
Psychogenic ataxia
Postconcussive ataxia
Yes
Consider: Lumbar puncture
Abnormal
Identify:
Encephalitis
Miller Fisher variant of Guillain-Barré
ADEM
Multiple sclerosis
Normal
Opsoclonus/myoclonus
Present
Consider:
Urine HVA/VMA
Chest/abd/pelvis CT or MRI
PET scan
MIBG scan
Identify:
OMA syndrome
Neuroblastoma
Absent
Identify:
Seizure
Psychogenic ataxia
Episodic ataxia
Syndromes
Abnormal
Identify:
Posterior fossa tumor
Acute hydrocephalus
Hematoma
Hemorrhage
Stroke
White matter lesions
Chronic
Nonprogressive
Identify:
Cerebellar malformation
Consider:
Imaging
–Brain MRI scan ±MRA
Progressive
Identify:
Cerebellar atrophy
Generalized atrophy
White matter abnormalities
Vascular malformation
Normal
Consider:
IgA level and AFP level
Urine for organic acids
Serum for amino acids
Ammonia
Lactate and pyruvate
Vitamin E level
LP for glucose, OCB, IgG index, lactate, pyruvate, neurotransmitters, amino acids
Specific genetic tests based on history and examination
Identify:
Ataxia telangiectasia
Friedreich ataxia
Glut-1 deficiency
Mitochondrial disorder
Metabolic disorder
Vitamin E deficiency
Inflammatory disorder

Ataxia is not treatable with medications. When it is due to an underlying treatable disorder, the symptoms of ataxia may improve with treatment of that condition. If it is due to a static or progressive condition, the lack of effective medications is often frustrating and disappointing for parents, patients, and physicians. Physical therapy may be modestly helpful for improving balance and patients should be referred for this. When other comorbidities are present, especially in the genetic ataxias, these should be addressed.

Table 6. **Causes of Acute and Chronic Ataxia**

Acute Onset	Chronic
Drug ingestion or medication toxicity	**Progressive**
Postinfectious cerebellitis	Hartnup disease
Basilar migraine	Maple syrup urine disease
Opsoclonus-myoclonus ataxia syndrome	Pyruvate dehydrogenase deficiency
Psychogenic ataxia (conversion)	Glut-1 deficiency syndrome
Brainstem encephalitis	Friedreich ataxia
Benign paroxysmal vertigo	Ataxia telangiectasia
Trauma	Ataxia with vitamin E deficiency
Hematoma	Abetalipoproteinemia
Postconcussive	Ataxia-oculomotor apraxia type 1 or 2
Vertebrobasilar artery occlusion	Ataxia with diffuse CNS hypomyelination
Inflammatory	Juvenile GM2 gangliosidosis
Multiple sclerosis	Adrenoleukodystrophy
• Miller Fisher variant of Guillain-Barré	Metachromatic leukodystrophy
• Kawasaki disease	Marinesco-Sjögren
Cerebellar hemorrhage	Ramsay Hunt syndrome
Episodic ataxias	Refsum disease
Seizure	Sea-blue histiocytosis
	Multiple carboxylase deficiency
	Mitochondrial disorders
	Dentatorubropallidoluysian atrophy (DRPLA)
	HARP
	Spinocerebellar ataxias
	Leber hereditary optic neuropathy
	Pelizaeus–Merzbacher disease
	Hereditary spastic ataxias
	Nonprogressive
	Congenital lesions
	Remote stroke

HARP, hypobetalipoproteinemia, acanthocytosis, retinitis pigmentosa and palliative degeneration syndrome.

CHOREA

C. Chorea is a jerky, irregular movement that occurs randomly and with unpredictable timing. It is present at rest, even when the patient is trying to hold completely still (as opposed to ataxia, which is a perturbation of purposeful movements only) and increases with voluntary movements. It may appear to randomly flow from one body part to another, but this is not required for diagnosis. It may be seen together with athetosis, which is a slow, writhing, continuous movement, and in that case is termed *choreoathetosis*, which is actually quite rare. There is typically no preceding feeling of restlessness or underlying urge, with the notable exception of Sydenham chorea. The movements are involuntary and uncontrollable, and may be incorporated into purposeful movements. Chorea is not suppressible. When it is mild and distal, it may appear only as jerks of the fingers or toes. Chorea of moderate severity appears to be constant fidgeting and a dance-like quality to the gait. Large-amplitude proximal chorea is called *ballismus.* It may be located anywhere in the body, and may be symmetric or asymmetric.

The differential diagnosis includes tics, which are more patterned and have a preceding urge; akathisia, which has an intense sense of inner restlessness; psychogenic abnormal movements; and, in young children, shaking and shuddering spells, spasmus nutans, and masturbation. Useful historical features include triggers, such as arising quickly from a chair (suggests a paroxysmal kinesigenic dyskinesia), foods or illness (which suggest an underlying metabolic disorder), medical history such as streptococcal infections, and comorbidities such as diabetes, epilepsy, or mental retardation. The causative factors are diverse and include fixed brain injuries, brain malformations, electrolyte abnormalities, vascular brain lesions, paroxysmal dyskinesias, drugs or medications, genetic and degenerative conditions, immune-mediated or postinfectious chorea, postsurgical and idiopathic (see Table 7). The most common diagnoses in a previously healthy, otherwise neurologically normal child are immune-mediated diseases and medications or drugs. If there is an accompanying severe encephalopathy, consider neuropsychiatric lupus or anti–*N*-methyl-D-aspartate (anti-NMDA) antibody-mediated encephalopathy.

The first step in evaluation is to exclude underlying medications or toxins and perform a laboratory workup including a throat culture for streptococcal infection, electrolytes, calcium, magnesium, phosphorous, glucose, thyroid function studies, ammonia, erythrocyte sedimentation rate (ESR), C-reactive protein, antinuclear antibody (ANA), anti-streptolysin O (ASO), anti-DNAse B, antiphospholipid antibodies, complete blood cell count (CBC), and medication levels or a urine toxicology screen. Consider an MRI scan with MRA if the earlier studies are unrevealing or the patient is not neurologically normal. Additional studies to consider for a child with a long-standing history of developmental delay and/or neurologic abnormalities include a metabolic workup with serum quantitative amino acids, urine organic acids, lactate and pyruvate, ammonia, serum copper and ceruloplasmin, and lumbar puncture for glucose, lactate, and pyruvate, neurotransmitters, amino acids, oligoclonal bands, IgG index, and anti-NMDA antibodies.

Lack of sleep, hunger, anxiety, stress, anger, and intercurrent illness may all increase chorea temporarily. Addressing these underlying conditions may be the best first step. Benzodiazepines or antiepileptics such as levetiracetam or valproic acid may reduce chorea. If it is severe, consider treatment with tetrabenazine, a dopamine-depleting medication without the risk for tardive dyskinesia present with dopamine receptor-blocking medications. If tetrabenazine is ineffective, or has untoward side effects, neuroleptics may be used, but the risk for significant adverse effects, acute dystonic reactions, akathisia, and tardive dyskinesia, a potentially permanent irreversible movement disorder, requires that the chorea be significantly disabling to the child before neuroleptics are considered.

Sydenham chorea may be seen anywhere from 1 to 6 months after a pharyngeal group A β-hemolytic streptococcal infection. It is seen in 10% to 30% of acute rheumatic fever cases. It typically occurs in children 5 to 15 years of age, with a peak at 8 to 9 years of age. There is a female predominance in 60% to 70% of cases. The chorea is typically moderate to severe, develops suddenly over several days, and is often asymmetric. It may be associated with behavioral changes including irritability, aggressiveness, and inattentiveness. Rarely, there may be an associated dystonia with twisting postures. Children often describe sensory abnormalities that are somewhat vague but involve an urge to move. In contrast with tics, making the movements does not provide a clear sense of relief, and tics

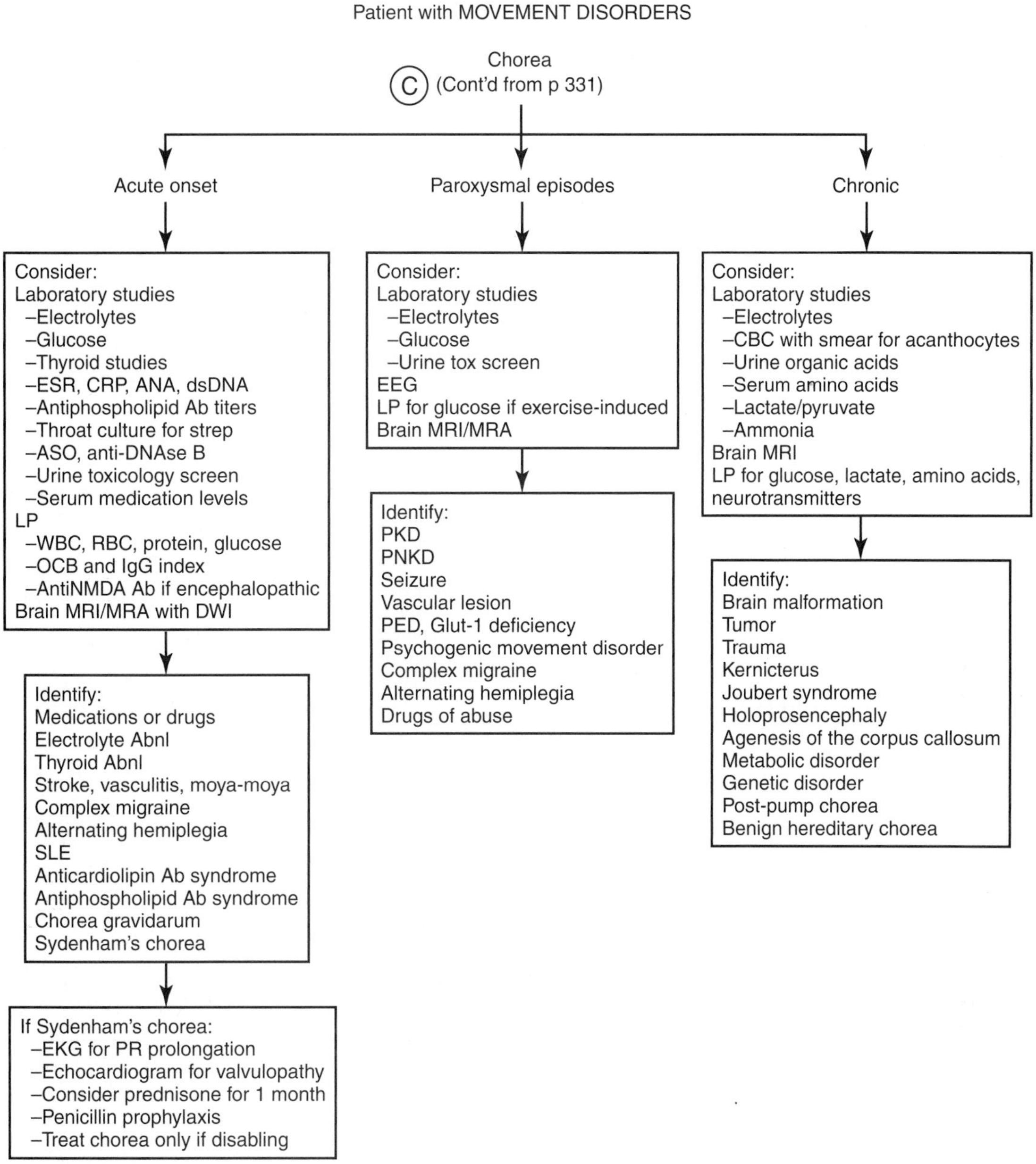
Patient with MOVEMENT DISORDERS
Chorea
C (Cont'd from p 331)
Acute onset
Paroxysmal episodes
Chronic
Consider:
Laboratory studies
–Electrolytes
–Glucose
–Thyroid studies
–ESR, CRP, ANA, dsDNA
–Antiphospholipid Ab titers
–Throat culture for strep
–ASO, anti-DNAse B
–Urine toxicology screen
–Serum medication levels
LP
–WBC, RBC, protein, glucose
–OCB and IgG index
–AntiNMDA Ab if encephalopathic
Brain MRI/MRA with DWI
Identify:
Medications or drugs
Electrolyte Abnl
Thyroid Abnl
Stroke, vasculitis, moya-moya
Complex migraine
Alternating hemiplegia
SLE
Anticardiolipin Ab syndrome
Antiphospholipid Ab syndrome
Chorea gravidarum
Sydenham's chorea
If Sydenham's chorea:
–EKG for PR prolongation
–Echocardiogram for valvulopathy
–Consider prednisone for 1 month
–Penicillin prophylaxis
–Treat chorea only if disabling
Consider:
Laboratory studies
–Electrolytes
–Glucose
–Urine tox screen
EEG
LP for glucose if exercise-induced
Brain MRI/MRA
Identify:
PKD
PNKD
Seizure
Vascular lesion
PED, Glut-1 deficiency
Psychogenic movement disorder
Complex migraine
Alternating hemiplegia
Drugs of abuse
Consider:
Laboratory studies
–Electrolytes
–CBC with smear for acanthocytes
–Urine organic acids
–Serum amino acids
–Lactate/pyruvate
–Ammonia
Brain MRI
LP for glucose, lactate, amino acids, neurotransmitters
Identify:
Brain malformation
Tumor
Trauma
Kernicterus
Joubert syndrome
Holoprosencephaly
Agenesis of the corpus callosum
Metabolic disorder
Genetic disorder
Post-pump chorea
Benign hereditary chorea

typically start in the head and neck. Diagnosis is made when the ASO and/or anti-DNAse B is significantly increased (at least three to four times the upper limit of normal), or a presumptive diagnosis is made when all other causes have been excluded. Mild increases of these antibodies reflect streptococcal pharyngeal or nasal carriage, and likely are not related to the underlying chorea. A mild increase of the ESR may also be seen. Sydenham chorea alone is sufficient for the diagnosis of rheumatic fever without fulfilling any other Jones criteria. It is uncommon to have an associated arthritis as a manifestation of rheumatic fever when Sydenham chorea is present. An electrocardiogram must be obtained to exclude prolongation of the P-R interval, and even if no murmur is auscultated on clinical examination, an echocardiogram should be performed to exclude a valvulopathy. One third of patients will have a murmur on examination, and up to 84% of patients will have rheumatic valve disease on echocardiogram. Penicillin prophylaxis should be started and continued until the age of 18, or 5 years, whichever is longer. The goal is to prevent recurrent streptococcal infections to prevent cardiac disease. Penicillin prophylaxis does not affect the course of the chorea. The chorea may persist for several months and even up to a year in mild form. Treatment with oral prednisone 2 mg/kg/day at a dosage maximum of 60 mg/day for 1 month followed by a taper over 2 weeks shortens the course of Sydenham chorea by about 50%. The chorea itself may be treated as any other type of chorea if it is severe and interfering with the child's function. A female patient with prior Sydenham chorea may have recurrence of chorea if she takes oral contraceptive pills or becomes pregnant (chorea gravidarum). Recurrence of chorea in a patient with a history of Sydenham should prompt an investigation for a recurrent streptococcal infection, other infections, pregnancy, oral contraceptive use, medication, or toxin ingestion.

(Continued on page 340)

Table 7. **Causes of Chorea**

Fixed Injury

Asphyxia (birth or subsequent)
Encephalitis or postencephalitic
Trauma
Tumors
Kernicterus

Malformations

Joubert syndrome
Holoprosencephaly
Agenesis of the corpus callosum

Chemical

Hyponatremia or hypernatremia
Hypomagnesemia
Hypocalcemia
Hypoglycemia or hyperglycemia
Hypoparathyroidism
Hyperthyroidism

Genetic and Degenerative

Ataxia telangiectasia
Acyl-CoA dehydrogenase deficiency
Basal ganglia calcification (Fahr disease)
Behçet disease
Biopterin-dependent hyperphenylalaninemia
Canavan disease
Ceroid lipofuscinosis
Dentatorubropallidoluysian atrophy (DRPLA)
Friedreich ataxia
Galactosemia
Gangliosidosis
Glutaric aciduria
Huntington disease
Lesch-Nyhan disease
Metachromatic leukodystrophy
Methylmalonic aciduria
Mitochondrial cytopathies
Neuroacanthocytosis
Niemann–Pick type C
Nonketotic hyperglycinemia
Pelizaeus–Merzbacher disease
Phenylketonuria
Propionic acidemia
PKAN and HARP syndrome
Rett syndrome
Vitamin E deficiency or malabsorption
Wilson disease

Vascular

Basal ganglia stroke
Cerebral vasculitis
Moyamoya disease
Complex migraine
Alternating hemiplegia

Acute and Paroxysmal

Paroxysmal kinesigenic dyskinesia
Paroxysmal nonkinesigenic dyskinesias
Paroxysmal exercise-induced chorea

Idiopathic

Benign hereditary chorea

Drug-Induced

Amphetamines and Stimulants

Amphetamine (with dextroamphetamine is Adderall)
Atomoxetine (Strattera)
Dexmethylphenidate (Focalin)
Dextroamphetamine (Dexedrine)
Methamphetamine (Desoxyn)
Methylphenidate (Ritalin)

Anticholinergics

Trihexyphenidyl (Artane)
Diphenhydramine (Benadryl)

Antiemetics

Prochlorperazine (Compazine)
Metoclopramide (Reglan)

Antiepileptics

Phenytoin (Dilantin)
Carbamazepine (Tegretol)
Valproic acid (Depakote)
Phenobarbital (Luminal)

HARP, hypobetalipoproteinemia, acanthocytosis, retinitis pigmentosa, and pallidal degeneration syndrome; *PKAN*, pantothenate kinase associated neurodegeneration.

Table 7. **Causes of Chorea—cont'd**

Benzodiazepines

Alprazolam (Xanax)
Chlordiazepoxide (Librium)
Clonazepam (Klonopin)
Clorazepate (Tranxene)
Diazepam (Valium)
Lorazepam (Ativan)

Calcium Channel Blockers

Amlodipine (Norvasc)
Diltiazem (Cardizem)
Nicardipine (Cardene)
Nimodipine (Nimotop)
Verapamil (Calan)

Neuroleptics

Aripiprazole (Abilify)
Haloperidol (Haldol)
Olanzapine (Zyprexa)
Pimozide (Orap)
Risperidone (Risperdal)
Ziprasidone (Geodon)

Tricyclic Antidepressants

Amitriptyline (Elavil)
Clomipramine (Anafranil)
Desipramine (Norpramin)
Imipramine (Tofranil)
Nortriptyline (Pamelor)

Other

Amantadine (Symmetrel)
Bismuth (ingredient in Maalox, Pepto-Bismol, Kaopectate)
Clonidine (Catapres)
Levodopa (Sinemet)
Lithium (Lithobid, Eskalith)
Oral contraceptives

Immune-Mediated

Systemic lupus erythematosus
Henoch–Schönlein Purpura
Anticardiolipin and antiphospholipid antibody syndrome
Sydenham chorea (poststreptococcal infection)
Chorea gravidarum

Postsurgical

Postcardiac bypass (postpump syndrome)

DYSTONIA

D. Dystonia is abnormal twisting postures that may be sustained for varying lengths of time, from a split-second to a permanent posture with contractures if severe and unremitting. It is thought to occur from cocontraction of agonist and antagonist muscles (such as the biceps and triceps while trying to straighten the arm at the elbow). It is a patterned movement and observation over several minutes and with different examination maneuvers demonstrates this point.

Historical features that are helpful in determining an underlying cause include medication exposures, a family history of dystonia, diurnal variation and location of onset, inflammatory/autoimmune disease, other neurologic or psychiatric symptoms, history of trauma in the affected limb, and perinatal medical history. If there is no clear evidence of birth asphyxia with neonatal seizures, other organ involvement (liver, kidney, heart), or a prolonged neonatal hospital stay in a child with a diagnosis of "dystonic cerebral palsy," metabolic disorders including glutaric aciduria, a mitochondrial disorder, or Glut-1 transporter deficiency must be excluded.

On examination, assess the pattern of involvement, whether there is a jerky dystonic tremor that reduces or resolves in a position (a null point), whether there is overflow dystonia in other parts of the body (such as feet) with voluntary movements elsewhere (hands), presence at rest, with action and at rest, or only with action. Determine whether a sensory trick is present, in which touching a part of the body reduces the dystonia. For example, a patient with dystonia of the neck may find that touching the side of the jaw or face lightly allows them to hold the head in midline. Determine whether the dystonia is present with unfamiliar or different learned motor programs (running or walking backward if present with walking forwards, grasping an implement differently if involves the hand). Look for other neurologic abnormalities on examination.

Dystonia is often grouped into different causes including idiopathic (genetic), secondary (symptomatic), dystonia-plus syndromes, and heredodegenerative dystonia. In idiopathic (genetic) dystonia, the only abnormal feature is dystonia and requires the presence of a gene mutation and/or exclusion of secondary dystonia (see Table 8). Secondary (symptomatic) dystonia results from underlying brain disease, injury, or medication usage. Dystonia-plus syndromes are non-neurodegenerative genetic disorders with other neurologic features, such as parkinsonism or myoclonus. Heredodegenerative dystonias are hereditary, progressive neurodegenerative diseases where other neurologic symptoms and signs are present in addition to the dystonia. Features on examination may help distinguish between these possibilities. An idiopathic (genetic) dystonia is suggested by dystonia only with certain actions, absence at rest if not severe, lack of overflow dystonia, presence of a sensory trick, and absence or reduction with unfamiliar motor programs. Secondary dystonia, dystonia-plus, or heredodegenerative dystonias are suggested by dystonia present at rest and worse with action, overflow dystonia, lack of a sensory trick, other abnormalities present on examination, early involvement of speech, and hemidystonia. Acute dystonic reactions to medications are commonly seen in children and are discussed separately later.

The differential diagnosis of dystonia includes psychogenic dystonia, self-stimulatory behavior, dystonic tics, seizures, Sandifer syndrome, Chiari malformation, and paroxysmal kinesigenic or nonkinesigenic dyskinesias, which are episodic and paroxysmal disorders that are likely channelopathies. The evaluation should include a complete electrolyte panel, liver function studies, a vitamin E level, serum ceruloplasmin and copper, ESR, ANA, brain MRI/MRA and slit-lamp examination in cognitively normal children, and cognitively abnormal children should have the above plus the metabolic workup outlined in the chorea section. All children with dystonia should be referred to a pediatric neurologist and/or movement disorder specialist for evaluation and treatment.

The mainstays of treatment for dystonia include withdrawal of offending agents when medication induced, medications, and botulinum toxin injections. Every child with idiopathic dystonia should have a trial of carbidopa-levodopa (Sinemet), even if there is not a prominent diurnal variation or onset in the feet, because a clinical diagnosis of dopa-responsive dystonia can be made if there is a *complete* resolution of the dystonia at low doses of levodopa. Other drugs that are helpful to treat dystonia regardless of the cause include trihexyphenidyl, baclofen, and benzodiazepines. Botulinum toxin injections may be used for focal dystonia or to target specific muscles to allow for improved function or patient care. Deep brain stimulation surgery may also reduce dystonia and is better for mobile rather than fixed dystonias regardless of the cause. There is not a lot of evidence to support the use of baclofen pumps for dystonia when there is not a significant component of comorbid spasticity.

Acute dystonic reactions occur in response to treatment with dopamine-receptor blocking and dopamine-depleting medications. These include antiemetics such as prochlorperazine (Compazine), promethazine (Phenergan), promotility agents such as metoclopramide (Reglan), all antipsychotics, including the "atypical" antipsychotics, and tetrabenazine (Xenazine). The muscles of the face, mouth, neck, and eye are typically involved with a combination of dystonic movements including upward or lateral deviation of the eyes, arching backward of the neck (retrocollis), trismus, tongue protrusion, and occasionally backward or lateral flexion of the trunk. Rarely, laryngospasm may occur and cause airway compromise. About half of all cases of acute dystonic reactions occur within the first 24 hours of treatment, and about 90% occur within the first 5 days. Patients at increased risk include young age (children), male sex, previous dystonic reaction, and the presence of a primary psychotic disorder. Acute treatment includes diphenhydramine (Benadryl) orally (or intravenously if the patient is unable to swallow a pill) or benztropine (Cogentin). Intravenous diazepam (Valium) may also be effective. Because the half-life of anticholinergics and benzodiazepines may be shorter

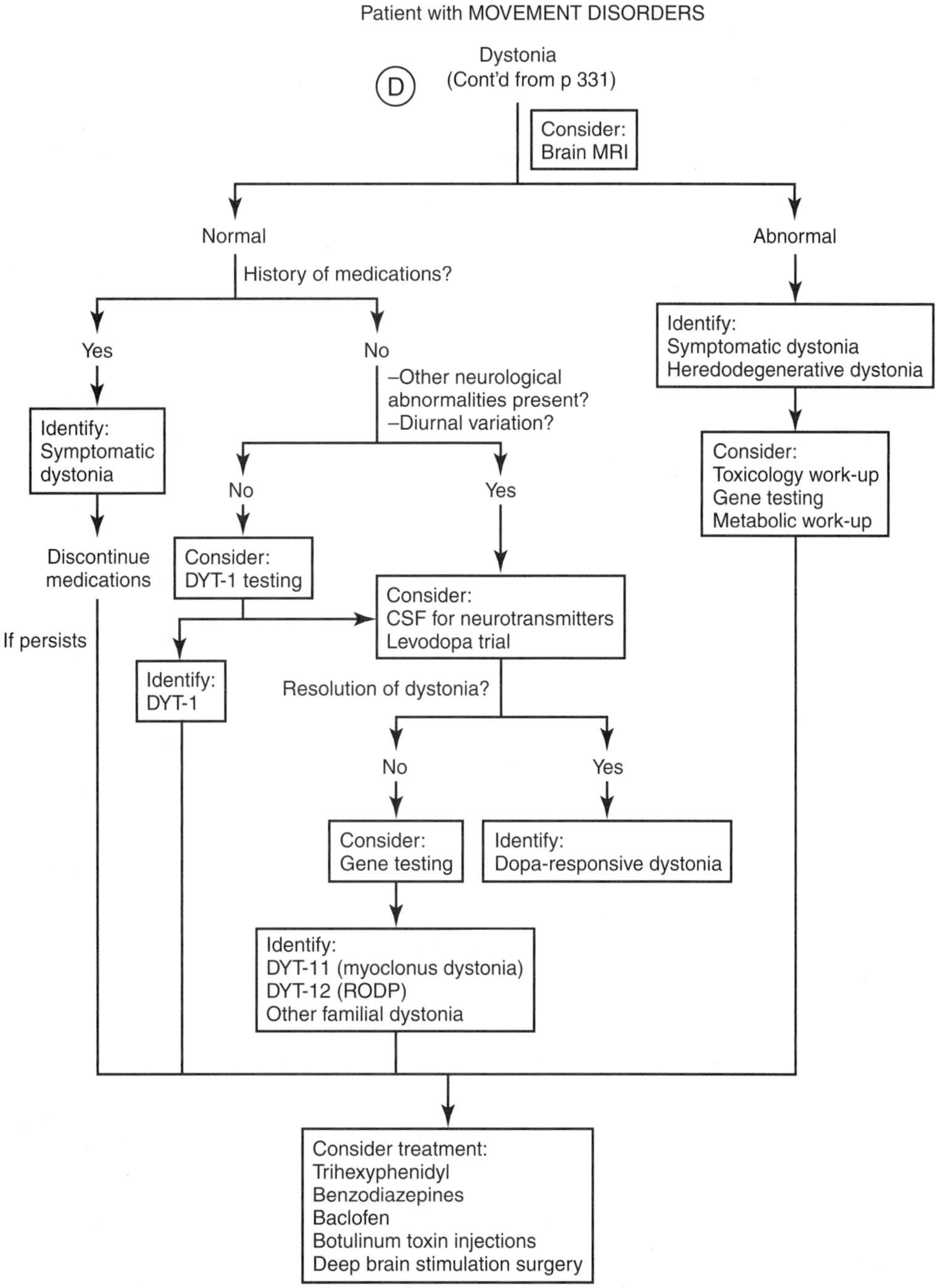
Patient with MOVEMENT DISORDERS
D
Dystonia
(Cont'd from p 331)
Consider: Brain MRI
Normal
Abnormal
History of medications?
Yes
No
Identify: Symptomatic dystonia
Discontinue medications
If persists
–Other neurological abnormalities present?
–Diurnal variation?
No
Yes
Consider: DYT-1 testing
Identify: DYT-1
Consider: CSF for neurotransmitters Levodopa trial
Resolution of dystonia?
No
Yes
Consider: Gene testing
Identify: Dopa-responsive dystonia
Identify: DYT-11 (myoclonus dystonia) DYT-12 (RODP) Other familial dystonia
Identify: Symptomatic dystonia Heredodegenerative dystonia
Consider: Toxicology work-up Gene testing Metabolic work-up
Consider treatment: Trihexyphenidyl Benzodiazepines Baclofen Botulinum toxin injections Deep brain stimulation surgery

than the half-life of dopamine receptor-blocking medications, it may be necessary to continue anticholinergics for 2 weeks. This is the one scenario in which stopping a neuroleptic medication abruptly is recommended, even though this may increase the risk for development of acute withdrawal dyskinesias or tardive dyskinesia. For children who require treatment with neuroleptic medications long term with a previous dystonic reaction, pretreating for several days with benztropine (Cogentin) and continuing this medication while taking neuroleptics may help reduce the recurrence of an acute dystonic reaction.

Table 8. **Causes of Dystonia**

Idiopathic	Symptomatic	Dystonia-plus	Heredodegenerative
DYT1 (idiopathic torsion dystonia)	Hypoxia or anoxia	Dopa-responsive dystonia (Segawa disease)	X-linked dystonia-parkinsonism (Lubag)
DYT6	Vascular malformations	Rapid-onset dystonia Parkinsonism (*DYT12*)	Huntington disease
DYT7	Brain tumors	Myoclonus-dystonia (*DYT11*)	Wilson disease
DYT2	Brainstem lesions		Neuroacanthocytosis
DYT4	Head injury		Rett syndrome
	Postinfectious		Juvenile parkinsonism
	Brain infections		PKAN
	Stroke		Ataxia telangiectasia
	Multiple sclerosis		Mitochondrial cytopathies
	Thalamotomy		Ceroid lipofuscinosis
	Cervical cord injury		DRPLA
	Lumbar stenosis		SCA3
	Peripheral trauma		Neuroaxonal dystrophy
	Hypoparathyroidism		Pelizaeus–Merzbacher disease
	Toxins		Fahr disease
	Carbon monoxide		Vitamin E deficiency
	Cyanide		Homocystinuria
	Manganese		Glutaric aciduria type I
	Methanol		Numerous metabolic disorders
	Medications		
	Phenytoin		
	Carbamazepine		
	Levodopa		
	Chlorpromazine (Thorazine)		
	Fluphenazine (Prolixin)		
	Haloperidol (Haldol)		
	Metoclopramide (Reglan)		
	Molindone (Moban)		
	Prochlorperazine (Compazine)		
	Promethazine (Phenergan)		
	Thioridizine (Mellaril)		
	Thiothixene (Navane)		
	Trifluoperzine (Stelazine)		

TREMOR

E. Tremor is an oscillatory involuntary to and fro movement, typically about a joint, but may involve other muscle groups such as the chin or tongue muscles. In children it may occur with other abnormal movements, alone, or may be a result of underlying weakness. Steps to diagnose the type of tremor include identifying the body part or parts involved; presence at rest, action, or both; amplitude and frequency; regularity; and factors that make it better or worse. It is important to identify any other abnormal movements or examination abnormalities that are present, whether medications were started before the onset of the tremor, and presence of a family history (although examination of the parents is often more helpful).

The most common types of tremor are a familial essential tremor, enhanced physiologic tremor, or a psychogenic tremor (see Table 9). Cerebellar tremors are uncommon and tend to be large amplitude and slow, and when they involve proximal muscles are called a *rubral* tremor, distal muscles are an *intention tremor*, or *titubation* when the neck or trunk is affected. Other signs of ataxia and in-coordination should be present on examination. Tremor only at rest that disappears with action suggests parkinsonism and should prompt referral to a neurologist. Assess for other features of parkinsonism on examination including facial masking, decreased blink rate, a soft voice, flexed forward position, small, shuffling steps with decreased arm swing, and balance impairment that may present as spontaneous falls. A jerky, irregular tremor may represent a myoclonic tremor, or a dystonic tremor if there is a null point (position in which the tremor significantly improves) and dystonia with purposeful movements. Jitteriness or tremor with excitement may be seen in young infants up to 6 months of age normally. There is no specific treatment for cerebellar tremors. Myoclonic and dystonic tremors are treated with the same medications as the underlying conditions. Psychogenic tremors are discussed later in the Psychogenic Movement Disorders section.

Familial essential tremor is a highly heritable condition with incomplete penetrance that worsens gradually over time and may have onset as young as infancy. It is present with action, such as reaching, pouring, writing, and performing small maneuvers such as threading a bead. It characteristically worsens or emerges with anxiety, anger, stress, or caffeine, and in adult family members with tremor, improves with alcohol. It may be asymmetric, intermittent, and is a high-frequency, low-amplitude regular tremor. On examination, it is noted distally in the fingers and hands with holding the arms outstretched, and is present with finger to nose, but does not worsen as the target is approached (this suggests a cerebellar intention tremor). An essential tremor may involve the voice, neck and legs, or tongue, but typically only if the hands are also involved. It characteristically slows down in frequency with advancing age, and worsens in severity and amplitude. Excluding other forms of physiologic or action tremor is important when there is a negative family history, and a laboratory workup and brain MRI should be obtained if the tremor

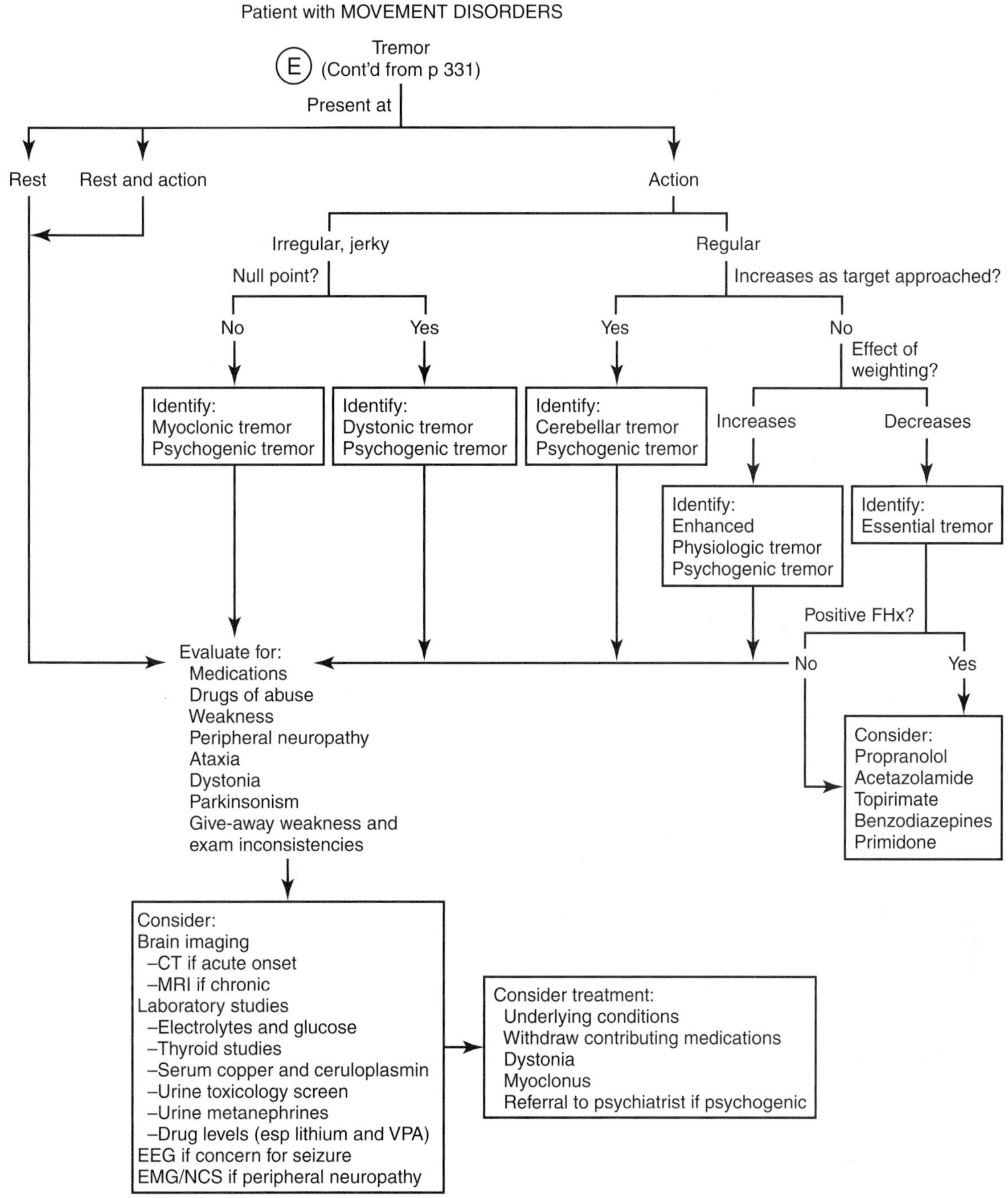
Patient with MOVEMENT DISORDERS
E
Tremor
(Cont'd from p 331)
Present at
Rest
Rest and action
Action
Irregular, jerky
Regular
Null point?
Increases as target approached?
No
Yes
Yes
No
Effect of weighting?
Identify: Myoclonic tremor Psychogenic tremor
Identify: Dystonic tremor Psychogenic tremor
Identify: Cerebellar tremor Psychogenic tremor
Increases
Decreases
Identify: Enhanced Physiologic tremor Psychogenic tremor
Identify: Essential tremor
Positive FHx?
No
Yes
Evaluate for: Medications Drugs of abuse Weakness Peripheral neuropathy Ataxia Dystonia Parkinsonism Give-away weakness and exam inconsistencies
Consider: Propranolol Acetazolamide Topirimate Benzodiazepines Primidone
Consider: Brain imaging –CT if acute onset –MRI if chronic Laboratory studies –Electrolytes and glucose –Thyroid studies –Serum copper and ceruloplasmin –Urine toxicology screen –Urine metanephrines –Drug levels (esp lithium and VPA) EEG if concern for seizure EMG/NCS if peripheral neuropathy
Consider treatment: Underlying conditions Withdraw contributing medications Dystonia Myoclonus Referral to psychiatrist if psychogenic

was sudden onset or there are any neurologic examination abnormalities.

Treatment will not affect the long-term course or severity of essential tremor. Nonmedication approaches such as bracing the arm, using wrist weights, weighted utensils, and writing implements may be the best first step. Medication choices for essential tremor (but not other forms of tremor) include propranolol, primidone, topiramate, acetazolamide, or benzodiazepines. Not every medication works for an individual patient with essential tremor, and the side-effect profile of each medication should guide choice. It may also be reasonable to use a short-acting benzodiazepine or propranolol on an as needed basis before a stressful or anxiety-provoking event known to worsen the tremor, such as performing on stage.

An enhanced physiologic tremor is an amplification of the physiologic tremor present in all individuals. It is an action tremor that may be present at any body site, but typically only occurs with a particular position at the joint or with loading of the muscles with a weight (in contrast with an essential tremor, which typically improves with loading). It may also be enhanced by stress, anxiety, medications, drugs of abuse, or weakness. This may be diagnosed by tremor analysis, but if this is not available in your region, it is important to exclude other causes of action tremor before making the diagnosis. If exacerbating factors are identified, they should be addressed, but there is otherwise no treatment for an enhanced physiologic tremor.

Table 9. **Causes of Action Tremor**

Familial essential tremor
Genetic
Myoclonus-dystonia syndrome
Dystonias
Cerebellar tremor
Psychogenic tremor
Enhanced physiologic tremor caused by:
Medications, drugs, and toxins: albuterol, amiodarone, amphetamines, arsenic, caffeine, cocaine, cyanide, cyclosporine, ethanol, lead, lindane, lithium, manganese, mercury, naphthalene, nicotine, thyroxine, toluene, tricyclic antidepressants, valproic acid
Metabolic: hepatic encephalopathy, hyperthyroidism, hypocalcemia, hypoglycemia, hypomagnesemia, pheochromocytoma
Weakness
Peripheral neuropathy

OTHER MOVEMENT DISORDERS

Psychogenic Movement Disorders

Psychogenic movement disorders are quite common and include nonepileptic seizures, weakness, dystonia, chorea, tremor, abnormal movements, and ataxia. The history is typically one of abrupt onset and spontaneous remissions, often with a combination of abnormal movements, weakness, ataxia, and sensory abnormalities. There is often a waxing and waning quality, with varying frequency, amplitude, and triggers. They may occur in children with true neurologic disorders but do not follow the course or respond to medications as expected. Psychogenic movements often occur in children who are high achievers and do not express stress or their emotions easily. It may also be a manifestation of underlying anxiety, depression, sexual or emotional abuse, and these must be carefully screened to ensure proper treatment. On examination, there may be "give-away" weakness, lack of findings when the patient is unaware he or she is being observed, inconsistencies of findings including distractibility and presence of abnormal movements on examination but not with spontaneous movements, and affect inconsistencies such as extreme effort when performing simple maneuvers or indifference to an apparently significant abnormality. With time and continued observation, inconsistencies may become more apparent. If a patient recently had neuroleptic medications discontinued, a tardive withdrawal syndrome must be excluded. (For key features, see Table 10.)

Table 10. **Features Suggestive of a Psychogenic Movement Disorder**

Sudden onset and spontaneous remissions
Multiple different types of abnormal movements
Inconsistencies with aggravating and alleviating factors
Atypical response to medications
Obvious psychiatric disturbance
Multiple somatizations
Prominent pain out of proportion to the movements
Functional disability out of proportion to examination findings
Ability to trigger or relieve movements with unusual or nonphysiologic interventions
Lack of movements when not aware that is being observed, or with spontaneous movements
Affect inconsistencies:
• Extreme effort with performing simple maneuvers
• Unconcerned affect with apparently significant weakness or movements (la belle indifference)
Suggestive examination findings:
• Give-away weakness
• Abnormal movements are inconsistently present with same activity over time
• Distractibility on examination (try having them name the months of the year backward, or backward tandem gait)

Psychogenic movement disorders fit into the spectrum of somatoform disorders, specifically conversion disorder. Patients are not consciously producing the movements and should not be blamed or accused of "making it up." Parents often unwittingly reinforce the condition by giving lots of attention to the child when the abnormal movements are present and allowing the child to avoid school or activities that he or she may no longer find enjoyable. After a brief evaluation to exclude a true underlying neurologic disorder, a straightforward explanation to the child and family should be given, calling it a *stress-induced movement disorder, conversion disorder,* or a *psychogenic movement disorder.* Explaining it as an unconscious bodily response to stress, similar to diarrhea, stomachaches, or migraines, is often an easily understandable analogy. Present the diagnosis as a positive one, emphasizing that there is no underlying progressive neurologic disorder, and that a stress-induced movement disorder has known and effective treatments. Parents and patients are often resistant to the diagnosis initially but must understand that treating with medications that are not indicated and have potentially dangerous side effects is inappropriate. Physicians should not waste months or years of the patient's life evaluating for rare or unusual conditions if the history and examination are consistent with a psychogenic movement disorder, because this only delays recovery. Referral to a psychologist or psychiatrist experienced in treating somatoform disorders with a focus on uncovering the underlying stressors and making internal conflicts conscious, with an emphasis on learning alternative methods for dealing with stress (such as stress reduction techniques) is key to a successful recovery. Treatment for underlying anxiety disorders or depression may be warranted. Referral to occupational and/or physical therapy for muscle "retraining" is often helpful in conjunction with treatment by a psychiatrist or psychologist, but the therapists must be made aware of the diagnosis ahead of time and feel comfortable designing a treatment program for conversion disorder. Untreated, spontaneous remissions may occur, but it can persist for years and lead to school and possible occupational failure as an adult.

Self-Stimulatory Behavior

Self-stimulatory behavior, also called *infantile masturbation or gratification disorder,* typically occurs in female more than male individuals, and often begins in the first year or two of life. The classic history is recurrent episodes of fairly rhythmic drawing up and/or stiffening of the legs, often accompanied by rocking of the pelvis that occurs when the child is seated in a car seat or high chair, when seated on the floor in a "W" position, or with lying down prone or on the side. The "triggering" location is usually consistent for an individual child. Accompanying features often include a "glassy"-eyed appearance or "faraway look," facial flushing or redness, heavy breathing, and/or grunting. The movements may go on for several minutes to hours a day. Parents report that they can interrupt the movements if they pick up or distract the child, but placing the child back in the preferred position for self-stimulation often results in resumption of the movements. Parents are often quite concerned that their child is in pain, but typically report that interrupting the child results in protestations and crying. It is important to exclude any features suggestive of seizure, such as a postictal period. If there is any uncertainty, obtaining a prolonged video-EEG that captures the movements is helpful to exclude an underlying seizure, and reassure both the clinician and parents. The neurologic examination should be normal, and any abnormalities should prompt a referral to a neurologist. In addition to seizures, the differential diagnosis includes dystonia, but the differentiating feature on history is that dystonia typically occurs with action such as walking, running, or crawling, and not in a particular environmental location or body position. Urinary tract infections should also be excluded because this may trigger or increase the behavior, especially if a previously continent child is now having urinary accidents.

Parents should be reassured that this is a normal *voluntary* human behavior, not a movement disorder, and that there is nothing wrong with the child. There are no medications to treat or prevent it. If the child engages in this behavior in a setting that is socially unacceptable, parents should distract the young child, and for older children, limit the environmental location where this behavior is allowed (e.g., to their bedroom). For parents who are very bothered by the behavior, providing a reward system to eliminate the unwanted behavior often works better than punitive measures. For example, they could put a sticker on the calendar for every day the child does not self-stimulate in public with a special treat, such as a trip to the zoo, for an agreed-on number of accumulated stickers. Children should not be shamed for engaging in self-stimulatory behavior because they do not understand the moral or religious implications of it, and long-term shaming can have a negative impact on self-image and future sexuality. Reassurance of the parents and encouraging them to manage it with positive reinforcement as for any other unwanted behavior usually has the best outcome. Many children do not actually "outgrow" the behavior but learn to limit it to an acceptable location.

Stereotypies

Stereotypies are commonly seen in children of normal intelligence, as well as children with autistic spectrum disorders and mental retardation. The typical history includes repetitive highly stereotyped movement (or collection of movements), typically involving the hands and arms that are made voluntarily by the child when they are excited, bored, upset, or engaged in imaginative play. The movements are typically bilaterally symmetric and involve extension and stiffening, or flexion toward the midline of the arms, often with twiddling or clenching of the fingers, or rotary movements of the wrists and occasionally ankles. Drawing up toward the chest or face is highly characteristic. Other types of stereotypies include hand flapping, foot peddling, spinning, rocking, and pressing down on surfaces. These movements typically start before 3 years old, often before 18 months, and do not change bodily location over time, or wax and wane in severity. Parents can usually demonstrate exactly what the movements look like. Older children do not describe a preceding urge (as opposed to tics) and explain that it is something they do because it feels good. Children may engage in these behaviors for hours on end but are easily interrupted once parents get their attention. Children will often stop what they are doing, perform the stereotypy, and then resume their previous activities. It is never superimposed on purposeful movements, such as would be expected with chorea or dystonia. Often, children are not even aware that they are making the movements. Parents may become concerned about them because others have raised the possibility of an autism spectrum diagnosis or because they are concerned that they are socially embarrassing. If the child has no other features consistent with autism, and a normal neurologic examination, parents should be reassured that this is common and does not indicate an underlying neurologic disorder. It is essentially an excessive habit or mannerism. It does not develop into anything else, and as the child gets negative attention for it by parents or peers, he often becomes aware of the behavior and either stops it altogether or performs it in a more subtle, socially acceptable way. It may persist into adulthood. There are no medications to treat it, and parents should manage it as any other unwanted behavior (for suggestions, see Self-Stimulatory Behavior section).

References

Demiroren K, Yavuz H, Cam L, et al. Sydenham's chorea: a clinical follow-up of 65 patients. J Child Neurol 2007;22:550–4.

Fahn S, Jankovic J. Principles and practice of movement disorders. Philadelphia: Churchill, Livingstone, Elsevier; 2007.

Fenichel GM. "Ataxia" in clinical pediatric neurology: a signs and symptoms approach. 4th ed. Philadelphia: WB Saunders Company; 2001. p. 223–42.

Fernandez-Alvarez E, Aicardi J. Movement disorders in children. London: Mac Keith Press; 2001.

Kirsch DB, Mink JW. Psychogenic movement disorders in children. Pediatr Neurol 2004;30:1–6.

Maricich SM, Zoghbi HY. The cerebellum and the hereditary ataxias. In: Swaiman, Ashwal, and Ferriero, editors. Pediatric neurology: principles and practice. 4th ed. St. Louis, MO: Mosby Elsevier; 2006. p. 1241–63.

Paz JA, Silva CA, Marques-Dias MJ, et al. Randomized double-blind study with prednisone in Sydenham's chorea. Pediatr Neurol 2006;34:264–9.

Rodnitzky RL. Drug-induced movement disorders in children. Semin Pediatr Neurol 2003;10:80–7.

We Move (Worldwide Education and Awareness for Movement Disorders). <www.wemove.org> [accessed April 12, 2011].

Tics and Tourette Syndrome

Abigail Collins, MD, and Paul G. Moe, MD

Tics are brief, sudden, repetitive abnormal movements (motor tics) or sounds (phonic or vocal tics) that are involuntary or semivoluntary. They mimic fragments of normal movements, sounds, or speech, and are categorized as simple or complex. Simple motor tics involve one muscle group, whereas complex motor tics involve multiple groups. Simple vocal tics are simple sounds, whereas complex vocal tics include meaningful components of speech (see Table 1 for examples). Motor tics may be further subdivided into clonic tics, which are brief jerking movements such as a quick neck movement, tonic tics, which are isometric contractions of a muscle group such as abdominal tensing, or dystonic tics, which are abnormal postures such as sustained eye closure. Many neurologists consider simple vocal tics not involving the vocal cords (such as sniffing or coughing) to be simple motor tics, and importantly, they often respond to medications that complex vocal tics do not. Motor tics almost always start in the head and neck, and may later involve other body parts including the abdomen or extremities with a rostral to caudal progression. Vocal tics typically begin as simple sounds and may later progress to complex vocal tics, and usually have a later onset than motor tics.

A. History and Physical Examination: Interestingly, tics may start as a purposeful movement or sound, such as sniffing with allergies, which then develops into a tic even once the underlying symptoms have resolved. Commonly, children will have been evaluated by an otolaryngologist, allergist, or pulmonologist for frequent eye blinking, sniffing, or coughing before the possibility of a tic diagnosis is raised. Tics may start suddenly after an intercurrent illness or with initiation of stimulants for treatment of attentional disorders. This does not mean that the illness (such as a streptococcal infection) or medication caused the tics, but rather that the underlying predisposition to development of tics was unmasked by the illness or medication. In this situation, tics continue once the illness resolves or medication is withdrawn.

Tics wax and wane in severity, and change body location over time. They are preceded by abnormal sensations such as tightness, tension, dryness, or burning, called a sensory "urge," in about 80% of patients. Not every tic is associated with an urge, even in patients who report sensory urges, and young children may not be able to clearly describe the urge. Performance of the tic provides relief from the sensory urge, albeit a temporary one. The urge then builds again until the tic is performed, and this cycle of urge-tic-relief repeats itself over and over, often in bouts. Tics are suppressible for a period ranging from seconds to hours. Suppression typically occurs during school or in the doctor's office, and the tics are often much worse at home. During a period of suppression, the sensory urge continues to build, leading to an exaggerated release of tics once they are no longer suppressed. Parents and teachers may mistake suppression with voluntary control over tics. Tics are increased by anxiety, stress, fatigue, or relaxation after an active period (such as while watching TV at home after school), or with discussion about the tics. Tics can occur during sleep. They tend to be decreased by distraction (especially concentration), or with performing purposeful movements involving the body part affected by tics, which is helpful in making the diagnosis in the examination. See Table 2 for key historical features of tics.

Motor tics typically start between the ages of 3 and 8, with 96% of patients having onset by age 11, although earlier or later onset does occur. Vocal tics tend to develop 1 to 2 years after the onset of motor tics, but not every child with motor tics will develop of vocal tics. It is unusual for a child to have vocal tics without a preceding history of motor tics. Tics can be thought of as occurring on a spectrum of severity ranging from simple, transient tics that may not even come to medical attention to Tourette syndrome with coprolalia. Up to 25% of kindergarten-age children have simple and transient motor tics, but only about 1% of the population develop Tourette syndrome with persistent chronic motor and vocal tics (specific diagnostic criteria outlined in Table 3). Of those patients with Tourette syndrome, less than 10% have coprolalia. It is not possible to predict which children will progress from transient motor tics to development of the full symptom complex of Tourette syndrome, but males are three to five times more likely to have Tourette syndrome than females. Tics tend to peak in severity at ages 3 to 5, and again at 10 to 12 years of age. By early adulthood, about one third of children with chronic tics disorders will have complete remission of tics, one third will have persistence of mild tics, typically motor, and one third will continue to have severe tics requiring treatment. Factors that may be associated with persistence of tics into adulthood include lower extremity involvement, coprolalia, a high number of tics at one time, or comorbid attention-deficit/hyperactivity disorder (ADHD). Medication treatment does not influence the outcome of tics or Tourette syndrome.

There is often a family history of tics, Tourette syndrome, attentional disorders, or obsessive-compulsive disorder (OCD) in the extended family members of the patient with tics or Tourette syndrome. Parents may not be aware that they had tics in childhood unless they ask their parents, and simple motor tics may be present in parents without recognition that they are tics. Asking about a family history of tics using specific examples of what tics are (sniffing, coughing, eye blinking, etc.) is

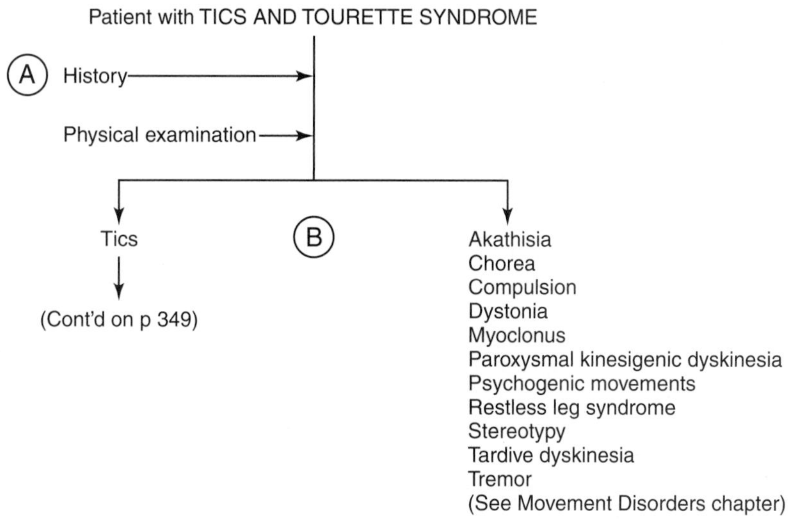
Patient with TICS AND TOURETTE SYNDROME
A
History
Physical examination
Tics
B
(Cont'd on p 349)
Akathisia
Chorea
Compulsion
Dystonia
Myoclonus
Paroxysmal kinesigenic dyskinesia
Psychogenic movements
Restless leg syndrome
Stereotypy
Tardive dyskinesia
Tremor
(See Movement Disorders chapter)

important to obtain an accurate history. It may also be helpful to watch the parents during the course of the interview to see whether they have any tics.

B. The neurologic examination should be normal in a child with a tic disorder, apart from the presence of tics. A useful feature of tics that can be helpful when trying to determine whether an abnormal movement is a tic on examination is the reduction of tics with purposeful movements of the involved body part and/or distraction (concentration). This examination feature is shared with tardive dyskinesia; however, other abnormal movements in the differential diagnosis of tics, such as chorea, dystonia, paroxysmal kinesigenic dyskinesia, psychogenic movement disorders, or myoclonus are often worsened with volitional movement (Table 4). Stereotypies have key historical differences in that they are highly stereotyped movements typically involving both hands (flapping, twisting, twiddling, or postures) that do not change up over time and usually start before the age of 3. With akathisia, there is an intense urge to move that typically manifests as pacing, rubbing the legs, and rocking. Patients are able to sit still, but it is extremely uncomfortable to do so. Restless leg syndrome tends to occur in the evening, with an uncomfortable feeling in the legs when recumbent that is relieved by standing up or walking around. See the Movement Disorders chapter for more information about these disorders. Workup for a diagnosis of tics is not indicated if the history is classic and the examination is normal. Neurologic abnormalities or an atypical history should prompt a laboratory, imaging, and/or electrographic evaluation and should suggest alternative underlying causative factors or diagnoses of the abnormal movements.

Tic disorders and Tourette syndrome are a clinical diagnosis, and there are no laboratory, imaging, or electrographic tests to confirm it. Diagnostic criteria for tic disorders are outlined by the DSM-IV-TR (see Table 3) and more stringently by the Tourette's Syndrome Classification Study Group. In addition to the criteria outlined by the DSM, the Study Group requires a changing anatomic location, frequency, type, number, complexity, or severity of tics over time; the tics must be witnessed directly by the examiner or recorded on video; and they must have onset before the age of 21.

Table 1. **Examples of Motor and Vocal Tics**

Simple Motor Tics	**Complex Motor Tics**
Eye blinking	Burping
Eye deviation	Head shaking
Eye closure	Finger drumming
Jaw opening or thrusting	Hitting
Nose wrinkling	Jumping
Facial grimacing	Twirling
Neck jerking	Smelling objects
Extremity jerking or snapping	Throwing
Trunk jerk	Bending
Abdominal tensing	Copropraxia (obscene gestures)
	Echopraxia (imitating another's gestures)
	Holding unusual postures
Simple Vocal Tics	***Complex Vocal Tics***
Sniffing	Repeated sounds
Grunting	Single words or phrases
Barking	Meaningless changes in pitch, volume, or emphasis of speech
Huffing	Speech blocking (stuttering or other interruption of fluency of speech)
Throat clearing	Palilalia (repeating one's own words or sounds)
Coughing	Echolalia (repeating the last heard word, sound, or phrase)
Snorting	Coprolalia (socially unacceptable obscenities or slurs)
Squealing	
Chirping	
Clicking	
Sucking or screaming sounds	

Table 2. **Key Historical Features of Tics**

Waxing and waning severity
Onset in head and neck region
Changing location over time
Sensory urge
Relief of urge with performance of tic
Increase tics with anxiety, fatigue, excitement, or relaxation
Decrease tics with distraction (concentration) or purposeful movement

C. Comorbidities are common in children with tics or Tourette syndrome, occurring in about 90% of patients with Tourette syndrome (Table 5). More than 50% of patients with Tourette syndrome have ADHD, whereas 20% to 60% have OCD. Children with ADHD have an enduring pattern of inattentive and/or hyperactive and impulsive behavior with onset before the age of 7, often before the emergence of tics. The behaviors cause significant impairment at home, with peers, and in academic settings. Obsessions are recurrent, intrusive, unwanted thoughts that are difficult to dislodge, whereas compulsions are meaningless, irrational, repetitive behaviors or rituals that one feels compelled to perform to ward off negative consequences (as opposed to tics, in which behaviors are made to obtain relief from the sensory urge). Although many children with chronic tics or Tourette syndrome have obsessive thoughts and compulsive behaviors, the diagnosis of OCD can only be made if the obsessions or compulsions occupy at least 1 hour of the day and interfere with daily living. The onset of OCD is typically 1 to 2 years after the onset of motor tics. Anxiety and depression are also common, as are learning problems. Comorbidities must be evaluated in every patient with tics or Tourette syndrome because they affect self-esteem, academic performance, and the approach to treatment of tics.

It is not known what causes tics or Tourette syndrome. The current model of pathophysiology for tics suggests an inherited developmental disorder of neurotransmission. Nerve cells in different areas of the brain communicate with each other using circuits linking the basal ganglia, prefrontal cortex, other cortical regions, and the thalamus. These circuits both use and are regulated by neurotransmitters, including dopamine. One primary role of the circuit is to filter information to refine responses of the brain, such as movement, thoughts, and behaviors. With Tourette syndrome and its comorbidities, information that should be filtered out is instead transmitted because of faulty dopamine regulation at critical checkpoints in the circuit. This results in disinhibition of thoughts, sensory experiences, organization of intellectual processes, and behavior, producing the phenomena of tics, obsessive thoughts and compulsions, and impulsive behaviors. The failure, then, is of filtering out unwanted or excessive signals.

(Continued on page 350)

Table 3. ***Diagnostic and Statistical Manual of Mental Disorders,* Fourth Edition, Text Revision (DSM-IV-TR) Diagnostic Criteria for Tic Disorders**

Transient Tic Disorder	Chronic Tic Disorder	Tourette Syndrome
Onset before 18 years	Onset before 18 years	Onset before 18 years
Single or multiple motor *and/or* vocal tics	Multiple motor *or* vocal tics	Multiple motor *and* vocal tics, although need not be simultaneously present
Tics occur many times a day, nearly every day for *at least 4 weeks, but not more than 12 consecutive months*	Tics occur many times a day, nearly every day for *longer than 1 year, with no more than three consecutive tic-free months* during that period	Tics occur many times a day, nearly every day for *longer than 1 year, with no more than three consecutive tic-free months* during that period
Not caused by the effect of a substance (e.g., stimulants) or general medical condition (such as Huntington disease)	Not caused by the effect of a substance (e.g., stimulants) or general medical condition (such as Huntington disease)	Not caused by the effect of a substance (e.g., stimulants) or general medical condition (such as Huntington disease)
Does not fulfill criteria for chronic tic disorder or Tourette syndrome	Does not fulfill criteria for Tourette syndrome	

Table 4. **Differential Diagnosis of Tics**

Akathisia
Chorea
Compulsions
Dystonia
Myoclonus
Paroxysmal kinesigenic dyskinesia
Psychogenic movements
Restless leg syndrome
Stereotypies
Tardive dyskinesia

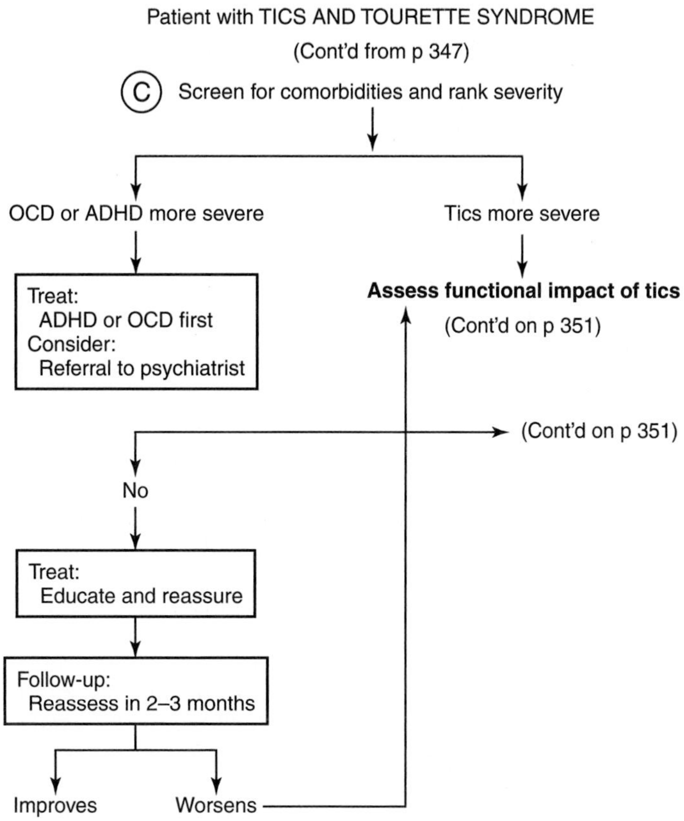
Patient with TICS AND TOURETTE SYNDROME
(Cont'd from p 347)
C
Screen for comorbidities and rank severity
OCD or ADHD more severe
Tics more severe
Treat:
ADHD or OCD first
Consider:
Referral to psychiatrist
Assess functional impact of tics
(Cont'd on p 351)
(Cont'd on p 351)
No
Treat:
Educate and reassure
Follow-up:
Reassess in 2–3 months
Improves
Worsens

Table 5. **Comorbidities of Tics and Tourette Syndrome**

ADD or ADHD	Hyperactivity Impulsiveness Inattention
OCD	Obsessions: • Unfounded fears • Excessive worries • A need for exactness, symmetry, evenness, neatness • Excessive religious thoughts • Perverse sexual thoughts • Intrusions of words, phrases, or music Compulsions: • Checking • Counting • Cleaning • Washing • Touching • Smelling • Hoarding • Rearranging
Learning disorders	Math Written language
Mood disorders	Anxiety Depression
Sleep disorders	
Executive dysfunction	
Self-injurious behavior	
Oppositional defiant disorder	
Personality disorders	

ADD, attention-deficit disorder; *ADHD,* attention-deficit/hyperactivity disorder; *OCD,* obsessive-compulsive disorder.

D. The decision to treat tics should be based on whether the tics are causing academic or social impairment, and not simply because they are present. Often, educating the family and teachers that the movements are tics, explaining that the child does not have complete control over them, and that the best approach is not to call attention to them is sufficient at first diagnosis. The child can explain that it is a "habit" or "just something I do" when other children ask what the movements are. When a child is impaired, determining whether the tics themselves or whether other comorbidities are causing the problem is vital to target the treatment appropriately. For example, if a 5-year-old is having frequent tics but is not paying attention in class because of comorbid ADHD, the attention problem should be addressed first. Asking the parents and patient to rank the problems in order of severity is helpful in designing your treatment plan. Children with significant comorbidities should be evaluated by a psychiatrist and/or neuropsychologist to address these issues appropriately.

Tics should be treated when a child is having a lot of difficulty with teasing from peers; when the child is spending a great deal of effort suppressing them in school and consequently not paying attention to the teacher, producing a reduction of grades or scores; or when the tics have the potential to cause self-injury, such as a violent neck flinging tic. Nonmedication approaches to treatment include brief "tic breaks" during the day if needed so that the child can release the tics in a private place. Home should be a safe place for the child to tic and parents should be counseled not to focus attention on their child's tics. Emotional support should be provided for the child and family members dealing with tics and Tourette syndrome, and a support group such as the local chapter of the Tourette's Syndrome Association or Internet-based group for families in rural areas may be beneficial. Cognitive-behavioral therapy or stress-reduction techniques for children in whom stress or anxiety significantly aggravates the tics may be useful (see Table 6 and the algorithm).

If these measures are not sufficient, the tics are severe, or continue to cause a functional impairment, it is appropriate to use medications. Setting realistic expectations for the benefit that medications can provide is important for both the child and parent to understand before embarking on medication management. Medications typically produce a 25% to 50% reduction in tics, and at best 90% reduction, but the response to any tic medication is variable from individual to individual. Medication choice is based on the severity and type of tics, the likelihood of a medication to reduce tics, common adverse effects, and potential for serious or possibly irreversible side effects. For this reason, we recommend a tiered approach to the medications used to treat tics, starting with medications that may not be as effective for reducing tics but have few serious adverse effects, and reserving dopamine-receptor blocking medications as a last resort when other medications have failed (see Table 7 and the algorithm). The general treatment strategy is to titrate one medication up slowly to a dose that provides sufficient reduction in tics, adverse effects, or no benefit at a maximal recommended dose. Ineffective or intolerable medications should be discontinued over 1 to 2 weeks (unless there are serious adverse effects, in which case they may be discontinued more quickly) while a new medication is gradually introduced. Given that there is no way to predict an individual's response to tic medications, trials of multiple medications in the Tier 2 category should be considered before using Tier 3 category medications. Rarely, a patient may need to be on multiple medications to provide sufficient tic control. If a child has been tic-free or had good control of tics for about 3 to 6 months, especially in late adolescence, it may be appropriate to taper off medication to determine whether it is still needed. The best time to do this is during a prolonged school break (such as summer) so that any recurrence of tics will not have academic consequences. Botulinum toxin injections may be helpful for reducing the sensory urge of specific chronic tics, such as eye blinking or shoulder shrugging. Deep brain stimulation surgery, although potentially beneficial for the treatment of severe, refractory tic disorders, should be considered only after the age of 25 because of the high potential for tic remission in the third decade of life, and the significant, potentially irreversible risks this procedure entails, including stroke, hemorrhage, and death. Ideally, a neurologist experienced at treating movement disorders should be involved in care when Tier 3 medications, deep brain stimulation surgery, or botulinum toxin injections are being considered.

(Continued on page 353)

Table 6. **Nonmedication Approaches to Tic Treatment**

Educate patient, family, school teachers and coaches
Tic breaks
Habit reversal training
Stress reduction techniques:
- Self-hypnosis
- Progressive relaxation
- Measured breathing
- Visualization

Vitamin supplements:
- Magnesium
- Riboflavin
- Coenzyme Q10

Patient with TICS AND TOURETTE SYNDROME

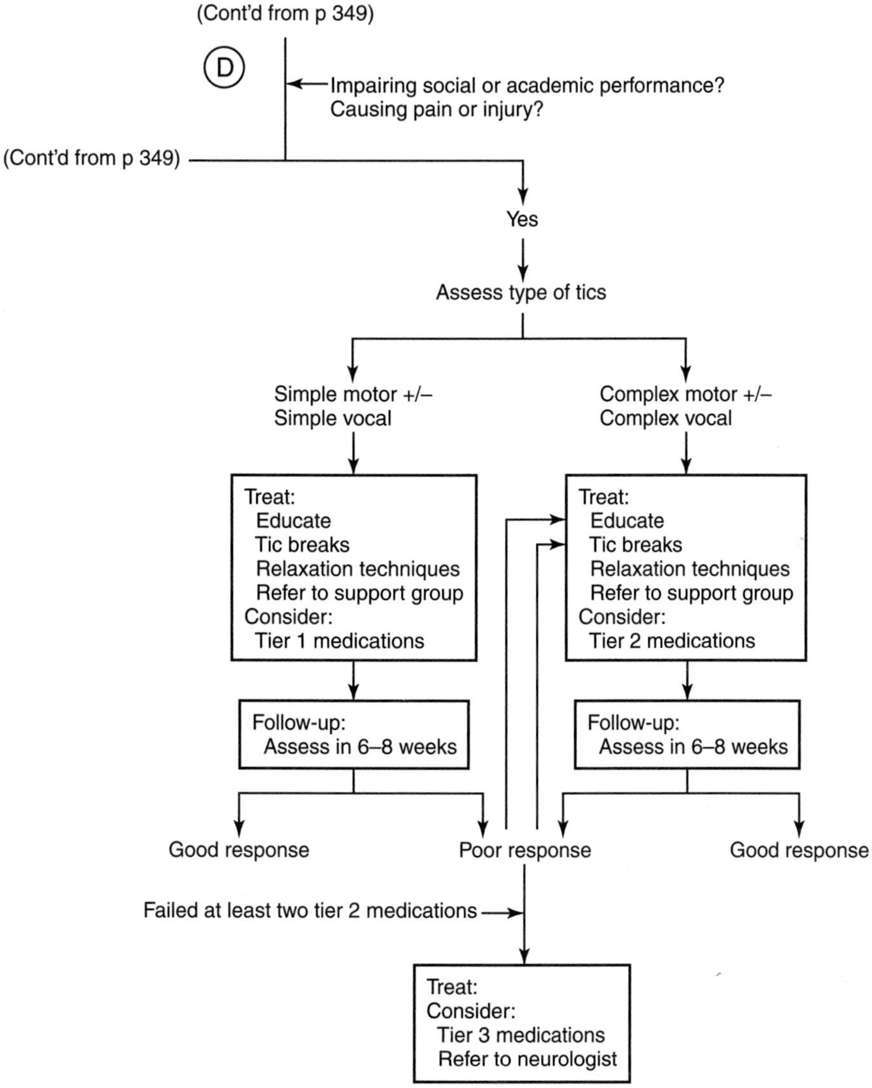
(Cont'd from p 349)
D
Impairing social or academic performance?
Causing pain or injury?
(Cont'd from p 349)
Yes
Assess type of tics
Simple motor +/–
Simple vocal
Complex motor +/–
Complex vocal
Treat:
Educate
Tic breaks
Relaxation techniques
Refer to support group
Consider:
Tier 1 medications
Treat:
Educate
Tic breaks
Relaxation techniques
Refer to support group
Consider:
Tier 2 medications
Follow-up:
Assess in 6–8 weeks
Follow-up:
Assess in 6–8 weeks
Good response
Poor response
Good response
Failed at least two tier 2 medications
Treat:
Consider:
Tier 3 medications
Refer to neurologist

Table 7. **Medications for Treatment of Tics**

Medication	Starting Dose	Titration Schedule	Goal and Maximum Doses	Adverse Effects	Comments
Tier 1: α_2-Adrenergic Agonists					
Clonidine, 0.1-mg tablets	0.05 mg at bedtime	Increase by 0.05 mg every 3–7 days	Goal: 0.05 mg in morning, 0.05 mg midday, and 0.1 mg at bedtime Maximum: 0.4 mg/day	Sleepiness, light-headedness, irritability, ataxia	• May benefit ADHD, aggression, and insomnia • May be used with stimulants Also comes in patch formulation
Guanfacine, 1-mg tablets	0.5 mg at bedtime	Increase by 0.5 mg every 3–7 days	Goal: 1 mg twice per day Maximum: 2 mg twice per day	Sleepiness, light-headedness, irritability	• May benefit ADHD, aggression, and insomnia • May have less irritability than clonidine
Tier 2: Benzodiazepines, Antiepileptics, Dopamine Agonists, Muscle Relaxants, SSRIs, and Selective Norepinephrine Reuptake Inhibitors					
Clonazepam	0.25 mg at bedtime	Increase by 0.25 mg every 3–7 days	Goal: 0.5 mg three times per day Maximum: 2 mg three times per day	Sleepiness, irritability	• Sleepiness usually resolves after 2 weeks • Do not stop abruptly or may result in withdrawal seizures
Levetiracetam	10–20 mg/kg/day divided three times per day	Increase by 10 mg/kg/day every 3–7 days	Goal: 30–50 mg/kg/day divided three times per day Maximum: 100 mg/kg/day divided three times per day	Sleepiness, irritability, hyperkinesis	• Does not have cognitive slowing • Weight neutral • Irritability may improve over time or with addition of 50–100 mg B_6 per day
Topiramate	25 mg at bedtime	Increase by 25 mg every 3–7 days	Goal: 50 mg two times per day Maximum: 100 mg two times per day	Insomnia, cognitive slowing, anorexia	• Can help with migraine prevention • May be useful if bipolar present
Ropinirole	0.25 mg at bedtime	Increase by 0.25 mg every 2 weeks	Goal: 0.5 mg two times per day Maximum: 12 mg twice per day	Nausea, sleepiness, compulsions, light-headedness, peripheral edema	• May cause sudden sleep attacks • Must monitor for compulsive eating, spending, organizing, sexual behaviors, gambling • May help with comorbid restless leg syndrome
Baclofen	5 mg at bedtime	Increase by 5 mg every 3–7 days	Goal: 10–20 mg three times per day Maximum: 40 mg three times per day	Sleepiness	• May help with comorbid spasticity • May increase underlying weakness if present
Sertraline	25 mg at bedtime	Increase by 25 mg every 1–2 weeks	Goal: 50–150 mg/day Maximum: 200 mg/day	Suicidality, mania, insomnia, stomach upset, dizziness, tremor, headache, anxiety	• Useful if significant anxiety or OCD
Fluoxetine	10 mg at bedtime	Increase by 10 mg every 1–2 weeks	Goal: 40–60 mg/day Maximum: 80 mg/day	Suicidality, mania, insomnia, stomach upset, dizziness, tremor, headache, anxiety	• Useful if significant anxiety or OCD
Atomoxetine	0.5 mg/kg at breakfast	Increase to goal after minimum of 3 days	Goal: 1.2 mg/kg/day Maximum: 1.8 mg/kg/day or 100 mg/day, whichever is lower	Weight loss, sedation, insomnia, nervousness, anxiety, depression, suicidality, mania, sudden cardiac death	• May be used if ADHD also present • May give at bedtime if sedation occurs • Divide twice daily if nausea occurs

Table 7. **Medications for Treatment of Tics—cont'd**

Medication	Starting Dose	Titration Schedule	Goal and Maximum Doses	Adverse Effects	Comments
Tier 3: Dopamine Reuptake Inhibitors and Dopamine-Receptor Blockers					
Tetrabenazine	12.5 mg at bedtime	Increase by 12.5 mg weekly	Goal: 25 mg three times per day Max: 50 mg three times per day	Sedation, anxiety, akathisia, weight gain, depression, psychosis, suicidality, acute dystonic reaction, parkinsonism	• NO RISK for tardive dyskinesia • If any depression, should have close monitoring in conjunction with a psychiatrist
Risperidone	0.25–0.5 mg at bedtime	Increase by 0.5 mg every 1–2 weeks	Goal: 1 mg two times per day Maximum: 4 mg/day	Weight gain, insomnia or sedation, anxiety, headache, parkinsonism, gynecomastia, acute dystonic reaction, tardive dyskinesia	• May prolong QTc
Olanzapine	1.25 mg at bedtime	Increase by 1.25 mg every 1–2 weeks	Goal: 2.5 mg two times per day Maximum: 5 mg twice per day	Weight gain, sedation, orthostatic hypotension, edema, GI upset, gynecomastia, parkinsonism, acute dystonic reaction, tardive dyskinesia	• May prolong QTc
Ziprasidone	20 mg at bedtime	Increase by 20 mg every 1–2 weeks	Goal: 40 mg/day Maximum: 80 mg/day	Sedation, weight gain, anxiety, depression, parkinsonism, acute dystonic reaction, tardive dyskinesia	• May prolong QTc
Haloperidol	0.25–0.5 mg at bedtime	Increase by 0.25–0.5 mg every 5–7 days	Goal: 0.05–0.075 mg/kg/day in 2–3 divided doses Maximum: 0.15 mg/kg/day	Weight gain and bulimia, sedation, anxiety, depression, dysphoria, parkinsonism, intellectual impairment, school and social phobia, tardive dyskinesia	• May prolong QTc • May also cause acute dystonic reaction • High risk for extrapyramidal symptoms • Very effective for reducing tics
Pimozide	0.25–0.5 mg at bedtime	Increase by 0.5 mg every 1–2 weeks	Goal: 1 mg two times per day Maximum: 5 mg two times per day	Weight gain, sedation, anxiety, depression, parkinsonism, tardive dyskinesia	• May also cause acute dystonic reaction • Can cause fatal arrhythmias because of prolonged QTc, especially when combined with some OTC medications • Very effective for reducing tics

ADHD, attention-deficit/hyperactivity disorder; *GI,* gastrointestinal; *OCD,* obsessive-compulsive disorder; *OTC,* over-the-counter; *QTc;* corrected *QT* interval; *SSRI,* selective serotonin reuptake inhibitor.

References

Coffey BJ, Biederman J, Geller DA, et al. The course of Tourette's disorder: a literature review. Harvard Rev Psychiatry 2000;8:192–8.

Gilbert D. Treatment of children and adolescents with tics and Tourette syndrome. J Child Neurol 2006;21:690–700.

Jankovic J. Tourette's syndrome. N Engl J Med 2001;345(16):1184–92.

Jimenez-Jimenez FJ, Garcia-Ruiz PJ. Pharmacological options for the treatment of Tourette's disorder. Drugs 2001;61(15):2207–20.

Kenney C, Kuo SH, Jimenez-Shahed J. Tourette's syndrome. Am Fam Physician 2008;77(5):651–8.

Leckman JF, Bloch MH, Scahill L, King RA. Tourette syndrome: the self under siege. J Child Neurol 2006;21:642–9.

Mink JW, Walkup J, Frey KA, et al. Patient selection and assessment recommendations for deep brain stimulation in Tourette syndrome. Mov Disord 2006;21(11):1831–8.

Swain JE, Scahill L, Lombroso PJ, et al. Tourette syndrome and tic disorders: a decade of progress. J Am Acad Child Adolesc Psychiatry 2007;46(8):947–68.

Zinner SH. Tourette syndrome—much more than tics. Moving beyond misconceptions to diagnosis. Contemp Pediatr 2004;21(8):22–36.

Zinner SH. Tourette syndrome—much more than tics. Management tailored to the entire patient. Contemp Pediatr 2004;21(8):38–49.

Seizure Disorders: Febrile

Daniel Arndt, MD, MA, Paul Levisohn, MD, and Stephen Berman, MD

A febrile seizure is defined as a seizure associated with a febrile illness without a central nervous system infection or other cause (such as electrolyte imbalance) in a child not known to have epilepsy. Simple febrile seizures are solitary, brief (several minutes in length at most), and generalized. In contrast, complex febrile seizures are prolonged (>15 minutes), occur multiple times during the same day, or are focal. Although a prolonged febrile seizure does not increase the risk for recurrence, the likelihood of another prolonged seizure is greater if there is a recurrence. Febrile seizures represent the most common type of childhood seizures, occurring in 2% to 5% of children younger than 5 years in Western Europe and North America. Approximately one third of children who have febrile seizures will experience recurrent episodes. Younger age (<18 months old), family history of febrile seizures, low peak temperature, and shorter duration of fever are associated with increased risk for recurrent febrile seizures. Risk factors for subsequent epilepsy include neurodevelopmental abnormality, complex febrile seizure, family history of epilepsy, and shorter duration of fever. The recurrence of episodes of febrile seizures in a child does not increase the risk for subsequent epilepsy. Whereas febrile seizures are a common problem, children with uncomplicated febrile seizures carry a low risk for subsequent epilepsy.

A. Focus the initial history on the nature of the seizure. Was it generalized or focal at onset? What was its length? Differentiate between the seizure itself and the postictal state. What was the child's condition immediately after the seizure? Lateralized weakness, difficulties with speech, and other localizing signs indicate a complex seizure, not a simple febrile seizure. Is there a history of prior seizures with fever? Without fever? Did more than one seizure occur in 24 hours?

Second, determine the nature of the illness and the relation of the seizure to the illness. Was the temperature elevated before the seizure, and if so, for how long? Often, the parents' first awareness of the illness is the occurrence of a seizure. Determine whether there is evidence of possible central nervous system infection (meningitis or encephalitis) suggested by altered mental status, severe headache, or focal neurologic signs before the seizure. Was there evidence of acute increase in intracranial pressure? What treatment, if any, has the child received for the illness, and could the seizure be caused by inappropriate use of over-the-counter medications? Ask about a family history of epilepsy or neurodevelopmental abnormalities in the child. Immediate, appropriate telephone communication can often prevent the 911 call and ambulance dispatch for an emergency department service, neither of which is necessary for a simple febrile seizure.

B. In the physical examination, identify the source of fever. Assess children for the symptoms and signs of meningitis (see p. 638). Consideration of meningitis remains key (missed meningitis not only may be devastating but remains a continual source of malpractice litigation). Although bacterial meningitis is present in only a small minority (2%–5%) of children with apparent febrile seizures, a high level of suspicion is important, especially in the young infant; meningismus is absent in about one third of infants with meningitis. Does the child complain of significant headache or is there persistence of altered mental status subsequent to the seizure? Are there signs of increased intracranial pressure, such as abnormal eye movements (e.g., "setting sun" sign), excessive vomiting, unstable vital signs, or even papilledema? Identification of a source of infection, although reassuring, does not eliminate concurrent central nervous system infection. For example, an intracranial abscess may be secondary to sinusitis. Other common sites of infection include ears, urinary tract, lungs, and less commonly, gastrointestinal tract and blood. Note any signs suggestive of child abuse and shaken baby syndrome. Perform a careful neurologic examination (see p. 306) to identify focal neurologic signs and seizures caused by acute intracranial disease.

C. Laboratory studies are of limited usefulness in the child with simple febrile seizures and should focus on determining the source of fever (see p. 178). Consider a blood culture, urine culture, and occasionally stool culture (for *Shigella/Salmonella*). For patients with complex seizures, obtain a complete blood cell count (CBC), electrolyte values, blood urea nitrogen (BUN) and creatinine concentrations (especially if gastroenteritis is present), and urinalysis. Calcium, phosphorus, and magnesium concentrations are rarely helpful. A low threshold for lumbar puncture is appropriate, particularly in the infant younger than 12 months. Computed tomography of the brain acutely is indicated if there are neurologic abnormalities suggesting a space-occupying lesion, such as abscess or intracranial hemorrhage. Electroencephalography has little prognostic significance and is of limited utility.

(Continued on page 356)

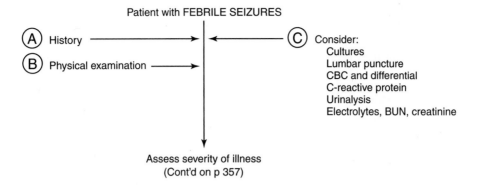

Patient with FEBRILE SEIZURES

(A) History

(B) Physical examination

(C) Consider:
- Cultures
- Lumbar puncture
- CBC and differential
- C-reactive protein
- Urinalysis
- Electrolytes, BUN, creatinine

Assess severity of illness
(Cont'd on p 357)

D. The child with simple febrile seizures rarely needs acute intervention other than treatment of the underlying illness and fever. Parents need counseling and reassurance. Many children, especially those older than 18 months, will not require an emergency department visit if the child can be seen in a timely fashion in the office to define the nature of the precipitating illness. However, ongoing seizure activity requires emergent intervention.

E. When necessary, manage febrile seizures with benzodiazepines. Manage status epilepticus as a medical emergency (see p. 370). Consider rectal diazepam in the home setting because it is rapidly absorbed and is safe and effective. Persistent alteration of mental status may require emergency department observation and subsequent hospitalization.

F. Intermittent prophylaxis with benzodiazepines, given at the time of fever, can significantly decrease the recurrence rate of febrile seizures. Two doses of oral diazepam, 0.3 to 0.5 mg/kg body weight given 8 hours apart, have been shown to decrease the risk for recurrent febrile seizures and should be considered in children with complex, frequent, or prolonged febrile seizures. Alternatively, rectal diazepam (dose, 0.2–0.5 mg/kg) may be given at the first evidence of fever. More practically, rectal diazepam can be given for prolonged seizures. Rectal diazepam gel (Diastat) provides an easy-to-use and safe method of administration. Unfortunately, antipyretic therapy given at the time of fever has not proved effective in preventing febrile seizures. Continuous prophylactic therapy for febrile seizures is generally not indicated given the benign nature of febrile seizures and the potential cognitive and systemic toxicity of the two medications—phenobarbital and valproate—proven successful in preventing recurrence.

G. Monitor for recurrences and subsequent epilepsy. Complex febrile seizures, that is, seizures that are prolonged (>15 minutes), focal, or repeated within 1 day, increase the risk for subsequent epilepsy. The presence of all three factors increases the risk for subsequent epilepsy to more than 20%.

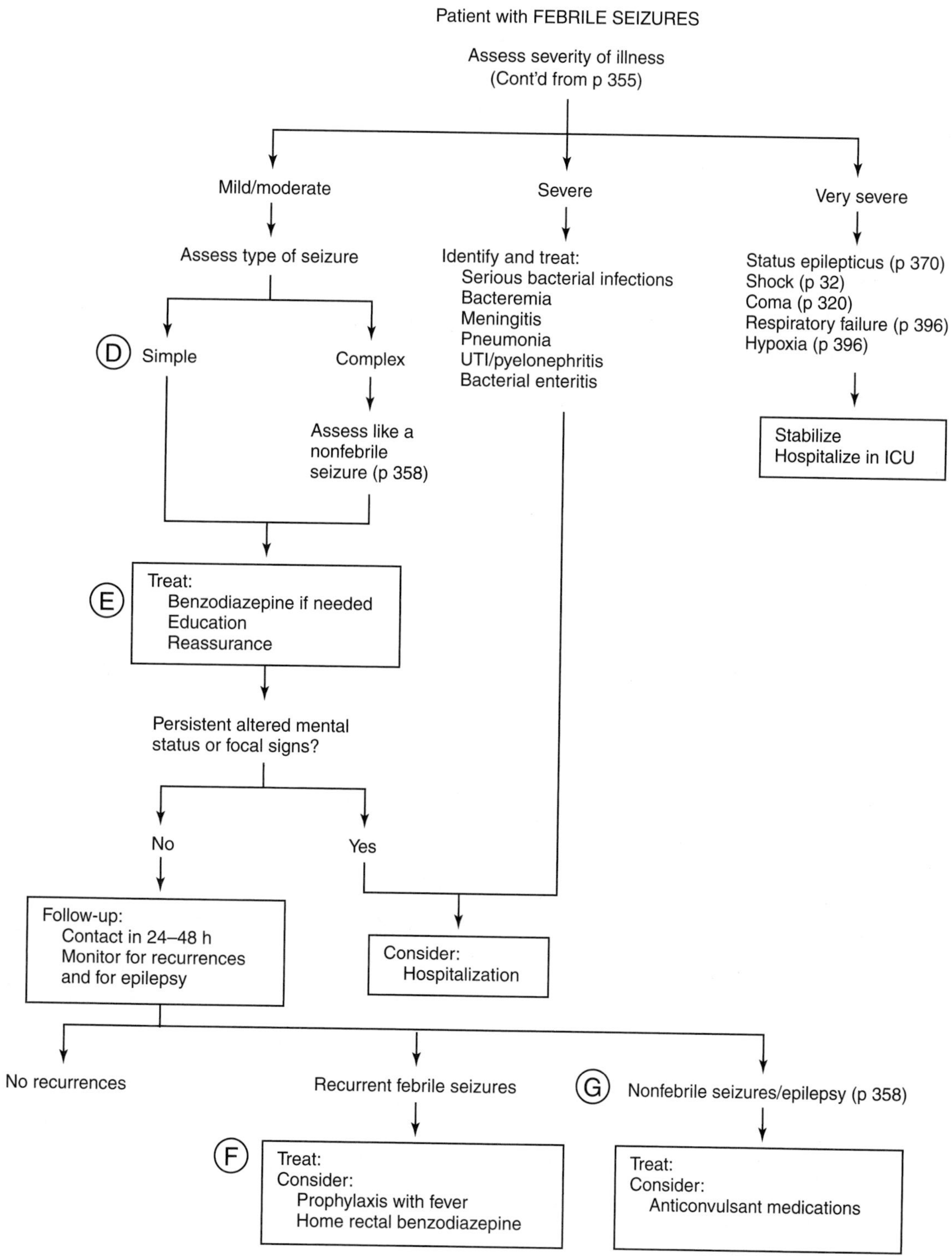
Patient with FEBRILE SEIZURES
Assess severity of illness
(Cont'd from p 355)
Mild/moderate
Severe
Very severe
Assess type of seizure
Identify and treat:
Serious bacterial infections
Bacteremia
Meningitis
Pneumonia
UTI/pyelonephritis
Bacterial enteritis
Status epilepticus (p 370)
Shock (p 32)
Coma (p 320)
Respiratory failure (p 396)
Hypoxia (p 396)
D
Simple
Complex
Assess like a nonfebrile seizure (p 358)
Stabilize
Hospitalize in ICU
E
Treat:
Benzodiazepine if needed
Education
Reassurance
Persistent altered mental status or focal signs?
No
Yes
Follow-up:
Contact in 24–48 h
Monitor for recurrences and for epilepsy
Consider:
Hospitalization
No recurrences
Recurrent febrile seizures
G
Nonfebrile seizures/epilepsy (p 358)
F
Treat:
Consider:
Prophylaxis with fever
Home rectal benzodiazepine
Treat:
Consider:
Anticonvulsant medications

References

American Academy of Pediatrics, Committee on Quality Improvement, Subcommittee on Febrile Seizures. Practice parameter: long-term treatment of the child with simple febrile seizures. Pediatrics 1999;103:1307–9.

American Academy of Pediatrics, Provisional Committee on Quality Improvement, Subcommittee on Diagnosis and Treatment of Febrile Seizures. Practice parameter: the neurodiagnostic evaluation of the child with a first simple febrile seizure. Pediatrics 1996;97:769–75.

Baram TZ, Shinnar S, editors. Febrile seizures. San Diego: Academic Press; 2001.

Berg AT, Shinnar S, Darefsky AS, et al. Predictors of recurrent febrile seizures. A prospective cohort study. Arch Pediatr Adolesc Med 1997;151:371–8.

Knudsen FU. Febrile seizures: treatment and prognosis. Epilepsia 2000;41:2–9.

Pellock JM, Bourgeois BFD, Dodson WE, et al. Pediatric epilepsy. New York: Demos Medical Publishing, LLC; 2008. p. 293–301.

Seizure Disorders: Nonfebrile

Daniel Arndt, MD, MA, Paul G. Moe, MD, Paul Levisohn, MD,
and Stephen Berman, MD

A seizure is a sudden, transient disturbance of brain function manifested by involuntary motor, sensory, autonomic, or psychic phenomena, alone or in any combination, often accompanied by alteration or loss of consciousness. Generalized seizures involve both hemispheres; 90% are convulsive (tonic, clonic, myoclonic), whereas 10% are nonconvulsive (absence, atypical absence, atonic). Focal or partial seizures involve a localized area of the brain and are classified as simple partial or complex partial seizures. Patients can rarely be in electrical status diagnosed by electroencephalography without having signs of seizures (electroclinical dissociation). Seizures are also described as symptomatic when a cause is identified or presumed, and idiopathic or unprovoked when a cause is unknown or thought to be genetic. Identifiable causes include acute events or disorders, such as fever, trauma, dehydration, and infection, as well as more chronic processes, such as tumors, metabolic disorders, and structural abnormalities. Unprovoked seizures occur commonly; every year, 25,000 to 40,000 children experience an unprovoked seizure. Whereas the child without identified risk factors for epilepsy who experiences a first unprovoked seizure has only about a 30% chance of a recurrence, a second unprovoked seizure carries a significant recurrence risk and usually heralds the diagnosis of epilepsy.

A. In the history, elicit a careful description of the seizure/event. The initial manifestations are the most important in defining the type of seizure, although observers will often focus on the more dramatic convulsive (tonic and clonic activity) aspects of the seizure. Incontinence of urine and tongue biting confirm the generalized nature of the seizure but are not necessary for the diagnosis. Note the time of day the seizure occurred and whether the child was awake, drowsy, or asleep. A school-aged child who has a partial seizure arising in sleep may have benign epilepsy of childhood with centrotemporal spikes (benign rolandic epilepsy). Ask about any behaviors before the seizure that suggest partial seizures or auras. An adolescent presenting with an early-morning tonic-clonic seizure may be able to relate a history of early-morning myoclonus (brief extension or flexion body jerks), consistent with the diagnosis of juvenile myoclonic epilepsy. Define the duration of the seizure, differentiating the seizure from postictal somnolence or agitation. Unilateral postictal weakness (Todd paresis) or difficulties with speech help establish the focal nature of the event. Ask about possible precipitating causes, including exposure to toxins or drugs. Elicit a family history of epilepsy, which suggests the diagnosis of genetic epilepsy presenting with a first seizure. Ask about any preexisting developmental or neurologic disorder.

B. When a seizure persists for more than 30 minutes, status epilepticus is present and requires immediate management (see p. 370). When a patient is seizing, immediately assess the vital signs with particular attention to adequate ventilation. Assess mental status; confusion and agitation may be noted during the postictal period. Focus on determining the potential cause of the seizure, as well as possible seizure-induced trauma. Perform a careful neurologic examination as described on page 306. Ophthalmoscopic examination may have findings that suggest an acute subdural hematoma from nonaccidental trauma. Examine the scalp carefully for evidence of head trauma. A stiff neck suggests meningitis or intracranial hemorrhage. Examination of the skin may reveal the stigmata of neurofibromatosis (café-au-lait spots), tuberous sclerosis (ash-leaf lesions), or Sturge–Weber syndrome (facial hemangioma). Postictal neurologic examination may reveal Todd paresis, helpful in defining the localized onset of the seizure. Persistent obtundation suggests the possibility of subclinical seizure activity that requires confirmation by electroencephalography. Neurologic examination may reveal persistent focal findings or evidence of a static neurologic dysfunction, such as cerebral palsy.

C. Although it is common to obtain laboratory studies, such as complete blood cell count, electrolyte values, glucose level, calcium and magnesium concentrations, and blood urea nitrogen (BUN) and creatinine concentrations, these evaluations are rarely helpful when seizures appear to be unprovoked and the patient lacks systemic signs and symptoms suggestive of an associated disorder such as uremia, meningitis, or dehydration. Younger children are more likely to have symptomatic seizures with a cause identified. Therefore, perform only those laboratory tests that are consistent with the specific clinical presentation of the patient. Consider toxicologic screening if there is concern about possible drug exposure or abuse. In the afebrile child with a first seizure, a lumbar puncture is of limited value unless other findings suggest meningitis or encephalitis. Consider metabolic studies when infants experience development of seizures and in patients with mental retardation or other neurologic findings.

D. Patients with a routine febrile seizure, absence seizure, focal seizures consistent with benign rolandic epilepsy, or a nonfebrile generalized seizure with normal examination findings rarely need a computed tomographic (CT) scan. Perform imaging studies of the child's brain when clinical symptoms or focal signs suggest an intracranial hemorrhage, increased intracranial pressure (closed-head trauma), or space-occupying lesion (focal neurologic signs or papilledema), or when there is difficulty controlling seizures, prolonged postictal

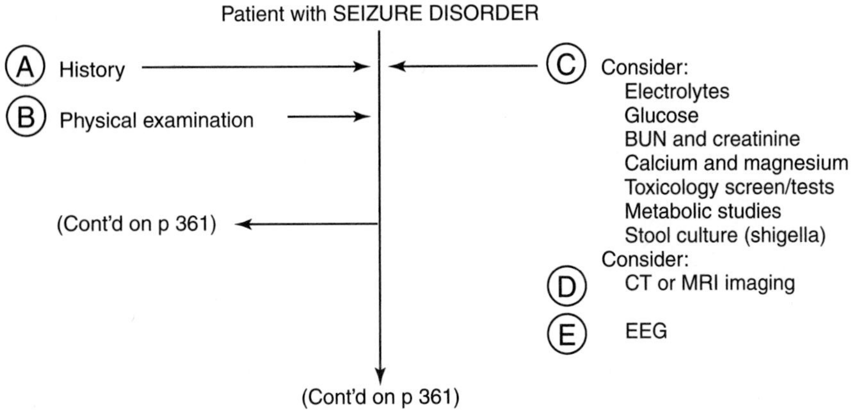
Patient with SEIZURE DISORDER
(A) History
(B) Physical examination
(C) Consider:
Electrolytes
Glucose
BUN and creatinine
Calcium and magnesium
Toxicology screen/tests
Metabolic studies
Stool culture (shigella)
Consider:
(D) CT or MRI imaging
(E) EEG
(Cont'd on p 361)
(Cont'd on p 361)

unresponsiveness, or progressing neurologic findings. CT is preferred for acute assessment of hemorrhage, edema, or other emergent mass effect, but magnetic resonance imaging (MRI) is the study of choice for evaluating seizure cause when possible and clinically feasible.

E. The clinical usefulness of electroencephalography after a first unprovoked seizure is controversial. An electroencephalogram (EEG) can help document ongoing seizure, alert the clinician to an underlying cerebral structural process, identify patients at greatest risk for recurrence, or even assist in diagnosing an epilepsy syndrome. An EEG is recommended as part of the neurodiagnostic evaluation of the child with an apparent first unprovoked seizure. However, some advocate an alternative approach of obtaining an EEG only if a second seizure occurs because a majority of children with a first seizure will not have a recurrence, and only a minority will have a diagnostic finding on electroencephalography.

F. A careful history will help differentiate seizures from other nonepileptic paroxysmal events, such as breath holding, infantile syncope, sleep disorders, tics, shuddering, benign nocturnal myoclonus, gastroesophageal reflux, conversion reaction, masturbation, temper tantrums, benign paroxysmal vertigo, and conversion reactions/pseudoseizures (Table 1).

G. Immediately treat and hospitalize children who present in status epilepticus (see p. 370). Consider hospitalization when a patient presents with two or more spontaneous seizures within a short time frame (24–48 hours), a prolonged seizure that resolved spontaneously, or prolonged altered mental status. Consider observing the child while an anticonvulsant therapy is initiated. Protect the seizing patient against self-injury and aspiration of vomitus. Avoid interventions such as inserting tongue depressors into the mouth or trying to restrain tonic-clonic movements.

H. Counseling and education are essential in the management. Most parents witnessing a first seizure in their child are extremely anxious and need reassurance, when it is appropriate, that their child is not gravely ill. In particular, the fear of the child's dying needs to be allayed. Provide education about seizure precautions for all children with a first seizure. In particular, discuss water safety and avoidance of heights (high diving and high climbing). For adolescents, discuss the need to avoid alcohol and restrictions on driving, which requires the clinician to be familiar not only with clinical risks but also with state laws. Educational information is available through the Epilepsy Foundation of America (4351 Garden City Drive, Landover, MD 20785, 800-EFA-1000).

I. Anticonvulsant therapy is not usually needed for the first unprovoked generalized seizure with normal findings on neurologic examination. When medications are necessary, the decision about the appropriate anticonvulsant depends on the seizure type, age of the patient, associated clinical factors including causal factors, and matching specific adverse effect profiles best suited for each patient. Table 2 reviews seizure types, clinical presentation, causes, electroencephalographic findings, diagnostic studies, and treatment. Table 3 provides a guide to therapy.

J. Monitor the patient carefully for response (seizure control), adverse effects, and toxicity (see Table 3). The sedation associated with many anticonvulsants can be reduced by working up to a therapeutic dose during 3 to 4 weeks. When adverse effects or drug toxicity other than serious allergic reactions become apparent in well-controlled patients, consider simply reducing the dose by 25% to 30%.

K. Factors that affect the recurrence of seizures after withdrawal of medications include: (1) the presence of associated neurologic signs/disorders and mental retardation, (2) the age at onset of the seizure disorder, (3) the electroencephalogram at the time medications are stopped, (4) the number of seizures experienced before control is achieved with medications, and (5) the type of seizures. However, treat most patients until they are free of seizures for 1 to 2 years unless the earlier listed factors preclude weaning medications.

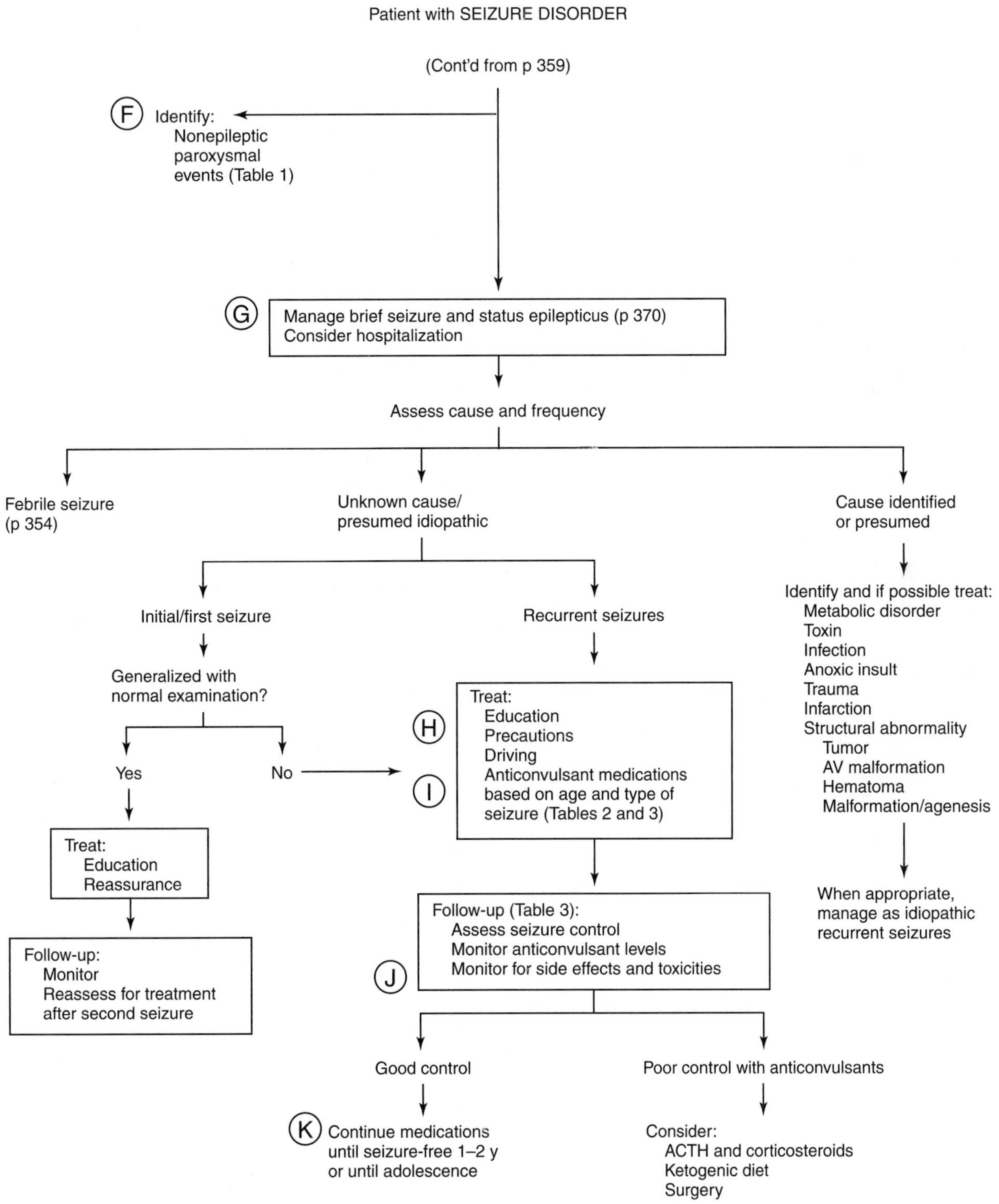

Patient with SEIZURE DISORDER
(Cont'd from p 359)
F Identify:
Nonepileptic paroxysmal events (Table 1)
G Manage brief seizure and status epilepticus (p 370)
Consider hospitalization
Assess cause and frequency
Febrile seizure (p 354)
Unknown cause/ presumed idiopathic
Cause identified or presumed
Initial/first seizure
Recurrent seizures
Generalized with normal examination?
Yes
No
Treat:
Education
Reassurance
Follow-up:
Monitor
Reassess for treatment after second seizure
H
I
Treat:
Education
Precautions
Driving
Anticonvulsant medications based on age and type of seizure (Tables 2 and 3)
J
Follow-up (Table 3):
Assess seizure control
Monitor anticonvulsant levels
Monitor for side effects and toxicities
Good control
Poor control with anticonvulsants
K Continue medications until seizure-free 1–2 y or until adolescence
Consider:
ACTH and corticosteroids
Ketogenic diet
Surgery
Identify and if possible treat:
Metabolic disorder
Toxin
Infection
Anoxic insult
Trauma
Infarction
Structural abnormality
Tumor
AV malformation
Hematoma
Malformation/agenesis
When appropriate, manage as idiopathic recurrent seizures

Table 1. **Nonepileptic Paroxysmal Events**

Breath-Holding Attacks

Age 6 months to 3 years. Always precipitated by trauma, frustration, or fright. Cyanosis; sometimes followed by stiffening, tonic (or jerking-clonic) convulsion (anoxic seizure). Patient may sleep after attack. Family history positive in 30%. Electroencephalogram (EEG) normal. Treatment is interpretation and reassurance. Consider iron deficiency screening.

Infantile Syncope (Pallid Breath Holding)

No external precipitant (perhaps internal pain, cramp, or fear). Pallor may be followed by seizure (anoxic-ischemic). Vagally (heart-slowing) mediated, like adult syncope. EEG normal; may see cardiac slowing with vagal stimulation (cold cloth on face) during EEG.

Tics or Tourette Syndrome

Simple or complex stereotyped (the same time after time) jerks or movements, coughs, grunts, sniffs. Worse at repose or with stress. May be suppressed during physician visit. Family history often positive. EEG negative. Approximately 40% incidence of comorbidities of attention-deficit disorders and/or obsessive-compulsive disorder with Tourette syndrome. Nonanticonvulsant drugs may benefit.

Night Terrors, Sleep Talking, Walking, "Sit-ups"

Age 3–10. Usually occur in first sleep cycle (30–90 minutes after going to sleep), with crying, screaming, and "autonomic discharge" (pupils dilated, perspiring). Lasts minutes. Child goes back to sleep and has no recall of event next day. Sleep studies (polysomnogram and EEG) are normal. Disappears with maturation. Sleep talking and walking and short "sit-ups" in bed are fragmentary arousals. If a spell is recorded, EEG shows arousal from deep sleep, but the behavior seems wakeful. Protect from injury, gradually settle down, and take back to bed.

Nightmares

Nightmares or vivid dreams occur in subsequent cycles of sleep, often in the early-morning hours, and generally are partially recalled the next day. The bizarre and frightening behavior may sometimes be confused with complex partial seizures. Typically occur during rapid eye movement (REM) sleep; epilepsy usually does not occur during REM sleep. In extreme or difficult cases, an all-night sleep EEG may help to differentiate seizures from nightmares.

Migraine

One variant of migraine can be associated with an acute confusional state. There may be the usual migraine prodrome with spots before the eyes, dizziness, visual field defects, and then agitated confusion. A history of other, more typical migraine with severe headache and vomiting but without confusion may aid in the diagnosis. Other seizure manifestations are practically never seen (e.g., tonic-clonic movements, falling, and complete loss of consciousness). Ocular migraines can be differentiated from occipital seizures in that they are longer duration (most seizures <1–2 min), black or white coloring (seizures are multicolored), and rudimentary shapes such as lines, zigzags, or circles (seizures are abstract images). The EEG in migraine is usually normal and seldom has epileptiform abnormalities often seen in patients with epilepsy. Last, migraine and epilepsy are infrequently linked: migraine-caused ischemia on the brain surface sometimes leads to later epilepsy.

Benign Nocturnal Myoclonus

Common in infants and may last even up to school age. Focal or generalized jerks (the latter also called *hypnic* or *sleep jerks*) may persist from onset of sleep on and off all night. A video record for physician review can aid in diagnosis. Routine or sleep EEG taken during jerks is normal, proving that these jerks are not epilepsy. Treatment is reassurance.

Shuddering

Shuddering or shivering attacks can occur in infancy and be a forerunner of essential tremor in later life. Often, the family history is positive for tremor. They are usually first noticed at mealtime. The spells may be very frequent. EEG is normal. There is no clouding or loss of consciousness. Peak incidence is between 9 and 11 months of age, and spells commonly begin to resolve after this time.

Table 1. **Nonepileptic Paroxysmal Events—cont'd**

Gastroesophageal Reflux

Seen more commonly in children with cerebral palsy or brain damage, reflux of acid gastric contents may cause pain that cannot be described by the child. At times, there may be unusual reflexive posturings (dystonic or other) of the head and neck or trunk, an apparent attempt to stretch the esophagus or close the opening. There is no loss of consciousness, but there may be eye rolling, nystagmus, apnea, and occasional vomiting that may simulate a seizure. An upper gastrointestinal series, cine of swallowing, sometimes even an EEG (which is always normal) may be necessary to distinguish this from seizures.

Masturbation

Rarely in infants, repetitive rocking or rubbing motions may simulate seizures. The youngster may look out of contact, be poorly responsive to the environment, and have autonomic expressions (e.g., perspiration, dilated pupils) that may be confused with seizures. Observation by a skilled individual, sometimes even in a hospital situation, may be necessary to distinguish this from seizures. EEG is, of course, normal between or during attacks. Interpretation and reassurance are the only necessary treatment.

Conversion Reaction/Nonepileptic Seizures (NES; Formerly Pseudoseizures)

As many as 50% of patients with NES have epilepsy. Episodes may be writhing, intercourse-like movements, tonic episodes, bizarre jerking and thrashing around, or even apparently sudden unresponsiveness. Often, there is ongoing psychological trauma. Often, but not invariably, the patients are developmentally delayed. The spells must often be seen or recorded on videotape in a controlled situation to distinguish them from epilepsy. A normal EEG during a spell is a key diagnostic feature. Often, the spells are so bizarre that they are easily distinguished. Sometimes NES can be precipitated by suggestion with injection of normal saline in a controlled situation. Combativeness is common; self-injury and incontinence are rare.

Temper Tantrums and Rage Attacks

These are sometimes confused with epilepsy. Amnesia or at least claims of amnesia for events during the spell can be reported. The attacks are usually precipitated by frustration or anger and are often directed either verbally or physically and subside with behavior modification and isolation. EEGs are generally normal but unfortunately seldom obtained during an attack. Anterior temporal leads may be helpful in ruling out temporal or lateral frontal abnormalities, the latter sometimes seen in partial complex seizures. Improvement of the attacks with psychotherapy, milieu therapy, or behavioral modification helps rule out epilepsy. A key differential diagnosis is postictal psychosis, but the psychosis is preceded by epileptic phenomenon.

Benign Paroxysmal Vertigo

These are brief attacks of vertigo in which the youngster often appears frightened and pale and clutches the parent. The attacks last 5–30 seconds. Sometimes nystagmus is identified. There is no loss of consciousness. Usually the child is well and returns to play immediately afterward. The attacks may occur in clusters, then disappear for months. Attacks are usually seen in infants and preschoolers aged 2–5. EEG is normal. If caloric tests can be obtained (often very difficult in this age group), abnormalities with hypofunction of one side are sometimes seen. Medications are usually not desirable or necessary.

Staring Spells

Teachers often make referral for absence seizures in children who stare or seem preoccupied at school, but their staring is behavioral or due to attention-deficit disorders. Helpful in the history is the lack of these spells at home (e.g., before breakfast, a common time for absence seizures). A lack of other epilepsy in the child or family history often is helpful. Sometimes these children have difficulties with school and a cognitive or learning disability. The child can generally be brought out of this spell by a firm command. An EEG is sometimes necessary to confirm that absence seizures are not occurring. A 24-hour ambulatory EEG to record attacks during the child's everyday school activities is occasionally necessary.

Table 2. **Seizure Category and Specific Clinical Information**

Age Group and Seizure Type	Age at Onset	Clinical Manifestations	Causative Factors	Electroencephalographic Pattern	Other Diagnostic Studies	Treatment and Comments (Anticonvulsants by Order of Choice)
Neonatal seizures	Birth to 2 weeks	Often atypical; sudden limpness or tonic posturing, brief apnea, and cyanosis; odd cry; eyes rolling up; fixed eye deviation, blinking, or mouthing or chewing movements; nystagmus, twitchiness, or clonic movements—focal, multifocal, or rarely generalized Some seizures are nonepileptic-decerebrate, or other posturings; release from forebrain inhibition; poor response to drugs	Neurologic insults (hypoxia/ischemia; intracranial hemorrhage) present more in first 3 days or after eighth day; metabolic disturbances alone between third and eighth days; hypoglycemia, hypocalcemia, hypernatremia, and hyponatremia Drug withdrawal Pyridoxine dependency and other metabolic causes CNS infections and structural abnormalities	May correlate poorly with clinical seizures Focal spikes or slow rhythms, multifocal discharges Electroclinical dissociation may occur; EEG electrical seizure without clinical manifestations and vice versa	Lumbar puncture: PCR of CSF for herpes, enterovirus; serum calcium, phosphorus, glucose, magnesium, BUN, amino acid screen, blood ammonia, organic acid screen, TORCHES IgM Ultrasound or CT scan for suspected intracranial hemorrhage and structural abnormalities	Phenobarbital, IV or IM; if seizures not controlled, add phenytoin IV (loading dose, 20 mg/kg each) Diazepam 0.3 mg/kg Treat underlying disorder Seizures caused by brain damage often resistant to anticonvulsants When cause in doubt, stop protein feedings until enzyme deficiencies of urea cycle or amino acid metabolism ruled out
West syndrome, infantile spasms (see also Lennox–Gastaut syndrome)	3–18 months; occasionally up to 4 years	Sudden, usually symmetric adduction and flexion of limbs with concomitant flexion of head and trunk; also abduction and extensor movements like Moro reflex Tendency for spasms to occur in clusters, on waking or falling asleep or when fatigued, or may be noted particularly when the infant is being handled, is ill, or is otherwise irritable Tendency for each patient to have own stereotyped pattern	Prenatal or perinatal brain damage or malformation in approximately one third; biochemical, infectious, degenerative causes in approximately one third, unknown in approximately one third With early-onset, pyridoxine deficiency, amino or organic aciduria Tuberous sclerosis in 5%–10% Chronic inflammatory disease and toxoplasmosis Aicardi syndrome (females with mental retardation, agenesis of corpus callosum, ocular and vertebral anomalies)	Hypsarrhythmia; chaotic high-voltage slow waves, random spikes, all leads (90%); other abnormalities in rest Rarely normal EEG normalization usually correlates with reduction of seizures; not helpful prognostically regarding mental development	Funduscopic and skin examination, trial of pyridoxine Amino and organic acid screen Chronic inflammatory disease: TORCHES screen CT or MRI scan should be done to (1) establish definite diagnosis (2) aid in genetic counseling SPECT or PET scan may identify focal lesion	Dosing of ACTH to: varied protocols, usually 40–60 U/day, then slow withdrawal Some prefer oral corticosteroids or vigabatrin, topiramate, zonisamide, clonazepam, valproic acid, or pyridoxine In resistant cases, ketogenic or medium-chain triglyceride diet Retardation of varying degree in approximately 90% of cases Occasionally, surgical extirpation of focal lesion may be curative Chronic B_6 (pyridoxine) popular treatment in Japan

Febrile seizures	6 months to 6 years old; usually 6–18 months	Usually single generalized seizures, less than 15 minutes; rarely focal in onset May lead to status epilepticus, usually benign Recurrence risk for second febrile seizure 30%; 50% if younger than 1 year; recurrence risk is same after status	Non-neurologic febrile illness (temperature increases to $\geq 39°$ C); family history frequently positive for febrile convulsions Some genetic sites identified; 2q, 8q, 19p	Normal interictal EEG, especially when obtained 8–10 days after seizure	Lumbar puncture in infants or whenever suspicion of meningitis exists. Consider neuroimaging if complex febrile seizure	Treat underlying illness, fever Diazepam orally or rectally as needed, 0.3–0.5 mg/kg three times daily during illness Chronic prophylaxis is not usually recommended as potential adverse effects outweigh benefits; considerations include prolonged seizures or family anxiety
Myoclonic-astatic spectrum (Doose syndrome to Lennox–Gastaut syndrome)	Any time in childhood; normally 2–7 years	Shocklike violent contractions of one or more muscle groups, singly or irregularly repetitive; may fling patient suddenly to side, forward, or backward Usually no or only brief loss of consciousness Half of patients or more also have generalized grand mal seizures Drop attacks (tonic, atonic, myoclonic)	Multiple causes, usually resulting in diffuse neuronal damage History of West syndrome; prenatal or perinatal brain damage; viral meningoencephalitides; CNS degenerative disorders, lead, or other encephalopathies; structural cerebral abnormalities (e.g., migrational abnormalities) Idiopathic (genetic)	Atypical slow (1–2.5 Hz) spike-wave complexes, generalized spikes, and/or polyspikes and bursts of high-voltage generalized spikes, often with diffusely slow background frequencies	As dictated by index of suspicion Lumbar puncture with measles, antibody titer, and CSF-IgG index Nerve conduction studies Skin biopsy for electron microscopy, MRI scan, WBC lysosomal enzymes if metabolic degenerative disease suspected Funduscopic examination	Difficult to treat Valproic acid, clonazepam, topiramate; felbamate, zonisamide, retigabine Ketogenic or medium-chain triglyceride diet ACTH or corticosteroids as in West syndrome Perhaps lamotrigine, topiramate, vigabatrin Protect head with helmet and chin padding
Absence (petit mal); also juvenile and myoclonic absence	3–15 years	Lapses of consciousness or vacant stares, lasting about 10 seconds, often in "clusters" Automatisms of face and hands; clonic activity in 30%–45% Often confused with complex partial seizures but no aura or postictal confusion	Unknown Genetic component: probably an autosomal dominant gene	3/s bilaterally synchronous, symmetric, high-voltage spikes and waves EEG normalization correlates closely with control of seizures	Hyperventilation when patient on inadequate or no medication often provokes attacks Imaging is rarely of value	Valproic acid or ethosuximide; lamotrigine (Lamictal); with latter, add or substitute valproate if major motor seizures In resistant cases, ketogenic diet, lamotrigine, topiramate, acetazolamide
Simple partial or focal seizures (motor/sensory/jacksonian)	Any age	Seizure may involve any part of body; may spread in fixed pattern (jacksonian march), becoming generalized In children, epileptogenic focus often "shifts" and epileptic manifestations may change concomitantly	Often secondary to birth trauma, inflammatory process, vascular accidents, meningoencephalitis, etc. If seizures are coupled with new or progressive neurologic deficits, a structural lesion (e.g., brain tumor) is likely	Focal spikes or slow waves in appropriate cortical region; sometimes diffusely abnormal or even normal	If seizures are difficult to control or progressive deficits occur, neurodiagnostic studies, particularly MRI brain scan, imperative	Carbamazepine, phenytoin, oxcarbazepine Valproic acid useful adjunct Also used lamotrigine, gabapentin, and topiramate

Continued

Table 2. **Seizure Category and Specific Clinical Information—cont'd**

Age Group and Seizure Type	Age at Onset	Clinical Manifestations	Causative Factors	Electroencephalographic Pattern	Other Diagnostic Studies	Treatment and Comments (Anticonvulsants by Order of Choice)
Complex partial seizures (psychomotor, temporal lobe, or limbic seizures)	Any age	Aura may be a sensation of fear, epigastric discomfort, odd smell or taste (usually unpleasant), visual or auditory hallucination (either vague and "unformed" or well-formed image, words, music) Aura and seizure stereotyped for each patient Seizure may consist of vague stare; facial tongue, or swallowing movements and throaty sounds; or various complex automatisms Unlike absences, complex partial seizures tend not to occur in clusters, but singly and to last longer ($\geq$1 minute) followed by confusion History of aura (or child running to adult from "vague fear") and of automatisms involving more than face and hands establish diagnosis	As in previous entry Temporal lobes especially sensitive to hypoxia; thus, this seizure type may be a sequela of birth trauma, febrile convulsions, etc. Also especially vulnerable to certain viral infections, especially herpes simplex Remediable or other causes are small cryptic tumors or vascular malformations	As in previous entry, but occurring in temporal lobe and its connections (e.g., frontotemporal, temporoparietal, temporo-occipital regions)	MRI when structural lesions suspected PCR of CSF in acute febrile situation for herpes; rarely, temporal lobe biopsy Carotid amobarbital injection when lateralization of speech dominance in question and surgical extirpation of epileptogenic area is contemplated	Oxcarbazepine, levetiracetam, topiramate, zonisamide, lamotrigine, valproic acid, phenobarbital, felbamate, gabapentin, tiagabine More than one drug may be necessary Valproic acid may be useful In cases refractory to at least two drugs, consider referral for epilepsy surgery evaluation Adjunctive psychotherapy required frequently Gabapentin, topiramate, levetiracetam, and tiagabine (for >12-year-olds)
Benign epilepsy of childhood (with centrotemporal or rolandic foci)	5–16	Partial motor or generalized seizures Similar seizure patterns may be observed in patients with focal cortical lesions Usually nocturnal simple partial seizures of face, tongue, hand	Seizure history of abnormal EEG findings in relatives of 40% of affected probands and 18%–20% of parents and siblings, suggesting transmission by a single autosomal dominant gene, possibly with age-dependent	Centrotemporal spikes or sharp waves ("rolandic discharges") appearing paroxysmally against a normal EEG background	Seldom need CT or MRI scan	Carbamazepine, oxcarbazepine, levetiracetam, lamotrigine, topiramate Often, no medication is necessary, especially if seizure is exclusively nocturnal and infrequent

Juvenile myoclonic epilepsy (of Janz)	Late childhood and adolescence, peaking at 13 years	Mild myoclonic jerks of neck and shoulder flexor muscles after awakening Intelligence usually normal Often absence seizures and GTCS as well	40% of relatives have myoclonias, especially in female individuals; 15% have the abnormal EEG pattern with clinical attacks Genetic loci: 6p, 15q14	Interictal EEG shows fast variety of spike-and-wave sequences or 4- to 6-Hz multispike and wave complexes Photosensitive responses common	Differentiate from progressive myoclonic encephalopathy of Unverricht–Lafora and other degenerative disorders by appropriate biopsies (muscle, liver, etc.)	Valproic acid, lamotrigine (Lamictal), levetiracetam, zonisamide, topiramate
GTCS	Any age	Loss of consciousness; tonic-clonic movements, often preceded by vague aura or cry Bladder and bowel incontinence in approximately 15% Postictal confusion; sleep Often mixed with or masking other seizure patterns	Often unknown Genetic component May be seen with metabolic disturbances, trauma, infection, intoxication, degenerative disorders, brain tumors	Bilaterally synchronous, symmetric multiple high-voltage spikes, spikes and waves, mixed patterns Often normal before age 4	As in entry above	Phenobarbital in infants; consider topiramate and levetiracetam (Keppra), Carbamazepine, lamotrigine (Lamictal), phenytoin, topiramate, valproic acid, zonisamide (Zonegran) More than one drug may be necessary

ACTH, adrenocorticotropic hormone; *BUN*, blood urea nitrogen; *CNS*, central nervous system; *CSF*, cerebrospinal fluid; *CT*, computed tomography; *EEG*, electroencephalogram; *GTCS*, generalized tonic-clonic seizures (grand mal); *IM*, intramuscular; *IV*, intravenous; *MRI*, magnetic resonance imaging; *PCR*, polymerase chain reaction; *PET*, positron emission tomography; *SPECT*, single-photon emission computed tomography; *WBC*, white blood cell.

Table 3. **Guide to Pediatric Anticonvulsant Drug Therapy**

Drug	Average Total Dosage	Steady State	Effective Blood Levels*	Side Effects and Precautions	Directions and Remarks
Adjunctive or Secondary Drug					
Acetazolamide	5–20 mg/kg/day in two or three divided doses	1–2 days	10–14 μg/ml	Anorexia; numbness and tingling Urinary frequency, so do not give in evening Renal stones	Supplement to other (Acetazolamide [Diamox]) medications, especially in absence and complex partial seizures Also in female patients 4 days before and in the first 2 or 3 days of menstrual period for catamenial seizures
Levetiracetam (Keppra)	30–80 mg/kg/day during 2–6 weeks	1–3 days	20–40 μg/ml	Somnolence, dizziness, headache, asthenia, behavioral agitation/psychosis Rare: decreased WBC	Complex partial seizures, myoclonic Little effect on other drugs
Clorazepate (Tranxene)	0.3 mg/kg/day in two divided doses	Not known (approximately 21 days)	0.2–1.5 μg/ml (>2)	Lethargy, drooling, ataxia Behavior changes	May be useful adjunct in generalized tonic-clonic, partial, and astatic seizures Not for children younger than 9 years
Felbamate (Felbatol)	15–45 mg/kg/day in three or four divided doses	5–7 days	30–50 μg/ml	Anorexia, vomiting, insomnia, headache, somnolence Rash in 1% Aplastic anemia and hepatic failure are significant hazards	Used in children with Lennox–Gastaut syndrome; in adults with complex partial seizures Obtain informed consent Drug interactions: effect decreased by phenytoin, carbamazepine
Vigabatrin	20–100 mg/kg/day in two or three divided doses	Not known	Not known	Drowsiness, confusion, weight gain, retinal changes	Infantile spasms, especially tuberous sclerosis Add-on drug for partial seizures Not licensed by FDA in United States as of 2008
Gabapentin (Neurontin) >12 years	30–60 mg/kg/day in three divided doses (900–1800 mg total per day)	1–2 days	12–25 μg/ml	Drowsiness, dizziness, ataxia, weight gain	Add-on drug for partial seizures; no effect on other anticonvulsant drug levels
Topiramate (Topamax)	Start 0.5–1 mg/kg/day to 10 mg/kg/day in two divided doses (maximum: 500 mg/day)	Not known	8–25 μg/ml	Somnolence, slowed mentation, dizziness, language problems (word finding), rarely kidney stones, anorexia	Adjunctive drug for partial seizures Minimal effect on other drug levels Lennox–Gastaut syndrome, West syndrome
Tiagabine	0.1–1.5 mg/kg/day in three or four divided doses	1–2 days	20–70 μg/ml	Dizziness, tremor, abnormal thinking	Adjunctive drug for partial seizures
Zonisamide	1–2 mg/kg/day to maximum 8–12 mg/kg/day in two divided doses/day (only 100-μg capsules in United States)	5–7 days	20–30 μg/ml	Drowsiness, anorexia, gastrointestinal symptoms, weight loss, behavior changes, renal stones (0.2%–2%), hypohidrosis, rash	Effects in multiseizure types A sulfonamide widely used in Japan
Lamotrigine (Lamictal)	5–15 mg/kg/day in two to four divided doses (1–5 mg if taking valproic acid); 5–400 mg/day total	8–15 day	10–20 μg/ml	Dizziness, headaches, diplopia, ataxia, nausea Rash in 5%–10%, 1% Stevens–Johnson usually in first 4–8 wk	Add-on drug for children with partial and complex partial seizures, Lennox–Gastaut syndrome, absence seizures, primary or secondary generalized tonic-clonic seizures Valproate increases drug half-life Increase dose slowly during 2 months

Table 3. **Guide to Pediatric Anticonvulsant Drug Therapy—cont'd**

Drug	Average Total Dosage	Steady State	Effective Blood Levels*	Side Effects and Precautions	Directions and Remarks
Treatment of Status Epilepticus†					
Diazepam (Valium)	0.3 mg/kg IV Repeat dose: 0.1–0.3 mg/kg IV			Administer slowly Monitor pulse and blood pressure May cause respiratory depression in presence of phenobarbital	May need to be repeated every 3–4 h Follow with phenytoin or phenobarbital for long-range control Note: Intramuscular administration for status epilepticus ineffective
Phenobarbital	5–20 mg/kg IV initially Repeat dose: 5–10 mg/kg IV			See above	Rule out pyridoxine deficiency In neonatal seizures, load with 15–20 mg/kg IV
Phenytoin (Dilantin) (fosphenytoin newer, safer)	10–20 mg/kg IV initially Repeat dose: 5–10 mg/kg IV			Administer IV during a 5-minute period Administer IM only if no IV access Monitor blood levels	Adjunct in neonatal seizures (20 mg/kg IV) if phenobarbital alone fails Fosphenytoin, new safe preparation; same dose; may give rapidly IV during 5 minutes
Lorazepam (Ativan)	0.05–0.2 mg/kg IV May repeat			Mild respiratory depression	May be more effective than diazepam Longer acting
Midazolam (Versed)	0.1–0.3 mg/kg IM or IV 0.2 mg/kg as nasal spray IV drip 1–5 μg/kg/min			See other benzodiazepines	Short acting
Valproate sodium (Depacon)	5–60 mg/min IV (maximum: 20 mg/min)			Administer slowly Dizziness, nausea, and injection-site pain	Half-life 16 hours Useful when child cannot take valproate orally

Treatment of infantile spasms is detailed.
*In parentheses are shown the levels at which clinical toxicity becomes manifest in monotherapy.
†General anesthesia if other measures fail.

References

Greenwood RS, Tennison RS. When to start and stop anticonvulsant therapy in children. Arch Neurol 1999;56:1073–77.

Hirtz D, Ashwal S, Berg A, et al. Practice parameter: evaluating a first nonfebrile seizure in children. Report of the Quality Standards Subcommittee of the American Academy of Neurology, the Child Neurology Society, and the American Epilepsy Society. Neurology 2000;55:616–23.

Hirtz D, Berg A, Bettis D, et al. Practice parameter: treatment of the child with a first unprovoked seizure. Report of the Quality Standards Subcommittee of the American Academy of Neurology and the Practice Committee of the Child Neurology Society. Neurology 2003;60:166–75.

Moe P, Benke TA, Bernard TJ, Levisohn P. Neurologic and muscular disorders. In: Hay W, Levin M, Deterding R, Sondheimer J, editors. Current diagnosis and management: pediatrics. 19th ed. New York: McGraw-Hill Companies; 2009. p. 679–728.

Shinnar S, O'Dell C. Treatment decisions in childhood seizures. In: Pellock JM, Bourgeois BFD, Dodson WE, Nordli DR Jr, Sankar R, editors. 2nd eds. Pediatric epilepsy: diagnosis and therapy. 3rd ed. New York: Demos Medical Publishing; 2008. p. 401–12.

Status Epilepticus

Carter Wray, MD, and Kelly Knupp, MD

Status epilepticus is a medical emergency defined by the International League Against Epilepsy as a "seizure which shows no clinical signs of arresting after a duration encompassing the great majority of seizures of that type in most patients or recurrent seizures without resumption of baseline central nervous system function interictally." Much debate exists about the minimum time required to determine whether a patient meets the definition of status epilepticus. Most experts use a timeframe between 5 and 30 minutes, or recurrent seizures, between which the patient does not regain consciousness. The use of the shorter time of 5 minutes is based on findings that the majority of seizures stop in less than 5 minutes, especially in children older than 5 years. Others reserve status epilepticus for seizures that last more than 30 minutes. The latter definition may be more accurate for new-onset seizures in children, which are often longer than those captured in epilepsy monitoring units, especially given that parental recall of the duration of a first seizure often seems longer than the actual spell. Status epilepticus can be associated with partial or generalized convulsive seizures or a prolonged fugue state ("spike and wave stupor"). If it is sufficiently prolonged, status epilepticus can lead to a coma with subtle or no clinical symptoms, sometimes called *nonconvulsive status epilepticus.* No cause can be identified in about half of children with status epilepticus. The mortality risk rate of 2% to 5% and morbidity depend largely on the cause of the seizure. However, prolonged status epilepticus itself can cause severe central nervous system sequelae because of hypoxemia, acidosis, and hypotension.

A. As soon as a duration of seizure longer than 5 minutes has been ascertained, seizure abortion needs to be initiated as described later, even as history is being obtained. The history needs to focus on finding a possible recent or remote precipitating cause for the seizure. Acute symptomatic causes include, but are not limited to, fever, sepsis, meningitis, encephalitis, gastroenteritis, anoxia, metabolic and electrolyte disorders, toxins, encephalopathies, malignancy, vascular disorders, and head trauma. Remote symptomatic causes include prior neurologic conditions such as birth asphyxia, traumatic brain injury, and prior central nervous system infection, or developmental delay that might suggest such an insult. Determine whether the child has any acute or chronic illness, especially diabetes, renal disease, or metabolic disease. If there is a known diagnosis of epilepsy, have prior status episodes of status epilepticus occurred? Determine current anticonvulsant medications and ascertain whether medications have been missed or there has been a change in formulation or dosing. Ask whether the seizure was focal or generalized at the onset of the status. Most importantly, determine whether management has been instituted for this seizure, such as rectal diazepam at home or parenteral medications provided by emergency response teams.

B. Physical examination needs to include vital signs such as heart rate, blood pressure, respirations, and temperature. Pulse oximetry may be inaccurate in a seizing child. Evaluate for focality: eye deviation, paresis, tonic (stiffening) or clonic (rhythmic jerking) activity, and signs of preexisting abnormalities such as prior neurologic injury or a genetic syndrome. Note evidence of trauma, as well as systemic illness. Perform a careful ophthalmoscopic examination to identify signs of increased intracranial pressure or retinal hemorrhage associated with an acute intracranial bleed or trauma. Examine the skin and mucous membranes for signs of dehydration, needle marks from intravenous injection of drugs in an adolescent, or skin lesions suggesting a neurocutaneous disorder. Note signs of heart disease that might suggest the possibility of emboli to the central nervous system.

C. Consider obtaining blood for initial laboratory evaluations when intravenous access is obtained. The workup should be guided by the history and physical you have obtained. In a meta-analysis, the cause of status epilepticus was classified acute symptomatic in 26%, remote symptomatic in 33%, remote symptomatic with an acute precipitant in 1%, a part of a progressive encephalopathy in 3%, febrile status in 22%, and cryptogenic in 15%. Given this diversity of causes, the value of any test to evaluate a child is dependent on its pretest probability. Of the following evaluations, none received a higher recommendation in the American Academy of Neurology's Practice Parameter than level B, meaning "probably effective, ineffective, or harmful for the given condition in the specified population." Determine antiepileptic medication blood levels when appropriate. Serum glucose level can be checked at the bedside. If a child is hypoglycemic, administer a bolus of dextrose possibly followed by a continuous infusion if appropriate. Serum chemistries can be checked such as electrolytes, blood urea nitrogen, creatinine, calcium, liver function tests, phosphorus, and magnesium. Blood gas analysis is of little use in the actively seizing child unless there is concern for prolonged respiratory compromise. Other diagnostic tests, such as imaging of the brain, must wait until the end of the convulsive activity but is appropriate in most children presenting for the first time with status epilepticus.

D. Many of the antiepileptic drugs used in status are listed in Table 1. The most effective route of administration requires obtaining intravenous access, although this can be difficult to obtain. If intravenous access cannot be quickly achieved, intramuscular, rectal, or nasal administration of benzodiazepines can result in therapeutic blood levels within several minutes. Most regimens for management of status use benzodiazepines first, followed by a longer acting antiepileptic drug, such as phenytoin, if necessary, or in small children without central access, preferably fosphenytoin given the caustic pH of traditional phenytoin. Of the benzodiazepines,

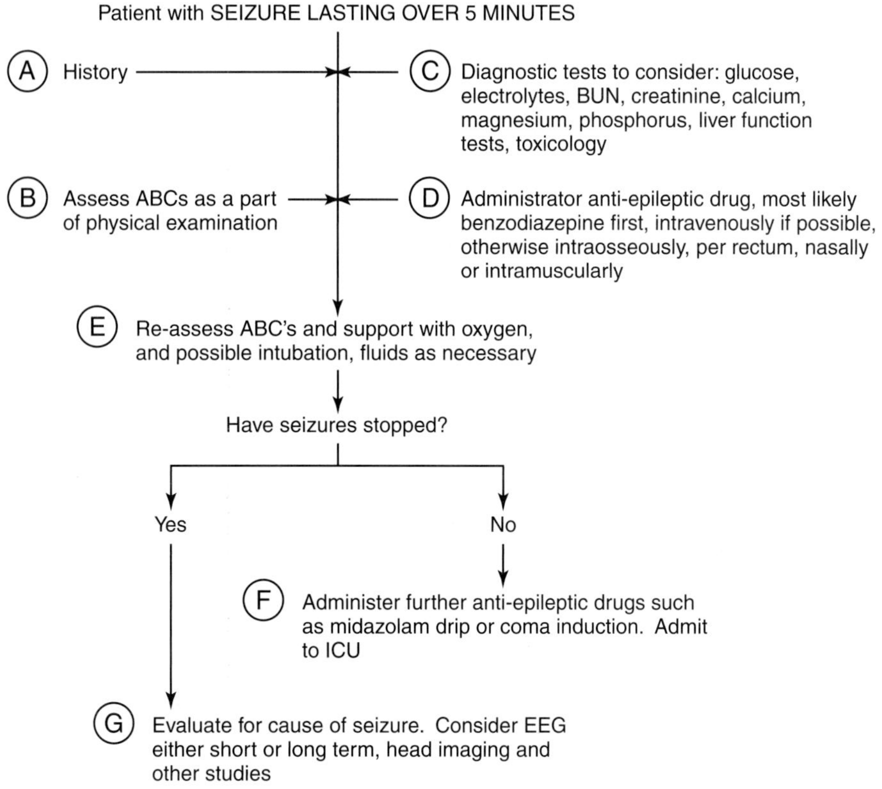
Patient with SEIZURE LASTING OVER 5 MINUTES
(A) History
(C) Diagnostic tests to consider: glucose, electrolytes, BUN, creatinine, calcium, magnesium, phosphorus, liver function tests, toxicology
(B) Assess ABCs as a part of physical examination
(D) Administrator anti-epileptic drug, most likely benzodiazepine first, intravenously if possible, otherwise intraosseously, per rectum, nasally or intramuscularly
(E) Re-assess ABC's and support with oxygen, and possible intubation, fluids as necessary
Have seizures stopped?
Yes
No
(F) Administer further anti-epileptic drugs such as midazolam drip or coma induction. Admit to ICU
(G) Evaluate for cause of seizure. Consider EEG either short or long term, head imaging and other studies

lorazepam has a longer duration of action than diazepam or midazolam. Intravenous infusion of fosphenytoin or phenytoin may cause cardiac arrhythmia, but both share an advantage of not suppressing respiratory drive as much as barbiturates. The most frequently used barbiturate in the United States is phenobarbital, and it may be more effective than other options. Other intravenous options for treating status that are not severely sedating are valproate and levetiracetam.

E. Reassess vital signs, as the goal of treatment is first to ensure adequate oxygenation and cardiac function, then to terminate the clinical and electrical seizure activity. Stabilize the patient to maintain adequate tissue oxygenation. Respiratory support includes establishment of an adequate airway by repositioning the child's head and, if necessary, placing an oral or nasopharyngeal airway. Administer oxygen by mask to all patients. If air exchange is poor, institute bag and mask ventilation; if necessary, intubate. Circulatory support with intravenous fluids and possibly pressors may be necessary if signs of shock or hypotension are present. Protect the patient from injury by placing the child on a soft, flat area free of hard or sharp objects. If the child is on a bed, table, or stretcher, prevent the child from falling. The risks of placing a nasogastric tube should be considered in relation to the risks from aspiration and may be safer if the patient is intubated.

F. Seizures that do not stop with two of the earlier treatments are referred to as refractory status epilepticus and bode a poor prognosis, with mortality rate as high as 32% in children. Pharmacologically induced coma with midazolam or pentobarbital for refractory status epilepticus is the treatment with the most data to support its use in children. Midazolam has fewer adverse effects, in part, because it is more rapidly cleared. In adults, response rates were best with pentobarbital, but it is associated with a far greater incidence of significant hypotension. It also requires continuous electroencephalographic (EEG) monitoring with titration to a burst-suppression pattern, with a goal of 1 second of burst to 5 to 10 seconds of suppression. Other barbiturates such as thiopental or phenobarbital can be used. General anesthetics such as propofol and ketamine may also be used but carry significant risks in this setting; however, they may be useful in certain cases.

G. Unless there is a rapid return to baseline mental status, children with status epilepticus should be hospitalized in the intensive care unit to provide ongoing support to cardiovascular and respiratory systems, as well as seizure management. The child who responds to intervention with cessation of seizures may not need EEG until he or she is recovered. The postictal EEG will usually contain slow activity as a result of both the episode of status and any artifact from benzodiazepines or barbiturates used to stop it. As such, it often has limited clinical use. For the child with persistent alteration of mental status, strongly consider performing EEG to identify subtle or nonconvulsive status epilepticus. EEG monitoring can be particularly helpful if a child requires neuromuscular blockade to provide airway support. Other diagnostic tests, such as imaging of the brain, must wait until the end of the convulsive activity but are appropriate in most children presenting for the first time with status epilepticus. Consider more occult causes of prolonged seizures such as underlying genetic or metabolic disorders. For further evaluation of seizures, see Seizure Disorders: Febrile (p. 354) and Seizure Disorders: Nonfebrile (p. 358).

Table-1. **Drug Therapy of Status Epilepticus in Children and Adolescents**

Drug	Dosage	Maximum Rate of Infusion	Other Information
Benzodiazepines			
Diazepam (Valium)	PR 0.2–0.5 mg/kg IV 0.1–0.3 mg/kg (maximum: 10 mg)	5 mg/min	May repeat q10min × 2
Lorazepam (Ativan, Alzapam)	0.1 mg/kg IV (maximum: 4 mg)	2 mg/min	May repeat q10min × 2
Midazolam (Versed)	Nasal, IM 0.2 mg/kg IV 0.2 mg/kg, then 0.75–10 μg/kg/min = 0.05–2 mg/kg/hr	"Bolus" vs. administer over 2–5 min	
Barbiturates			
Phenobarbital (Luminal)	10–20 mg/kg IV	2 mg/kg/min	
Pentobarbital (Nembutal)	2–20 mg/kg, then 0.5–5 mg/kg/hr IV	Load over 1–2 hours	Continuous EEG needed
Thiopental (Pentothal)	5 mg/kg	Administer over 20–30 seconds	
Others			
Phenytoin (Dilantin)	15–20 mg/kg IV	50 mg/min	Monitor blood level
Fosphenytoin (Cerebyx)	IV or IM 15–20 PE (phenytoin mg equivalents)/kg	150 mg/min	Monitor blood level
Valproate (Depacon)	20–40 mg/kg IV	5 mg/kg/min	
Levetiracetam (Keppra)	20–30 mg/kg IV	5 mg/kg/min	
Propofol (Diprivan)	1–2 mg/kg in 5 minutes, then 5–10 mg/kg/hr	25–75 μg/kg/min	
Ketamine (Ketalar)	7.5 mg/kg IV q12h	0.5 mg/kg/min	
Lidocaine	2 mg/kg, then 4 mg/kg/hr	20–50 μg/kg/min	

EEG, electroencephalogram; *IM*, intramuscularly; *IV*, intravenously, can also be given intraosseously; *PR*, per rectum.

References

Abend NS, Dlugos DJ. Treatment of refractory status epilepticus: literature review and a proposed protocol. Pediatr Neurol 2008;38:377–90.

Blume WT, Lüders HO, Mizrahi E, et al. Glossary of descriptive terminology for ictal semiology. <http://www.ilae-epilepsy.org/ctf/gloss_frame.html>; 2004 [accessed 01.04.10].

Claassen J, Hirsch LJ, Emerson RG, Mayer SA. Treatment of refractory status epilepticus with pentobarbital, propofol, or midazolam: a systematic review. Epilepsia 2002;43(2):146–53.

Lowenstein DH, Bleck T, Macdonald RL. It's time to revise the definition of status epilepticus. Epilepsia 1999;40:120–2.

Raspall-Chaure M, Chin RF, Neville BG, Scott RC. Outcome of paediatric convulsive status epilepticus: a systematic review. Lancet Neurol 2006; 5:769–79.

Riviello JJ, Ashwal S, Hirtz D, et al. Practice parameter: diagnostic assessment of the child with status epilepticus (an evidence-based review): report of the Quality Standards Subcommittee of the American Academy of Neurology and the Practice Committee of the Child Neurology Society. Neurology 2006;67(9):1542–50.

Sahin M, Menache CC, Holmes GL, Riviello JJ. Outcome of severe refractory status epilepticus in children. Epilepsia 2001;42(11): 1461–7.

Shaner DM, McCurdy SA, Herring MO, Gabor AJ. Treatment of status epilepticus: a prospective comparison of diazepam and phenytoin versus phenobarbital and optional phenytoin. Neurology 1988; 38:202–7.

Shinnar S, Berg AT, Moshe SL, Shinnar R. How long do new-onset seizures in children last? Ann Neurol 2001;49:659–64.

van Gestel J, Blussé van Oud-Alblas HJ, Malingré M, et al. Propofol and thiopental for refractory status epilepticus in children. Neurology 2005;65(4):591–2.

Wheless J, Venkataraman V. Safety of high intravenous valproate doses in epilepsy patients. J Epilepsy 1999;11:319–24.

Wolfe TR. Intranasal midazolam therapy for pediatric status epilepticus. Am J Emerg Med 2006;24(3):343–6.

Working Group on Status Epilepticus, Epilepsy Foundation of America. Treatment of convulsive status epilepticus. JAMA 1993;270:854–9.

Acute Weakness in Childhood

Britt Stroud, MD, and Timothy J. Bernard, MD

Acute onset of weakness in a child is a neurologic emergency and should be evaluated in a hospital setting where subspecialists are available. A systematic approach to diagnosis is provided in the algorithm. The essential component to establishing a diagnosis is localization of the lesion. Unlike adult neurology, however, localization can be challenging (and sometimes misleading) in a pediatric patient, especially infants and toddlers. For this reason, we suggest an initial workup that is based on localization, but rapid expansion of the differential is essential in cases where the workup is initially unrevealing.

A. History and Physical Examination: When weakness is accompanied by central nervous system abnormalities—such as a seizure, headache, encephalopathy, brisk reflexes, hypertonia, or an upgoing Babinski—there is likely a cortical component to the underlying disease state. For this reason, the workup of weakness associated with these abnormalities is usually initiated with imaging of the brain. In contrast, patients with preserved levels of cognition and signs of peripheral disease (such as hyporeflexia, hypotonia, and a down-going Babinski) are often initially evaluated for nerve, muscle, and neuromuscular junction pathology. Patients with spinal cord disease often present with specific signs and symptoms of spinal cord dysfunction, such as incontinence and a sensory level on examination.

For the purposes of this chapter, we have divided the evaluation of acute-onset weakness into four categories: (1) unilateral or bilateral weakness with evidence of cortical involvement, (2) unilateral weakness without cortical involvement, (3) bilateral weakness without cortical involvement, and (4) weakness with signs of spinal cord involvement.

B. Unilateral or Bilateral Weakness with Evidence of Cortical Involvement: In patients with weakness and evidence of cerebral dysfunction (mental status change, seizures, upper motor neuron signs, or meningismus), localization of disease almost uniformly implicates the cerebral cortex. Initial management of these patients usually consists of urgent brain imaging and consideration of a lumbar puncture (LP; after brain imaging), as for the majority of these diseases, rapid diagnosis and initiation of therapy improves outcome. The most common causes of this presentation are ischemic stroke, tumor, hemorrhagic stroke, acute demyelinating encephalomyelitis, multiple sclerosis (MS), infection, Todd's paralysis, or complicated migraine.

1. Ischemic stroke: Childhood arterial ischemic stroke is increasingly recognized as a significant cause of morbidity and mortality in the pediatric population. Typically, unless the cerebral insult is large, a child's consciousness is preserved. Certainly, any child who presents with acute onset of weakness or acute changes in sensation, speech, vision, or coordination should be urgently evaluated for the possibility of an arterial ischemic stroke. A known history of coagulopathy, sickle cell disease, lupus, drug use, heart disease, infection, metabolic disorder, or neck trauma may raise suspicion for an arterial ischemic stroke.
2. Tumor: Although supratentorial unilateral tumors are not as common as posterior fossa tumors in children, a tumor can present acutely with weakness, especially if there is associated hemorrhage. Early in the presentation, a child with a brain tumor may present with a history of head tilt, ataxia, vision loss, decline in school performance, persistent new-onset headache, or a change in personality.
3. Hemorrhagic stroke: Children with hemorrhagic stroke need to be identified urgently to perform the initial management, which may include mannitol, surgical resection, and/or blood pressure control. For this reason, urgent brain imaging is indicated in a patient with suspected hemorrhagic stroke. Underlying causative factors include arteriovenous malformation, aneurysm, hemophilia, trauma, and nonaccidental trauma. Workup should be based on identifying one of these causes.
4. Demyelinating disease: Differentiating between acute disseminated encephalomyelitis and MS can be challenging. Patients with acute disseminated encephalomyelitis tend to be younger and usually present with encephalopathy. Magnetic resonance imaging (MRI) demonstrates T2 hyperintense lesions that are often multifocal and consistent with demyelination. Mimickers of demyelinating disease (such as infection, neoplasm, metabolic derangements, sarcoidosis, and vasculitis) must be considered. Treatment usually consists of high-dose steroids.
5. Central nervous system infection: Unilateral infection of the brain can present with confusion, meningismus, seizure, and/or hemiparesis. Abscess and herpes simplex virus (classically affecting the temporal lobe) are the most common causes of unilateral presentation, although any meningoencephalitis can present asymmetrically. Fever should raise suspicion for central nervous system infection, and antibiotics should be administered as quickly as possible when meningitis is suspected. After neuroimaging to exclude increased intracranial pressure, an LP should be obtained.
6. Todd's paralysis: Patients with focal seizures will often have a postictal hemiparesis associated with their seizure. Typically, Todd's paralysis manifests as

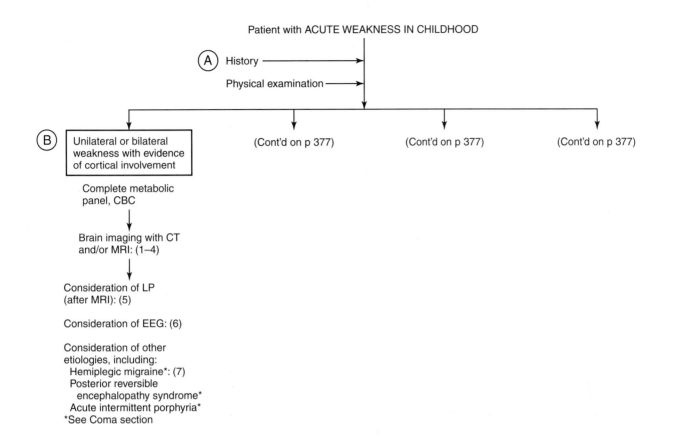

Patient with ACUTE WEAKNESS IN CHILDHOOD

(A) History →

Physical examination →

(B) **Unilateral or bilateral weakness with evidence of cortical involvement**

Complete metabolic panel, CBC

↓

Brain imaging with CT and/or MRI: (1–4)

↓

Consideration of LP (after MRI): (5)

Consideration of EEG: (6)

Consideration of other etiologies, including:
- Hemiplegic migraine*: (7)
- Posterior reversible encephalopathy syndrome*
- Acute intermittent porphyria*

*See Coma section

(Cont'd on p 377)

(Cont'd on p 377)

(Cont'd on p 377)

a hemiparesis contralateral to the seizure focus, lasting less than 24 hours (although atypical cases can last longer). Patients are initially hypotonic and may have asymmetric reflexes. In patients with a known history of Todd's paralysis and seizure, the diagnosis is confirmed, and watchful resolution of the paralysis is all that is indicated as long as the typical resolution pattern is observed. In patients without a known seizure disorder or an atypical course, caution must be taken, as seizures can be associated with a structural abnormality such as stroke or tumor.

7. Hemiplegic migraine: Hemiplegic migraine is a common cause of hemiparesis. As the majority of these channelopathies are inherited in an autosomal dominant pattern, a family history aids in confirming the diagnosis. The high morbidity of alternative considerations underscores the importance of urgent brain imaging and further evaluation if the diagnosis is uncertain.

C. Unilateral Weakness without Cortical Involvement: Acute onset of unilateral weakness without evidence of brain or spinal cord disease may be caused by lower motor neuron dysfunction involving the peripheral nerve, plexus, or nerve root. There is often a suggestive history of trauma or compressive injury at the affected site. The distinct pattern of motor/sensory changes should localize the abnormality, and reflexes are often depressed in lower motor neuron diseases. Imaging of the spine and nerve roots, as well as electromyogram/nerve conduction studies (EMG/NCS), should be considered. In contrast, brisk reflexes, upgoing plantar reflex, seizures, and speech or mental status changes should prompt consideration of cortical involvement. Acute bilateral weakness with bowel/bladder changes should prompt emergent evaluation for spinal cord disease.

1. Neuropathy: Decreased reflexes, weakness, and hypotonia suggest peripheral nerve involvement, especially when the distribution of weakness and sensory findings follow a known nerve distribution. In addition, the mechanism of injury may also be suggestive. Common presentations of focal neuropathy in children include wrist drop from radial injury and foot drop in peroneal nerve injury.
2. Plexopathy: Plexopathies present with similar signs and symptoms as a neuropathy but are often more extensive and more painful. Common causes include hematoma, tumor (i.e., neurofibroma), radiation, or trauma. Diffuse weakness presents in the distribution of the plexus with associated pain and sensory changes. If the cause is unclear, MRI should be considered. The most common cause of plexopathy in the pediatric population is birth trauma. Erb palsy (upper brachial plexus injury) should be considered in large infants born with shoulder dystocia. An infant may show an asymmetric Moro reflex with flaccid monoparesis. The arm is extended at the elbow with a classic "waiter's tip" appearance. Most neonates improve without intervention.
3. Radiculopathy: Radiculopathy is often caused by spondylosis or disc herniation in adults, but is more often associated with tumor or other space-occupying lesions in children. Dysfunction of the nerve root typically causes partial (not complete) weakness of a limb and sensory changes that follow a dermatomal pattern. Examination reveals decreased reflexes in the roots involved. Injury that extends into the cord may cause brisk reflexes at the levels below the roots involved. Imaging of the cord should be considered in all radiculopathies.
4. Bell's palsy: Unilateral facial weakness is a unique and frequent cause of focal neurologic deficit in children, usually caused by an idiopathic, postinfectious entity termed *Bell's palsy.* The diagnosis of Bell's palsy has three key features: (1) involvement of the eye to assure that the lesion is truly a VIIth nerve abnormality, (2) a lack of any other cranial nerve involvement, and (3) consideration of another systemic condition (such as Guillain-Barré syndrome or Lyme disease) that can cause a VIIth nerve palsy. Examination reveals a unilateral weakness of the face that involves a unilaterally asymmetric smile and decreased nasolabial fold. Impaired eye closed on the affected side is essential to the diagnosis, and if not present should lead to urgent consideration of a central process. History usually reveals a sudden onset. If there is fever, diminished reflexes, or additional focal neurologic symptoms/signs (such as diplopia and a VIth nerve palsy), an alternative diagnosis must be made. Treatment is controversial, although if the child presents within 72 to 96 hours, the practitioner should strongly consider the use of prednisone and acyclovir (especially if there are herpetic lesions in the ear canal) therapy. Patching and the use of artificial tears in the affected eye are essential if the eye cannot be fully closed.

D. Bilateral Weakness without Cortical Involvement: Acute bilateral weakness, without signs or symptoms of cortical or spinal cord involvement, often localizes to nerve, neuromuscular junction, or muscle. The preservation of reflexes suggests a myopathic or neuromuscular junction disease, although reflexes are sometimes preserved in the early phase of neuropathic disease. In many of these diseases, such as myasthenia gravis, botulism, and spinal muscular atrophy, close monitoring for respiratory compromise is essential.

1. Nerve: The most common cause of acute bilateral weakness in children is acute inflammatory demyelinating polyradiculoneuropathy, also known as Guillain-Barré syndrome. Typically, children present with symmetric, ascending weakness and decreased or absent reflexes. Dysesthesias and bilateral facial weakness may also be seen, especially in sensory or Miller Fisher variants. A thorough history may reveal a recent respiratory or gastrointestinal infection, and LP classically shows an increase of protein in the absence of pleocytosis. Other considerations for this presentation include new-onset chronic inflammatory demyelinating polyradiculoneuropathy or spinal muscular atrophy in infants.
2. Neuromuscular junction: Patients with neuromuscular junction disease typically present with diffuse weakness that worsens throughout the day and with exercise. The two most common causes of neuromuscular weakness in children are myasthenia gravis and botulism toxin. In myasthenia gravis, the initial presentation may be associated with intercurrent illness. Most commonly, patients present with a combination of cranial nerve weakness and fluctuating/fatigable weakness. Observation in the evening hours and maneuvers that facilitate fatigue may demonstrate increasing weakness. Serum acetylcholine receptor antibody is specific for myasthenia gravis. In botulism, facial weakness, ophthalmoplegia, and poorly responsive pupils accompany diffuse descending weakness.
3. Muscle: Patients with acute myopathic disease usually present with diffuse weakness, accompanied by preserved (or slightly diminished) reflexes and increased muscle enzymes. Bilateral symmetric weakness with

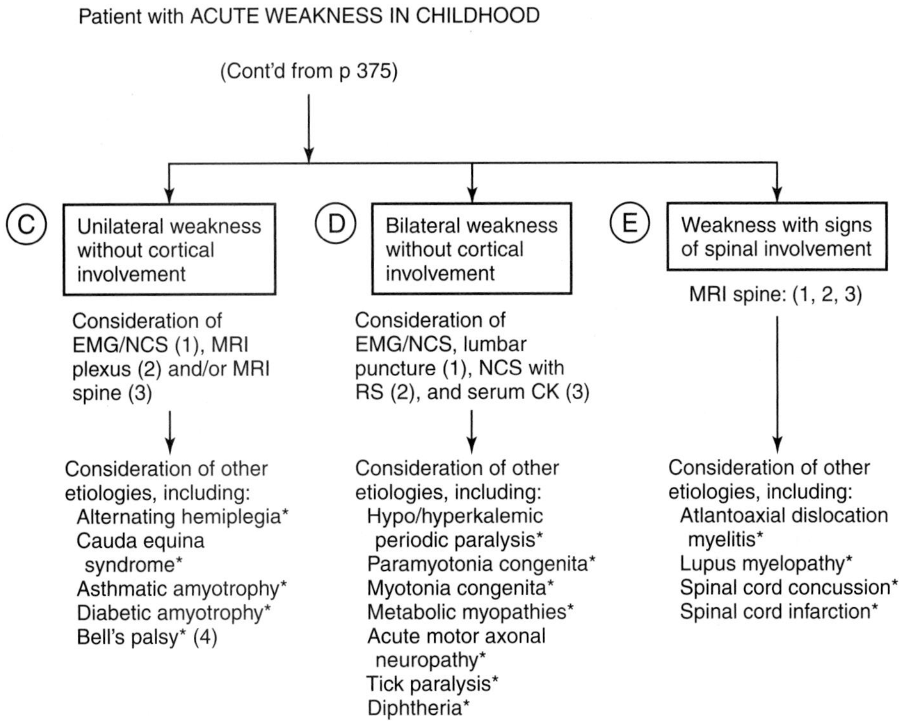
Patient with ACUTE WEAKNESS IN CHILDHOOD
(Cont'd from p 375)
C
Unilateral weakness without cortical involvement
Consideration of EMG/NCS (1), MRI plexus (2) and/or MRI spine (3)
Consideration of other etiologies, including:
Alternating hemiplegia*
Cauda equina syndrome*
Asthmatic amyotrophy*
Diabetic amyotrophy*
Bell's palsy* (4)
D
Bilateral weakness without cortical involvement
Consideration of EMG/NCS, lumbar puncture (1), NCS with RS (2), and serum CK (3)
Consideration of other etiologies, including:
Hypo/hyperkalemic periodic paralysis*
Paramyotonia congenita*
Myotonia congenita*
Metabolic myopathies*
Acute motor axonal neuropathy*
Tick paralysis*
Diphtheria*
E
Weakness with signs of spinal involvement
MRI spine: (1, 2, 3)
Consideration of other etiologies, including:
Atlantoaxial dislocation myelitis*
Lupus myelopathy*
Spinal cord concussion*
Spinal cord infarction*

myalgia should prompt consideration of a myositis. In acute infectious myositis, a history of preceding infection may be elicited and creatine kinase (CK) values are increased. Symmetric, proximal muscle weakness associated with myalgias and skin changes (Gottron papules along knuckles, malar rash or heliotropic rash on upper eyelids) should prompt evaluation for dermatomyositis.

E. Weakness with Signs of Spinal Involvement: Patients with acute bilateral weakness caused by spinal cord disease classically show reflexes that are increased in the lower extremities, an upgoing Babinski, and incontinence of bowel or bladder. Spinal shock and diseases of the conus medullaris can diverge from this pattern. A sensory level following dermatomal patterns may also be seen, and if the lesion is above T10, abdominal reflexes are absent. Children with weakness may refuse to walk or stand. Asymmetric spinal cord disease, as well as epidural disease, may present with unilateral weakness.

1. Myelopathy: Patients with intrinsic spinal cord disease often present with bilateral weakness and a sensory level. Imaging of the spinal cord should readily identify an abnormality (often a T2 hyperintensity with cord swelling), but it is often challenging to differentiate between transverse myelitis, MS, and neuromyelitis optica. These conditions are often preceded by viral illness, and cerebrospinal fluid studies sometimes show a lymphocytic pleocytosis with normal glucose and increased protein. Infections, intramedullary tumors, and cord infarction can also have a similar presentation and appearance on MRI. MRI of the brain and a cerebrospinal fluid profile with oligoclonal bands may be helpful in the diagnosis of MS, whereas serum neuromyelitis optica IgG antibodies are specific for neuromyelitis optica.

2. Epidural: Diseases of the epidural space initially cause symptoms attributable to nerve root irritation such as back pain and dermatomal sensory loss. However, these signs and symptoms may evolve to include symptomatology reflective of progressive extrinsic spinal cord compression (i.e., weakness, sensory level, and bowel and bladder dysfunction). Symptoms often present asymmetrically and may evade prompt localization. Caution should be used as tumors, infection, and hemorrhage can invade the epidural space, causing a neurologic emergency. MRI confirms the diagnosis.

3. Conus medullaris: Lesions in the conus medullaris are somewhat atypical of spinal cord disease because they may present with diminished reflexes and perianal numbness. For this reason, bowel and/or bladder incontinence is often the pertinent historical feature. Tumors, myelitis, and demyelinating disease can all present in the conus.

References

Bradley WG, Daroff RB, et al. Neurology in clinical practice: principles of diagnosis and management. 4th ed. Philadelphia: Butterworth Heinemann; 2004.

Brinar VV, Habek M, Brinar M, et al. The differential diagnosis of acute transverse myelitis. Clin Neurol Neurosurg 2006;108(3):278–83.

Compeyrot-Lacassagne S, Feldman BM. Inflammatory myopathies in children. Rheum Dis Clin North Am 2007;33:525.

Darouiche RO. Spinal epidural abscess. N Engl J Med 2006;355(19): 2012–20.

Fenichel G. Clinical pediatric neurology: a signs and symptoms approach. 4th ed. Philadelphia: WB Saunders Company; 2001.

Francisco AM, Arnon SS. Clinical mimics of infant botulism. Pediatrics 2007;119:826.

Hahn JS, Pohl D, Rensel M, Rao S. Differential diagnosis and evaluation in pediatric multiple sclerosis. Neurology 2007;68:S13.

Hay WW, Hayward AR, Levin MJ, et al. Current pediatric diagnosis and treatment. 16th ed. New York: McGraw-Hill Company; 2003.

Korinthenberg R, Schessl J, Kirschner J. Clinical presentation and course of childhood Guillain-Barré syndrome: a prospective multicentre study. Neuropediatrics 2007;38:10.

Ophthalmology

Evaluation of Poor Vision

Carolyn K. Pan, MD, and Scott C. N. Oliver, MD

A. History: A detailed history of present illness is imperative to determine time of onset of vision loss. This helps to distinguish between congenital and acquired causative factors. Medical history is always important, and one must be sure to include prenatal, perinatal, and postnatal development. Ocular history can be difficult to obtain in younger children. Parents' observations can reveal valuable information. Some questions that may be useful to ask include: Does your child seem to see well? Do your child's eyes appear straight, or do they seem to cross or drift or seem lazy? Have you noticed anything unusual in the appearance of your child's eyes? Do the eyelids droop, or does one eyelid tend to close? Has there been any trauma to your child's eyes? A family ocular history is essential (i.e., neoplasms, early use of glasses in parents or siblings, poor night vision), and a family history of general developmental problems, systemic abnormalities, neurologic disorders, and medication use is also helpful.

B. Physical Examination: The first part to any eye examination is to simply observe the child. Inspect the lids and periorbital area for swelling, redness, and drainage. Be sure to note any asymmetry in palpebral fissures. Discoloration of the conjunctiva and sclera, corneal opacities, and iris abnormalities should also be noted.

C. Assess Visual Acuity Changes with the Age of the Child:

1. In newborns, presence of vision may be demonstrated by pupil responses or by aversion to bright lights.
2. Children younger than 3 years (but older than 3 months of age) or any nonverbal child are examined by evaluating the child's ability to fixate and follow objects. A sign of poor vision in one eye is objection to covering the fellow (better) eye.
3. Children older than 3 years can be evaluated with picture tests and Allen cards. In school-aged children, wall charts containing Snellen letters/numbers, tumbling Es, and the HOTV test may be used.
4. Each eye should be tested individually with occlusion of the fellow eye.

D. Examine Ocular Motility: If misalignment is a concern, the corneal light reflex (Hirschberg test) should be performed. A penlight is held 2 feet in front of the face with the child fixating on the light. The corneal light reflex should be symmetric and appear in the center of both pupils. The pupils should be equal, round, and reactive to light in both eyes. Red reflex examination should also be performed to detect any opacities in the visual axis. In a darkened room, the direct ophthalmoscope (set at *zero*) held 12 to 18 inches away from the eye should be focused on each pupil. Then both eyes are viewed simultaneously at a distance of 3 feet. The red reflex should be bright red-yellow and identical in both eyes. Asymmetry of the red reflex, lack of red reflex, or presence of a white reflex are all indications for ophthalmic consultation. Ophthalmoscopy at a distance of 6 to 12 inches should be attempted on children older than 3 years to evaluate the optic nerve and retinal vasculature in the posterior pole of the eye.

E. The visual pathway continues to develop throughout early childhood. Many childhood eye problems can affect the development and result in vision loss. Therefore, early detection and referral to a pediatric ophthalmologist is imperative.

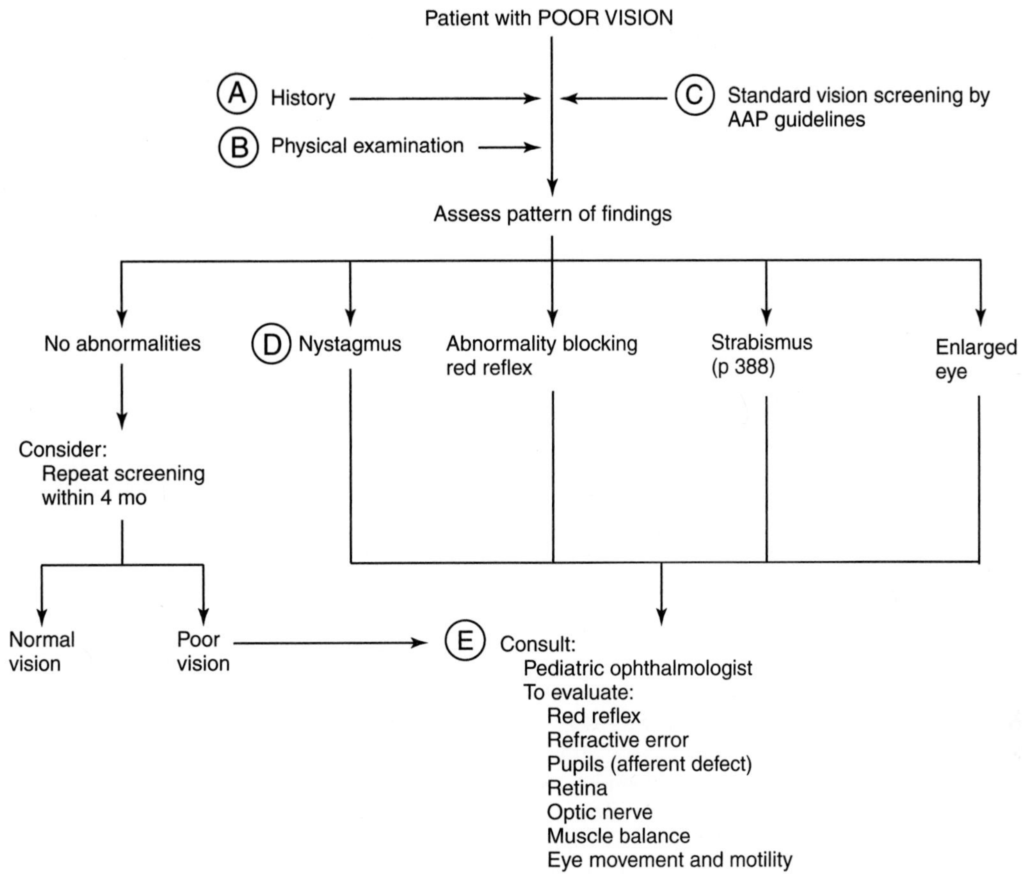
Patient with POOR VISION
A History
B Physical examination
C Standard vision screening by AAP guidelines
Assess pattern of findings
No abnormalities
D Nystagmus
Abnormality blocking red reflex
Strabismus (p 388)
Enlarged eye
Consider: Repeat screening within 4 mo
Normal vision
Poor vision
E Consult: Pediatric ophthalmologist
To evaluate:
Red reflex
Refractive error
Pupils (afferent defect)
Retina
Optic nerve
Muscle balance
Eye movement and motility

References

American Academy of Pediatrics Policy Statement. Eye Examination in Infants, Children, and Young Adults by Pediatricians. Ophthalmology 2003;110:860–5.

Pediatric ophthalmology and strabismus. 2008-2009 ed. Vol. 6, Basic and clinical science course. San Francisco: American Academy of Ophthalmology; 2008.

Prentiss K, Dorfman D. Pediatric ophthalmology in the emergency department. Emerg Med Clin North Am 2008;26:181–98.

Periorbital (Preseptal) Cellulitis

Carolyn K. Pan, MD, and Scott C. N. Oliver, MD

Periorbital (preseptal) cellulitis is defined as inflammation and infection confined to the eyelids and periorbital structures anterior to the orbital septum. It usually results from direct inoculation of pathogen after trauma. It can also result from an associated skin infection (i.e., hordeolum [stye] or blepharitis [lid margin inflammation]). It may also result from nasolacrimal duct obstruction, leading to dacryocystitis and subsequent cellulitis. *Staphylococcus aureus* and *Streptococcus* are the most common pathogens. *Haemophilus influenzae* may be associated with an upper respiratory infection; however, it is less common in areas with high rates of immunization.

A. History and Physical Examination: Edema, erythema, induration, tenderness, and/or warmth of the periorbital area are frequently seen. A patient may have a history of trauma, insect bites, or hordeolum. A fluctuant abscess near the medial canthus is suspicious for dacryocystitis. There is no proptosis of the globe, no decreased vision, no restriction of extraocular motility, and no pain with eye movement. A patient may present with a fever, but other signs of systemic illness are often absent (See Table 1).

B. Evaluation: Consider complete blood cell count (CBC) with differential and Gram stain and culture any open wound or drainage. Perform computed tomographic (CT) scan of the brain and orbits (with both axial and coronal views) with and without intravenous (IV) contrast if there is suspicion for orbital cellulitis or history of trauma with suspected retained orbital foreign body. If patient appears toxic, a full systemic evaluation for sepsis should be performed.

C. Treatment: Outpatient therapy is usually appropriate. Treatment includes broad-spectrum oral antibiotics targeted against Gram-positive bacteria and *H. influenzae* (i.e., amoxicillin-clavulanate). A 7- to 10-day course of treatment is appropriate. Criteria for admission and intravenous antibiotics (ampicillin/sulbactam is usually initial therapy): Patient appears toxic, may be noncompliant with outpatient treatment and follow-up, failure to respond to oral antibiotic therapy after 24 to 48 hours, and patient younger than 5 years. In penicillin-allergic patients, trimethoprim/sulfamethoxazole and moxifloxacin may be reasonable alternatives. If there is uncertainty about antibiotic coverage, consult local pharmacist or infectious disease specialist to assist in the selection of an appropriate antimicrobial agent. Surgical drainage may be required if a fluctuant mass/abscess is present (See Table 2).

Table 1. **Degree of Illness in Periorbital Cellulitis**

Moderate	Severe	Very Severe
Temperature <38.5°C without associated systemic symptoms	Temperature ≥38.5°C or systemic symptoms or severe pain or headache	Altered mental status or signs of meningitis or focal neurologic, signs or seizures or signs of shock

Table 2. **Antibiotic Therapy for Periorbital Cellulitis in Children**

Drug	Dosage	Product Availability
Oral Antibiotics		
Amoxicillin-clavulanate (Augmentin) ES	25–30 mg/kg/dose tid	Liquid: 600 mg/5 ml Tablets (slow-release 2 g)
Cefdinir (Omnicef)	7 mg/kg/dose bid (maximum dose: 600 mg)	Suspension: 125 mg/5 ml Capsules: 300 mg Tablets: 200, 400 mg
Cefpodoxime (Vantin)	5 mg/kg/dose bid	Suspension: 50 mg/5 ml, 100 mg/5 ml 100-mg tabs
Intravenous Antibiotics for Hospitalized Patients		
Cefotaxime (Claforan)	50 mg/kg/dose q8h	Vials: 0.5, 1, 2 g
Ceftriaxone (Rocephin)	50 mg/kg/dose q12-24h	Vials: 0.25, 0.5, 1 g
Clindamycin (Cleocin)	10 mg/kg/dose q6-8h	Ampules: 0.15, 0.3, 0.6 g
Nafcillin	25–50 mg/kg/dose q6h (maximum: 12 g)	Vials: 0.5, 1, 2 g
Oxacillin (Prostaphlin)	50 mg/kg/dose q6h	Vials: 500 mg, 1 g

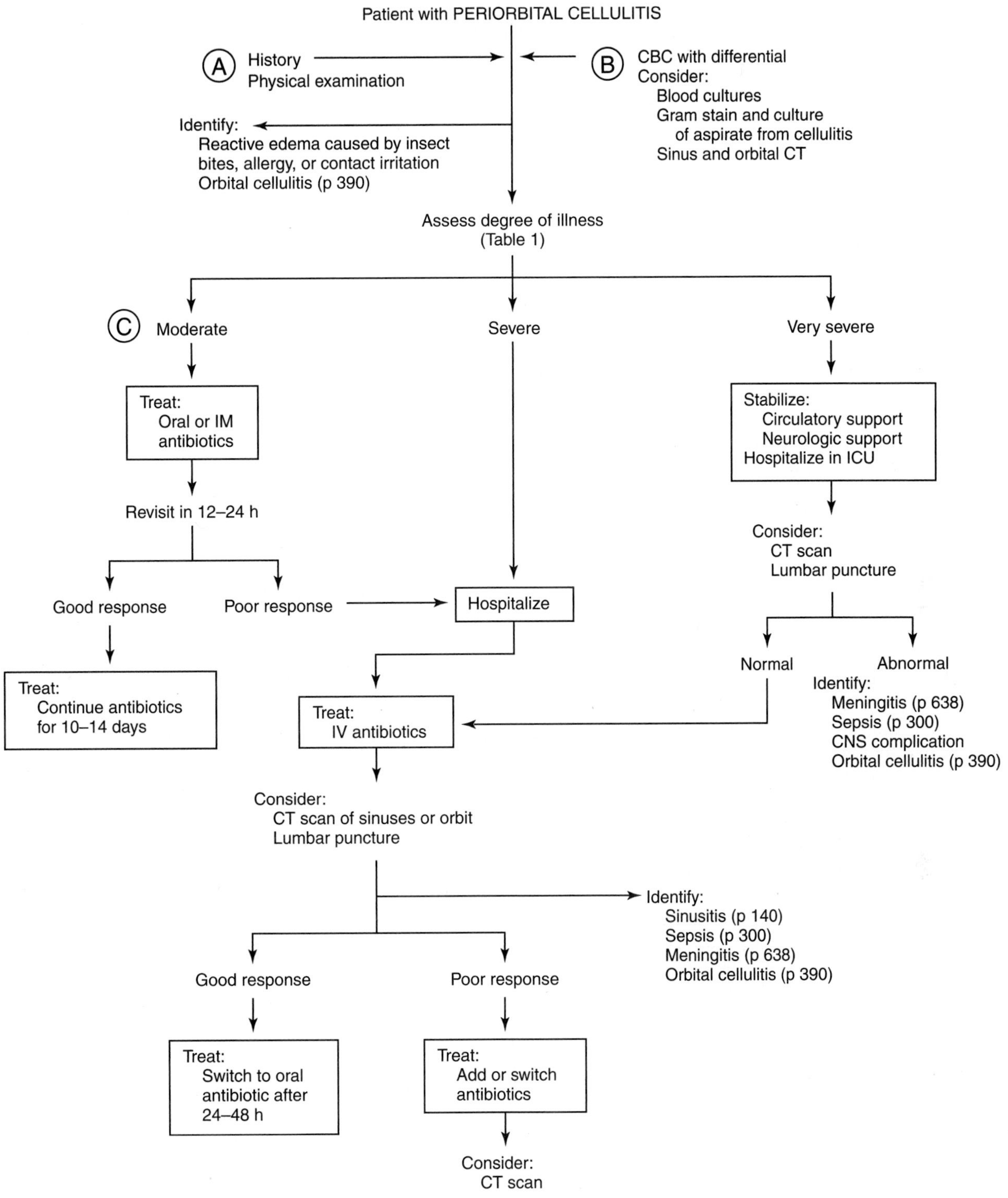
Patient with PERIORBITAL CELLULITIS
A History
Physical examination
B CBC with differential
Consider:
Blood cultures
Gram stain and culture
of aspirate from cellulitis
Sinus and orbital CT
Identify:
Reactive edema caused by insect
bites, allergy, or contact irritation
Orbital cellulitis (p 390)
Assess degree of illness
(Table 1)
C Moderate
Severe
Very severe
Treat:
Oral or IM
antibiotics
Revisit in 12–24 h
Good response
Poor response
Treat:
Continue antibiotics
for 10–14 days
Hospitalize
Stabilize:
Circulatory support
Neurologic support
Hospitalize in ICU
Consider:
CT scan
Lumbar puncture
Normal
Abnormal
Identify:
Meningitis (p 638)
Sepsis (p 300)
CNS complication
Orbital cellulitis (p 390)
Treat:
IV antibiotics
Consider:
CT scan of sinuses or orbit
Lumbar puncture
Identify:
Sinusitis (p 140)
Sepsis (p 300)
Meningitis (p 638)
Orbital cellulitis (p 390)
Good response
Poor response
Treat:
Switch to oral
antibiotic after
24–48 h
Treat:
Add or switch
antibiotics
Consider:
CT scan

References

Ehlers JP, Shah CP, Fenton GL, Hoskins EN. Wills Eye manual office and emergency room diagnosis and treatment of eye disease. Philadelphia: Lippincott Williams & Wilkins; 2008.

Givner L. Periorbital versus orbital cellulitis. Pediatr Infect Dis J 2002;21(12):1157–8.

Jain A, Rubin P. Orbital cellulitis in children. Int Ophthalmol Clin 2001;41(4):71–86.

Prentiss K, Dorfman D. Pediatric ophthalmology in the emergency department. Emerg Med Clin North Am 2008;26:181–98.

Tovilla-Canales J, Nava A, Tovilla y Pomar JL. Orbital and periorbital infections. Curr Opin Ophthalmol 2001;12:335–41.

Conjunctivitis/Red, Painful Eyes

Leo K. Seibold, MD, and Scott C. N. Oliver, MD

Conjunctivitis is a general term used to describe any inflammation of the conjunctiva that typically results in a red eye. There are numerous causative factors, such as bacterial, viral, chlamydial, allergic, vernal/atopic, drug/toxin/chemical reaction, scleritis/episcleritis, trauma, foreign body, nasolacrimal duct obstruction and subconjunctival hemorrhage.

The most frequent pathogens are:

- Bacterial: *Staphylococcus aureus, Staphylococcus epidermidis, Streptococcus pneumonia, Haemophilus influenzae, Neisseria gonorrhoeae*
- Viral: adenovirus, enterovirus, herpes simplex virus, herpes zoster virus
- Chlamydial: *Chlamydia trachomatis*
- Ophthalmia neonatorum: chemical (<24 hours from birth), *N. gonorrhoeae* (<1 week of age), *C. trachomatis* (1–3 weeks of age)

A. History and Physical Examination: All forms of conjunctivitis present with conjunctival hyperemia or "red eye." They may have varying degrees of tearing, discomfort, chemosis, discharge, foreign body sensation, and duration. Severe ocular pain, photophobia, and profoundly decreased vision are not typical findings in conjunctivitis and suggest a more serious cause. The initial diagnostic approach to a patient with conjunctivitis should begin by eliminating other causes of a red eye including trauma, iritis, keratitis, glaucoma, corneal abrasion, measles, Kawasaki disease, scleritis/episcleritis, and others. A complete history and physical examination should be performed including a detailed ocular examination. Important aspects of the history include age of child, duration of symptoms, sick contacts, prior episodes, allergy symptoms, presence of pain or photophobia, recent trauma, and drug/chemical exposures. Important examination findings to look for include decreased visual acuity, elevated intraocular pressure, corneal opacity or fluorescein uptake, follicles/papillae along palpebral conjunctiva, discharge/tearing, anterior chamber inflammation, eyelid edema/erythema, skin lesions or vesicles, and palpable preauricular lymph nodes.

Some clues to the cause include:

- Bacterial: Foreign body sensation, purulent yellow-white discharge, minimal itching
- Gonococcal: Severe purulent discharge, sudden onset (<12–24 hours), chemosis, papillae
- Viral: Foreign body sensation, itching, follicles, watery discharge, membranes/pseudomembranes, subepithelial infiltrates, palpable preauricular lymph node, and history of recent upper respiratory infection symptoms or sick contact
- Chlamydial: Newborns aged 1 to 4 weeks or sexually active teenagers, inferior follicles, palpable preauricular node, stringy mucous discharge
- Allergic: Intense itching, watery discharge, chemosis, papillae, and a history of allergies
- Vernal/Atopic: Intense itching, thick/ropy discharge, large conjunctival papillae, superior corneal "shield ulcer," and seasonal recurrence in young male individuals
- Herpetic: Pain, photophobia, watery discharge, vesicular skin rash, and history of previous episodes or cold sores
- Toxin/Drug/Chemical: Follicles and history of topical medication use or chemical/toxin exposure
- Ophthalmia neonatorum: Onset <1 month of age, purulent or mucoid discharge
- Subconjunctival hemorrhage: Usually asymptomatic with deep red blood under the conjunctiva completely obscuring view of the sclera, usually in one sector
- Nasolacrimal duct obstruction: Copious tearing, medial eyelid erythema/redness/swelling, reflux of mucopurulent material from punctum with pressure to the lacrimal sac, onset within first 2 months of life
- Gonococcal conjunctivitis: Conjunctival scrapings for urgent Gram stain and culture/sensitivities (blood and chocolate agar)
- Chlamydial conjunctivitis: Conjunctival scrapings for polymerase chain reaction or immunofluorescent antibody test and Giemsa stain looking for basophilic intracytoplasmic inclusion bodies
- Nasolacrimal duct obstruction: Digital palpation of lacrimal sac looking for purulent reflux from punctum, which is diagnostic; placement of fluorescein dye in both eyes and monitoring for disappearance of dye; dye will remain in eye after 10 minutes if obstruction is present
- Ophthalmia neonatorum: Gram stain, Giemsa stain, polymerase chain reaction or antibody tests for chlamydia, conjunctival cultures (chocolate and blood agar), and viral cultures

TREATMENT

B. Hordeolum/Chalazion: Includes warm compresses and can consider lid scrubs.

C. Herpes Simplex: Immediate pediatric ophthalmologist consultation for evaluation and initiate treatment with acyclovir.

D. Viral: Usually self-limited but highly contagious. Cool compresses, artificial tears, and topical antihistamine

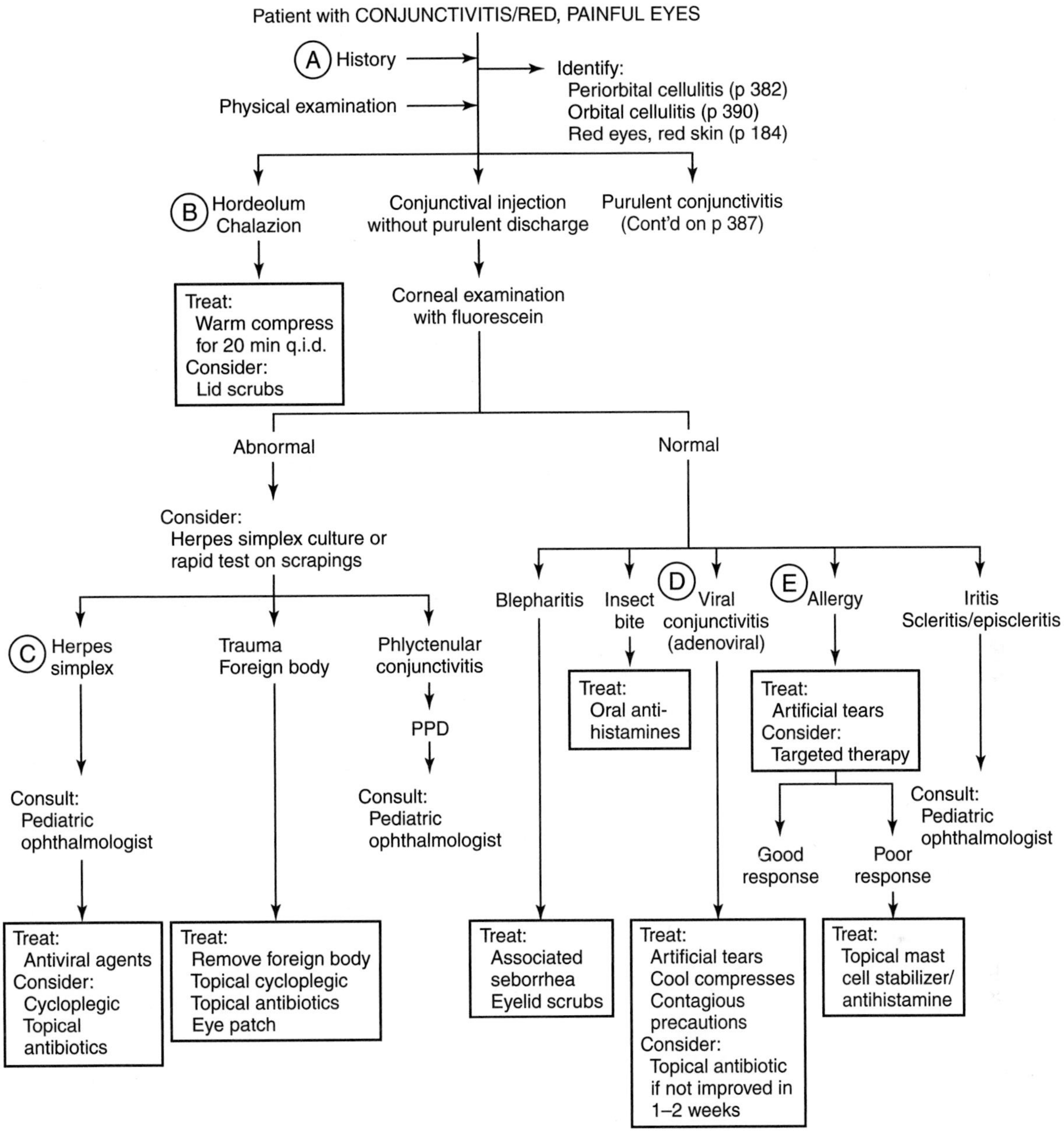
Patient with CONJUNCTIVITIS/RED, PAINFUL EYES
A History
Physical examination
Identify:
Periorbital cellulitis (p 382)
Orbital cellulitis (p 390)
Red eyes, red skin (p 184)
B Hordeolum
Chalazion
Conjunctival injection
without purulent discharge
Purulent conjunctivitis
(Cont'd on p 387)
Treat:
Warm compress
for 20 min q.i.d.
Consider:
Lid scrubs
Corneal examination
with fluorescein
Abnormal
Normal
Consider:
Herpes simplex culture or
rapid test on scrapings
C Herpes simplex
Trauma
Foreign body
Phlyctenular
conjunctivitis
PPD
Consult:
Pediatric
ophthalmologist
Consult:
Pediatric
ophthalmologist
Treat:
Antiviral agents
Consider:
Cycloplegic
Topical
antibiotics
Treat:
Remove foreign body
Topical cycloplegic
Topical antibiotics
Eye patch
Blepharitis
Insect
bite
D Viral
conjunctivitis
(adenoviral)
E Allergy
Iritis
Scleritis/episcleritis
Treat:
Oral anti-
histamines
Treat:
Artificial tears
Consider:
Targeted therapy
Consult:
Pediatric
ophthalmologist
Good
response
Poor
response
Treat:
Associated
seborrhea
Eyelid scrubs
Treat:
Artificial tears
Cool compresses
Contagious
precautions
Consider:
Topical antibiotic
if not improved in
1–2 weeks
Treat:
Topical mast
cell stabilizer/
antihistamine

for symptomatic relief. Patient/parent education on frequent hand washing, avoidance of touching/rubbing eyes, shaking hands, and so forth.

E. Allergic: Elimination/avoidance of inciting agent if possible, cool compresses, artificial tears, topical antihistamines (olopatadine, epinastine, ketotifen, etc.). Moderate to severe cases may require mild topical steroid (fluorometholone, loteprednol) and oral antihistamines (diphenhydramine, loratadine). Vernal/Atopic: Similar treatment as allergic conjunctivitis. Patients should be given prophylactic mast cell stabilizer (lodoxamide or pemirolast) and/or antihistamine 2 to 3 weeks before inciting season starts. If a shield ulcer is present, a topical steroid, antibiotic, and cycloplegic agent should be added.

F. Drug/Toxin/Chemical Reaction: Discontinue/avoid inciting agent and artificial tears PRN to treat irritation.

G. Chlamydia: Oral (PO) antibiotics (azithromycin or erythromycin), topical erythromycin, and treatment of sexual partners if applicable.

H. Ophthalmia Neonatorum: If chemical suspected, observation with artificial tears. If chlamydia suspected, erythromycin PO for 14 days and treatment of mother/sexual partner. If gonorrhea suspected, hospitalize patient and monitor for systemic disease, frequent saline irrigation, intravenous or intramuscular ceftriaxone, bacitracin ointment, and treat chlamydial coinfection.

I. Nasolacrimal Duct Obstruction: Digital pressure to lacrimal sac qid, topical antibiotic if mucopurulent discharge is present, and systemic antibiotics if acute dacryocystitis (red, swollen, painful sac). Ninety percent of cases will resolve by 1 year of age. If conservative treatment fails, nasolacrimal duct probing or surgery may be performed.

J. Bacterial: Topical antibiotics qid (trimethoprim/polymyxin B or fluoroquinolone) for 1 week with adjustment of regimen based on cultures, if taken. *H. influenzae* should be treated with amoxicillin/clavulanate because of possible extraocular involvement.

K. Ophthalmologic consultation is always warranted for nasolacrimal duct obstruction, ophthalmia neonatorum, and gonococcal, herpes zoster, or herpes simplex conjunctivitis.

References

Ehlers JP, Shah CP, Fenton GL, Hoskins EN. Wills Eye manual office and emergency room diagnosis and treatment of eye disease. Philadelphia: Lippincott Williams & Wilkins; 2008.

Pediatric ophthalmology and strabismus. 2008-2009 ed. Vol. 6, Basic and clinical science course. San Francisco: American Academy of Ophthalmology; 2008.

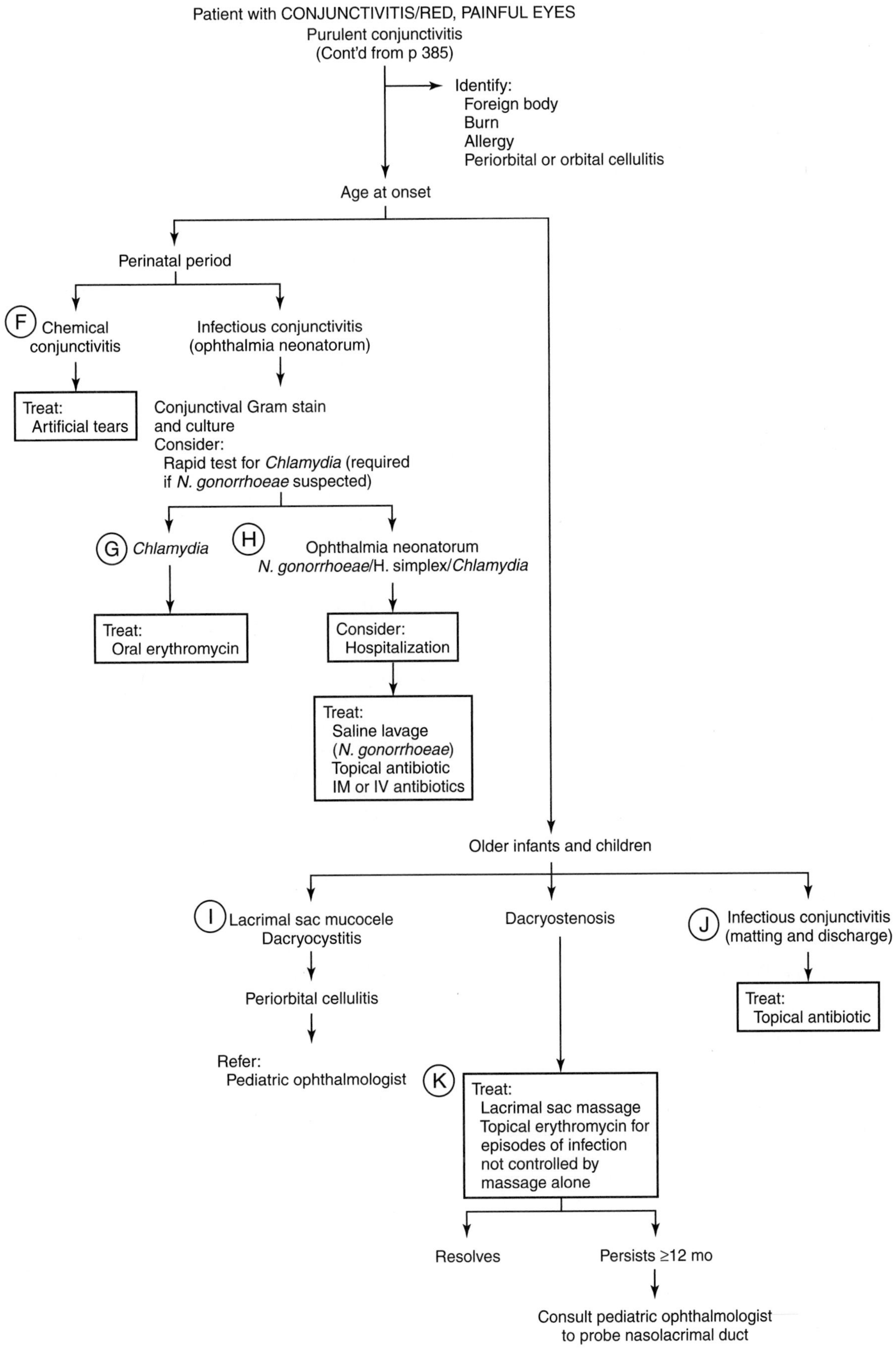
Patient with CONJUNCTIVITIS/RED, PAINFUL EYES
Purulent conjunctivitis
(Cont'd from p 385)
Identify:
Foreign body
Burn
Allergy
Periorbital or orbital cellulitis
Age at onset
Perinatal period
F
Chemical conjunctivitis
Treat:
Artificial tears
Infectious conjunctivitis (ophthalmia neonatorum)
Conjunctival Gram stain and culture
Consider:
Rapid test for *Chlamydia* (required if *N. gonorrhoeae* suspected)
G
Chlamydia
Treat:
Oral erythromycin
H
Ophthalmia neonatorum
N. gonorrhoeae/H. simplex/*Chlamydia*
Consider:
Hospitalization
Treat:
Saline lavage (*N. gonorrhoeae*)
Topical antibiotic
IM or IV antibiotics
Older infants and children
I
Lacrimal sac mucocele
Dacryocystitis
Periorbital cellulitis
Refer:
Pediatric ophthalmologist
Dacryostenosis
K
Treat:
Lacrimal sac massage
Topical erythromycin for episodes of infection not controlled by massage alone
Resolves
Persists ≥12 mo
Consult pediatric ophthalmologist to probe nasolacrimal duct
J
Infectious conjunctivitis (matting and discharge)
Treat:
Topical antibiotic

Strabismus (Eye Misalignment)

Leo K. Seibold, MD, and Scott C. N. Oliver, MD

Strabismus is defined as any deviation of ocular alignment that may be caused by abnormal neuromuscular control of ocular motility or by abnormalities in binocular vision. An esodeviation describes any inward turning of the eye. An exodeviation describes any outward turning of the eye. Strabismus should be differentiated from amblyopia, which is a loss of vision that results from the failure of visual pathway development. Extraocular muscle immaturity (<3–4 months of age) is often seen.

Strabismus is often divided into the following categories:

- Comitant (nonparalytic): The amplitude of misalignment is constant in all directions of gaze
  - Congenital: Deviation manifests before 6 months of age
  - Accommodative: Esodeviation stimulated by the accommodative reflex
  - Intermittent: Deviation is intermittently controlled by fusion of images
  - Sensory deprivation: Secondary to poor vision in one or both eyes
  - Divergence or convergence insufficiency: Deviation that only occurs during distance or near fixation
  - Pseudoesotropia: Wide nasal bridge simulates esodeviation
- Incomitant (paralytic): The amplitude of misalignment changes with the direction of gaze
  - Serious neurologic disorder: Hydrocephalus, tumor, increased intracranial pressure
  - Muscle restriction: Entrapment in orbital wall fracture
  - Cranial nerve palsy: III, IV, or VI
  - Inflammation: Pseudotumor, thyroid disease, myositis, myasthenia gravis

A. History and Physical Examination: A detailed history is crucial in the evaluation and management of a child with strabismus. Pertinent questions to ask parents include:

1. Age of first onset (pictures may help)?
2. Is the deviation constant or intermittent?
3. If intermittent, under what conditions does the deviation occur?
4. Does it occur during distance or near vision?
5. Which eye is affected or does it alternate?
6. Any prior history of glasses, patching, eye drops, or eye muscle surgery?
7. Was onset associated with any trauma or illness?
8. Any family history of strabismus, amblyopia, patching, eye muscle surgery, or "lazy eye."

Complete ocular examination looking for decreased visual acuity, abnormal ocular motility, ocular misalignment (Hirschberg and cover-uncover test), proptosis, lid ptosis, nystagmus, and pupillary abnormalities. Complete cranial nerve examination and focused neurologic examination should be done. Either eye can be constantly or intermittently deviated from primary gaze. During cover-uncover test, the uncovered eye moves from deviated position to midline to fixate. Asymmetry of corneal light reflex can be seen on Hirschberg test. Subnormal vision in one eye unexplained by ocular disease can be seen. Ocular motility is limited in one or more directions of gaze. This evaluation can help determine whether strabismus is comitant or incomitant.

B. Evaluation: Laboratory workup for myasthenia gravis or thyroid disease as history/examination warrants. Consider brain/orbit imaging in cases associated with trauma, nerve palsies, or neurologic findings.

C. Treatment: All strabismus cases in children older than 4 months should be referred to a pediatric ophthalmologist on an outpatient basis. Neurologic consultation should be considered for any new-onset cranial nerve palsy or signs/symptoms of increased intracranial pressure. Treatment is usually dependent on the nature and frequency of the deviation, as well as the presence of amblyopia. Both surgical and nonsurgical interventions are used. Nonsurgical options include glasses, bifocals, patching, pharmacologic penalization, eye exercises (orthoptic therapy), and Botox injections. Eye muscle surgery is usually performed in conditions not likely to respond to conservative treatment. This usually involves tightening or loosening one or more rectus muscles to restore ocular alignment.

References

Ehlers JP, Shah CP, Fenton GL, Hoskins EN. Wills Eye manual office and emergency room diagnosis and treatment of eye disease. Philadelphia: Lippincott Williams & Wilkins; 2008.

Pediatric ophthalmology and strabismus. 2008-2009 ed. Vol. 6, Basic and clinical science course. San Francisco: American Academy of Ophthalmology; 2008.

Prentiss K, Dorfman D. Pediatric ophthalmology in the emergency department. Emerg Med Clin North Am 2008;26:181–98.

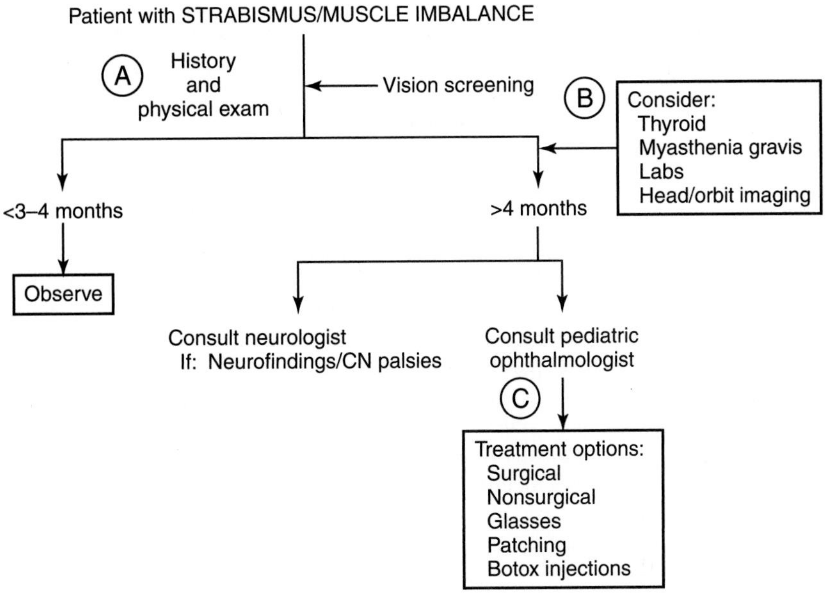
Patient with STRABISMUS/MUSCLE IMBALANCE
A
History and physical exam
Vision screening
B
Consider:
Thyroid
Myasthenia gravis
Labs
Head/orbit imaging
<3–4 months
Observe
>4 months
Consult neurologist
If: Neurofindings/CN palsies
Consult pediatric ophthalmologist
C
Treatment options:
Surgical
Nonsurgical
Glasses
Patching
Botox injections

Orbital Cellulitis or Abscess

Carolyn K. Pan, MD, and Scott C. N. Oliver, MD

In contrast with periorbital (preseptal) cellulitis, orbital cellulitis involves infection or inflammation posterior to the orbital septum. Greater than 90% of cases occur as secondary extension of bacterial sinusitis and can be either complications of orbital trauma, orbital surgery, or paranasal sinus surgery, or more commonly from vascular extension (i.e., from systemic bacteremia or septic thrombophlebitis from veins draining the sinuses). Multiple organisms have been identified as disease-causing pathogens, including gram-positive cocci *(Staphylococcus, Streptococcus), Haemophilus influenzae, Moraxella catarrhalis,* anaerobes, and fungi in immunocompromised patients (i.e., mucormycosis, aspergillus).

A. History and Physical Examination: Proptosis, chemosis, ptosis, fever, and restriction of and pain with ocular motility are frequently seen. Patient may have signs of compressive optic neuropathy, which includes decreased visual acuity, color vision, or pupillary abnormalities. There may also be resistance to retropulsion of the affected eye, as well an afferent papillary defect and elevation of intraocular pressure.

B. Evaluation: Computed tomography (CT) scan of the orbits and sinuses (axial and coronal views) with and without intravenous (IV) contrast should be obtained before ophthalmology consultation. Systemic workup with complete blood cell count (CBC; to assess for leukocytosis) and blood cultures should be obtained. It is recommended that a Gram stain and culture is sent from any drainage.

C. Obtain lumbar puncture if meningitis is suspected. Brain CT may also be required if brain abscess or cavernous sinus thrombosis is suspected.

D. Treatment: Integrated care with early involvement of ophthalmology, ear, nose, and throat (ENT), and infectious disease as needed. Most patients will need admission and inpatient monitoring. Criteria for mandatory admission include diplopia, proptosis, or ophthalmoplegia; reduced visual acuity; abnormal pupillary reflexes or abnormal swinging light test (presence of afferent pupillary defect); signs of central nervous system involvement; or systemic toxicity. Broad-spectrum IV antibiotics are used to cover gram-positive, gram-negative, and anaerobic organisms. Use a nasal decongestant spray if there is sinusitis on history/physical or imaging.

E. If there are signs of compressive optic neuropathy, immediate canthotomy/cantholysis should be performed by emergency department staff. Surgical decompression by ophthalmology and/or ENT may also be required if poor response to antibiotics.

References

Ehlers JP, Shah CP, Fenton GL, Hoskins EN. Wills Eye manual office and emergency room diagnosis and treatment of eye disease. Philadelphia: Lippincott Williams & Wilkins; 2008.

Givner L. Periorbital versus orbital cellulitis. Pediatr Infect Dis J 2002;21(12):1157–8.

Howe L, Jones NS. Guidelines of the management of periorbital cellulitis/abscess. Clin Otolaryngol 2004;29:725–8.

Jain A, Rubin P. Orbital cellulitis in children. Int Ophthalmol Clin 2001;41(4):71–86.

Orbit, eyelids, and lacrimal system. 2008-2009 ed. Vol. 7, Basic and clinical science course. San Francisco: American Academy of Ophthalmology; 2008.

Prentiss K, Dorfman D. Pediatric ophthalmology in the emergency department. Emerg Med Clin North Am 2008;26:181–98.

Tovilla-Canales J, Nava A, Tovilla y Pomar JL. Orbital and periorbital infections. Curr Opin Ophthalmol 2001;12:335–41.

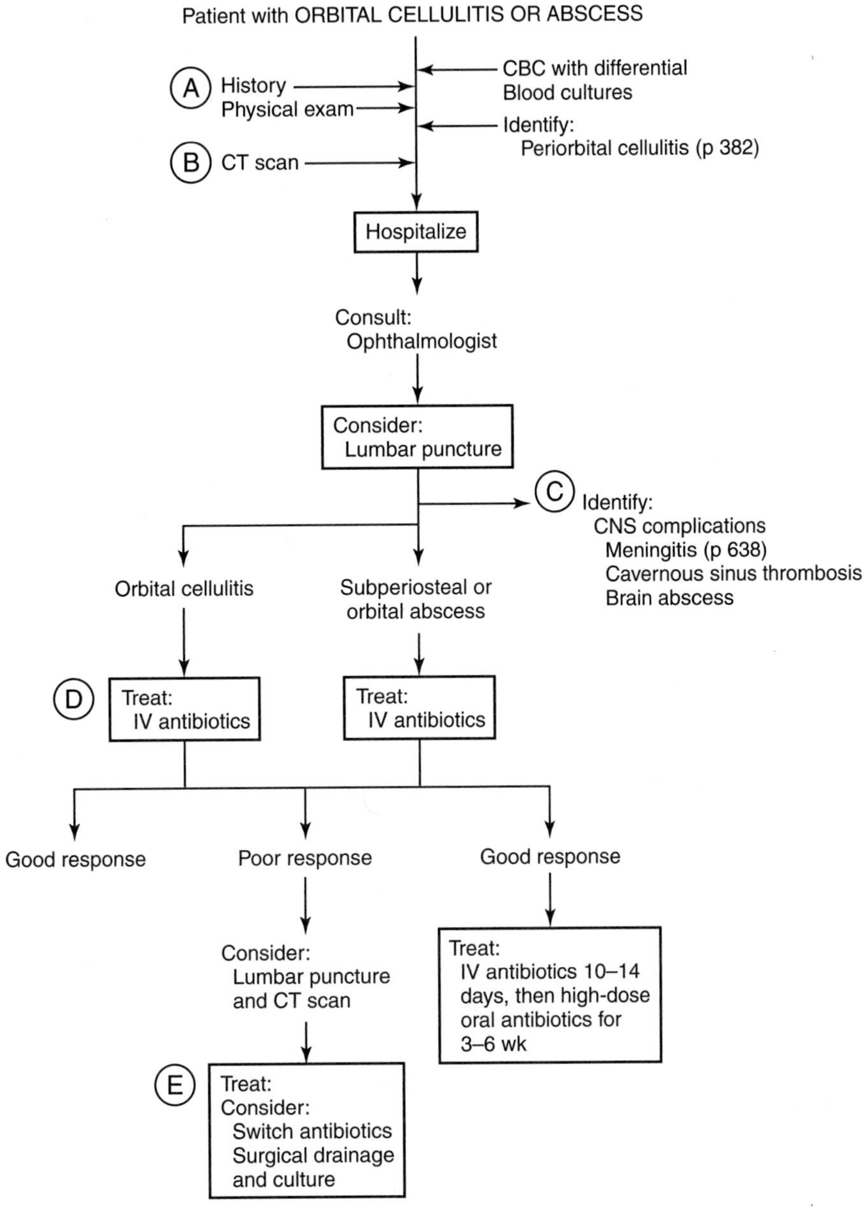
Patient with ORBITAL CELLULITIS OR ABSCESS
A
History
Physical exam
B
CT scan
CBC with differential
Blood cultures
Identify:
Periorbital cellulitis (p 382)
Hospitalize
Consult:
Ophthalmologist
Consider:
Lumbar puncture
C
Identify:
CNS complications
Meningitis (p 638)
Cavernous sinus thrombosis
Brain abscess
Orbital cellulitis
Subperiosteal or orbital abscess
D
Treat:
IV antibiotics
Treat:
IV antibiotics
Good response
Poor response
Good response
Consider:
Lumbar puncture and CT scan
Treat:
IV antibiotics 10–14 days, then high-dose oral antibiotics for 3–6 wk
E
Treat:
Consider:
Switch antibiotics
Surgical drainage and culture

PULMONARY

Evaluation of Cough and Pulmonary Disorders

Edith T. Zemanick, MD, MSCS, and Monica J. Federico, MD

A. In the history, ask the following: When did the cough begin? How long has the cough been present? Is it difficult for your child to breathe? Is there fast breathing? Wheezing or noisy breathing? Is there chest indrawing with breathing? Has your child turned blue or appeared very pale? Did you notice any time when your child stopped breathing? Is your child too weak to feed or play? Has your child had seizures or convulsions? Ask about the following: (1) presence and duration of upper respiratory symptoms, including runny nose (color), nasal congestion, earache, ear drainage, sore throat, difficulty swallowing, and hoarseness; (2) systemic symptoms, including fever, headache, muscle aches, malaise, vomiting, and diarrhea; (3) current use of medications and allergies to medications; (4) underlying pulmonary (asthma, bronchopulmonary dysplasia, cystic fibrosis, tracheomalacia), immunodeficiency (human immunodeficiency virus infection), or cardiac disease; and (5) immunization status. Ask about access to a telephone and transportation to the hospital, and assess the ability of the family to manage the child at home.

B. During the physical examination, count the respirations for 1 minute. Look for agitation or restlessness, chest indrawing or retractions, cyanosis, pallor, nasal flaring, drooling, purulent rhinorrhea, and ear discharge. Listen for hoarseness, stridor, wheezing, and grunting. With a stethoscope, identify signs of (1) bronchiolitis or asthma (wheezing, poor air exchange, prolongation of the expiratory phase of respiration); (2) pneumonia (rales, crepitations, tubular or decreased breath sounds); and (3) cardiac disease, such as an irregular heart rate (arrhythmia), abnormal heart sounds, a heart murmur, or a pericardial friction rub. Percuss the chest for dullness. Palpate and percuss the liver because hepatomegaly suggests right-sided heart failure. Use pneumatic otoscopy to assess tympanic membrane color, mobility, and landmarks. Use a tongue blade to examine the pharynx and tonsils for size, exudate, ulcerations, and other lesions. Examine the nares for purulent secretions, mucosal erythema or swelling, and nasal polyps. Evaluate the extremities for clubbing and cyanosis.

C. Mild illness has no findings of bacterial upper airway infection (acute sinusitis, otitis media) or lower respiratory involvement (no rales, wheezing, chest indrawing [retractions], stridor at rest, cyanosis, or apnea). Children with mild illness have good air exchange and respiratory rate less than 60 per minute in infants younger than 2 months, less than 50 per minute in infants 2 to 11 months, and less than 40 per minute in children 12 months and older. Treatment for mild upper respiratory infections is supportive. Recently, the U.S. Food and Drug Administration (FDA) recommended that over-the-counter cold and cough medicines not be used for children younger than 2 years because of lack of efficacy and risk for adverse effects. The FDA is now examining the use of these medicines in children 2 to 11 years of age. Some cold medication manufacturers voluntarily changed labeling to recommend medication not be given to children younger than 4 years.

D. Moderate illness presents with signs of lower respiratory tract involvement including wheezing, rales, mild retractions, stridor when agitated or feeding, and oxygen saturations greater than 90%. Possible diagnoses include pneumonia, bronchiolitis, croup, and asthma. Prolonged purulent nasal discharge (>10–14 days), fever, and sinus tenderness suggests acute bacterial sinusitis. Children at high risk for deterioration who need close follow-up not available at home include immunocompromised children; children with sickle cell disease, immunodeficiency disorders (steroid-treated or immunosuppressed children), severe malnutrition, and underlying cardiac or pulmonary disease (especially premature infants with bronchopulmonary dysplasia); and premature infants younger than 8 weeks with documented respiratory syncytial virus infection. Early in the course of illness, infants and children living in families with little or no means of communication or transportation who are at risk for deterioration should be considered severely ill.

E. Severe illness includes signs of respiratory distress: stridor at rest, respiratory rate more than 70 per minute, severe chest indrawing (marked retractions), cyanosis, grunting respirations, and oxygen saturation below 90% by pulse oximetry. Signs of respiratory distress in wheezing patients include poor response to inhaled bronchodilators and poor aeration. Signs of systemic toxicity include mental status changes (inability to feed or drink, lethargy and inability to arouse, disorientation) and dehydration with vascular instability (mottling, poor capillary refill, low blood pressure). Radiographic findings of pleural fluid, abscess, pneumatoceles, or extensive infiltrate indicate severe bacterial disease.

F. Very severe illness includes respiratory arrest or signs of impending respiratory failure, such as recurrent apnea, cyanosis unresponsive to oxygen, inability to maintain Pa_{O_2} greater than 55 mm Hg or oxygen saturation above 86% despite 100% oxygen through a nonrebreather face mask and inability to maintain P_{CO_2} less than 50 mm Hg. Signs of impending upper airway obstruction that signal very severe illness include stridor at rest with air hunger, restlessness, cyanosis, severe retractions, minimal air exchange, and a clinical presentation suggesting acute epiglottitis (severe sore throat with drooling, sniffing posture, muffled voice, red swollen epiglottis).

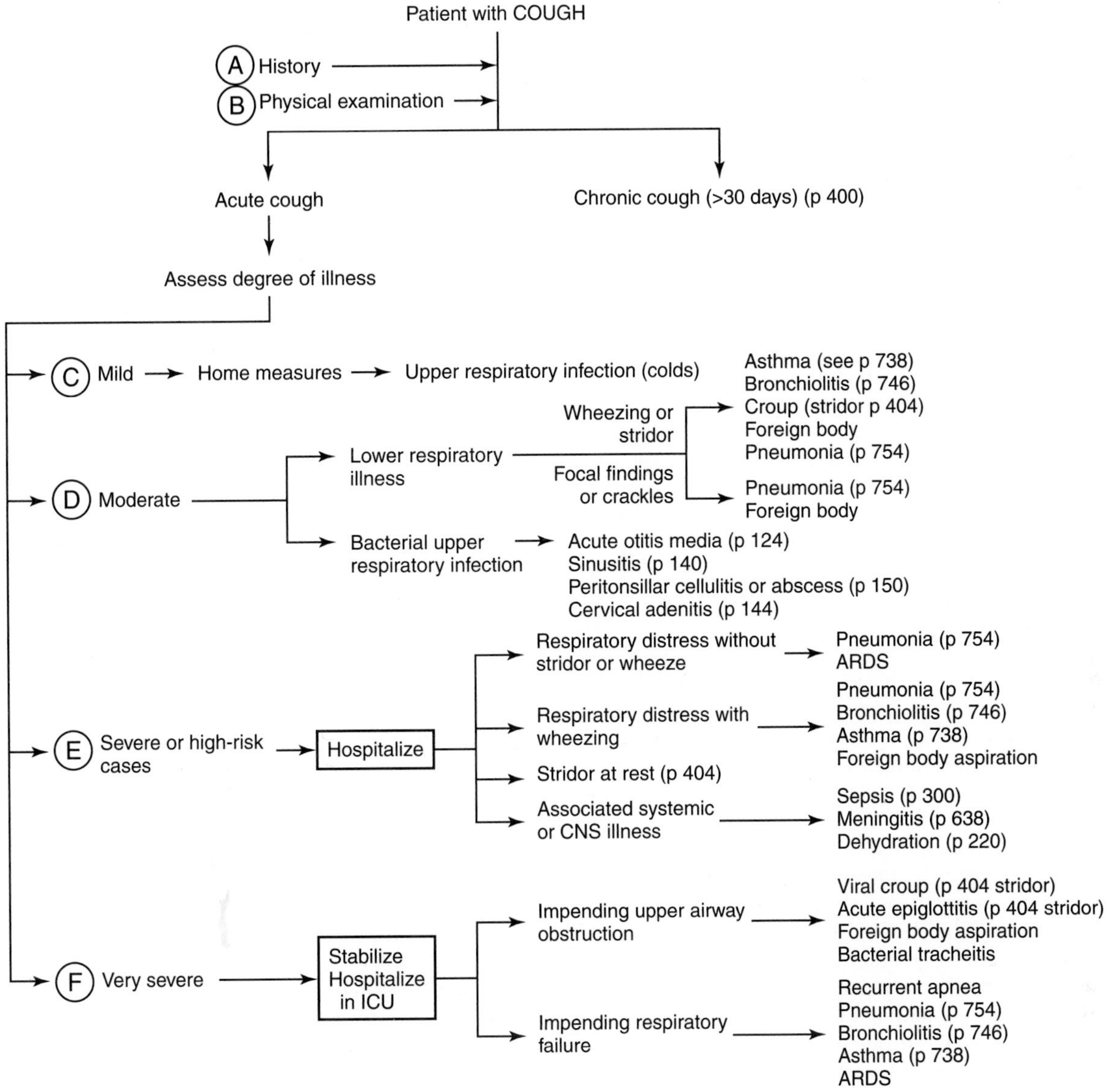
Patient with COUGH
A History
B Physical examination
Acute cough
Chronic cough (>30 days) (p 400)
Assess degree of illness
C Mild
Home measures
Upper respiratory infection (colds)
D Moderate
Lower respiratory illness
Wheezing or stridor
Asthma (see p 738)
Bronchiolitis (p 746)
Croup (stridor p 404)
Foreign body
Pneumonia (p 754)
Focal findings or crackles
Pneumonia (p 754)
Foreign body
Bacterial upper respiratory infection
Acute otitis media (p 124)
Sinusitis (p 140)
Peritonsillar cellulitis or abscess (p 150)
Cervical adenitis (p 144)
E Severe or high-risk cases
Hospitalize
Respiratory distress without stridor or wheeze
Pneumonia (p 754)
ARDS
Respiratory distress with wheezing
Pneumonia (p 754)
Bronchiolitis (p 746)
Asthma (p 738)
Foreign body aspiration
Stridor at rest (p 404)
Associated systemic or CNS illness
Sepsis (p 300)
Meningitis (p 638)
Dehydration (p 220)
F Very severe
Stabilize Hospitalize in ICU
Impending upper airway obstruction
Viral croup (p 404 stridor)
Acute epiglottitis (p 404 stridor)
Foreign body aspiration
Bacterial tracheitis
Impending respiratory failure
Recurrent apnea
Pneumonia (p 754)
Bronchiolitis (p 746)
Asthma (p 738)
ARDS

References

Acute Respiratory Infections in Children. Case Management in Small Hospitals in Developing Countries. A Manual for Doctors and Other Senior Health Workers. WHO/ARI 90.5. Geneva: World Health Organization; 1991.

Acute Respiratory Infections Case Management Charts. Programme for Control of Acute Respiratory Infections. Geneva: World Health Organization; 1990.

Berman S. Epidemiology of acute respiratory infections in children of developing countries. Rev Infect Dis 1991;13(Suppl 6):S454.

Berman S, Shanks MB, Feiten D, et al. Acute respiratory infections during the first three months of life: clinical and physiologic predictors of etiology. Pediatr Emerg Care 1990;6:179.

Lozano JM, Steinhoff M, Ruiz JG, et al. Clinical predictors of acute radiological pneumonia and hypoxaemia at high altitude. Arch Dis Child 1994;71:323.

Simoes EAF, Roark R, Berman S, et al. Respiratory rate: measurement variability over time and accuracy at different counting periods. Arch Dis Child 1991;66:1199.

Slavin RG, Spector SL, Bernstein IL, et al. The diagnosis and management of sinusitis: a practice parameter update. J Allergy Clin Immunol 2005;116:S13–47.

Subhi R, Smith K, Duke T. When should oxygen be given to children at high altitude? A systematic review to define altitude-specific hypoxaemia. Arch Dis Child 2009;94:6–10.

U.S. Food and Drug Administration, Center for Drug Evaluation and Research. FDA public health advisory: nonprescription cold and cough medicine use in children. <http://www.fda.gov/CDER/drug/advisory/cough_cold_2008.htm>; 2008 [accessed 17.01.08; updated 10.10.08].

Hypoxemia Related to Pulmonary Disease/Respiratory Distress

Marc Chester, MD, and Robin R. Deterding, MD

Hypoxemia is defined as a low partial pressure of oxygen ($Pa{O_2}$) in the arterial blood. Hypoxemia has four main causes: (1) alveolar hypoventilation, (2) diffusion impairment, (3) right-to-left shunting of blood, and (4) ventilation/perfusion mismatch ($\dot{V}/Q$). The most common cause is $\dot{V}/Q$ mismatch, and the least common in children is diffusion impairment. Occasionally, a fifth cause, reduction of the inspired $Pa{O_2}$, needs to be considered if, for example, the patient resides at high altitude. Pulse oximetry is a noninvasive measure of the percentage of hemoglobin molecules that are saturated with oxygen at a given partial pressure. Normal oxygen saturation is between 95% and 100% at sea level. Perfoming an arterial blood gas is slightly more invasive but provides a direct measure of the $Pa{O_2}$. The relation between $Pa{O_2}$ and oxygen saturation is explained by the oxygen dissociation curve. Cyanosis, bluish coloring of the skin, and mucous membranes from excessive amounts of reduced hemoglobin in capillary blood usually occurs at $Pa{O_2}$ less than 60 mm Hg or oxygen saturations between 85% and 90%.

A. Physical examination may demonstrate signs of distress including tachypnea, tachycardia, retractions, use of accessory muscles, nasal flarring, grunting, stridor, cyanosis, or clubbing. Vital signs may also demonstrate hypertension or increased temperature. Auscultate for poor air exchange, wheezing, crackles, tubular breath-sounds, or prolongation of expiration. Absences of breathsounds may indicate a pneumothorax or pleural effision, which can be distinguished by percussion. Dullness on percussion may indicate fluid in pleural space or consolidation. Abscent or poor bowel sounds may suggest ileus, commonly seen with bilateral pneumonia. An irregular heart rate, murmur, gallop, or friction rub may suggest cardiac disease. Hepatomegaly may suggest right-sided heart failure.

B. Pulmonary disease, such as asthma, bronchiolitis, and pneumonia with $\dot{V}/Q$ mismatch are suggested when the administration of 100% oxygen causes a significant increase in the $Pa{O_2}$ compared with the room air value. Electrocardiogram (ECG) and echocardiogram are useful in confirming cardiac disease and pulmonary hypertension. Echocardiogram is most reliable with the exception of heart catheterization. A polysomnogram may identify central and obstructive apnea, periodic breathing, or central hypoventilation. A lung biopsy is required in children to demonstrate a diffusion impairment that can be seen in children with interstitial lung disease.

C. Aspiration is common in premature infants with incomplete development of coordination between suck, swallow, and breathing. Full-term newborns with compromised ventilation, tachypnea, and increased work of breathing after respiratory illnesses are also at significant risk for aspiration. Aspiration must also be considered in those with significant gastroesophageal reflux disease, Down syndrome, developmental delay, as well as in those with congenital anatomic abnormalities of their upper airway. Diagnostic studies to confirm aspiration include 24-hour esophageal pH or impedence monitoring (reflux), barium swallow study, and bronchoalveolar lavage (presence of lactose or lipid-laden macrophages). However, none of these tests is 100% diagnostic for aspiration. Treatment may require antireflux medication, thickening feeds, or if severe, Nissen fundoplication and gastrostomy tube placement.

D. Pulmonary edema is an abnormal accumulation of fluid in the extravascular spaces and tissues of the lung. Circulatory overload can result from renal failure, SIADH, excessive intravenous infusions, pulmonary venous disease, as well as left-heart dysfunction. Hypoproteinemia usually makes pulmonary edema worse but alone will not cause pulmonary edema. Direct pulmonary capillary damage can occur from toxic inhalation, aspiration, or pneumonia. High-altitude pulmonary edema can occur in children living at lower altitudes who ascend to more than 8500 feet, in residents of high altitude who return home from low altitudes, and in residents of high altitude who experience development of viral upper respiratory infections. Treatment of high-altitude pulmonary edema is oxygen and descent to lower altitude. Clinical signs of pulmonary edema may include hypoxemia, dyspnea, cough, and frothy sputum. Chest radiograph may demonstrate an enlarged heart with prominent pulmonary vessels along with septal lines, peribronchial cuffing, and bilateral patchy consolidation in a perihilar distribution.

E. Space-occupying pulmonary lesions include those associated with an air leak, pneumothorax, pneumomediastinum, pneumopericardium, as well as pulmonary interstitial emphysema secondary to high ventilatory pressures. Space-occupying lesions also include congenital thoracic malformations, diaphragmatic hernias, congenital lobar emphysema, cystic adenomatoid malformations, pulmonary sequestations, and bronchogenic cysts. Other space-occupying lesions include complicated pneumonia with empyema, lung abscess, and tumors. Pneumothoraces that are symptomatic are usually treated by chest tube placement. Surgical removal is usually the treatment of choice for congenital space-occupying lesions.

(Continued on page 398)

Patient with HYPOXEMIA RELATED TO PULMONARY DISEASE/RESPIRATORY DISTRESS

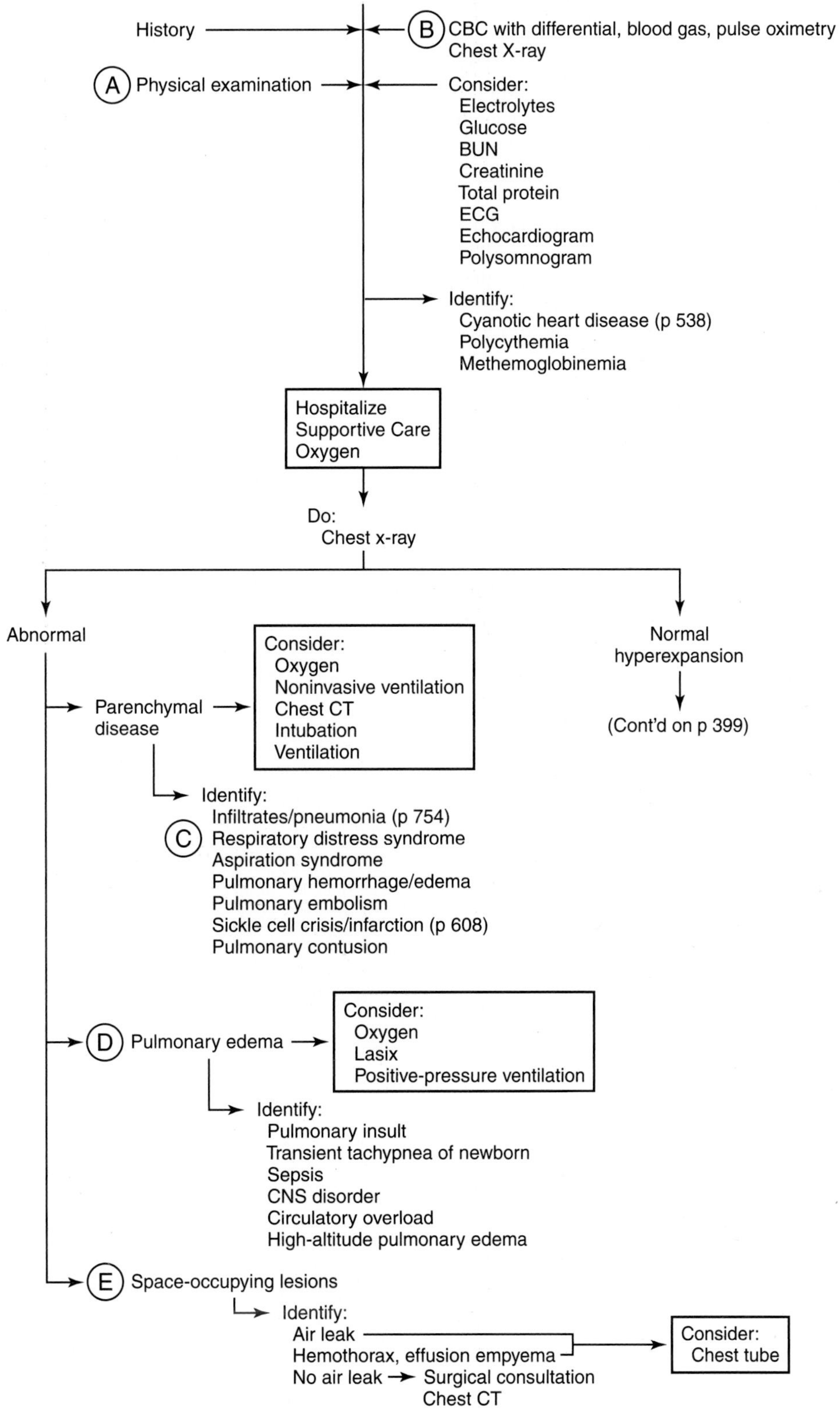
History
(A) Physical examination
(B) CBC with differential, blood gas, pulse oximetry
Chest X-ray
Consider:
Electrolytes
Glucose
BUN
Creatinine
Total protein
ECG
Echocardiogram
Polysomnogram
Identify:
Cyanotic heart disease (p 538)
Polycythemia
Methemoglobinemia
Hospitalize
Supportive Care
Oxygen
Do:
Chest x-ray
Abnormal
Normal hyperexpansion
(Cont'd on p 399)
Parenchymal disease
Consider:
Oxygen
Noninvasive ventilation
Chest CT
Intubation
Ventilation
Identify:
(C)
Infiltrates/pneumonia (p 754)
Respiratory distress syndrome
Aspiration syndrome
Pulmonary hemorrhage/edema
Pulmonary embolism
Sickle cell crisis/infarction (p 608)
Pulmonary contusion
(D) Pulmonary edema
Consider:
Oxygen
Lasix
Positive-pressure ventilation
Identify:
Pulmonary insult
Transient tachypnea of newborn
Sepsis
CNS disorder
Circulatory overload
High-altitude pulmonary edema
(E) Space-occupying lesions
Identify:
Air leak
Hemothorax, effusion empyema
Consider:
Chest tube
No air leak
Surgical consultation
Chest CT

F. Obstructive lesions of the upper airway and trachea may be acute as in angioedema, foreign body aspiration, epiglottitis, croup, peritonsillar abscess, and tracheitis. Obstruction of the airway also occurs from congenital anatomic abonormalities including choanal atresia, laryngomalacia, tracheomalacia, tracheal stenosis, congenital webs or cysts, vascular rings and slings, as well as in those with Pierre Robin syndrome. Obstructive lesions are sometimes the result of previous surgery or endotracheal intubation, as in vocal cord paralysis, subglottic stenosis, and subglottic cysts. Other less common causes of airway obstruction include airway hemangiomas and neoplasms. Laryngoscopy and bronchoscopy should be considered.

G. Hemoglobinopathies including sickle cell disease and thalassemia must be considered in the differential of hypoxemia. These are genetic defects that lead to either a quantitative deficiency or structural abnormality of the globin portion of hemoglobin causing anemia. Acute treatment includes oxygen administration and possibly transfusion.

References

Chernick V, Boat TF, Wilmott RW, Bush A, editors. Kendig's disorders of the respiratory tract in children. 7th ed. Philadelphia: Saunders; 2006.

West JB. Pulmonary pathophysiology: the essentials. 5th ed. Philadelphia: Lippincott Williams & Wilkins; 1998.

(Cont'd from p 397)

Identify:
- Asthma (p 738)
- Bronchiolitis (p 746)
- Cystic fibrosis

↓

(F) Obstructive lesions of upper airway
- Consider:
  - Laryngoscopy
  - Bronchoscopy
  - Barium swallow

(G) Hemoglobinopathies
Intrapulmonary right-to-left shunt
Hypoventilation

↓

Consider:
- High resolution chest
- Echocardiogram
- Polysomnogram
- Pulmonary consultation

Chronic Cough

Edith T. Zemanick, MD, MSCS, and Monica J. Federico, MD

Chronic cough is defined as persistent cough longer than 4 weeks. Although the differential diagnosis for chronic cough is extremely broad, a thorough history and physical examination often leads to the underlying cause without the need for exhaustive testing. "Specific cough" is defined as cough with an identifiable underlying causative factor. The initial evaluation of chronic cough looks for specific pointers that suggest the cause. "Nonspecific cough" typically presents as isolated, dry, chronic cough with no associated symptoms or underlying respiratory disorders.

The type of cough may indicate the cause: productive (asthma, bronchiolitis, bronchiectasis, cystic fibrosis [CF]), brassy (habit cough, tracheitis), barky (croup, tracheitis, tracheomalacia, subglottic or glottic foreign body), paroxysmal (foreign body, pertussis, *Mycoplasma* infection, *Chlamydia* infection, CF), bizarre, or honking (habit cough). The pattern can be helpful: nocturnal (sinusitis, rhinitis, asthma, gastroesophageal reflux), early morning (CF, bronchiectasis), exercise induced (asthma, CF, bronchiectasis), or absent during sleep (habit cough).

A. In the patient's history, ask about the onset, duration, precipitating factors, nature (dry, wet, barky), and pattern of the cough. Distinguish recurrent episodes of upper respiratory infections from continuous cough. Ask about family history of asthma, allergies, atopic dermatitis, or other chronic respiratory illness. Ask about growth and development; perinatal history; exposure to illness at home, school, or daycare; and exposure to passive or active smoking. Ask about sputum production, hemoptysis, or history of choking. Note symptoms of sinusitis, chronic rhinitis, atopic conditions, asthma, gastroesophageal reflux, and sleep disorders (snoring, sleep disruption from cough, obstructive sleep apnea) Ask about previous treatment with antibiotics, allergy medication, bronchodilators, steroids, or other medications. Ask about immunizations and environmental exposures (allergens, molds, tuberculosis).

B. In the physical examination, note fever, respiratory rate, retractions, and prolonged expiration. Measure oxygen saturation by pulse oximetry. Examine the upper airway carefully, and note sinus tenderness, nasal polyps, mouth-breathing, tonsillar hypertrophy, postnasal drip, foul breath, tracheal position, and signs of atopy. Note chest wall deformities. Auscultate the chest to identify stridor, wheezing, rales, or differential air entry. Differentiate monophonic from polyphonic wheeze. Auscultate the heart for murmurs or gallops. Note digital clubbing (chronic hypoxia, CF, heart disease).

C. Obtain a chest film and spirometry (children 5 years and older) in the initial evaluation. Evaluate for symptoms and signs *(specific pointers)* of underlying causative factor. Cough is classified as "specific" or "nonspecific" based on the presence or absence of specific pointers. Specific pointers include wheezing (asthma), failure to thrive (CF, immunodeficiency), feeding difficulties (gastroesophageal reflux, aspiration, tracheoesophageal fistula [TEF]), allergy/nasal symptoms (postnasal drip, sinusitis), productive cough (infectious, CF, primary ciliary dyskinesia), paroxysmal cough (pertussis), barky or brassy cough with or without stridor (airway anomalies), constitutional symptoms such as fever, weight loss (lymphoma, tuberculosis, *Mycoplasma pneumoniae*), hemoptysis (bronchiectasis, CF, vascular abnormalities), recurrent pneumonia (CF, immunodeficiency, aspiration, TEF, congenital lung lesion), evidence of cardiac disease (associated airway anomalies, pulmonary edema). Rapid diagnostic tests are available for respiratory syncytial virus, chlamydia, and pertussis. Perform a sweat test of children with diarrhea, failure to thrive, or a history of recurrent respiratory infections (sinusitis, bronchitis, pneumonia).

D. In children with nonspecific cough, approach can include further observation for spontaneous resolution or a trial of bronchodilator and anti-inflammatory therapy with reassessment in 3 to 4 weeks. Asthma that causes chronic cough without wheezing (cough-variant asthma) is often exercise induced. In older children before and after exercise, spirometry may suggest asthma. Patients who fail to respond to this therapy should be re-evaluated for specific pointers and underlying causative factors including sinusitis, gastroesophageal reflux, CF, aspiration, foreign body or airway anomalies, and/or referred to a pediatric pulmonologist.

(Continued on page 402)

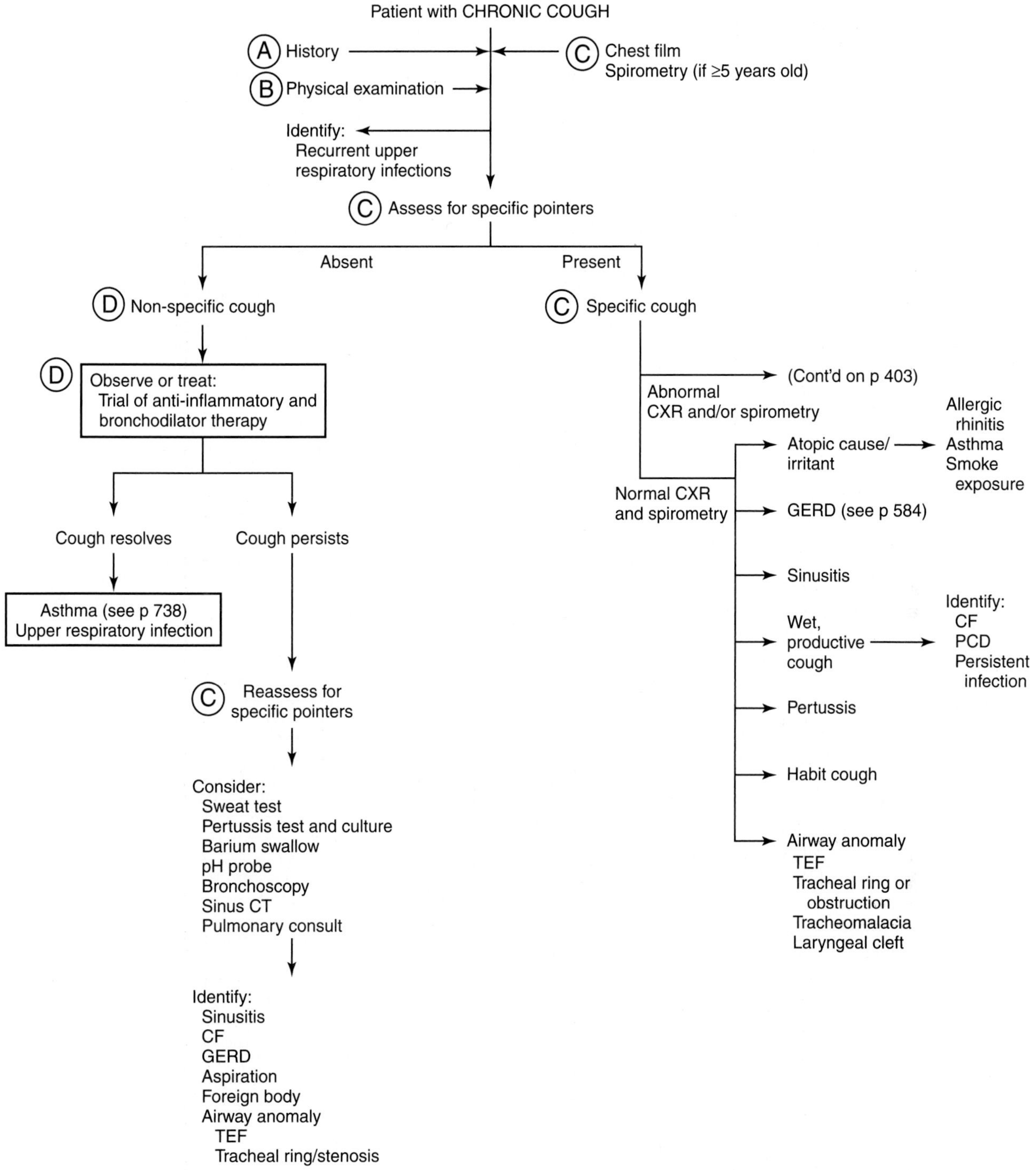
Patient with CHRONIC COUGH
A History
B Physical examination
C Chest film
Spirometry (if ≥5 years old)
Identify:
Recurrent upper respiratory infections
C Assess for specific pointers
Absent
Present
D Non-specific cough
D Observe or treat:
Trial of anti-inflammatory and bronchodilator therapy
Cough resolves
Cough persists
Asthma (see p 738)
Upper respiratory infection
C Reassess for specific pointers
Consider:
Sweat test
Pertussis test and culture
Barium swallow
pH probe
Bronchoscopy
Sinus CT
Pulmonary consult
Identify:
Sinusitis
CF
GERD
Aspiration
Foreign body
Airway anomaly
TEF
Tracheal ring/stenosis
C Specific cough
Abnormal CXR and/or spirometry
(Cont'd on p 403)
Normal CXR and spirometry
Atopic cause/ irritant
Allergic rhinitis
Asthma
Smoke exposure
GERD (see p 584)
Sinusitis
Wet, productive cough
Identify:
CF
PCD
Persistent infection
Pertussis
Habit cough
Airway anomaly
TEF
Tracheal ring or obstruction
Tracheomalacia
Laryngeal cleft

E. Investigate diffuse pulmonary infiltrates for an infectious causative factor with skin tests, rapid diagnostic tests, and cultures for bacterial disease (tuberculosis, pertussis, *Mycoplasma* infection, and *Chlamydia* infection), fungal disease (monilia, histoplasmosis, coccidioidomycosis), parasitic disease *(Pneumocystis, Echinococcus),* and viral infection (respiratory syncytial virus, cytomegalovirus, adenovirus, influenza virus, parainfluenza virus). Obtain a pulmonary consultation and pulmonary function testing to diagnose restrictive lung disease. Obtain a high-resolution chest computed tomographic scan. Consider bronchoscopy with bronchoalveolar lavage to obtain culture and stain specimens for lipid-laden and hemosiderin-laden macrophages. Consider other causative factors including hypersensitivity pneumonitis, pulmonary edema, pulmonary hemorrhage, pulmonary alveolar proteinosis, and interstitial lung disease. Consider evaluation for immune deficiency for children with recurrent or unusual infections.

F. Causes of bronchiectasis include CF, immunodeficiency syndrome, primary ciliary dyskinesia, foreign body aspiration, aspiration of oral or gastric contents, allergic bronchopulmonary aspergillosis, chronic infection (bacterial pneumonia, pertussis, measles, influenza, adenovirus), and defects of tracheobronchial cartilage. Spirometry may show reversible or fixed airflow obstruction. Workup includes sweat chloride test, high-resolution chest computed tomographic scan, immune evaluation, swallow study, sputum culture and/or bronchoscopy, and evaluation for primary ciliary dyskinesia.

G. The workup for mediastinal masses includes computed tomographic scan, magnetic resonance imaging, and pulmonology, oncology, and surgical consultation for management. Spirometry may show fixed airflow obstruction or restriction. The most common mediastinal mass is a normal thymus (anterior). The most common abnormal masses (and their usual location in the mediastinum) are neurogenic tumors (33%, posterior), lymphoma (14%, anterior or middle), teratoma (10%, anterior), thymic lesion (9%, anterior), bronchogenic cyst (7.5%, middle), angioma (7%, anterior), duplication cyst (7%, posterior), and lymph node infection (4%, middle). Patients with mediastinal mass may be at risk for severe, life-threatening complications with sedation and should be evaluated thoroughly by an experienced anesthesiologist before sedation.

H. Causes of pulmonary masses include pulmonary sequestration, bronchogenic cyst, congenital lung cyst, eventration of the diaphragm, cystic adenomatoid malformation, lung abscess, massive atelectasis, and tumor. The workup for pulmonary masses includes computed tomographic scan, magnetic resonance imaging, and surgical consultation. Consider skin tests, bronchoscopy, and angiography.

I. Investigate chest radiography findings of tracheal deviation, localized infiltrate, or localized hyperexpansion with additional studies to diagnose a foreign body, infection, or mass lesion obstructing the airway (intrinsic or extrinsic obstruction). Spirometry may show fixed airflow obstruction and/or inspiratory loop flattening. Consider bronchoscopy when a foreign body or obstructing mass is suspected. Manage patients with localized infection with a trial of antibiotic therapy combined with chest physiotherapy.

References

Brooke AM, Lambert PC, Burton PR, et al. Recurrent cough: natural history and significance in infancy and early childhood. Pediatr Pulmonol 1998;26:256–61.

Chang AB. Cough, cough receptors, and asthma in children. Pediatr Pulmonol 1999;28:59–70.

Chang AB. Cough. Pediatr Clin North Am 2009;56(1):19–31, ix.

Chang AB, Glomb WB. Guidelines for evaluating chronic cough in pediatrics. Chest 2006;129:260S-83S.

Hack HA, Wright NB, Wynn RF. The anesthetic management of children with anterior mediastinal masses. Anaesthesia 2008;63(8):837–46.

Hart MA, Kercsmar CM. Chronic cough in children: a systemic approach. J Respir Dis Pediatrician 2001;3:155–63.

Ing AJ. Cough and gastroesophageal reflux. Am J Med 1997;103:91S-6S.

Kamei RK. Chronic cough in children. Pediatr Clin North Am 1991;38:593–605.

Leigh MW, Zariwala MA, Knowles MR. Primary ciliary dyskinesia: improving the diagnostic approach. Curr Opin Pediatr 2009;21:320–5.

Parks DP, Ahrens RC, Humphries CT, Weinberger MM. Chronic cough in childhood: approach to diagnosis and treatment. J Pediatr 1989;115:856–62.

Perez CR, Wood RE. Update on pediatric flexible bronchoscopy. Pediatr Clin North Am 1994;41:401–24.

Reisman JJ, Canny GJ, Levinson H. The approach to chronic cough in childhood. Ann Allergy 1988;61:163–9.

Shields MD, Bush A, Everard L, et al. Recommendations for the assessment and management of cough in children. Thorax 2008;63:iii1–15.

Wright AL, Holberg CJ, Morgan WJ, et al. Recurrent cough in childhood and its relation to asthma. Am J Respir Crit Care Med 1996; 153:1259–65.

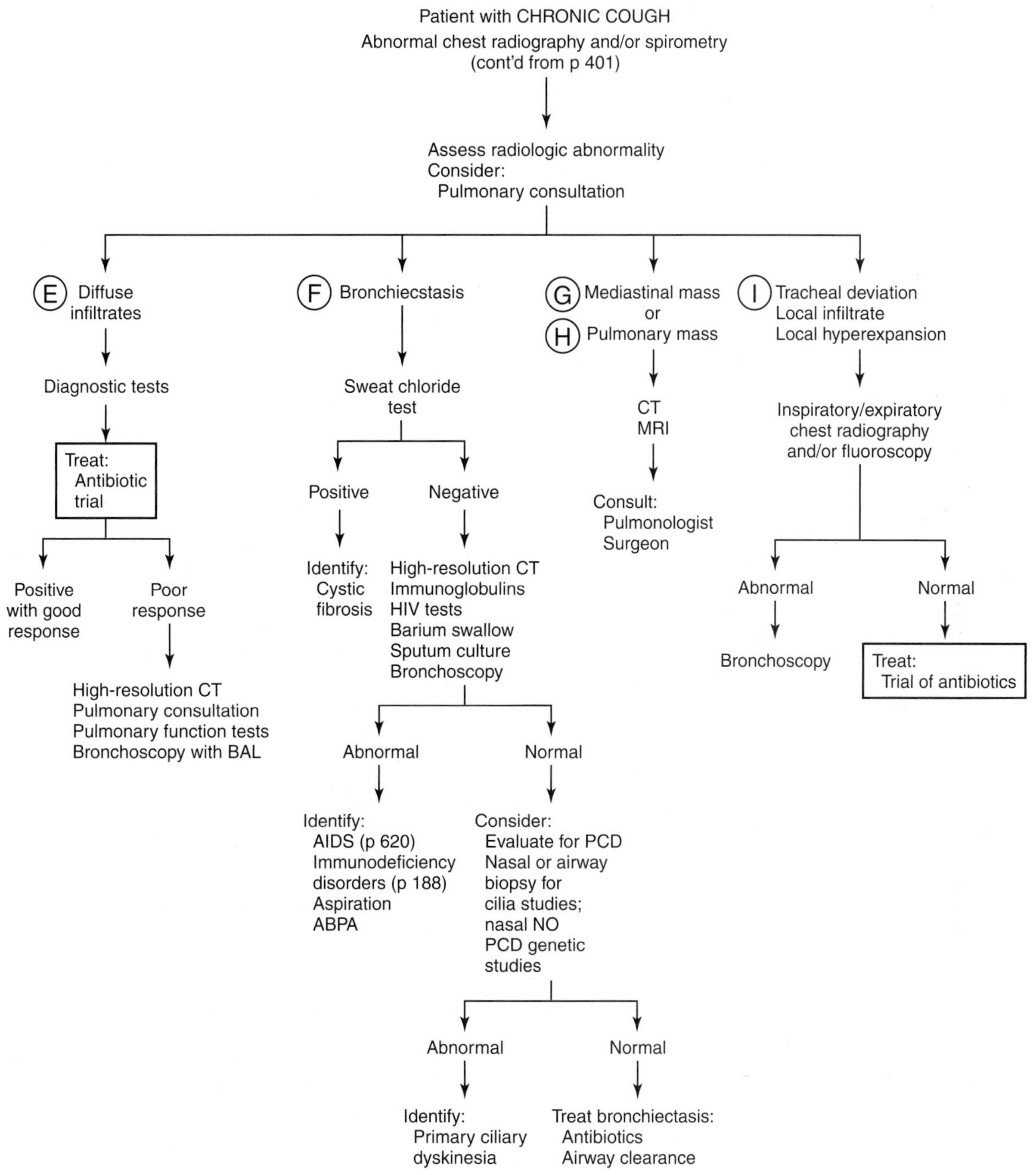
Patient with CHRONIC COUGH
Abnormal chest radiography and/or spirometry
(cont'd from p 401)
Assess radiologic abnormality
Consider:
Pulmonary consultation
E Diffuse infiltrates
Diagnostic tests
Treat:
Antibiotic trial
Positive with good response
Poor response
High-resolution CT
Pulmonary consultation
Pulmonary function tests
Bronchoscopy with BAL
F Bronchiecstasis
Sweat chloride test
Positive
Negative
Identify:
Cystic fibrosis
High-resolution CT
Immunoglobulins
HIV tests
Barium swallow
Sputum culture
Bronchoscopy
Abnormal
Normal
Identify:
AIDS (p 620)
Immunodeficiency disorders (p 188)
Aspiration
ABPA
Consider:
Evaluate for PCD
Nasal or airway biopsy for cilia studies;
nasal NO
PCD genetic studies
Abnormal
Normal
Identify:
Primary ciliary dyskinesia
Treat bronchiectasis:
Antibiotics
Airway clearance
G Mediastinal mass
or
H Pulmonary mass
CT
MRI
Consult:
Pulmonologist
Surgeon
I Tracheal deviation
Local infiltrate
Local hyperexpansion
Inspiratory/expiratory chest radiography and/or fluoroscopy
Abnormal
Normal
Bronchoscopy
Treat:
Trial of antibiotics

Stridor

Theresa Laguna, MD, MSCS

Stridor is a vibratory noise caused by turbulent air flow and airway obstruction. Stridor can be heard on inspiration (extrathoracic obstruction), expiration (intrathoracic obstruction), or during both phases of the respiratory cycle (fixed obstruction) depending on the location of the lesion. Stridor can be classified as acute, chronic, or recurrent in nature.

CAUSATIVE FACTORS

Inflammation, edema, compression, or intraluminal obstruction of the respiratory tract above the larynx (uvula, epiglottis, and arytenoid cartilages), at the level of the larynx (false cords, vocal cords, and arytenoepiglottic folds), or in the trachea causes narrowing of the airway and signs of airway obstruction. **1.** Infection is a main cause of acute stridor in children. Croup is the most common cause of acute inspiratory stridor in children between 6 months and 3 years of age. Croup is a clinical respiratory syndrome characterized by the sudden onset of a barky cough, respiratory distress, and inspiratory stridor usually secondary to viral pathogens, most commonly parainfluenza types 1 and 3, respiratory syncytial virus, influenza virus, adenovirus or human metapneumovirus. In unimmunized children, laryngeal diphtheria and measles are important infectious causative factors of croup to consider. Spasmodic croup is similar to viral croup; however, its symptoms usually occur without a viral prodrome and tend to be more short-lived. A rare cause of inspiratory stridor, epiglottitis, is usually caused by *Haemophilus influenzae* type b, although *Streptococcus pneumoniae* and *Streptococcus pyogenes* can rarely cause acute epiglottitis. Immunization against H. influenzae type b has dramatically decreased the cases of epiglottitis seen in the United States. Bacterial tracheitis, either caused by *Staphylococcus aureus, S. pneumoniae, H. influenzae* or influenza viruses has emerged as a leading cause of life-threatening airway infection in children, surpassing epiglottis and viral croup. **2.** Acute stridor can also be secondary to noninfectious causes. Etiologies to consider include angioedema, foreign body aspiration, peritonsillar abscess, retropharyngeal abscess, and trauma. **3.** Recurrent or chronic stridor can be caused by intrinsic lesions such as laryngomalacia, tracheomalacia, masses and foreign bodies, or extrinsic lesions such as vascular rings or slings.

MEDICAL MANAGEMENT AND APPROACH

A. In the patient's history, ask the following questions: When did the stridor begin? Does the child have symptoms of an upper respiratory infection or cold, such as coughing or rhinitis? When did the cold symptoms begin? Is it difficult for the child to breathe? Is there fast breathing? Did the child recently choke on something and have difficulty breathing or turn blue? Does the child have a sore throat, hoarseness, or a change in voice? Can the child swallow? Is there drooling or fever?

B. In the physical examination, count the respiratory rate, note the heart rate, and assess the oxygen saturation for signs of impending respiratory failure. Listen for stridor at rest when the child is calm or an increase in stridor during crying or coughing. Note the phase of the breathing cycle that stridor is heard (during inspiration, expiration, or both). Most cases of acute stridor are inspiratory in nature. Listen for hoarseness, a barky cough, or a muffled voice. Look for retractions, cyanosis, extreme anxiety or confusion, restlessness, drooling, or a sniffing-type posture. With a stethoscope, note air exchange, wheezing, and rales. Determine whether the stridor is acute or chronic.

C. Angioedema usually presents with facial swelling, urticaria, and a history of similar allergic reactions. Foreign body aspiration can cause stridor, asymmetric breath sounds, or wheezing. The onset is sudden, and upper respiratory infection symptoms and fever are not usually present. An ingested foreign body can rarely lodge in the esophagus and cause upper airway obstruction. A forced expiratory chest film may demonstrate air trapping and possibly a shift of the mediastinum. Bronchoscopy is diagnostic and therapeutic, and should be performed if foreign body is suspected. Assess carefully for tonsillitis or peritonsillar abscess.

D. Assess the degree of respiratory distress and determine whether it is mild/moderate, severe, or very severe (Table 1). Antibiotics play no role in uncomplicated viral croup. Early corticosteroid treatment appears to modify the course of even mild/moderate viral croup and should be used to reduce the progression of the inflammation and to prevent return for care and/or hospitalization. Corticosteroids may be given orally, intramuscularly, or parenterally. Nebulized corticosteroids may be useful, although oral or intramuscular routes are preferred.

E. Encourage parents to give fluids to the child with uncomplicated, mild/severe viral croup. Instruct the parents to call or seek medical care if the child develops stridor at rest, has evidence of respiratory distress (retractions), or becomes too ill to drink. Children with croup whose stridor resolves after treatment with nebulized racemic epinephrine in an ambulatory setting should be observed for at least 3 hours before returning home because stridor and respiratory distress frequently recur.

F. When stridor is moderate to severe and does not respond to traditional therapy, hospitalization in a pediatric ward or pediatric intensive care unit (ICU) should be considered. If acute epiglottitis is suspected, it should be

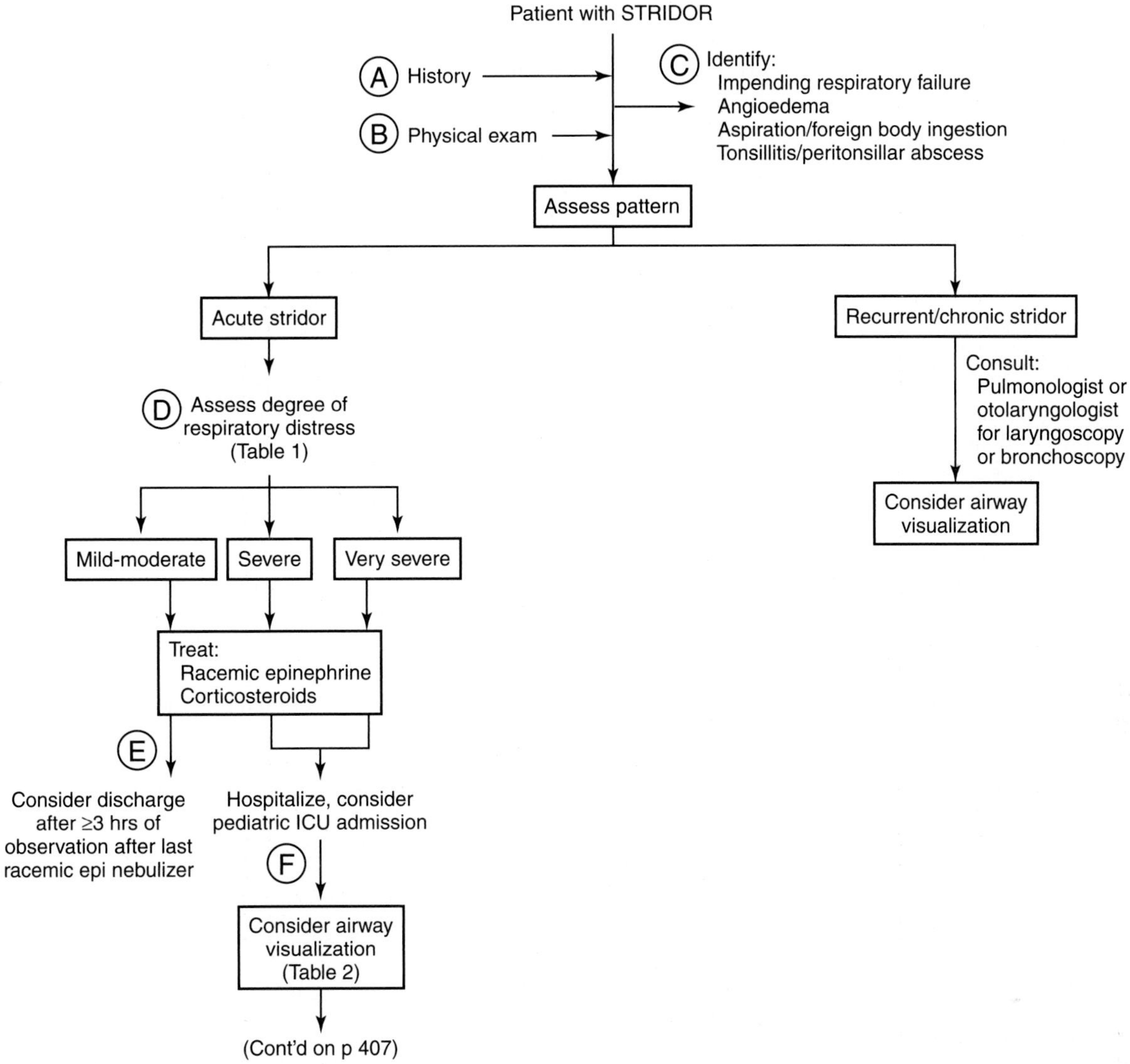

Patient with STRIDOR
A History
B Physical exam
C Identify:
Impending respiratory failure
Angioedema
Aspiration/foreign body ingestion
Tonsillitis/peritonsillar abscess
Assess pattern
Acute stridor
Recurrent/chronic stridor
Consult:
Pulmonologist or
otolaryngologist
for laryngoscopy
or bronchoscopy
Consider airway
visualization
D Assess degree of
respiratory distress
(Table 1)
Mild-moderate
Severe
Very severe
Treat:
Racemic epinephrine
Corticosteroids
E
Consider discharge
after ≥3 hrs of
observation after last
racemic epi nebulizer
Hospitalize, consider
pediatric ICU admission
F
Consider airway
visualization
(Table 2)
(Cont'd on p 407)

considered an airway emergency and airway visualization should be considered (Figure 1). It is important to assess the risk for acute airway obstruction before attempting to visualize the epiglottis in any patient suspected of having acute epiglottitis to allow for adequate preparation (Table 2). When there is severe distress, inspection of the epiglottis should be done in the operating room by an anesthesiologist whenever possible, with an otolaryngologist or pediatric surgeon available for emergency intubation and/or tracheostomy. In visualizing the epiglottis, it is important to have oxygen, a self-inflating Ambu bag, a laryngoscope, and an appropriately sized endotracheal tube (0.5–1 mm less than expected for the child's age) available in case the examination precipitates acute upper airway obstruction. Never force a distressed sitting child to lie down. This may compromise the airway and cause immediate obstruction. Lateral neck radiographs should not be taken initially in patients at high risk for acute epiglottitis because of the danger of acute obstruction in the radiology department and the delay in diagnosis and treatment while waiting for the film. The value of lateral neck films as an alternative to direct visualization in cases with a moderate risk for epiglottitis is controversial.

G. Suspect bacterial tracheitis when croup is complicated by high fever, purulent tracheal secretions, and increasing respiratory distress. This may be the presenting pattern (resembling epiglottitis), or it may present after several days of stridor (secondary bacterial tracheitis). Endotracheal intubation is often necessary. Tracheal secretions should be cultured to allow for appropriate antibiotic therapy. Abundant purulent secretions and pseudomembrane formation require aggressive pulmonary toilet.

H. In hospitalized children, manage respiratory distress and stridor associated with viral croup with racemic epinephrine and corticosteroids. Corticosteroid treatment shortens the hospital stay. Although humidified mist therapy is used routinely in many centers, its efficacy has not been documented, and tents are a barrier to observation. Viral croup rarely requires endotracheal intubation, although extreme vigilance is required. Heliox (70% helium and 30% oxygen) may prevent intubation in severe cases, although there is not enough evidence to recommend its regular use. Ribavirin therapy is not indicated for viral croup. Always continue to reassess the patient if incomplete response to therapy for secondary infections such as bacterial tracheitis.

I. Manage acute epiglottitis with intubation in a controlled setting because of the high risk for acute airway obstruction. Initiate antibiotic therapy with an appropriate cephalosporin antibiotic (Table 3). Blood cultures will be positive in more than 50% of the cases caused by *H. influenzae* type b. Identify extraepiglottic foci of infections, such as pneumonia, septic arthritis, pericarditis, and meningitis. Consider bacterial pathogens other than *H. influenzae* in a child immunized against *H. influenzae* type b.

J. Causes of stridor identified by direct laryngoscopy or bronchoscopy include laryngomalacia, laryngeal web, laryngeal papilloma, redundant folds in the glottic area, and supraglottic masses. Diagnoses associated with pharyngeal or retropharyngeal masses include enlarged adenoids; abscess or cellulitis; benign neoplasms, such as cystic hygroma, hemangioma, goiter, and neurofibroma; and malignant neoplasms, such as neuroblastoma, lymphoma, and histiocytoma. Bronchoscopy can further identify tracheomalacia and/or tracheal compression from a variety of lesions including vascular malformations. Esophagram or barium swallow can also aid in the diagnosis of intrathoracic lesions, which often are characterized by expiratory or fixed stridor.

K. Discharge children from the hospital when stridor at rest and respiratory distress has resolved and they no longer need oxygen. They should be afebrile, eating well, and appropriately active. Schedule a follow-up visit 24 to 48 hours after discharge. Consider a visiting nurse referral. Instruct the parents to call the physician immediately if stridor or signs of respiratory distress (fast breathing or chest indrawing) return.

(Continued on page 408)

Table 1. **Degree of Respiratory Distress**

	Mild/Moderate	Severe	Very Severe
Stridor	Intermittent stridor with crying and/or coughing, no audible stridor at rest	Stridor at rest, often both inspiratory and expiratory	Stridor at rest, cyanosis
Air exchange	Good air exchange with minimal or no retractions	Decreased air entry with marked retractions	Minimal air exchange with severe retractions
Volume status	No signs of dehydration	Signs of dehydration including increased heart rate and decreased urine output	Signs of dehydration including increased heart rate and decreased urine output
Ability to take PO	Able to drink without drooling	Impaired ability to drink	Inability to drink
Mental status	Normal mental status	Altered mental status	Agitation and anxiety secondary to air hunger, or lethargic
Oxygen saturation	Normal	Normal or slightly decreased	Hypoxemic

Table 2. **Risk for Acute Airway Obstruction and Guidelines for Visualization of the Epiglottis in Children with Stridor and Suspected Epiglottitis**

Risk for Acute Obstruction	Clinical Manifestations	Location and Personnel for Visualization
High	Drooling, muffled voice, severe sore throat, sniffing posture, high fever, dehydration, anxiety, toxicity, no URI or cough	Operating room with airway specialist (anesthesia, otolaryngologist, pulmonologist) and surgeons
Moderate	Stridor (intermittent or constant) with minimal URI signs, high fever, age >5 years old without other signs of epiglottitis	Emergency department with airway specialist
Low	Stridor at rest associated with URI symptoms for 3–4 days, low-grade fever	Visualization usually not necessary; if done in emergency department or in patient ward, have physician present experienced with pediatric resuscitation
Minimal	Intermittent stridor with 2–4 days of URI, low-grade to absent fever, no toxicity, no respiratory distress	Visualization not necessary

URI, upper respiratory infection.

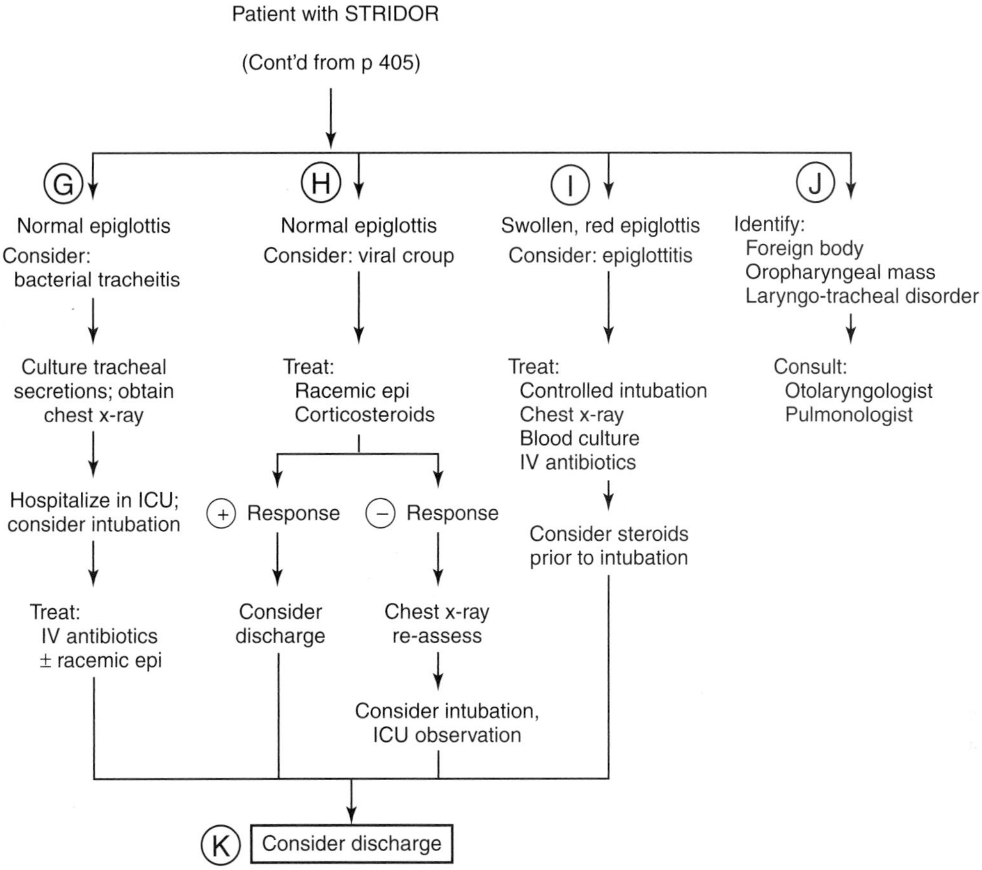
Patient with STRIDOR
(Cont'd from p 405)
G
Normal epiglottis
Consider:
bacterial tracheitis
Culture tracheal secretions; obtain chest x-ray
Hospitalize in ICU; consider intubation
Treat:
IV antibiotics
± racemic epi
H
Normal epiglottis
Consider: viral croup
Treat:
Racemic epi
Corticosteroids
+ Response
Consider discharge
– Response
Chest x-ray re-assess
Consider intubation, ICU observation
I
Swollen, red epiglottis
Consider: epiglottitis
Treat:
Controlled intubation
Chest x-ray
Blood culture
IV antibiotics
Consider steroids prior to intubation
J
Identify:
Foreign body
Oropharyngeal mass
Laryngo-tracheal disorder
Consult:
Otolaryngologist
Pulmonologist
K
Consider discharge

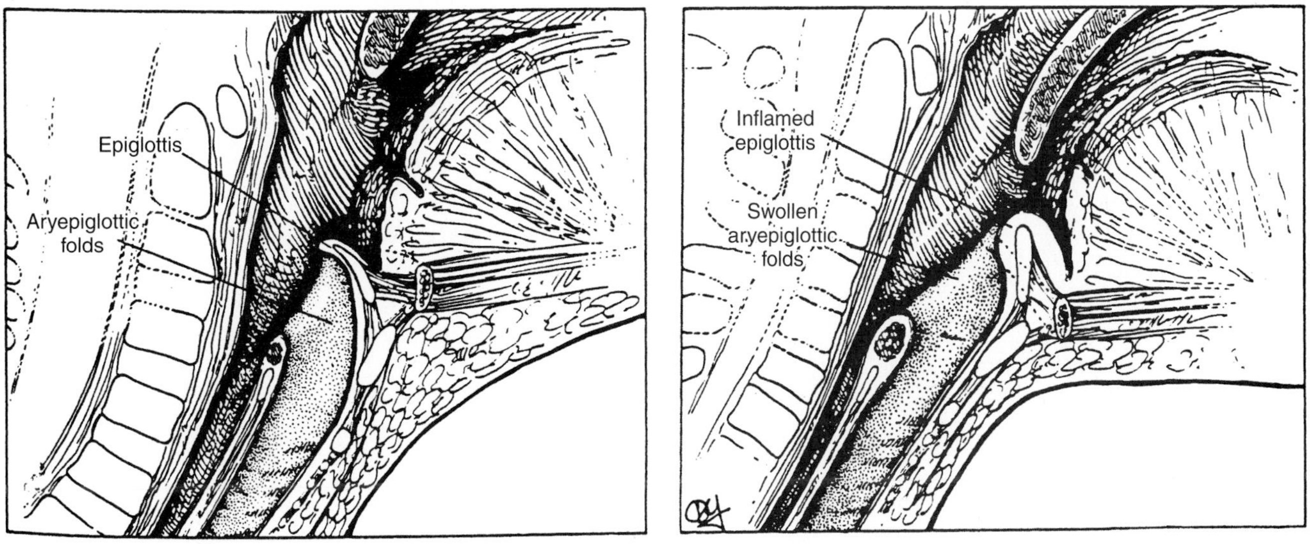
Epiglottis
Aryepiglottic folds
Inflamed epiglottis
Swollen aryepiglottic folds

Figure 1. Diagram of the lateral neck region in a normal child (left) and in a child with epiglottitis (right). *(From Fleisher GR, Ludwig S, editors. Textbook of pediatric emergency medicine. 3rd ed. Baltimore: Williams & Wilkins; 1993. p. 619.)*

Table 3. **Drugs Used in the Treatment of Viral Croup, Bacterial Tracheitis, or Epiglottitis in Children**

Drug	Dosage
Racemic epinephrine	0.5 ml in 2.5 ml normal saline by nebulization every 1–6 h PRN (2.25% solution)
Methylprednisolone (Solu-Medrol)	1 mg/kg/dose every 12h; may repeat as needed
Dexamethasone	0.6 mg/kg/dose given PO or IM × 1; may repeat as needed
Ceftriaxone	50–75 mg/kg/day IM/IV divided every 12–24h for mild/moderate infections, 80–100 mg/kg/day IM/IV divided every 12–24h for severe infections; maximum: 2 g/24 hr
Cefotaxime	50 mg/kg IM/IV divided every 6–8h; maximum: 12 g/day; alternative: 50–75 mg/kg IM/IV divided every 6–8h for PCN-resistant pneumococci
Oxacillin	100–200 mg/kg/day IM/IV every 4–6h; maximum: 12 g/day
Nafcillin	50–100 mg/kg/day IV divided every 6h or 100–200 mg/kg/day IV divided every 4–6h if severe infection; maximum: 12 g/day

IM, intramuscularly; *IV*, intravenously; *PCN*, penicillin; *PO*, orally; *PRN*, as needed.

References

Ausejo M, Saenz A, Pham B, et al. The effectiveness of glucocorticoids in treating croup: meta-analysis. BMJ 1999;319:595.

Bjornson CL, Johnson DW. Croup. Lancet 2008;371:329–39.

Daines CL, Wood RE, Boesch RP. Foreign body aspiration: an important etiology of respiratory symptoms in children. J Allergy Clin Immunol 2008;121:1297–8.

Doshi J, Krawiec ME. Clinical manifestations of airway malacia in young children. J Allergy Clin Immunol 2007;120:1276–8.

Epocrates online. <https://online.epocrates.com/noFrame/>.

Fitzgerald D, Mellis C, Johnson M, et al. Nebulized budesonide is as effective as nebulized adrenaline in moderately severe croup. Pediatrics 1996;97:722.

Guillemaud JP, El-Hakim H, Richards S, Chauhan N. Airway pathology abnormalities in symptomatic children with congenital cardiac and vascular disease. Arch Otolaryngol Head Neck Surg 2007;133:672–6.

Hopkins A, Lahiri T, Salerno R, Heath B. Changing epidemiology of life-threatening upper airway infections: the reemergence of bacterial tracheitis. Pediatrics 2006;118:1418–21.

Leung AK, Kellner JD, Johnson DW. Viral croup: a current perspective. J Pediatr Health Care 2004;18:297–301.

Moore M, Little P. Humidified air inhalation for treating croup. Cochrane Database Syst Rev 2006;3:CD002870.

Scolnik D, Coates AL, Stephens D, et al. Controlled delivery of high vs. low humidity vs. mist therapy for croup in emergency departments. JAMA 2006;295:1274–80.

Smith RJH, Coombe WT. When congenital vascular anomalies cause airway problems. Contemp Pediatr 1985;94–106.

Sparrow A, Geelhoed G. Prednisolone versus dexamethasone in croup: a randomised equivalence trial. Arch Dis Child 2006;91: 580–3.

Vorwerk C, Coats TJ. Use of helium-oxygen mixtures in the treatment of croup: a systemic review. Emerg Med J 2008;25:547–50.

Wheeze

Monica J. Federico, MD

Wheezing is a high-pitched, expiratory noise most commonly audible only with a stethoscope. Wheezing can be detected acutely or can recur depending on the cause.

The evaluation of a child with a wheeze can be based either on the kind of wheeze the provider detects or on the recurrence of the finding. There are at least two types of wheeze: 1) monophonic, the same sound throughout the chest or 2) polyphonic, or heterogeneous sounds heard throughout the chest. Monophonic wheeze is generally due to obstruction or compression of a large, central airway, and polyphonic wheeze is most likely heard in the setting of diffuse, small airway obstruction or compression. Unfortunately, it can be difficult to determine the quality of the wheeze and the finding may be variable depending on the cause. Therefore, this algorithm will help the provider move through a differential diagnosis of wheeze based upon whether the wheeze is acute versus chronic/recurrent.

A. In the patient's history, document any signs or symptoms of airway obstruction and/or respiratory distress, including: cough, chest tightness, wheeze, shortness of breath, ability to talk in complete sentences, tachypnea, difficulty with activities, and trouble laying flat. Work through a comprehensive differential and include questions about gestational age and newborn course to evaluate for chronic lung disease of infancy; foreign body aspiration; pneumonia or infection indicated by fevers and chest pain; response to a beta agonist suggesting asthma; a cough with feeding indicating aspiration; a mass or lymphadenopathy causing airway compression as indicated by weight loss, night sweats, positional trouble breathing, or poor response to bronchodilators; or a different chronic illness as indicated by chronic increased work of breathing, failure to thrive, and/or hypoxemia. Ask about sinusitis, headaches, bad breath, facial pain, and fever.

B. In the physical examination, take a full set of vital signs including oxygen saturation, and note signs of respiratory distress, including tachypnea, retractions, dyspnea, nasal flaring, use of accessory muscles, ability to talk, wheezing, prolongation of the expiratory phase, forced expiratory phase, and decreased breath sounds. Signs of severe respiratory distress include markedly decreased or absent breath sounds, cyanosis, and increased pulsus paradoxus (exaggeration of the normal variation of cardiac output with the respiratory cycle). An altered mental status (lethargy, restlessness, disorientation, and air hunger) indicates severe hypoxemia. Treat the child with oxygen if needed to keep saturations greater than 90%.

C. Evaluate acute wheeze by evaluating for foreign body aspiration by history and then by forced exhalation on a chest radiograph if the history is positive or even suspicious. If the chest radiograph is positive or inconclusive in the setting of a clear history of aspiration, otolaryngology should be consulted for a bronchoscopy and removal. The most common foreign bodies aspirated in children are peanuts and hot dogs.

1. If there is no concern for foreign body and the child is younger than 2 years *and* has symptoms of an upper respiratory infection (URI), consider bronchiolitis (see p. 746) for management.
2. If the child is older than 2 years or the child is younger than 2 years and does not have an URI, try a dose of an inhaled beta agonist (see Asthma, p. 738). If there is a clear response, and the child has no history consistent with chronic pulmonary disease such as failure to thrive or a history of hypoxemia, consider the diagnosis of asthma (see p. 738) for further management. If the child responds to albuterol and has symptoms of chronic disease such as failure to thrive, clubbing, or a history of prolonged hypoxemia, treat the acute wheeze and work through the differential of the acute wheeze and chronic disease. If the child is older than 2 years and has symptoms consistent with a respiratory tract infection, and the child is stable with low-grade fevers and a symmetric examination, the most likely cause is viral pneumonia (see p. 754); if the examination is asymmetric or the child is ill-appearing, check a chest radiograph to rule out pneumonia, a mass, or lymphadenopathy compressing the airway. If the child has no URI symptoms, check chest radiograph to rule out a mass or evidence of extrinsic compression and consider consulting pulmonary for evaluation for any evidence of endobronchial or extrinsic compression or possible inhalation injury.

D. If there is no concern for foreign body and the wheeze is chronic or recurrent, try a dose of an inhaled beta agonist (see Asthma chapter, p. 738). If there is a clear response, and the child has no history consistent with chronic pulmonary disease such as failure to thrive, clubbing, or a history of hypoxemia, consider the diagnosis of asthma (see p. 738) for further management. If the child responds to albuterol but the history is concerning for a chronic lung disease other than asthma, treat the acute wheeze and respiratory distress with beta agonist as needed, consider systemic corticosteroids (asthma p. 738), and work through the differential of recurrent wheeze and chronic disease: a chest radiograph and pulmonary function testing if possible to evaluate for obvious airway compression or evidence of fixed airway obstruction; consider a sweat test for cystic fibrosis (CF); a barium swallow and possibly a

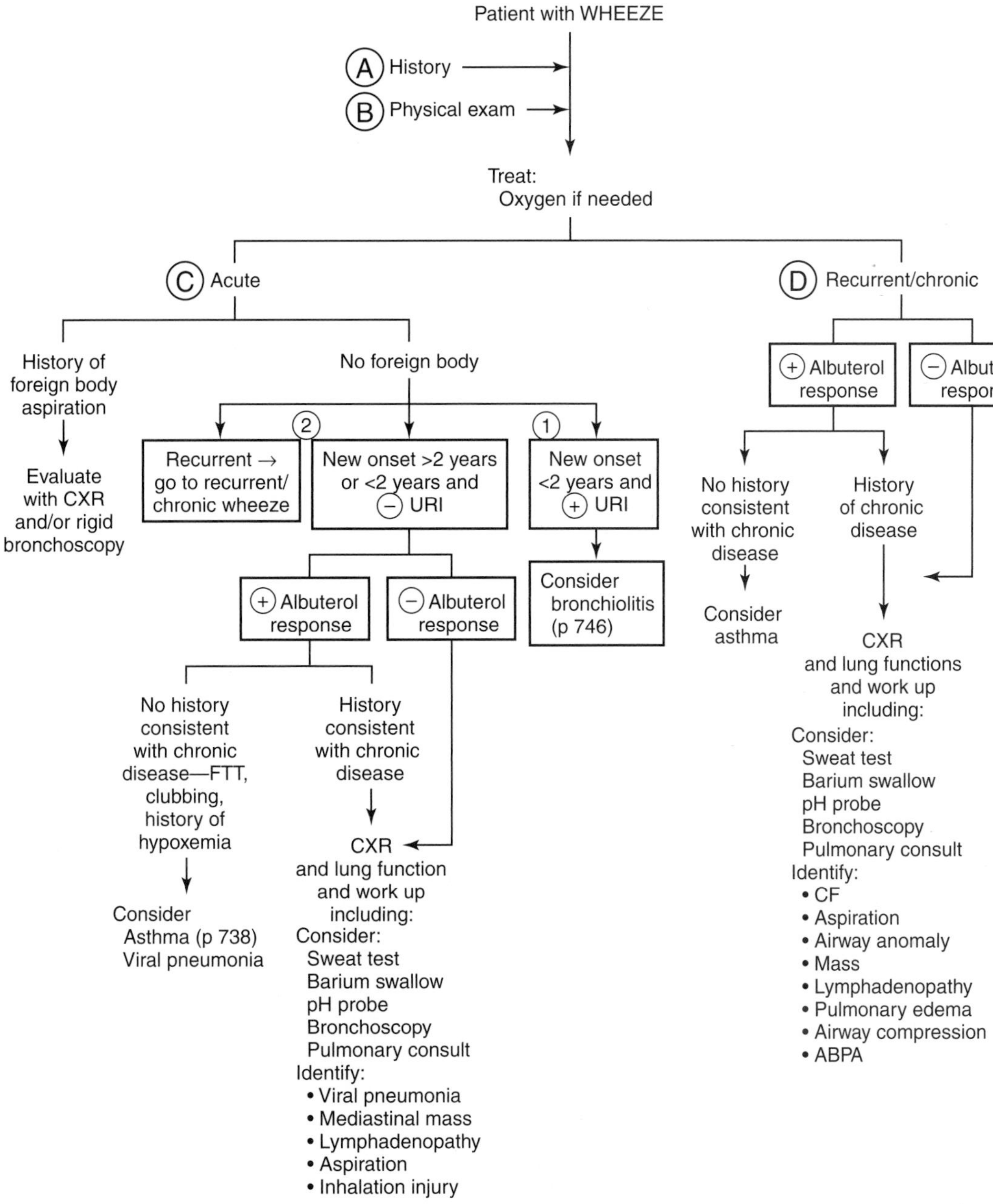
Patient with WHEEZE
A History
B Physical exam
Treat:
Oxygen if needed
C Acute
D Recurrent/chronic
History of foreign body aspiration
Evaluate with CXR and/or rigid bronchoscopy
No foreign body
2
1
Recurrent → go to recurrent/ chronic wheeze
New onset >2 years or <2 years and − URI
New onset <2 years and + URI
Consider bronchiolitis (p 746)
+ Albuterol response
− Albuterol response
No history consistent with chronic disease—FTT, clubbing, history of hypoxemia
Consider Asthma (p 738) Viral pneumonia
History consistent with chronic disease
CXR and lung function and work up including:
Consider: Sweat test Barium swallow pH probe Bronchoscopy Pulmonary consult
Identify: • Viral pneumonia • Mediastinal mass • Lymphadenopathy • Aspiration • Inhalation injury
+ Albuterol response
− Albuterol response
No history consistent with chronic disease
Consider asthma
History of chronic disease
CXR and lung functions and work up including:
Consider: Sweat test Barium swallow pH probe Bronchoscopy Pulmonary consult
Identify: • CF • Aspiration • Airway anomaly • Mass • Lymphadenopathy • Pulmonary edema • Airway compression • ABPA

bronchoscopy to evaluate for vascular compression of the trachea and the esophagus; a speech therapy evaluation for recurrent aspiration; if the chest radiograph does not show a mass or lymphadenopathy, consider a bronchoscopy to evaluate for airway malacia, endobronchial lesions, or evidence of extrinsic compression; a cardiology evaluation if there is evidence of pulmonary edema or cardiomegaly by chest radiograph; and finally, consider a complete blood cell count (CBC), an IgE, and a chest computed tomographic (CT) scan for further evaluation for allergic bronchopulmonary aspergillosis (ABPA). If the wheeze does not respond to albuterol, consider a work up for other causes of recurrent wheeze including: A CXR to evaluate for a mediastinal mass, cardiac enlargement or lymphadenopathy, pulmonary function testing, a barium swallow to evaluate for vascular airway compression, a bronchoscopy for airway anomalies or compression not previously identified, and for a bronchoalveolar lavage.

References

Divisi D, Di Tommaso S, Garramone M, et al. Foreign bodies aspirated in children: role of bronchoscopy. Thorac Cardiovasc Surg 2007;55(4):249–52.

Guidelines for the Diagnosis and Management of Asthma. National Asthma Education Program, Expert Panel Report 2. Bethesda, MD: U.S. Department of Health and Human Services, Public Health Service, National Institutes of Health, National Heart, Lung, and Blood Institute; 1997.

Pasterkamp H. The history and physical examination. In: Chernick V, Boat TF, Kendig EL Jr, editors. Kendig's disorders of the respiratory tract in children. Philadelphia: Elsevier; 1998. p. 99–100.

Shuh S. Evaluation of the utility of radiography in acute bronchiolitis. J Pediatr 2007;150(4):429–33.

Zerella JT, Dimler M, McGill LC, Pippus KJ. Foreign body aspiration in children: value of radiography and complications of bronchoscopy. J Pediatr Surg 1998;33(11):1651–4.

TRAUMA

PREHOSPITAL BASIC LIFE SUPPORT
HEAD INJURY
NECK INJURY
CHEST TRAUMA
ABDOMINAL TRAUMA
GENITOURINARY TRAUMA
UPPER EXTREMITY TRAUMA
LOWER EXTREMITY TRAUMA
OCULAR INJURY
DENTAL AND ORAL TRAUMA
HAND INJURIES
LACERATIONS
BITES
THERMAL INJURY (FROSTBITE/BURNS)
CHILD ABUSE: PHYSICAL ABUSE
CHILD ABUSE: SEXUAL ABUSE

Prehospital Basic Life Support

Lara Rappaport, MD, MPH, and Maria Mandt, MD

The goal of pediatric basic life support is to restore adequate tissue oxygenation and perfusion when a child has a respiratory or cardiopulmonary arrest. Basic life support requires a rapid assessment of responsiveness, airway, breathing, and circulation. Limited data exist to characterize out-of-hospital pediatric cardiac arrest, but outcomes in general are poor with survival-to-discharge rates ranging from 8% to 12%. Sustained return of spontaneous circulation is obtained in 28% of victims. Witnessed arrests have a comparatively greater chance of survival, as do patients with nontraumatic causes of arrest. The best predictor of survival-to-discharge is correlated with a short duration (20 minutes or less) of cardiopulmonary resuscitation (CPR).

RESPONSIVENESS

A. Assess the responsiveness by tapping the child and speaking loudly. For a lone rescuer, if the patient is unresponsive and there was a witnessed sudden collapse, first call Emergency Medical Services (EMS) and, if possible, get an automated external defibrillator (AED). Then return to the victim, defibrillate as soon as the AED is available, and initiate CPR. If there is not a witnessed collapse, stay with the victim to provide CPR for 2 minutes, then call EMS, get the AED, and defibrillate when available. If there are two rescuers, one person should activate EMS and get the AED, whereas the other starts CPR.

AIRWAY

B. A health care provider should use the head-tilt/chin-lift maneuver to open the airway of a victim without evidence of head or neck trauma. If a cervical spine injury is suspected, jaw thrust with spine immobilization without head tilt is recommended. If a cervical spine injury is suspected and the jaw thrust does not open the airway, it is acceptable to use a head-tilt/chin-lift maneuver to achieve adequate ventilation.

BREATHING

C. If the child is not breathing or has only occasional gasps, give two rescue breaths at 1 second per breath, and continue to give one breath every 3 to 5 seconds. Equal chest rise is an absolute marker of effectiveness of rescue breathing. In infants, it is acceptable to use both mouth-to-mouth and mouth-to-nose techniques. In children, use only the mouth-to-mouth technique. Barrier devices have not reduced the risk for transmission of infection and may increase the resistance to flow. Although not encouraged, barrier devices are acceptable as long as there is not a time delay to rescue breathing.

CIRCULATION

D. The pulse check should take no longer than 10 seconds. In a child, the femoral or carotid sites are used; in an infant, the brachial site is preferred. Several studies have shown that health care providers have difficulty in detecting the presence of a pulse and often think one is present when there is none. Therefore, if you are not certain there is a pulse, start compressions. Chest compressions should be initiated in children with heart rates less than 60 beats/min if there are also signs of poor perfusion.

(Continued on page 416)

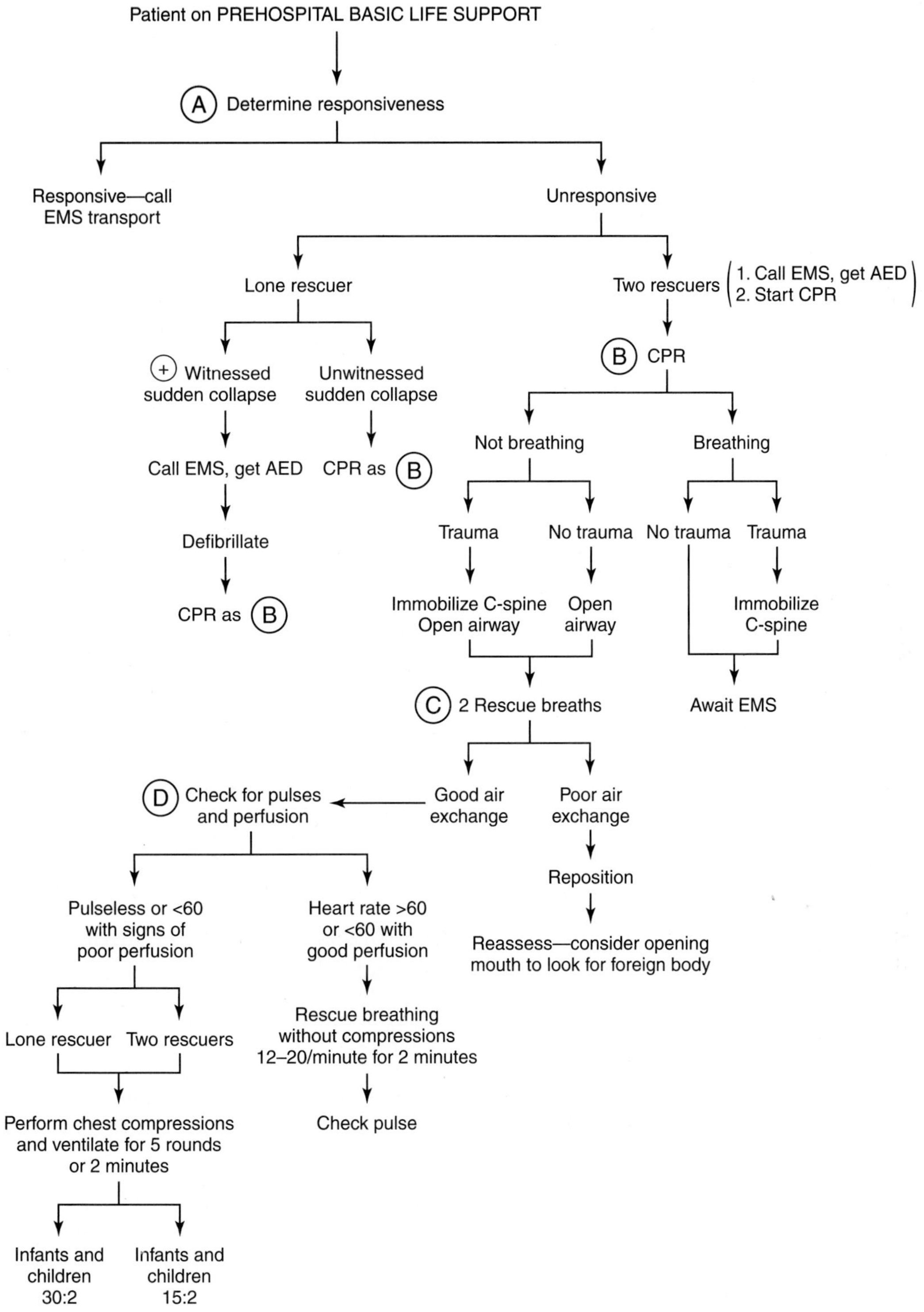
Patient on PREHOSPITAL BASIC LIFE SUPPORT
(A) Determine responsiveness
Responsive—call EMS transport
Unresponsive
Lone rescuer
Two rescuers
1. Call EMS, get AED
2. Start CPR
(+) Witnessed sudden collapse
Unwitnessed sudden collapse
Call EMS, get AED
CPR as (B)
Defibrillate
CPR as (B)
(B) CPR
Not breathing
Breathing
Trauma
No trauma
No trauma
Trauma
Immobilize C-spine Open airway
Open airway
Immobilize C-spine
(C) 2 Rescue breaths
Await EMS
(D) Check for pulses and perfusion
Good air exchange
Poor air exchange
Reposition
Reassess—consider opening mouth to look for foreign body
Pulseless or <60 with signs of poor perfusion
Heart rate >60 or <60 with good perfusion
Lone rescuer
Two rescuers
Rescue breathing without compressions 12–20/minute for 2 minutes
Perform chest compressions and ventilate for 5 rounds or 2 minutes
Check pulse
Infants and children 30:2
Infants and children 15:2

OTHER IMPORTANT ISSUES

Bag Mask Ventilation

For children requiring airway control for short periods in the prehospital setting, bag-valve-mask ventilation (BVM) is the method of choice. An out-of-hospital pediatric, prospective, randomized, control study showed that BVM compared with tracheal intubation has equivalent survival to hospital discharge rates and neurologic outcome. A two-person technique may be optimal for providing the appropriate chest rise, tidal volume, and peak pressures as compared with a single-rescuer technique. The two-person technique is performed by one rescuer using both hands to maintain an open airway with a jaw thrust and a tight mask-to-face seal, whereas the other compresses the ventilation bag. Both rescuers should observe chest rise.

Compression/Ventilation Ratio

For health care providers providing two-rescuer CPR, a compression/ventilation ratio of 15:2 is recommended. A universal rate of 30:2 is recommended for the lone rescuer responding to children and adults. For newborns, the 3:1 recommendation has not changed. A mnemonic that is helpful is "squeeze-release-release" at a normal speaking rate.

Excessive ventilation may be harmful. Complications such as air trapping and barotrauma are widely recognized. Excessive ventilation has been shown to increase intrathoracic pressure and decrease venous return, ultimately reducing cardiac output.

Compressions

Chest compressions consist of rhythmic applications of pressure over the lower half of the sternum. Blood flow generated by chest compressions delivers a small, but critical, amount of oxygen and substrate to the brain and myocardium. There has been an increased emphasis placed on performing rigorous, high-quality chest compressions. The important principles are reviewed: (1) "push hard" with sufficient force to compress one third to half the anterior-posterior depth of the chest; (2) "push fast," compress at a rate of 100 compressions per minute; and (3) allow the chest to recoil fully with each compression. In other words, make certain that your hands are lifted slightly off the chest at the end of each compression.

Use the heel of one or two hands to compress the chest on the lower half of the sternum at the nipple line. No outcome studies show a preference for a one-hand versus two-hand technique. For infants, the two-thumb encircling hands technique is preferred over the two-finger chest compression technique in infants when there are two rescuers. The two-thumb encircling hands technique showed higher coronary perfusion pressures and more consistently correct depth and force of compression than the two-finger technique. The two-finger technique is preferred for single-rescuer infant resuscitation to allow for quick transition between compressions. It is essential to perform continuous CPR without interruption.

Achieving a rate of 100 compressions per minute can be challenging. Devices are available that monitor compression and ventilation rates, and metronomes can be purchased and set to 100 beats/min. Another method of pacing is to choose a song that has a bass line of 100 beats/min and sing it to yourself as you do compressions. Ironically, two such songs are the Bee Gees' "Stayin' Alive" and "Another One Bites the Dust" by Queen. Matlock et al. showed that listening to "Stayin' Alive" assisted providers in performing chest compressions on manikins at the proper rate.

Rescuer fatigue may lead to inadequate compression rates or depth. Significant fatigue and shallow compressions are seen after 1 minute of CPR, despite rescuers denying that fatigue is present. Exhaustion can lead to failure of the rescuer to "push hard" and not allow for compete chest wall recoil between compressions. When two or more rescuers are available, it is reasonable to switch the compressor about every 2 minutes. Effort should be made to accomplish this switch in less than 5 seconds.

Compression-Only Cardiopulmonary Resuscitation

It has been shown that ventilation during the first few minutes of ventricular fibrillation in adult cardiac arrest may not be essential. However, this is not true for most pediatric arrests, which are much more likely to be asphyxial and prolonged. The key difference is that during asphyxia, blood continues to flow to the tissues, causing oxygen saturation to decrease and carbon dioxide to increase. Pediatric patients need both prompt ventilation and chest compressions. However, if there is resistance to performing prompt ventilation, chest compression-only ventilation is better than doing no CPR.

References

2005 American Heart Association Guidelines for Cardiopulmonary Resuscitation and Emergency Cardiovascular Care. Part 12: Pediatric Advanced Life Support. Circulation 2005;112:IV-167–87.

Donoghue AJ, Nadkarni VM, Berg RA, et al. Out-of-hospital pediatric cardiac arrest: an epidemiologic review and assessment of current knowledge. Ann Emerg Med 2005;46(6):512–22.

Gausche M, Lewis RJ, Stratton SJ. Effect of out-of-hospital pediatric endotracheal intubation on survival and neurologic outcome: a controlled clinical trial. JAMA 2000;283:783–90.

Gerein RB, Osmond MH, Stiell IG, et al. What are the etiology and epidemiology of out-of-hospital pediatric cardiopulmonary arrest in Ontario, Canada? Acad Emerg Med 2006;13:653–8.

Haque IU, Udassi JP, Zaritsky AL. Outcome following cardiopulmonary arrest. Pediatr Clin North Am 2008;55(4):969–87.

Lopez-Herce J, Garcia C, Dominguez P, et al. Outcome of out-of-hospital cardiorespiratory arrest in children. Pediatr Emerg Care 2005;21(12): 807–15.

Matlock D. 'Stayin' alive:' a pilot study to test the effectiveness of a novel mental metronome in maintaining appropriate compression rates in simulated cardiac arrest scenarios. Abstracts of the American College of Emergency Physicians (ACEP) Research Forum 2008, Scientific Assembly. October 27–28, 2008. Chicago, Illinois, USA. Ann Emerg Med 2008;52(4 suppl):S41–172, (abstract 83).

Samson RA, Nadkarni VM, Meaney PA, et al. Outcomes of in-hospital ventricular fibrillation in children. N Engl J Med 2006;354(22): 2328–39.

Young KD, Gausche-Hill M, McClung CD, et al. A prospective, population-based study of the epidemiology and outcome of out-of-hospital pediatric cardiopulmonary arrest. Pediatrics 2004;114(1):157–64.

Head Injury

Joseph Grubenhoff, MD

Acute head injury is common in pediatric patients. It is responsible for more than 500,000 emergency department visits annually. Of those, there are approximately 60,000 hospitalizations and 7000 deaths. However, most children suffer only mild traumatic brain injury (mTBI; concussion). There is considerable controversy in the medical literature about how best to assess and manage victims of mild, moderate, and severe head injury. This algorithm is designed for practitioners in the office, urgent care, or community hospital setting.

A. Airway, breathing, and circulation should be addressed first. Immobilize the cervical spine when significant forces or altered mental status are involved. Evaluate for irregular respirations, hypertension, and bradycardia (Cushing triad) indicating the presence of increased intracranial pressure (ICP). Note any asymmetry of pupils and the Glasgow Coma Scale (GCS) score (Table 1). A score less than 9 suggests severe injury and the loss of airway protective reflexes; consider endotracheal intubation. Expose the patient to identify any other evidence of trauma. Treat increased ICP and any life-threatening conditions.

B. Once stabilized, obtain a focused history and perform a complete physical examination. History should include the mechanism and time of injury; use of any protective equipment; presence, severity, and duration of symptoms associated with brain injury (Table 2); identification of underlying medical conditions such as central nervous system (CNS) abnormalities, bleeding diatheses, and the use of intoxicants. Abusive head trauma is a leading cause of death in children younger than 1 year. Examine the head for the following findings: bruises, abrasions, lacerations, hematomas, bony depressions, and full or bulging fontanelle. Note pupil size and reactivity, optic disc margins, and the presence of retinal hemorrhages. The absence of retinal hemorrhages on a nondilated examination does not exclude them. Note any periorbital bruising (raccoon sign), mastoid bruising (Battle sign), hemotympanum, otorrhea, or rhinorrhea; these findings suggest basilar skull fracture. A neurologic examination should focus on extraocular movements, motor strength, reflexes, pain sensation and proprioception, station, and gait.

C. Assess severity of injury (Table 3). The GCS provides a uniform assessment of severity that can be used to facilitate communication between physicians and institutions.

D. Children 2 years or older with normal mental status at the time of evaluation, a normal neurologic examination, less than 5 seconds of loss of consciousness, no vomiting, absence of severe headache, minor mechanism, no evidence of basilar skull fracture, and no concerns for multisystem trauma do not require a computed tomographic (CT) scan. Observation of symptomatic children with mTBI (GCS $\geq$13) in the emergency department until it is clear their symptoms are dissipating is a reasonable alternative to obtaining head CT.

Children younger than 2 years with minor mechanisms, who are acting normally per caregiver, have a normal neurologic examination and mental status, less than 5 seconds of loss of consciousness, no scalp hematoma or evidence of skull fracture, no concerns for multisystem trauma or abuse, and who have a reliable caregiver at home do not require imaging.

E. Most children with blunt head injury will suffer mTBI (concussion) defined as a transient alteration in mental status that *may or may not involve a loss of consciousness*. Loss of consciousness is an unreliable tool for identifying mTBI and is not predictive of the severity of injury. Post-traumatic amnesia is a better predictor of severity and the likelihood of development of postconcussion syndrome. The symptoms listed in Table 2 are typical of mTBI. Concussions cause somatic, cognitive, and emotional disturbances. Informal orientation questions are poor at detecting these disturbances. Consider using a standardized concussion evaluation tool that focuses on orientation, concentration, memory, and recall, such as the Standardized Assessment of Concussion. Many commonly used concussion grading scales with return-to-play guidelines exist. None is evidence based, and there is considerable variation in recommendations. Most authors agree that children should not return to sports until they are free of symptoms both at rest and with exertion. For children with postconcussive symptoms persisting past 48 hours, consider referral to a neurologist or pediatric rehabilitation specialist for more detailed assessment.

F. The use of imaging should be directed by the history and physical examination. Skull radiographs are of limited value in the evaluation of children with head injury. Negative findings do not rule out intracranial injury. Positive findings often lead to obtaining more detailed studies. Noncontrast head CT is the study of choice in acute head injury. Indications for head CT include evidence of depressed or basilar skull fracture, significant alteration or sudden deterioration in mental status, focal neurologic findings, persistent or worsening symptoms, concern for foreign body, the presence of a bleeding diathesis, or if there is a concern for abuse. Some authors recommend imaging for any infant younger than 3 months because of the greater likelihood of occult intracranial injury.

G. Evidence of intracranial bleeding, presence of a foreign body, depressed or basilar skull fracture, GCS score of 8 or less, anemia or a significant decline in hematocrit, the presence of a bleeding diathesis, or intracranial instrumentation (e.g., ventriculoperitoneal shunt) should prompt immediate referral for neurosurgical

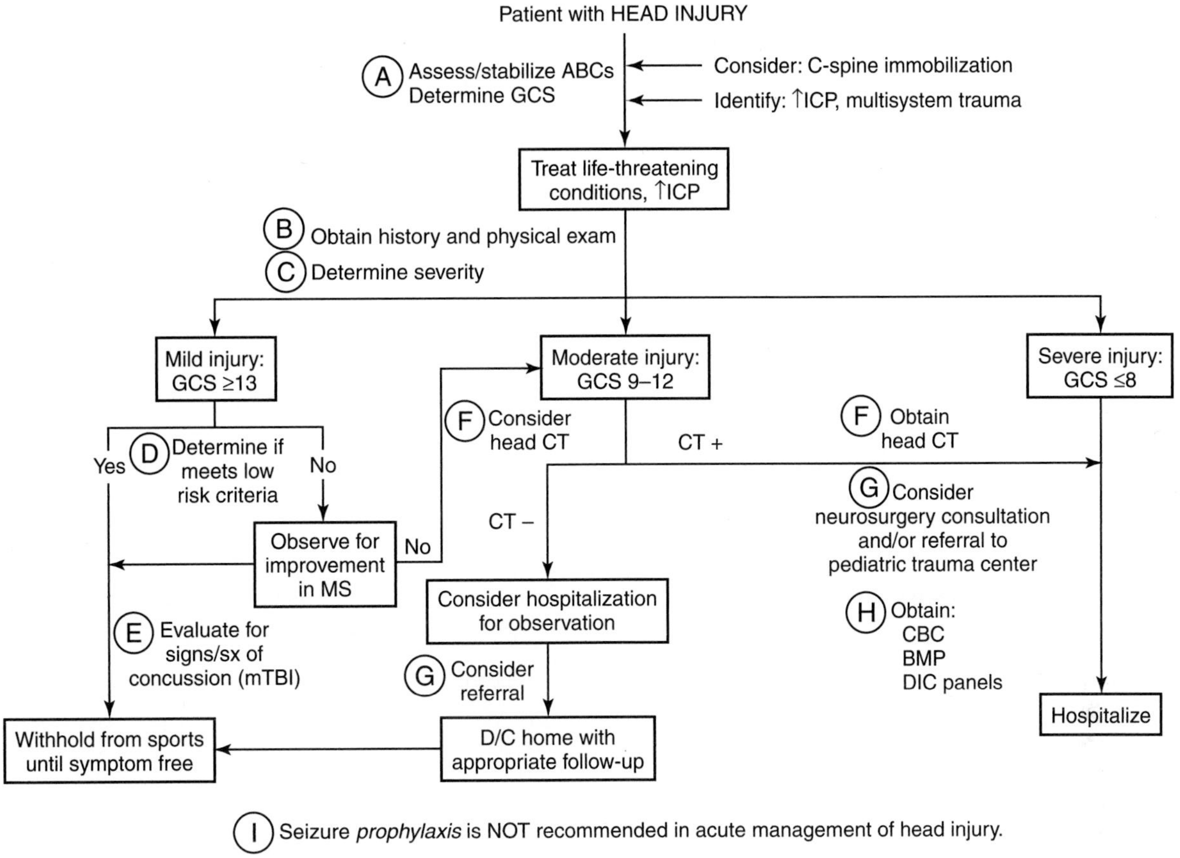

Patient with HEAD INJURY
A Assess/stabilize ABCs
Determine GCS
Consider: C-spine immobilization
Identify: ↑ICP, multisystem trauma
Treat life-threatening conditions, ↑ICP
B Obtain history and physical exam
C Determine severity
Mild injury: GCS ≥13
Moderate injury: GCS 9–12
Severe injury: GCS ≤8
D Determine if meets low risk criteria
Yes
No
Observe for improvement in MS
No
F Consider head CT
CT +
CT –
F Obtain head CT
G Consider neurosurgery consultation and/or referral to pediatric trauma center
H Obtain:
CBC
BMP
DIC panels
Consider hospitalization for observation
G Consider referral
E Evaluate for signs/sx of concussion (mTBI)
Withhold from sports until symptom free
D/C home with appropriate follow-up
Hospitalize
I Seizure prophylaxis is NOT recommended in acute management of head injury.

evaluation. Consider referral for children with moderate injury (GCS score, 9–12) or whose mental status is not improving.

H. Patients with moderate-to-severe brain injury are at risk for electrolyte disturbances (syndrome of inappropriate antidiuretic hormone secretion, diabetes insipidus) and disseminated intravascular coagulation (DIC); consider obtaining a basic metabolic panel and DIC screen. Infants with an open fontanelle are at risk for anemia caused by hemorrhage. Consider obtaining a complete blood cell count (CBC). Children younger than 1 year with linear skull fractures are at risk for development of a leptomeningeal cyst. Outpatient follow-up evaluation by a neurosurgeon is recommended.

I. Post-traumatic seizures occur in about 10% of all cases of blunt head trauma, with significantly greater rates in the moderately to severely injured child; 95% occur in the first 24 hours. Studies of postinjury prophylaxis irrespective of age show reduction of seizure rates by up to 66%; there is no improvement in neurologic outcomes or risk for death. Subsequent randomized, controlled trials in children do not show this dramatic reduction in seizure rates. Given the potential risks associated with antiepileptic drugs (e.g., Stevens–Johnson syndrome), seizure prophylaxis is not recommended. Children with persistent or recurrent seizure activity warrant intracranial imaging. Benzodiazepines are the first choice for acute management. Consider fosphenytoin (or phenobarbital for infants <1 year) for ongoing seizures not responsive to benzodiazepines. Obtain a head CT for recurrent or prolonged seizures.

Table 1. **Glasgow Coma Scale**

Subscale	Response (verbal child)	Response (infant, young child)	Score
Best eye opening	Spontaneous	Spontaneous	4
	To voice	To voice/sound	3
	To pain	To pain	2
	None	None	1
Best verbal response	Oriented	Coos, babbles, interacts	5
	Confused	Irritable cry; consolable	4
	Inappropriate words	Cries to pain; inappropriate words	3
	Inappropriate sounds	Moans to pain; incomprehensible words	2
	None	None	1
Best motor response	Obeys commands	Spontaneous	6
	Localizes pain	Withdraws to touch; localizes pain	5
	Withdraws from pain	Withdraws from pain	4
	Flexor posturing	Flexor posturing	3
	Extensor posturing	Extensor posturing	2
	None	None	1

Table 2. **Symptoms of Head Injury**

Headache
Nausea/vomiting
Blurry vision/diplopia
Tinnitus
Photophobia
Phonophobia
Irritability
Depression, feelings of sadness
Sleep disturbance
Slowed thinking
Memory disturbance/amnesia
Difficulty concentrating
Ataxia
Easily frustrated
Feeling like in a fog

Table 3. **Severity of Injury Based on Glasgow Coma Scale Score**

Severity of Injury	Score
Mild	13–15
Moderate	9–12
Severe	3–8

GCS, Glasgow Coma Scale.

References

Ahmed S, Bierley R, Sheikh JI, et al. Post-traumatic amnesia after closed head injury: a review of the literature and some suggestions for future research. Brain Injury 2000;14(9):765–80.

American Academy of Neurology Quality Standards Subcommittee. Practice parameter: the management of concussion in sports (summary statement). Neurology 1997;48:581–5.

American Academy of Pediatrics Committee on Quality Improvement. The management of minor closed head injury in children. Pediatrics 1999;104(6):1407–15.

Dias M. Traumatic brain and spinal cord injury. Pediatr Clin North Am 2004;51(2):271–303.

Hahn YS, Fuchs S, Flannery AM, et al. Factors influencing posttraumatic seizures in children. Neurosurgery 1988;22:864–7.

Kuppermann N, Holmes JF, Dayan PS, et al. Identification of children at very low risk of clinically important brain injuries after head trauma: a prospective cohort study. Lancet 2009;374:1160–70.

Langlois JA, Rutland-Brown W, Thomas KE. Traumatic brain injury in the United States: emergency department visits, hospitalizations, and deaths. Atlanta, GA: Centers for Disease Control and Prevention, Nation Center for Injury Prevention and Control; 2006.

Martin C, Falcone RA. Pediatric traumatic brain injury: an update of research to understand and improve outcomes. Curr Opin Pediatr 2008;20(3):295–9.

McCrea M, Kelly JP, Randolph C, et al. Standardized assessment of concussion (SAC): on-site mental status evaluation of the athlete. J Head Trauma Rehabil 1998;13(2):27–35.

Palchak MJ, Holmes JF, Vance CW, et al. A decision rule for identifying children at low risk for brain injuries after blunt head trauma. Ann Emerg Med 2003;42(4):492–506.

Schierhout G, Roberts I. Prophylactic antiepileptic agents after head injury: a systematic review. J Neurol Neurosurg Psychiatry 1998;64:108–12.

Schutzman SA, Branes P, Duhaime A, et al. Evaluation and management of children younger than two years old with apparently minor head trauma: proposed guidelines. Pediatrics 2001;107(5):983–93.

Teasdale G, Jennett B. Assessment of coma and impaired consciousness. A practical scale. Lancet 1974;2:81–4.

Young KD, Okada PJ, Sokolove P, et al. A randomized, double-blinded, placebo-controlled trial of phenytoin for the prevention of early post-traumatic seizures in children with moderate to severe blunt head injury. Ann Emerg Med 2004;43(4):435–46.

Neck Injury

Joseph Grubenhoff, MD

Pediatric cervical spine injury is uncommon, seen in only 1% to 2% of all pediatric trauma victims. The leading cause of injury for all age groups is motor vehicle collisions followed by sports-related mechanisms in children older than 8 years and falls in younger children. However, children are at substantial risk for morbidity and mortality if a cervical spine or spinal cord injury is present. Children are at risk for spinal cord injury without radiographic abnormality (SCIWORA) because of the differences in the pediatric cervical spine. There is considerable controversy in the medical literature regarding the use of corticosteroids in children with spinal cord injuries. This algorithm is designed for practitioners in the office, urgent care, or community hospital setting.

A. Airway, breathing, and circulation (ABCs) should be addressed first. Immobilization of the cervical spine with a rigid age-appropriate collar is critical, especially when significant forces or altered mental status is involved. Expose the patient to identify any other evidence of trauma including penetrating neck trauma. It is important to recognize and treat spinal shock (hypotension and bradycardia, autonomic dysregulation). Fluids, and epinephrine if refractory to fluids, is the treatment of choice for spinal shock. Special attention to body temperature is required. Helmets should be removed if there are any indications that respiratory failure or airway compromise is present or imminent. Maintain in-line cervical spine immobilization; bivalving the helmet can aid in removal. Otherwise, it is acceptable to leave helmets in place until someone experienced in removal is available.

B. Once stabilized, obtain a focused history and perform a complete physical examination. History should include the mechanism and time of injury; use of any protective equipment; presence, severity, and duration of symptoms associated with neck injury; identification of underlying medical conditions such as central nervous system (CNS) abnormalities, spine anomalies (Down syndrome, Arnold–Chiari malformation, Marfan syndrome, etc.), or the use of intoxicants. Examine the neck for the following: tenderness in the posterior midline, step-off, crepitus, and paraspinous tenderness. A neurologic examination should focus on blood pressure, heart rate, respiratory effort and mechanics, motor strength, reflexes, and pain sensation. Every effort must be made to remove children from spine boards as soon as possible to prevent pressure ulcers, especially if spinal cord injury is suspected. Patients presenting more than 24 hours from time of injury or with delayed onset of neck pain are unlikely to have a serious cervical spine or spinal cord injury. In those who do, most were involved in motor vehicle accidents or falls from significant heights, had distracting injuries, or were intoxicated at time of initial presentation.

C. Penetrating trauma to the neck should prompt referral to a pediatric trauma center.

D. In certain instances, the cervical spine can be "cleared" clinically and immobilization discontinued without obtaining radiographs. The following criteria must be satisfied: (1) no midline cervical spine tenderness or step-off; (2) no focal neurologic findings; (3) no distracting painful injuries (fractures, substantial lacerations, abdominal injuries, etc.); (4) normal mental status; and (5) no intoxicants, narcotics present. Caution should be exercised in applying these rules to children younger than 9 years and especially younger than 2 years.

Often trauma patients will receive narcotics in the field or will have appendicular skeletal fractures requiring reduction. If there is low suspicion of cervical spine injury and no focal neurologic deficit or evidence of spinal shock, it is reasonable to repeat an examination after the effects of narcotics have worn off and fractures are appropriately splinted. If there is no midline cervical tenderness at that time, immobilization may be safely discontinued assuming the other criteria noted earlier have been met.

E. If the earlier criteria cannot be met, consider imaging the cervical spine. Plain radiographs are usually adequate. A minimum of three views is required to achieve a sensitivity of 95%: (1) a lateral projection that includes C1-7 and the C7-T1 junction; (2) an anteroposterior (AP) projection; and (3) open mouth odontoid. Additional images such as oblique films, swimmer's view, or flexion-extension views may be necessary to complete the evaluation. Consultation with a radiologist is strongly encouraged given the radiologic differences of the pediatric cervical spine (Table 1).

F. Computed tomographic (CT) scans provide more detail of the cervical vertebral anatomy, especially when AP and coronal reconstructions are performed. However, they administer a substantially greater dose of radiation, and plain radiographs can usually provide adequate evaluation of the cervical spine. Indications for CT include possible but poorly defined fracture identified on plain films; delineation of complex fractures; inability to obtain adequate plain films because of patient factors (e.g., C1-2 evaluation in infants and toddlers). Given the cumulative risk for radiation exposure and expense, routinely performing CT of the neck in conjunction with a head CT is not recommended.

(Continued on page 424)

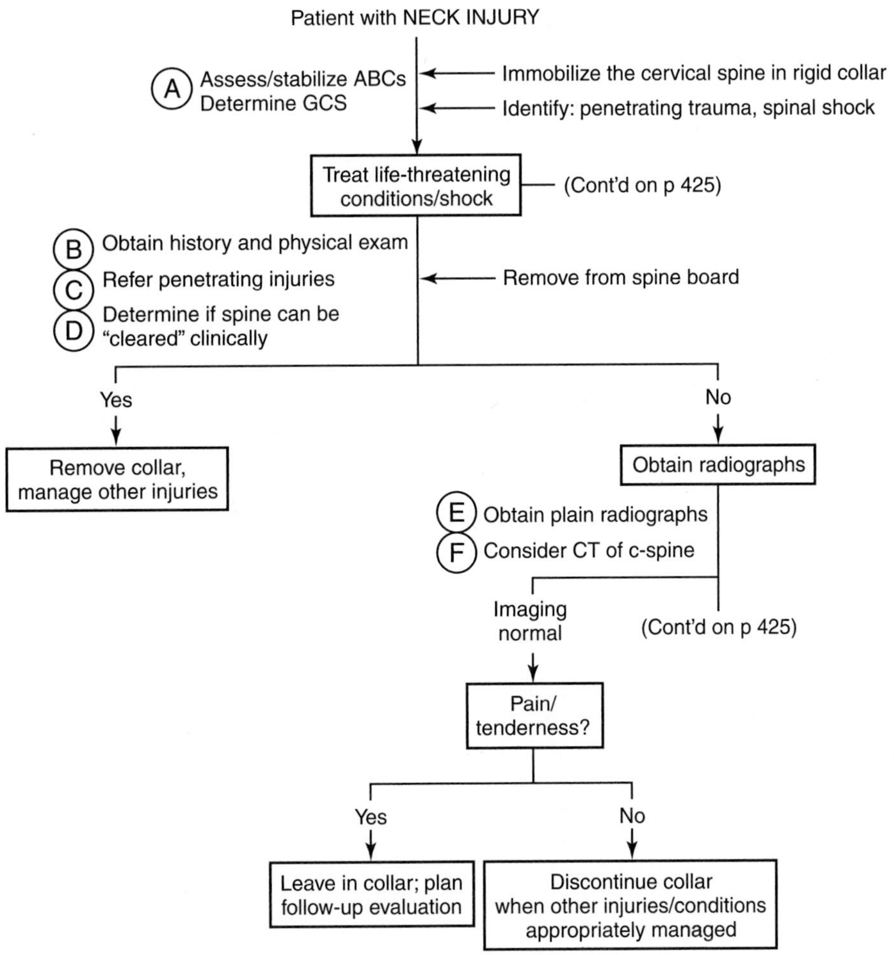
Patient with NECK INJURY
A
Assess/stabilize ABCs
Determine GCS
Immobilize the cervical spine in rigid collar
Identify: penetrating trauma, spinal shock
Treat life-threatening conditions/shock
(Cont'd on p 425)
B
Obtain history and physical exam
C
Refer penetrating injuries
D
Determine if spine can be "cleared" clinically
Remove from spine board
Yes
No
Remove collar, manage other injuries
Obtain radiographs
E
Obtain plain radiographs
F
Consider CT of c-spine
Imaging normal
(Cont'd on p 425)
Pain/ tenderness?
Yes
No
Leave in collar; plan follow-up evaluation
Discontinue collar when other injuries/conditions appropriately managed

Table 1. **Differences in the Pediatric Cervical Spine (Children <8 Years)**

Greater ligamentous laxity
Higher fulcrum (C2-3 at 1 year; C3-4 at 5–6 years; C5-6 at 8 years)
Weaker paraspinous musculature
More shallow angles of facet joints
Proportionally larger head
Incomplete ossification

G. Children with negative radiographic findings of cervical spine injury who continue to have pain may be discharged in a rigid collar with recommendations for follow-up for repeat examination by their primary care physician.

Children with positive findings should be referred for pediatric neurosurgical or orthopedic evaluation. Consider vascular imaging.

H. Children with focal neurologic deficits or spinal shock require magnetic resonance imaging (MRI) once stabilized. Children can have SCIWORA because of differences in anatomy. SCIWORA accounts for approximately 20% of all cervical spine injuries in children, but only 0.5% of all pediatric trauma victims. Because children undergoing MRI often require sedation, the practitioner must carefully consider the risks of sedation with the benefit of gaining information regarding cord injury. This study can be deferred until the patient arrives at a regional pediatric trauma center and should not delay transfer.

I. When spinal cord injury is present, practitioners have the *option* to start high-dose corticosteroids. A recent review of the literature concluded that methylprednisolone is not an evidence-based standard of care for patients with spinal cord injury. No study has evaluated the role of methylprednisolone in pediatric patients younger than 14 years. Based on the lack of evidence in pediatrics and the potential adverse effects of high-dose corticosteroids, methylprednisolone treatment is not recommended for pediatric patients with spinal cord injury.

References

Brown RL, Brunn MA, Garcia VF. Cervical spine injuries in children: a review of 103 patients treated consecutively at a level 1 pediatric trauma center. J Pediatr Surg 2001;36:1107–14.

Cirak B, Ziegfeld S, Knight VM, et al. Spinal injuries in children. J Pediatr Surg 2004;39:607–12.

Cox GR, Barish RA. Delayed presentation of unstable cervical spine injury with minimal symptoms. J Emerg Med 1991;9(3):123–7.

Kokoska E, Keller MS, Rallo MC, Weber TR. Characteristics of pediatric cervical spine injuries. J Pediatr Surg 2001;36:100–5.

Martin BW, Dykes E, Lecky FE. Patterns and risks in spinal trauma. Arch Dis Child 2004;89:860–5.

Patel JC, Tepas JJ, Mollitt DL, Pieper P. Pediatric cervical spine injuries: defining the disease. J Pediatr Surg 2001;32:373–6.

Platzer P, Jaindl M, Thalhammer G, et al. Cervical spine injuries in pediatric patients. J Trauma 2007;62:394–6.

Sayer FT, Kronvall E, Nilsson OG. Methylprednisolone treatment in acute spinal cord injury. Spine 2006;31:S16–21.

Shah VM, Marco RA. Delayed presentation of cervical ligamentous instability without radiologic evidence. Spine 2007;32(5):E168–74.

Viccellio P, Simon H, Pressman BD, et al. A prospective multicenter study of cervical spine injury in children. Pediatrics 2001;108:e20.

Woodward GA. Neck trauma. In: Fleisher GR, Ludwig S, Henretig FM, editors. Textbook of pediatric emergency medicine. 5th ed. New York: Lippincott Williams & Wilkins; 2005. p. 1412.

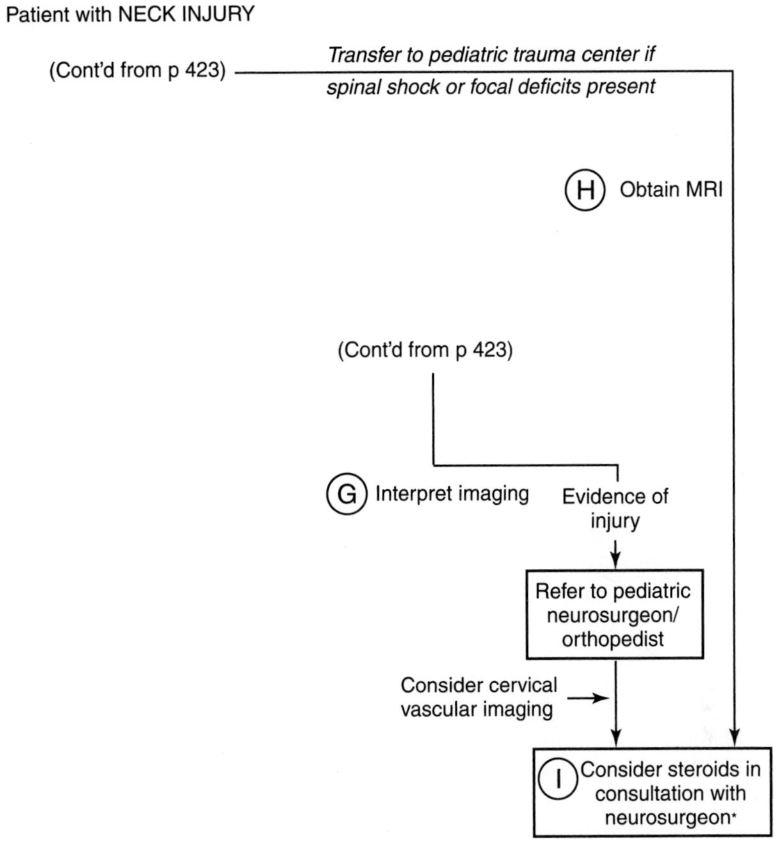
Patient with NECK INJURY
(Cont'd from p 423)
Transfer to pediatric trauma center if spinal shock or focal deficits present
H Obtain MRI
(Cont'd from p 423)
G Interpret imaging
Evidence of injury
Refer to pediatric neurosurgeon/ orthopedist
Consider cervical vascular imaging
I Consider steroids in consultation with neurosurgeon*

(I) *Because of the lack of demonstrable benefit and potential adverse effects, high-dose methylprednisolone is NOT routinely recommended for treatment of spinal cord injury in children.

Chest Trauma

George S. Wang, MD

Approximately 4% to 6% of hospitalized children with trauma have chest injuries. The presence of chest injuries increases the mortality of trauma patients twentyfold and accounts for 14% of trauma-related deaths, only second to head injuries. The majority of pediatric chest injuries (greater than 80%) are attributed to blunt trauma, and motor vehicle-related injuries account for at least 75% of chest injuries.

A. The physiology of the pediatric chest wall is quite different from the adult chest wall. Pediatric chest wall is highly compliant because of the greater amount of cartilage; thus, there can be intrathoracic injuries without rib fractures or chest wall injury. The mediastinum is mobile and cardiac function is primary preload and rate dependent. In addition, infants and young children have lower functional residual capacity and are preferential diaphragm breathers, so abdominal injuries can affect ventilation. Intra-abdominal injuries should be investigated to any injuries at the level of the sixth rib or below. Initial management of a chest trauma patient begins with the initial assessment per Pediatric Advance Life Support and Advanced Trauma Life Support: airway, breathing, and circulation (ABCs). Initial primary survey is then followed by secondary survey and obtaining history from witnesses and Emergency Medical Services (EMS).

B. During physical examination, inspection for chest wall rise, position of airway, respiratory rate, and cardiopulmonary auscultation can provide information about potential injuries. Pulse oximetry will help in your evaluation of oxygenation. Circulatory status must be evaluated after airway and breathing has been stabilized. The physical examination is not always reliable in determining thoracic injury, so a high index of suspicion should be maintained. Signs of injury include tachypnea, tachycardia, jugular venous distention, pallor, narrow pulse pressure or pulsus paradoxus, nasal flaring, grunting, retractions, decreased breath sounds/heart sounds, poor or asymmetric chest wall rise, crepitus, hypoxia, ecchymosis, or abrasions.

C. Laboratory and imaging studies depend on the suspicion of injury. CBC can help evaluate for hemorrhage, and a blood gas can evaluate ventilation. Chest radiograph helps identify 60% to 90% of injuries. However, chest CT is more helpful in further delineation of injuries noted on chest radiograph or high clinical suspicion despite normal chest radiograph. Even though ECG can be helpful, echocardiography is more definitive, and cardiac enzymes can also aid in diagnosis for cardiac injuries. The majority (>90%) of chest trauma can be managed nonoperatively.

D. Immediate life-threatening injuries such as airway obstruction, tension pneumothorax, hemothorax, and pericardial tamponade must be treated before further imaging/evaluation.

E. Pulmonary injuries consist of contusions, lacerations, pneumothoraces, hemothoraces, or pneumohemothoraces. Cardiac injury is rare; contusions are more common than lacerations. Great vessel injury is also rare but has a high mortality. The aorta is most commonly injured. Chest wall injuries such as rib fractures, sternal fractures, scapular fractures, and flail chest must be investigated. Lastly, diaphragmatic, esophageal, and tracheobronchial injuries are often overlooked but must be considered in thoracic injury.

F. Surgical intervention is needed for suspicion or evidence of the following injuries: persistent hemorrhage, pneumothorax, hemothorax or hemopneumothorax, pneumomediastinum, cardiac injury, tracheobronchial injury, esophageal injury, diaphragmatic injury, or major vascular injury.

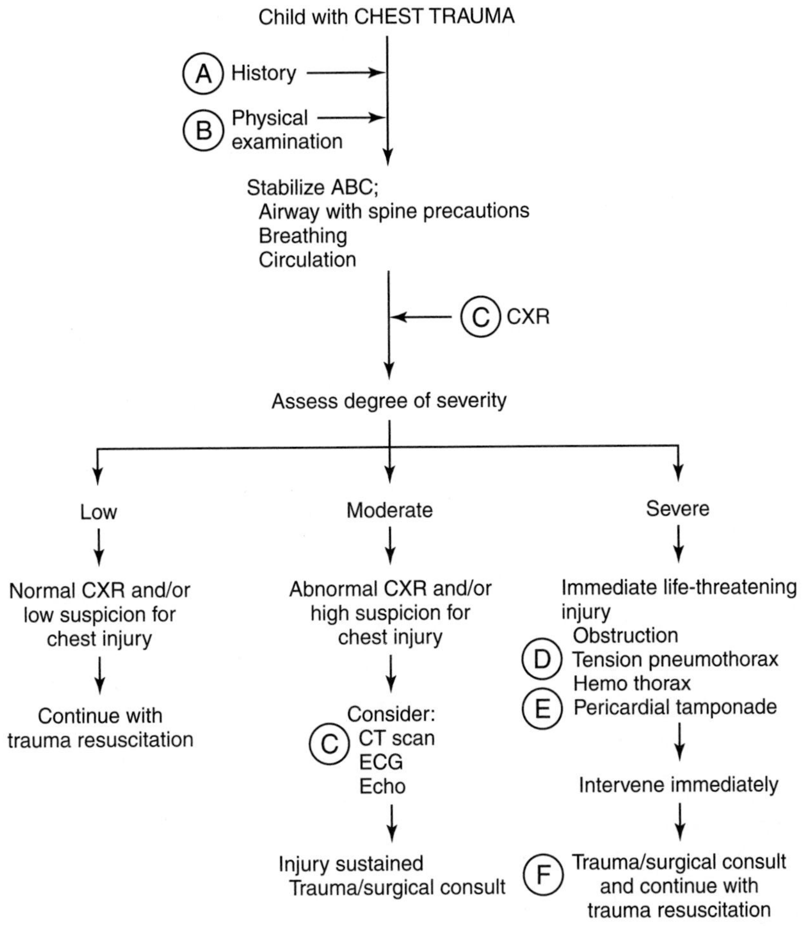
Child with CHEST TRAUMA
A History
B Physical examination
Stabilize ABC;
Airway with spine precautions
Breathing
Circulation
C CXR
Assess degree of severity
Low
Moderate
Severe
Normal CXR and/or low suspicion for chest injury
Continue with trauma resuscitation
Abnormal CXR and/or high suspicion for chest injury
Consider:
C CT scan
ECG
Echo
Injury sustained
Trauma/surgical consult
Immediate life-threatening injury
Obstruction
D Tension pneumothorax
Hemo thorax
E Pericardial tamponade
Intervene immediately
F Trauma/surgical consult and continue with trauma resuscitation

References

Avarello JT, Cantor RM. Pediatric major trauma: an approach to evaluation and management. Emerg Med Clin North Am 2007;25:3.

Holmes, JF, Sokolove PE, Brant WE, Kuppermann N. A clinical decision rule for identifying children with thoracic injuries after blunt torso trauma. Ann Emerg Med 2002;39(5):4929.

Kadish HA. Thoracic trauma. In: Fleisher GR, Ludwig S, Henretig FM, editors. Textbook of pediatric emergency medicine. 5th ed. 2006. Philadelphia: Lippincott, Williams & Wilkins; 2006. p.1433.

Sartorelli KH, Vane DW. The diagnosis and management of children with blunt injury of the chest. Semin Pediatr Surg 2004;13(2): 98–105.

Abdominal Trauma

Joe Wathen, MD

Intra-abdominal trauma occurs from blunt forces in about 90% of the cases, most commonly from motor vehicle collisions, auto-pedestrian accidents, falls, sports, bike, and child abuse. Multisystem injuries are common. Pediatric abdomen is more susceptible to abdominal trauma because of decreased musculature and fat, as well as more exposed solid organs and bladder. Abdominal trauma is the most common unrecognized cause of fatal injuries. Hypovolemic shock can occur from "hidden" intra-abdominal sources.

A. Historical items that are important to consider in all traumas include when the injury occurred, the mechanism, surrounding environment, and the severity of the forces. Obtaining a history can be difficult because of the urgency of the situation, associated intracranial injuries, a preverbal child, alcohol or drug use, and unavailable parents. In vehicular trauma, inquire about the speed of the collision, damage to the automobile, and whether proper restraint devices were used. In penetrating trauma, attempt to determine the type of weapon, number of shots or stab wounds inflicted, and approximate blood loss. Note symptoms including abdominal pain, low chest pain, back pain, pelvic pain, vomiting, and hematuria.

B. Assess the patient for multiple trauma. The primary survey is conducted first, addressing the airway with cervical spine immobilization, breathing and ventilation, circulation and hemorrhage control, disability, and exposure/environment. During the primary survey, identify and manage life-threatening injuries. Give oxygen and obtain intravenous or intraosseous access. Identify shock initially by tachycardia and signs of inadequate tissue perfusion. Hypotension represents a late finding. If significant head trauma has occurred, consider the need for immediate neurosurgical intervention. In severe or multiple trauma situations, stabilize by addressing any compromise of airway, breathing, and circulation, and involve a trauma surgeon promptly. Consider referral to an appropriate trauma facility.

The evaluation for intra-abdominal injuries begins with a high index of suspicion in any traumatized patient. Blunt injuries may initially have subtle findings on physical examination. Inspect the abdomen, lower chest, back, flanks, and pelvis for abrasions, ecchymosis, lacerations, or signs of a penetrating injury. Abdominal wall ecchymosis is the hallmark finding for the lap belt complex (i.e., associated intra-abdominal injury and lumbar spine fracture). Auscultate for absent bowel sounds suggestive of an ileus. Gently palpate the entire abdomen to localize tenderness while noting the presence of involuntary guarding and rebound tenderness (Table 1). Abdominal tenderness, distention, and shock suggest intra-abdominal injuries. A rectal examination should be performed to look for blood that may indicate a bowel perforation and to assess sphincter tone for spinal cord integrity. Examine the genitourinary (GU) structures for urethral blood, scrotal swelling and pain, or vaginal bleeding. Intra-abdominal injury may initially exist in the absence of any physical examination findings; therefore, serial examinations are important.

C. Laboratory evaluation includes a hematocrit or complete blood cell count (CBC), urinalysis (UA), and in some cases, a type and cross match. Gross hematuria is often a mark of intra-abdominal injury. Radiographic studies include a cervical spine series and chest and pelvis films. Abdominal computed tomography (CT) is an excellent imaging study for solid organ injury, with indications listed (Table 2). Repeat abdominal CT may be needed (i.e., in 6 hours) when clinical findings are significant and the initial CT is negative. Focused abdominal sonography in trauma (FAST) is used in many institutions as a rapid diagnostic tool detecting hemoperitoneum and hemopericardium. Ultrasound has only modest sensitivity in detecting hemoperitoneum (76–84%), with better specificity (95–97%) in excluding hemoperitoneum. It cannot be used as the sole test to exclude intra-abdominal injury and should be an adjunct to clinical suspicion. Positive findings on abdominal ultrasound warrants further computed tomography. Diagnostic peritoneal lavage has fallen out of favor as a screening tool on children in most instances. Pediatric diagnostic peritoneal lavage should be performed only by experienced surgeons because of its invasive nature, with associated increased risk for injuries to the intra-abdominal organs. Retrograde urethrogram may occasionally be indicated to detect bladder and urethral injury.

(Continued on page 430)

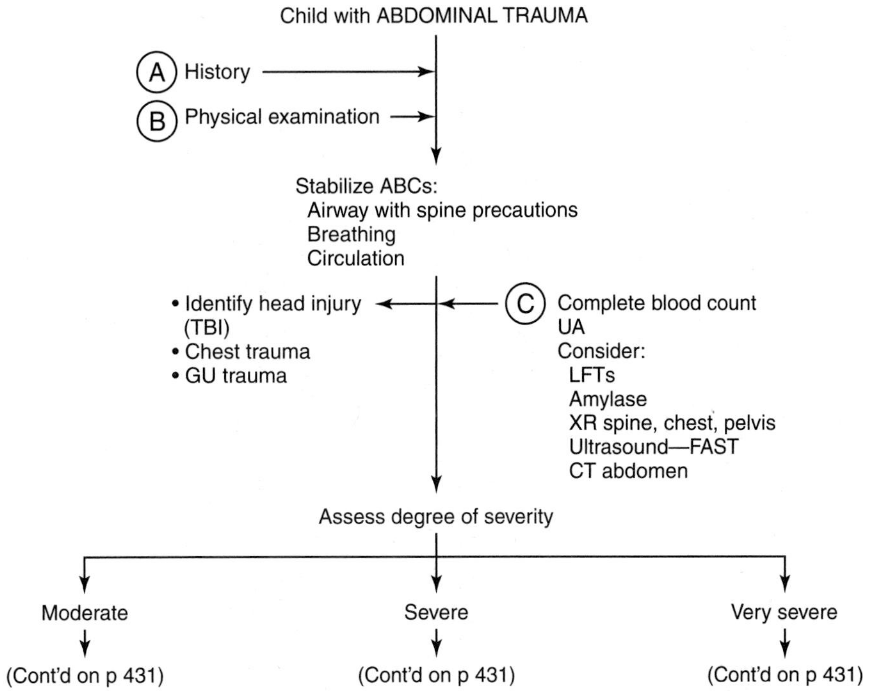
Child with ABDOMINAL TRAUMA
A History
B Physical examination
Stabilize ABCs:
Airway with spine precautions
Breathing
Circulation
• Identify head injury (TBI)
• Chest trauma
• GU trauma
C Complete blood count
UA
Consider:
LFTs
Amylase
XR spine, chest, pelvis
Ultrasound—FAST
CT abdomen
Assess degree of severity
Moderate
Severe
Very severe
(Cont'd on p 431)
(Cont'd on p 431)
(Cont'd on p 431)

Table 1. **Degree of Severity in Abdominal Trauma**

Mild to Moderate	Severe	Very Severe
Minor mechanism	Mechanism—substantial force with risk for intestinal injury	Multisystem trauma, penetrating injury
Asymptomatic with severe hemodynamic stability	Abdominal tenderness—not resolving; abdominal distention, guarding, or rebound	Abdominal tenderness—with hemodynamic instability
Minor or no abdominal pain	Able to maintain hemodynamic stability	Rapidly falling hematocrit
	Fracture of lower six ribs, lumbar spine	Massive hemoperitoneum
		Pneumoperitoneum
		Hematuria

Table 2. **Indications for Abdominal Computed Tomography**

Mechanism of injury suggesting abdominal trauma
History or physical examination findings suggestive of liver, spleen, or renal injury (abdominal tenderness, distention, guarding, rebound, abdominal wall ecchymosis)
Hemodynamic compromise
Slowly declining hematocrit
Unaccountable fluid or blood requirements
Hematuria
Unreliable physical examination because of head injury, drugs, or general anesthesia
Persistent abdominal tenderness

D. Most patients with suspected abdominal injury need admission for re-evaluation and repeat or additional diagnostic studies. The early diagnosis of intestinal injuries is difficult and can be missed with computed tomography. In particular, lap belt injuries can cause a hollow viscus injury that is difficult to diagnose. In children with a seat belt ecchymosis or otherwise at risk for intestinal injury, a period of observation and re-evaluation is warranted. Monitor for signs and symptoms of increasing abdominal pain, fever, tachycardia, and increased white blood cell (WBC) count. The timely treatment of this injury relies on a high index of suspicion and serial examinations, with involvement of a trauma surgeon.

E. Home follow-up includes instructions to the parents to observe for signs of delayed presentation of an intra-abdominal injury. Late findings of an intestinal stricture caused by localized ischemia and fibrosis can occur even several weeks after injury. Post-traumatic intestinal obstructions should be suspected in children who develop signs and symptoms consistent with a partial small bowel obstruction. A common scenario is a duodenal hematoma after a bicycle handlebar injury to the abdomen. Parents should monitor for nausea, bilious vomiting, abdominal pain, and distention. Consider an upper gastrointestinal study with small bowel follow-through in this situation.

F. Indications for immediate laparotomy include multisystem trauma with need for a craniotomy in the presence of a positive result of diagnostic peritoneal lavage or radiographic or other evidence of significant intra-abdominal injury, hemodynamic instability without evidence of extra-abdominal injury, penetrating injuries to the abdomen, pneumoperitoneum, and significant abdominal distention associated with hypotension.

References

Boulanger BR, Kearney PA, Brennenman FD, et al. Utilization of FAST (focused assessment with sonography for trauma) in 1999: results of a survey of North American trauma centers. Am Surg 2000;66:1049–55.

Cantor RM, Leaming JM. Evaluation and management of pediatric major trauma. Emerg Med Clin North Am 1998;16:229–56.

Garcia VF, Brown RL. Pediatric trauma: beyond the brain. Crit Care Clin 2003;19:551–61.

Jaffe D, Wesson D. Emergency management of blunt trauma in children. N Engl J Med 1991;324:1477–82.

Mooney DP. Multiple trauma: liver and spleen injury. Curr Opin Paediatr 2002;14:482–5.

Nadler EP, Patoka DA, Schultz BL. The high morbidity associated with handlebar injuries. J Trauma 2005;58:1171–4.

Newman KD, Bowman LM, Eichelberger MR, et al. The lap belt complex: intestinal and lumbar spine injury in children. J Trauma 1990;30:1133–40.

Patel JC, Tepas JJ. The efficacy of focused abdominal sonography for trauma (FAST) as a screening tool in the assessment of injured children. J Pediatr Surg 1999;34:44–7.

Rothrock SG, Green SM, Morgan R. Abdominal trauma in infants and children: prompt identification and early management of serious and life-threatening injuries. Part 1: injury patterns and initial assessment. Pediatr Emerg Care 2000;16:106–15.

Rothrock SG, Green SM, Morgan R. Abdominal trauma in infants and children: prompt identification and early management of serious and life-threatening injuries. Part 2: specific injuries and ED management. Pediatr Emerg Care 2000;16:189–95.

Taylor GA, Eichelberger MR, Potter BM. Hematuria: a marker of abdominal injury in children after blunt trauma. Ann Surg 1988;208:688–93.

Wegner S, Colletti JE, Van Wie D. Pediatric blunt abdominal trauma. Pediatr Clin North Am 2006;53:243–56.

Winston FK, Shaw KN, Kreshak AA, et al. Hidden spears: handlebars as injury hazards to children. Pediatrics 1998;102:596–601.

Child with ABDOMINAL TRAUMA

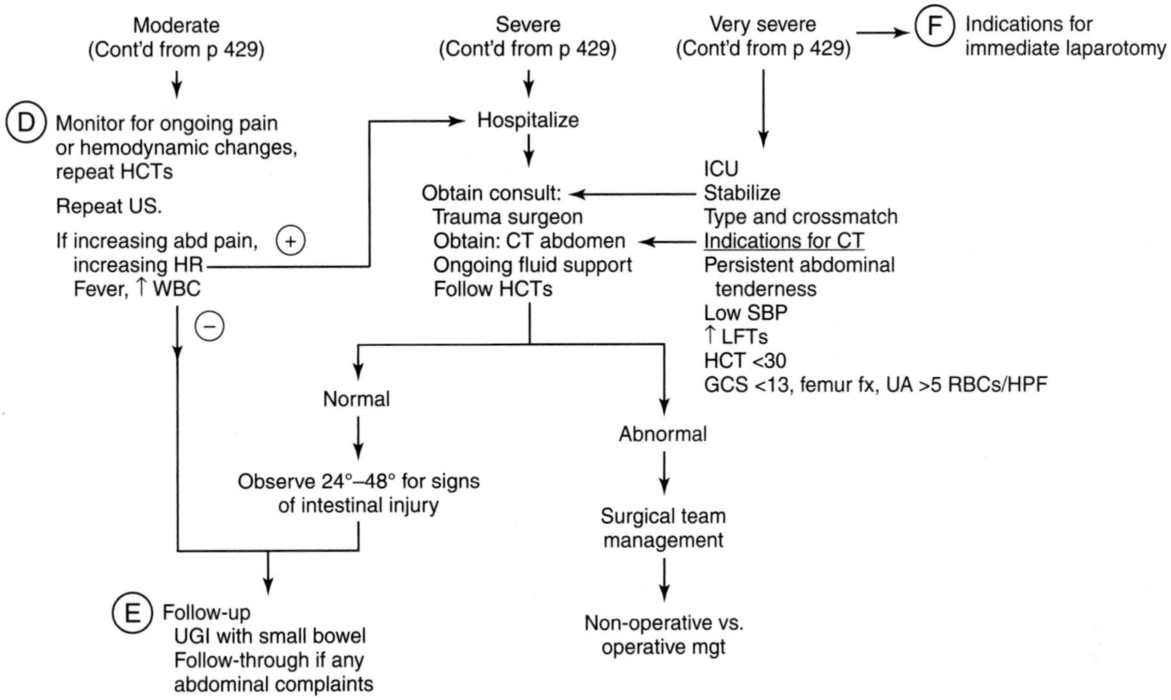
Moderate
(Cont'd from p 429)
D
Monitor for ongoing pain or hemodynamic changes, repeat HCTs
Repeat US.
If increasing abd pain, increasing HR
Fever, ↑ WBC
+
−
Severe
(Cont'd from p 429)
Hospitalize
Obtain consult:
Trauma surgeon
Obtain: CT abdomen
Ongoing fluid support
Follow HCTs
Very severe
(Cont'd from p 429)
F
Indications for immediate laparotomy
ICU
Stabilize
Type and crossmatch
Indications for CT
Persistent abdominal tenderness
Low SBP
↑ LFTs
HCT <30
GCS <13, femur fx, UA >5 RBCs/HPF
Normal
Observe 24°–48° for signs of intestinal injury
Abnormal
Surgical team management
Non-operative vs. operative mgt
E
Follow-up
UGI with small bowel Follow-through if any abdominal complaints

Genitourinary Trauma

Sarah Halstead, MD

Genitourinary (GU) and pelvic trauma results from blunt trauma about 80% of the time, most commonly from motor vehicle collisions (MVCs), falls from height, saddle injuries, and direct blows to the torso or external genitalia. Penetrating injuries, including gunshot wounds and stabbings, are less common in children than in adults. GU injuries include injuries to the external genitalia, urethra, bladders, ureters, and kidney. The kidney is the most common GU injury encountered in children, accounting for greater than 47% of GU trauma, and after liver and spleen injuries is the third most common solid-organ injury seen in children. Simultaneous upper and lower tract injuries are rare, and often incompatible with survival, whereas isolated urologic injuries are rarely the cause of death. Injuries to the GU area are often associated with pelvic fractures. Pelvic fractures with greatest risk for associated GU injuries include concomitant fractures of all four pubic rami or fractures of both ipsilateral rami accompanied by massive posterior disruption through the sacrum, sacroiliac joint, or ilium. Low-risk injuries include single ramus fractures and ipsilateral rami fractures without posterior ring disruption. The risk for urethral injury approaches zero with isolated fractures of the acetabulum, ilium, and sacrum. Overall, urethral disruption accompanies pelvic fracture in approximately 5% of cases in women and up to 25% in men, with risk varying depending on the fracture.

A. Determine the time, circumstance, and severity of the trauma. As with all traumas, inquiring about forces of blunt trauma (i.e., speed of collision, damage to the automobile) or penetrating trauma (i.e., number of stab wounds) will help risk stratify the patient. Because GU/pelvic injuries are rarely life threatening and often associated with head and abdominal trauma, it is important to stabilize the patient and manage all life-threatening conditions first. In severe or multiple trauma, make sure airway, breathing, and circulation (ABCs) are managed before performing secondary survey. In an unstable patient, consult with a trauma surgeon promptly and consider referral to an appropriate trauma facility. Identify predisposing conditions (i.e., GU surgeries, pregnancy, bleeding disorders).

B. Once the primary survey is complete and airway, breathing, and circulation are secure, evaluate the patient for intra-abdominal or pelvic injuries that might raise the concern for GU injury. Because blunt injuries are often subtle, it is important to closely inspect the abdomen, flank, back, and pelvis for bruising, deformities, lacerations, or abrasions. Flank tenderness, flank hematoma, or palpable flank mass should raise the concern for significant renal injuries, although they might not be present initially. With both significant renal injuries and pelvic fractures, blood loss can be considerable, so monitoring for tachycardia, inadequate tissue perfusion, and hypotension need to be on ongoing process. An enlarging flank mass in the absence of retroperitoneal bleeding suggests urinary extravasation and should raise the concern for ureteral injury. Ureteral injuries, however, are often asymptomatic initially and therefore missed. The inability to void, especially if accompanied by lower abdominal tenderness, should raise concerns for bladder or urethral injury. After a thorough abdominal and pelvic examination, an external genitalia examination should be performed. Upward blows to the scrotum can result in testicular dislocation, so palpation of both testicles is essential in this type of injury. Ecchymosis, swelling, or pallor of the testicles/scrotum may be signs of torsion, rupture, or displacement. Looking for blood at the meatus/introitus is important when evaluating for a urethral injury, although it is not always present. If blood is seen at the urethral meatus, catheterization must be avoided. Perineal ecchymosis (especially if in the shape of a butterfly) is typical for anterior urethra injury.

C. Laboratory evaluation includes hematocrit and urine analysis. Gross hematuria, although considered the hallmark sign of GU injury, may be absent even in severe injuries. Greater than two thirds of blunt bladder injuries present with gross hematuria, with microhematuria, defined here as ≥25 red blood cells (RBCs)/high-powered field (HPF), is present in nearly all remaining cases. Ureteral injuries, however, will present with hematuria only 70% of the time. Plain films of pelvis are often obtained in patients who sustain pelvic or lower abdominal trauma. Although the American College of Surgeons Committee on Trauma recommends the use of pelvic radiography for all patients who have sustained a multisystem blunt traumatic injury, pelvic fractures remain uncommon in pediatrics. Patients who are older than 9 years, patients who were in an MVC, or pedestrians struck by a vehicle have a greater likelihood of having pelvic fractures.

D. If a child presents with significant trauma and/or gross hematuria, CT abdomen/pelvis is indicated. If CT scan is not available or the patient is unstable, an intravenous pyelogram can be preformed to assess for renal injury. An intravenous pyelogram is preformed by administering 2 ml/kg (maximum: 100 ml) nonionic contrast agent intravenously and obtaining a flat plate plain film 10 minutes later. Indications of renal injury include delayed excretion of contrast by the injured kidney, nonvisualization of the caliceal system, or extravasation of contrast into the perinephric tissues. If there are concerns for a bladder injury, and there is no pelvic fracture or blood seen at the meatus, a retrograde cystogram can be performed. The urethra is catheterized, making sure that the bladder is full. A cystogram is then obtained with anteroposterior and

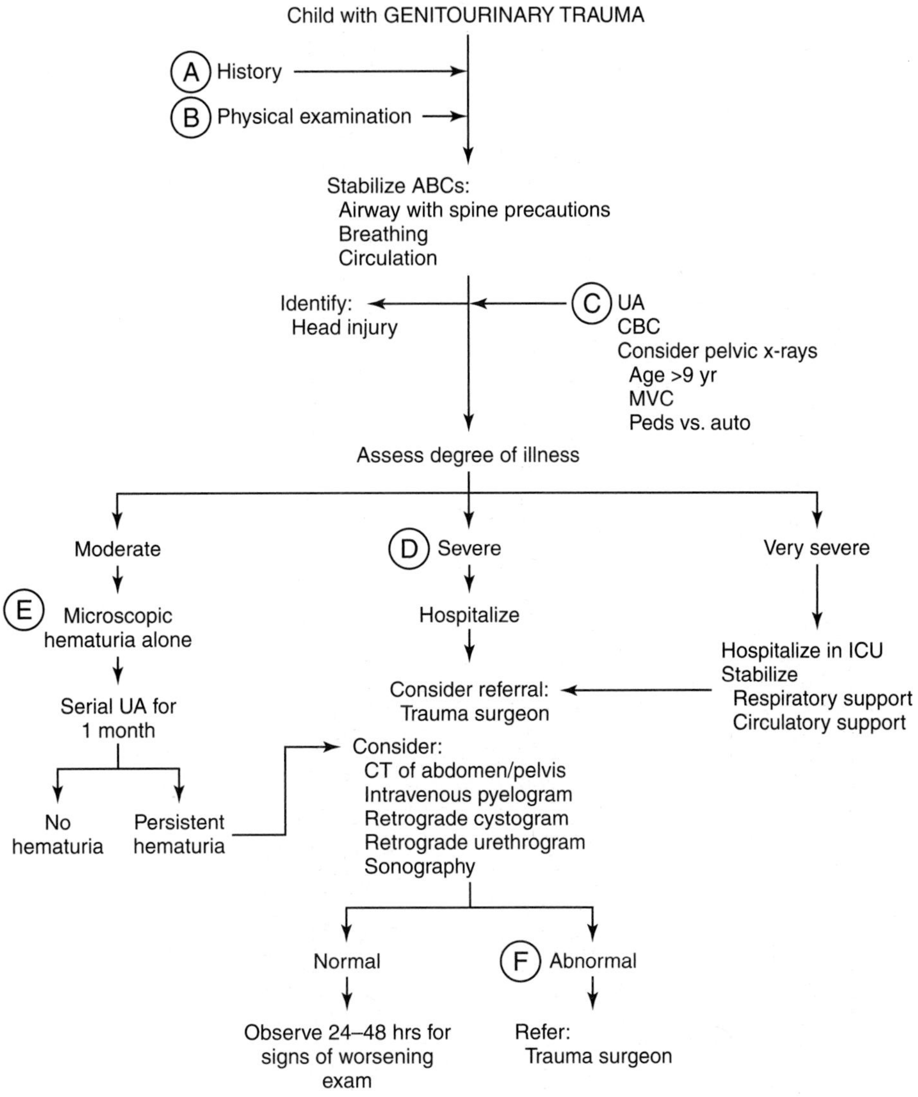

Child with GENITOURINARY TRAUMA
A History
B Physical examination
Stabilize ABCs:
Airway with spine precautions
Breathing
Circulation
Identify:
Head injury
C UA
CBC
Consider pelvic x-rays
Age >9 yr
MVC
Peds vs. auto
Assess degree of illness
Moderate
D Severe
Very severe
E Microscopic hematuria alone
Hospitalize
Hospitalize in ICU
Stabilize
Respiratory support
Circulatory support
Serial UA for 1 month
Consider referral:
Trauma surgeon
Consider:
CT of abdomen/pelvis
Intravenous pyelogram
Retrograde cystogram
Retrograde urethrogram
Sonography
No hematuria
Persistent hematuria
Normal
F Abnormal
Observe 24–48 hrs for signs of worsening exam
Refer:
Trauma surgeon

oblique views as well as a postdrainage film. If there are concerns for a urethral injury or catheterization of the bladder is unsuccessful or contraindicated, then a retrograde urethrogram should be completed. Because bladder catheterization could turn a partial urethral tear into a complete transection, a urethrogram would ideally be obtained before bladder catheterization. However, urethral injuries, especially in female patients without significant pelvic fractures, are uncommon. For concerns for scrotal or testicular injury, ultrasound remains the gold standard, and these, together with urethral injuries, are often missed on CT scanning alone.

E. Pediatric patients who have microscopic hematuria and no other associated injuries may be suspected of having isolated renal contusions, and may be followed with serial urinalysis with no immediate imaging. If microscopic hematuria persists for more than 1 month, imaging is then recommended.

F. Management: In cases of blunt trauma and grade 1–3 renal injuries, conservative management is acceptable. Strict bed rest, analgesia, and prophylactic antibiotics are used until gross hematuria resolves and limited activity until microscopic hematuria resolves. In patients with penetrating injuries or grade 4–5 renal injuries, trauma surgery evaluation should be obtained. Although most penetrating renal injuries are managed surgically, many blunt renal injuries are being managed expectantly. Patients treated without surgery have a complication rate up to 50% (recurrent hemorrhage, extravasation, urinoma formation, infection, infarction, and segmental hydronephrosis) but a slightly lower nephrectomy rate.

KIDNEYS

The Organ Injury Scaling Committee of the American Association for the Surgery of Trauma:

- Grade 1: Injuries include contusions or subcapsular nonexpanding hematomas (60%–90%)
- Grade 2: Nonexpanding hematomas confined to the retroperitoneum or lacerations less than 1 cm in depth without urinary extravasation
- Grade 3: Lacerations extending more than 1 cm into the renal cortex without collecting system rupture or urinary extravasation
- Grade 4: Lacerations extending into the collecting system or renal vascular injuries with contained hemorrhage
- Grade 5: Completely shattered kidneys or avulsions of renal hilum with devascularized kidneys (3% of renal injuries)

References

Avey G, Blackmore CC, Wessells H, et al. Radiographic and clinical predictors of bladder rupture in blunt trauma patients with pelvic fracture. Acad Radiol 2006;13:573.

Morey AF, Iverson AJ, Swan A, et al. Bladder rupture after blunt trauma: guidelines for diagnostic imaging. J Trauma 2001;51:683–6.

Morgan DE, Nallamala LK, Kenney PJ, et al. CT cystography: radiographic and clinical predictors of bladder rupture. AJR Am J Roentgenol 2000; 174:89.

Upper Extremity Trauma

Julia Fuzak, MD

Upper extremity injuries are common in pediatric patients. A careful history will help determine the nature of the injury, with simple falls resulting in mild or moderate injuries, and high-energy trauma such as motor vehicle accidents and falls from heights causing severe injuries. Repetitive movements may lead to overuse syndromes. Most injuries to the upper extremity in the pediatric patient result from a fall onto the arm or an outstretched hand. Common fractures include the clavicle, elbow, forearm, and distal radius.

A. Assess the degree of injury. The signs of injuries in the upper extremity include swelling, point tenderness, deformity, and possible reluctance to move the extremity. Mild injuries often result in diffuse, poorly localized pain without evidence of joint effusion. Gross deformity, point tenderness, rapid onset of effusion, and obvious ligamentous instability suggest a severe injury. Gross deformity, point tenderness, and crepitus indicate a fracture. Open wounds in the vicinity of the injury indicate a possible open fracture, which requires immediate treatment and consultation with an orthopedist. Pulses and sensation distal to the injury should be assessed to determine whether there is a nerve or vascular injury necessitating emergent evaluation and treatment. If the extremity appears grossly deformed and pulses are not present, the arm should be repositioned and the deformity corrected immediately. All fractures should be splinted before transfer of the patient. Always be alert for signs of nonaccidental trauma, including a history that is inconsistent with the injury, a delay in treatment, multiple fractures, metaphyseal fractures, posterior rib fractures, and fractures in nonambulatory patients. Treat acute injuries with rest, ice, elevation, and mild compression for the first 24 to 36 hours to help control pain and swelling. Apply ice (not in direct contact with skin) for 20 minutes at a time. If the injury is chronic or associated with repetitive actions such as pitching, playing tennis, swimming, or gymnastics training, it should initially be treated with rest, ice, and elevation, and followed by a rehabilitation program. This should include gentle range-of-motion exercises and muscle strengthening and stretching before a gradual resumption of activities. This regimen should also be followed for sprains and strains.

B. The most common shoulder injury is clavicle fracture, which often occurs secondary to fall onto an outstretched arm, fall onto the lateral shoulder, or direct blow to the clavicle. This injury may also be seen in the newborn period after a difficult delivery. Fractures typically occur in the middle to lateral third of the clavicle and cause mild swelling over this area with point tenderness. A bony deformity or crepitus can often be palpated. Neurovascular complications are rare with clavicle fractures, but a detailed examination of the affected upper extremity is suggested. In children, clavicle fractures do not require reduction and can be managed by immobilizing the shoulder girdle with a sling and swath or figure-of-eight dressing. Clavicle fractures generally heal in 3 to 4 weeks, and patients can expect return to function in 4 to 8 weeks. Adolescent patients should be referred to orthopedics within 2 to 3 days.

C. Fractures of the humerus may cause injury to the radial nerve. The patient should be assessed for numbness over the dorsal hand or weakness of the hand and wrist. Most simple fractures to the radius heal without surgery. Casting is not possible with most types of humerus fractures. If the elbow is not involved, the arm should be placed in a sling and the fracture will heal with time.

D. Elbow injuries may be complex. A careful history of the injury will delineate simple injuries from fractures that require referral to an orthopedist. Nursemaids' elbow is a simple and common childhood injury that results from traction on the upper extremity such as lifting the child by one arm. The injury consists of subluxation of the radial head caused by displacement of the annular ligament. This occurs in toddler-aged children who present with refusal to use an arm. The affected arm is often held at the patient's side with the elbow slightly flexed and the forearm pronated. If the history of injury is consistent with a traction mechanism, a nursemaids' elbow can be easily reduced in the primary care setting. This is accomplished by gentle, quick, complete flexion of the elbow with simultaneous supination of the forearm. The elbow should be cupped firmly during this maneuver because successful reduction is usually accompanied by a click felt over the area of the radial head. The child will usually regain function with several minutes. If function does not return promptly, the arm should be placed in a posterior long-arm splint for several days, and radiographs should be considered to rule out other injury. If reduction is successful, the family should be counseled on the mechanism of this injury and risk for recurrence. Elbow fractures are more severe injuries and should be suspected in any child with swelling around the elbow, refusal to flex or straighten the joint, and history of fall. If these symptoms are present, radiographs should be obtained. Attention should be paid to the ossification centers and the order in which they appear (Figures 1 and 2). An anterior fat pad is normal, but a posterior fat pad is pathologic. If supracondylar or epicondylar fracture of the

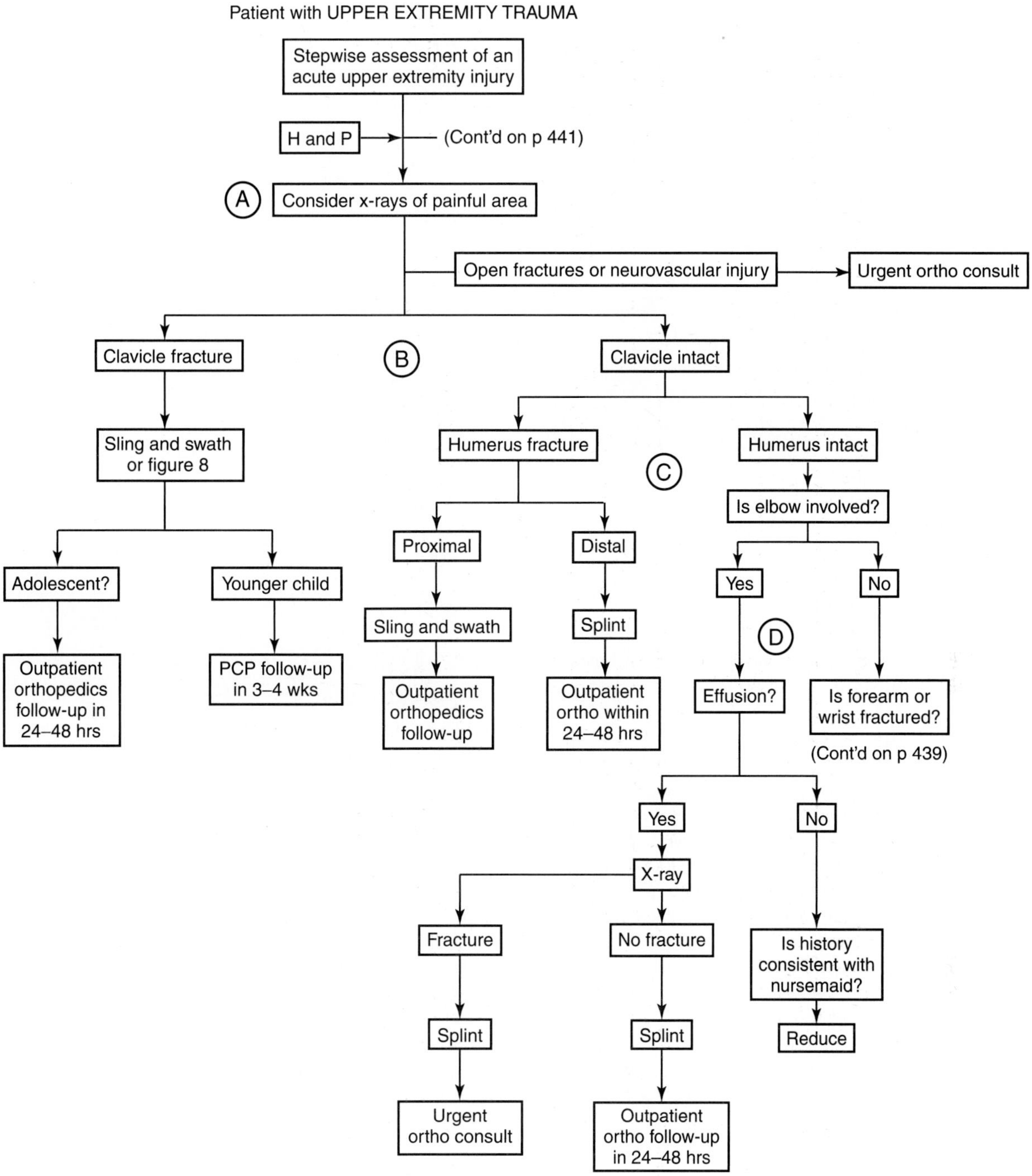
Patient with UPPER EXTREMITY TRAUMA
Stepwise assessment of an acute upper extremity injury
H and P
(Cont'd on p 441)
A
Consider x-rays of painful area
Open fractures or neurovascular injury
Urgent ortho consult
Clavicle fracture
B
Clavicle intact
Sling and swath or figure 8
Humerus fracture
C
Humerus intact
Is elbow involved?
Adolescent?
Younger child
Proximal
Distal
Yes
No
Sling and swath
Splint
D
Outpatient orthopedics follow-up in 24–48 hrs
PCP follow-up in 3–4 wks
Outpatient orthopedics follow-up
Outpatient ortho within 24–48 hrs
Effusion?
Is forearm or wrist fractured?
(Cont'd on p 439)
Yes
No
X-ray
Fracture
No fracture
Is history consistent with nursemaid?
Splint
Splint
Reduce
Urgent ortho consult
Outpatient ortho follow-up in 24–48 hrs

humerus is suspected, the arm should be placed in a posterior long arm splint for stabilization, and an orthopedic surgeon should be consulted. These injuries generally require operative repair. Injuries to or distal to the elbow should prompt a careful neurovascular examination. This should include sensory testing with two-point discrimination. Motor function of the radial nerve can be tested by extension of the fingers and wrist against resistance. The median nerve can be tested by having the patient make an "OK" sign, and the ulnar nerve can be assessed by having the patient separate the fingers against resistance.

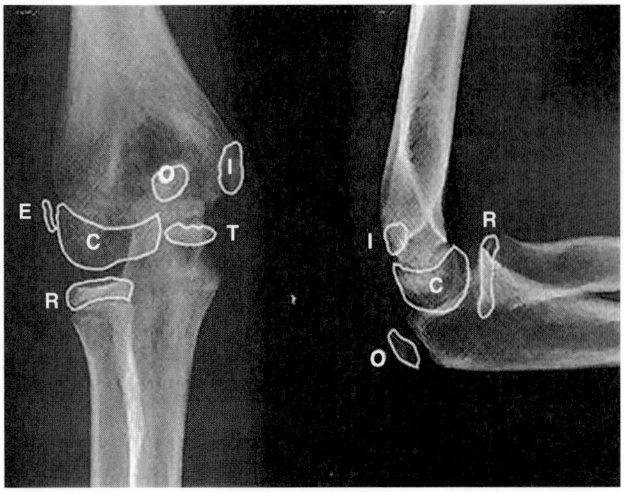
E
C
R
O
I
T
I
C
R
O

Figure 1. The capitellum (C) appears first, followed by the radial head (R), internal (medial) epicondyle (I), trochlea (T), olecranon (O), and external (lateral) epicondyle (E). From www.radiologyassistant.nl.

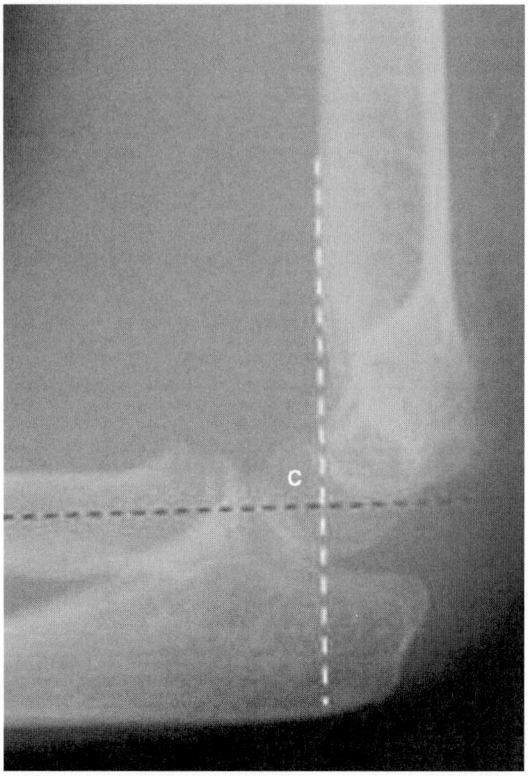
C

Figure 2. A true lateral view with the elbow flexed to 90 degrees is essential. On lateral view, an hourglass figure can be seen at the distal radius. Both the anterior humeral line and radiocapitellar line should bisect the capitellum (C). From http://i225.photobucket.com/albums/dd253/drkmliau/elbow%20x%20ray/Elbow7.jpg

E. Forearm fractures are common in children and usually result from a fall onto an outstretched hand but may also occur secondary to a direct blow to the forearm. Buckle (greenstick or torus) fractures with less than 20 degrees of angulation are stable and can be splinted with follow-up in 3 to 4 weeks. A Monteggia fracture (fracture of the proximal third of ulna with associated dislocation of the radial head) or Galeazzi fracture (radial shaft fracture with associated dislocation of the distal radioulnar joint) requires immediate reduction. If no fractures of the upper extremity are seen on radiograph but the child continues to have point tenderness over the radial and ulnar physis, the arm should be placed in a splint with follow-up in 7 days to re-evaluate for Salter–Harris type I fracture.

F. Wrist injuries are also common in children and are also often associated with a fall onto an outstretched hand. If point tenderness or pain with range of motion is noted, radiographs should be obtained. The child should be carefully examined for scaphoid fracture because these are at risk for avascular necrosis and poor healing. Findings suggestive of scaphoid fracture include tenderness over the "snuff box" area or pain with axial load on the thumb. If scaphoid fracture is suspected, the patient should be placed in a thumb spica splint and referred to orthopedics in 1 week.

(Continued on page 440)

Patient with UPPER EXTREMITY TRAUMA

(Cont'd from p 437)

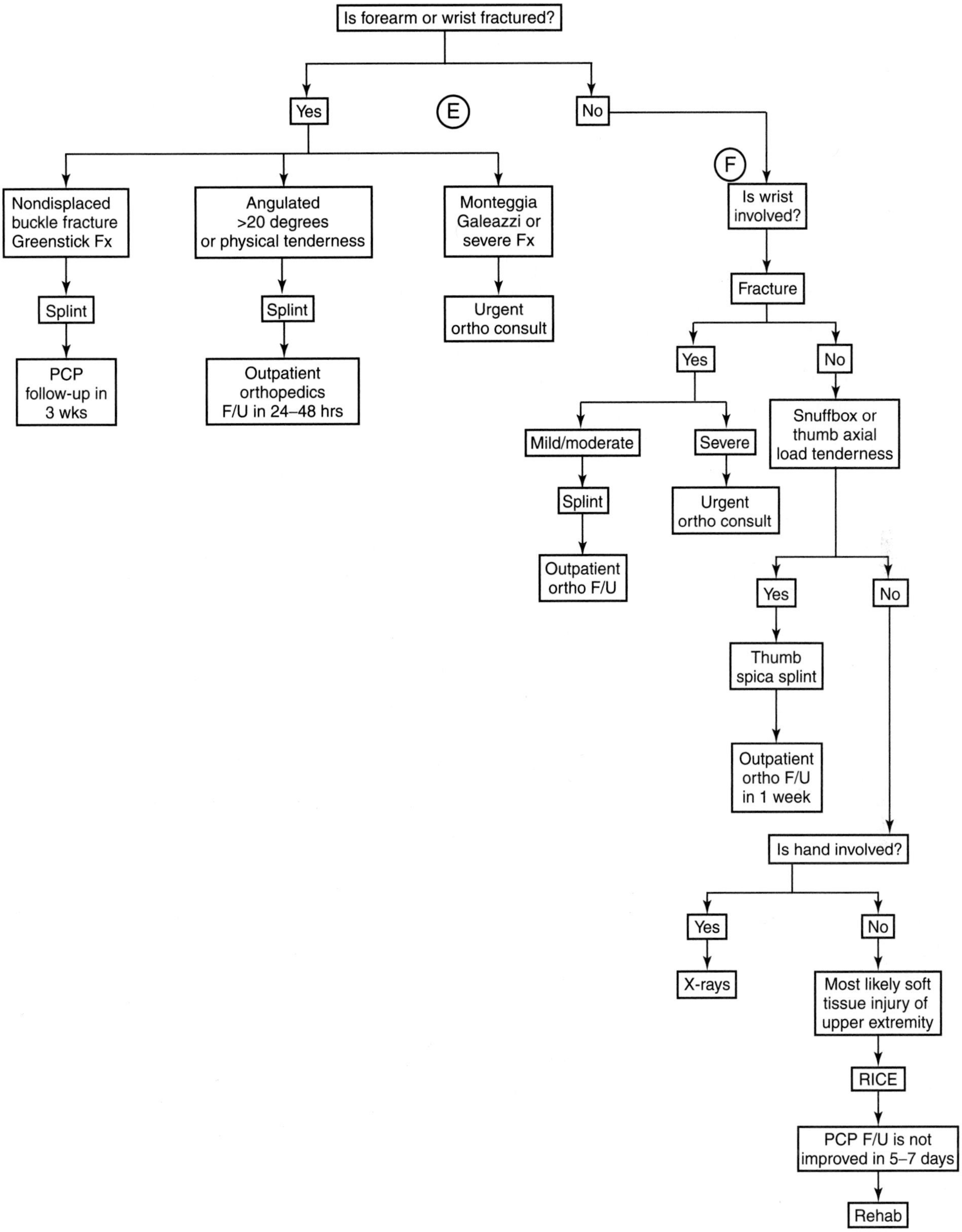
Is forearm or wrist fractured?
Yes
E
No
Nondisplaced buckle fracture Greenstick Fx
Splint
PCP follow-up in 3 wks
Angulated >20 degrees or physical tenderness
Splint
Outpatient orthopedics F/U in 24–48 hrs
Monteggia Galeazzi or severe Fx
Urgent ortho consult
F
Is wrist involved?
Fracture
Yes
No
Mild/moderate
Splint
Outpatient ortho F/U
Severe
Urgent ortho consult
Snuffbox or thumb axial load tenderness
Yes
No
Thumb spica splint
Outpatient ortho F/U in 1 week
Is hand involved?
Yes
No
X-rays
Most likely soft tissue injury of upper extremity
RICE
PCP F/U is not improved in 5–7 days
Rehab

G. Lacerations to the upper extremity can be repaired after copious irrigation and assessment for neurovascular or tendon injury. Deep sutures should be avoided in the wrist and the hand.

H. Shoulder dislocation occurs more frequently in adolescents than in younger children because epiphyseal growth plate fractures tend to occur before dislocation in this age group. Anterior shoulder dislocations are far more common than posterior dislocations (~97% vs. 3%) and result from abduction, extension, and external rotation, such as when preparing for a volleyball spike. The dislocated arm is held in slight abduction and external rotation. The shoulder appears "squared off" or boxlike with loss of the deltoid contour, and the humeral head is usually palpable anteriorly. The patient will resist movement. Axillary nerve injury should be assessed by testing for sensation over the deltoid muscles. Sensory and motor function of the radial and musculocutaneous nerves should also be evaluated. Prereduction and postreduction radiographs including axillary Y view are recommended to evaluate for fracture. The patient may require procedural sedation to achieve adequate muscle relaxation for reduction. The shoulder can usually be reduced with the following method: Stabilize the elbow against the trunk with one hand. With the elbow flexed at 90 degrees, gradually allow the forearm to move laterally to the extent that muscle relaxation allows, pausing for pain. Never use force. The shoulder will likely reduce before the forearm reaches the coronal plane. If not, proceed slowly with abduction of the humerus until forearm is over head. The arm should then be immobilized in a sling and neurovascular examination should be repeated.

References

Barkin R. Pediatric emergency medicine. 2nd ed. St. Louis, MO: Mosby; 1997.

Fleisher G, Ludwig S, Henretig F. Textbook of pediatric emergency medicine. 5th ed. Philadelphia: Lippincott Williams & Wilkins; 2006.

Patient with UPPER EXTREMITY TRAUMA

(Cont'd from p 437)

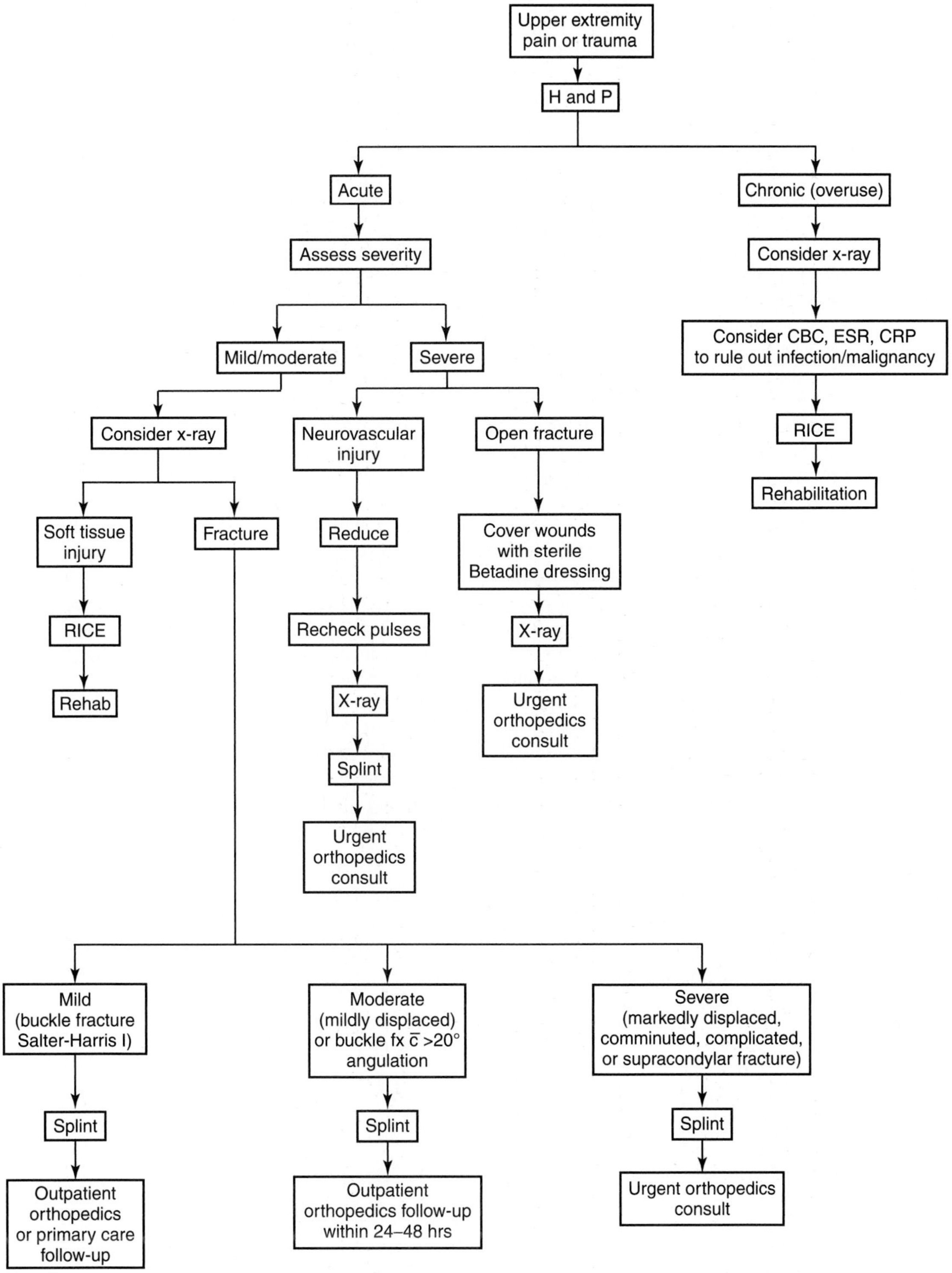
Upper extremity pain or trauma
H and P
Acute
Chronic (overuse)
Assess severity
Consider x-ray
Mild/moderate
Severe
Consider CBC, ESR, CRP to rule out infection/malignancy
Consider x-ray
Neurovascular injury
Open fracture
RICE
Rehabilitation
Soft tissue injury
Fracture
Reduce
Cover wounds with sterile Betadine dressing
RICE
Recheck pulses
X-ray
Rehab
X-ray
Urgent orthopedics consult
Splint
Urgent orthopedics consult
Mild (buckle fracture Salter-Harris I)
Moderate (mildly displaced) or buckle fx c̄ >20° angulation
Severe (markedly displaced, comminuted, complicated, or supracondylar fracture)
Splint
Splint
Splint
Outpatient orthopedics or primary care follow-up
Outpatient orthopedics follow-up within 24–48 hrs
Urgent orthopedics consult

Lower Extremity Trauma

Patrick Mahar, MD

A. The first step in determining the cause of the lower extremity trauma is a complete history. An abrupt onset of pain and/or decreased ability to use the effected extremity would suggest an acute injury, whereas a more insidious onset of pain may suggest a chronic injury. A history of a distinct traumatic event, such as a fall, a twisting of involved joint, or being struck by something can help dictate the workup and treatment of the injury. The physical examination will also be helpful in determining the workup and the diagnosis of the traumatic lower extremity injury. It is important to examine not only the joint/area where the patient is reporting pain, but also to pay special attention to the joint above and below the site of injury. The nature and severity of the injury can often be predicted by the events of the injury. Injuries that involve a direct high-energy force (such as being struck by an automobile), may be an indication of long bone and/or pelvic fractures, whereas a simple twisting injury (such as an ankle inversion injury) may predict a simple sprain. In cases where there is not a clear story to the injury, one must consider an overuse injury in older children/adolescents and nonaccidental trauma in infants and toddlers. If there is no history, the history changes, and/or the degree of injury does not fit the history, one must look for signs of nonaccidental trauma by having patient fully undressed and look for bruising or other signs of injuries. If an injury is thought to be secondary to nonaccidental trauma, the proper authorities must be notified (including police and social services). Findings such as multiple fractures of differing ages, metaphyseal lesions, posterior rib fractures, and long-bone fractures in children younger than 2 years are often associated with nonaccidental trauma.

B. The findings on physical examination should dictate whether and what types of radiographic studies are called for. A patient with severe pain, point tenderness, gross deformity, and/or inability to ambulate will most likely require an x-ray film to try to identify any fractures or dislocations. Temporary splinting of the injured area can provide pain relief and protection from further injury when moving the patient to obtain radiographic studies. No x-ray film would be needed if the physical examination shows a patient with the ability to bear weight and ambulate, together with minimal soft-tissue swelling and full range of motion. Severe injuries, such as an unstable pelvis, open fracture, and/or loss of distal pulses, should lead to an immediate orthopedic consult. In the acute setting, x-ray films are the most available and inexpensive radiographic test. The downside of x-ray films is that they cannot give a true picture of tendons, ligaments, and cartilage. For patients with injuries chronic in nature, x-ray films may provide only a limited amount of information, but are usually obtained before more expensive radiographic studies such as magnetic resonance imaging (MRI) or bone scans.

(Continued on page 444)

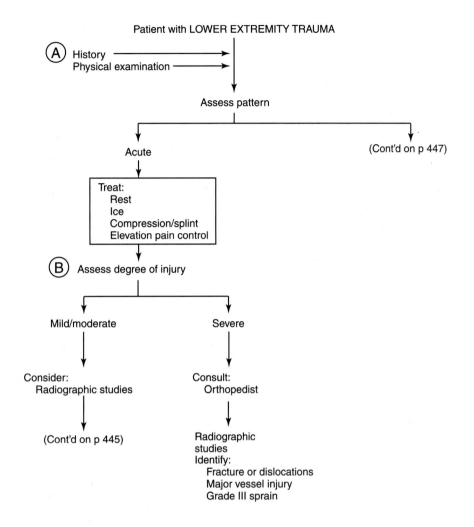

Patient with LOWER EXTREMITY TRAUMA

(A) History
Physical examination

Assess pattern

- Acute
  - Treat:
    - Rest
    - Ice
    - Compression/splint
    - Elevation pain control
  - (B) Assess degree of injury
    - Mild/moderate
      - Consider:
        - Radiographic studies
      - (Cont'd on p 445)
    - Severe
      - Consult:
        - Orthopedist
      - Radiographic studies
      - Identify:
        - Fracture or dislocations
        - Major vessel injury
        - Grade III sprain
- (Cont'd on p 447)

C. A majority of the lower extremity fractures seen in children and adolescents are nondisplaced tibial fractures or torus (buckle) fractures. These fractures present pain with ambulation or inability to bear weight and mild swelling with point tenderness on examination. The radiographic findings are usually minimal. In young children learning to walk, a common fracture seen is a nondisplaced distal tibia spiral fracture (i.e., toddler fracture). Most children with toddler's fractures are brought to a medical provider with complaint of refusing to bear weight on the affected extremity. In many cases, there is no history of significant trauma or history of only a minor fall. Often, the physical examination shows a normal examination with the exception of patient refusing to bear weight on affected leg and possible local tenderness with palpitation of distal tibia. When x-ray films are obtained, the radiographic findings are subtle, and initial radiographs may be normal in as many as 43% of cases. These injuries do not require immediate orthopedic evaluation, as treatment in the acute setting is splinting. The ankle should be splinted at 90 degrees (i.e., neutral position) to provide support and control pain. A posterior short-leg splint is sufficient, and a sugar-tong (i.e., coaptation) splint can be added for additional mediolateral support. These patients should follow up with orthopedist or sports medicine physician in 1 week for re-evaluation and possible casting. It is important to have significant amounts of cast padding in place, especially over any potential pressure points, and to stress to patient/caregivers that these splints are not made to be used for ambulation and doing so could lead to extensive skin breakdown and complications. In toddlers, another cause for acute onset of not bearing weight without a known precipitating event is a foreign body in foot; thus, close examination of the bottom of feet is important.

D. Soft-tissue injuries are a common diagnosis when a patient presents with an acute lower extremity trauma. This would include injuries involving ligaments, tendons, cartilage, and/or muscles. The ankle and knee are the joints most often associated with soft-tissue injuries. Physical examination findings associated with acute lower extremity joint injuries include significant joint effusion, joint instability, and point tenderness. The severity of the ligament injury (sprain) is graded based on severity of injury from the least (grade I) to the most severe (grade III).

1. Grade I: There is pain and no laxity with testing. There may be small tears in the ligament, yet the majority of the ligament is intact.
2. Grade II: There is a partial tear in the ligament, yet the majority of the ligament is intact. There is increased ligamentous laxity and an end point with provocative testing.
3. Grade III: There is complete disruption of the ligament. There is gross laxity with provocative testing and no end point.

The grades of sprains are easiest to determine in the immediate postinjury period before the onset of swelling and secondary muscle spasm. A severe ligamentous injury will most likely have significant hemarthrosis immediately after injury and instability of the joint. To test the integrity of the knee ligaments, one would start with testing the anterior cruciate ligament (ACL). This is done via anterior drawer test, Lachman test, or both. The anterior drawer test is performed with the knee flexed to 90 degrees and the foot stabilized, the proximal tibia is grasped firmly with both hands, and the tibia is forcibly pulled anteriorly, noting any pain, laxity, or abnormal movement compared with the opposite side. The Lachman test is similar to the anterior drawer test, except that the knee is flexed only to 20 degrees and the examiner's knee is placed under the patient's knee. The distal thigh is grasped above the patella with one hand and pressed down on the examiner's knee to stabilize the thigh, and the proximal tibia is grasped with the other hand to pull the tibia forward. As with the anterior drawer test, the Lachman test is positive if there is excessive anterior glide of the tibia compared with the opposite knee, or if there is no sharp end point to the anterior motion. The posterior cruciate ligament (PCL) is rarely injured in pediatric/adolescent patients. PCL integrity is evaluated with the posterior sag test and the posterior drawer test. In the posterior sag test, the patient is supine, with hips flexed to 45 degrees, knees flexed to 90 degrees, and the feet flat on the table. In a positive test, the tibia sags backward. A positive posterior drawer test also suggests PCL injury. Laxity of the medial collateral ligament (MCL) is evaluated with the valgus stress test, in which the examiner places one above the knee along the lateral thigh to stabilize the leg while the other hand applies valgus stress on the calf. If this valgus stress to the knee reveals laxity with the knee flexed to 30 degrees, it is suggestive of an isolated MCL sprain. The lateral collateral ligament (LCL) is tested in a similar manner, except this time the examiner applies a varus stress to the lower leg. Meniscus injuries are often associated with ligament injuries. Although these, too, are a rare injury in children, one must consider a meniscus injury in an adolescent patient with knee effusion and joint line tenderness. To grade an ankle sprain, one must test the integrity of the ankle joint. The anterior drawer test evaluates stability of the anterior talofibular ligament (ATFL) and is performed by stabilizing the lower leg and applying stress with opposite hand from the heel to pull the foot anteriorly. In cases of complete disruption of the ATFL, the anterior drawer test will result in anterior subluxation of the calcaneus and talus. The fibulocalcaneal ligament

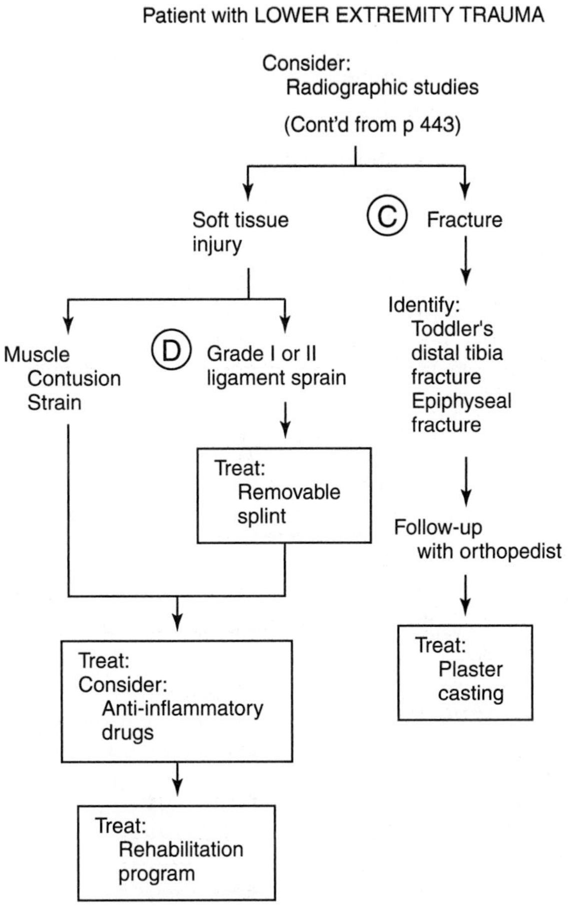
Patient with LOWER EXTREMITY TRAUMA
Consider:
Radiographic studies
(Cont'd from p 443)
Soft tissue injury
C
Fracture
Muscle
Contusion
Strain
D
Grade I or II ligament sprain
Identify:
Toddler's distal tibia fracture
Epiphyseal fracture
Treat:
Removable splint
Follow-up with orthopedist
Treat:
Consider:
Anti-inflammatory drugs
Treat:
Plaster casting
Treat:
Rehabilitation program

integrity can be tested by inverting the heel and palpating for tenderness and laxity over the ligament (i.e., the lateral aspect of the ankle). It is important to note that, in children, the ligaments are often stronger than the growing/developing bone; thus, epiphyseal fractures are more common than ligament ruptures in young children. For this reason, even if there is no fracture on x-ray film, if there is point tenderness over the physis, a Salter type I fracture is diagnosed. The acute treatment for all sprains should be include RICE (rest, ice, compression, elevation), together with nonsteroidal anti-inflammatory drugs. Grade III sprains (and some grade II sprains) will also require immobilization via splinting and orthopedic referral.

E. Insidious onset of pain is suggestive of a chronic/overuse injury. When evaluating for chronic/overuse injuries, it is important to remember to closely examine both the joint above and below the site of pain. Knee pain can be secondary to hip injury or foot/ankle problems. Serious nontraumatic hip abnormalities, such as Legg–Perthes syndrome and slipped capital femoral epiphysis, often have knee pain as the initial symptom. The same is true for hip pain that can be directly related to knee issues. Determining what, if any, tests are indicated is a challenge with overuse injuries. If there is a history of fevers and/or weight loss, one must consider nontraumatic causative factors such as infection (osteomyelitis or septic joint) or malignancy. Often plain x-ray films will not be beneficial, and thus should not be obtained; history and physical examination may be enough to make a diagnosis. In other cases, more specialized radiographic studies such as MRI or bone scan may be indicated.

F. Knee pain is a common lower extremity complaint in adolescent patients. This is especially true for patients starting a new activity or with excessive training. The patients often describe pain that has slowly increased in intensity. Patellofemoral pain syndrome (PFPS) is a frequently encountered overuse injury. PFPS presents most often as anterior knee pain. PFPS is the most common cause of knee pain seen by primary care physicians (PCPs), orthopedic surgeons, and sports medicine specialists, and is more common in female than male patients. Typically, knee pain associated with PFPS is exacerbated by squatting, running, prolonged sitting, or when going up or down stairs. Physical examination may show a small effusion and mild crepitus. Like PFPS, Osgood-Schlatter disease is related to the overuse of one component of the extensor mechanism of the knee. The typical patient with Osgood-Schlatter is an active adolescent who recently has undergone a rapid growth spurt. The anterior knee pain increases gradually over time and may be exacerbated by direct trauma, running, jumping, or kneeling. The characteristic physical finding is considerable tenderness over the tibial tuberosity with an otherwise completely normal knee examination. Another source of knee pain is iliotibial band syndrome. The iliotibial band runs from the ilium along lateral aspect of thigh to the fibula. Patients present with pain at the site where the band passes over the lateral femoral condyle and, occasionally, the pain radiates up the thigh toward the hip. Iliotibial band syndrome has been associated with a varus alignment of the knee, excessive running mileage, worn shoes, or continuous running on uneven terrain.

G. Pain in the lower leg is often related to overuse or repetitive exercise. Shin splints syndrome (medial tibial stress syndrome) is the name given to a complex of pain and discomfort in the lower leg occurring after repetitive overuse. The mechanism of this syndrome is a tibial stress reactions result from a progressive process of injury and may result in a cortical stress fracture. Patients have pain involving the anterior aspect of the lower leg that is worsened by activity. A stress fracture occurs when a bone breaks after being subjected to repeated tensile or compressive stresses. Stress fractures are characterized by pain with activity and point tenderness. A recent increase in activity level is frequent. Common areas of stress fracture are the metatarsals, distal fibula, proximal tibia, and femoral neck. All female patients with suspected or confirmed stress fracture should raise concern for the "female athlete triad." The female athlete triad is a combination of decreased bone density, abnormal eating and/or exercise habits, and amenorrhea (primary or secondary). Female individuals who fit this description are at a greatly increased risk for stress fractures. When working up potential stress fractures, the initial radiographs may be normal, and thus may need the bone scan or MRI to make radiographic diagnosis. Calcaneal apophysitis (Sever disease) is a common cause of heel pain in young athletes, particularly those who play soccer and basketball or participate in gymnastics or running. The calcaneal apophysis is located on the posterior inferior aspect of the calcaneus and is where the Achilles tendon inserts into the os calcis apophysis. Inflammation at the calcaneal apophysis is the cause of the heel pain and can be seen with increased metabolic activity in the growth plate during periods of rapid growth, footwear (particularly soccer cleats) that lacks heel cushioning may provide inadequate protection, and repetitive microtrauma seen with overuse in sports that involve jumping and running. Pain in bottom of foot, especially on first getting out of bed in the morning, is suggestive of plantar fasciitis. Although much more common in adults, it can also be seen in adolescent patients.

H. Treatment of most overuse lower extremity injuries involves initially reducing/stopping the activity involved in the mechanism of injury. This may mean a brief period of complete rest, followed by a slow return to activity once completely pain free. In short term, nonsteroidal anti-inflammatory drugs may help decrease inflammation and reduce pain. Physical therapy may be indicated in many cases to help improve range of motion, muscle strengthening, and flexibility. Referral to sports medicine physician and physical therapy may be indicated in athletes wanting to return to sports.

References

Gregg JR, Das M. Foot and ankle problems in preadolescent athlete. Clin Sports Med 1982;1:131.

Halsey MF, Finzel KC, Carrion WV, Haralabatos SS. Toddler's fracture: presumptive diagnosis and treatment. J Pediatr Orthop 2001;21:152.

Katz JW, Fingeroth RJ. The diagnostic accuracy of ruptures of the anterior cruciate ligament comparing the Lachman test, the anterior drawer sign, and the pivot shift test in acute and chronic knee injuries. Am J Sports Med 1986;14:88.

Reid DC. Sports injury assessment and rehabilitation. New York: Churchill Livingstone; 1992.

Tanner SM. Putting children with knee injuries back in the game. Contemp Pediatr 1995;12:114.

Patient with LOWER EXTREMITY TRAUMA

(Cont'd from p 443)

↓

Chronic trauma (overuse)

↓

(E) Consider:
- Radiographic studies
- Bone scan
- CBC with differential
- Sedimentation rate

↓

(G) Lower leg

↓

Identify:
- Stress fracture
- Shin splints
- Achilles tendinitis
- Sever syndrome

(F) Knee

↓

Identify:
- Patellofemoral pain
- Osgood-Schlatter syndrome

↓

Treat:
- Reduce painful activity
- Ice
- Massage

↓

(H) Treat:
- Rehabilitation program
- Progress to full activity

Ocular Injury

Carolyn K. Pan, MD, and Scott C. N. Oliver, MD

A. History and Physical Examination: A detailed history including the timing, mechanism, and location of injury is imperative. Visual symptoms such as decreased vision, flashes, floaters, pain, double vision, and discharge should be noted. The mnemonic AMPLE should be used: *a*llergies, *m*edications, *p*revious medical/surgical history, *l*ast meal, *e*vents/environment surrounding the injury. Triage concomitant injuries. Life- and limb-threatening injuries should be addressed first. Physical examination should be performed in a systematic fashion. (Refer to Evaluation of Poor Vision chapter, p. 380) In the setting of trauma, performing a detailed physical examination may be difficult, especially if there is periorbital edema. Cotton-tipped applicators can be used to gently open the eyelids. Take extra care not to place pressure on the globe. If it is not possible to visualize the globe, continue with assessment of the fellow eye, complete the physical examination, order imaging and ancillary testing as needed, and wait for an official ophthalmology consult. If possible, a slit-lamp examination should be performed. Staining of the ocular surface with fluorescein and subsequent examination with a Wood's lamp or cobalt blue filter (available on most direct ophthalmoscopes and slit lamps) can reveal any disruptions of the ocular surface epithelium (abrasions, lacerations, or retained foreign bodies).

B. The radiologic examination most readily available and useful in the emergency department is a computed tomographic (CT) scan of the orbits (both axial and coronal views) without contrast. This is a noninvasive method of assessing for orbital fractures, intraocular foreign bodies, and a limited examination of soft-tissue processes. An ultrasound may also be useful if available.

C. Foreign body: Patients often present with pain, photophobia, and tearing. Patients may complain of a foreign body sensation even when there is no retained foreign body. Foreign bodies not located in the visual axis may be removed with a 30-gauge needle or ophthalmic drill. Evert the upper lid to assess for any retained foreign body under the lid.

D. Corneal Abrasions: Patients often present with pain, photophobia, and tearing. These can be identified with administration of fluorescein dye and examination via Wood's lamp or cobalt blue light on the direct ophthalmoscope or slit lamp. Assess depth of abrasion at the slit lamp to rule out a laceration or penetrating injury. Also check for an anterior chamber reaction and corneal infiltrate. Loose epithelium should be gently débrided with a cotton-tipped applicator soaked with topical anesthetic.

E. Treatment is dictated by offending agent (plant and vegetable matter require broader coverage) and whether the patient is a contact lens wearer. Contact lens wearers require antipseudomonal coverage. A cycloplegic may be necessary if associated with traumatic iridocyclitis (presence of anterior chamber reaction).

(Continued on page 450)

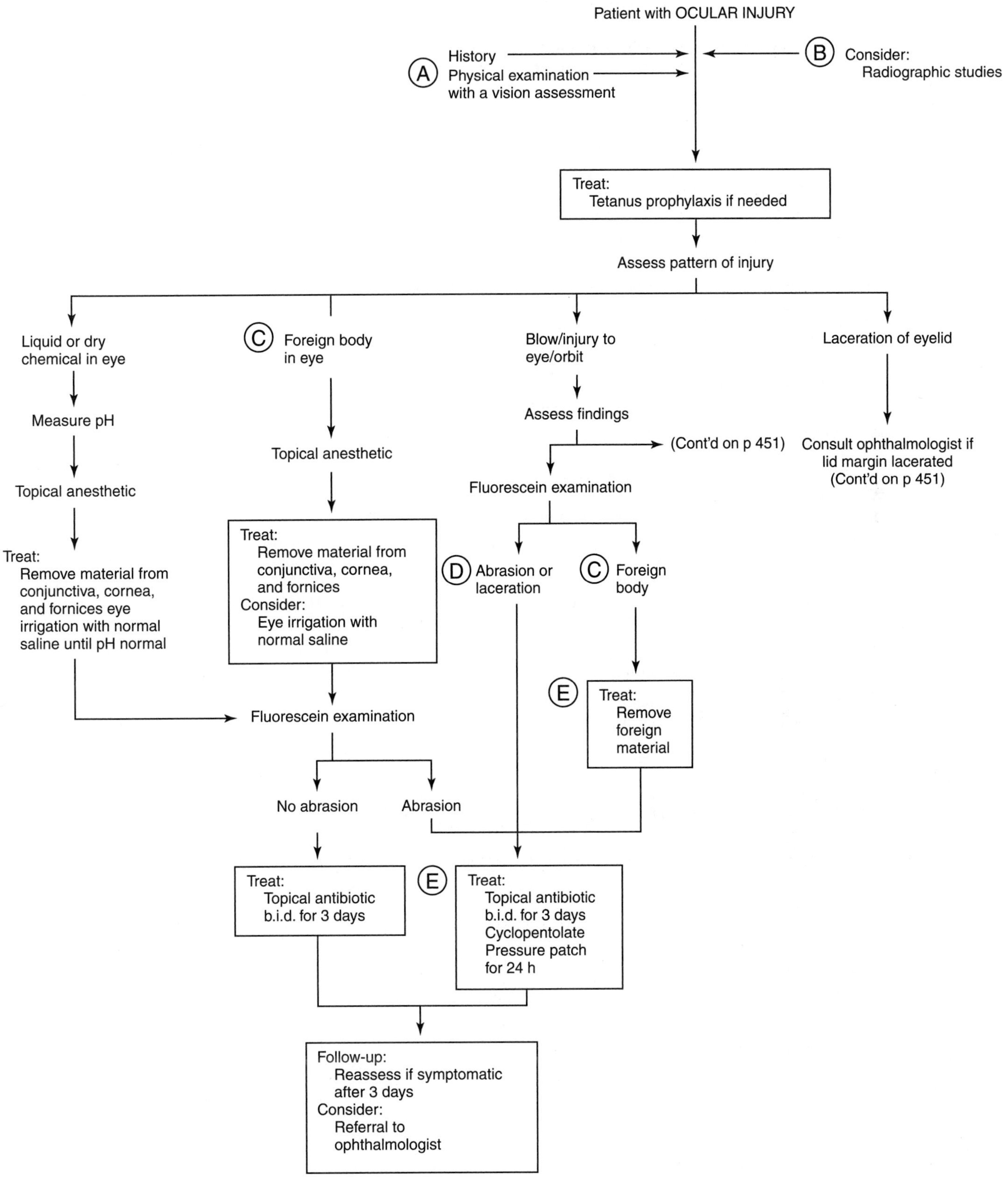

Patient with OCULAR INJURY
A History
Physical examination with a vision assessment
B Consider:
Radiographic studies
Treat:
Tetanus prophylaxis if needed
Assess pattern of injury
Liquid or dry chemical in eye
Measure pH
Topical anesthetic
Treat:
Remove material from conjunctiva, cornea, and fornices eye irrigation with normal saline until pH normal
C Foreign body in eye
Topical anesthetic
Treat:
Remove material from conjunctiva, cornea, and fornices
Consider:
Eye irrigation with normal saline
Fluorescein examination
No abrasion
Abrasion
Treat:
Topical antibiotic b.i.d. for 3 days
Blow/injury to eye/orbit
Assess findings
(Cont'd on p 451)
Fluorescein examination
D Abrasion or laceration
C Foreign body
E Treat:
Remove foreign material
E Treat:
Topical antibiotic b.i.d. for 3 days
Cyclopentolate
Pressure patch for 24 h
Follow-up:
Reassess if symptomatic after 3 days
Consider:
Referral to ophthalmologist
Laceration of eyelid
Consult ophthalmologist if lid margin lacerated
(Cont'd on p 451)

F. Traumatic Hyphema: Blood can be seen overlying the iris. Place the patient upright to allow blood to layer inferiorly. Examine carefully to rule out a ruptured globe. Obtain complete medical and family history, especially regarding any bleeding disorders. Obtain immediate ophthalmology consult.

G. Ruptured Globe: An open globe may be obvious if intraocular contents are visualized. Signs of an occult rupture include bullous 360-degree subconjunctival hemorrhage, deep or shallow anterior chamber, an irregularly shaped pupil (usually peaked toward wound), low intraocular pressure, or exposed uveal tissue. Once a ruptured globe is confirmed, further examination of the globe should be deferred and a protective shield should be placed immediately over the affected eye. Patient should be kept NPO. Antiemetics, analgesics, and systemic antibiotics should be administered. Orbital CT should be obtained to rule out retained foreign bodies. Urgent ophthalmology consultation should be obtained.

H. Orbital Fractures: Patient may present with periorbital edema/ecchymosis, diplopia, anesthesia along the maxillary division of the trigeminal nerve (V2), epistaxis, ptosis, enophthalmos, or exophthalmos. The diagnosis is confirmed with CT scan of the orbits. Orbital fractures are not considered an ophthalmologic emergency unless there is visual impairment, globe injury, or evidence of muscle entrapment. Orbital roof fractures require neurosurgical evaluation. Extensive concomitant facial fracture/injuries may also require evaluation by ENT (ear, nose, and throat), plastics, or maxillofacial surgery. Surgical repair may be necessary if there is persistent diplopia or enophthalmos and is usually performed 7 to 10 days after the injury, to allow edema to subside. Patients should be instructed to avoid nose blowing or Valsalva maneuvers. Prophylactic antibiotics are recommended only if there is known history of or radiologic evidence of sinusitis.

I. Orbital Compartment Syndrome: In the setting of trauma, retrobulbar hemorrhage may result in orbital compartment syndrome. This is usually seen in association with nondisplaced fractures because the blood cannot drain into the sinuses and accumulates within the orbit. This can lead to acute increase in intraorbital pressure, which then affects the optic nerve and globe, resulting in optic nerve ischemia and central retinal artery occlusion. Patients may present with proptosis, acute vision loss, an afferent pupillary defect on the swinging flashlight test, resistance to retropulsion, and increased intraocular pressure. The emergency department staff should perform immediate lateral canthotomy and inferior cantholysis. An urgent ophthalmology consult should then be placed. Imaging may help with diagnosis; however, treatment should not be delayed for radiologic studies.

J. Subconjunctival Hemorrhage: This occurs secondary to ruptured small conjunctival blood vessels. Physical examination reveals a painless, smooth, bright red area over the bulbar conjunctiva and is sharply demarcated by the limbus. Examine carefully with the slit lamp to rule out any underlying scleral injury. Reassure the patient. Artificial tears and cool compresses may improve any symptoms of mild irritation. These usually resolve spontaneously in 2 to 4 weeks.

K. Chemical Burns: After placement of topical proparacaine, immediate copious irrigation with saline should proceed for at least 30 minutes to 1 hour. Clark cups connected to intravenous tubing will maximize fluid contact with the ocular surface. Be sure to irrigate both superior and inferior fornices. Wait 5 to 10 minutes after irrigation is stopped. Then check the pH in the inferior fornix with litmus paper. Continue irrigation until a neutral pH is reached. Examine and treat as described earlier for corneal abrasion.

L. Traumatic Mydriasis and Miosis: Blunt injury may damage iris sphincter. Rule out cranial nerve palsy and brain herniation.

References

Bord SP, Linden J. Trauma to the globe and orbit. Emerg Med Clin North Am 2008;26:97–123.

Ehlers JP, Shah CP, Fenton GL, Hoskins EN. Wills eye manual office and emergency room diagnosis and treatment of eye disease. Philadelphia: Lippincott Williams & Wilkins; 2008.

Juang P, Rosen P. Ocular examination techniques for the emergency department. J Emerg Med 1997;15(6):793–810.

Patient with OCULAR INJURY

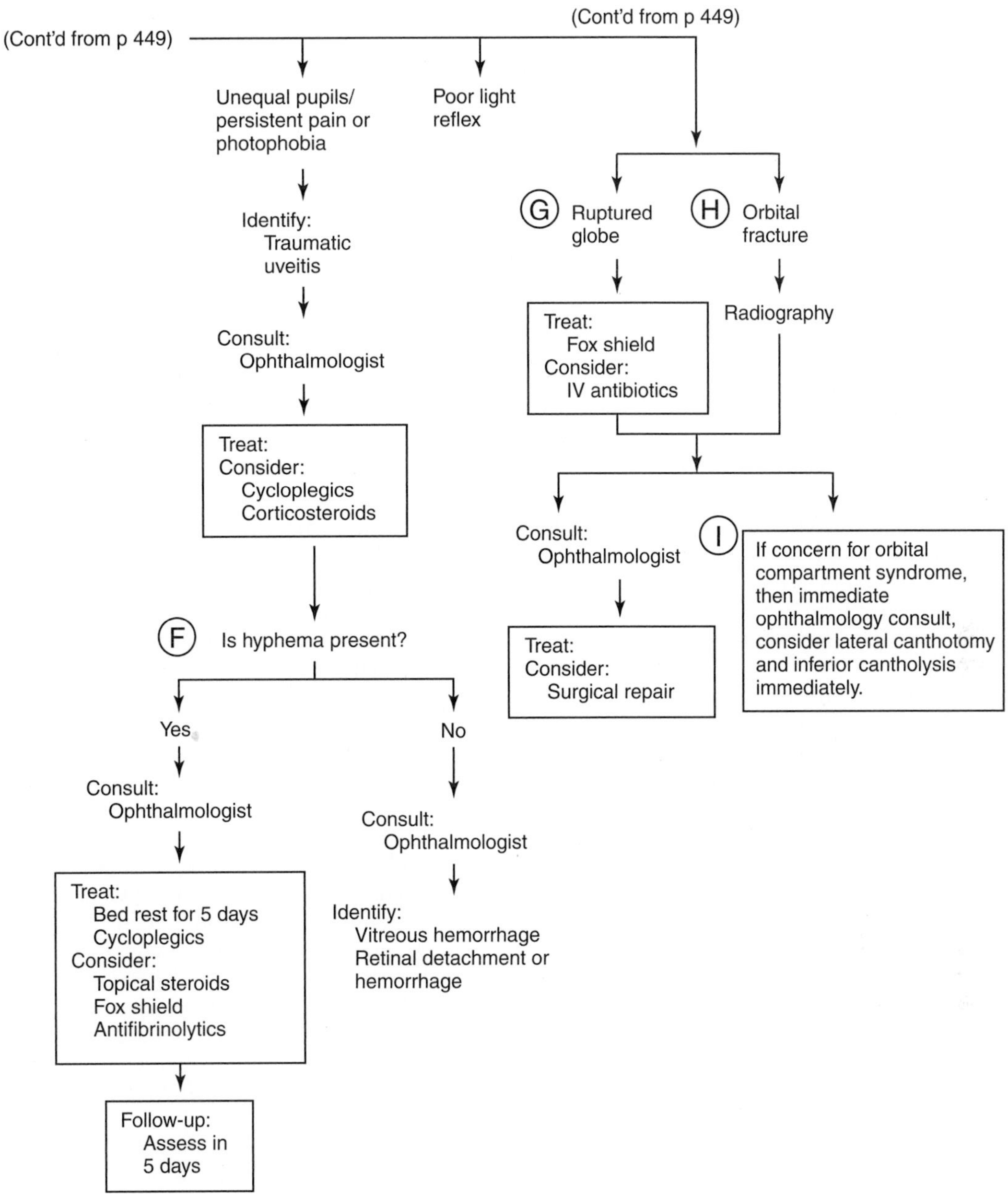
(Cont'd from p 449)
(Cont'd from p 449)
Unequal pupils/ persistent pain or photophobia
Poor light reflex
Identify: Traumatic uveitis
Consult: Ophthalmologist
Treat: Consider: Cycloplegics Corticosteroids
F Is hyphema present?
Yes
No
Consult: Ophthalmologist
Treat: Bed rest for 5 days Cycloplegics Consider: Topical steroids Fox shield Antifibrinolytics
Follow-up: Assess in 5 days
Consult: Ophthalmologist
Identify: Vitreous hemorrhage Retinal detachment or hemorrhage
G Ruptured globe
H Orbital fracture
Treat: Fox shield Consider: IV antibiotics
Radiography
Consult: Ophthalmologist
Treat: Consider: Surgical repair
I If concern for orbital compartment syndrome, then immediate ophthalmology consult, consider lateral canthotomy and inferior cantholysis immediately.

Dental and Oral Trauma

Anne Wilson, DDS, MS

Dental injuries occur commonly in childhood; incidence peaks at ages 2 to 3 years as motor coordination is developing, at ages 9 to 10, and during adolescence. For school-aged children, maxillary incisors are at most risk for trauma, particularly if the incisors are protrusive. Falling is the most common cause of injuries, followed by traffic accidents, violence, and sports. To prevent sport-related injuries, use of protective gear, mouth guards, and decreasing the level of aggression has been effective. Children with conditions that affect neurologic and motor coordination such as cerebral palsy are also at greater risk for orofacial trauma. Evidence of bite marks, orodental trauma, infection, and disease may be caused by child abuse or neglect. In physically abused children, orodental trauma including burns, contusions, lacerations, and fractured, displaced, or avulsed teeth occurs in more than 50% of cases. Immediate assessment involving a thorough history and systematic evaluation is essential.

A. Injury assessment requires a complete history including loss of consciousness, altered neurologic status, headache, nausea/vomiting, pain history including location and severity, previous related trauma, date of the last tetanus inoculation, and when, where, and how the injury occurred. Are the involved teeth primary or secondary, and are all lost teeth and tooth fragments accounted for? Dental pain or sensitivity to temperature may indicate pulp inflammation or exposure. Determine time elapsed until injuries are treated because prognosis worsens with delayed care, particularly for avulsed permanent teeth.

B. Physical assessment for nondental injuries includes evaluation for facial fractures, lacerations/abrasions, contusions, swelling, hemorrhage, asymmetry and deviation of the temporomandibular joint, and presence of foreign bodies. Intraorally inspect the tongue, lips, frena, mucosa, gingivae, palate, floor of the mouth, oropharynx, and the occlusal relation and position of teeth. Diagrams and photographs of injuries are helpful.

C. Fracture and injuries of teeth are complicated if the pulp is involved and uncomplicated if only enamel and dentin are involved. Traumatized permanent teeth commonly feature fractures, whereas primary teeth commonly feature displacement. Traumatic exposure of the pulp results in bleeding at the site of injury and requires prompt recognition. Refer all tooth injuries to a dentist able to manage trauma in children; however, complicated tooth fractures require immediate consultation. Treatment is aimed at preventing pulp necrosis and unnecessary loss of teeth.

D. Treatment for dental injuries varies depending on tooth type (primary, permanent with partial or full root development), and injury extent of teeth, periodontium, and associated structures. Teeth are held in bone by the periodontal ligament. Trauma to the periodontal ligament may cause teeth to loosen or even avulse (complete displacement from the bony socket). Injury or damage to supporting structures may result in tooth tenderness with palpation or percussion, sulcular bleeding, mobility, and displacement. Trauma can cause intrusive luxation of teeth into the socket, with full intrusion appearing as a missing tooth. If previously existing teeth are missing, evaluate for aspiration or ingestion of teeth. Intruded primary teeth that are positioned against the developing permanent tooth germ require extraction. Intruded permanent teeth may require repositioning and endodontic treatment depending on the extent of root formation. Immediate dental consultation is recommended.

E. If a permanent tooth has been avulsed, immediate reimplantation should be attempted to maintain vitality of the periodontal ligament for reattachment and healing. The avulsed tooth should be held by the crown to prevent damage to the periodontal ligament. Gently rinse debris using saline or water. If immediate reimplantation is not possible, place the tooth in one of the following (listed from most preferred): cell culture medium such as Hank's Balanced Salt Solution or commercially available tooth-preserving systems, cold milk, oral vestibule, physiologic saline, or water. Healing capacity is unlikely when the extraoral dry time exceeds 60 minutes. Immediately refer to a dental professional for emergent care; teeth reimplanted within 5 minutes have an 85% likelihood of healing. Do not reimplant an avulsed primary tooth because of subsequent infection and damage to the developing permanent tooth germ.

F. Tooth mobility from injury to the supporting structures requires dental consultation. Trauma may result in displaced teeth, with the type of injury determining urgency. Obtain urgent dental consultation when excessive mobility, extrusion, or malposition causes interference with function. Teeth with minimal or no movement may be evaluated by a dental professional within days.

G. Thoroughly evaluate soft tissue for injuries including the lips, gingivae, tongue, palate, posterior pharyngeal and retropharyngeal areas, floor of the mouth, and mucosa. Lip lacerations involving the vermillion border require careful approximation and consultation with a plastic surgeon when indicated. Lacerations of the tongue require repair if they are gaping, edges are involved, or bleeding cannot be controlled with ice or pressure. Hematomas on the floor of the mouth suggest mandibular fracture. Injury to the frenulum rarely requires suturing but may reflect child abuse. Inflicted injuries from abuse most commonly involve the lips followed by oral mucosa, gingivae, and the tongue. Multiple injuries, different stages of healing, and discrepancies in injury histories heighten suspicion of physical abuse.

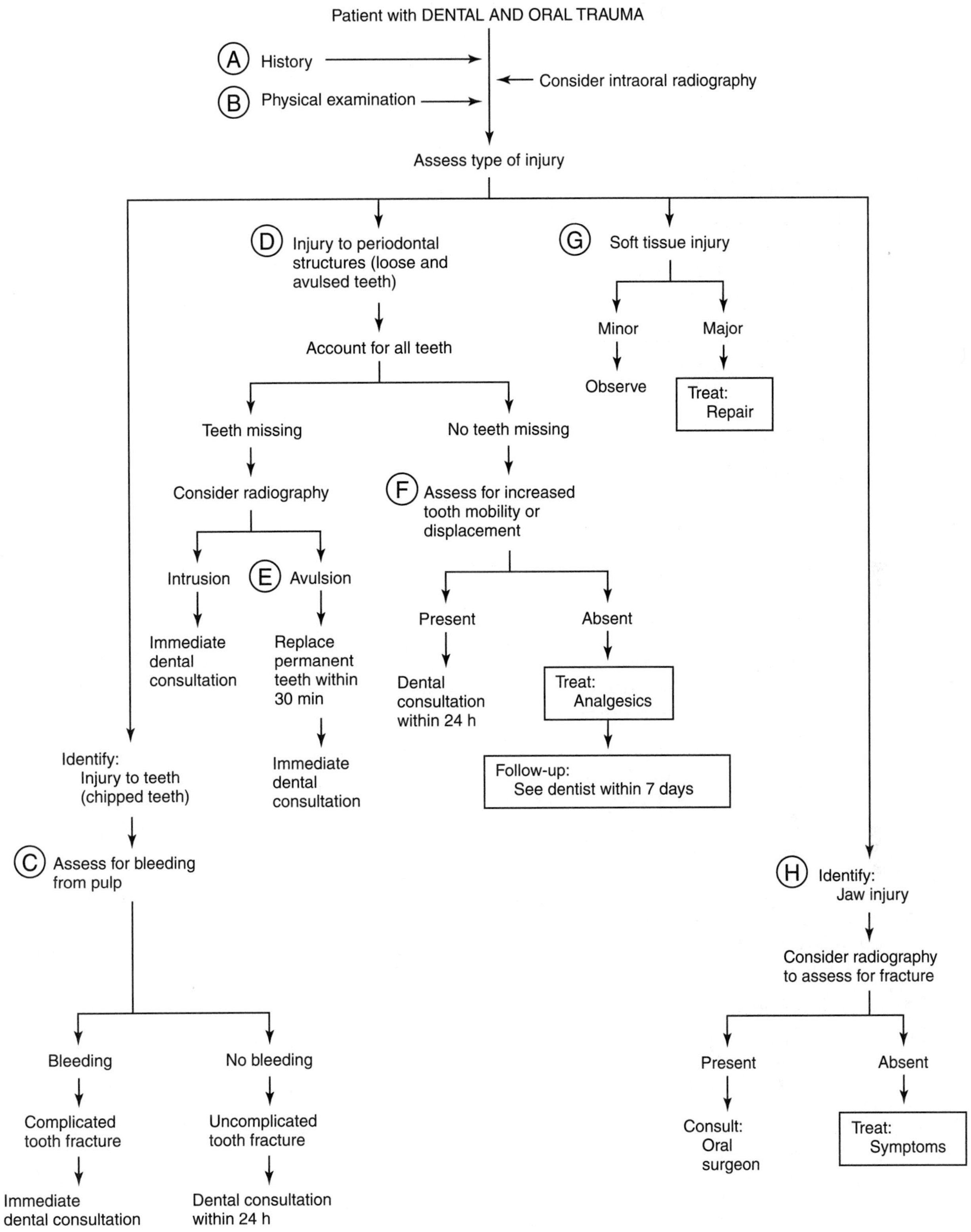
Patient with DENTAL AND ORAL TRAUMA
A History
B Physical examination
Consider intraoral radiography
Assess type of injury
D Injury to periodontal structures (loose and avulsed teeth)
G Soft tissue injury
Minor
Major
Observe
Treat: Repair
Account for all teeth
Teeth missing
No teeth missing
Consider radiography
F Assess for increased tooth mobility or displacement
Intrusion
E Avulsion
Immediate dental consultation
Replace permanent teeth within 30 min
Immediate dental consultation
Present
Absent
Dental consultation within 24 h
Treat: Analgesics
Follow-up: See dentist within 7 days
Identify: Injury to teeth (chipped teeth)
C Assess for bleeding from pulp
Bleeding
No bleeding
Complicated tooth fracture
Uncomplicated tooth fracture
Immediate dental consultation
Dental consultation within 24 h
H Identify: Jaw injury
Consider radiography to assess for fracture
Present
Absent
Consult: Oral surgeon
Treat: Symptoms

H. Evaluate for alveolar and facial bone fractures. Symptoms include pain, swelling, impaired opening of the mouth, mandibular deviation on opening, malocclusion, mobility of alveolar segments, and facial asymmetry. Trauma to the chin may result in fracture of mandibular condyles. Radiographic evaluation is critical. Obtain prompt oral surgery consultation for facial bone fractures.

Reference

Andreasen JO, Andreasen FM, Bakland LK, Flores MT. Traumatic dental injuries: a manual. 2nd ed. Copenhagen, Denmark: Blackwell Munksgaard; 2003. p. 8–9.

Hand Injuries

Lester Young, MD, and Kyros Ipaktchi, MD

Hand injuries are the most common musculoskeletal injuries encountered in pediatric patients. In this patient group, obtaining a thorough history and detailed hand examination can be exceedingly difficult to impossible. Therefore, time must be taken to observe digital posture and unobserved usage of hand and fingers to diagnose underlying injuries. Deep lacerations overlying the course of tendinous or neurovascular structures mandate exploration in the operating room. In these cases, until proved otherwise, one must assume injury to aforementioned structures. Whenever possible, the injured pediatric hand should receive comprehensive treatment on first presentation. This includes potential referral to a hand surgical service for single-stage repair of sustained injuries.

A. History: Determine injury mechanism (laceration, crush, burn, direct trauma, indirect trauma, or combination hereof) and involved energy. Establish a high level of suspicion for inconspicuous injuries. Within the tight confines of the hand, combined injuries to diverse anatomic structures are possible, involving soft tissue, bone, and epiphyseal plates. Penetrating lacerations may involve nerves, vessels, tendons, and joints. High-energy crush injuries may seriously damage hand intrinsic musculature and lead to compartment syndrome. Fractures and dislocations are the result of direct impact (blunt/penetrating trauma) or indirect trauma (extreme flexion/extension, bending/torquing). Open fractures and joint injuries mandate urgent operative intervention.

B. Physical Examination: In the physical examination, observe for swelling, contusions, lacerations, bone deformity, and vascularity. Assess digital posture at rest, during active ranging, and on passive wrist flexion-extension (tenodesis effect) to diagnose tendon injuries and assess motor function. Be alert for pain on passive stretch potentially indicative of a compartment syndrome (crush) or pyogenic flexor tenosynovitis (Kanavel signs), and perform a sensory and motor examination. Consult a hand surgeon for all suspicious findings to assess need for surgical exploration.

C. Imaging: In fractures, dislocations, penetrating lacerations, or potential retained foreign body, radiographs are indicated. Obtain standard three-view films (anteroposterior, lateral, oblique). When suspecting organic foreign body material (e.g., wood splinter, plant thorns) or an abscess, consider additional ultrasound. In unclear radiologic findings, consider obtaining contralateral images.

D. Laceration: When evaluating lacerations, consider the potential involvement of neurovascular and tendinous structures, and focus the physical examination accordingly. Superficial lacerations can be safely sutured in the emergency department after the wound has been properly cleaned and intact tendon function and neurovascular status are documented. If compromised, questionable, or if a foreign body presence is suspected, surgical consultation for operative exploration is warranted. Always consider the trauma of suture removal in children and use resorbable sutures.

E. Fracture/Dislocation: Phalangeal fractures are most commonly seen, followed by metacarpal and carpal fractures. Specific fracture types are related to mechanism of injury and force distribution.

Though carpal bone fractures are uncommon in younger children, scaphoid fractures occur in adolescence with increasing frequency. Similarly, metacarpal fractures occur more commonly in older children from falls or punching injuries (boxer's fracture). Acceptable deformity of metacarpal neck fractures range from 10 degrees at the index metacarpal to 40 degrees at fifth metacarpal. Reduction should be attempted and splinting performed. Rotational deformity is unacceptable and should be referred to a hand surgeon. Phalangeal fractures commonly occur in falls or by catching the finger on an object (Figure 1). Most proximal and middle phalanx fractures are intra-articular or periarticular and usually involve the base of the phalanx. Check for rotational deformity by evaluating the fingers in semiflexed position. Distal phalanx fractures can result from crush injuries. Reduction should be attempted and splinting performed.

Diagnosed or suspected scaphoid fractures should be immobilized in a thumb spica splint and followed up by a hand surgeon.

Dislocations of proximal and distal interphalangeal joints are often associated with athletic activities. Dislocation should be reduced and splinted. A reduction maneuver should be attempted before initial radiograph. Fractures in adjacent bones must be ruled out.

F. Crush: Crush injury is the most common mechanism in pediatric hand injuries. Most apical crush injuries occur when fingers are caught in closing doors. A more serious entity is the whole-hand crush injury as seen in falling furniture. Apical crush injuries typically result in subungual hematoma presenting as a painful, throbbing fingertip with nail discoloration. If the hematoma occupies less than 50% of the nail bed and is not significantly painful, it may be treated with cold packs. However, if there is significant hematoma-induced pain, then decompression using a heated paperclip or a hypodermic needle is necessary. In extensive hematomas and/or associated nail injuries, surgical consult is warranted for exploration and possible nail-bed repair. Tuft fractures resulting from crush injury should be splinted and followed up by a hand surgeon.

Whole-hand crush injuries need a detailed, repeated neurovascular examination. A compartment syndrome needs to be ruled out. In this case, typical findings are a swollen hand held in clawlike position,

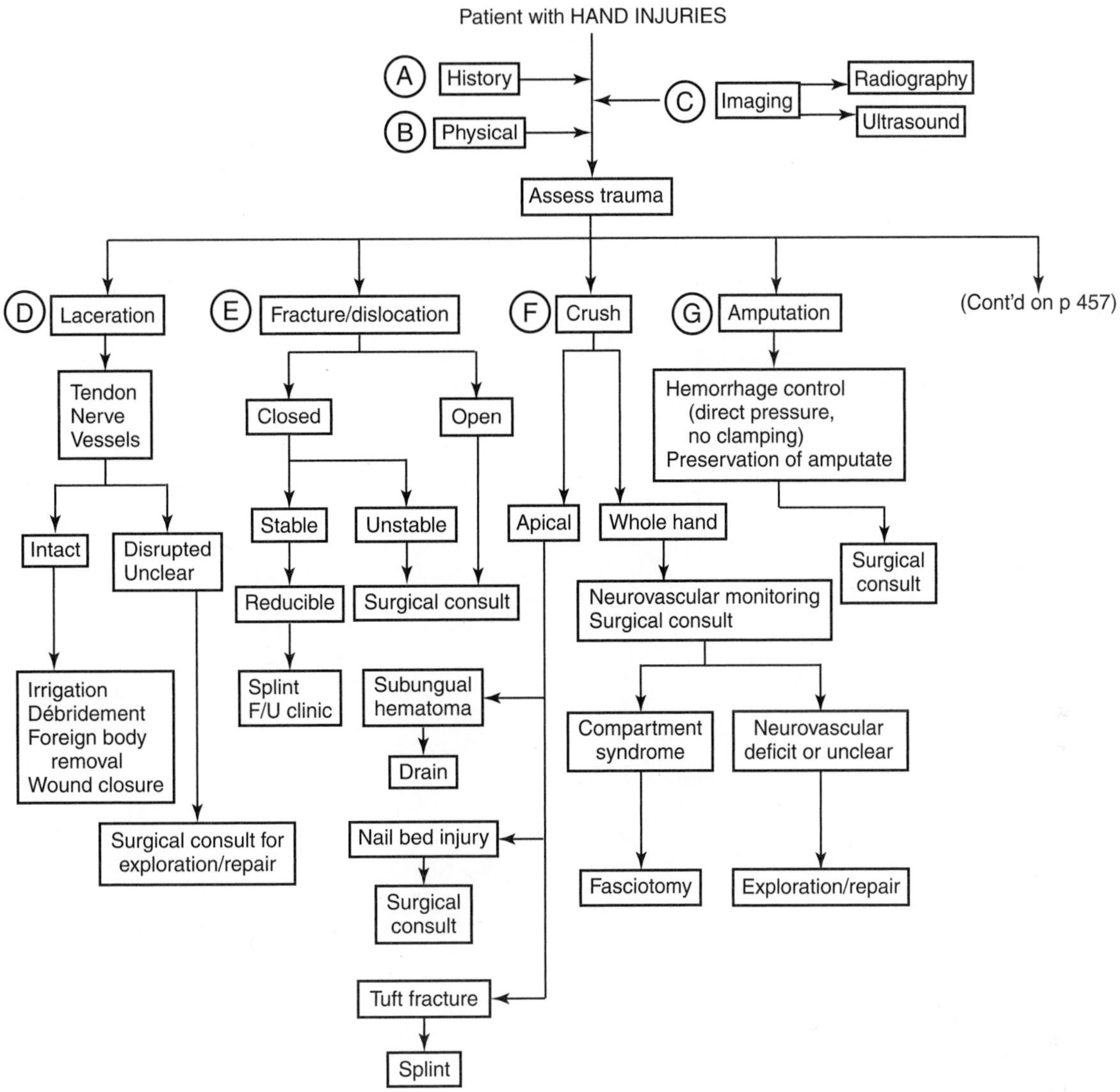
Patient with HAND INJURIES
A
History
B
Physical
C
Imaging
Radiography
Ultrasound
Assess trauma
D
Laceration
E
Fracture/dislocation
F
Crush
G
Amputation
(Cont'd on p 457)
Tendon
Nerve
Vessels
Intact
Disrupted
Unclear
Irrigation
Débridement
Foreign body
removal
Wound closure
Surgical consult for
exploration/repair
Closed
Open
Stable
Unstable
Reducible
Surgical consult
Splint
F/U clinic
Apical
Whole hand
Subungual
hematoma
Drain
Nail bed injury
Surgical
consult
Tuft fracture
Splint
Neurovascular monitoring
Surgical consult
Compartment
syndrome
Neurovascular
deficit or unclear
Fasciotomy
Exploration/repair
Hemorrhage control
(direct pressure,
no clamping)
Preservation of amputate
Surgical
consult

with exquisite tenderness on passive finger extension. Surgical consultation has to be ordered to assess need for emergent fasciotomies.

G. Amputations: Pediatric amputations occurring at any level or location should be considered for replantation. Outcomes are generally favorable, as epiphyseal growth continues after replantation and function can be regained. Hemorrhage must be controlled by means of direct pressure only. Haphazard clamping of bleeding vessels may result in irreparable crushing of neurovascular structures. The amputate should be placed on saline-moistened gauze inside a clean plastic bag, which, in turn, is placed in an ice-filled container. The amputate should not be directly placed on ice. A surgical replantation team should be contacted immediately. Successful replantation of digits can be achieved up to 24 hours after injury if the amputate is properly cooled.

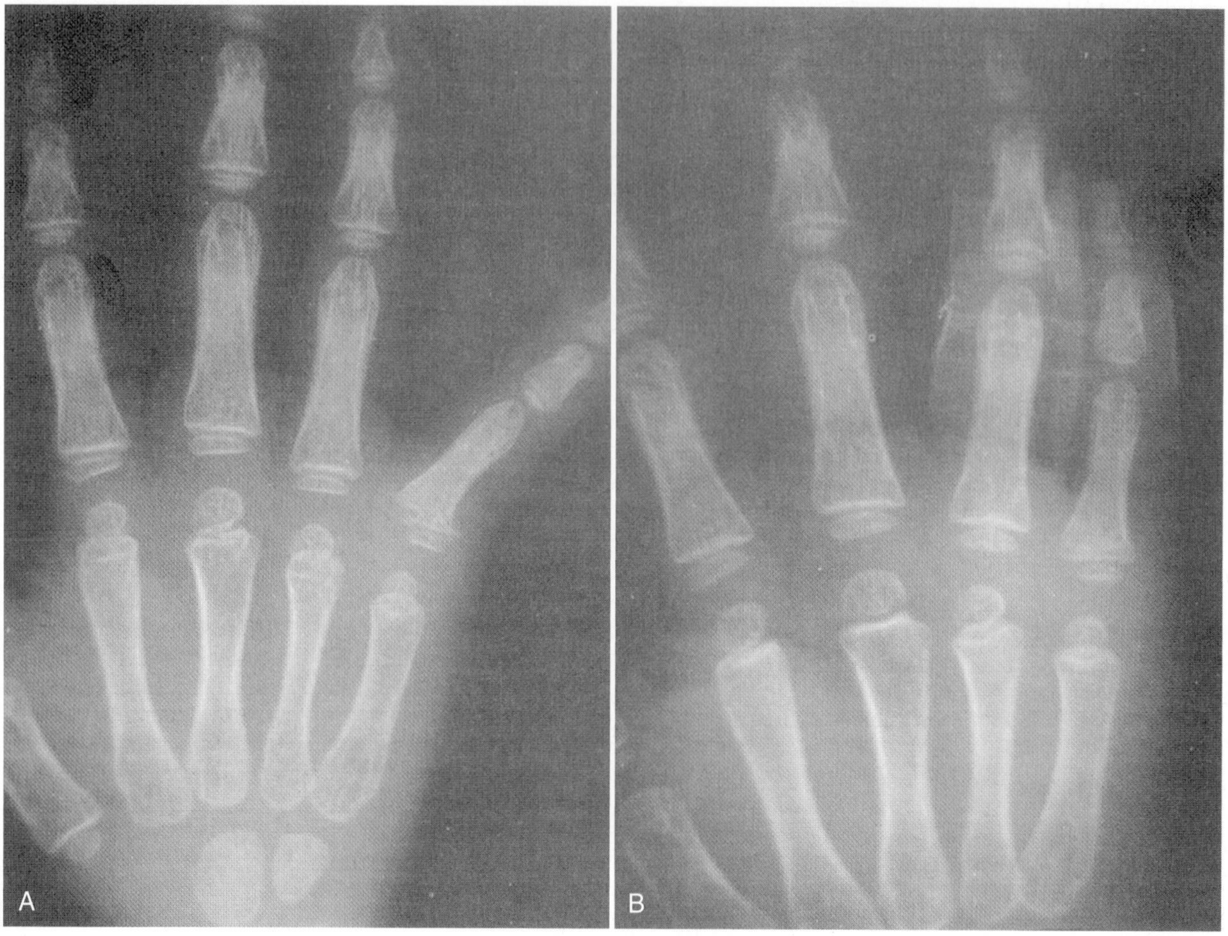
A
B

Figure 1 Proximal phalanx fracture of fifth digit. A, Prereduction. B, Postreduction.

H. Burn: Burn injuries to the hands pose a special problem in young children. Scald burns are the most common types of burns in the pediatric population younger than 3 years, whereas flame burns are more prevalent in older children. The depth and extent of the burn must be assessed. Burns that are superficial partial thickness may be dressed with topical antimicrobials and followed up in a clinic. Indeterminate, deep partial thickness, or full-thickness burns warrant surgical consultation and possible transfer to a burn center for evaluation and possible excision and skin grafting.

References

American Society for Surgery of the Hand; Burgess L, editors. The hand: examination and diagnosis. New York: Churchill Livingstone; 1990.

Armstrong MB, Adeogun BS. Tendon injuries in the pediatric hand. J Craniofac Surg 2009;20(4):1005–10.

Bhende MS, Dandrea LA, Davis HW. Hand injuries in children presenting to a pediatric emergency department. Ann Emerg Med 1993;22:1519.

Garcia-Moral CA, Green NE, Fox JA. Hand and wrist. In: Sullivan JA, Anderson SJ, editors. Care of the young athlete. Rosemont, IL: American Academy of Pediatrics/American Academy of Orthopaedic Surgeons; 2000.

Gellman H. Fingertip & nail bed injuries in children: current concepts and controversies of treatment. J Craniofac Surg 2009;20(4): 1033–5.

Green DP, Hotchkiss RN, Pederson WC, Wolfe SW. Green's operative hand surgery. 5th ed. Philadelphia: Elsevier Churchill Livingstone; 2005.

Kaufman Y, Cole P, Hollier L. Peripheral nerve injuries of the pediatric hand: issues in diagnosis and management. J Craniofac Surg 2009;20(4):1011–5.

Nofsinger CC, Wolfe SW. Common pediatric hand fractures. Curr Opin Pediatr 2002;14(1):42–5.

Patient with HAND INJURIES

(Cont'd from p 455)

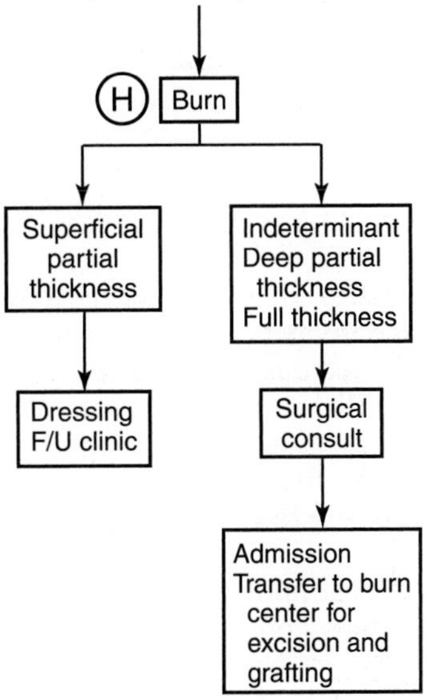
H
Burn
Superficial partial thickness
Indeterminant
Deep partial thickness
Full thickness
Dressing
F/U clinic
Surgical consult
Admission
Transfer to burn center for excision and grafting

Lacerations

Kelley Roswell, MD

A. Obtain a thorough history from the patient and parents, including the mechanism of injury, age of the wound, and possibility of foreign body. Assess the environment of the wound for infection and tattooing. Inquire about the general health status of the patient, including diabetes and immunocompetence, allergies to medicines and latex, and tetanus immunization status. If the wound is caused by a bite, see the Bites chapter (see p. 460); if the wound is a burn, see the Burns chapter (see p. 462).

B. Evaluate the adequacy of the airway, breathing, and circulation (ABCs), including control of bleeding. Perform a primary and secondary survey with attention to associated injuries. Assess the location and depth of the wound before administering local anesthetics. Assess for vascular damage; control venous and arterial bleeding initially with direct pressure. Avoid blind clamping of a bleeding artery when it is close to nerves. Assess for nerve damage, including motor and sensory evaluations with two-point discrimination. Assess for tendon injury including range of motion, but do not test range of motion against resistance because a partial tendon laceration can be converted to a complete tendon laceration with resistance to movement; also make sure to assess for tendon damage in the anatomic position in which the injury occurred. Further inspection of the wound for foreign material may take place with local anesthesia after the neurovascular examination is complete.

C. If the history or physical examination suggests a radiopaque foreign body, obtain a radiograph. Radiopaque foreign bodies may include metals, bone, gravel, stone chips, most glass, and some plastics. A radiograph may be especially important in assessing a wound caused by glass because deeply embedded glass may be missed without radiographs. Some authors recommend obtaining radiographs in all cases in which glass is involved except for the most superficial wound in which the bottom of the wound is clearly visualized. Ultrasonography may also be helpful in localizing some types of foreign objects. Also obtain radiographs if there is the possibility of a fracture (i.e., a crush injury to a distal digit with accompanying laceration).

D. Administer local anesthesia before wound cleansing. Use wound irrigation as the primary method for cleansing wounds. For the average 2-cm wound, irrigate with approximately 250 ml normal saline by use of a large syringe (20–60 ml) and an 18- to 19-gauge needle or intravenous catheter. When held 2 cm above the wound, a 35-ml syringe and 19-gauge needle or intravenous catheter delivers approximately 8 pounds per square inch (psi), which is effective in removing bacteria and particulate debris. Larger or dirty wounds may need increased volume of saline for irrigation. Scrubbing of wounds should be done only for particularly dirty wounds in which irrigation alone is not effective. Povidone-iodine (Betadine) "scrub" should not be used because it is toxic to tissues. Alcohol or hydrogen peroxide is not recommended in cleaning wounds. It may be necessary to débride the wound with forceps or by scraping with a scalpel blade to remove embedded dirt and to prevent a "traumatic tattoo." Shaving the hair around the wound is not recommended because it may increase the infection risk. Eyebrows should never be shaved. If hair must be removed, clip the hair with scissors or use petroleum jelly to keep the hair out of the way during suturing.

E. With minor, clean wounds, immunize for tetanus if the patient has had three previous tetanus immunizations and the last immunization was more than 10 years ago (Table 1). Immunize if the wound is not a minor, clean wound and if the last tetanus immunization was more than 5 years ago. If the wound is not clean or minor and the patient's tetanus immunization status is unknown or the patient has received fewer than 3 tetanus immunizations, administer tetanus toxoid and tetanus immunoglobulin.

F. Refer a patient with vascular, nerve, or tendon injury to a surgical specialist for further evaluation. Refer wounds involving the cartilage of the ear or nose to an otolaryngologist or plastic surgeon, and refer eyelid lacerations to an ophthalmologist. Deep or extensive wounds to the face or a foreign body that is unable to be retrieved may need referral to a surgical specialist for possible exploration and repair in the operating room.

G. Assess the wound for primary closure. The risk for infection increases with delay in primary closure. The length of time before the risk for infection is significant is variable. Most authors suggest wound closure within 6 to 12 hours. Many "clean" wounds (wounds to the face or scalp) may be closed up to 24 hours after the injury occurred. Puncture wounds and most bites should not undergo primary closure (see p. 460 for more information on bites). Options for wound closure include suturing with absorbable or nonabsorbable material, staples, and tissue adhesive such as Dermabond. Dermabond should be used only to close superficial wounds. Do not use tissue adhesive to close wounds that are deep, irregularly shaped, subject to tension (such as over joints or hands), or at high risk of infection, such as bites. Apply an antibiotic ointment to wounds (except those closed with Dermabond) and dress with dry sterile gauze. Follow-up visits should occur between 3 and 14 days, depending on anatomic location and type of wound closure (Table 2).

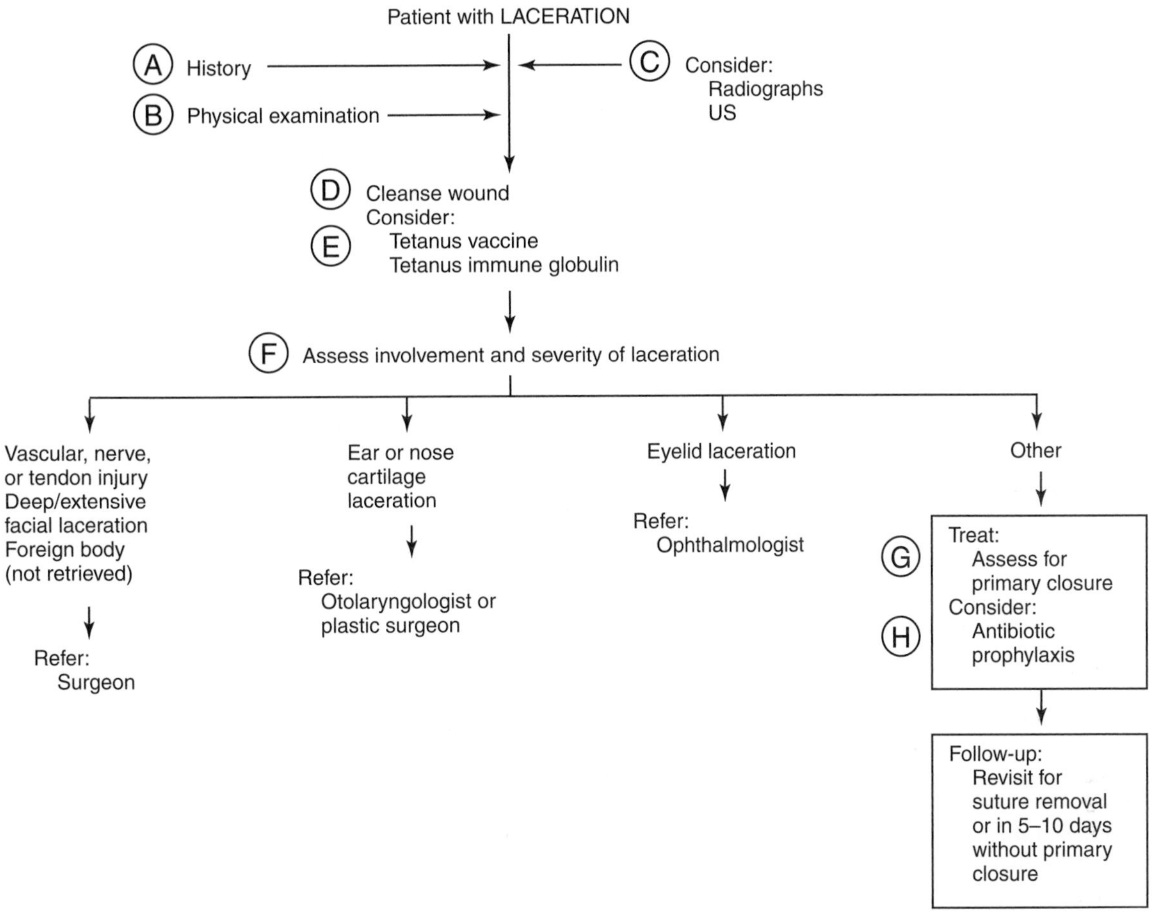
Patient with LACERATION
A History
B Physical examination
C Consider: Radiographs US
D Cleanse wound
Consider:
E Tetanus vaccine
Tetanus immune globulin
F Assess involvement and severity of laceration
Vascular, nerve, or tendon injury
Deep/extensive facial laceration
Foreign body (not retrieved)
Refer: Surgeon
Ear or nose cartilage laceration
Refer: Otolaryngologist or plastic surgeon
Eyelid laceration
Refer: Ophthalmologist
Other
G Treat: Assess for primary closure
H Consider: Antibiotic prophylaxis
Follow-up: Revisit for suture removal or in 5–10 days without primary closure

Table 1. **Tetanus Immunization Recommendations**

Prior Tetanus Immunizations	Clean, Minor Wounds	Other Wounds
<3 (or unknown)	Tetanus only	Tetanus and tetanus Immunoglobulin
≥3, last >10 years	Tetanus only	Tetanus only
≥3, last <5 years	None	None
≥3, last 5–10 years	None	Tetanus only

Adapted from Selbst SM, Attia M. Minor trauma—lacerations. In: Fleisher GR, Ludwig S, editors. Textbook of pediatric emergency medicine. 4th ed. Philadelphia: Lippincott Williams & Wilkins; 2000. p. 1490.

Table 2. **Suture Removal**

Area of Body	Number of Days
Face	3–4
Neck	5
Scalp	6–7
Chest or abdomen	7
Arms and backs of hands	7
Legs and tops of feet	10
Back	10
Palms of hands or soles of feet	14

H. Prophylactic antibiotics are not routinely recommended for most sutured lacerations, and their use remains controversial. Decontamination with appropriate irrigation is more efficacious than use of antibiotics to prevent wound infection. Consider antibiotics if the wound is a sutured dog or cat bite (see Bites chapter, p. 460, for more information), heavily contaminated, or a crush wound. In addition, wounds of hands, feet, and perineum are at a greater risk for infection. Immunocompromised patients may also benefit from prophylactic antibiotics. Treat with a first-generation cephalosporin or penicillinase-resistant penicillin for prophylaxis in most wounds. Amoxicillin-clavulanic acid is the recommended antibiotic for human and animal bites.

References

Berk WA, Welch RD, Bock BF. Controversial issues in clinical management of the simple wound. Ann Emerg Med 1992;21:72.

Bruns TB, Simon HK, McLario DJ, et al. Laceration repair using a tissue adhesive in a children's emergency department. Pediatrics 1996;98:673.

Callhan JM, Baker MD. General wound management. In: Henretig FM, King C, editors. Textbook of pediatric emergency procedures. Baltimore: Williams & Wilkins; 1997. p. 1125–39.

Edlich RF, Rodeheaver GT, Morgan RF, et al. Principles of emergency wound management. Ann Emerg Med 1988;17:1284.

Grisham J. Principles of wound healing. In: Dieckmann RA, Fiser DH, Selbst SM, editors. Illustrated textbook of pediatric emergency and critical care procedures. St. Louis, MO: Mosby; 1997. p. 665–8.

Grisham J, Perro M. Laceration repair. In: Dieckmann RA, Fiser DH, Selbst SM, editors. Illustrated textbook of pediatric emergency and critical care procedures. St. Louis, MO: Mosby; 1997. p. 669–79.

Hollander JE, Singer AJ. Laceration management. Ann Emerg Med 1999;34(30):356–67.

McNamara R, Loiselle J. Laceration repair. In: Henretig FM, King C, editors. Textbook of pediatric emergency procedures. Baltimore: Williams & Wilkins; 1997. p. 1141–68.

Red Book 2009: Report of the Committee on Infectious Diseases. 28th ed. Elk Grove Village, IL: American Academy of Pediatrics; 2009. p. 187–91, 657–8.

Selbst SM, Attia M. Minor trauma—lacerations. In: Fleisher GR, Ludwig S, editors. Textbook of pediatric emergency medicine. 6th ed. Philadelphia: Lippincott Williams & Wilkins; 2010. p. 1266.

Simon HK, McLario DJ, Bruns TB, et al. Long-term appearance of lacerations repaired using a tissue adhesive. Pediatrics 1997;99:193.

Bites

Catherine C. Ferguson, MD

Animal bites are a common problem in the United States and account for approximately 1% of all emergency department visits and more than $30 million dollars in health care costs each year. Ten percent of those who seek medical attention require wound repair, and 1% to 2% require hospitalization. Fatalities are rare, but the majority of the 10 to 20 people who die as a result of animal bites each year are children.

About 85% to 90% of animal bites are inflicted by dogs; 15% to 30% of these bites are inflicted by the family pet. Dogs are capable of causing severe penetrating wounds and crush injuries because of the tremendous force generated by their jaws. Dog bites most often affect the extremities; however, in children younger than 5 years, a dog will strike the head more than 80% of the time, increasing the potential for fractures of the skull and facial bones and intracranial hemorrhage. The overall rate of infection from dog bites is relatively low at approximately 2% to 5%. Cats are responsible for an additional 5% to 10% of all animal bites. Cat bites are problematic because cat's slender, sharp fangs create deep puncture wounds that are difficult to adequately irrigate and are at high risk for infection. Human bites account for a small portion of all animal bites, approximately 2% to 3%. Human bites in adolescents and adults usually occur as a result of clenched-fist or "fight bite" injury and can result in metacarpal-phalangeal joint capsule perforation and possibly septic arthritis and osteomyelitis. Occlusive human bites occurring anywhere else than the hand seem to be at no greater risk for infection than any other bite.

A. History: A complete history should include a description of how the injury occurred, including where and at what time the injury took place, the type of offending animal and its health status, the name and address of the animal's owner (if known), and whether local law enforcement has been involved. In addition, the patient's medical history, specifically whether the patient is immunosuppressed by medication or disease, the patient's tetanus immune status, and allergies to medications are important to guide decisions regarding antibiotic and/or tetanus prophylaxis. Finally, particularly in the case of injuries related to human bites, assess for nonaccidental trauma.

B. Physical Examination: Perform a thorough physical examination remembering that the bite wound may be a distracting injury. Assess the depth of the wound and any related crush injury. Assess the function of the local nerves, tendons, and vascular supply. If the wound overlies a joint, consider evaluating for penetration of the joint capsule.

C. Laboratory/Radiologic Evaluation: If the wound appears to be infected, obtain both aerobic and anaerobic cultures from deep within the wound. Evidence of a wound infection that develops within a few hours after a bite wound strongly suggests a *Pasteurella multocida* infection. Consider plain films for suspected fracture and/or to evaluate for the presence of a foreign body.

D. Local Wound Care: The most important step in preventing infection is careful local wound care as soon as possible after the injury. The skin may be cleaned with 1% povidone-iodine, and the depths of the wound, including puncture wounds, should be irrigated with at least 200 ml normal saline under high pressure, best achieved by using an 18-gauge needle or plastic catheter attached to a large-volume syringe. Carefully débride devitalized tissue and foreign material. Do not débride puncture wounds.

E. Tetanus Prophylaxis: Tetanus can result from animal and human bites. Children younger than 3 years and children whose immunization status is unknown should receive both Td (tetanus diphtheria toxoid) or Tdap (tetanus, diphtheria, and pertussis) and tetanus immunoglobulin (TIG). Tdap is preferred to Td for adolescents who have never received Tdap. Intravenous immunoglobulin (IVIG) should be used when TIG is not available. Children 3 years and older should receive Td or Tdap if it has been 5 or more years since the last tetanus-containing vaccine dose.

F. Rabies Prophylaxis: Human rabies infection in the United States is rare; only 19 rabies-related deaths were reported in the United States from 2000 to 2006. Seventeen of those deaths were associated with bites from or direct contact with bats. Because rabies infection is nearly always fatal without appropriate prophylaxis before the development of clinical signs of disease, animal bites should at least raise the possibility of rabies exposure. Children who have been bitten by a dog or cat should receive both active and passive rabies immunoprophylaxis if the offending animal is rabid or develops signs of rabies during a 10-day period of observation. If the animal is not able to be observed, contact public health officials for advice. No case of human rabies in the United States has been attributed to a dog or cat that remained healthy throughout a standard 10-day period of confinement.

G. Evaluate Wound: Consider hospitalizing those patients with bite wounds that require reconstructive surgery, patients whose bite wounds are at greatest risk for infection (immunocompromised host; significant bites to the hand; likelihood for patient noncompliance; penetration of joint, bone, or tendon), and patients with infected bite wounds that are refractory to outpatient therapy. Begin parenteral antibiotics (ampicillin-sulbactam, or an extended-spectrum cephalosporin or trimethoprim-sulfamethoxazole, plus clindamycin) and consult with general surgery and/or an infectious disease specialist. Clenched-fist injuries should be evaluated by an orthopedic hand surgeon. All other bite wounds should receive local wound care and be assessed for their risk for infection to determine further course of action, including repair and antibiotic prophylaxis.

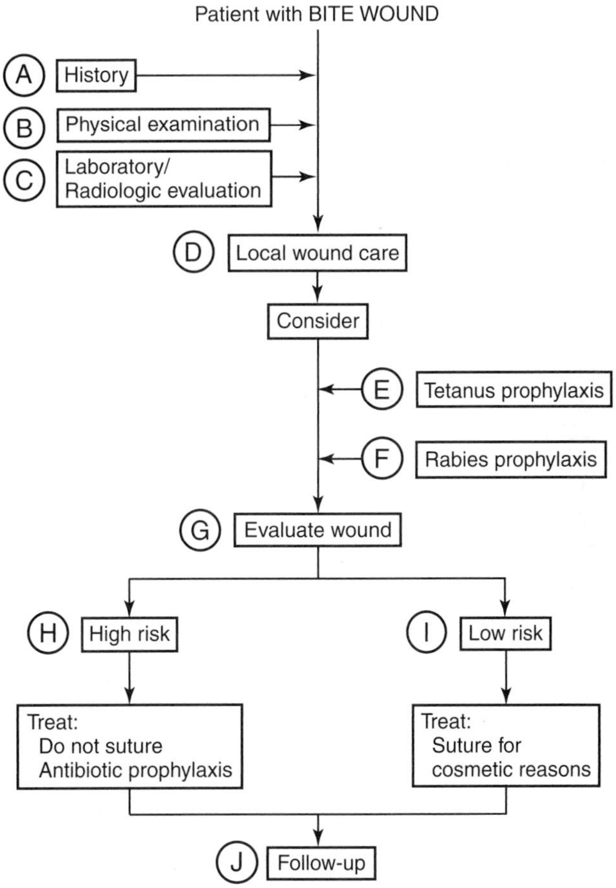

Patient with BITE WOUND
A
History
B
Physical examination
C
Laboratory/
Radiologic evaluation
D
Local wound care
Consider
E
Tetanus prophylaxis
F
Rabies prophylaxis
G
Evaluate wound
H
High risk
I
Low risk
Treat:
Do not suture
Antibiotic prophylaxis
Treat:
Suture for
cosmetic reasons
J
Follow-up

H. High Risk: Crush injuries, puncture wounds, bites involving the hand, dog bite wounds presenting greater than 12 hours after the injury, cat or human bites (except those to the face), and bite wounds in immunocompromised hosts are at greater risk for infection and should not be sutured. Instead, these wounds should receive meticulous local wound care, be left open, and be re-examined frequently. Although controversial, current indications for antibiotic prophylaxis include human bites, all cat bites, and high-risk dog bites (hand wounds, deep puncture wounds, wounds requiring surgical débridement, wounds in immunocompromised hosts, bite wounds near or in a prosthetic joint, and bite wounds in an extremity with underlying vascular compromise). The organisms most likely to cause infection as a result of dog or cat bites include *Pasteurella* species, *Staphylococcus aureus,* streptococci, anaerobes, *Capnocytophaga* species, *Moraxella* species, *Corynebacterium* species, and *Neisseria* species. The organisms most likely to cause infection from a human bite include streptococci, *S. aureus, Eikenella corrodens, Haemophilus* species, and anaerobes. Amoxicillin-clavulanate for 3 to 5 days is an effective first-line oral therapy for human, cat, and dog bite wounds. For penicillin-allergic children, an extended-spectrum cephalosporin or trimethoprim-sulfamethoxazole plus clindamycin is an acceptable alternative.

I. Low Risk: Most low-risk bite wounds can be sutured within 12 hours of the injury. Infection of bite wounds to the face and head is uncommon because of good vascular supply, and these wounds should be closed to minimize scarring. Bite wounds should be closed with percutaneous nonabsorbable sutures; deep sutures should be avoided to minimize infection risk.

J. Follow-up: All patients should be instructed to follow-up within 24 to 48 hours for a wound check and to seek medical attention earlier if there are signs of infection including worsening pain, warmth, or redness, puslike discharge, or fever. Patients should also be instructed to keep the involved area elevated to minimize edema. Finally, keep in mind that children who have suffered animal bites may be at risk for the development of post-traumatic stress disorder; therefore, referral for psychologic intervention should be considered.

References

Brogan TV, Bratton SL, Dowd D, Hegenbarth MA. Severe dog bites in children. Pediatrics 1995;96:947–50.

Griego RD, Rosen T, Orengo IF, Wolf JE. Dog, cat, and human bites: a review. J Am Acad Dermatol 1995;33(6):1019–29.

Nakamura Y, Daya M. Use of appropriate antimicrobials in wound management. Emerg Med Clin North Am 2007;25:159–76.

Pickering LK, editor. Red Book 2006: Report of the Committee on Infectious Diseases. Elk Grove Village, IL: American Academy of Pediatrics; 2006.

Rupprecht CE, Gibbons RV. Prophylaxis against rabies. New Engl J Med 2004;351:2626–35.

Wyatt J. Rabies—update on a global disease. Pediatr Infect Dis J 2007; 26:351–2.

Thermal Injury (Frostbite/Burns)

Joe Wathen, MD, and Kathryn D. Emery, MD

Thermal injury describes damage by extremes of either cold or heat. The degree of injury depends on temperature and time of exposure. Children are unique in that their skin is more susceptible (larger surface area, thinner) and their developmental status increases their risk for a thermal injury (more likely to pull hot water down from the stove, or inability to protect or remove themselves from a cold environment or burning building).

FROSTBITE

Definition

Frostbite is a tissue injury caused by exposure to temperatures below the freezing point of intact skin. The most frequent areas affected are the hands and feet (90%), followed by the face (ears, nose, and cheeks). Symptoms of frostbite occur on rewarming. The range of frostbite injuries is illustrated in Table 1.

Pathophysiology

Frostbite includes both reversible and irreversible tissue damage. Two mechanisms are responsible for this tissue damage: (1) direct cellular damage, and (2) indirect cellular damage with progressive dermal ischemia. Direct cellular damage results when exposure to the cold freezes the tissues, leading to the formation of both intracellular and extracellular ice crystals. Ice crystal formation leads to cell dehydration and shrinkage, abnormal intracellular electrolyte concentrations, and lipid-protein denaturation. Indirect cellular damage results from progressive microvascular insults with initial cycles of vasoconstriction and vasodilatation, followed by a progressive thrombosis. Microthrombi produce tissue ischemia with resulting local metabolic acidosis, endothelial cell injury, inflammatory mediator release, and edema. The tissue edema further reduces blood flow, creating more thrombosis leading to a spiraling effect. If the process is not interrupted in time, necrosis and tissue losses occur.

A. In the patient's history, determine the circumstances of the injury. Factors that predispose a person to injury include poor circulation caused by previous cold injury, constrictive clothing, cigarette smoking, alcohol consumption, diabetes mellitus, hypothermia, diseases of the blood vessels, immobility, and developmental delay. Wind-chill contributes markedly to frostbite.

B. In the initial physical examination, most injuries appear similar, making it difficult to determine the severity until after rewarming. The extent of the freezing and tissue loss may not be apparent for 4 to 5 days. Frostbite injuries can be classified as either superficial or deep. Superficial injuries may appear as either a numb central white plaque with surrounding erythema, or as blisters filled with clear or milky fluid with surrounding erythema and edema. Deep frostbite injuries are characterized by either hemorrhagic blisters that develop into a black eschar in 2 weeks or by complete tissue loss and necrosis. Final tissue demarcation may take 3 to 4 weeks to establish. Note the appearance of the skin, sensation to pinprick, and whether the vesicles are clear or hemorrhagic. Identify signs of dehydration, hypothermia, altitude effects (pulmonary edema), and exhaustion.

C. During transport, replace wet clothing with dry, loose clothing followed by padding and splinting. Do not allow the affected area to thaw and refreeze. Once at a medical facility, initially treat systemic hypothermia to a temperature of at least 34°C. Systemic effects may include arrhythmias, depressed cardiac output, hypoventilation with hypoxia and acidosis, decreased mentation, and altered coagulation system. After systemic effects are treated, the focus is on rapidly rewarming the frostbite areas in warm water at the specific range of 40°C to 42°C (104–108°F) for 15 to 30 minutes until thawing is complete (skin becomes red/purple in appearance with pliable texture). Do not massage the area. Do not initiate thawing if there is a chance of the area refreezing.

(Continued on page 464)

Table 1. **Degree of Illness in Frostbite Injury**

Moderate/First- and Second-Degree Superficial (No Tissue Loss)	Severe/Third-Degree Deep (Tissue Loss)	Very Severe/Fourth Degree
White plaque, erythema, clear or milky blister, deforming skin, edema	Dark fluid blister, nonblanching cyanosis, hard nondeforming skin, frozen appearance, absence of edema Progress to black eschar over 2 weeks	Severe frostbite with systemic signs: hypothermia, altitude illness, dehydration, associated trauma Produces complete necrosis and tissue loss
Initial numbness progresses to intact sensation, "burning sensation"	Absent sensation, "electric current-like shock"	Absent sensation

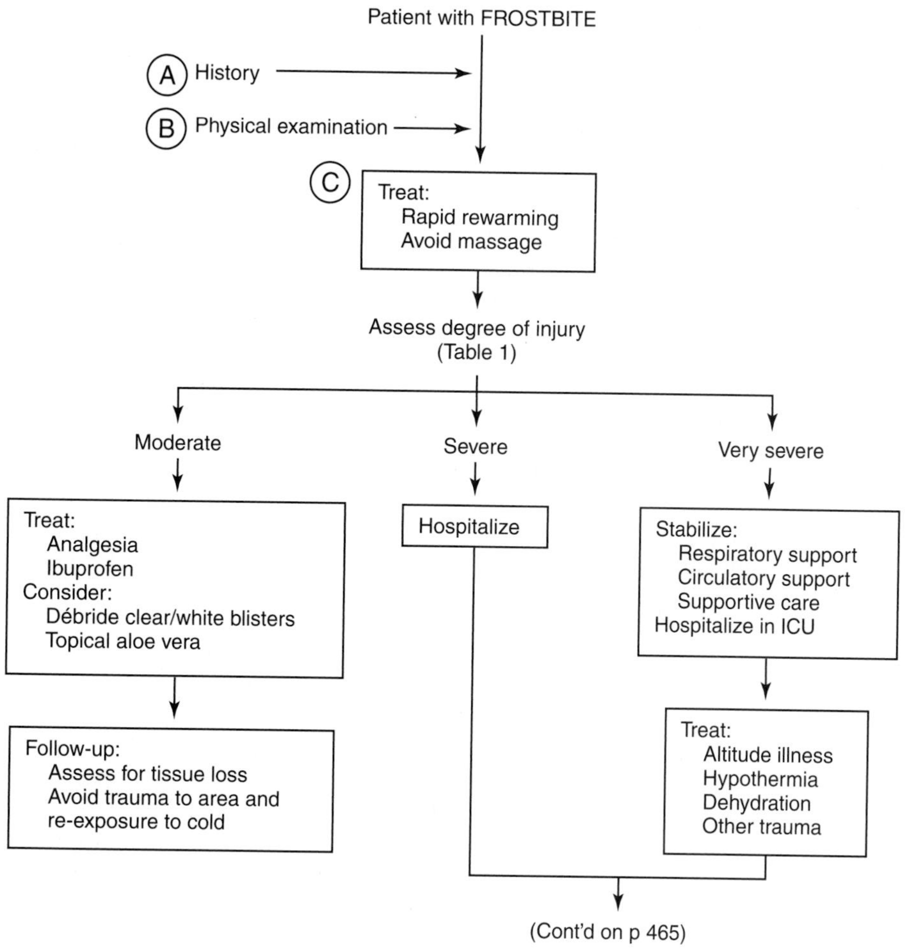
Patient with FROSTBITE
A History
B Physical examination
C Treat:
Rapid rewarming
Avoid massage
Assess degree of injury
(Table 1)
Moderate
Severe
Very severe
Treat:
Analgesia
Ibuprofen
Consider:
Débride clear/white blisters
Topical aloe vera
Follow-up:
Assess for tissue loss
Avoid trauma to area and
re-exposure to cold
Hospitalize
Stabilize:
Respiratory support
Circulatory support
Supportive care
Hospitalize in ICU
Treat:
Altitude illness
Hypothermia
Dehydration
Other trauma
(Cont'd on p 465)

D. Post-thaw care begins with débridement of clear or white blisters, leaving hemorrhagic blisters intact. Apply topical aloe vera every 6 hours on any affected areas. Elevate the affected areas with splinting as feasible to reduce edema. Administer tetanus prophylaxis as indicated. Adequate analgesia is important. Administer opiates such as morphine or meperidine intravenously (IV) or intramuscularly (IM). All patients should receive ibuprofen or another nonsteroidal anti-inflammatory agent to reduce inflammation. Adjunctive therapies for extensive injuries require subspecialist involvement. These therapies may include volume expanders (low-molecular-weight dextran), anticoagulation (heparin, aspirin), vasodilators (Priscoline [generic name: tolazoline], pentoxifylline, reserpine), hyperbaric oxygen, and thrombolytic enzymes (streptokinase, tissue plasminogen activator). Some evidence exists that the use of tissue plasminogen activator and heparin after rapid rewarming is safe and reduced considerably the predicted digit amputation rate. Otherwise, only limited animal studies support these adjunctive therapies.

E. Daily hydrotherapy for 30 to 45 minutes at 40°C aids débridement of devitalized tissue and aids in range of motion. Monitor the injury closely for signs of infection. The use of prophylactic antibiotics is unclear. Surgical treatment is normally reserved for late treatment of frostbite. Only fasciotomy/escharotomy may be needed early on to treat a compartment syndrome and ischemia. Amputation is not performed until the tissue ischemia is complete and final demarcation occurs (over 1–3 months). The use of angiography, technetium scintigraphy, or magnetic resonance imaging/angiography may allow for earlier assessment of the tissue viability and encourage earlier surgical involvement such as tissue graft coverage over injured deeper tissues (bone and tendon).

F. Late sequelae of frostbite include infection, increased cold sensitivity, increased tissue sweating, numbness, abnormalities of the nails, joint stiffness, and premature closure of physeal growth plate.

(Continued on page 466)

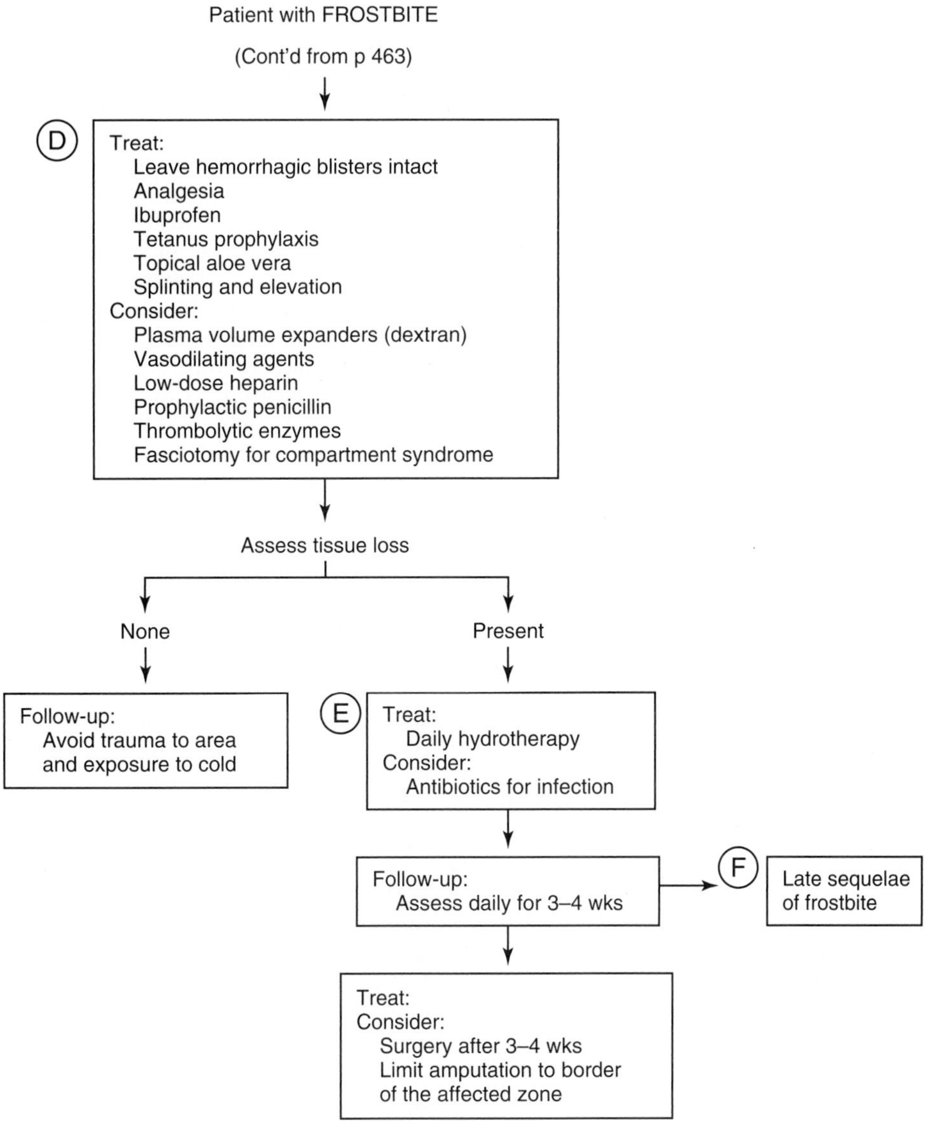
Patient with FROSTBITE
(Cont'd from p 463)
D
Treat:
Leave hemorrhagic blisters intact
Analgesia
Ibuprofen
Tetanus prophylaxis
Topical aloe vera
Splinting and elevation
Consider:
Plasma volume expanders (dextran)
Vasodilating agents
Low-dose heparin
Prophylactic penicillin
Thrombolytic enzymes
Fasciotomy for compartment syndrome
Assess tissue loss
None
Present
Follow-up:
Avoid trauma to area
and exposure to cold
E
Treat:
Daily hydrotherapy
Consider:
Antibiotics for infection
Follow-up:
Assess daily for 3–4 wks
F
Late sequelae
of frostbite
Treat:
Consider:
Surgery after 3–4 wks
Limit amputation to border
of the affected zone

BURNS

Definition

Burns are classified by depth of the burn and body surface area (BSA) involved. First-degree burns are limited to the epidermis and characterized by redness and a mild inflammatory response. They usually heal without scarring. First-degree burns are not included in the calculation of burn surface area used for therapeutic decisions. Second-degree or partial-thickness burns involve destruction of the epidermis and a portion of the dermis, sparing the sweat glands, sebaceous glands, and hair follicles. Superficial second-degree burns are characterized by pain, erythema, blister formation, and a surface that is moist and blanching. These usually heal without scarring. Deep second-degree burns involve the deep dermal layer. Deep second-degree burns are often difficult to distinguish from third-degree burns. They may be characterized by a blistered and moist surface or a dry, white, nonblanching surface. These burns usually result in scarring. Full-thickness or third-degree burns involve destruction of the epidermis and all of the dermis, including the dermal appendages. Destruction of the cutaneous nerves in the dermis makes them nontender. These burns result in scarring and contractures. Fourth-degree burns are those full-thickness injuries that involve underlying fascia, muscle, or bone.

Pathophysiology

A. The first step in the evaluation of the burned child is careful attention to adequacy of airway, breathing, and circulation (ABCs). Remove smoldering clothing or other sources of continued burning. Assess the child for associated injuries. Consider child abuse when the history is inconsistent with the examination findings or there is an unusual burn pattern. Consult a surgeon familiar with pediatric burns in all but the most minor cases.

B. Burns are considered severe to very severe (major burn) if any of the following criteria are met: second- and third-degree burns of more than 10% BSA in patients younger than 10 years; second- and third-degree burns of more than 20% BSA in other age groups; third-degree burns of more than 5% BSA; involvement of the face, eyes, ears, hands, feet, perineum, or major joints with second- or third-degree burns; associated major trauma; inhalation burns; significant electrical burns, including lightning injury; circumferential burn of the extremities or chest; and chemical injuries with serious threat of functional or cosmetic impairment. The palm of the child's hand is approximately 1% BSA and can be used as a rough guide to estimate burned area. Transfer children with major burns to a pediatric burn center.

C. Mild or moderate (minor) burns are usually treated on an outpatient basis. Cleanse the wound with a dilute mild soap and rinse it with saline. Débride ruptured vesicles. Intact blisters are generally left alone. Apply a thin layer of 1% sulfadiazine cream or Neosporin (especially for the face) and a sterile dressing. Give a tetanus booster if needed. Some children require codeine for pain control. Most burns should be re-examined and redressed in 24 hours.

D. In children with major burns, the first priority is to maintain a patent airway. Respiratory distress, cyanosis, facial burns, singed facial hairs, cough, or voice changes suggest the need for aggressive airway management. Administer oxygen in all such cases or if the history suggests smoke inhalation. Continually assess for the need for intubation when the child is at risk for airway edema and progressive obstruction.

E. Vigorous fluid administration is indicated for patients with major burns. Children with extensive burns have difficulty in retaining body fluids and regulating body temperature. Initial therapy is normal saline or lactated Ringer solution, 20 ml/kg IV, repeated until perfusion is adequate. Subsequent fluid is given at 4 ml/kg per BSA percentage burned, with half of that amount given during the first 8 hours. Calculate maintenance fluid as usual and add it to this replacement. A Foley catheter will help monitor urine output, with a goal of at least 1 ml/kg urine output per hour. Consider IV morphine for pain control. Cover burns loosely with clean sheets.

F. Baseline laboratory tests include complete blood cell count (CBC), arterial blood gas analysis, carboxyhemoglobin level, type and crossmatch of blood, electrolyte values, blood urea nitrogen (BUN) and creatinine concentrations, and urinalysis. Obtain a baseline chest radiograph.

G. Several preventive strategies can reduce the risk for burns to children. Decreasing the temperature of water heaters to 120°F increases the time required for full-thickness scalding to occur (10 minutes at 120°F, 30 seconds at 130°F). Smoke detectors and sprinkler systems can reduce deaths if they are properly installed and maintained.

References

Barker JR, Haws MJ, Brown RE, et al. Magnetic resonance imaging of severe frostbite. Ann Plast Surg 1997;38:476–9.

Bracker MD. Environmental and thermal injury. Clin Sports Med 1992;11:419.

Britt LD, Dascombe WH, Rodriguez A. New horizons in the management of hypothermia and frostbite injury. Surg Clin North Am 1991;71:345.

Fleisher G, Ludwig S, editors. Textbook of pediatric emergency medicine. 4th ed. Baltimore: Lippincott Williams & Wilkins; 2000.

Foray J. Mountain frostbite: current trends in prognosis and treatment (from results concerning 1261 cases). Int J Sports Med 1992; 13:S193.

Greenwald D, Cooper B, Gottlieb L. An algorithm for early aggressive treatment of frostbite with limb salvage directed by triple-phase scanning. Plast Reconstr Surg 1998;102:1069.

Heggers JP, Robson HC, Manavalen K, et al. Experimental and clinical observations on frostbite. Ann Emerg Med 1987;161:1056–62.

Murphy JV, Banwell PE, Roberts AH, et al. Frostbite: pathogenesis and treatment. J Trauma 2000;48:171–8.

Petrone P, Kuncir E, Asensio J. Surgical management and strategies in the treatment of hypothermia and cold injury. Emerg Med Clin N Am 2003;21:1165–78.

Shonfeld N. Outpatient management of burns in children. Pediatr Emerg Care 1990;6:249–53.

Twomey J, Peltier G, Zera R. An open-label study to evaluate the safety and efficacy of tissue plasminogen activator in treatment of severe frostbite. J Trauma 2005;59:1350–5.

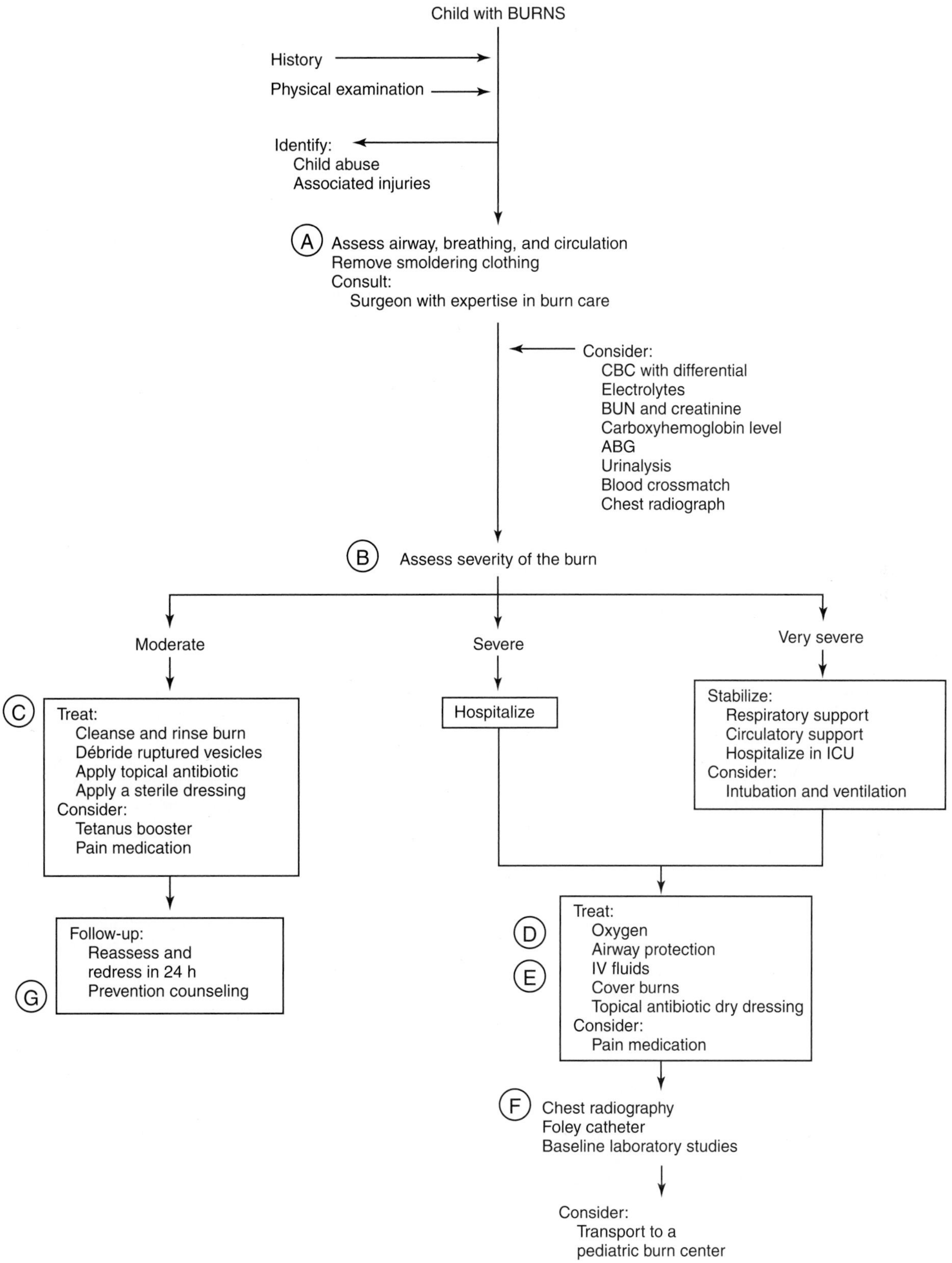

Child with BURNS
History
Physical examination
Identify:
Child abuse
Associated injuries
A
Assess airway, breathing, and circulation
Remove smoldering clothing
Consult:
Surgeon with expertise in burn care
Consider:
CBC with differential
Electrolytes
BUN and creatinine
Carboxyhemoglobin level
ABG
Urinalysis
Blood crossmatch
Chest radiograph
B
Assess severity of the burn
Moderate
Severe
Very severe
C
Treat:
Cleanse and rinse burn
Débride ruptured vesicles
Apply topical antibiotic
Apply a sterile dressing
Consider:
Tetanus booster
Pain medication
Hospitalize
Stabilize:
Respiratory support
Circulatory support
Hospitalize in ICU
Consider:
Intubation and ventilation
Follow-up:
Reassess and
redress in 24 h
Prevention counseling
G
D
E
Treat:
Oxygen
Airway protection
IV fluids
Cover burns
Topical antibiotic dry dressing
Consider:
Pain medication
F
Chest radiography
Foley catheter
Baseline laboratory studies
Consider:
Transport to a
pediatric burn center

Child Abuse: Physical Abuse

Kathryn Wells, MD, FAAP, and Andrew Sirotnak, MD

A. In the patient's history, ask how the injury happened, including sequence of events, people present, and assess for any possible delay in seeking medical attention. Record the parent's explanation of each positive physical finding in quotations whenever possible. If the child is older than 2 years, try to elicit the child's history in a private setting and compare it with the parent's version, again using quotations. Use adult translators who are not relatives or friends if there is a language barrier. Obtain at least a detailed 48-hour history of the feeding, sleeping, and behavior patterns. A complete medical, pregnancy, and family history should be obtained. The child's temperament, behavior history, and developmental level should all be assessed. Check for growth failure, previous injuries to child or siblings, death of siblings, and risk for abuse to siblings or the spouse. Social factors (such as substance abuse) and stressors (such as financial) should be identified.

B. The physical examination should consist of a thorough head-to-toe assessment including evaluation of all growth parameters that need to be plotted and compared with any previous measurements. Document all bruises, abrasions, and scars by site, size, shape, and color; note their resemblance to identifiable objects. Pay special attention to the scalp, retinas, eardrums, pinnae, oral cavity, and genitals including anus for signs of occult trauma. One study showed that approximately 60% of abused children had injuries to the head, face, and neck. Whenever possible, color photographs are helpful documentation. Consider referral of bite marks to a forensic dentist for further documentation and potential evaluation. Acute bites should be swabbed for potential DNA evidence. Bruises cannot be accurately dated. Palpate all bones for tenderness and test joints for full range of motion. Unexplained change in level of consciousness or focal neurologic signs should prompt consideration of abusive head injury, even in infants without external signs of trauma. Abdominal injury may also be present without external bruises.

C. Systemic or organic diseases can mimic physical abuse. Consider diagnoses mimicking bone (osteogenesis imperfecta, congenital syphilis, metaphyseal chondrodysplasia, infection, metabolic disease), skin (coagulopathies, vasculitides, Mongolian pigmentation, bullous impetigo, purpura), and intracranial (meningitis, sepsis, metabolic disease) injuries. Medical conditions that predispose to unrecognized accidental trauma, such as spina bifida and spasticity, require sensitive but careful investigation to ensure that the child has not experienced inadequate care or abuse.

D. Order a bleeding disorder screen in children with bruises when you suspect a bleeding disorder, if the case is expected to go to court, if the parents deny inflicting the injuries and claim easy bruising, or if there is a family history of easy bleeding. A bleeding disorder screen includes a complete blood cell count (CBC), including platelet count, partial thromboplastin time, and prothrombin time. In addition, fibrinogen level, von Willebrand factor, ristocetin cofactor, and assays for factors II, V, VII, VIII, IX, X, XI, and XIII should be considered. Finally, a study of platelet function such as a PFA-100 is preferable to bleeding time and may also be obtained. Consultation with other disciplines to evaluate hematologic, metabolic, or other diagnostic considerations may be helpful.

E. Bone trauma is found in 11% to 55% of physically abused children; young children are most vulnerable. An absence of bruising does not exclude abusive skeletal injury. In any child younger than 2 years who presents with findings concerning for abuse, a skeletal survey should be obtained. In children between 2 and 5 years, a skeletal survey (which needs to include oblique rib films) can be obtained in those with evidence of severe abuse or concerning findings on examination. After age 5 years, obtain radiographs only if there is bone tenderness or limited range of motion. Ask the radiologist to estimate age of healing positive radiographic findings. Metaphyseal chip fractures, rib fractures, or multiple injuries at different stages of healing are highly suspicious. A radionuclide bone scan may assist in identifying acute rib fractures, as well as subtle nondisplaced long-bone fractures. If underlying bone disease is suspected, calcium, alkaline phosphatase, phosphorus, 25-OH vitamin D, and parathyroid hormone levels can be obtained. Consider repeating the skeletal survey minus the skull films in 2 to 3 weeks for high-risk cases. If osteogenesis imperfecta is a consideration, a genetics consultation should be obtained. Always consider the possibility of head and/or abdominal injury when children have suspicious fractures.

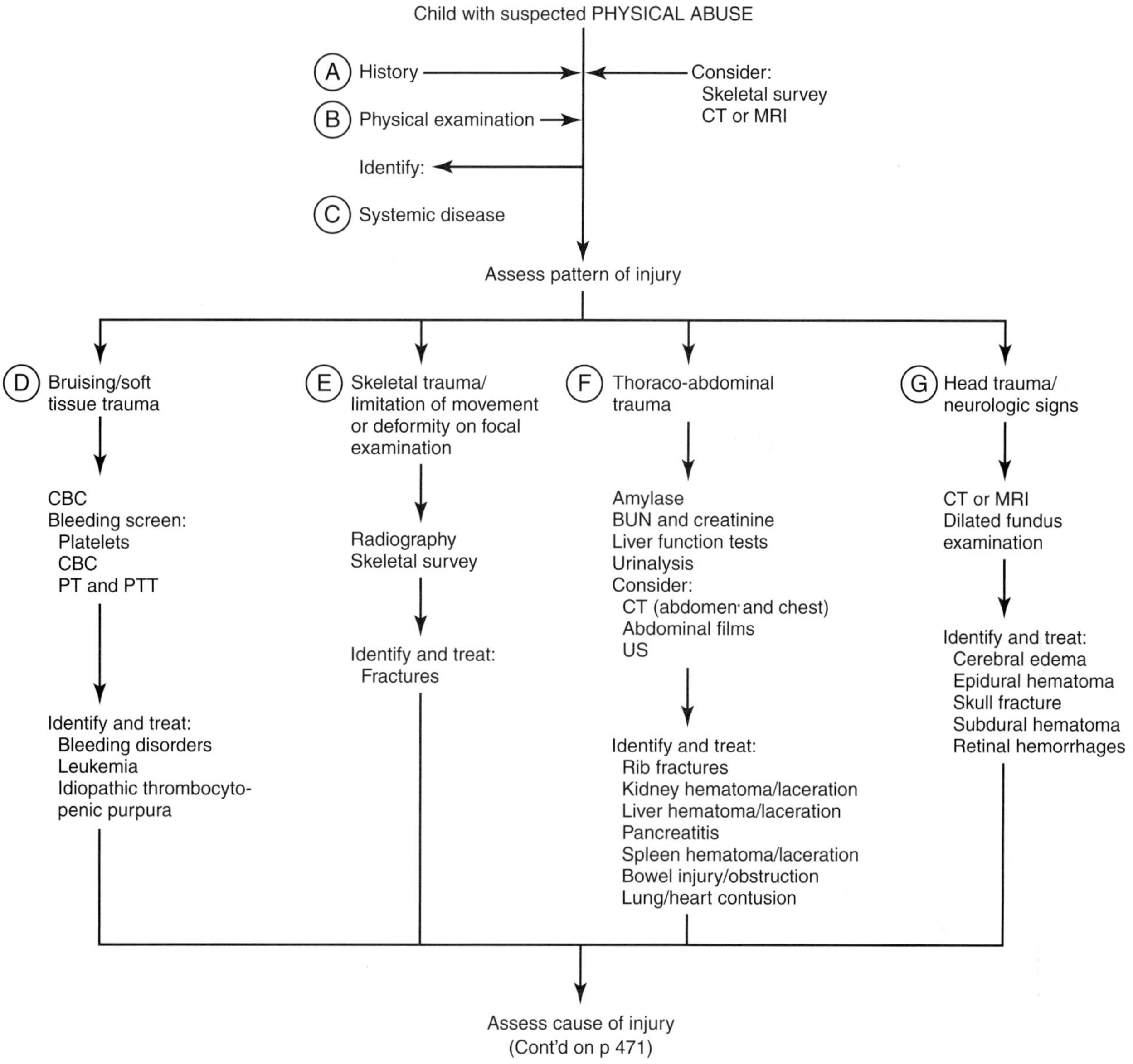
Child with suspected PHYSICAL ABUSE
A History
B Physical examination
Consider:
Skeletal survey
CT or MRI
Identify:
C Systemic disease
Assess pattern of injury
D Bruising/soft tissue trauma
CBC
Bleeding screen:
Platelets
CBC
PT and PTT
Identify and treat:
Bleeding disorders
Leukemia
Idiopathic thrombocytopenic purpura
E Skeletal trauma/limitation of movement or deformity on focal examination
Radiography
Skeletal survey
Identify and treat:
Fractures
F Thoraco-abdominal trauma
Amylase
BUN and creatinine
Liver function tests
Urinalysis
Consider:
CT (abdomen and chest)
Abdominal films
US
Identify and treat:
Rib fractures
Kidney hematoma/laceration
Liver hematoma/laceration
Pancreatitis
Spleen hematoma/laceration
Bowel injury/obstruction
Lung/heart contusion
G Head trauma/neurologic signs
CT or MRI
Dilated fundus examination
Identify and treat:
Cerebral edema
Epidural hematoma
Skull fracture
Subdural hematoma
Retinal hemorrhages
Assess cause of injury
(Cont'd on p 471)

F. Evaluate thoracoabdominal injuries with laboratory tests of the pancreas, liver, and kidneys (amylase, lipase, liver function tests, creatinine, blood urea nitrogen [BUN], and a urinalysis). In addition to a chest radiograph evaluating for rib fractures, imaging studies such as chest and abdominal computed tomographic (CT) scanning to identify injury to lungs, heart, esophagus, spleen, bladder, and bowels may also be indicated.

G. Head injury is the leading cause of child abuse fatalities. In one study, it was found that 31% of children and infants with abusive head trauma were initially misdiagnosed, so there should be a low index of suspicion for head injury especially in an infant with evidence of physical abuse. A head CT scan is a good initial method to assess head injury and should be done in infants less than 6 months old with findings suggestive of abuse; magnetic resonance imaging (MRI) may be considered when symptoms do not fit CT findings. MRI technology can identify early cerebral edema, as well as shearing tears of axonal injury. Cervical spine MRI should be considered as further evaluation of an identified intracranial injury. Head-injured children may require emergent measures to control intracranial pressure and shock. Children with evidence of chronic intracranial bleeding should be screened for metabolic disease with urine organic acids and serum amino acids. A dilated funduscopic examination optimally by a pediatric ophthalmologist, for identification, documentation, and description of retinal hemorrhages, is standard of care.

H. Many cases of physical abuse are first suspected because the injury is unexplained or the explanation is implausible and incompatible with the physical findings. An injury may be inconsistent with developmental ability of the child. A verbal child may confirm that a particular adult hurt him or her. The diagnosis of physical abuse (nonaccidental trauma) is based on whether the physical findings are consistent with the history given. Many patterned bruises, burns, and scars are pathognomonic of physical abuse. Bruises on the buttocks and lower back are frequently related to spanking; fingerprints and thumbprints can be found where a child has been forcefully grabbed such as on the upper arms or legs; hard pinching leaves curvilinear bruises; slapping leaves a bruise with parallel lines running through it that represent the spaces between the fingers; attempts to silence a screaming child or force-feeding may bruise the upper lip and/or tear the frenulum; human bite marks are distinctive paired, crescent-shaped bruises facing each other; a bruise or welt often resembles the blunt instrument used. The most common sites of accidental bruises are the forehead, anterior tibia, and bony prominences. Inflicted immersion burns usually produce a water line and may spare surfaces touching the porcelain surface of the bathtub (e.g., the buttocks) or flexed surfaces (e.g., intertriginous areas or the closed palm). Surface tension properties of liquids can help to explain patterns of scalds. Intentional cigarette burns should be distinguished from usually more superficial nonintentional burns and from skin trauma and infections. A medical provider should suspect child abuse when life-threatening injuries result from reportedly short falls or stairway falls.

I. Accidents are results of unexpected and unintentional forces. Reasonably prudent parents allow their children to be exposed to some risks that are generally low in injury potential or very low in frequency. Supervisional neglect should be considered when a parent has failed to meet the safety needs of the child or when a child has had sustained repeated serious injuries because of poor supervision.

J. Some cases are obvious; others are confusing. If you cannot decide whether the injuries are accidental or inflicted, seek immediate consultation. Consider consulting a pediatric orthopedist, radiologist, neurosurgeon, or forensic dentist for help. Whenever a medical provider suspects abuse or neglect, they are legally obligated to report suspicious injuries to the local Child Protection Services for investigation and follow-up observation.

K. Hospitalize children with severe injuries or for safety of the child, and immediately report to the local Child Protection Services. Include in the report details of injury, treatment plans, and recommendations for protection of the child and follow-up. Child abuse–trained pediatricians may be available in local children's hospitals for consultation, referral, or both. Be available to the juvenile court when necessary. Child abuse cases may involve criminal investigation and court. Report any concerns about the safety of siblings and other nonviolent caregiver. Siblings may need to be medically evaluated as well. Reports should be made to law enforcement agencies so that they can assist in the investigation. Often a scene investigation may uncover an implement used to cause an injury or other important information. For example, in immersion burns, the temperature of water in the home can be measured with properly standardized chemistry thermometers.

L. Child abuse produces psychological distress. Manifestations of abuse span the spectrum of child and adult psychopathology. Immediate psychological resources may be needed. Avoidance or denial of need of psychological resources does not indicate the absence of distress. Long-term follow-up of school functioning, behavior, and long-term relationships is important. Coordination and case management of community-based services for children and parents is important. Follow-up is critical to address any ongoing needs. It is also important to assure that regular medical care has been established for the child as well as that any needed mental health services have been initiated.

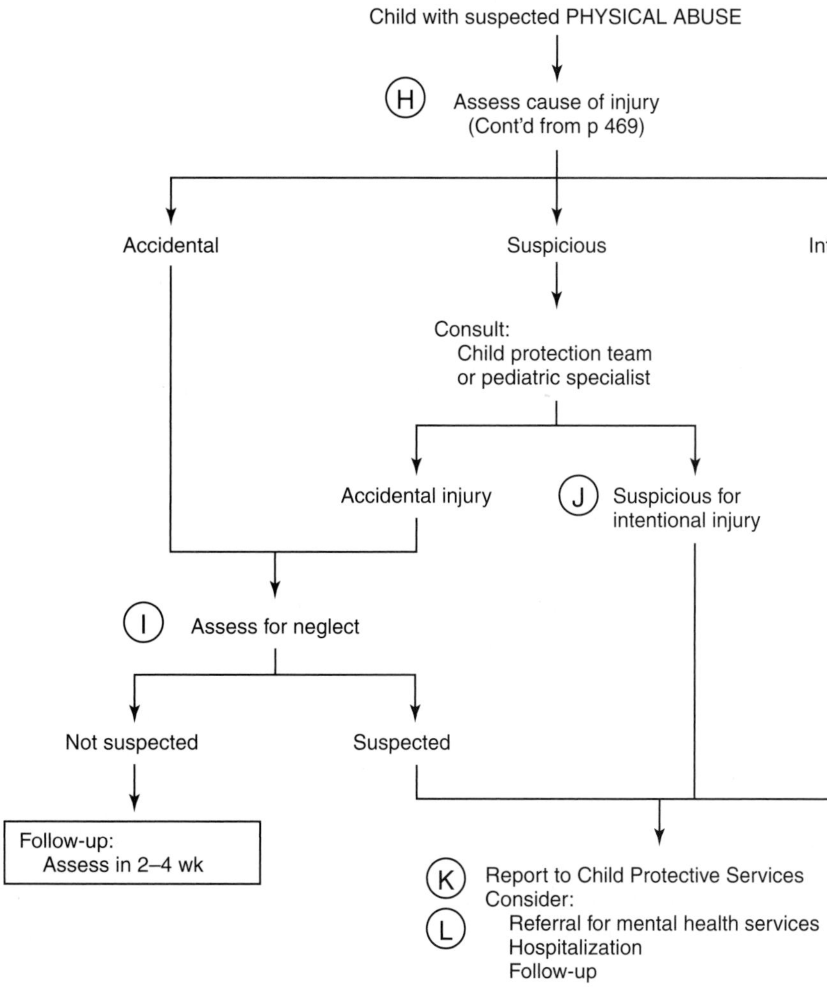
Child with suspected PHYSICAL ABUSE
H
Assess cause of injury
(Cont'd from p 469)
Accidental
Suspicious
Inflicted
Consult:
Child protection team
or pediatric specialist
Accidental injury
J
Suspicious for intentional injury
I
Assess for neglect
Not suspected
Suspected
Follow-up:
Assess in 2–4 wk
K
Report to Child Protective Services
Consider:
L
Referral for mental health services
Hospitalization
Follow-up

References

American Academy of Pediatrics. Visual diagnosis of child abuse [CD-ROM]. 3rd ed. Chicago, IL: American Academy of Pediatrics; 2009.

Cairns AM, Mok JY, Welbury RR. Injuries to the head, face, mouth and neck in physically abused children in a community setting. Int J Paediatr Dent 2005;15:310–8.

Frasier LD, et al, editors. Abusive head trauma in infants and children: a medical, legal, and forensic reference. St. Louis, MO: G.W. Medical Publishing; 2006.

Helfer ME, Kempe R, Krugman R, editors. The battered child. 5th ed. Chicago, IL: University of Chicago Press; 1997.

Jenny C, Hymel KP, Ritzen A, et al. Analysis of missed cases of abusive head trauma. JAMA 1999;281:621–6 [published erratum appears in JAMA 1999;282:29].

Kellogg ND, American Academy of Pediatrics Committee on Child Abuse and Neglect. Evaluation of suspected child physical abuse. Pediatrics 2007;119(6):1232–41.

Kleinman PK. Diagnostic imaging of child abuse. 2nd ed. Baltimore: Williams & Wilkins; 1998.

Reece RM, editors. Treatment of child abuse: common ground for mental health, medical, and legal practitioners. Baltimore, MD: Johns Hopkins University Press; 2000.

Reece RM, Christian C, editors. Child abuse: medical diagnosis and management. 3rd ed. Elk Grove Village, IL: American Academy of Pediatrics; 2009.

Child Abuse: Sexual Abuse

Andrew Sirotnak, MD, and Antonia Chiesa, MD

Children are sexually mistreated most commonly by family members, less frequently by friends and acquaintances, and least commonly by strangers. A child may present to medical care after specific disclosure by the child, with either specific or nonspecific behavioral changes or medical complaints. A detailed account of sexual experiences, unexplained vaginal bleeding, other genital symptoms, compulsive masturbation, precocious sexual behaviors, specific examination findings, sexually transmitted disease (STD), rectal or vaginal foreign body, or vaginitis should prompt consideration of the diagnosis of sexual abuse.

A. Take a careful history; few sexual abuse victims have physical or laboratory findings. Interview parents and children separately. Children older than 3 years can provide an accurate description to a skillful interviewer. Coordination with Child Protection Services or law enforcement for the medical examination of a child who has previously disclosed sexual abuse is important, as details of an interview and type of sexual contact may be known. Repeated questioning of such a child is not indicated.

When a nondisclosing child suspected of being sexually abused presents for care, an experienced clinician should do a nonleading, unbiased interview. Establish rapport; be supportive, not authoritarian; be nonjudgmental and honest with the child about the visit. Allow the child the opportunity to stop the interview (or examination). Observe and document the child's affect.

Ask open-ended and nonleading questions, such as "Tell me more about that," or "What happened next?" Progress to more specific questions if the child discloses sexual abuse. Document all details concerning type and frequency of sexual contact. Note the child's special names for body parts. Document date, time, place, person, and sites of sexual abuse. In older children, record menstrual history, whether force was involved, the patient's concept of intercourse, and whether penetration or ejaculation occurred. Refer the patient to a child psychiatrist or psychologist for additional evaluation if there is a possibility of unintentional or intentional suggestion (induced memory or coached disclosure).

B. Examine the body surface for signs of nongenital trauma. Examine the mouth and rectum for signs of acute trauma. Visually examine the external genitals for signs of trauma or vaginal discharge. Use labial traction (grasp the labia and protract them directly away and posteriorly from the child) and labial separation to examine the hymen and posterior fourchette areas. Although hymen width measurement and measurement of the posterior hymenal rim in abused and nonabused populations have been studied, the overall appearance of the tissue is more important than these measurements. When attempted, hymen width measurement is best done by colposcope with standardized optical measuring devices, noting, however, that measurements have not been shown to be a reliable diagnostic tool. In prepubertal children, vaginal speculum examination or surgical exploration under anesthesia is not indicated unless acute bleeding is unexplained or a foreign body is expected. Consider magnification and photographic documentation of the genitalia with use of a colposcope if injuries are found. Most penetrating hymenal injuries occur posteriorly, between the 3- and 9-o'clock positions. Acute trauma of the genitals, rectum, or mouth usually has epithelial closure within about a week and complete restoration of the tissues within a few weeks. Acute injuries appear as lacerations, contusions, fissures, and abrasions. Anal laxity leading to dilation greater than 20 mm without stool present is not necessarily specific for sexual abuse, but some authors have suggested there may be an association with a history of rectal penetration. Female genital injuries frequently heal without any residua of prior trauma. When apparent, healed injuries can appear as transections completely through the posterior hymen and hymenal attenuation. Healed anal injuries usually leave no discernible findings; however, scars or anal skin tags outside the midline suggest previous injury.

C. Consider consultation with a local child protection team or physician or nurse experienced in child sexual abuse evaluations. The female genitalia and anal examination have normal variability, and reliable evaluation requires some practiced skill. Some conditions can be misdiagnosed as resulting from trauma (e.g., lichen sclerosus, urethral prolapse, group A streptococcal infection). If forensic evidence collection is indicated, care should be taken to ensure the appropriate handling of specimens and maintenance of chain of evidence. Attention to proper completion of forms that accompany the collection of evidence kits is also required. Report to Child Protection Services if you are uncertain whether the concerns warrant a finding of abuse. Child abuse will produce psychological distress that can span the spectrum of child psychopathology, so consider the need for immediate psychological resources.

D. Two categories of sexual abuse can be distinguished: (1) nonpenetrating contact (viewing or fondling the child's genitals, asking the child to fondle or masturbate the adult's genitals, exposure to pornography); and (2) penetrating sexual contact, including attempted and actual vaginal, oral, or rectal penetration. Evaluate each case individually for the following: (1) the degree of force, threat, or coercion; (2) the psychological response of the parents and child; and (3) the need for laboratory investigation.

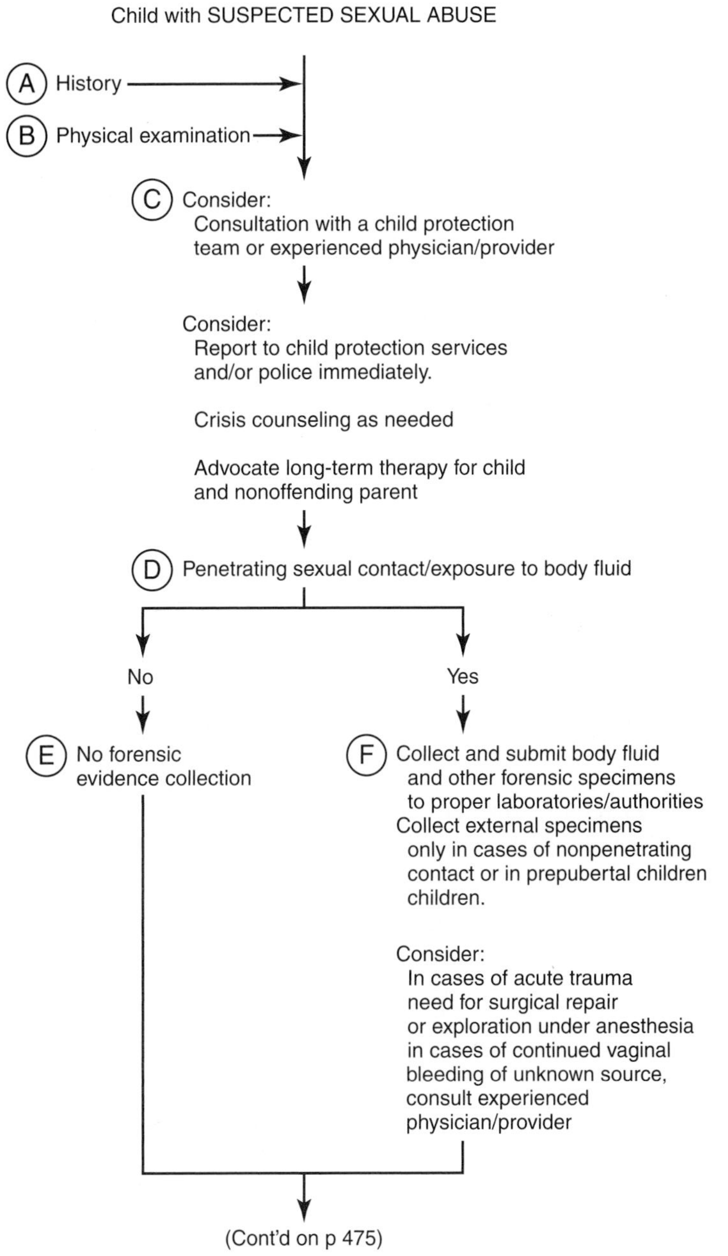
Child with SUSPECTED SEXUAL ABUSE
A History
B Physical examination
C Consider:
Consultation with a child protection team or experienced physician/provider
Consider:
Report to child protection services and/or police immediately.
Crisis counseling as needed
Advocate long-term therapy for child and nonoffending parent
D Penetrating sexual contact/exposure to body fluid
No
Yes
E No forensic evidence collection
F Collect and submit body fluid and other forensic specimens to proper laboratories/authorities
Collect external specimens only in cases of nonpenetrating contact or in prepubertal children children.
Consider:
In cases of acute trauma need for surgical repair or exploration under anesthesia in cases of continued vaginal bleeding of unknown source, consult experienced physician/provider
(Cont'd on p 475)

E. For nonpenetrating contact, collect specimens as appropriate to test for semen or saliva on skin or clothing. Data suggest that in prepubertal children, swabs from the body are unlikely to reveal forensic evidence outside of 24 hours, and that there is a much higher yield of DNA evidence from clothing and linens. Follow chain-of-evidence possession procedures.

F. If penetration has occurred, collect specimens from the clothing and body (semen, pubic hair, scalp hair, fingernail and debris scrapings, saliva, blood samples) that help to identify the perpetrator. Forensic evidence collection kits are helpful only if collected within 72 hours of alleged sexual contact or assault (up to 120 hours for adolescents with a disclosure of rape). Use protocols to guide specimen collection. Adhere to chain-of-evidence possession procedures. When there has been trauma or significant exposure to body fluid, collect a serum sample for immediate baseline testing for hepatitis B and C, human immunodeficiency virus, and syphilis, as well as for comparison with follow-up sera.

G. For the postpubertal patient, assess the possibility of pregnancy. Medication to prevent pregnancy can be given to girls who are postmenarchal and have had vaginal intercourse within 72 hours. Recent studies have suggested that this window of treatment may be extended to 120 hours. If the pregnancy test result is negative, U.S. Food and Drug Administration–approved products can be prescribed to prevent pregnancy. Although not specifically labeled for emergency contraception, there are also well-described, safe, and effective regimens that use combination oral hormonal contraceptives. There are multiple mechanisms by which emergency contraception prevents pregnancy. Unlike mifepristone (RU-486), an antiprogestin, hormonal emergency contraception is not an abortifacient. Regardless, carefully document decision-making process with family about these drugs.

H. After obtaining initial culture and wet mount specimens, treat adolescent victims of penetrating assault prophylactically with ceftriaxone (gonorrhea), azithromycin or doxycycline (chlamydia infection), and metronidazole (trichomonas infection). Nucleic acid amplification tests for the diagnosis of gonorrhea and chlamydia are increasingly used in sexually active adolescents and adults; however, their use in forensic cases of child sexual abuse has not yet been determined, and culture remains the preferred test. If culture is not available, two different nucleic acid amplification tests may be an alternative for testing. Consider postexposure prophylaxis for hepatitis B and human immunodeficiency virus (HIV) infection if trauma is present and an exchange of blood or body fluid occurred. HIV prophylaxis is costly and carries significant risk for adverse effects from the medication; compliance to prescribed regimens can be poor in pediatric and adolescent populations, so prescribing decisions should be based on risk for infection and the ability to monitor follow-up. Before initiating HIV prophylaxis, baseline serum chemistry should be drawn for safety and adverse effect monitoring. Make the decision to evaluate prepubertal children for STDs on an individual basis (type of assault, symptoms, risk of STD in the alleged perpetrator). Routine testing for STDs in every prepubertal child with a suspicion of sexual abuse is not indicated. When necessary, collect suspicious discharge, or specimens from the vagina or urethral meatus. Cervical or urethral swabs are not indicated in the prepubertal patient.

I. Follow-up examination for STDs should be done at 2 weeks after assault. Inquire about the effects of postcoital pregnancy prophylaxis. Repeat culture and wet mount tests. Repeat serologic testing for HIV, hepatitis B (unless vaccinated), hepatitis C, and rapid plasma reagin should be arranged at this time. Obtain recent menstrual history. Examine for genital warts and consider routine health screen for adolescents (Pap smear, sexual activity counseling). Evaluate all victims for signs of psychological and emotional sequela. Refer to counseling as needed. Avoidance or denial of a need for psychological resources does not indicate the absence of distress. Long-term follow-up, especially of development, school function, and sustained relationships, is important. Research in the field indicates that childhood sexual abuse is strongly associated with multiple types of future adult health and psychosocial problems.

(Continued on page 476)

Child with SUSPECTED SEXUAL ABUSE

(Cont'd from p 473)

↓

(G) Treat:
- Assess need for pregnancy/STD diagnosis and prophylaxis

Consider:
- Emergency contraception
- Ceftriaxone
- Azithromycin or doxycycline
- HIV prophylaxis (collect baseline serum)
- Hepatitis B prophylaxis
- Metronidazole

Arrange follow-up for any necessary infectious serology monitoring

↓

(H) Follow-up: 2 week visit

Consider:
- Culture and wet mount
- Monitor tolerance/compliance with any prophylactic medications
- Schedule repeat infectious serology testing at appropriate intervals

↓

(I) Evaluate all victims for emotional sequela of abuse

Refer to counseling as necessary

References

Adams JA, Kaplan RA, Starling SP, et al. Guidelines for medical care of children who may have been sexually abused. J Pediatr Adolesc Gynecol 2007;20:163.

American Academy of Pediatrics Committee on Adolescence. Emergency contraception. Pediatrics 2005;116:1038.

Babl FE, Cooper ER, Damon B, et al. HIV postexposure prophylaxis for children and adolescents. Am J Emerg Med 2000;18:282.

Berkoff MC, Zolotor AJ, Makoroff KL, et al. Has this prepubertal girl been sexually abused? JAMA 2008;300:2779.

Centers for Disease Control and Prevention, Workowski KA, Berman SM. Sexually transmitted diseases treatment guidelines, 2006. MMWR Recomm Rep 2006;55(RR-11):1–94.

Christian CW, Lavelle JM, DeJong AR, et al. Forensic evidence findings in prepubertal victims of sexual assault. Pediatrics 2000;106:100.

De Jong. Sexually transmitted infections in child sexual abuse. In: Reece RM, Christian CW, editors. Child abuse: medical diagnosis and management. Elk Grove Village, IL: American Academy of Pediatrics; 2009.

Dube SR, Anda RF, Whitfield CL, et al. Long-term consequences of childhood sexual abuse by gender of victim. Am J Prev Med 2005;28:430.

Finkel MA. Medical aspects of prepubertal sexual abuse. In: Reece RM, Christian CW, editors. Child abuse: medical diagnosis and management. Elk Grove Village, IL: American Academy of Pediatrics; 2009.

Finkel MA, Giardino AP. Medical evaluation of child sexual abuse: a practical guide. 3rd ed. Elk Grove Village, IL: American Academy of Pediatrics; 2009.

Girardet RG, Lemme S, Biason TA, et al. HIV post-exposure prophylaxis in children and adolescents presenting for reported sexual assault. Child Abuse Negl 2009;33:173.

Havens PL, Committee on Pediatric AIDS. Postexposure prophylaxis in children and adolescents for nonoccupational exposure to human immunodeficiency virus. Pediatrics 2003;111:1475.

Heger AH, Emans SJ, Muram D, editors. Evaluation of the sexually abused child: a medical textbook and photographic atlas. 2nd ed. New York: Oxford University Press; 2000.

Heger AH, Ticson L, Guerra L, et al. Appearance of the genitalia in girls selected for nonabuse: review of hymenal morphology and nonspecific findings. J Pediatr Adolesc Gynecol 2002;15:27–35.

Kellogg N, Committee on Child Abuse and Neglect. The evaluation of sexual abuse in children. Pediatrics 2005;116:506.

Lowen D, Reece RM. Visual diagnosis of child abuse on CD-ROM for Macintosh and Windows [CD-ROM]. 3rd ed. Elk Grove Village, IL: American Academy of Pediatrics; 2008.

McCann J, Miyamoto S, Boyle C, Rogers K. Healing of nonhymenal genital injuries in prepubertal and adolescent girls: a descriptive study. Pediatrics 2007;120:1000.

McCann J, Voris J. Perianal injuries resulting from sexual abuse: a longitudinal study. Pediatrics 1993;91:390.

TOXICOLOGY

Evaluation of Acute Poisoning and Overdose

Suzan Mazor, MD

Acute poisoning may result from ingestion, eye or topical exposure, inhalation, or envenomation. The types of substances most often reported to cause poisoning are cleaning products, analgesics, cosmetics, plants, decongestant and antihistamine cold drugs, pesticides, hydrocarbons, topical medications, bites, venoms, and foreign bodies.

A. If initial contact is by telephone, quickly obtain the patient's telephone number and address in case contact is broken. Ask about the product and amount ingested, time of ingestion, current symptoms, and medical history. Note toxins with a delayed onset of serious effects, such as acetaminophen, iron, lithium, and diphenoxylate with atropine (Lomotil). Contact the poison center by calling 1-800-222-1222.

B. In the physical examination, rapidly assess the airway, breathing, circulation (ABCs), and level of consciousness with the Glasgow Coma Scale (see p. 321) or other age-appropriate scale. Carefully assess the eyes for pupil size and responsiveness, nystagmus, and extraocular eye movements, and visualize the fundi. Note corrosive lesions and bleeding in the mouth. Assess airway-protective reflexes. Count respirations and listen for air exchange; note retractions, grunting, and nasal flaring (signs of distress). Assess the peripheral perfusion, and note heart rate and rhythm. Note skin color and any lesions such as bites, burns, or blisters, or topical patches. Note unusual odors.

C. Initial decontamination may include saline eye lavage, removal of contaminated clothing and washing the skin with soap and water, or gastrointestinal interventions. Options for gastric decontamination include syrup of ipecac, gastric lavage, activated charcoal, or whole-bowel irrigation. The choice of gastric decontamination depends on the poison ingested, time since ingestion, and clinical presentation (Table 1). Current recommendations for decontamination have an increased focus on the use of activated charcoal with a decreased emphasis on syrup of ipecac and gastric lavage. Toxins not adsorbed well to charcoal include iron, mineral acids or bases, alcohol, cyanide, solvents, hydrocarbons, and other water-insoluble compounds. Most poisoned children who are not critically ill are managed safely and effectively in the emergency department or office setting with activated charcoal alone. Activated charcoal may be given with a cathartic agent on the first dose. After the first dose, coadministration of cathartic with charcoal should be avoided because of the possibility of causing fluid and electrolyte abnormalities. The dose of activated charcoal is 1 g/kg; it may be administered orally, by nasogastric tube, or by orogastric tube.

Whole-bowel irrigation should be considered for potentially toxic ingestions of iron, sustained-release medications, and lead, as well as packets of illicit drugs. Consider gastric lavage only when the patient has ingested a potentially life-threatening amount of a poison and the procedure can be undertaken within 60 minutes of the ingestion. An absolute contraindication to gastric lavage is the ingestion of caustic agents because of the increased risk for esophageal or gastric perforation by this procedure. Gastric lavage is also contraindicated in hydrocarbon ingestions because of an increased risk for aspiration. The role of syrup of ipecac is limited, and recommendations for its use have been on the decline. Because of the emetogenic effect of syrup of ipecac, administration of activated charcoal or other gastric decontamination techniques may be more difficult. Syrup of ipecac may still be useful in some poisonings that occur at locations distant from medical care. All gastric decontamination may cause emesis, which puts the patient at risk for aspiration, and care must be taken in patients who have ingested caustic agents or hydrocarbons, have a compromised or unprotected airway, or have an altered mental status.

D. Simple maintenance of the airway, ventilation, oxygenation, attention to intravascular fluid status, and appropriate cardiovascular support may contribute more to survival than any other specific antidotes in the care of the poisoned patient. When hypoglycemia is identified, give 0.25 to 1 g/kg glucose as 10% to 25% dextrose in water. Hypoglycemia can be associated with poisoning by ethanol, insulin, salicylates, oral hypoglycemics, and beta-blocking agents. If a patient presents with coma, bradycardia, and miosis, suspect an opioid toxin and administer 0.4 to 2 mg naloxone (Table 2). Treat adolescent patients with a history of opioid intoxication with a 2-mg bolus every 2 minutes up to five times (total of 10 mg) if necessary for a response.

(Continued on page 480)

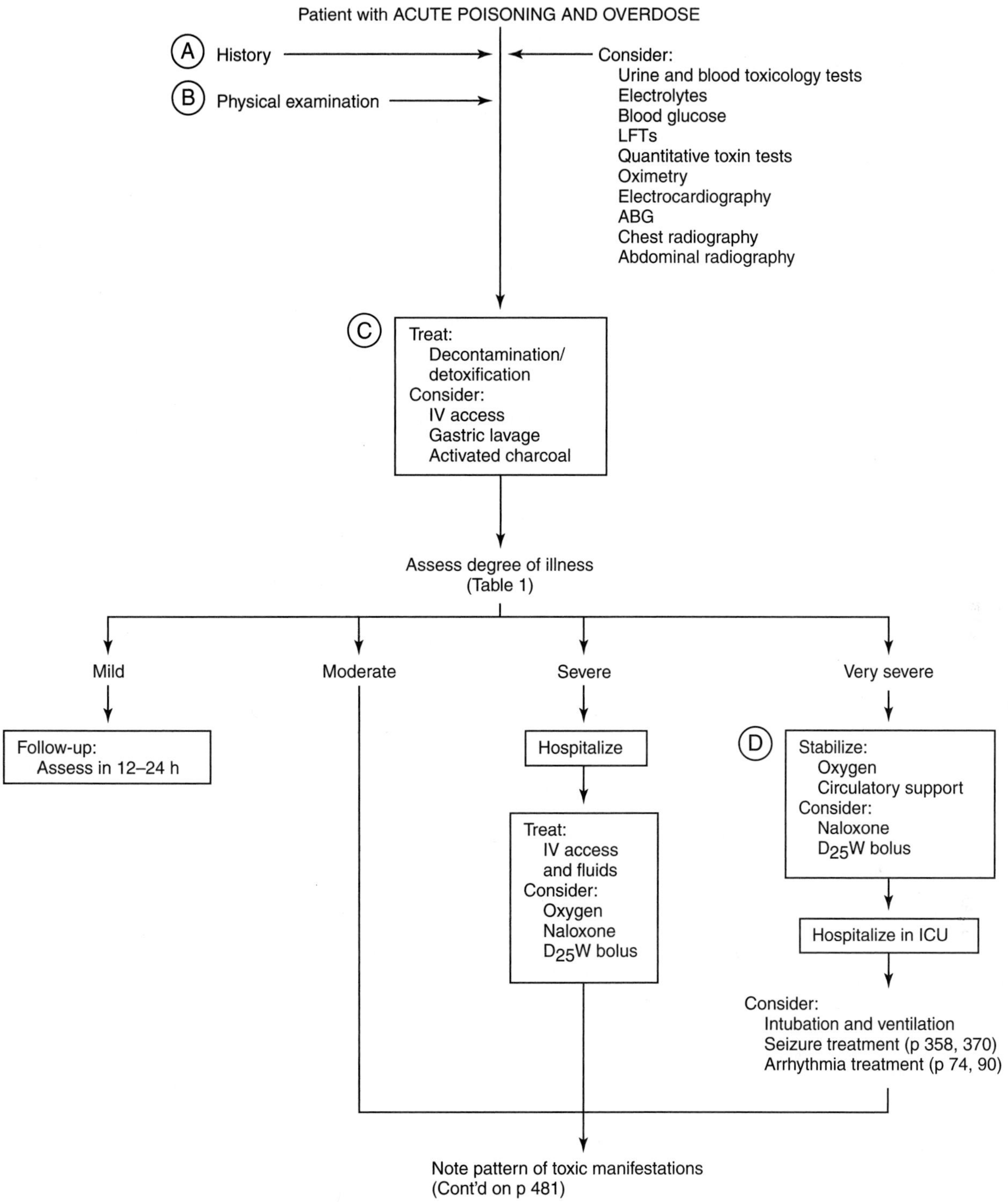
Patient with ACUTE POISONING AND OVERDOSE
A History
B Physical examination
Consider:
Urine and blood toxicology tests
Electrolytes
Blood glucose
LFTs
Quantitative toxin tests
Oximetry
Electrocardiography
ABG
Chest radiography
Abdominal radiography
C Treat:
Decontamination/
detoxification
Consider:
IV access
Gastric lavage
Activated charcoal
Assess degree of illness
(Table 1)
Mild
Moderate
Severe
Very severe
Follow-up:
Assess in 12–24 h
Hospitalize
Treat:
IV access
and fluids
Consider:
Oxygen
Naloxone
D25W bolus
D Stabilize:
Oxygen
Circulatory support
Consider:
Naloxone
D25W bolus
Hospitalize in ICU
Consider:
Intubation and ventilation
Seizure treatment (p 358, 370)
Arrhythmia treatment (p 74, 90)
Note pattern of toxic manifestations
(Cont'd on p 481)

Table 1. **Degree of Illness in Poisoning and Overdose**

Mild	Moderate	Severe	Very Severe
Asymptomatic No risk for deterioration	Benign, self-limited toxic effects	Altered mental state (lethargy) or signs of toxicity that may worsen and become life threatening	Unstable vital signs (shock, respiratory depression, arrhythmia) *or* Coma *or* Stupor *or* Seizures

Table 2. **Specific Antidotes to Acute Poisoning in Children and Adolescents**

Poison	Antidote
Acetaminophen	*N*-acetylcysteine; intravenous (IV)—150 mg/kg over 1 h, then 12.5 mg/kg/h for 4 h, then 6.25 mg/kg/hr; enteral—140 mg/kg, then 70 mg/kg every 4 h.
Anticholinergics	Physostigmine (adult, 0.5 to 2 mg; child, 0.02 mg/kg) slow IV; may repeat in 15 min until desired effect is achieved; subsequent doses every 2–3 h PRN *(Caution: May cause seizures, asystoles, cholinergic crisis; discuss with medical toxicologists)*
Anticholinesterases	Atropine, 2–5 mg (adults); 0.05–0.1 mg/kg (children) intramuscular (IM) or IV, repeated every 10–15 min until atropinization is evident
Organophosphates	Pralidoxime chloride 1–2 g (adults); 25–50 mg/kg (children) IV; repeat dose in 1 h PRN, then every 6–8 h for 24–48 h (consider also constant infusion; see text)
Carbamates	Atropine, as above; pralidoxime for severe cases (see text)
Benzodiazepines	Flumenazil, 0.01 mg/kg IV (estimated pediatric dose; see text)
β-Adrenergic blockers	Glucagon, 0.1 mg/kg IV, followed by 0.05 mg/kg/h
Calcium channel blockers	Calcium chloride 10%, 10 mL (adult); 0.2 mL/kg (pediatric) IV Insulin (see text) Or Calcium gluconate 10%, 30 ML (adult); 0.6 mL/kg (pediatric) IV
Carbon Monoxide	Oxygen 100% inhalation, consider hyperbaric for severe cases
Cyanide—cyanide antidote kit	*Adult:* Amyl nitrite inhalation (inhale for 15–30 s every 60 s) pending administration of 300 mg sodium nitrite (10 mL of a 3% solution) IV slowly (over 2–4 min); follow immediately with 12.5 g sodium thiosulfate (2.5–5 mL/min of 25% solution) IV *Children:* (Na nitrite should not exceed recommended dose because dangerous methemoglobinemia may result): Hemoglobin / Initial dose 3% Na nitrite / Initial dose 25% Na thiosulfate IV 8 g / 0.22 mL (6.6 mg)/kg / 1.10 mL/kg 10 g / 0.27 mL (8.7 mg)/kg / 1.35 mL/kg 12 g (normal) / 0.33 mL (10 mg)/kg / 1.65 mL/kg 14 g / 0.39 mL (11.6 mg)/kg / 1.95 mL/kg
Cyanide—hydroxycobalamin	*Adult:* 5g IV; *Child:* 70 mg/kg IV
Digitalis	Fab antibodies (Digibind): dose based on amount ingested and/or digoxin level (see package insert)
Isoniazid (INH)	Pyridoxine 5%–10%, 1 g per gram of INH ingested (70 mg/kg up to 5 g if dose unknown) IV slowly over 30–60 min
Methanol/ethylene glycol	Fomepizole: load 15 mg/kg; maintenance 10 mg/kg q12h 4 doses, then 15 mg/kg q 12h (dose should be adjusted during dialysis; ethanol may be used if fomepizole unavailable) Ethanol loading dose: 0.75 g/kg infused over 1 h (fomepizole is preferred) Ethanol maintenance: 0.1–0.2 g/kg/h infusion; adjust as needed with target level 100 mg/dL Folate 1 mg/kg IV every 6 h (methanol) Thiamine 0.5 mg/kg and pyridoxine 2 mg/kg (ethylene glycol)
Methemoglobinemic agents	Methylene blue 1%, 1–2 mg/kg (0.1–0.2 mL/kg) IV slowly over 5–10 min if cyanosis is severe or methemoglobin level >40%
Opioids	Naloxone 0.4–2 mg IV, IM, sublingual or by ETT; may repeat up to total 8–10 mg in adolescent/adult (see text)
Phenothiazines (dystonic reaction)	Diphenhydramine, 1–2 mg/kg IM or IV; or Benztropine, 1–2 mg IM or IV (adolescents)
Sulfonylureas	Octreotide 1–2 μg/kg/dose subcutaneous (SC) or IV every 6–12 h
Tricyclic antidepressants	Sodium bicarbonate, 1–2 mEq/kg IV
Warfarin (and "superwarfarin" rat poisons")	Vitamin K, 10 mg (adult); 1–5 mg (pediatric) IV, IM, SC, PO

Modified from Osterhoudt KC, Ewald MB, Shannon M. Toxicologic emergencies. In: Fleisher GR, Ludwig S, eds. Textbook of Pediatric Medicine. 6th ed. Baltimore, MD: Lippincott Williams & Wilkins; 2010

E. Narcotic-sedative-hypnotic toxic syndrome is characterized by depressed mental state, depressed respirations, and hypotension. Narcotics, excluding meperidine, produce miosis. Central nervous system sedatives, such as alcohol, barbiturates, ethchlorvynol, chlordiazepoxide, diazepam, meprobamate, and methaqualone, can be associated with small or normal pupils. Glutethimide (Doriden) overdose causes fixed pupils. Naloxone reverses narcotic overdose but rarely helps overdose of other sedative-hypnotic drugs.

F. Anticholinergic toxic syndrome is characterized by altered mental state (confusion, agitation, delirium, hallucinations, seizures, coma), dry skin and mucous membranes, mydriasis, tachycardia, urinary retention, fever, and decreased bowel sounds. Anticholinergic drugs include antihistamines, antiparkinsonian agents, belladonna alkaloids, haloperidol, tricyclic antidepressants, and toxic mushrooms and plants. Physostigmine should be considered only when symptoms are life-threatening because its use may cause seizures, asystole, and cholinergic crisis. Physostigmine is contraindicated in patients with asthma, vascular compromise, or urinary obstruction.

G. Cholinergic toxic syndrome is characterized by miosis, increased salivation, lacrimation, muscle fasciculations and weakness, sweating, vomiting, sneezing, and bradycardia. The central nervous system effects include irritability, headache, confusion, seizures, and coma. Chemicals and drugs that cause this syndrome include organophosphate and carbamate insecticides, physostigmine, neostigmine, and edrophonium.

H. Toxins that produce an increased anion gap metabolic acidosis include salicylates, methanol (treat with ethanol or fomepizole), ethylene glycol (treat with ethanol or fomepizole), carbon monoxide (treat with oxygen),

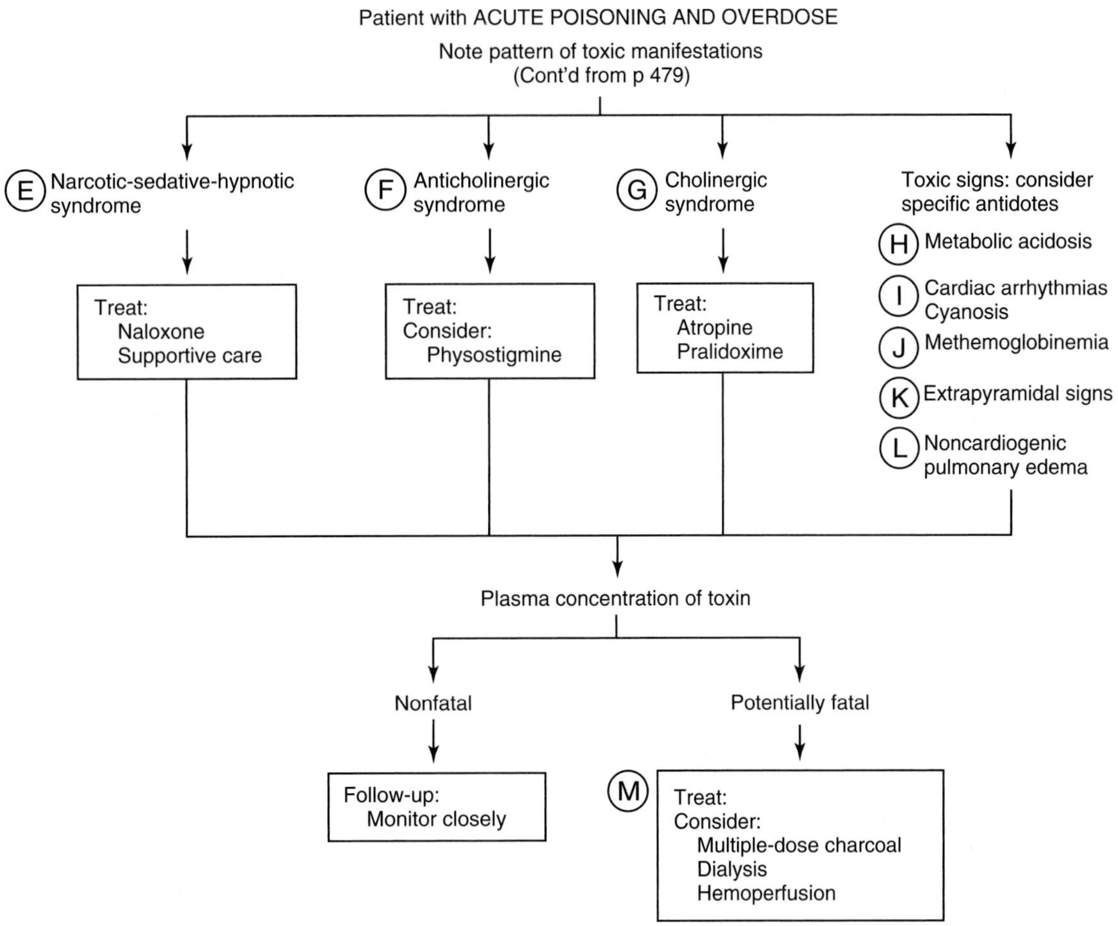

Patient with ACUTE POISONING AND OVERDOSE
Note pattern of toxic manifestations
(Cont'd from p 479)
E Narcotic-sedative-hypnotic syndrome
F Anticholinergic syndrome
G Cholinergic syndrome
Toxic signs: consider specific antidotes
H Metabolic acidosis
I Cardiac arrhythmias Cyanosis
J Methemoglobinemia
K Extrapyramidal signs
L Noncardiogenic pulmonary edema
Treat: Naloxone Supportive care
Treat: Consider: Physostigmine
Treat: Atropine Pralidoxime
Plasma concentration of toxin
Nonfatal
Potentially fatal
Follow-up: Monitor closely
M
Treat: Consider: Multiple-dose charcoal Dialysis Hemoperfusion

cyanide (treat with cyanide antidote kit or hydroxocobalamin), paraldehyde, isoniazid, and iron.

I. Toxins most frequently associated with cardiac arrhythmia are cyclic antidepressants, amphetamines, anticholinergics, arsenic, beta-blockers, calcium channel blockers, chloral hydrate, cyanide, theophylline, digitalis, phenothiazines, quinidine, and lithium.

J. Toxins that can induce methemoglobinemia and cyanosis unresponsive to oxygen include nitrates, nitrites, aniline, phenacetin, phenols, local anesthetics, sulfonamides, phenazopyridine, antimalarials, sulfones, naphthalene, and *p*-aminosalicylic acid.

K. Toxins that produce extrapyramidal central nervous system effects (dystonic reactions or oculogyric crisis) include phenothiazines and butyrophenones. Treat with an antiparkinsonian agent (Cogentin) or an antihistamine.

L. Toxins that produce noncardiogenic pulmonary edema may be inhaled (carbon monoxide, phosgene, hydrogen sulfide, chlorine, nitrogen oxides, and beryllium) or ingested (narcotics, salicylates, sedative hypnotics).

M. Consider additional therapies when the risk for a serious complication or a poor outcome is high. These include multiple-dose activated charcoal, dialysis and hemoperfusion. Multiple-dose activated charcoal is used for serious ingestions of phenobarbital, carbamazepine, dapsone, quinine, salicylates, and theophylline. Hemodialysis may be indicated for potentially fatal poisonings with lithium, ethylene glycol, methanol, and salicylates. Hemoperfusion may benefit poisonings with phenobarbital, theophylline, paraquat, glutethimide, methaqualone, ethchlorvynol, or meprobamate.

References

Bond GR. The poisoned child—evolving concepts in care. Emerg Med Clin North Am 1995;13:343.

Brent J, McMartin K, Phillips S, et al. Fomepizole for the treatment of ethylene glycol poisoning. N Engl J Med 1999;340:832.

Chyka PA, Seger D. Position statement: single-dose activated charcoal. American Academy of Clinical Toxicology; European Association of Poisons Centres and Clinical Toxicologists. J Toxicol Clin Toxicol 1997;35:721.

Henretig FM. Special considerations in the poisoned pediatric patient. Emerg Med Clin North Am 1994;12:549.

Howland MA. Antidotes in Depth. In: Nelson L, Lewin N, Howland MA, Hoffman R, Goldfrank L, Flomenbaum N, eds. Goldfrank's Toxicologic Emergencies. 9th ed. New York: McGraw-Hill; 2011.

Osterhoudt KC, Ewald MB, Shannon M. Toxicologic emergencies. In: Fleisher GR, Ludwig S, eds. Textbook of Pediatric Medicine. 6th ed. Baltimore, MD: Lippincott Williams & Wilkins; 2010.

Phillips S, Gomez H, Brent J. Pediatric gastrointestinal decontamination in acute toxin ingestion. J Clin Pharmacol 1993;33:497.

Tenenbein M. Position statement: whole bowel irrigation. American Academy of Clinical Toxicology; European Association of Poisons Centres and Clinical Toxicologists. J Toxicol Clin Toxicol 1997;35:753.

Vale JA. Position statement: Gastric lavage. American Academy of Clinical Toxicology; European Association of Poisons Centres and Clinical Toxicologists. J Toxicol Clin Toxicol 1997;35:711.

Vernon DD, Gleich MC. Poisoning and drug overdose. Crit Care Clin 1997;13:647.

Lead Exposure and Intoxication in Children

Mark E. Anderson, MD

CURRENT STATE

No level of lead in a child's blood is safe. Despite the current "action level" of 10 μg lead/dl blood, research consistently demonstrates a dose–response relation between blood lead levels and IQ (intelligence quotient) testing at levels both above and below the action level. The same research demonstrates a greater relative decrement in IQ at levels less than 10 μg/dl. Granted, great progress has been made with environmental lead, such as with lead additives in gasoline. However, the United States still has an estimated 1% to 2% of children with lead levels greater than 10 μg/dl and 14% with lead levels between 5 and 9 μg/dl. Average childhood blood lead levels have declined precipitously from an average of 15 μg/dl 30 years ago to now less than 2 μg/dl, but disparities remain, especially for the urban poor. Housing quality is an important risk factor for lead exposure via poorly maintained paint. Many more children have levels of blood lead that fall below the threshold action level but who experience effects from the exposure.

Given these successes, casefinding ideally should shift from testing of children to testing of environments, but this goal has not been realized. Much is known about the interaction of lead and biological systems, most of which is subclinical and, therefore, argues for lead screening. Subclinical effects include transplacental transfer and decreased IQ at levels less than 10 μg/dl, and alterations in heme synthesis, vitamin D metabolism, and nerve conduction velocity at higher levels. Clinically evident effects are seen at levels greater than 50 μg/dl and include frank anemia, colic, nephropathy, and encephalopathy. Death may occur at levels greater than 100 μg/dl.

Lead exposure can be viewed as a lifetime exposure even after blood lead levels decline. Serum lead is bound into bones, which are metabolically active and serve as an ongoing source of lead over an individual's lifetime. Chelation will reduce serum lead levels but will not directly affect lead already incorporated into bone. Cognitive outcomes after chelation are inconsistent between studies, but if a clinically apparent effect exists, it is likely small and should be balanced with the fact that chelation therapy imparts significant risks, including death. The potential high cost to individuals of lead exposure and the lack of an effective, outcomes-based intervention argues for prevention of lead exposure. Identifying and remediating environments harmful to children before the exposure occurs may be the most reasonable lead policy approach.

A. History: An appropriate patient history for possible lead exposure is essentially the environmental history, which should include questions about the home, such as its age and renovation history, and questions regarding activities within the home such as hobbies that may use lead or occupations that expose children to special risk, like scrap-metal recycling. The patient history includes work in which the child or adolescent may engage and also the parent's type of work. History of known or suspected exposure should prompt screening, as should the presence of another occupant in the home with an increased blood lead level. Children with pica behaviors are at increased risk for lead intoxication, and the presence of anemia may be a marker for increased blood lead. Many miscellaneous exposure pathways are known such as use of lead-glazed ceramics, storage of food in lead-containing packages or containers, folk remedy use, and use of imported cosmetics.

B. Sampling Procedures: Lead screening is usually done with a capillary specimen, typically a finger prick with blood blotted onto a testing paper. Testing in this manner requires that the skin surface be clean and is prone to false-positive test results. Therefore, elevated capillary screening should be followed by venipuncture testing to confirm a true elevation of blood lead. However, in cases where the screening test demonstrates an elevated lead level and the venipuncture follow-up test does not, recognize that the child still has an exposure to lead in the environment.

C. Routine and Specific Recommendations: In the early 1990s, U.S. screening was recommended at ages 1 and 2 years or at least once for all children younger than 6 years. More recently, targeted screening is recommended. The Centers for Medicaid and Medicare Services (CMS) mandates screening at 1 and 2 years, but screening is not universal even in the high-risk populations covered by Medicaid. Practitioners should know their local lead epidemiology because departments of health may have unique screening programs in place based on local lead issues. As part of lead screening, consider screening for and treatment of anemia.

In general, a diet with adequate calcium and iron is thought to have a protective effect against lead absorption, but this recommendation should not replace lead screening.

D. Other Resources: Many communities have governmental and nongovernmental resources to offer both providers and children living in the community. Governmental examples include local, county, and state departments of public/environmental health that may include expertise in environmental lead exposure and cleanup. In the United States, the Environmental Protection Agency (EPA) has specific programs dealing with lead, and each EPA region has a "Children's Health Representative" whose responsibilities include

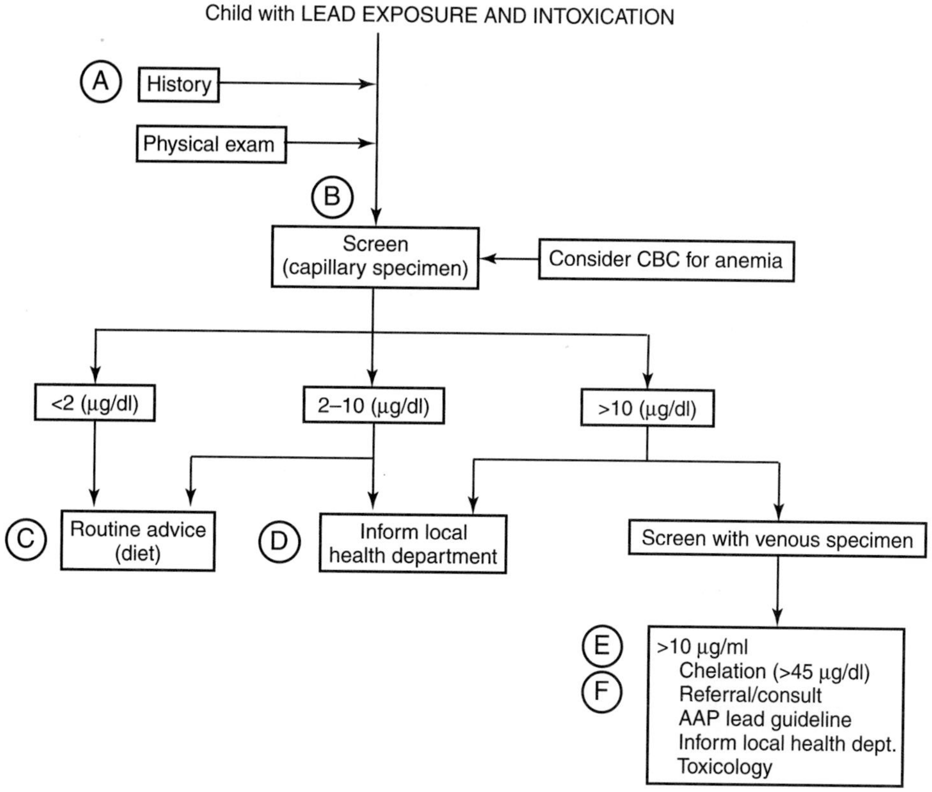
Child with LEAD EXPOSURE AND INTOXICATION
A
History
Physical exam
B
Screen (capillary specimen)
Consider CBC for anemia
<2 (μg/dl)
2–10 (μg/dl)
>10 (μg/dl)
C
Routine advice (diet)
D
Inform local health department
Screen with venous specimen
E
F
>10 μg/ml
Chelation (>45 μg/dl)
Referral/consult
AAP lead guideline
Inform local health dept.
Toxicology

an awareness regarding resources and programs that exist locally and regionally. Outside government, local grassroots organizations may exist that focus on housing safety and quality. Such organizations typically operate under public funding sources and include programs such as the U.S. Healthy Homes Initiative. Knowledge of and access to specific resources speaks to the role of the pediatric provider in the community and a need for activism in support of children and their environmental health.

E. Chelation: At levels greater than 45 μg/dl, chelation therapy is a reasonable consideration and can be administered on an outpatient basis. At greater levels, such as those more than 70 μg/dl, inpatient therapy should be considered. The decision to chelate and/or to hospitalize a patient for lead intoxication involves consideration of many variables, such as the safety of the home, isolation of the lead source, the family social situation, and the chronicity of the exposure. Recognize that chelation has adverse effects that range from foul odor and taste with succimer to death subsequent to intravenous chelation therapy.

F. National Guidelines: In 2005, the American Academy of Pediatrics (AAP) published its most recent policy statement on lead exposure in children. The Statement from the AAP's committee on Environmental Health attempts to cover the current state of the science of lead epidemiology, screening, and therapy for children. The statement charges government and the medical/research community to further understand the effects of lead on IQ at lower levels and to establish the use of "low-tech" prevention interventions such as simple hand washing and the use of high-chairs for mealtimes. Current casefinding techniques may need to evolve from testing of children to include clearer identification of high-risk areas, minimizing further entry of lead into the environment, and work with public (and private) health individuals and housing representatives such as landlords.

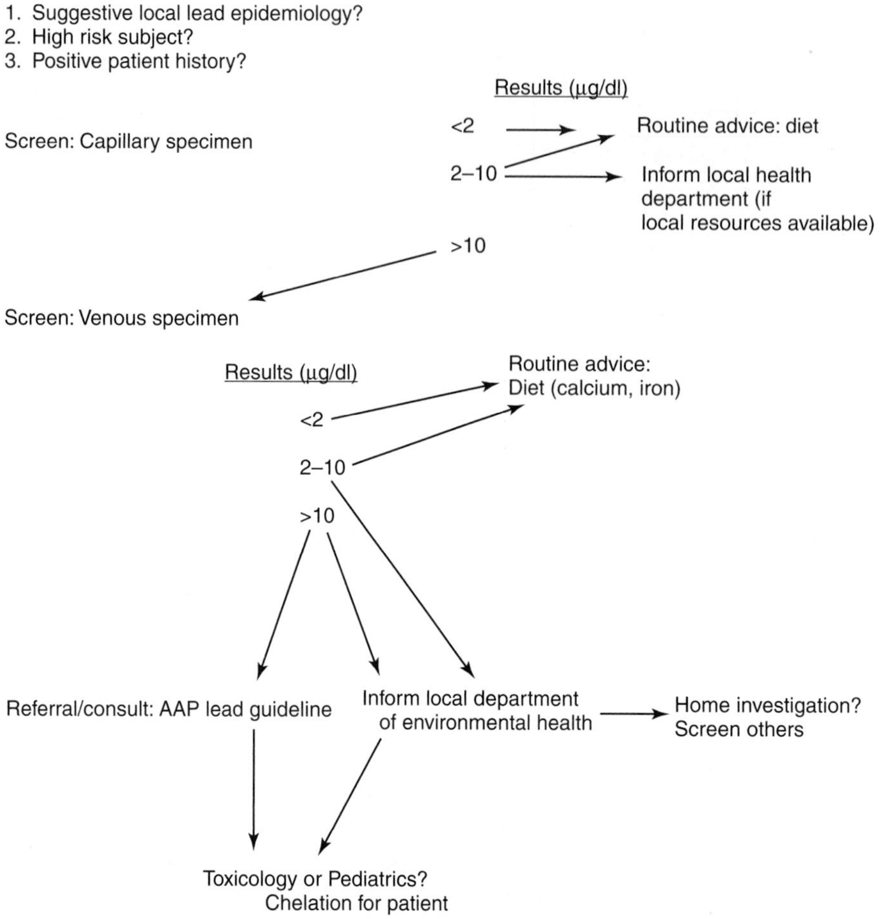
1. Suggestive local lead epidemiology?
2. High risk subject?
3. Positive patient history?
Results (μg/dl)
Screen: Capillary specimen
<2
Routine advice: diet
2–10
Inform local health department (if local resources available)
>10
Screen: Venous specimen
Results (μg/dl)
Routine advice: Diet (calcium, iron)
<2
2–10
>10
Referral/consult: AAP lead guideline
Inform local department of environmental health
Home investigation? Screen others
Toxicology or Pediatrics? Chelation for patient

Figure 1 Screening, confirmation, and treatment guideline for lead exposure in children. *AAP,* American Academy of Pediatrics.

References

American Academy of Pediatrics Committee on Environmental Health. Lead exposure in children: prevention, detection, and management. Pediatrics 2005;116:1036–46.

Canfield R, Henderson C Jr, Cory-Slechta D, et al. Intellectual impairment in children with blood lead concentrations below 10 micrograms per deciliter. N Engl J Med 2003;348(16):1517–26.

Committee on Environmental Health, Etzel R, Balk S, editors. Pediatric environmental health. 2nd ed. Elk Grove Village, IL: American Academy of Pediatrics; 2003.

Jusko T, Henderson C, Lanphear B, et al. Blood lead concentrations <10 μcg/dl and child intelligence at 6 years of age. Environ Health Perspect 2008;116(2):243–8.

Levin R, Brown MJ, Kashtock M, et al. Lead exposure in US children, 2008: implications for prevention. Environ Health Perspect 2008;116(10):1285–93.

SPECIFIC DISORDERS

Adolescent Medicine

Contraception (Including Emergency Contraception)

Amy E. Sass, MD, MPH

Almost half of high-school students reported having had sexual experience, and one third reported being currently sexually active according to the Centers for Disease Control 2007 Youth Risk Behavior Survey. Most adolescents have sex for the first time at about age 17, but do not marry until their middle or late 20s. This means that young adults are at risk for unwanted pregnancy and sexually transmitted infections (STIs) for nearly a decade. A sexually active teen who does not use contraceptives has almost a 90% chance of becoming pregnant within a year. In the United States, approximately 750,000 adolescents younger than 19 become pregnant every year. The majority of teen pregnancies is unintended. The United States has the highest rate of teen pregnancy in the developed world. Pregnancy rates for female Hispanic and non-Hispanic black adolescents aged 15 to 19 years are much greater (132.8/1000 and 128.0/1000 population, respectively) than their non-Hispanic white peers (45.2/1000 population). Lower socioeconomic status and lower maternal education are risk factors for teen pregnancy regardless of racial or ethnic group (Table 1).

A. The American Academy of Pediatrics endorses a comprehensive approach to sexuality education that incorporates encouraging abstinence while providing appropriate risk reduction counseling regarding sexual behaviors. Adolescents often delay seeing a clinician for contraceptive services after initiating sexual activity. Concern about lack of confidentiality is an important reason for this delay. Regularly talking with teenagers about sexual intercourse and its implications in a nonjudgmental manner can help teens make informed decisions regarding engaging in intimate behaviors. The goals of counseling adolescents about contraception include promoting safe and responsible sexual behavior through delaying the initiation of sexual activity, reinforcing consistent condom use for those who are sexually active, and discussing other contraceptive methods and emergency contraception (EC) to provide additional protection from unwanted pregnancy. The routine health care visit is an opportune time to conduct a comprehensive social history and have these discussions. Some authors have suggested that the date of the female patient's last menstrual period should be the "fifth vital sign." This is an intriguing idea because it quickly provides information about the possibility of pregnancy regardless of the reason for the visit. An extension of this is inquiring about sexual activity at all office visits to provide access to reproductive health counseling and medications that the teen might not otherwise have because many adolescents do not seek routine well care. Minors can consent for family planning and contraceptive services in most states under explicit statutes and in every state in a site funded by the federal Title X Family Planning Program. Minors can consent for testing and treatment services for STIs in every state. Providers should familiarize themselves with their state policies regarding the ability of minors to consent for sexual and reproductive health care services. These data are accessible on the Internet from the Guttmacher Institute (http://www.guttmacher.org) and the Center for Adolescent Health and the Law (http://www.adolescenthealthlaw.org).

B. The evaluation of a female adolescent requesting contraception should include a review of current and past medical conditions, current medications and allergies, menstrual history, confidential social history including sexual history, and family medical history. Important components of a sexual history include age at first intercourse, number of partners in lifetime, history of STIs and pelvic inflammatory disease, condom use, current and past use of other contraceptives and reasons for discontinuation, and pregnancy history and outcomes. This visit also provides an opportunity to screen for partner violence. Refer the patient to appropriate social and support services if violence is identified.

C. It is helpful to have a baseline weight, height, body mass index (BMI), and blood pressure. A pelvic examination is not necessary before initiating contraception. However, if the woman is sexually active and has missed menstrual periods or has symptoms of pregnancy, a pregnancy test is warranted. Screening for STIs should be offered if a sexually experienced woman is asymptomatic, and testing for STIs is indicated if she is symptomatic.

(Continued on page 488)

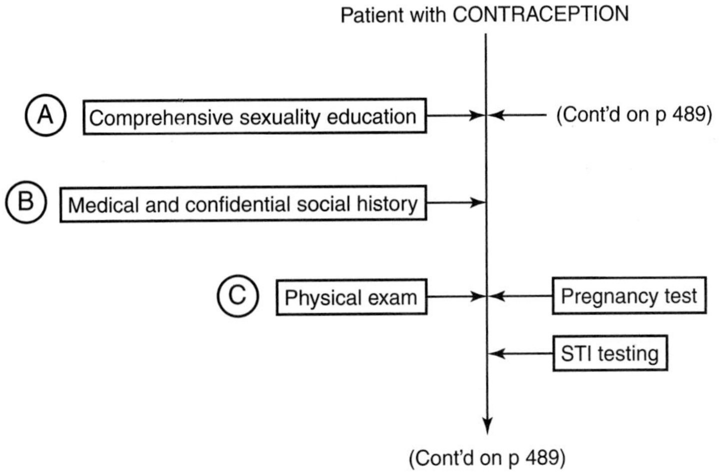
Patient with CONTRACEPTION
A
Comprehensive sexuality education
(Cont'd on p 489)
B
Medical and confidential social history
C
Physical exam
Pregnancy test
STI testing
(Cont'd on p 489)

Table 1. **Percentage of Women in the United States Experiencing an Unintended Pregnancy during the First Year of Typical Use and the First Year of Perfect Use**

	Contraceptive Efficacy: % of Women Experiencing an Unintended Pregnancy within the First Year of Use	
Method	**Typical Use**	**Perfect Use**
No method	85	85
Withdrawal	27	4
Male condom	15	2
Combined oral contraceptive pill	8	0.3
Depo-medroxyprogesterone acetate	3	0.3
Transdermal patch	8	0.3
Intravaginal ring	8	0.3
Intrauterine device	0.8	0.6
Intrauterine system	0.2	0.2
Contraceptive implant	0.05	0.05

Adapted from Trussell J. Contraceptive efficacy. In: Hatcher RA, Trussell J, Nelson AL, et al, editors. Contraceptive technology. 19th revised ed. New York: Ardent Media; 2007.

D. It is important to assess patients for possible risk factors for venous thromboembolic events before initiating any contraceptive product containing estrogen. Given the low population risk of venous thromboembolic events, it is not cost-effective to screen all reproductive aged women for inherited thrombophilia (factor V Leiden; prothrombin mutation; protein S, protein C, and antithrombin deficiencies). If a first-degree relative had a venous thromboembolic event, determine whether testing for inherited thrombophilia was conducted. If a specific defect was identified, testing the patient for that defect before initiating a product containing estrogen should be considered. If testing is unknown but the family history is highly suggestive of inherited thrombophilia, consulting pediatric hematology and/or testing for all of the inherited thrombophilic disorders before initiating estrogen is recommended. In addition, if testing is indicated but not possible, providers should consider alternative contraceptive products that do not contain estrogen.

Patients with underlying medical conditions such as systemic lupus erythematosus may be at risk for having acquired risk factors for thromboembolism such as the presence of antiphospholipid antibodies, and the use of exogenous estrogen in contraceptive products for these women should be avoided. The World Health Organization's publication *Improving Access to Quality Care in Family Planning: Medical Eligibility Criteria for Contraceptive Use* (http://www.who.int/reproductivehealth/publications/family_planning/9789241563888/en/index.html) is an evidence-based guide providing criteria for initiating and continuing contraceptive methods based on a risk assessment of an individual's characteristics or known preexisting medical condition. Table 2 lists absolute (a condition that represents an unacceptable health risk if the contraceptive method is used) and relative (a condition where the theoretical or proven risks usually outweigh the advantages of using the method) contraindications to using combined hormonal birth control pills. These contraindications can be extended to other combined hormonal products that contain estrogen and progestins including the transdermal patch and intravaginal ring.

E. The primary mechanism of action for combined hormonal contraceptives containing estrogen and progestin (combined oral contraceptive pills, transdermal patch, intravaginal ring) and the progestin-only methods (progestin-only pills and depot medroxyprogesterone acetate) is inhibition of ovulation. Thickening of the cervical mucus makes sperm penetration more difficult, and atrophy of the endometrium diminishes the chance of implantation. Starting all birth-control methods during the menstrual period (either first day of bleeding or first Sunday of bleeding) produces the most reliable suppression of ovulation. "Quick start" is an alternative approach to starting a contraceptive method that allows the patient to start the method on the day of the appointment after a negative pregnancy test regardless of menstrual cycle day. These women need to be counseled that they may not have immediate protection from pregnancy, as suppression of ovulation cannot be guaranteed when starting a method outside of the first week of the menstrual cycle.

Studies evaluating compliance with contraceptive methods during adolescence have shown generally poor long-term adherence in this age group. This makes the use of long-acting, reversible contraceptive methods such as the contraceptive implant, which contains etonogestrel, the levonorgestrel-releasing intrauterine system (IUS), and the copper T 380A intrauterine device (IUD) appealing for use with adolescents. All of these methods can be used with nulliparous women and provide contraception for 3, 5, and 10 years, respectively. A common misconception about IUS and IUD use is that they increase the risk for pelvic inflammatory disease. Current research shows that the risk for pelvic inflammatory disease is increased above baseline only at the time of insertion. Ideally, adolescents should be screened for STIs before insertion of an IUS or IUD. IUS and IUD have also not been shown to increase the risk for tubal infertility or ectopic pregnancy.

It is important to thoroughly review the advantages, disadvantages, potential adverse effects, and instructions for use of contraceptive methods in a concise and age-appropriate manner with adolescent patients. Written instructions that are clear and at an appropriate educational level can also be helpful (http://www.youngwomenshealth.org) as a useful source for instructions. Some offices use consent forms to further ensure that the adolescent has a full understanding of the chosen contraceptive method. Teens need to be reminded that hormonal contraception will not protect them from STI transmission, and condoms need to be used consistently. Encouraging teens to be creative about personal reminders such as setting a cell phone alarm to take a pill can help with compliance. Teens often discontinue birth control for nonmedical reasons or minor adverse effects and should be encouraged to contact their providers if any questions or concerns about the chosen method arise to avoid unintentional pregnancy. Frequent follow-up visits every few months with a provider may also improve adherence. These visits also provide opportunities for further reproductive health education and STI screening. In general, contraceptive adverse effects are mild and improve or lessen during the first 3 months of use. Table 3 shows the most common adverse effects of various methods.

F. EC refers to the use of hormonal medications within 72 hours of unprotected or underprotected intercourse for the prevention of pregnancy (Table 4). EC has been studied up to 120 hours after unprotected intercourse; however, its efficacy diminishes with time from the event. EC is 90% effective if used within 24 hours, 75% effective if used within 72 hours, and approximately 60% effective if used within 60 hours. It is, therefore, important to counsel patients to take the medication as soon as possible after unprotected intercourse or contraception failure. EC is also used following sexual assault. EC could potentially prevent approximately 80% of unintended pregnancies and should be part of anticipatory guidance given to sexually active adolescents of both sexes. Advanced prescription for EC at health maintenance visits should be considered

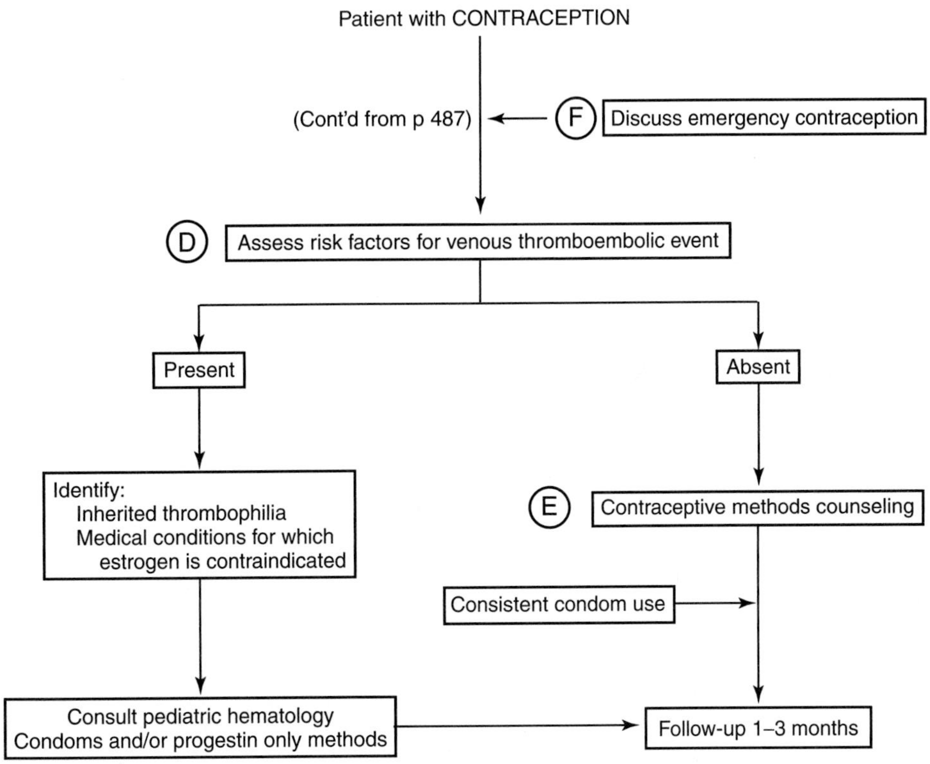

Patient with CONTRACEPTION
(Cont'd from p 487)
F
Discuss emergency contraception
D
Assess risk factors for venous thromboembolic event
Present
Absent
Identify:
Inherited thrombophilia
Medical conditions for which estrogen is contraindicated
E
Contraceptive methods counseling
Consistent condom use
Consult pediatric hematology
Condoms and/or progestin only methods
Follow-up 1–3 months

in sexually active teens. The exact mechanism of EC is unknown but is thought to disrupt follicular development or interfere with the maturation of the corpus luteum. EC is not teratogenic and does not interrupt a pregnancy that has already implanted in the uterine lining. Plan B is a two-pill method delivering 0.75 mg levonorgestrel per pill. It was initially prescribed with instructions to take one pill immediately after unprotected intercourse, followed by a second pill 12 hours later. Current studies have shown that taking two pills simultaneously has the same efficacy, and a newer product, Plan B One-Step, which is a one-pill regimen that contains 1.5 mg levonorgestrel, was approved in July 2009. Both products are available over the counter for patients older than age 17 years. A prescription is required for adolescents younger than 17. If Plan B is not available, certain combined oral contraceptive pills containing levonorgestrel or norgestrel can be used for EC with the Yuzpe method (see Table 4). An antiemetic drug taken 30 minutes before pills containing estrogen may help control nausea. A pregnancy test is not required before prescription and administration of EC. A follow-up appointment should be held in 10 to 14 days for pregnancy testing, STI screening, and counseling regarding reproductive health and contraceptive use.

Table 2. **Contraindications to Combined Oral Contraceptive Pills**

Absolute Contraindications

Pregnancy
Breast-feeding (within 6 weeks of childbirth)
Hypertension: SBP >160 mm Hg or DBP >100 mm Hg
History of thrombophlebitis; current thromboembolic disorder, cerebrovascular disease, or ischemic heart disease
Known thrombogenic mutations (factor V Leiden; prothrombin mutation; protein S, protein C, and antithrombin deficiencies)
Systemic lupus erythematosus
Complicated valvular heart disease (with pulmonary hypertension; atrial fibrillation; history of bacterial endocarditis)
Diabetes with nephropathy; retinopathy; neuropathy
Liver disease: active viral hepatitis; severe cirrhosis; tumor (hepatocellular adenoma or hepatoma)
Breast cancer (current)
Migraine headaches with aura
Major surgery with prolonged immobilization

Relative Contraindications

Postpartum (first 3 weeks)
Breast-feeding (6 weeks to 6 months after childbirth)
Hypertension (adequately controlled HTN; any history of HTN where BP cannot be evaluated; SBP 140–159 mm Hg or DPB 90–99 mm Hg)
Migraine headache without aura (for continuation of COC)
Breast cancer history with remission for 5 years
Active gallbladder disease or history of COC-induced cholestasis
Use of drugs that affect liver enzymes (rifampin, phenytoin, carbamazepine, barbiturates, primidone, topiramate, oxcarbazepine, lamotrigine, ritonavir-boosted protease inhibitors)

BP, blood pressure; *COC,* combined oral contraceptive; *DBP,* diastolic blood pressure; *HTN,* hypertension; *SBP,* systolic blood pressure.

Table 3. **Common Adverse Effects of Contraceptive Methods**

Combined oral contraceptive pill	Irregular menstrual bleeding, nausea, abdominal pain, breast tenderness and/or enlargement, weight changes, mood changes
Depo-medroxyprogesterone acetate	Irregular menstrual bleeding, abdominal pain, weight gain, headache; black box warning for risk for decreased bone density with prolonged use
Transdermal patch	Breast pain and/or swelling, headache, nausea, and skin irritation; may be less effective in women weighing >90 kg and those with skin conditions preventing absorption
Intravaginal ring	Vaginal discharge, headache, weight gain, and nausea
Intrauterine device	Menstrual pain, menorrhagia
Intrauterine system	Irregular menstrual bleeding amenorrhea, abdominal/pelvic pain, ovarian cysts
Contraceptive implant	Irregular menstrual bleeding, headache, weight gain, acne, breast pain, emotional lability; efficacy is not established in women with body mass index >130% ideal, and use is not recommended for women who chronically take drugs that are potent hepatic enzyme inducers

Table 4. **Emergency Contraception Regimens**

Pill	Dose
Progestin Only	**One Dose**
Plan B	2 pills
Plan B One-Step	1 pill
Estrogen and Progestin	Repeat dose in 12 hours
Ovral, Ogestrel	2 white pills
Levlen, Nordette	4 orange pills
Lo/Ovral, Low-ogestrel, Levora, Quasense, Cryselle	4 white pills
Jolessa, Portia, Seasonale, Trivora	4 pink pills
Triphasil, Tri-Levlen	4 yellow pills
Seasonique	4 light blue-green pills
Enpresse	4 orange
Alesse, Lessina, Levlite	5 pink pills
Aviane	5 orange pills
Lutera	5 white

References

ACOG Committee. Intrauterine device and adolescents. Opinion No. 392, December 2007. Obstet Gynecol 2007;110:1493–5.

American Academy of Pediatrics Committee on Adolescence; American College of Obstetricians and Gynecologists Committee on Adolescent Health Care, Diaz A, Laufer MR, Breech LL. Menstruation in girls and adolescents: using the menstrual cycle as a vital sign. Pediatrics 2006;118:2245–50.

American Academy of Pediatrics Committee on Adolescence, Blythe MJ, Diaz A. Contraception and adolescents. Pediatrics 2007;120:1135–48.

Cheng L, Gülmezoglu AM, Piaggio G, et al. Interventions for emergency contraception. Cochrane Database Syst Rev 2008;(2):CD001324.

Eaton DK, Kann L, Kinchen S, et al. Youth risk behavior surveillance—United States, 2007. Surveillance summaries 2008. Centers for Disease Control and Prevention (CDC). MMWR Surveill Summ 2008;57:1–131.

Gavin L, MacKay AP, Brown K, et al. Centers for Disease Control and Prevention (CDC). Reproductive health of persons aged 10–24 Years—United States, 2002–2007. Surveillance Summaries, July 17, 2009. MMWR Surveill Summ 2009;58:1–58.

Kaplan DW, Sass AE. Adolescence. In: Hay W, et al, editors. Current pediatric diagnosis and treatment. 20th ed. New York: McGraw-Hill Companies; 2011.

Sass AE, Neufeld EJ. Risk factors for thromboembolism in teen: when should I test? Curr Opin Pediatr 2002;14:370–8.

Tolaymat LL, Kaunitz AM. Long-acting contraceptives in adolescents. Curr Opin Obstet Gynecol 2007;19:453–60.

Trussell J. Contraceptive efficacy. In: Hatcher RA, Trussell J, Nelson AL. et al, editors. Contraceptive technology. 19th revised ed. New York: Ardent Media; 2007.

Venous thromboembolic disease and combined oral contraceptives: results of international multicentre case-control study. World Health Organization Collaborative Study of Cardiovascular Disease and Steroid Hormone Contraception. Lancet 1995;346:1575–82.

Westhoff C, Heartwell S, Edwards S, et al. Initiation of oral contraceptives using a quick start compared with a conventional start: a randomized controlled trial. Obstet Gynecol 2007;109:1270–6.

World Health Organization. Improving access to quality care in family planning: medical eligibility criteria for contraceptive use. Geneva, Switzerland: World Health Organization; 2004. <http://whqlibdoc.who.int/publications/2004/9241562668.pdf>; 2004 [accessed 07.02.10].

Eating Disorders

Eric J. Sigel, MD

Anorexia nervosa (AN) has the following characteristics: (1) weight being less than 85% of healthy body weight, (2) fear of fatness or fat-containing food, (3) distorted body image, and (4) primary or secondary amenorrhea in female individuals. AN may be either restricting or purging type. Bulimia nervosa (BN) occurs when the following behaviors are present: (1) repeated bingeing at least twice a week for 3 or more months, (2) patient's perceiving eating to be out of control, (3) recurrent purging behavior (vomiting; use of laxatives, diuretics, emetics, nutritional supplements; excessive exercise; severely restricted intake) to prevent weight gain, and (4) overconcern with body image. In some instances, both diagnoses may coexist, or a patient may have AN at one point and then BN later. The most common eating disorder is actually known as eating disorder not otherwise specified (EDNOS); components of AN or BN may be present, but full criteria are not met for either one. Adolescents may present early in the evolution of their eating disorder, so full criteria are not met. For example, subclinical AN may be diagnosed if weight is only 10% less than expected or the patient has not yet missed three consecutive menstrual cycles. The adolescent who restricts and purges but does not binge (as needed for BN) and is not sufficiently underweight (as needed for AN) would have a diagnosis of EDNOS.

A. Elicit the history from the parent and adolescent together and then the adolescent alone. Inquire about how patients feel about their bodies: Do they think they are about the right weight, underweight, or overweight? Is there anything they would like to change? If there is concern for being overweight/too fat, have they tried to lose weight? How so? Ask about specific indicators of an eating disorder: weight history (including maximum, minimum, and desired weight); dietary intake (changes in types of foods they eat, what foods they avoid, specifics of intake throughout the day, binges, unusual eating behaviors); purging history (vomiting, diuretics, laxatives, emetics, excessive exercise), and menstrual history (irregular cycles, primary or secondary amenorrhea). In addition, direct the review of systems toward other diseases in the differential diagnosis and symptoms secondary to malnutrition or purging (dizziness, syncope, fatigue, muscle cramps, epigastric pain, reflux, hair loss, lanugo hair). The adolescent with an eating disorder may present with constitutional symptoms without an overt complaint about weight.

B. The physical examination findings are often normal, especially in bulimics who are generally within 10 pounds of their healthy body weight. Healthy body weight is assessed by using the 50th percentile BMI as the denominator. For reliability, weigh the patient in a gown only after voiding.

Orthostatic vital signs should be obtained. Hypothermia, bradycardia, hypotension, or postural hypotension may be present if the patient is malnourished or dehydrated. Anorexics may appear emaciated, with scaphoid abdomen, prominent ribs and joints, and loss of subcutaneous tissue. In addition, there may be loss of shine and curl of scalp hair; downy lanugo hair on the body; excoriation over the spine from excessive sit-ups; hard stool in the rectal vault; and acrocyanosis, coldness, and edema of the extremities. The patient who has been vomiting may have lost tooth enamel, either from the molars or the posterior aspect of the front teeth, or have calluses on the dorsum of their index finger.

C. The clinical presentation guides the laboratory evaluation. Malnutrition can affect virtually every organ system (Table 1). Abnormalities can include electrolyte alterations (present with malnutrition alone or with persistent vomiting and diuretic or laxative use), compromised renal function, bone marrow suppression, mild liver inflammation, suppressed thyroid function with low free thyroxine (T4) and thyroid-stimulating hormone (TSH) levels, and hypothalamic-pituitary suppression. Perform an electrocardiogram if a patient is hypokalemic or bradycardic, evaluating for long QT syndrome. Consider determination of follicle-stimulating hormone (FSH), luteinizing hormone (LH), TSH, prolactin, and human chorionic gonadotropin (hCG) levels to rule out other causes of amenorrhea. If amenorrhea has persisted for 6 months or longer, there is a significant risk for osteoporosis. Approximately 50% of patients have osteopenia after 6 months, and by 2 years, nearly all patients have osteoporosis. Consider bone densitometry in male patients (total body and L2–4 region) 6 months after onset of illness, and in female patients with 6 months of amenorrhea.

(Continued on page 494)

Patient with EATING DISORDER
(Anorexia Nervosa, Bulimia Nervosa, or Eating Disorder NOS)

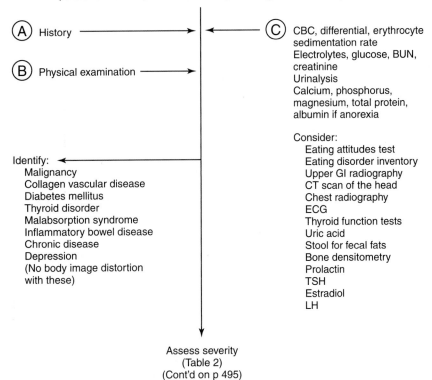

(A) History →

(B) Physical examination →

← (C) CBC, differential, erythrocyte sedimentation rate
Electrolytes, glucose, BUN, creatinine
Urinalysis
Calcium, phosphorus, magnesium, total protein, albumin if anorexia

Consider:
- Eating attitudes test
- Eating disorder inventory
- Upper GI radiography
- CT scan of the head
- Chest radiography
- ECG
- Thyroid function tests
- Uric acid
- Stool for fecal fats
- Bone densitometry
- Prolactin
- TSH
- Estradiol
- LH

Identify:
- Malignancy
- Collagen vascular disease
- Diabetes mellitus
- Thyroid disorder
- Malabsorption syndrome
- Inflammatory bowel disease
- Chronic disease
- Depression
- (No body image distortion with these)

↓

Assess severity
(Table 2)
(Cont'd on p 495)

Table 1. **Complications of Anorexia Nervosa and Bulimia**

Cardiovascular

Bradycardia
Postural hypotension
Arrhythmia, sudden death
Congestive heart failure (during refeeding)
Pericardial effusion
Mitral value prolapse
ECG abnormalities (prolonged QT, low voltage, T-wave abnormalities, conduction defects)

Endocrine

↓ LH, FSH
↓ T3, ↑ rT3; normal T4, TSH
Irregular menses
Amenorrhea
Hypercortisolism
Growth retardation
Short stature
Delayed puberty

Gastrointestinal

Dental erosion
Parotid swelling
Esophagitis, esophageal tears
Delayed gastric emptying
Gastric dilatation (rarely rupture)
Pancreatitis
Constipation
Diarrhea (laxative abuse)
Superior mesenteric artery syndrome
Hypercholesterolemia
↑ Liver function tests (fatty infiltration of the liver)

Hematologic

Leukopenia
Anemia
Thrombocytopenia
↑ ESR
Impaired cell-mediated immunity

Metabolic

Dehydration
Acidosis
Hypokalemia
Hyponatremia
Hypochloremia
Hypochloremic alkalosis
Hypocalcemia
Hypophosphatemia
Hypomagnesemia
Hypercarotenemia

Neurologic

Cortical atrophy
Peripheral neuropathy
Seizures
Thermoregulatory
Abnormalities
↓ REM and slow-wave sleep
Renal
Hematuria
Proteinuria
↓ Renal concentrating ability

Skeletal

Osteopenia
Fractures

ECG, electrocardiogram; *ESR,* erythrocyte sedimentation rate; *FSH,* follicle-stimulating hormone; *LH,* luteinizing hormone; *REM,* rapid eye movement; *TSH,* thyroid-stimulating hormone.

D. Mildly ill patients may begin to show eating disorder behavior but have not experienced the physical consequences, including significant weight loss (Table 2). Explaining to the family and child that the behavior could develop into a full-blown eating disorder raises the appropriate level of concern. Nutritional and behavioral changes at home may be enough to reverse the trend. Consider nutritional counseling alone or in conjunction with psychological intervention, taking into account both the patient's and the parents' interests. Consistent medical follow-up is needed to determine whether more aggressive intervention is necessary.

E. Explain to the patient and family that the patient may be struggling with emotional issues; the focus on eating and weight may be the patient's attempt to maintain a sense of control in life when feeling overwhelmed. The resulting physical symptoms reflect the underlying psychiatric disorder. Psychotherapy involving the patient and family may be necessary for a healthy outcome. The patient should be reassured that the aim is restoring health and regaining control, not gaining excess weight.

F. Manage patients with moderately severe illness with an aggressive intervention consisting of psychiatric evaluation, psychological counseling, nutrition counseling, and close medical monitoring. If the behavior continues, it is likely to lead to medical instability and eventual hospitalization. Medical monitoring must continue on a regular basis, initially weekly. Weights in gown only after voiding, vital signs, urine specific gravity, and specific questioning about dietary intake and physical symptoms must be done weekly until the patient is steadily gaining weight. Medical visits may then spread out to every 2 weeks until 90% to 95% of healthy body weight is reached, then monthly until menses return. This phase can take 4 to 8 months. Bulimics should be monitored weekly until weight and electrolytes are stable and psychotherapy is under way. Antacids may be useful in preventing and treating reflux esophagitis and gastritis. Consider a selective serotonin reuptake inhibitor when the patient is depressed, but be aware that this medication may not be effective when the patient is malnourished. Consider fluoxetine (60 mg) for patients with bulimia. Starting hormone replacement for osteoporosis is controversial. No studies have shown that hormone replacement improves bone density, although some suggest that it keeps osteopenia and osteoporosis from worsening.

G. A dietitian can monitor intake, dispel food and calorie myths, and assist in developing well-balanced meal plans. The focus should be taken off calories or fat grams. A supplement such as Ensure or Boost may be given if meals are not finished. Patients may benefit from a multivitamin, as well as calcium and zinc supplement. Using family-based intervention, parents should be given responsibility for meal planning, preparing food, and supervising all meals and snacks.

H. A behavioral contract signed by the patient, parents, and caregivers is useful. For patients with AN, it might include long-term goal weight range, expected rate of weight gain, consequences of failure to meet weight goals, or even specifics of dietary intake. For patients with BN, the contract might address a maintenance weight range, honesty about frequency of bingeing and purging, and gradually delaying purge behavior until more than an hour after meals. Address the patient's exercise regimen in the behavioral contract. Patients are often excessive exercisers and need to decrease or stop their exercise to reverse weight loss and to establish a positive nutrition balance. Exercise can then be steadily incorporated back into a patient's life as weight gain continues.

I. Individual, family, or group psychotherapy may be appropriate. Family involvement is critical with adolescents. The therapist should be skilled in working with adolescents and familiar with eating disorders. A recent advance in psychotherapy uses a manualized family-based treatment approach, which empowers parents to take control of their adolescent's nutrition. Regular communication between the treatment team is essential to prevent splitting. Cognitive restructuring, a technique in which the patient's beliefs and attitudes are challenged with alternative healthier views, can be practiced by all members of the team. Group therapy with peers can be a helpful adjunct to recovery.

J. A day treatment facility is often associated with general psychiatric day treatment programs, although some may be eating disorder specific. This level of care falls in between outpatient and inpatient management, and can be used as an initial intervention if the patient has borderline medical symptoms or does not meet criteria for inpatient admission. It can also be used as a transition from the inpatient setting to outpatient treatment to support the patient's recovery chances. Consider a residential level of care, which includes eating disorder-specific treatment centers, if inpatient management is not successful or a patient relapses quickly after aggressive intervention. The decision to access residential care should involve the patient, family, therapist, and primary care provider. Residential treatment often lasts 2 to 4 months.

(Continued on page 496)

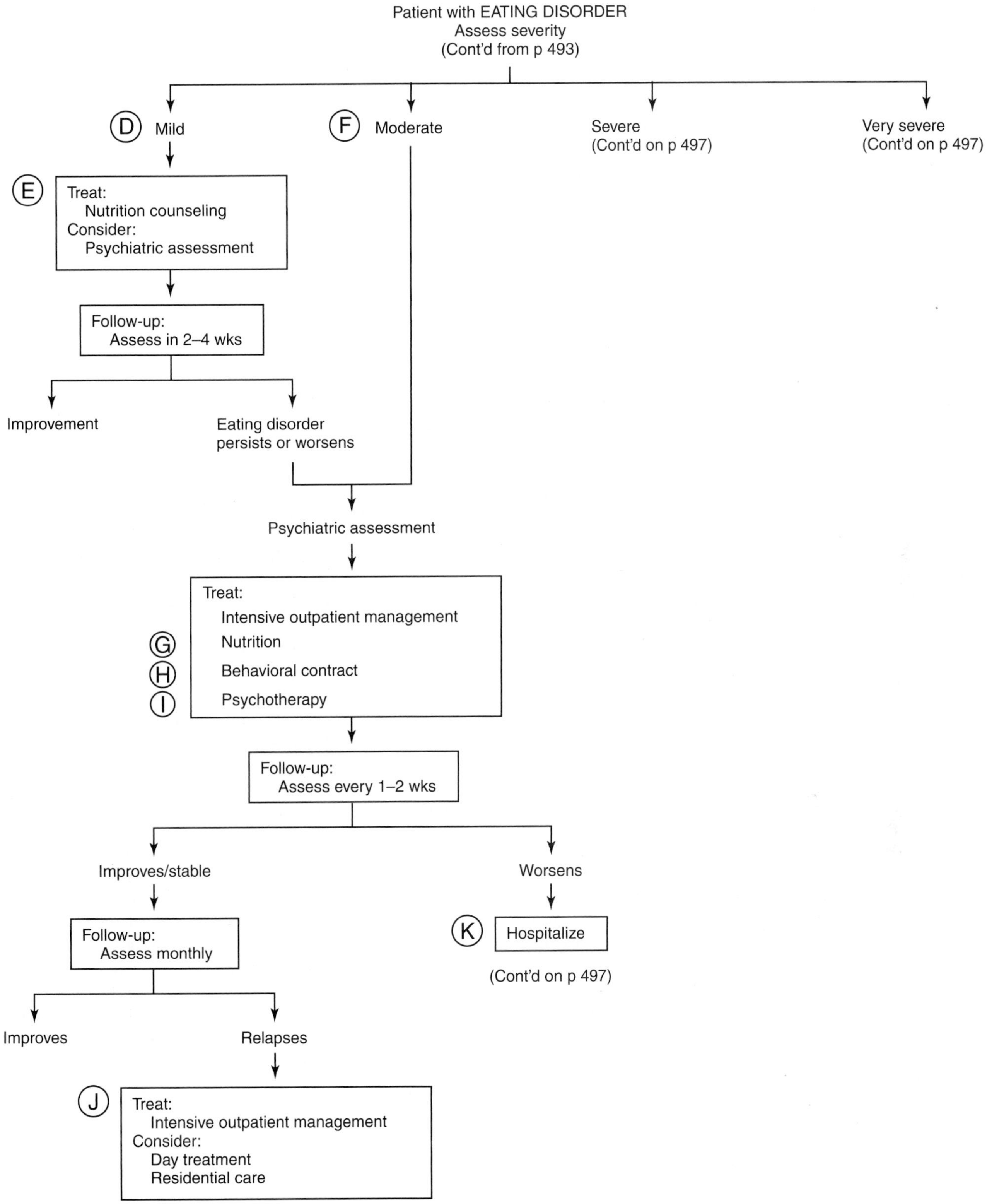
Patient with EATING DISORDER
Assess severity
(Cont'd from p 493)
D
Mild
F
Moderate
Severe
(Cont'd on p 497)
Very severe
(Cont'd on p 497)
E
Treat:
Nutrition counseling
Consider:
Psychiatric assessment
Follow-up:
Assess in 2–4 wks
Improvement
Eating disorder
persists or worsens
Psychiatric assessment
Treat:
Intensive outpatient management
G
Nutrition
H
Behavioral contract
I
Psychotherapy
Follow-up:
Assess every 1–2 wks
Improves/stable
Worsens
Follow-up:
Assess monthly
K
Hospitalize
(Cont'd on p 497)
Improves
Relapses
J
Treat:
Intensive outpatient management
Consider:
Day treatment
Residential care

Table 2. **Severity of Eating Disorders**

Mild	Moderate	Severe	Very Severe
Recent onset of symptoms and physiologically stable *and* Not less than 85% of ideal body weight	Moderate physiologic abnormality, e.g., slight hypothermia or hypokalemia amenable to oral replacement *and* Not less than 75% of ideal body weight or depression without suicidal ideation	<75% ideal body weight *or* Evidence of metabolic disturbance: Heart rate <40 Temperature <36°C (96.8°F) Systolic blood pressure <70 mm Hg Significant orthostatic hypotension Serum potassium <3.0 Dehydration or syncopal episodes *or* Severe bingeing and purging *or* Refusal of minimal oral intake *or* Severe depression with suicidal ideation or psychosis *or* Family crisis *or* Inadequate response to outpatient treatment	Dehydration *or* Electrolyte imbalance (depressed serum phosphorus or magnesium) *or* Arrhythmia <65% ideal body weight Serum potassium <2.0 Serum phosphorus <1.5

K. Hospitalization may be necessary for medical or psychiatric reasons. Short-term stays, for example, to correct electrolyte abnormalities, may be best accomplished on a medical unit. Patients may need medical hospitalization for bradycardia (heart rate <45), for severe malnutrition (<75% healthy body weight), and to monitor for refeeding syndrome. Intermediate-length hospitalization to establish weight gain and to institute psychotherapy may also be accomplished on a medical unit with a team including physician, therapist, dietitian, and nursing staff. Dedicated eating disorder units, if available, can be used when a patient is expected to benefit from a longer stay with milieu therapy. Adolescent psychiatric hospitalization may be appropriate if a patient has suicidal ideation.

L. Medical stabilization is the first goal. Correct fluid and electrolyte status with careful monitoring of vital signs. For malnourished patients, begin refeeding. Initial caloric level should be about 250 kcal more than what the patient had been eating. It is essential to work closely with a nutrition expert to help monitor calories and administer food. In general, patients can tolerate oral feeding, especially in a structured setting. Consider giving nutritional supplements if a patient is overwhelmed by eating solid food. On occasion, a patient may need to be fed by a nasogastric tube or rarely by total parenteral nutrition. One can safely increase calories to 125 to 250 kg/day until patients are gaining weight steadily, from 0.1 to 0.2 kg/day. Administer multivitamins with iron, as well as zinc supplementation. All staff must remain firm in the goal to restore the patient to health. This often requires supervising meals, use of the bathroom, and free time.

M. Refeeding syndrome occurs when a patient takes in calories too rapidly. An increase in insulin prompts potassium to move intracellularly, placing the patient at risk for hypokalemia. Phosphorus levels can decrease as the Krebs cycle makes adenosine triphosphate. Fluid shifts and increased metabolism in the presence of a weakened heart may potentiate congestive heart failure and edema. The patient is most at risk for refeeding syndrome during the initial 4 to 6 days of admission. Carefully examine the patient for rales, a gallop, and edema. Check potassium and phosphorus levels daily to identify refeeding syndrome. Often the first sign of refeeding syndrome is a decrease in phosphorus levels. Phosphorus supplementation should occur if PO_4 <3.0 mg/dl. Once a patient is gaining weight steadily, the frequency of laboratory checks can decrease.

N. A thorough psychiatric evaluation should begin soon after medical admission. Patients with severe malnutrition may display cognitive slowing, and an accurate assessment of psychiatric pathology may not be reliable until positive nutrition balance has been established. A psychologist can be instrumental in tailoring an individualized behavioral contract with the underlying principles of gradually reaching a goal weight range, interrupting bingeing and purging behaviors, developing more healthful coping strategies, understanding underlying issues, and restoring the appropriate level of control to the patient. The entire treatment team must support the contract. Weekly staff meetings are useful for discussing progress and plans, any splitting, and issues that arise in caring for difficult patients. When psychotherapy begins, family involvement is crucial. Group therapy can also be helpful. Several open-label trials using atypical antipsychotics have shown promise in treating adolescents with AN and are used frequently, though these findings have not been replicated in a randomized, controlled trial. High-dose SSRIs, such as fluoxetine 60 mg can be of benefit to patients with BN. It is important to evaluate and treat other common comorbidities, such as depression and anxiety disorders.

(Continued on page 498)

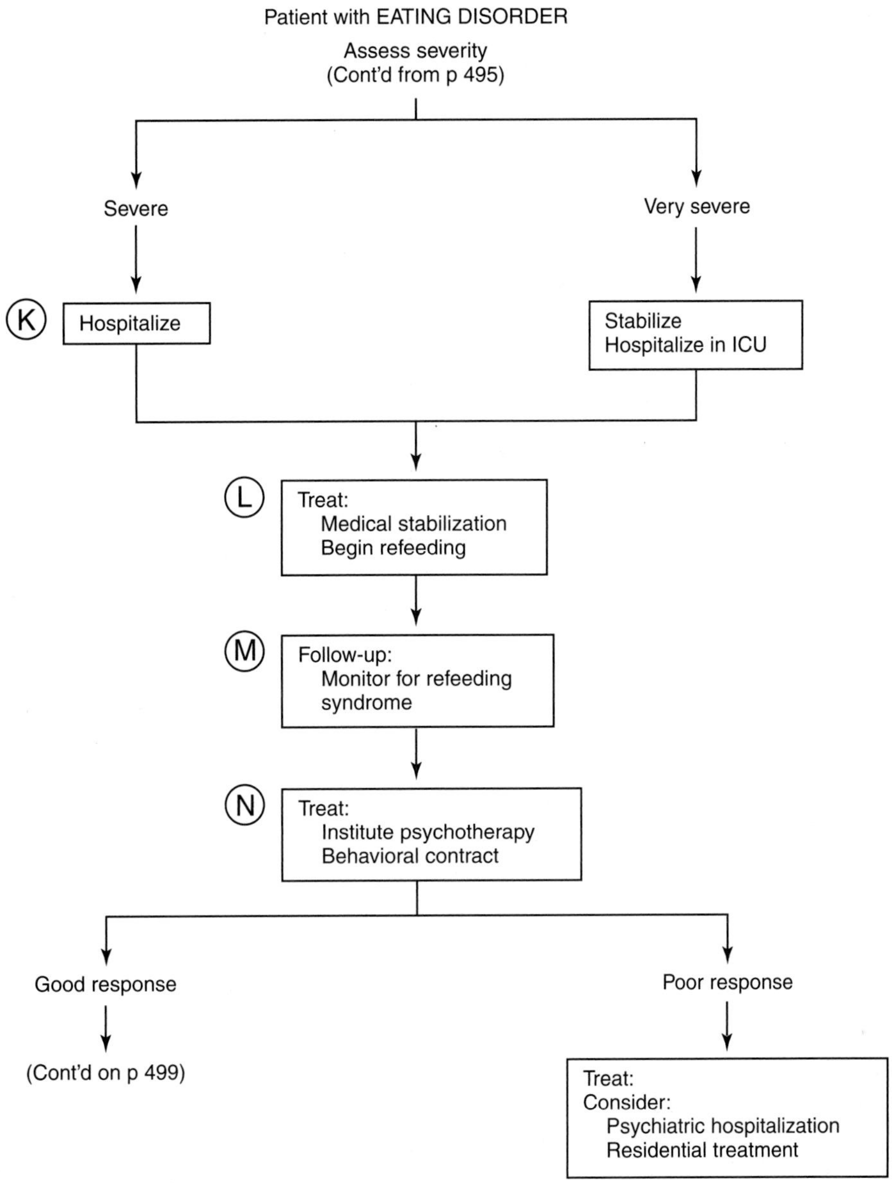
Patient with EATING DISORDER
Assess severity
(Cont'd from p 495)
Severe
Very severe
K
Hospitalize
Stabilize
Hospitalize in ICU
L
Treat:
Medical stabilization
Begin refeeding
M
Follow-up:
Monitor for refeeding syndrome
N
Treat:
Institute psychotherapy
Behavioral contract
Good response
(Cont'd on p 499)
Poor response
Treat:
Consider:
Psychiatric hospitalization
Residential treatment

O. Consider discharge from an inpatient setting when medical stabilization is achieved with improved bradycardia (>40 at night), correction of electrolytes, interruption of purging behavior, ability to tolerate oral feedings, and steady weight gain. Patients should be at a minimum of 75% to 80% of their healthy body weight, depending on their admission weight. Some studies suggest that the likelihood of recovery is increased when the patient has a rapid return to healthy body weight, as well as a higher percentage body weight at discharge. Often patients benefit from stepping down from an inpatient unit, to day treatment, to outpatient level of care. Eating disorders have achieved a parity diagnosis in many states, though insurance plans may not pay for a prolonged hospitalization to achieve a 90% to 95% healthy body weight goal.

References

American Psychiatric Association. Diagnostic and statistical manual of mental disorders. 4th ed. Washington, DC: American Psychiatric Association; 1994.

Birmingham CL, Gritzner S. How does zinc supplementation benefit anorexia nervosa? Eat Weight Disord 2006;11:e109.

Dunican KC, Del Dotto D. The role of olanzapine in the treatment of anorexia nervosa. Ann Pharmacother 2007;41:111.

Golden NH. Osteopenia and osteoporosis in anorexia nervosa. Adolesc Med State Art Rev 2003;14:97.

LeGrange D, Binford R, Loeb KL. Manualized family-based treatment for anorexia nervosa: a case series. J Am Acad Child Adolesc Psychiatry 2005;44:41.

Rome E, Ammerman S, Rosen DS, et al. Children and adolescents with eating disorders: state of the art. Pediatrics 2003;111:e98.

Sigel EJ. Eating disorders: adolescent medicine state of the art reviews. American Academy of Pediatrics. Adolesc Med 2008;19:547–72.

Swenne I. Weight requirements for return of menstruations in teenage girls with eating disorders, weight loss, and secondary amenorrhea. Acta Paediatr 2004;93:1449.

Patient with EATING DISORDER

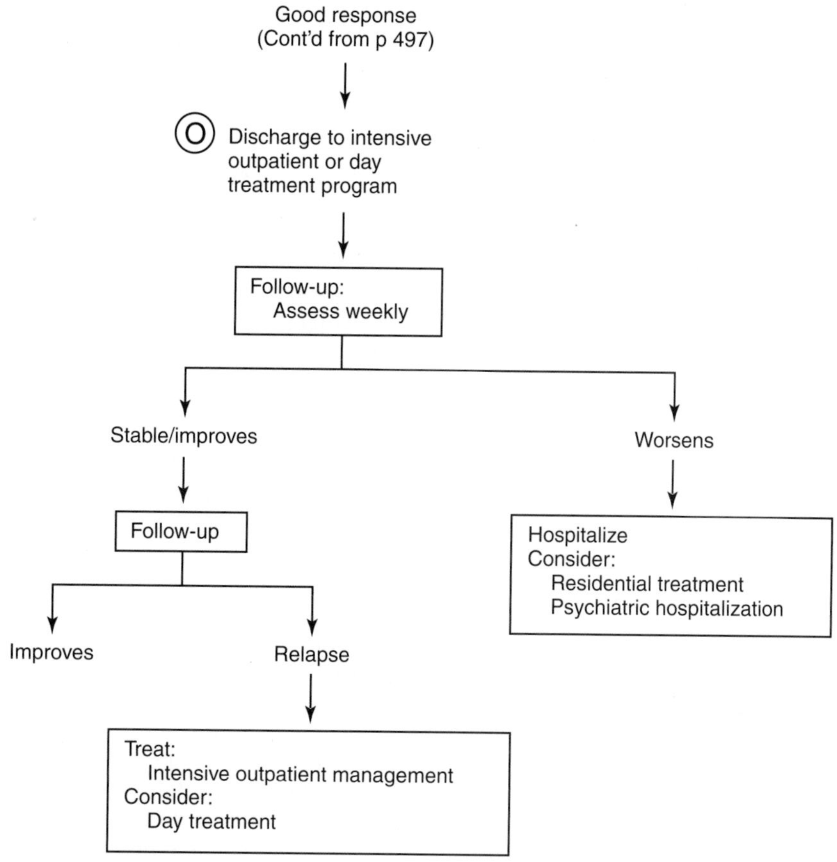
Good response
(Cont'd from p 497)
O
Discharge to intensive outpatient or day treatment program
Follow-up:
Assess weekly
Stable/improves
Worsens
Follow-up
Hospitalize
Consider:
Residential treatment
Psychiatric hospitalization
Improves
Relapse
Treat:
Intensive outpatient management
Consider:
Day treatment

Substance Abuse

Mary N. Cook, MD, and John Peterson, MD

Adolescent substance abuse continues to be a significant problem encountered in both clinical and community settings. Teenage substance abuse is associated with an increased risk for depression, suicide, violence, criminal behavior and incarceration, motor vehicle accidents, sexually transmitted infections (STIs), unwanted pregnancies, and other health, safety, and social concerns. In 2007, according to the Centers for Disease Control and Prevention (CDC), approximately 45% of U.S. high-school students reported current alcohol use, 26% engaged in "heavy drinking," and 20% reported current marijuana use. Although inquiring about alcohol and drug use in the primary care setting may be difficult, the following information outlines a brief framework for the understanding, assessment, and treatment of adolescent substance abuse.

A. A careful history elicited from both the adolescent patient and the parents will likely yield most of the information needed to diagnose a substance abuse disorder. Using a matter-of-fact, nonjudgmental demeanor may enhance self-reporting by youth. The clinician should inquire about the age at onset and progression of use, types of agents, circumstances, frequency, and variability of use. Assuming an adolescent uses, asking "How much do you drink?" rather than "Do you drink?" is more likely to facilitate discussion of use. Inquires should be made regarding consequences of use in all life domains, including exploration of family, school, vocational, social, psychological, and medical problems. Although not specific to substance abuse, adolescents who are actively using will likely exhibit marked changes in mood, behavior, and cognition. While intoxicated or even between bouts of drug use, adolescents might appear disinhibited, lethargic, agitated, or hypervigilant. Substance abuse is often accompanied by impaired concentration and distorted thoughts or perceptions, sometimes even including hallucinations and delusions. The effects of drugs are quite variable and depend on the type of substance, amount, context of use, degree of psychopathology at baseline, as well as an individual's experiences and expectations of the drug. Most adolescents do experiment with using substances such as alcohol and cigarettes, and a portion of them later advance to the use of marijuana; a smaller portion proceed to the use of other drugs. Risk factors include a history of disruptive behavior, anxiety and mood disorders, as well as parent use of drugs, alcohol, or tobacco. Childhood sexual abuse and other trauma increase the vulnerability, as does a family history of substance abuse disorders, low self-esteem, and involvement with drug-using peers.

B. Vital signs and a physical examination are important in conducting a thorough assessment of substance abuse problems. Findings may be subtle and are often nonspecific, such as an increased heart rate and blood pressure associated with amphetamine, cocaine, or stimulant abuse, as well as marijuana intoxication and/or alcohol withdrawal. Poor hygiene, injected sclera, upper respiratory symptoms, signs of trauma, and nasal septum changes are some of the nonspecific findings that may be associated with adolescent substance abuse. One helpful screening tool (Table 1) uses the letters CRAFFT as a mnemonic device for a series of screening questions specifically developed for adolescents.

C. Toxicologic screening (usually urine, but may include blood or hair samples) is a standard part of any formal evaluation of substance abuse problems. Urine toxicologic screening is usually obtained as part of the initial evaluation but may be used in an ongoing fashion to monitor treatment progress. Samples must be properly collected, results evaluated, and a specific course of action should be outlined in the event of a positive result. Rules of confidentiality regarding results should be established before testing. Drug screening should not be performed simply at the request of a parent or school staff, and such testing is likely to disrupt the patient–physician alliance. A negative drug screen does not definitively establish that a youth does not use, as drugs remain in urine only a limited time and samples may be subjected to tampering. Other laboratory tests may be indicated, depending on the clinical need. For instance, a complete blood cell count (CBC) and basic metabolic panel may be indicated when there are concerns about malnutrition and anemia associated with alcohol and/or cocaine/amphetamine use. Liver function tests (LFTs) should be considered when significant alcohol or inhalant use is suspected. A thyroid-stimulating hormone (TSH) level is useful when depressive symptoms accompany substance abuse problems.

(Continued on page 502)

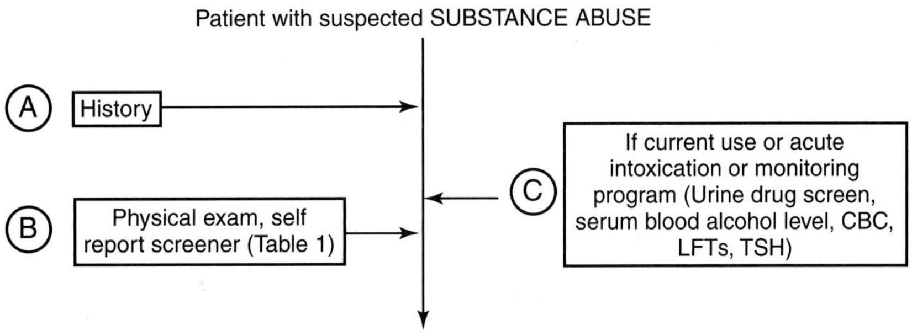
Patient with suspected SUBSTANCE ABUSE
A
History
B
Physical exam, self report screener (Table 1)
C
If current use or acute intoxication or monitoring program (Urine drug screen, serum blood alcohol level, CBC, LFTs, TSH)

(Cont'd on p 503)

Table 1. CRAFFT Substance Abuse Screening Test for Adolescents

C—Have you ever ridden in a CAR driven by someone (including yourself) who was "high" or had been using alcohol or drugs?
R—Do you ever use alcohol or drugs to RELAX, feel better about yourself, or fit in?
A—Do you ever use alcohol or drugs while you are by yourself, ALONE?
F—Do you ever FORGET things you did while using alcohol or drugs?
F—Does your family or FRIENDS ever tell you that you should cut down on your drinking or drug use?
T—Have you ever gotten into TROUBLE while you were using alcohol or drugs?
Two or more "yes" answers suggest a positive screen and that a more thorough assessment is needed.

From Knight JR, Sherritt L, Shrier LA, et al. Validity of the CRAFFT substance abuse screening test among adolescent clinic patients. Arch Pediatr Adolesc Med 2002;156:607–14.

D. Anticipatory guidance on substance abuse should begin in grade school and include discussions about risky situations and strategies for avoidance. Psychosocial skills training, including assertiveness, social skills, and problem solving, can help prevent the onset or progression of drug use. Primary care providers should routinely counsel youth and their parents about the hazards of substance use, paying special attention when risk factors are present, such as a family history of alcohol or substance abuse. Physicians possess unique knowledge, perspective, and training, which positions them well to support and consult around school and community substance abuse prevention efforts. Parents should also be provided with information about the signs of substance use and what they can do to help prevent their child from using alcohol or other drugs. Primary care providers should be able to recognize early signs and symptoms of substance abuse, and should screen all adolescents for substance use as part of the overall psychosocial history. If a youth has only experimented with alcohol or drugs, counseling the family about the seriousness of alcohol and drug abuse, together with providing guidance about communication, limit-setting, parental monitoring, and effective discipline, may be appropriate. Physicians might also forge contracts with youth who identify themselves as "experimental users," which typically would consist of careful monitoring and possibly drug screens. If progression of use is evident from escalating symptoms and impairment of functioning, further involvement with parents and a referral may become necessary.

E. In the event of progression of use, alliance building with parents and youth is fundamental to facilitating additional intervention. Motivational interviewing consists of a nonjudgmental, nondirective strategy designed to move the adolescent to a "stage of change," in which the youth is more receptive to treatment or behavior change. Self-help groups such as Alcoholics Anonymous (AA) or Narcotics Anonymous (NA) can provide drug-free peer group support and often serve as adjuncts to treatment. For the young person who has begun to experience adverse consequences of substance abuse, such as injuries associated with acute intoxication, trouble with the law, truancy, decline in school performance, or deterioration in physical or mental health, definitive treatment is indicated. Primary care providers should make referrals and work with the adolescent and family to accept and follow through with the referral. Primary care providers need to be aware of the substance abuse treatment programs and resources in their communities (including formal treatment programs and 12-step groups such as Alcoholics Anonymous and Narcotics Anonymous). If indicated by assessment, they should help the adolescent access these and other supports or mentors in the community (e.g., coaches, teachers, relatives, faith-based organizations). Screening for comorbid psychiatric disorders is appropriate, together with making related referrals, as indicated. A full and unbiased psychiatric assessment cannot be accurately completed until the youth has been abstinent at least 2 to 4 weeks.

F. After referral, the primary care physician should follow up with the youth and his/her parents to ensure procurement of treatment and progress, as well as to demonstrate interest. Substance abuse is commonly associated with other risky behaviors including sexual activity, truancy, violence, and criminal acts. Medical interventions such as provision of contraception might be indicated. Periodic monitoring and drug screens should occur together with frequent contact with therapists or others involved in treatment. Ongoing psychoeducation about substance abuse disorders can decrease patient and family resistance to treatment and increase motivation and engagement. Outpatient family therapy appears to be superior to other forms of outpatient treatment. Despite the importance of family interventions, treatment can be effective without participation of the adolescent. Similarly, interventions with the adolescent alone can also be effective. Treatment completion is the treatment variable most consistently related to positive outcome. Related variables are motivation and compliance, which are also related to better outcomes. Adolescent perceptions can contribute to whether the youth will be engaged in treatment, suggesting that specialized, adolescent-focused engagement interventions are necessary.

G. Severe and treatment refractory substance abuse might require detoxification in a hospital setting and treatment in a residential treatment facility or on an adolescent inpatient psychiatric unit. Treatment will involve attaining a significant period of sobriety, assessing and treating psychiatric comorbidities, addressing psychological and interpersonal issues, and family therapy, as well as aftercare planning. Programs with more comprehensive services such as vocational counseling, recreational activities, and medical services (including birth control) have better outcomes than programs without those services. Programs that deal with the social ecology or total life circumstances of the adolescent are likely to produce more lasting benefits than those that do not.

References

Barrett Waldron H, Turner CW. Evidence-based psychosocial treatments for adolescent substance abuse. J Clin Child Adol Psychol 2008;37:238–61.

Bukstein OG, Bernet W, Arnold V, et al, for the Work Group on Quality Issues. Practice parameter for the assessment and treatment of children and adolescents with substance use disorders. J Am Acad Child Adolesc Psychiatry 2005;44:609–21.

Eaton DK, Kann L, Kinchen S, et al. Youth risk behavior surveillance—United States, 2007. MMWR Surveill Summ 2008;57:1–131.

Griswold, KS, Aronoff H, Kernan KB, Kahn LS. Adolescent substance use and abuse: recognition and management. Am Fam Physician 2008;77:331–6.

Kaminer Y, Bukstein OG. Adolescent substance abuse: dual diagnosis and high risk behaviors. New York: Routledge/Taylor & Francis; 2008.

Knight JR, Sherritt L, Shrier LA, et al. Validity of the CRAFFT substance abuse screening test among adolescent clinic patients. Arch Pediatr Adolesc Med 2002;156:607–14.

Winters KC, Kaminer Y. Screening and assessing adolescent substance use disorders in clinical populations. J Am Acad Child Adolesc Psychiatry 2008;47:740–4.

Patient with suspected SUBSTANCE ABUSE

(Cont'd from p 501)

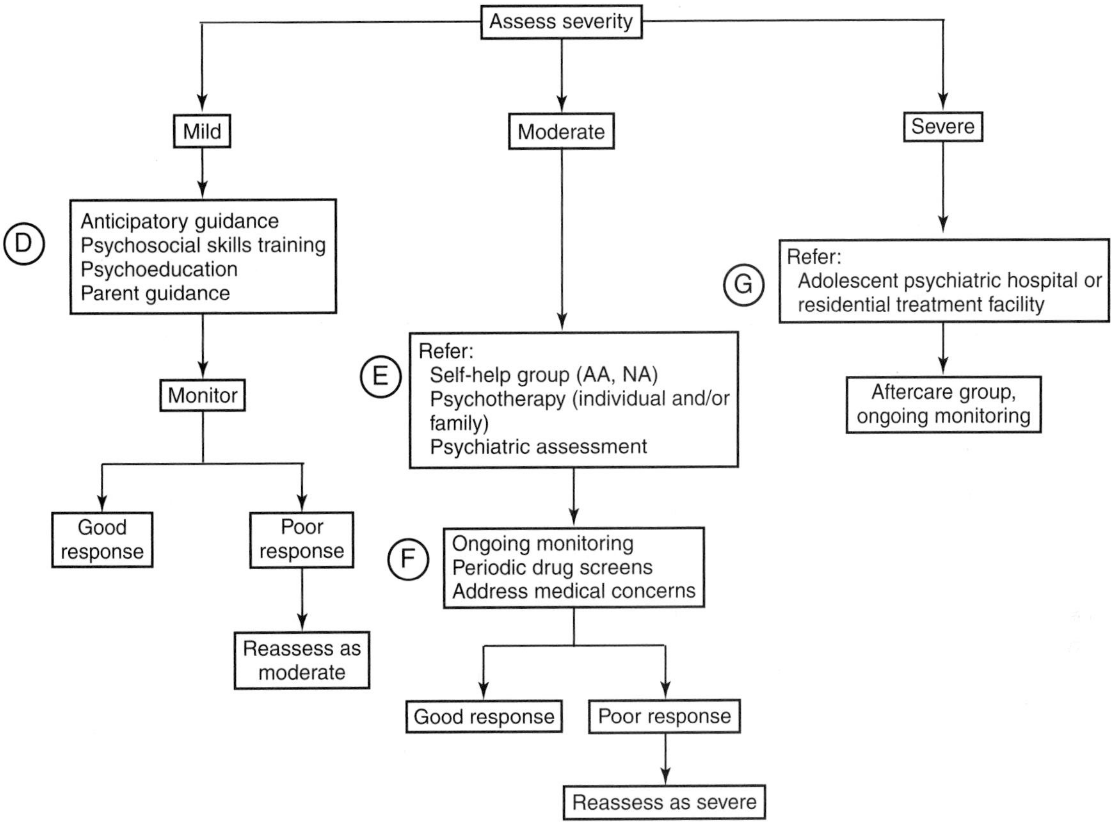

Assess severity
Mild
Moderate
Severe
D
Anticipatory guidance
Psychosocial skills training
Psychoeducation
Parent guidance
Monitor
Good response
Poor response
Reassess as moderate
E
Refer:
Self-help group (AA, NA)
Psychotherapy (individual and/or family)
Psychiatric assessment
F
Ongoing monitoring
Periodic drug screens
Address medical concerns
Good response
Poor response
Reassess as severe
G
Refer:
Adolescent psychiatric hospital or residential treatment facility
Aftercare group, ongoing monitoring

Behavioral/Developmental Disorders/Psychiatric Issues

Attention-Deficit/Hyperactivity Disorder

Joseph M. Smith, MD, FAAP

The current criteria for the diagnosis of attention-deficit/hyperactivity disorder (ADHD) are found in the *Diagnostic and Statistical Manual of Mental Disorders*, 4th Edition, Text Revision (DSM-IV-TR) and the *Diagnostic and Statistical Manual for Primary Care* (DSM-PC) (Table 1). The DSM-IV-TR defines ADHD by a list of symptoms that are grouped into three core areas: inattention, hyperactivity, and impulsivity. The core area of inattention includes nine symptoms, and a person is considered impaired in this area if six or more of these symptoms occur "often." The core areas of hyperactivity and impulsivity have a sum total of nine symptoms and, likewise, a person is considered impaired in these areas if six or more symptoms occur "often." These six symptom designations are arbitrary. An evaluator might consider four or five significant symptoms to be sufficient enough to make the diagnosis of ADHD if those symptoms are severe enough. Current DSM-IV-TR diagnostic criteria require the presence of symptoms before 7 years of age and the persistence of symptoms for more than 6 months. This age of onset for ADHD has been challenged for years and has no scientific basis and much evidence to the contrary. More recent research suggests that it would be more accurate to state that the onset of ADHD is in childhood or adolescence. The final DSM-IV-TR requirement is that impairment be present in at least two settings (i.e., school, home, work). Although this is an important consideration, it is essential that the evaluator take into account the quality of the observations being made in various settings. Lack of evidence for ADHD provided by a poor observer may prompt the need to seek out other, more scrupulous observers, particularly in the case of the inattentive type of ADHD where symptoms are less obvious. The DSM-IV-TR divides ADHD into three subtypes: the predominantly inattentive type (in which a person demonstrates impairment only in the area of inattention), the predominantly hyperactive-impulsive type (in which a person demonstrates impairment only in the areas of hyperactivity and impulsivity), and the combined type (in which impairment occurs in each of the three core areas). Although historically these three subtypes have been described, the existence of a hyperactive-impulsive subtype without inattention has been challenged. Furthermore, people can shift across subtypes as they grow, which makes the current subtyping of ADHD ineffective. It is more important to remember that the hallmark symptoms for ADHD are lack of sustained attention, poor persistence, distractibility, and impulsivity.

A. Prevalence rate of ADHD is estimated to be 6% to 8%. Because of this, it is recommended that screening for ADHD be part of every patient's mental health assessment. The assessment of ADHD should include direct evidence of symptomatology and impairment from parents, teachers, and in some cases, other observers (such as the individual being evaluated or that individual's employers). Parents and individuals who are evaluated should be asked for a detailed description of what they perceive the impairments to be.

B. A thorough review of medical history should include an assessment of medical, behavioral, mental health, developmental, and academic problems. A history of injuries, particularly head trauma, should be documented. Perinatal history including gestation at delivery, pregnancy, labor and delivery complications, and maternal medication and substance use during pregnancy should also be explored. A detailed review of systems including diet, exercise, sleep habits, history of depression, and history of anxiety should be obtained. It is also important to ask whether the patient has had a history of syncope, palpitations, or chest pain with exercise or exertion. A psychosocial history should evaluate family structure, psychosocial stressors, academic performance, grades, extracurricular activities, risk-taking behaviors, history of being bullied, and history of abuse.

C. ADHD is primarily a genetic-based disorder. To date, five to eight gene polymorphisms implicated in the cause of ADHD have been identified. Twelve or more additional genetic sites have been identified in genome scans that may play a role. Therefore, it is essential to obtain a detailed family history that includes all primary and secondary relatives. Assessment should identify the presence of all neurodevelopmental and mental health disorders within the family. This would include presence of ADHD, autism spectrum disorders, depression, anxiety, bipolar mood disorder, or other developmental disorders and syndromes. In addition, it is important to ask whether there is a family history of sudden, unexplained cardiac death.

D. Other nongenetic causes of ADHD include perinatal stress, low birth weight, head trauma, brain injury, maternal smoking during pregnancy, in utero alcohol or drug exposure, and severe early deprivation.

E. If available, any previous IQ testing or academic performance measures can be analyzed.

F. Review of any psychotropic medications that have been tried in the past and what their effects were can aid in formulation of a treatment plan. Efficacy of these treatments (or lack thereof), as well as ascertaining whether side effects occurred, can be informative.

G. Other medical problems that should be assessed include the presence of enuresis, encopresis, and tics, because each of these conditions is more prevalent in individuals with ADHD.

H. ADHD in and of itself does not have any characteristic physical or neurologic findings. However, a complete

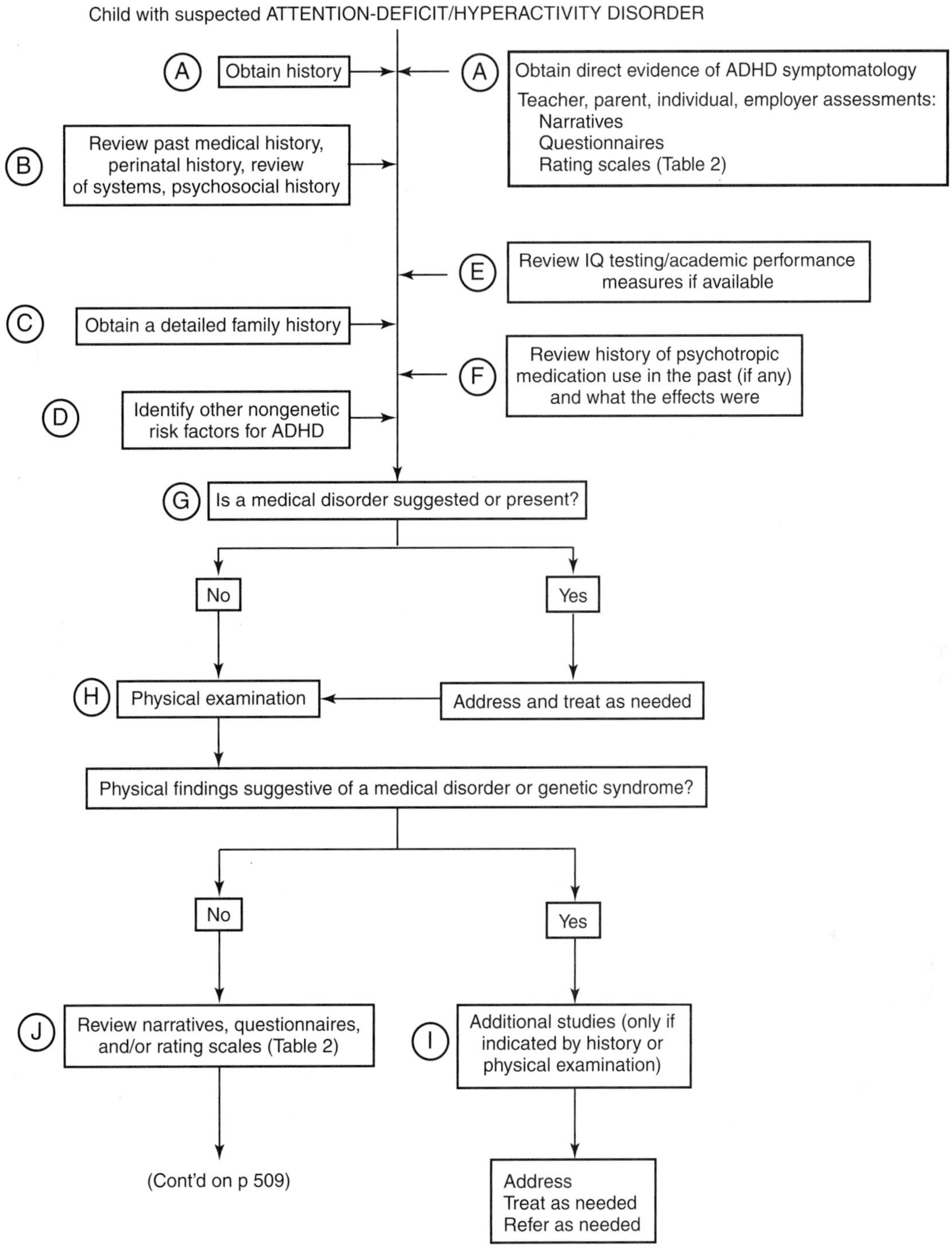
Child with suspected ATTENTION-DEFICIT/HYPERACTIVITY DISORDER
A
Obtain history
A
Obtain direct evidence of ADHD symptomatology
Teacher, parent, individual, employer assessments:
Narratives
Questionnaires
Rating scales (Table 2)
B
Review past medical history, perinatal history, review of systems, psychosocial history
E
Review IQ testing/academic performance measures if available
C
Obtain a detailed family history
F
Review history of psychotropic medication use in the past (if any) and what the effects were
D
Identify other nongenetic risk factors for ADHD
G
Is a medical disorder suggested or present?
No
Yes
H
Physical examination
Address and treat as needed
Physical findings suggestive of a medical disorder or genetic syndrome?
No
Yes
J
Review narratives, questionnaires, and/or rating scales (Table 2)
I
Additional studies (only if indicated by history or physical examination)
(Cont'd on p 509)
Address
Treat as needed
Refer as needed

physical examination can help to rule out other disorders that can masquerade as ADHD.

I. Laboratory and radiologic evaluation is seldom necessary in the workup of ADHD unless conditions are suggested by the medical history or physical examination. As noted in the DSM-IV-TR, evaluation of symptoms is based on observation alone. Currently, there are no laboratory, electroencephalogram, or radiological studies (including PET and SPECT scans) with sufficient normative data to be helpful in the diagnosis of ADHD. Continuous performance tests are likewise nonessential and are prone to false-negative results. Routine testing for blood lead levels and thyroid function is not recommended unless the history or physical examination suggests the need to do so.

J. Data can be gathered from parents, teachers, employers, and individuals by way of verbal or written narratives, questionnaires, and through the use of standardized rating scales. Many such scales exist and are listed in Table 2. The ideal rating scales are those that not only include assessments of the DSM-IV-TR criteria for ADHD, but also include screening questions for the most common comorbidities found in individuals who have ADHD (see section K).

K. ADHD rarely occurs in isolation. In 60% to 80% of cases, individuals will manifest symptoms of an associated comorbid (coexisting) condition. Because of this, all individuals with ADHD should be evaluated for comorbidities. The most common comorbidities of ADHD are oppositional defiant disorder (40%–80%), conduct disorder (20%–50%), mood disorders (15%–30%), language or learning disorders (25%–35%), anxiety disorders (30%), smoking (19%), and substance use disorder (15%). Encopresis and enuresis appear to be about twice as common in children with ADHD compared with their non-ADHD counterparts. Other disorders can present with prominent ADHD features. These include Tourette disorder, fragile X syndrome, fetal alcohol syndrome, autism spectrum disorders (particularly the higher functioning forms), obsessive-compulsive disorder, learning disabilities, attachment disorders, and genetic abnormalities. The coexistence of these problems and conditions can strongly influence treatment choices and outcomes. General behavior rating scales such as the Swanson, Nolan, and Pelham (SNAP-IV), the Child Behavior Checklist (CBCL), and the Behavior Assessment Scales for Children (BASC) can aid in the identification of these coexisting conditions. Primary care physicians may wish to have some of these comorbid conditions confirmed through referral.

L. Areas of impairment in children and adolescents with ADHD include abnormal family and peer relationships, delayed social skills, academic underperformance, impaired self-esteem, increased risk for antisocial behaviors, increased substance use and abuse, impaired driving skills, increased risk for sexually transmitted diseases and unwanted pregnancy, and increased risk for accidental injury. Identifying areas of impairment can help providers, parents, and educators to formulate plans that will best fit the individual needs of the child or adolescent with ADHD. ADHD is more impairing than most other disorders treated in the mental health outpatient setting and carries a substantial economic burden to society. Impairment in ADHD can be so significant that failure to treat (or failure to adequately treat) ADHD can carry substantial risk to the individual, including death from injury.

M. ADHD is thought to be a disorder that is caused by abnormalities of dopamine and norepinephrine in the dorsolateral prefrontal cortex, anterior cingulate, anterior corpus callosum, the striatum of the basal ganglia, and the vermis of the cerebellum. As such, the most effective intervention demonstrated for ADHD is medical intervention. In the largest empirical study on ADHD to date, intensely managed medication therapy with or without behavioral therapy produced superior results over behavioral therapy alone. Adding behavioral therapy to intensely managed medication therapy for the most part did not confer much additional advantage except in those individuals who had coexisting conditions such as anxiety.

N. Stimulant medications (methylphenidate, dexmethylphenidate, dextroamphetamine, mixed amphetamine salts, lisdexamfetamine dimesylate), as well as atomoxetine and extended-release guanfacine, are first-line treatments for ADHD. Psychopharmacologic treatment alone is adequate therapy for some individuals. The most widely used treatments have been the stimulant medications, which are well studied, work quickly, and are generally well tolerated. The long-acting stimulants confer the additional advantages of longer duration of action, improved adherence to therapy, decreased social stigmata (and increased confidentiality) as medication does not need to be administered at school, fewer adverse effects, decreased abuse potential, and management of evening symptoms. Only the long-acting stimulants have been shown to improve motor vehicle driving abilities in individuals with ADHD. Long-acting stimulant medications come in various forms that include tablets or capsules that are swallowed, capsules that can be sprinkled on applesauce or mixed in water, and a patch worn on the hip that releases medication transdermally. Some individuals respond preferentially to one stimulant class (methylphenidate vs. amphetamine derivatives), whereas others respond equally well to both. This is a known phenomenon, and an individual's symptoms do not predict which stimulant class will work best. A trial of both stimulant classes is reasonable to determine which class will provide the best response. Dosing of stimulant medication is not based on weight, but response. An individual should be started on a low dose of stimulant, and the dose should be titrated at weekly intervals until normalization of symptoms occurs or further titration is limited because of adverse effects. If an individual has a history of syncope, palpitations, chest pain with exercise or exertion, or a family history of sudden, unexplained cardiac death, consultation with a cardiologist may be indicated before starting a stimulant medication.

Atomoxetine may also be used and has a reasonable safety profile. With atomoxetine, improvement is usually noted within 3 weeks, with maximum improvement achieved by 10 weeks of therapy. Atomoxetine may be particularly helpful in individuals who have ADHD with comorbid anxiety, tic disorders, or who have not responded to stimulants. Dosing of atomoxetine is based on weight.

Extended-release guanfacine may also be used to treat individuals with ADHD and may be particularly beneficial in those who have oppositional symptoms, a comorbid tic disorder, or who have not responded to stimulants. Improvement in symptoms usually occurs within 2 to 4 weeks with extended-release guanfacine, and dosing is based on weight.

Less well-studied (and non–FDA-approved) therapies include bupropion, short-acting α_2-adrenergics, tricyclic antidepressants, and modafinil. Cardiotoxic effects of the tricyclic medications eliminate these therapies from consideration for most individuals as safer treatment modalities have emerged. Bupropion carries the risk for seizure induction, whereas modafinil carries the risk for Stevens–Johnson syndrome. Table 3 outlines current therapies for ADHD.

O. Other helpful interventions for children and adolescents with ADHD include providing self-esteem building techniques, teaching time management and organizational

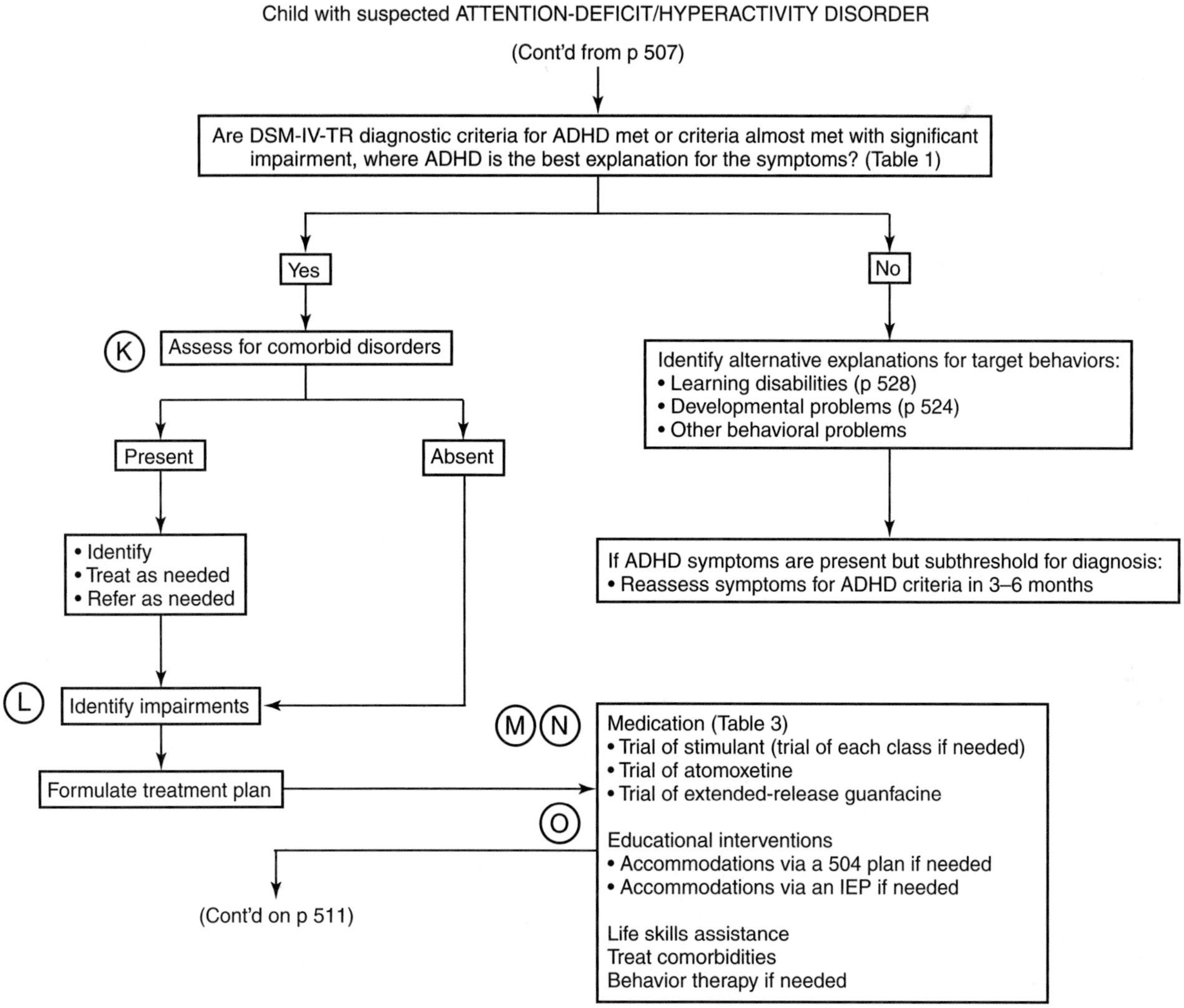
Child with suspected ATTENTION-DEFICIT/HYPERACTIVITY DISORDER
(Cont'd from p 507)
Are DSM-IV-TR diagnostic criteria for ADHD met or criteria almost met with significant impairment, where ADHD is the best explanation for the symptoms? (Table 1)
Yes
No
K
Assess for comorbid disorders
Present
Absent
• Identify
• Treat as needed
• Refer as needed
L
Identify impairments
Formulate treatment plan
Identify alternative explanations for target behaviors:
• Learning disabilities (p 528)
• Developmental problems (p 524)
• Other behavioral problems
If ADHD symptoms are present but subthreshold for diagnosis:
• Reassess symptoms for ADHD criteria in 3–6 months
M N
Medication (Table 3)
• Trial of stimulant (trial of each class if needed)
• Trial of atomoxetine
• Trial of extended-release guanfacine
O
Educational interventions
• Accommodations via a 504 plan if needed
• Accommodations via an IEP if needed
Life skills assistance
Treat comorbidities
Behavior therapy if needed
(Cont'd on p 511)

skills, establishing appropriate educational interventions, which may include an Individual Education Plan or a 504 plan, treating coexisting problems, treating ADHD and/or mental health disorders in parents, and aiding the individual in the development of coping strategies for ongoing problems. Behavior therapy may be helpful in some individuals, especially in those with comorbid conditions or those who have incomplete response to other treatment modalities. Interventions that have not been shown to be helpful for core ADHD symptoms include dietary modification, cognitive-behavioral therapy, electroencephalographic feedback, and formal social skills training.

P. Follow-up visits should include interim history, standardized reassessment of symptoms to objectively measure success of intervention, review of efficacy of interventions, as well as discussing possible adverse effects incurred by prescribed medication, adjustment of medication dosing, periodic screening for comorbid conditions, and review of home and school functioning, as well as social development. Ongoing education of the parent, educators, and the individuals about the disorder and the challenges that occur can be beneficial. Follow-up visits may be as frequent as every 1 to 4 weeks initially, followed by two to four times a year once goals are met. The presence of comorbidities may warrant more frequent monitoring. All follow-up visits should include measurement of height, weight, and vital signs (especially heart rate and blood pressure).

Q. If response to therapy is not satisfactory, different treatment modalities can be explored. If several therapies do not yield satisfactory results, the clinician should carefully review the diagnosis and consider other diagnoses instead of ADHD or comorbid conditions to ADHD that are interfering with treatment. Addition of behavioral therapy or referral to a developmental pediatrician, child and adolescent psychiatrist, or child neurologist may be indicated.

Table 1. **Diagnostic Criteria for Attention-Deficit/Hyperactivity Disorder**

A. Either criteria 1 or 2:

1. Six (or more) of the following symptoms of inattention have persisted for at least 6 months to a degree that is maladaptive and inconsistent with developmental level:

Inattention

- a. Often fails to give close attention to details or makes careless mistakes in schoolwork, work, or other activities
- b. Often has difficulty sustaining attention in tasks or play activities
- c. Often does not seem to listen when spoken to directly
- d. Often does not follow through on instructions and fails to finish schoolwork, chores, or duties in the workplace (not because of oppositional behavior or failure to understand instructions)
- e. Often has difficulty organizing tasks and activities
- f. Often avoids, dislikes, or is reluctant to engage in tasks that require sustained mental effort (such as schoolwork or homework)
- g. Often loses things necessary for tasks or activities (e.g., toys, school assignments, pencils, books, or tools)
- h. Is often easily distracted by extraneous stimuli
- i. Is often forgetful in daily activities

2. Six (or more) of the following symptoms of *hyperactivity-impulsivity* have persisted for at least 6 months to a degree that is maladaptive and inconsistent with developmental level:

Hyperactivity

- a. Often fidgets with hands or feet or squirms in seat
- b. Often leaves seat in classroom or in other situations in which remaining seated is expected
- c. Often runs about or climbs excessively in situations in which it is inappropriate (in adolescents or adults, may be limited to subjective feelings of restlessness)
- d. Often has difficulty playing or engaging in leisure activities quietly
- e. Is often "on the go" or often acts as if "driven by a motor"
- f. Often talks excessively

Impulsivity

- a. Often blurts out answers before questions have been completed
- b. Often has difficulty awaiting turn
- c. Often interrupts or intrudes on others (e.g., butts into conversations or games)

B. Some hyperactive-impulsive or inattentive symptoms that caused impairment were present before age 7 years.

C. Some impairment from the symptoms is present in two or more settings (e.g., at school [or work] and at home).

D. There must be clear evidence of clinically significant impairment in social, academic, or occupational functioning.

E. The symptoms do not occur exclusively during the course of a pervasive developmental disorder, schizophrenia, or other psychotic disorder and are not better accounted for by another mental disorder (e.g., mood disorder, anxiety disorder, dissociative disorder, or a personality disorder).

Table reprinted with permission from the AAP.

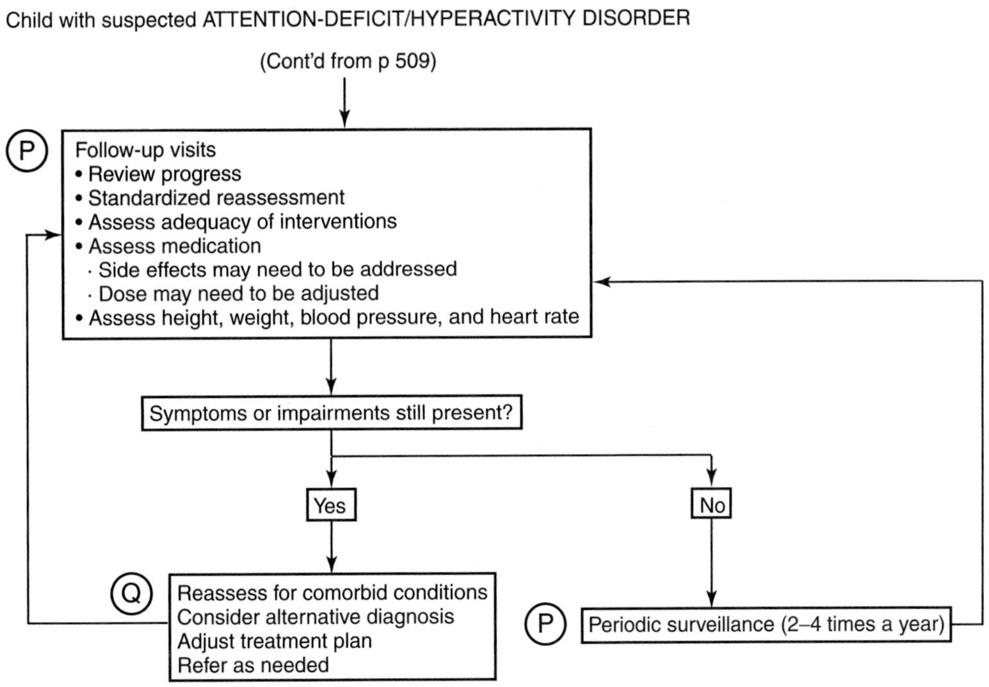
Child with suspected ATTENTION-DEFICIT/HYPERACTIVITY DISORDER
(Cont'd from p 509)
P
Follow-up visits
• Review progress
• Standardized reassessment
• Assess adequacy of interventions
• Assess medication
· Side effects may need to be addressed
· Dose may need to be adjusted
• Assess height, weight, blood pressure, and heart rate
Symptoms or impairments still present?
Yes
No
Q
Reassess for comorbid conditions
Consider alternative diagnosis
Adjust treatment plan
Refer as needed
P
Periodic surveillance (2–4 times a year)

Table 2. **Common Behavior Rating Scales Used in the Assessment of Attention-Deficit/Hyperactivity Disorder and Monitoring of Treatment**

Rating Scales	Description
Academic Performance Rating Scale (APRS)	The APRS is a 19-item scale for determining a child's academic productivity and accuracy in grades 1–6 that has six scale points; construct, concurrent, and discriminant validity data, as well as norms (n = 247) available (Barkley, 1990)
ADHD Rating Scales-IV	The ADHD Rating Scale-IV is an 18-item scale using DSM-IV criteria (DuPaul et al., 1998)
Brown ADD Rating Scales for Children, Adolescents, and Adults	Psychological Corporation, San Antonio, TX (www.drthomasebrown.com/assess_tools/index.html) (Brown, 2001)
Child Behavior Checklist (CBCL)	Parent-completed CBCL and Teacher-completed Teacher Report Form (TRF) (www.aseba.org/index.html)
Conners Parent Rating Scale—Revised (CPRS-R)*	Parent and adolescent self-report versions available (Conners, 1997)
Conners Teacher Rating Scale—Revised (CPRS-R)*	Conners, 1997
Home Situations Questionnaire—Revised (HSQ-R), School Situations Questionnaire—Revised (SSQ-R)	The HSQ-R is a 14-item scale designed to assess specific problems with attention and concentration across a variety of home and public situations; it uses a 0–9 scale and has test-retest, internal consistency, construct validity, discriminant validity, concurrent validity, and norms (n = 581) available (Barkley, 1990).
Inattention/Overactivity with Aggression (IOWA) Conners Teacher Rating Scale	The IOWA Conners is a 10-item scale developed to separate the inattention and overactivity ratings from oppositional defiance (Loney and Milich, 1982).
Swanson, Nolan, and Pelham (SNAP-IV) and SKAMP Internet site ADHD.NET *(obtainable from www.adhd.net)*	The SNAP-IV (Swanson, 1992) is a 26-item scale that contains DSM-IV criteria for ADHD and screens for other DSM diagnoses; the SKAMP (Wigal et al., 1998) is a 10-item scale that measures impairment of functioning at home and at school.
Vanderbilt ADHD Diagnostic Parent and Teacher Scales	Teachers rate 35 symptoms and 8 performance items measuring ADHD symptoms and common comorbid conditions (Wolraich et al., 2003a). The parent version contains all 18 ADHD symptoms, with items assessing comorbid conditions and performance (Wolraich et al., 2003b).

*The longer form should be used for initial assessment, whereas the shorter form is often used for assessing response to treatment, particularly when repeated administration is required.

ADD, attention-deficit disorder; *ADHD,* attention-deficit/hyperactivity disorder; *DSM-IV, Diagnostic and Statistical Manual of Mental Disorders,* Fourth Edition.
Italics added. Table reprinted with permission from AACAP.

Table 3. Medications Approved by the U.S. Food and Drug Administration for Attention-Deficit/Hyperactivity Disorder (Alphabetical by Class)

Generic Class/ Brand Name	Dose Form	Typical Starting Dose	FDA Max/Day	Off-label Max/Day	Comments
Amphetamine Preparations					
Short acting					Short-acting stimulants often used as initial treatment in small children (<16 kg), but have disadvantage of bid-tid dosing to control symptoms throughout day
Adderall°	5-, 7.5-, 10-, 12.5-, 15-, 20-, 30-mg tablets	3–5 yr: 2.5 mg qd; ≥6 yr: 5 mg qd to bid	40 mg	>50 kg: 60 mg	
Dexedrine°	5-mg capsules	3–5 yr: 2.5 mg qd			
DextroStat°	5-, 10-mg capsules	≥6 yr: 5 mg qd to bid			
Long acting					Longer acting stimulants offer greater convenience, confidentiality, and compliance with single daily dosing but may have greater problematic effects on evening appetite and sleep Adderall XR cap may be opened and sprinkled on soft food
Dexedrine Spansule	5-, 10-, 15-mg capsules	≥6 yr: 5–10 mg qd to bid	40 mg	>50 kg: 60 mg	
Adderall XR	5-, 10-, 15-, 20-, 25-, 30-mg capsules	≥6 yr: 10 mg qd	30 mg	>50 kg: 60 mg	
Lisdexamfetamine	30-, 50-, 70-mg capsules	30 mg qd	70 mg	Not yet known	
Methylphenidate Preparations					
Short acting					Short-acting stimulants often used as initial treatment in small children (<16 kg), as above, but have disadvantage of bid to tid dosing to control symptoms throughout day
Focalin	2.5-, 5-, 10-mg capsules	2.5 mg bid	20 mg	50 mg	
Methylin°	5-, 10-, 20-mg tablets	5 mg bid	60 mg	>50 kg: 100 mg	
Ritalin°	5, 10, 20 mg	5 mg bid	60 mg	>50 kg: 100 mg	
Intermediate acting					Longer acting stimulants offer greater convenience, confidentiality, and compliance with single daily dosing but may have greater problematic effects on evening appetite and sleep Metadate CD and Ritalin LA capsules may be opened and sprinkled on soft food
Metadate ER	10-, 20-mg capsules	10 mg every morning	60 mg	>50 kg: 100 mg	
Methylin ER	10-, 20-mg capsules	10 mg every morning	60 mg	>50 kg: 100 mg	
Ritalin SR°	20 mg	10 mg every morning	60 mg	>50 kg: 100 mg	
Metadate CD	10, 20, 30, 40, 50, 60 mg	20 mg every morning	60 mg	>50 kg: 100 mg	
Ritalin LA	10, 20, 30, 40 mg	20 mg every morning	60 mg	>50 kg: 100 mg	
Long acting					
Concerta	18-, 27-, 36-, 54-mg capsules	18 mg every morning	72 mg	108 mg	Swallow whole with liquids Nonabsorbable tablet shell may be seen in stool
Daytrana patch	10-, 15-, 20-, 30-mg patches	Begins with 10 mg patch qd, then titrate up by patch strength	30 mg	Not yet known	
Focalin XR	5-, 10-, 15-, 20-mg capsules	5 mg every morning	30 mg	50 mg	
Selective Norepinephrine Reuptake Inhibitor					
Atomoxetine					Not a schedule II medication. Consider if active substance abuse or severe adverse effects of stimulants (mood liability, tics); give every morning or divided doses bid (effects on late evening behavior); do not open capsule; monitor closely for suicidal thinking and behavior, clinical worsening, or unusual changes in behavior.
Strattera	10-, 18-, 25-, 40-, 60-, 80-, 100-mg capsules	Children and adolescents <70 kg; 0.5 mg/kg/day for 4 days, then 1 mg/kg/day for 4 days, then 1.2 mg/kg/day	Lesser of 1.4 mg/kg or 100 mg	Lesser of 1.8 mg/kg or 100 mg	

°Generic formulation available.
ADHD, attention-deficit/hyperactivity disorder; *FDA*, U.S. Food and Drug Administration; *max*, maximum.
Table reprinted with permission from AACAP.

References

American Academy of Child and Adolescent Psychiatry. Practice parameter for the assessment and treatment of children and adolescents with attention-deficit/hyperactivity disorder. J Am Acad Child Adolesc Psychiatry 2007;46:7.

American Psychiatric Association. Diagnostic and statistical manual of mental disorders. 4th ed [text revision]. Washington, DC: American Psychiatric Association; 2000.

Arnold LE. Methylphenidate vs amphetamine: Comparative review. J Atten Disord 2000;3:200–11.

Barkley RA. Attention-deficit hyperactivity disorder: a handbook for diagnosis and treatment. 3rd ed. New York: Guilford Press; 2006.

Barkley RA. Attention deficit hyperactivity disorder: A handbook for diagnosis and treatment. 1st ed. New York: Guilford; 1990.

Barkley RA, et al. ADHD in adults: what the science says. New York: Guilford Press; 2008.

Biederman J, et al. Comorbidity of attention deficit hyperactivity disorder with conduct, depressive, anxiety, and other disorders. Am J Psychiatry 1991;148:565–77.

Biederman J, et al. Is ADHD a risk factor for psychoactive substance use disorders? Findings from a four-year prospective follow-up study. J Am Acad Child Adolesc Psychiatry 1997;36:21–9.

Brown TE. The Brown attention deficit disorder scales. San Antonio, TX: Psychological Corporation; 2001.

Conners CK. Conners rating scales—Revised. Toronto, Canada: Multi-Health Systems; 1997.

DuPaul GJ, Power TJ, Anastopoulos AD, Reid R. ADHD rating scales–IV: Checklists, norms and clinical interpretation. New York: Guilford; 1998.

Faraone SV, et al. Molecular genetics of attention-deficit/hyperactivity disorder. Biol Psychiatry 2005;57:1313–23.

Jensen PS, et al. Findings for the NIMH multimodal treatment study of ADHD (MTA): Implications applications for primary care providers. J Dev Behav Pediatr 2001;22:60–73.

Kreppner JM, et al. Can inattention/overactivity be an institutional deprivation syndrome? J Abnorm Child Psychol 2001;29:513–28.

Loney J, Milich M. Hyperactivity, inattention, and aggression in clinical practice. In: Wolraich M, Routh DK, editors. Advances in Behavioral and Developmental Pediatrics, Vol. 3. Greenwich, CT: JAI; 1982. p. 113–47.

Milberger S, et al. Attention deficit hyperactivity disorder is associated with early initiation of cigarette smoking in children and adolescents. J Am Acad Child Adolesc Psychiatry 1997;36: 37–44.

MTA Cooperative Group. A 14 month randomized clinical trial of treatment strategies for children with attention-deficit hyperactivity disorder. Arch Gen Psychiatry 1999;56:1073–86.

Swanson JM. School-based assessments and intervention for ADD students. Irvine, CA: KC Publishing; 1992.

Wigal SB, Gupta S, Guinta D, Swanson JM. Reliability and validity of the SKAMP rating scale in a laboratory school setting. Psychopharmacol Bull 1998;34:47–53.

Wilens T. New research on ADHD and substance use disorders. Symposium presented at the 158th Annual APA Meeting; May 21, 2005; Atlanta, GA.

Wolraich ML, Lambert EW, Baumgaertel A, et al. Teachers' screening for attention deficit/hyperactivity disorder: Comparing multinational samples on teacher ratings of ADHD. J Abnorm Child Psychol 2003;31:445–55.

Wolraich ML, Lambert W, Doffing MA, Bickman L, Simmons T, Worley K. Psychometric properties of the Vanderbilt ADHD diagnostic parent rating scale in a referred population. J Pediatr Psychol 2003;28:559–67.

Autism Spectrum Disorders

William Campbell, MD

Autism spectrum disorders (ASDs) are also known as pervasive developmental disorders and include autistic disorder (autism), Asperger syndrome, and pervasive developmental disorder not otherwise specified (PDD-NOS). All of these involve impairments in reciprocal social interactions, impairments in verbal and nonverbal communication (including pretend play), and atypical, restricted, repetitive activities, interests, and behaviors (Table 1). ASD has been diagnosed with increasing frequency, and the prevalence is currently estimated to be about 1 in 110. The cause is most likely related to genetic differences influencing brain development. More than one gene is likely involved, given the variable phenotypes among individuals with ASDs. Early intervention may help improve functional outcomes.

A. Survey development and behavior at every well visit. Elicit concerns by asking questions such as "Do you have any questions or concerns about your child's development or behavior?" Use standardized general developmental screening instruments at recommended times (e.g., at the 9- or 12-month, 18-month, and 24- or 30-month visits). Look for unevenness in development, social and communication delays, and unusual interests, behaviors, or mannerisms. For young children, ask about interest in other children, pretend play, sharing interests and enjoyment with parents, following a parent's point, and imitation. For older children, ask about relationships (with peers and adults) and performance in school. The family history may be notable for language delay, poor social skills, cognitive impairment, and psychiatric illness. Behavioral observations may be significant for poor eye contact (or eye contact that is poorly integrated with vocalizations and pointing), poor joint attention (not paying attention to what the parent or examiner is trying to get the child to pay attention to), lack of pointing, and lack of pretend play.

B. Schedule a "problem-targeted" clinic visit if the parent has concerns or if the clinician has concerns about ASD or related issues.

C. Developmental surveillance is described in the chapter "Developmental Delay in Children Younger Than 6 Years," and more details can be found in the policy statement of the American Academy of Pediatrics ("Identifying Infants and Young Children with Developmental Disorders in the Medical Home: An Algorithm for Developmental Surveillance and Screening." Pediatrics 2006;118(1):405-20).

To survey for ASDs, score 1 point for "yes" answers to each of the following questions, and follow the algorithm accordingly:

1. Sibling with ASD?
2. Parent concern for ASD?
3. Other caregiver concern for ASD?
4. Clinician concern for ASD?

D. Autism-specific screening tools are recommended at the 18- and 24-month well visits.

E. Examples of ASD-specific screening tools include the Checklist for Autism in Toddlers (CHAT) and the Modified Checklist for Autism in Toddlers (M-CHAT). If doubt exists because of difficulty finding or interpreting an age-appropriate screening tool, it is acceptable to refer the patient for further evaluation.

F. Refer all children with suspected ASDs to their local early intervention systems or public school systems, depending on the age of the child. Appropriate services can often begin before the diagnostic ASD evaluation is completed.

G. Refer all children with suspected ASDs for a diagnostic ASD evaluation. Although some relatively small communities have, or are visited by, appropriate evaluation teams, most diagnostic ASD evaluations are done by specialists or specialty clinics in larger cities and are associated with tertiary care children's hospitals, medical schools, and University Centers for Excellence in Developmental Disabilities Education, Research, & Service (UCEDD).

H. Arrange appropriate follow-up, within a month or two, for children with ASD concerns, regardless of whether they were referred for further evaluation. If there were no concerns, continue routine health care maintenance.

(Continued on page 516)

Patient with AUTISM SPECTRUM DISORDERS

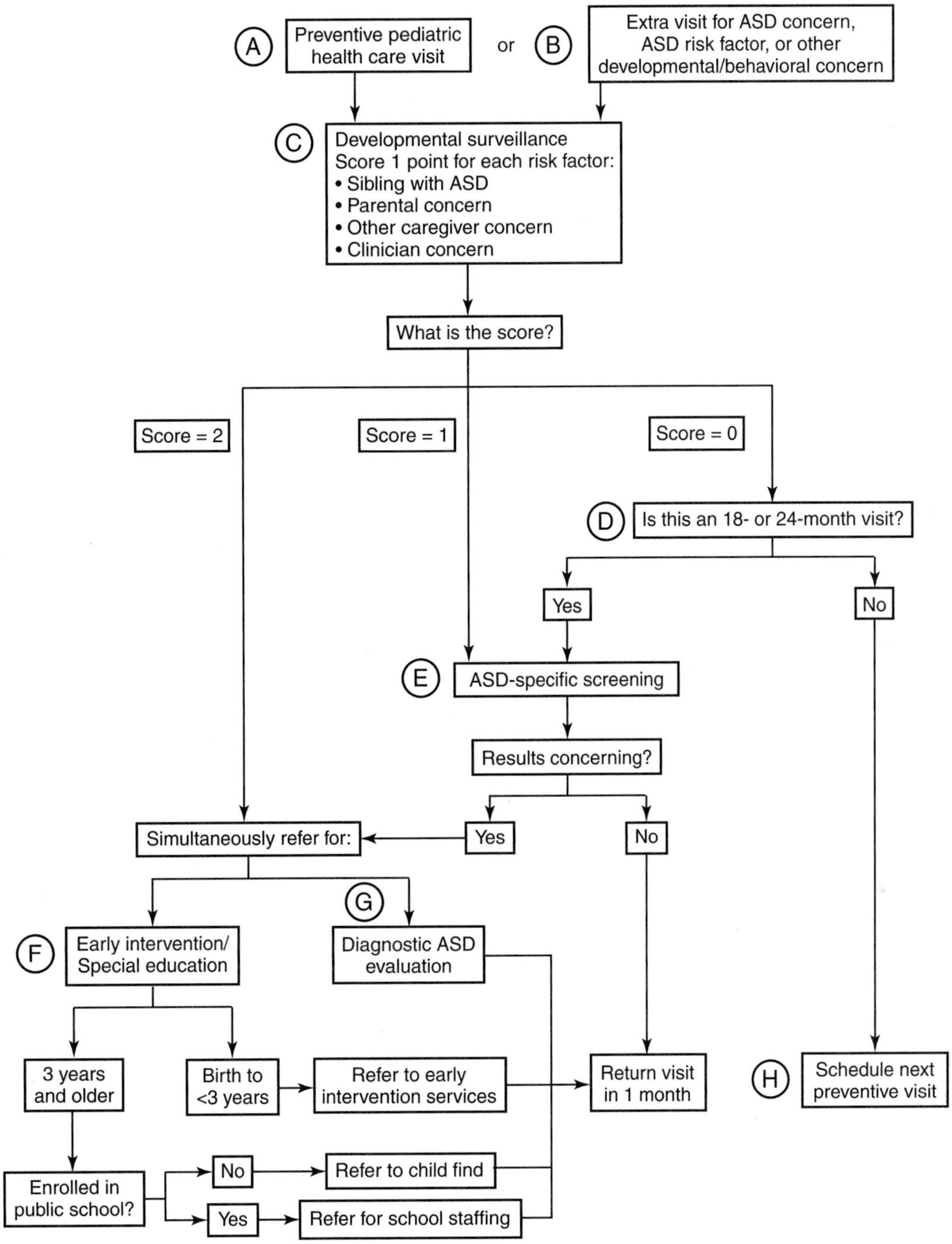
A
Preventive pediatric health care visit
or
B
Extra visit for ASD concern, ASD risk factor, or other developmental/behavioral concern
C
Developmental surveillance
Score 1 point for each risk factor:
• Sibling with ASD
• Parental concern
• Other caregiver concern
• Clinician concern
What is the score?
Score = 2
Score = 1
Score = 0
D
Is this an 18- or 24-month visit?
Yes
No
E
ASD-specific screening
Results concerning?
Yes
No
Simultaneously refer for:
F
Early intervention/ Special education
G
Diagnostic ASD evaluation
3 years and older
Birth to <3 years
Refer to early intervention services
Return visit in 1 month
H
Schedule next preventive visit
Enrolled in public school?
No
Refer to child find
Yes
Refer for school staffing

Table 1. **Signs and Symptoms of Autistic Spectrum Disorder**

<3 Years Old	3–6 Years Old	>6 Years Old
No babbling by 12 months No gestural communication (pointing, waving bye) by 12 months No single words by 16 months Failure to orient to own name by 12 months; diminished auditory attention No pretend play by 18 months No use of index finger to indicate interest in something (pointing to show or share) by 18 months Lack of gaze monitoring by 18 months No two-word spontaneous (not echolalic) phrases by 24 months Limited initiation of activity/play before 36 months	Same as for age <3: Language may be somewhat developed, but history of late development or atypical development such as much echolalia, memorization of strings of words, or scripts Diminished eye contact Diminished interest in other children or forming friendships Has repetitive, stereotyped, or odd motor behavior Attends more to parts of objects (e.g., wheels on toy car) Unable to understand others' emotional states Hypersensitive to sounds (often typical household noises such as vacuum cleaner, blender) or touch Unusual preoccupations or a narrow range of interests (e.g., letters, geography, street maps, time tables, *Star Wars*) Lack of shared enjoyment with peers Excessive routines or rituals Difficulty with transitions	Language appears "normal" but may have had some early delay Often cannot be clearly identified until school age Perseverative behavior may not appear until later Mild gross and fine motor clumsiness Odd prosody (rhythm, inflection) of speech, peculiar formal speech Cognitive skills more typically in the normal range Intense absorption in certain interests, often to exclusion of other activities and having a repetitive quality Difficulty with abstract language Often appears socially immature, lacks friends, disinterest in peers, or socially inappropriate behavior Poor nonverbal communication including limited gestures, limited facial expression

References

Johnson CP, Scott M. Myers, and the Council on Children With Disabilities. Identification and evaluation of children with autism spectrum disorders. Pediatrics 2007;120:1183–1215.

Identifying infants and young children with developmental disorders in the medical home: an algorithm for developmental surveillance and screening. Pediatrics 2006;118:405–20.

Adolescent with Depression

Mary N. Cook, MD, and John Peterson, MD

INTRODUCTION AND EPIDEMIOLOGY

Depressive symptoms are common in pediatric clinical settings, with 5% to 10% of children and adolescents presenting with subsyndromal symptoms of major depressive disorder (MDD). MDD is estimated to affect 2% of children, aged 6 to 12 years, and 4% to 8% of adolescents, aged 13 to 17 years. In children, the male/female ratio is 1:1, but in teens, the ratio changes to 1:2. Dysthymic disorder (DD), a more chronic, milder form of depression, has been reported to afflict 0.6% to 1.7% of children and 1.6% to 8% of adolescents. The risk for depression increases significantly after puberty (particularly in girls), and by age 18, the cumulative incidence rate is 20%. Suicidal ideation is common among depressed adolescents, with an estimated 60% of depressed teens experiencing suicidal thoughts and 30% reporting a suicide attempt. Adolescents with depression are at greater risk for substance abuse as well as depression in adulthood. In addition, it appears that pediatric-onset depression tends to be a more chronic and debilitating condition than depression that begins in adulthood.

A. Screening and Assessment: Primary care providers should screen all youths for depression by asking about key symptoms, including sad or irritable mood and anhedonia, the inability to experience pleasure and have fun. In youngsters, changes associated with onset of depression might include deteriorating academic performance, weight or appetite loss or gain, social withdrawal, changes in sleep, increased defiance (related to irritability), and discontinuation of previously preferred activities. Depression in youth may be accompanied by hallucinations or delusions, although rarely. Psychotic depression in children has been associated with a family history of bipolar disorder and depression with psychotic features, more severe depression, a worse prognosis, resistance to antidepressants, and increased risk for future onset of bipolar disorder. Youths with seasonal affective disorder mainly have symptoms of depression during seasons with less daylight. Seasonal affective disorder should be differentiated from depression triggered by school stress because both can coincide with the school calendar. Adolescents may not readily report emotional or behavioral manifestations of psychiatric disorders. They might deny the existence of these symptoms or behaviors or simply have difficulty articulating their thoughts and feelings. Open-ended or indirect questions are recommended in pediatric interviews, as the information is likely to be more comprehensive and reliable. Direct or closed-ended questions often elicit more limited and potentially biased responses from children and teens. Collateral information from parents, caregivers, teachers, and others is often essential for a complete evaluation. The onset and course of a depression may be determined through the use of a mood diary or timeline, using significant life events as anchors. A mood timeline can enable the provider, child, and parents to identify environmental triggers, as well as comorbid conditions.

B. Situational Problems: Careful assessment of current and past stressors is indicated. This should include identifying interpersonal or family conflicts, verbal, physical, and/or sexual abuse, as well as neglect or poverty. It is also important to assess for symptoms consistent with post-traumatic stress disorder, which can develop in response to traumatic events. Depression often occurs against a backdrop of family conflict. Depression is often associated with increased irritability, leading to increased interpersonal tension and estrangement of others. This may cause teens to perceive diminishing social support and experience loneliness. Involvement in deviant peer groups may lead to antisocial behavior, generating more stressful life events and increasing the likelihood of depression. Asking about family psychiatric history is important due to genetic predispositions and because parental psychopathology often predicts compliance with treatment, course of illness, and outcome. It is essential to assess for marital and family discord, impaired attachment, inadequate parent support, and controlling parent–child relationships, because these factors can worsen depressive symptoms and increase risk for substance abuse and conduct disorder.

C. Comorbidity: Clinicians need to screen for comorbidities. Both MDD and dysthymic disorder are typically accompanied by other psychiatric and medical conditions. They also can occur together, a condition termed *double depression.* Approximately 40% to 90% of youths with depression also meet criteria for an additional psychiatric disorder, with up to 50% manifesting two or more comorbid psychiatric diagnoses. The most frequent comorbid diagnoses are anxiety disorders, followed by disruptive disorders (e.g., ADHD, conduct disorder, and oppositional defiant disorder) and substance abuse disorders.

D. Differential Diagnosis: It is important to rule out other causative factors for depressive symptoms, because a variety of conditions can present as depression. Psychiatric illnesses that may overlap with depression include anxiety, disruptive, psychotic, and substance abuse disorders, to name a few. Bereavement and reactions to environmental stressors and trauma can also present with depressive symptoms. Various medical conditions, including hypothyroidism, anemia, autoimmune diseases, and chronic fatigue syndrome may mimic or occur coincidentally with depression. Symptoms shared between these conditions and depression might include fatigue, low energy, sleep and appetite disturbances, and impaired concentration. Demoralization and low self-esteem can manifest as part of a chronic medical

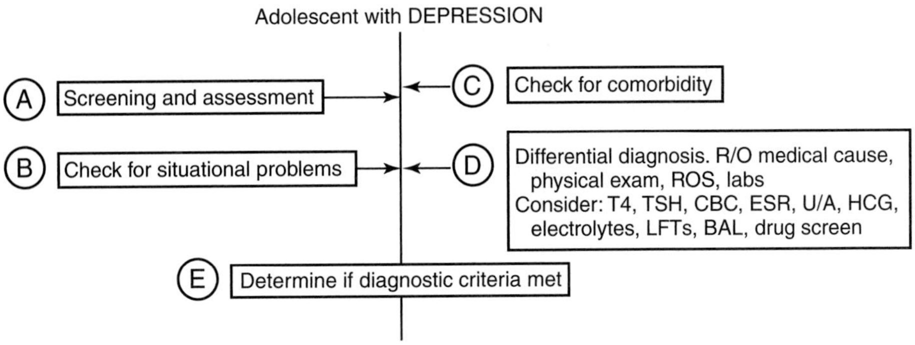
Adolescent with DEPRESSION
A
Screening and assessment
C
Check for comorbidity
B
Check for situational problems
D
Differential diagnosis. R/O medical cause, physical exam, ROS, labs
Consider: T4, TSH, CBC, ESR, U/A, HCG, electrolytes, LFTs, BAL, drug screen
E
Determine if diagnostic criteria met

(Cont'd on p 521)

illness. An extensive list of medications can produce depressive symptoms. For instance, stimulants, corticosteroids, and contraceptives are often associated with worsening mood lability or irritability. They can also disturb sleep and appetite, as well as induce weight changes. Children presenting for treatment are often experiencing their first episode of depression, making it difficult to ascertain whether they are experiencing unipolar depression or the first episode of a bipolar disorder. A strong family history of bipolar disorder, symptoms of psychosis in the child, and a history of pharmacologically induced mania or hypomania increase the likelihood of future onset of a bipolar disorder. It is prudent for clinicians to systematically screen for a history of manic or hypomanic symptoms because such a history predicts which youths are more likely to experience a medication-induced mania when treated with antidepressants.

E. Diagnostic Criteria: Depression is a spectrum disorder, ranging from subsyndromal to syndromal. Criteria for the full syndrome of MDD are listed in Table 1. The symptoms must be impairing, represent a change from baseline functioning, and not be attributable to another psychiatric or medical causative factor, bereavement, or substance abuse. MDD can also be manifested with atypical symptoms such as increased reactivity to rejection, lethargy (leaden paralysis), increased appetite, craving for carbohydrates, and hypersomnia. Dysthymic disorder consists of a persistent, long-term change in mood that generally is less intense but more chronic than in MDD. Because of its more subtle and chronic nature, dysthymic disorder is often overlooked or misdiagnosed. Although the symptoms of dysthymia are not as severe as in MDD, they nonetheless typically cause as much or more psychosocial impairment. Criteria for dysthymic disorder are listed in Table 1.

F. Suicidality: Assessment for risk for self-harm and suicidality is essential (Table 2), with suicide remaining the third leading cause of death in U.S. adolescents, claiming almost 2000 lives each year among youths aged 12 to 19 years. Almost 1 in 5 (17%) of U.S. high-school students have had suicidal thoughts in a given year, and almost 1 in 10 (8%) have attempted suicide. Current suicidal ideation is a risk factor for suicide, and having made a suicide attempt is the strongest predictor of future suicidal behavior. Other self-harming and suicide risk characteristics for adolescents include:

Psychiatric diagnosis: Diagnoses associated with adolescent suicide include major depression, substance abuse, and conduct disorder.

Sex: Female individuals attempt suicide more often, but male individuals complete suicide more often (4:1).

Older age: Suicide completion, suicide attempts, and nonsuicidal self-injury increase during adolescence; older teens are at greater risk.

Psychosocial factors: Relationship and situational stressors can contribute to self-harming and suicidal behavior (often with a psychiatric disorder present), and these include poor social supports, recent loss or rejection, family conflicts, living alone (e.g., running away/homeless), family suicidal behavior, poor communication with parents, availability of firearms, legal problems, academic difficulties, gender identity conflicts, history of maltreatment, being bullied and bullying others, risk-taking behaviors, and exposure to suicide in the community or media.

G. Pharmacologic Treatment: Antidepressant treatment may be indicated for moderate and especially for severe pediatric depression. However, the use of pharmacologic agents to treat pediatric depression has been shrouded in controversy in recent years. The controversy stems from a relative paucity of controlled data documenting efficacy for antidepressants in youth, and some data demonstrating a small but significant signal of increased suicidality associated with the initiation of some antidepressants. The lack of efficacy studies and the high potential for lethality in overdose have led to the consensus that tricyclic antidepressants are inappropriate for treating youths with depression. To date, only two agents, fluoxetine and escitalopram, have received U.S. Food and Drug Administration (FDA) approval for the indication of major depression in 8- to 17-year-olds. Other antidepressants are frequently still used for pediatric depression, but their use is considered "off label." Based on data from clinical trials, fluoxetine, at doses ranging from 20 to 40 mg, and escitalopram, at doses ranging from 20 to 40 mg, do appear to have efficacy in the treatment of pediatric depression, with the majority of controlled studies demonstrating positive results. Some studies, although not all, support efficacy for sertraline and paroxetine, but currently these medications have not been awarded FDA approval for treating depression in the pediatric population.

H. Informed Consent: Before initiating treatment with any psychotropic medication, the physician must first obtain informed consent from the parent or legal guardian, and in some states, assent from the adolescent. Informed consent involves informing the family about alternative treatment options, as well as the risks and benefits to the recommended treatment. In particular, common, as well as serious, adverse events should be reviewed. With selective serotonin reuptake inhibitor (SSRIs), nausea, diarrhea, insomnia, and akathisia should be mentioned as common adverse effects, as well as the rare but serious worries about associated increased suicidality, within the first few weeks of treatment. Patients and parents need to know that the FDA issued a black box warning about the potential for SSRIs to cause an increase in suicidality. Although there is a small increase in the risk for suicidality among adolescents taking SSRIs, compared with placebo (4% vs. 2%), the consensus among expert clinicians is that the benefits outweigh the potential risks in most teens with moderate to severe depression, at least with respect to treating with fluoxetine.

I. Psychotherapy Treatments:

Cognitive-Behavioral Therapy (CBT): Referral for psychotherapy, ideally CBT, is indicated for moderate to severe depression. Combination treatment involving CBT plus fluoxetine is more effective than monotherapy with either medication or psychotherapy alone. More severe depression is likely to respond preferentially to treatment that includes medication. In addition, CBT has been shown to be protective against the emergence of suicidality. CBT, which emphasizes that thoughts, feelings, and behaviors are interrelated, is considered a first-line treatment for pediatric depression, with a large body of literature demonstrating its efficacy in youth. CBT also emphasizes the development of improved psychosocial skills, such as communication, problem solving, and self-soothing skills.

Interpersonal Psychotherapy for Adolescents (IPT-A): Referral for IPT-A might also be considered and has been noted to be efficacious in the acute treatment of depressed adolescents. Studies have documented maintenance of improvement at 1-year follow-up, with associated reduction in hospitalization rates and suicidality. A central tenet of IPT-A is that clinical depression occurs in an interpersonal context, and that response to treatment is influenced by the relationship between the patient and significant others.

Family Therapy: Referral for family therapy is sometimes indicated and may be particularly helpful when family communication problems contribute to the youth's feelings of distress and inability to involve family in an adequate safety plan.

J. Clinical Course: It is recommended, for prevention of relapse, that antidepressant treatment be continued for 7 to 9 months. Clinically referred youths with major depression will have a median episode duration of 8 months, whereas community samples experience a median duration of 1 to 2 months. Nearly all children and adolescents will recover from their first depressive

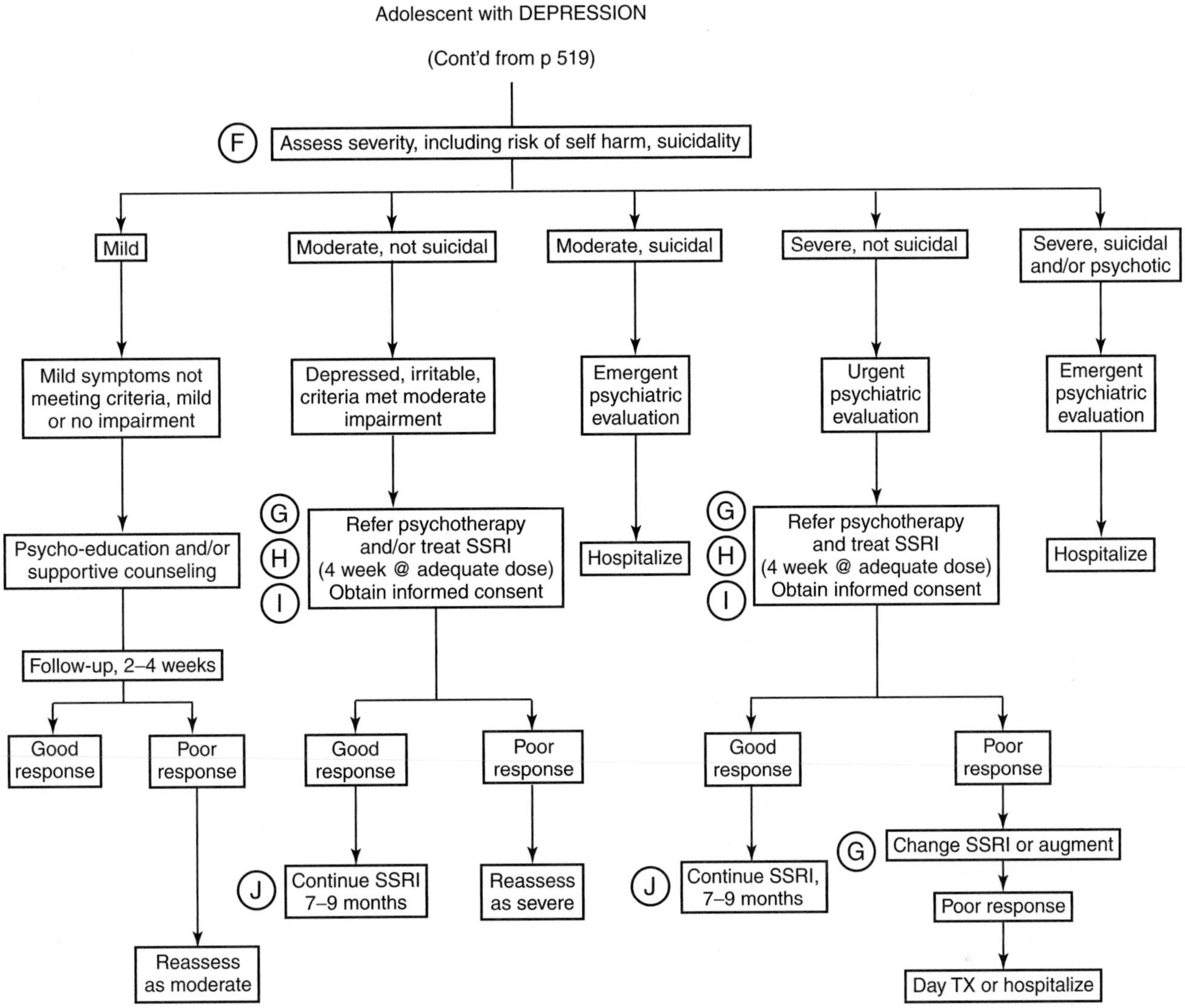
Adolescent with DEPRESSION
(Cont'd from p 519)
F
Assess severity, including risk of self harm, suicidality
Mild
Moderate, not suicidal
Moderate, suicidal
Severe, not suicidal
Severe, suicidal and/or psychotic
Mild symptoms not meeting criteria, mild or no impairment
Depressed, irritable, criteria met moderate impairment
Emergent psychiatric evaluation
Urgent psychiatric evaluation
Emergent psychiatric evaluation
Psycho-education and/or supportive counseling
G
H
I
Refer psychotherapy and/or treat SSRI (4 week @ adequate dose) Obtain informed consent
Hospitalize
G
H
I
Refer psychotherapy and treat SSRI (4 week @ adequate dose) Obtain informed consent
Hospitalize
Follow-up, 2–4 weeks
Good response
Poor response
Good response
Poor response
Good response
Poor response
J
Continue SSRI 7–9 months
Reassess as severe
J
Continue SSRI, 7–9 months
G
Change SSRI or augment
Poor response
Reassess as moderate
Day TX or hospitalize

episode, but long-term studies show recurrence rates increasing to 70% after 5 years. A significant proportion of youths with MDD will continue to suffer from MDD during adulthood. Between 20% and 40% of pediatric patients with depression will develop bipolar disorder at some point. Those especially at risk include patients with concomitant psychotic features, family histories of bipolar, and those with histories of pharmacologically induced mania or hypomania. Children with dysthymia are likely to experience a prolonged course of illness, with a mean episode length of 3 to 4 years for clinical and community samples. In addition, this disorder is further associated with increased risk for subsequent development of MDD and substance abuse. Poor outcomes are associated with greater severity, chronicity, or recurrence, comorbid conditions, hopelessness, residual subsyndromal symptoms, pessimism, family discord, low socioeconomic status, and chronic environmental stressors (e.g., abuse, family conflict).

Table 1. **DSM-IV-TR Criteria for Major Depressive Episode and Dysthymic Disorder**

Major Depressive Episode

Five (or more) of the following symptoms must be present during the same 2-week period and represent a change from previous functioning; at least one of the symptoms is either (1) depressed mood or (2) loss of interest or pleasure.

Note: Do not include symptoms that are clearly caused by a general medical condition, or mood-incongruent delusions or hallucinations.

1. Depressed or irritable mood most of the time
2. Diminished interest or pleasure in most activities
3. Weight (or appetite) loss or gain
4. Insomnia or hypersomnia nearly every day
5. Psychomotor agitation or retardation observed by others
6. Fatigue/energy loss nearly every day
7. Feelings of worthlessness or inappropriate guilt
8. Decreased concentration or indecisiveness
9. Recurrent thoughts of death or suicidal ideation

Dysthymic Disorder

Depressed or irritable mood for most of the time for at least 1 year. Presence, while depressed, of at least two of the following:

1. Poor appetite or overeating
2. Insomnia or hypersomnia
3. Fatigue or low energy
4. Low self-esteem
5. Poor concentration or difficulty making decisions
6. Feelings of hopelessness

Based on American Psychiatric Association. Diagnostic and statistical manual of mental disorders (DSM-IV-TR). 4th ed [text revision]. Washington, DC: American Psychiatric Association; 2000.

Table 2. **The Suicidal/Self-Harming Adolescent**

Complete a thorough psychiatric assessment, including:

- Interviewing teen separately from parents
- Adopting an empathic and nonjudgmental demeanor
- Observing for signs of acute self-harm, scarring, bruises
- Identifying significant psychiatric symptoms, particularly depression, psychosis, substance abuse
- Asking about acute stressors (e.g., breakup)
- Assessing recent and prior self-harming issues

  Self-injury: episodes, frequency, duration, precipitants

  Suicidal thoughts: plans, frequency, duration, precipitants

  Suicide attempts: previous attempts, methods, consequences

  Suicide intent: past and present desire to die
- Asking about homicidal thoughts and determining any "duty to warn"

Obtain additional information:

- From parents/family, caseworkers, teachers, and others
- By observing family interaction and identifying conflicts impacting safety
- Consider urine toxicology screen, pregnancy test, in addition to physical examination and "routine" labs

Consider outpatient treatment when there are <u>no</u> suicidal thoughts or plans, <u>no</u> prior suicide attempts, <u>no</u> medical problems requiring hospital care, <u>no</u> significant substance abuse problems, and <u>no</u> significant psychiatric disorders needing stabilization.

And there is a parent/guardian that will be home to monitor safety and relationship is positive and stable, a plan for the youth to communicate dangerous or overwhelmed feelings to the parent, stabilization of any precipitating conflicts, psychotherapy will begin or continue, parents are aware of alcohol/drug risks (e.g., increasing impulsivity and decreasing inhibitions) and will limit access, parent will remove lethal items (e.g., firearms) from home, parent and youth agree with a safety plan (including use of emergency services if the situation deteriorates), and follow-up services have been scheduled.

Consider inpatient treatment when there are continuing suicidal thoughts, specific suicidal plans, needs for further assessment in a safe environment, previous suicide attempts, severe depressive symptoms, significant psychiatric symptoms (e.g., psychosis), past impulsive and dangerous behaviors, substance abuse problems present with depression and/or self-harm, difficulties forming an alliance with the clinician, difficulties participating in the assessment of safety, and significant conflicts with family/significant other.

References

American Academy of Child and Adolescent Psychiatry. Practice parameter for the assessment and treatment of children and adolescents with depressive disorders. J Am Acad Child Adolesc Psychiatry 2007;46:1503–26.

American Academy of Child and Adolescent Psychiatry. Practice parameter for the assessment and treatment of children and adolescents with suicidal behavior. J Am Acad Child Adolesc Psychiatry 2001;40(Suppl 7):24S–51S.

American Psychiatric Association. Diagnostic and statistical manual of mental disorders (DSM-IV-TR). 4th ed [text revision]. Washington, DC: American Psychiatric Association; 2000.

Anderson RN. Deaths: leading causes for 2000. Natl Vital Stat Rep 2002;50:1–85.

Bridge J, Axelson D. The contribution of pharmacoepidemiology to the antidepressant-suicidality debate in children and adolescents. Int Rev Psychiatry 2008;20(2):209–14.

Brunstein Klomek A, Stanley B. Psychosocial treatment of depression and suicidality in adolescents. CNS Spectr 2007;12(2):135–44.

Centers for Disease Control and Prevention. Web-based injury statistics query and reporting system (WISQARS). <http://www.cdc.gov/ncipc/wisqars>; 2011 [accessed 30.06.08].

Emslie G, Kennard BD, Mayes TL, et al. Fluoxetine versus placebo in preventing relapse of major depression in children and adolescents. Am J Psychiatry 2008;165:459–67.

Emslie GJ, Ventura D, Korotzer A, Tourkodimitris S. Escitalopram in the treatment of adolescent depression: A randomized placebo controlled multisite trial. J Am Acad Child Adolesc Psychiatry 2009;48:721–729.

Hammad TA. Results of the analysis of suicidality in pediatric trials of newer antidepressants. Psychopharmacology Drugs Advisory Committee and the Pediatric Advisory Committee, September 13–14, 2004. <www.fda.gov/ohrms/dockets/ac/04/briefing/2004-4065b1-10-TAB08-Hammads-review.pdf>; 2004 [accessed 15.02.2009].

Hughes C, Emslie G, Crismon ML, et al. Texas children's medication algorithm project: update from Texas consensus conference panel on medication treatment of childhood major depressive disorder. J Am Acad Child Adolesc Psychiatry 2007;46(6):667–86.

Kratochvil C, Vitiello B, Walkup J, et al. Selective serotonin reuptake inhibitors in pediatric depression: is the balance between benefits and risks favorable? J Child Adolesc Psychopharm 2006;16(1):11–24.

Libby A, Brent DA, Morrato EH, et al. Decline in treatment of pediatric depression after FDA advisory on risk of suicidality with SSRIs. Am J Psychiatry 2007;164:884–91.

National Center for Health Statistics. Health, United States, 2006; Centers for Disease Control and Prevention. <http://www.cdc.gov/nchs/data/hus/hus06.pdf#062>; 2006 [accessed 13.03.08].

National Library of Medicine (NLM). DailyMed: current medication information. <http://dailymed.nlm.nih.gov/dailymed/about.cfm>; 2009 [accessed 29.06.09].

Physicians' desk reference 2009. 63rd ed. Montvale, NJ: Physician's Desk Reference Inc; 2008.

Sutton J. Prevention of depression in youth: a qualitative review and future suggestions. Clin Psychol 2007;27(5):552–71.

TADS Team. Fluoxetine, cognitive-behavioral therapy, and their combination for adolescents with depression: treatment for adolescents with depression study (TADS) randomized, controlled trial. JAMA 2004;292:807–20.

World Health Organization. International classification of diseases (ICD-10). 10th revision. Geneva, Switzerland: World Health Organization; 1992.

Developmental Delay in Children Younger Than 6 Years

William Campbell, MD

Developmental delay (DD) is a condition in which a child is delayed in achieving milestones in any of the major domains of development: motor, language, cognitive/problem solving, adaptive/self-help, and social skills. In this chapter, DD also refers to atypical development—that is, patterns of development not typical for a child of any age (e.g., as in autism spectrum disorders). About 12% of infants, toddlers, and preschoolers have significant delays in at least one area of development, and about 2% have delays in two or more domains (global DD).

Although DD in some young children appears to be temporary (i.e., they eventually "catch up" to normal), DD often is the first sign of a lifelong developmental disability (e.g., intellectual disability, formerly referred to as mental retardation). In many cases, children's delays are due to a combination of environmental and biological (including genetic) factors, resulting in chronic central nervous system dysfunction, with a slower rate of development. In addition to addressing health conditions contributing to DD, early intervention and early childhood special education services (under the Individuals with Disabilities Education Act [IDEA]) can help achieve optimal outcomes.

The American Academy of Pediatrics (AAP) has summarized specific recommendations in a policy statement ("Identifying Infants and Young Children with Developmental Disorders in the Medical Home: An Algorithm for Developmental Surveillance and Screening." Pediatrics 2006:118(1):405–20).

A. Survey development and behavior at every health care visit. Elicit parent concerns about development and behavior (e.g., "Do you have any questions or concerns about your child's development or behavior?"); document the developmental history; make accurate observations; identify risk factors and protective factors; and maintain accurate records of the process and findings.

B. Part C of IDEA requires states to provide early intervention services to infants and toddlers who have conditions of "established risk," defined as a "diagnosed physical or mental condition which has a high probability of resulting in developmental delay." These conditions include, but are not limited to, chromosomal abnormalities, genetic or congenital disorders, severe sensory impairments (including hearing and vision), inborn errors of metabolism, disorders reflecting disturbance of the development of the nervous system, congenital infections, disorders secondary to exposure to toxic substances (including fetal alcohol syndrome), and severe attachment disorders. Such infants and toddlers may be eligible for services by virtue of their diagnosis, regardless of whether a measurable delay is present.

Some biological/medical risk factors do not always lead to DD, but affected children warrant more frequent developmental screening and early referral. Examples include prematurity, low birth weight, intraventricular hemorrhage, chronic lung disease, failure to thrive, and a family history of developmental problems.

Environmental risk factors include child abuse or neglect, poverty, homelessness, family social disorganization, and parental age, educational attainment, developmental disability, and substance abuse.

Protective factors include child temperament (happy, easygoing), high self-esteem, a history of successful learning experiences, and a satisfactory emotional relationship with at least one parent/caregiver.

C. Screen for DD using appropriate standardized instruments if the young child has developmental risk factors. Do general screening at the 9-month (or 12-month) visit, 18-month visit, and 30-month (or 24-month) visit, and also do autism-specific screening (see Autism Spectrum Disorder, p. 514) at the 18- and 24-month visits, even if there are no risk factors or parent/clinical concerns. General developmental screening tools include the Ages & Stages Questionnaires (ASQ) and the Parents' Evaluation of Developmental Status (PEDS), although the latter is more of a prescreening, developmental surveillance instrument. Autism-specific screening tools include the Modified Checklist for Autism in Toddlers (M-CHAT) and the Social Communication Questionnaire (SCQ). Additional screening tools are listed in the AAP policy statement noted earlier.

D. If the results of developmental screening are concerning, or if there are parent or clinician concerns for DD, further evaluation is indicated. Such children should simultaneously (1) be referred to local early intervention or special education agencies, and (2) undergo appropriate medical evaluation.

E. The age of the child will determine where to refer for educational and developmental intervention services. Child Find is a component of IDEA that requires states to identify, locate, and evaluate all children with disabilities, aged birth to 21, who are in need of early intervention or special education services. In most states, children 3 years of age and older are served by their local public school districts, whereas infants and toddlers from birth to 36 months of age are served by their statewide system of early intervention services. Primary pediatric health care clinicians should be familiar with their local resources. It is helpful for the public school and early intervention teams to have copies of the standardized developmental screening instrument and results to avoid unnecessary rescreening and to help inform the assessment.

In general, early intervention and Child Find evaluation teams assess all areas of development. A delay in one domain suggests the possibility of delays in others. The developmental/educational assessment results are used to help determine eligibility for early intervention or special education services (Parts C and B of IDEA, respectively).

(Continued on page 526)

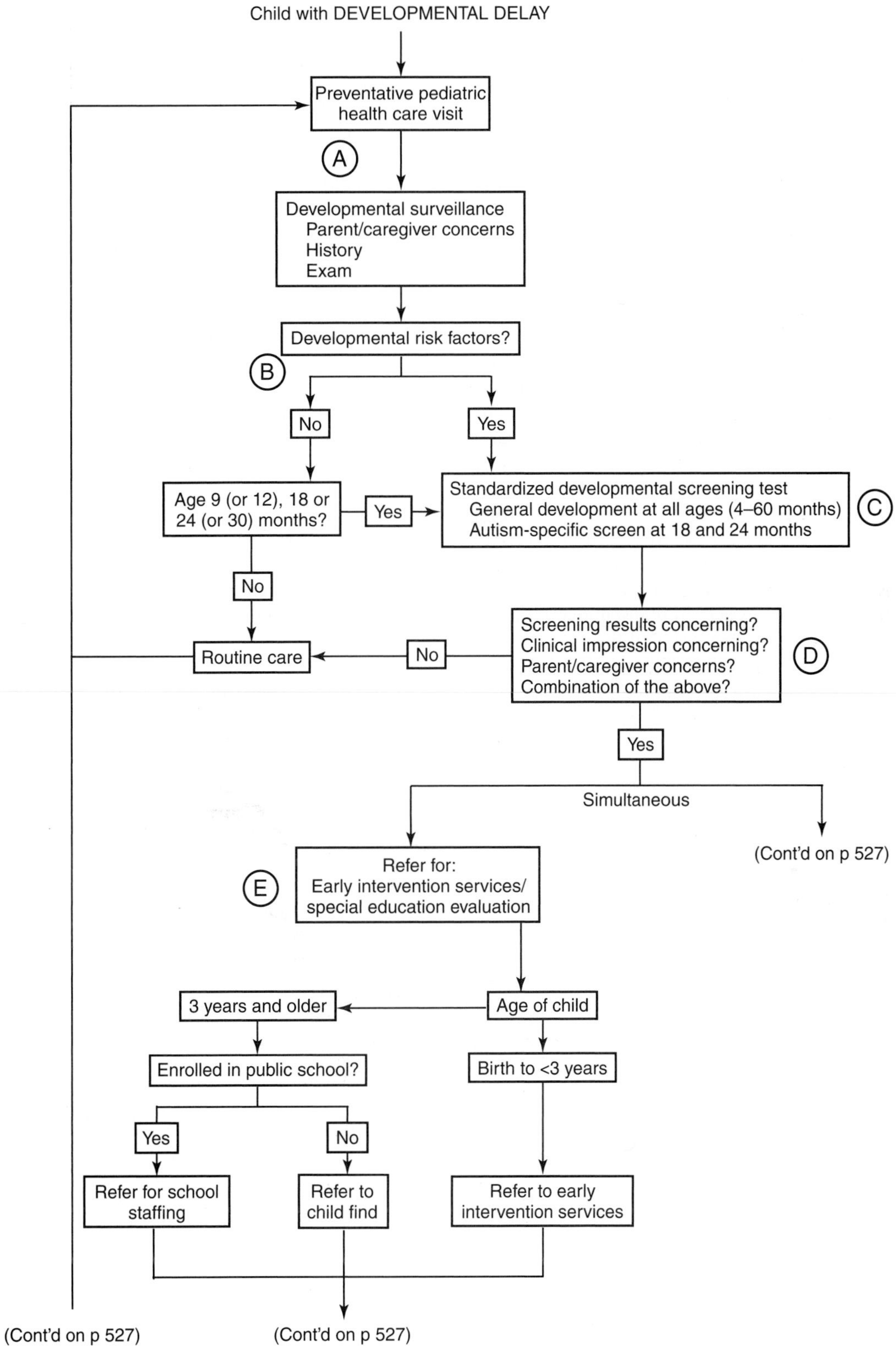
Child with DEVELOPMENTAL DELAY
Preventative pediatric health care visit
A
Developmental surveillance
Parent/caregiver concerns
History
Exam
Developmental risk factors?
B
No
Yes
Age 9 (or 12), 18 or 24 (or 30) months?
Yes
Standardized developmental screening test
General development at all ages (4–60 months)
Autism-specific screen at 18 and 24 months
C
No
Routine care
No
Screening results concerning?
Clinical impression concerning?
Parent/caregiver concerns?
Combination of the above?
D
Yes
Simultaneous
(Cont'd on p 527)
E
Refer for:
Early intervention services/
special education evaluation
3 years and older
Age of child
Enrolled in public school?
Birth to <3 years
Yes
No
Refer for school staffing
Refer to child find
Refer to early intervention services
(Cont'd on p 527)
(Cont'd on p 527)

F. Appropriate medical workup can begin as soon as there are significant developmental concerns but should not delay referral for early intervention or special education assessments and services. The health history and physical examination may reveal genetic risk factors, conditions associated with a high probability of delay, or conditions that might adversely affect development. Impairments of vision and hearing should be ruled out in all children with DD. Formal hearing evaluation (at least annually) by an audiologist is indicated for children with communication delay or impairment.

The medical workup may include not only a search for the cause of the delay, to help inform treatment and family recurrence risk, but also an evaluation to find one or more neurodevelopmental diagnoses, such as cerebral palsy, autism, particular genetic syndromes, or global DD. Some of these conditions are discussed elsewhere in this textbook.

For children with global DD, the workup will depend on the severity of delays, among other factors. Consultation from specialists is frequently warranted (e.g., neurology, genetics, metabolic disease, rehabilitation medicine, developmental pediatrics).

G. Even after a comprehensive multidisciplinary assessment by an early intervention or Child Find team, additional diagnostic developmental evaluation is often needed to further quantify the degree of delay and to help arrive at a medical diagnosis. The early intervention/Child Find assessments generally do not directly result in medical diagnoses such as autism or cerebral palsy, but the assessment results often help the primary health care clinician arrive at a diagnosis and/or determine additional workup and treatment needs.

The disciplines involved in the diagnostic developmental evaluation are often the same as those who participated in the early intervention/Child Find assessment, for example, Speech-Language Pathology, Child Psychology, and Occupational/Physical Therapy. These diagnostic developmental team evaluations can be done by local or visiting teams in relatively small communities, but are also done in larger communities in various clinics (high-risk infant follow-up clinics, physical medicine and rehabilitation, neurology, developmental pediatrics). Primary care clinicians should be familiar with local resources and referral centers. If in doubt about where to refer, it is generally best to ask a colleague or a specialist at the clinic under consideration, so that the appropriate evaluation is done as soon as possible.

H. Young children with DD should receive the same clinical consideration as children with chronic special health care needs and should be followed more frequently than healthy, typically developing children. Specific information about the medical workup of young children with global DD can be found on the American Academy of Neurology's Web site (http://www.aan.com) in the Practice Guidelines section.

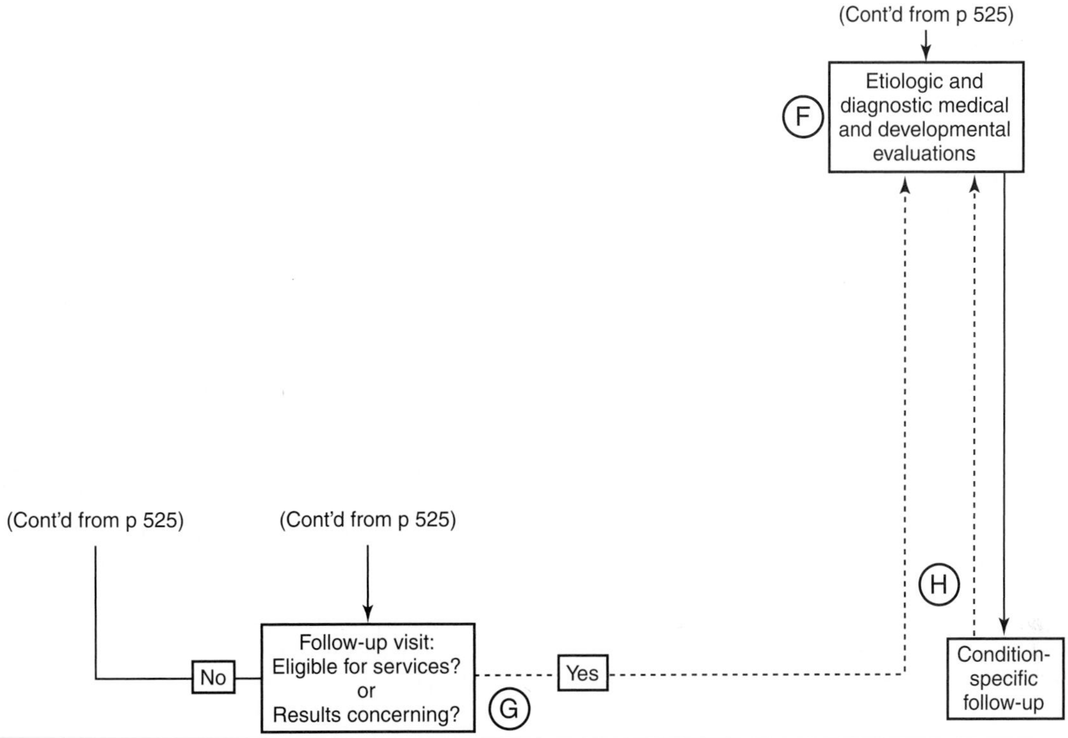
(Cont'd from p 525)
F
Etiologic and diagnostic medical and developmental evaluations
(Cont'd from p 525)
(Cont'd from p 525)
H
No
Follow-up visit: Eligible for services? or Results concerning?
Yes
G
Condition-specific follow-up

References

Council on Children With Disabilities; Section on Developmental Behavioral Pediatrics; Bright Futures Steering Committee; Medical Home Initiatives for Children With Special Needs Project Advisory Committee. Pediatrics 2006 Jul;118(1):405-20. Erratum in: Pediatrics 2006 Oct;118(4):1808–9.

American Academy of Pediatrics, Committee on Children with Disabilities. The pediatrician's role in development and implementation of an Individual Education Plan (IEP) and/or Individual Family Service Plan (IFSP). Pediatrics 1999 Jul;104(1 Pt 1): 124–7.

School Learning Problems

William Campbell, MD

A. About 11% of schoolchildren have learning disorders and/or school failure. The history may reveal family genetic risk factors, prenatal and perinatal exposures and events, acute or chronic health conditions (e.g., seizures, concussions, meningitis/encephalitis, insufficient sleep, anemia, lead), and psychosocial risk factors (e.g., low self-esteem, family conflict, bullying). Many children with learning difficulties have a history of early developmental delay. Screen for behavior and attention problems (especially attention-deficit/hyperactivity disorder [ADHD]).

B. The neurologic examination and general physical examination may point to acute or chronic conditions associated with poor academic performance. Especially if there has been a recent deterioration in behavior or academic performance, look for focal neurologic findings (e.g., acquired torticollis, strabismus, ataxia). Dysmorphic features may suggest a particular genetic syndrome; more than four minor dysmorphic features can be a nonspecific marker of learning problems.

C. Have the parent bring copies of report cards, and, if applicable, current (and prior) Individualized Education Program (IEP), early intervention records, and results of academic achievement testing, psychological/educational testing (e.g., intelligence quotient [IQ] and/or learning testing), and any other pertinent information. Ask for a letter from the classroom teacher summarizing the student's main school problems; how the student behaves, pays attention, and completes academic work; and how the student interacts with peers and staff. It is sometimes helpful to get an additional letter from the student's teacher from the prior school year. Arrange to have an ADHD-specific behavior rating scale completed by the teacher and returned for clinician review at the first or follow-up visit.

D. Look for discrepancies between (1) the current year and prior years, (2) performance and effort/behavior, (3) grades in various subject areas, (4) report card grades and achievement test scores, and (5) grades and cognitive scores. Significant discrepancies between ability and academic achievement suggest a learning disability. Clinicians should be aware that each state department of education uses its own discrepancy definition. Poor physical health, emotional disorders, difficult psychosocial circumstances, and neurobehavioral disorders such as ADHD may also account for discrepancies between ability and performance.

E. If a discrepancy is present, the family should request a formal meeting with the school staff, involving the classroom teacher, a school administrator, and special education staff, including professionals in the area of concern. The school teams involved in such meetings are variously referred to as Case Study Teams, Student Study Teams, Student Success Teams, and so on, depending on the locality.

It is important for parents to know that they have the right under special education law (the Individuals with Disabilities Education Act [IDEA]) to request a comprehensive educational evaluation, and that the school must do this within a specified amount of time. However, it is usually in the best interests of the student and everyone else to simply have the parents meet with the school staff, mention their concerns, and go from there. School staff will likely want to make further classroom observations and try one or more interventions to gain a better understanding of the student's strengths and weaknesses. This information will be important in developing an appropriate educational assessment plan.

Parents should also know that they are not required to pay out of pocket or use health insurance for any portion of the evaluation included on the school's assessment plan, even though the school is allowed to ask the parents to do so. In many cases, medical and clinical child psychological questions are not included on the school assessment plan, or the plan states that the parents will pursue these evaluations on their own.

F. Students functioning close to expectations may have cognitive abilities ranging from low-normal to disabled. "Intellectual disability" is a term that is replacing "mental retardation," although the latter is still in common use, including within state departments of human services. The clinician should help the family understand the student's slower rate of learning and help ensure that the student's education program is appropriate.

G. All children are entitled under IDEA to a free and appropriate public school education, including appropriate evaluations and services. Not all children with learning difficulties are eligible for (or need) an IEP; school staff may develop a 504 Plan (in accordance with Section 504 of the Americans with Disabilities Act) for children with disabling health conditions such as ADHD. Under Section 504, if parents believe their child has a disability (whether by ADHD or any other impairment) and if the school staff has reason to believe the child needs special education or related services, the school must evaluate the child to determine whether he or she is disabled as defined by Section 504.

H. Clinicians' schedules generally do not allow them to attend IEP meetings. But clinicians can still monitor the student's progress, screen for health and psychosocial conditions that might impede academic progress, and advocate for the student. Resources are available on the Internet and in print to help parents understand their rights under special education law.

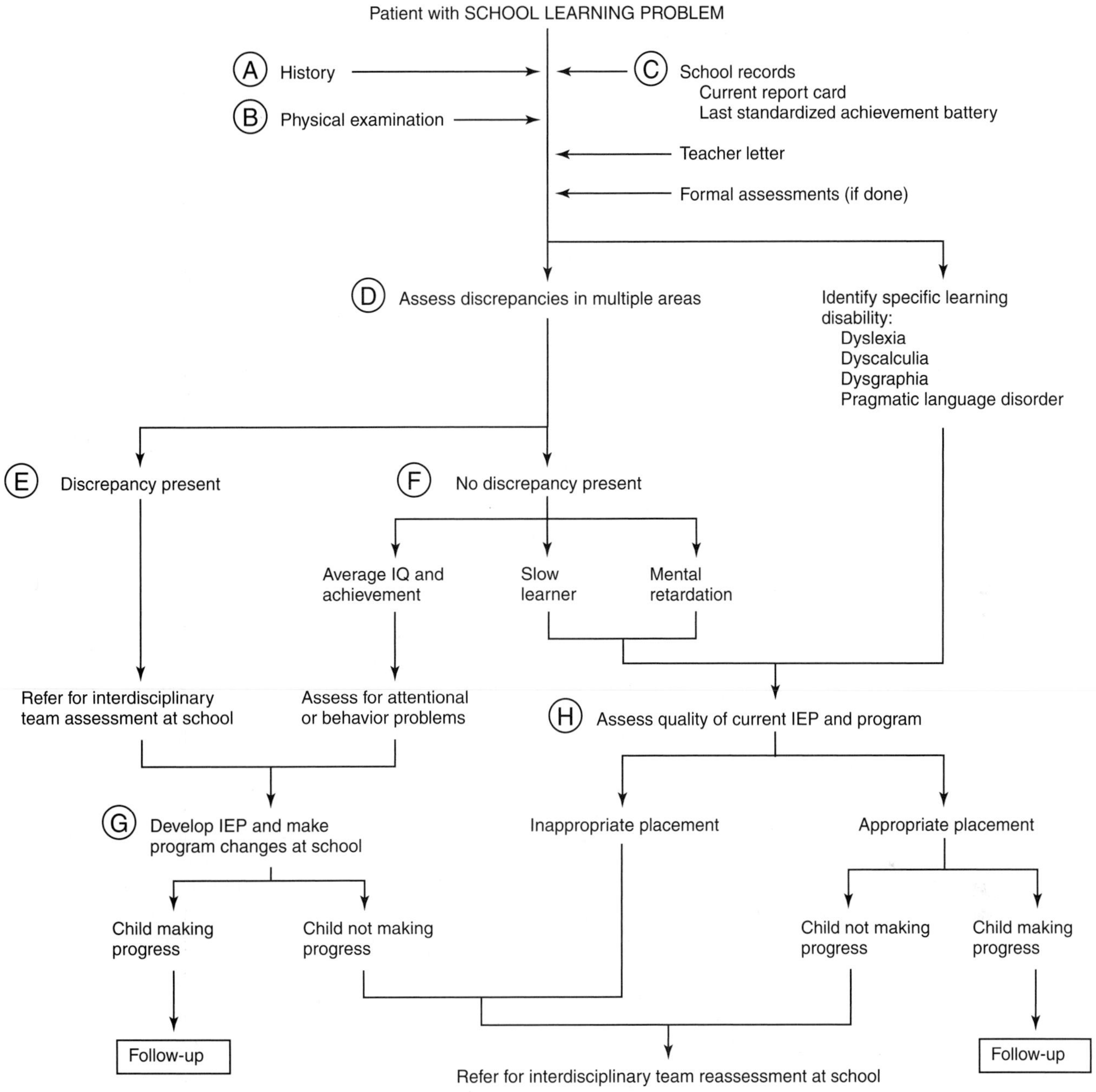
Patient with SCHOOL LEARNING PROBLEM
A History
B Physical examination
C School records
Current report card
Last standardized achievement battery
Teacher letter
Formal assessments (if done)
D Assess discrepancies in multiple areas
Identify specific learning disability:
Dyslexia
Dyscalculia
Dysgraphia
Pragmatic language disorder
E Discrepancy present
F No discrepancy present
Average IQ and achievement
Slow learner
Mental retardation
Refer for interdisciplinary team assessment at school
Assess for attentional or behavior problems
H Assess quality of current IEP and program
G Develop IEP and make program changes at school
Inappropriate placement
Appropriate placement
Child making progress
Child not making progress
Child not making progress
Child making progress
Follow-up
Refer for interdisciplinary team reassessment at school
Follow-up

References

American Academy of Pediatrics, Section on Ophthalmology, Council on Children with Disabilities; American Academy of Ophthalmology; American Association for Pediatric Ophthalmology and Strabismus; American Association of Certified Orthoptists. Joint statement—learning disabilities, dyslexia, and vision. Pediatrics 2009;124:837–44.

American Academy of Pediatrics, Committee on Children with Disabilities. The pediatrician's role in development and implementation of an Individual Education Plan (IEP) and/or Individual Family Service Plan (IFSP). Pediatrics 1999 Jul;104(1 Pt 1):124–7.

American Academy of Pediatrics Council on Children With Disabilities, Cartwright JD. Provision of educationally related services for children and adolescents with chronic diseases and disabling conditions. Pediatrics 2007 Jun;119(6):1218–23.

LD Online. www.ldonline.org; 2010 [accessed 01.04.2011].

Wrightslaw. www.wrightslaw.com; 2011 [accessed 01.04.2011].

Sleep Disturbances

Maida Lynn Chen, MD

One of the most common caregiver concerns in pediatric practices is sleep problems. Epidemiologic surveys have shown that up to 25% to 50% of preschool and 20% to 37% of elementary school children have some sort of caregiver-reported sleep problem. However, the definition of a "sleep problem" is highly subjective and often determined by the amount of disruption caused to the household. Regardless, children of all ages who have inadequate or disturbed sleep may or may not manifest with overt excessive daytime sleepiness; rather, many will have significant mood and behavioral problems (including hyperactivity), and neurocognitive performance impairments. Adult caregivers often also suffer from sleep deprivation and are at risk for significant sequelae including increased injuries (e.g., motor vehicle accident) and decreased ability to parent effectively and safely. Children with developmental delays are at greater risk for sleep disorders that go unrecognized and untreated. This chapter focuses primarily on the preschool- and elementary school-age child.

A. In the patient's history, include a review of any prenatal and perinatal problems, neurodevelopmental concerns, and respiratory problems including allergic rhinitis and asthma. To better characterize the sleep problem, consider using the BEARS questionnaire, which specifically assesses for *b*edtime problems, *e*xcessive daytime sleepiness, *a*wakenings at night, *r*egularity and duration of sleep, and *s*leep-disordered breathing. If caregivers are unable to give accurate reports, consider obtaining a 2-week sleep log/diary at this point before further assessments.

B. In the physical examination, focus on the otolaryngologic and respiratory examination, specifically looking at tonsils and nasal passages. Overall neurodevelopmental status and tone are important as well. Assess for mood and affect of the child, as well as close observation of the caregiver–child interaction.

C. If history is complex, or child has significant underlying comorbid conditions, consider referral to a sleep specialist.

D. Reports of snoring, neck hyperextension, mouth breathing, witnessed apneic pauses, or labored breathing during night, enuresis, or examinations revealing tonsillar hypertrophy, adenoidal facies, or other craniofacial abnormalities should prompt referral to a sleep specialist for diagnostic sleep study. Otolaryngology referral should also be considered.

E. Good sleep hygiene is the cornerstone of treatment for nearly all pediatric sleep problems. Ensure that the sleep environment is conducive to and associated with restful sleep: comfortable and appropriate bedding; quiet, darkened (nightlight acceptable); and set at a comfortable temperature (68°F to 72°F). Particular attention to "technology" (e.g., computers, cell phones, laptop computers, televisions, and video games) needs to be paid, and these should all be removed from the bedroom. Regular bedtimes and wake times should be enforced on school days with no more than an hour difference for nonschool days. Set a bedtime routine that includes quiet, relaxing activities that do not include high-energy physical exertion or any screen time (TV, videos, computers). Caffeinated products should be avoided altogether, but particularly in the afternoon hours. Regular exercise during the daytime (but not in the 2 hours before desired bedtime) should be a part of a child's daily routine. If possible, the bedroom, and specifically the bed, should be associated with sleep only; thus, do not use the room as a punishment or bed as a place to do homework

(Continued on page 532)

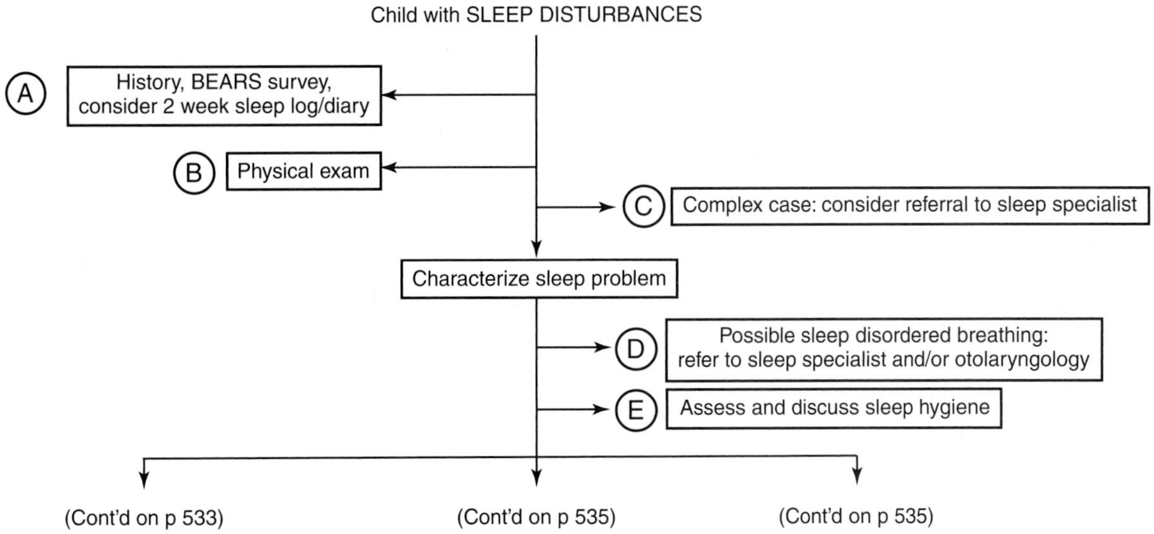
Child with SLEEP DISTURBANCES
A
History, BEARS survey, consider 2 week sleep log/diary
B
Physical exam
C
Complex case: consider referral to sleep specialist
Characterize sleep problem
D
Possible sleep disordered breathing: refer to sleep specialist and/or otolaryngology
E
Assess and discuss sleep hygiene
(Cont'd on p 533)
(Cont'd on p 535)
(Cont'd on p 535)

F. Restless legs syndrome is characterized by uncomfortable sensations in legs relieved by movement that occurs during periods of inactivity (sleep onset). There is often a strong family history. In young children, this may manifest by running, rubbing, complaining of "itchy" or "creepy/crawly" legs, and may be mislabeled as "growing pains." Eighty percent of those with restless legs syndrome also have periodic limb movements seen on a sleep study. Diagnosis and treatment should be directed by a sleep specialist, and may include treatment with supplemental iron based on low ferritin levels or dopamine agonists.

G. Behavioral insomnia of childhood has two subtypes. Sleep-onset association disorders, where the child learns to fall asleep only under certain condition (e.g., being rocked, fed, parental presence), can manifest both at the beginning of the night and after nocturnal arousals. Brief, physiologic arousals from sleep turn into prolonged episodes of wakefulness if the child's sleep-onset association is not present. Limit-setting disorders are the other subtype, which are characterized by bedtime resistance (e.g., curtain calls) primarily at the beginning of the night. This often is based on parental inability to enforce regular bedtime habits. Treatment techniques for both include extinction (systematic ignoring), graduated extinction (progressively decreasing parental contact during these awakenings with limited interaction), and positive reinforcement. Bedtime fading can be used, which allows the child to sleep at his/her desired bedtime (thus avoiding struggles and the associated resistant behaviors), but then gradually moving the bedtime earlier to the desired time. Importantly, the best prevention for these problems is to have parents start putting their children to bed awake but drowsy during infancy, so that the children will learn self-soothing skills that they can use during initial sleep onset and after nocturnal awakenings.

H. Insomnia can be caused by a developmentally appropriate nighttime fear (e.g., monsters under the bed). Treatment for benign nighttime fears is based on reassuring the child that he/she is safe in the bedroom and encouraging communication. Behavioral strategies of developmentally appropriate coping skills are also recommended, such as security objects, nightlights, and reinforcing positive behaviors (e.g., sticker rewards). Creative solutions such as "monster spray," magic wands, or protective stuffed animals can also be used. Limit media venues containing violence, which can be present even in cartoons.

I. Assess for pathologic fears (e.g., worried about harm when abuse is present), a conditioned fear of not being able to sleep, or anxiety associated with daytime stressors or associated with comorbid conditions. Rarely is insomnia idiopathic in childhood. Conditioned insomnia is less common in younger children, but relaxation techniques and stimulus control can be attempted. For concern of pathologic fears, severe conditioned insomnia or generalized anxiety disorders, referral to a mental health specialist may be warranted.

J. Circadian disorders involve problems with a body's natural timing for sleep cycles. Circadian problems need to be distinguished from developmentally inappropriate bedtimes. They fall into three major categories: delayed (night owl), advanced (morning lark), and irregular (catnappers). The latter two are rare. Delayed sleep onset is considered physiologic during adolescence, which conflicts with most school start times. Treatment for delayed sleep onset includes enforcing strict sleep schedules without weekend deviations, exposure to early morning light, regular daytime exercise, and consideration for evening melatonin. Bedtime fading (see section G) can be used in conjunction with a strict wake time every day. Severe cases leading to significant daytime dysfunctions may need chronotherapy and should be referred to a sleep specialist.

(Continued on page 534)

Child with SLEEP DISTURBANCES

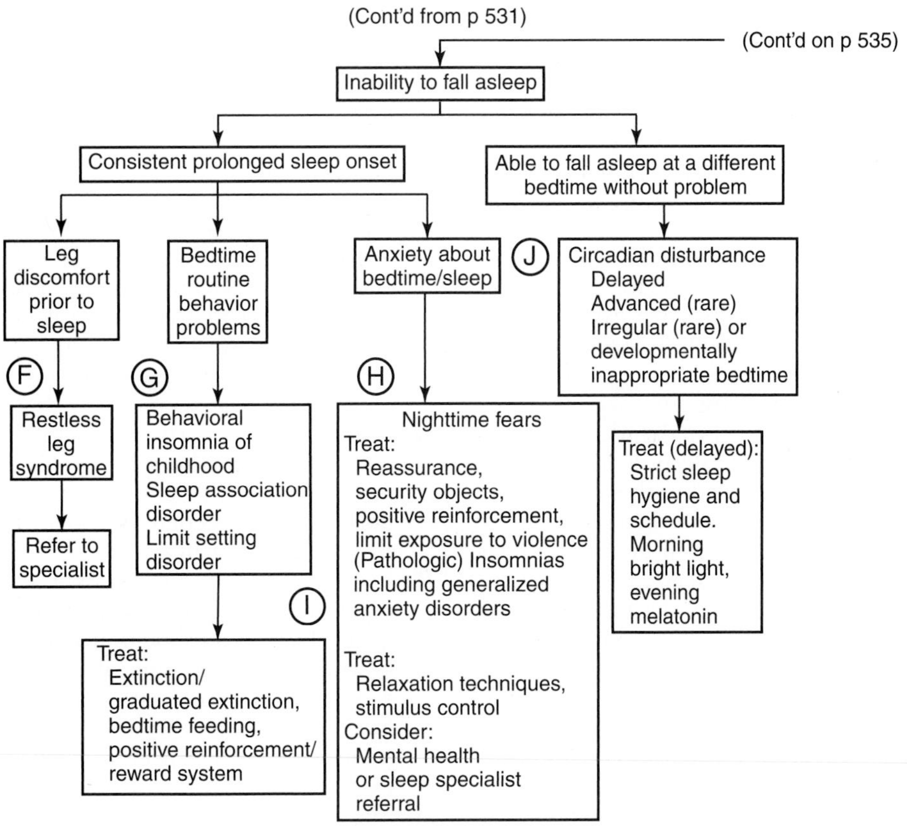
(Cont'd from p 531)
(Cont'd on p 535)
Inability to fall asleep
Consistent prolonged sleep onset
Able to fall asleep at a different bedtime without problem
Leg discomfort prior to sleep
Bedtime routine behavior problems
Anxiety about bedtime/sleep
J
Circadian disturbance
Delayed
Advanced (rare)
Irregular (rare) or developmentally inappropriate bedtime
F
G
H
Restless leg syndrome
Behavioral insomnia of childhood
Sleep association disorder
Limit setting disorder
Nighttime fears
Treat:
Reassurance, security objects, positive reinforcement, limit exposure to violence
(Pathologic) Insomnias including generalized anxiety disorders
Treat:
Relaxation techniques, stimulus control
Consider:
Mental health or sleep specialist referral
Treat (delayed):
Strict sleep hygiene and schedule.
Morning bright light, evening melatonin
Refer to specialist
I
Treat:
Extinction/ graduated extinction, bedtime feeding, positive reinforcement/ reward system

K. Assessments for medical conditions associated with nocturnal arousals should be pursued as indicated. Predisposing conditions include prematurity, in utero exposures including alcohol and illicit drugs, gastroesophageal reflux, seizures, neurobehavioral disorders such as attention-deficit/hyperactivity disorder and autism, atopic conditions including asthma, allergies, eczema, and congenital heart defects. Medications must also be considered such as steroids, beta agonists, psychoactive agents, and stimulants.

L. Parasomnias are episodic, partial arousals out of slow-wave sleep in the first third of the night, and include night terrors and sleep walking. Children have no recall of the events. Healthy, developmentally normal children may have these events, which can occur regularly in up to 4% of children. However, triggers may include a primary sleep disorder such as sleep disordered breathing, or be exacerbated by acute sleep deprivation. No specific treatment is usually needed, as these are usually self-limited. However, during these episodes, parents should be counseled to NOT awaken the child, which can prolong the agitation, but rather to focus on the child's safety (gates, alarms systems, locks, uncluttered floors) and sleep hygiene. Negative reinforcement should be avoided. Rarely, pharmacologic treatment is needed.

M. Rhythmic movement disorders include head banging and body rocking, which occur as self-soothing mechanisms during wake/sleep transitions. Both are frequent and can be present in some form in up to 15% of children. Treatment is based on minimizing the number of sleep/wake transitions by ensuring adequate sleep with good sleep hygiene, and also ensuring the child's safety. Evaluation for occult sleep-disordered breathing or other organic sleep disorder may need to be considered.

N. Restless sleep with frequent movements, position changes, or being a "light" sleeper may herald an otherwise undiagnosed sleep disorder such as sleep-disordered breathing or periodic limb movements. If history does not provide a clear diagnostic picture, consider referral to a sleep specialist for a sleep study to obtain more objective information.

O. Nightmares are "bad dreams," and children have full recall of them. They tend to occur during the later third of the night when rapid eye movement (REM) sleep is predominant. Nightmares are usually developmentally appropriate. Treatment includes child reassurance by parents that "it was only a dream" and encouraging the child to go back to sleep in his or her own bed. Using "dream catchers," magic wands, protective stuffed animals, or nightlights may also be comforting. Reducing exposure to violence, frightening or overstimulating images in media venues, increasing adequate sleep, encouraging relaxation before sleep, and good sleep hygiene all help to decrease the likelihood of nightmares.

P. Conditioned awakenings in the middle of the night likely fall under the behavioral insomnia category (see section G).

Q. Excessive daytime sleepiness may be primary or secondary. Should there be coexisting complaints of nocturnal disturbances, the excessive daytime sleepiness is likely secondary. Follow the algorithm for nocturnal complaints.

R. Excessive daytime sleepiness in the absence of overt nocturnal complaints, and in the presence of adequate sleep hours should prompt a referral to a sleep specialist for evaluation of an occult sleep disorder causing disturbed sleep or a hypersomnia including narcolepsy. Narcolepsy is rare in childhood but does occur and does not need accompanying cataplexy for diagnosis.

S. The most common cause of daytime sleepiness in children is inadequate sleep. Younger children outgrow daily naps at varying times, and if sleepy during the day, may still require a regular nap. Older children may have school and extracurricular demands that prevent adequate sleep; even adolescents still require 9 hours of sleep a night, but most obtain only 7. Parental work schedules may interfere with physiologically appropriate sleep and wake times, causing inadequate sleep. Children thrive on schedules and regularity, and particularly for those suffering the consequences of sleep deprivation, these schedules should be made a priority for the entire family.

(Continued on page 536)

Child with SLEEP DISTURBANCES

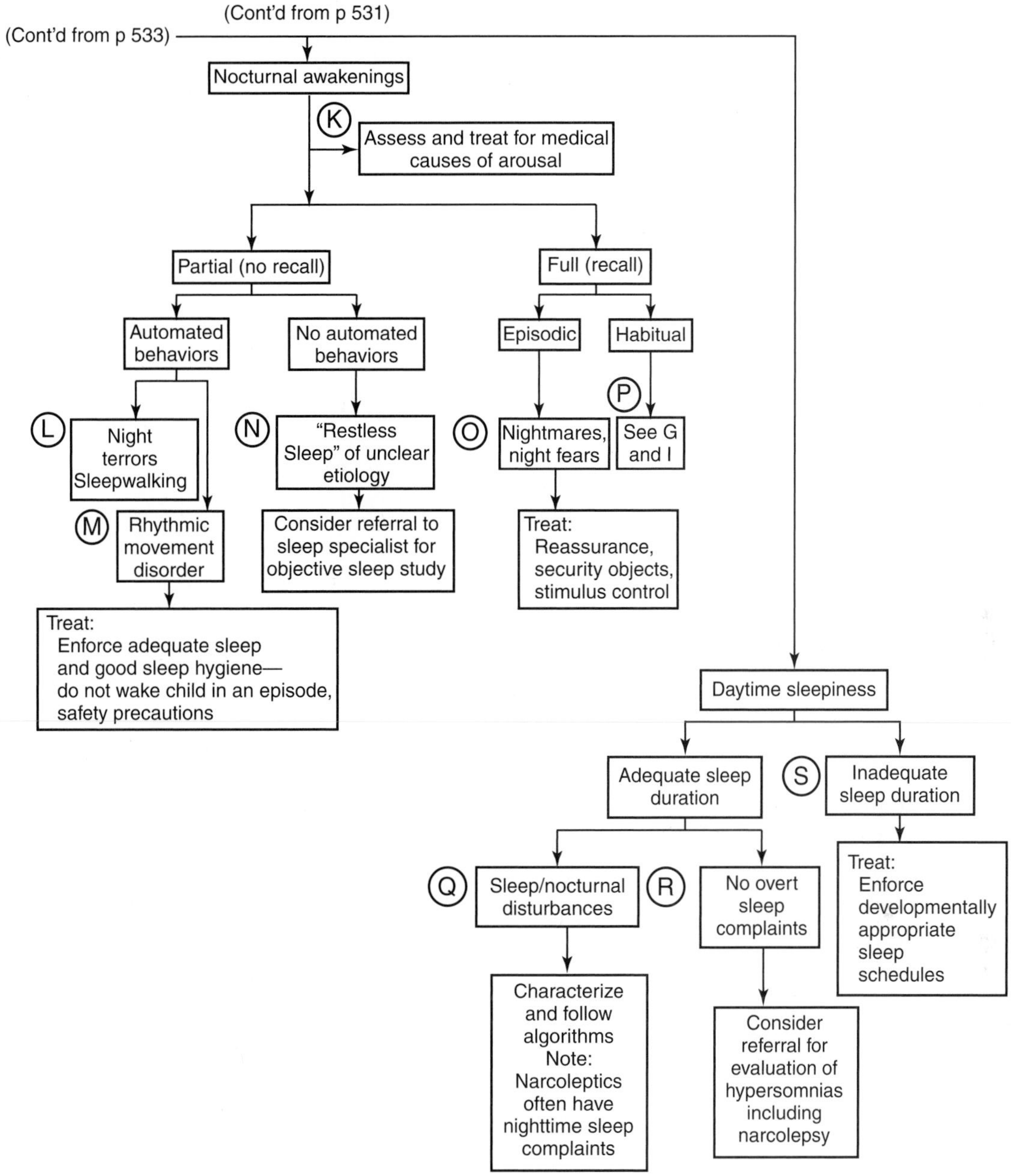
(Cont'd from p 531)
(Cont'd from p 533)
Nocturnal awakenings
K
Assess and treat for medical causes of arousal
Partial (no recall)
Full (recall)
Automated behaviors
No automated behaviors
Episodic
Habitual
P
L
Night terrors Sleepwalking
N
"Restless Sleep" of unclear etiology
O
Nightmares, night fears
See G and I
M
Rhythmic movement disorder
Consider referral to sleep specialist for objective sleep study
Treat: Reassurance, security objects, stimulus control
Treat: Enforce adequate sleep and good sleep hygiene— do not wake child in an episode, safety precautions
Daytime sleepiness
Adequate sleep duration
S
Inadequate sleep duration
Q
Sleep/nocturnal disturbances
R
No overt sleep complaints
Treat: Enforce developmentally appropriate sleep schedules
Characterize and follow algorithms Note: Narcoleptics often have nighttime sleep complaints
Consider referral for evaluation of hypersomnias including narcolepsy

References

Chervin R, Archbold K, Panahi P, Pituch K. Sleep problems seldom addressed in two general pediatric clinics. Pediatrics 2001;107:1375–80.

Kerr S, Jowett S. Sleep problems in pre-school children; a review of the literature. Child Care Health Dev 1994;20:379–91.

Mindell J, Owens J. A clinical guide to pediatric sleep: diagnosis and management of sleep problems in children and adolescents. Philadelphia: Lippincott Williams & Wilkins; 2003.

Owens J, Spirito A, Mguinn M, Nobile C. Sleep habits and sleep disturbance in school-aged children. J Dev Behav Pediatr 2000;21:27–36.

Owens J, Witmans M. Sleep problems. Curr Probl Pediatr Adolesc Health Care 2004;34:154–79.

Cardiovascular Disorders

Cyanotic Heart Disease

Rheumatic Fever

Cyanotic Heart Disease

Jesse Davidson, MD, and Michael S. Schaffer, MD

Cyanosis is a bluish discoloration of the skin and mucous membranes resulting from increased concentrations of deoxygenated hemoglobin in the circulation. In this chapter, cyanosis refers to central cyanosis (seen best in the mucous membranes), as opposed to peripheral or circumoral cyanosis, which are caused by changes in perfusion. Central cyanosis is observed when the absolute level of deoxygenated hemoglobin reaches 3 to 5 g per 100 ml blood. Clinical appearance of cyanosis therefore depends not only on the relative levels of oxygenated to deoxygenated hemoglobin but on the total number of grams of hemoglobin. For example, polycythemic patients may have a normal percentage of reduced hemoglobin but still have a cyanotic appearance because of an absolute increase in deoxygenated hemoglobin. Cyanosis due to a relative increase in deoxygenated hemoglobin may have several different etiologies: inadequate alveolar ventilation, ventilation-perfusion mismatch, abnormal hemoglobin, increased extraction of oxygen from the peripheral tissues, or right-to-left shunt (e.g., cyanotic heart disease, pulmonary arteriovenous malformations). All patients, especially neonates, with central cyanosis of unknown cause should be evaluated for the presence of congenital heart disease.

A. In the patient's history, document frequency, onset, and duration of cyanosis. Assess for any associated symptoms such as tachypnea, dyspnea, hypercyanotic spells, excessive fussiness or crying, sweating, or pallor. Ask about precipitating factors, such as feeding, exercise, bathing, apnea, or seizures. Review any abnormal obstetric or perinatal history. Note in the family history any genetic diseases and syndromes that have increased incidence of congenital heart disease.

B. In the physical examination, assess the general appearance of the patient. Decide whether the child shows evidence of significant respiratory distress (tachypnea with retractions or nasal flaring) or shock (pallor, lethargy, poor pulses/capillary refill). Obtain a full set of vital signs including heart rate, blood pressure (four extremities), respiratory rate, and preductal/postductal oxygen saturations. Next, differentiate central cyanosis from peripheral cyanosis. Assess the respiratory status for evidence of airway compromise, respiratory insufficiency, and pulmonary signs of heart failure (rales/wheezing/grunting). Perform a thorough cardiovascular examination including cardiac auscultation, assessment of peripheral pulses/perfusion, and examination of the neck and abdomen for evidence of right-heart failure (jugular venous distension or hepatomegaly). Pay particular attention to any murmurs, abnormalities of S2 (loud, fixed split, or single), gallops, and femoral pulses. Complete the remainder of the examination looking closely for evidence of dysmorphic features that might indicate the presence of a genetic syndrome. These findings may help determine a cause of the cyanosis.

C. Diagnostic tests for evaluating infants with cyanosis should include at minimum complete blood count (CBC) with differential, chest radiograph, and preductal/postductal oxygen saturation measurement with a pulse oximeter. If congenital heart disease is suspected, electrocardiogram (ECG), hyperoxia test, and/or echocardiogram should be performed.

D. Chest radiograph is best used for evaluating pulmonary blood flow, heart size, and any pulmonary causes of cyanosis. CBC assesses for anemia/polycythemia, as well as providing evidence of infection. ECG can be of significant value, but only in certain situations. Right ventricular predominance is normal in the neonate, so left ventricular predominance should raise concern for a small right ventricle (e.g., tricuspid atresia). Left-axis deviation in the presence of right-heart predominance is suggestive of an atrioventricular septal defect.

E. Pulse oximetry is being used with increasing frequency for routine neonatal screening for congenital heart disease. Studies have shown that at sea level, routine predischarge screening with pulse oximetry using a cutoff of 95% for preductal saturations or preductal/postductal difference of greater than 3% yielded excellent specificity and improved sensitivity over physical examination alone for the detection of congenital heart disease, especially ductal-dependent disease. Abnormal screenings were followed by echocardiography, with the results of 2.3 normal echoes performed for every abnormal echo.

F. A more traditional test for cyanotic heart disease is the hyperoxia test. This test compares the arterial partial pressure of oxygen (PaO_2) in the blood on breathing of room air with the PaO_2 on 100% inspired oxygen. If the child's PaO_2 does not increase to more than 150 mm Hg, a cardiovascular causative factor should be explored. If the PaO_2 does increase to more than 150 mm Hg with oxygen, the cause of the central cyanosis is likely to be pulmonary in origin. The biggest advantage of this test is its ability to safely exclude cyanotic congenital heart disease when the PaO_2 increases to more than 150 mm Hg. The disadvantage is that it is invasive and requires either the placement of an arterial line or two arterial punctures. Therefore, it is best used in a situation where cyanotic heart disease is less likely and exclusion could avoid echocardiogram or transfer to another facility. In situations where cyanotic heart disease is thought likely by examination, history, and noninvasive screening, an echocardiogram should be performed for definitive diagnosis.

G. When cyanotic congenital heart disease is suspected, obtain cardiology consultation and an echocardiograph. Many specific diagnoses can produce cyanosis (see Table 1 for a list of some of the more common

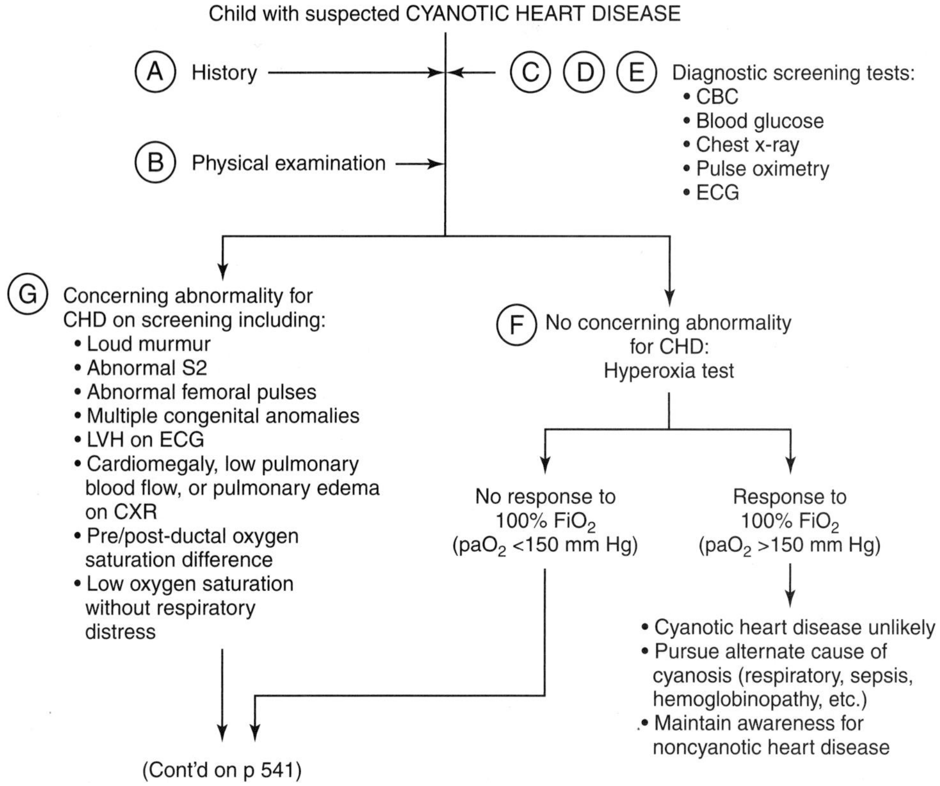
Child with suspected CYANOTIC HEART DISEASE
A History
B Physical examination
C D E Diagnostic screening tests:
• CBC
• Blood glucose
• Chest x-ray
• Pulse oximetry
• ECG
G Concerning abnormality for CHD on screening including:
• Loud murmur
• Abnormal S2
• Abnormal femoral pulses
• Multiple congenital anomalies
• LVH on ECG
• Cardiomegaly, low pulmonary blood flow, or pulmonary edema on CXR
• Pre/post-ductal oxygen saturation difference
• Low oxygen saturation without respiratory distress
F No concerning abnormality for CHD: Hyperoxia test
No response to 100% FiO_2 (paO_2 <150 mm Hg)
Response to 100% FiO_2 (paO_2 >150 mm Hg)
• Cyanotic heart disease unlikely
• Pursue alternate cause of cyanosis (respiratory, sepsis, hemoglobinopathy, etc.)
• Maintain awareness for noncyanotic heart disease
(Cont'd on p 541)

diagnoses); but in general, they can be grouped into four major groups:

1. *Transposition of the great arteries:* This results in separation of the pulmonary and systemic circulation. As a result, oxygenated blood returning from the lungs has difficulty reaching the systemic circulation, leading to cyanosis. Mixing occurs primarily at the atrial level, and lack of a significant atrial septal defect requires emergent transfer to a center capable of performing an atrial septostomy.
2. *Pulmonary outflow obstruction:* This leads to cyanosis from decreased pulmonary blood flow and right-to-left shunt. Specific diagnoses include tetralogy of Fallot, pulmonary atresia with intact ventricular septum, severe pulmonary stenosis with intact ventricular septum, severe Ebstein's anomaly, and tricuspid atresia with a small ventricular septal defect. Pulmonary hypertension with right-to-left shunting at the patent ductus arteriosus or foramen ovale can lead to cyanosis and mimic cyanotic heart disease.
3. *Complete mixing lesions:* These cause total mixing of systemic and pulmonary circulation before ejection from the heart without limitation to pulmonary blood flow. Such lesions include total anomalous pulmonary venous return, truncus arteriosus, and tricuspid atresia with a large ventricular septal defect. Presentations may vary, but many of these lesions present only initially with significant cyanosis while pulmonary pressures are still high. Once the pulmonary resistance declines, pulmonary blood flow increases dramatically, resulting in minimal cyanosis and a presentation of congestive heart failure.
4. *Left ventricular outflow tract obstruction/hypoplastic left-heart syndrome:* Left ventricular obstructive lesions include critical aortic stenosis, interrupted aortic arch, critical coarctation of the aorta, and hypoplastic left-heart syndrome. Most often these diseases present with hypoperfusion and shock once the ductus arteriosus closes. However, they can initially present with cyanosis (critical aortic stenosis or hypoplastic left-heart syndrome) or preductal/postductal saturation difference (coarctation or interrupted arch) because of mixing at the atrial level or right-to-left shunt at the patent ductus arteriosus (PDA), respectively. If the duct remains open, cyanosis will lessen as pulmonary blood flow increases in a similar manner to complete mixing lesions.

Table 1. **Neonatal Cyanotic Heart Disease, Clinical Findings**

Lesion	Auscultation	Chest Radiograph	Electrocardiogram	Presentation
Transposition	No murmur Loud single S2	Cardiomegaly, increased PBF	NL or RVH	Asymptomatic cyanosis, CHF late
Tetralogy of Fallot	SEM Loud single S2	Boot-shaped heart decreased PBF	RVH	Asymptomatic cyanosis, no CHF
TAPVR, nonobstructed	SEM Split S2	Cardiomegaly, including PBF "snowman"	RVH	Asymptomatic cyanosis, CHF late
TAPVR, obstructed	No murmur Loud single S2	NL heart; pulmonary venous congestion	RVH	Deep cyanosis, respiratory distress
Tricuspid atresia	SEM with/without single S2	NL heart size, variable PBF	LVH, LAD	Asymptomatic cyanosis, CHF late if no PS
Truncus arteriosus	Click, SEM or to and fro murmur	Cardiomegaly, increased PBF	BVH, ST-T changes	Asymptomatic cyanosis, CHF late
Pulmonary atresia intact vent septum	LLSB murmur (tricuspid regurgitation)	Cardiomegaly, decreased PBF	LVH, NL axis	Deep cyanosis, CHF if no ASD
Ebstein anomaly	LLSB murmur multiple systolic clicks	Massive cardiomegaly, decreased PBF	RAE, IVCD with/without WPW	Deep cyanosis, CHF in first days of life

BVH, biventricular hypertrophy; *CHF,* congestive heart failure; *IVCD,* intraventricular conduction delay; *LAD,* left axis deviation; *LLSB,* left lower sternal border; *LVH,* left ventricular hypertrophy; *PBF,* pulmonary blood flow; *RAE,* right atrial enlargement; *RVH,* right ventricular hypertrophy; *SEM,* systolic ejection murmur; *WPW,* Wolff–Parkinson–White.

H. After the lesion has been diagnosed, transfer to a pediatric cardiac center is usually indicated. Before transfer, prostaglandin E_1 (PGE_1) therapy should be initiated to maintain ductal patency either before diagnosis if the child is unstable or after diagnosis if the child is stable with either ductal-dependent pulmonary or systemic blood flow.

References

de-Wahl Granelli A, Wennergren M, Sandberg K, et al. Impact of pulse oximetry screening on the detection of duct dependent congenital heart disease: a Swedish prospective screening study in 39,821 newborns. BMJ 2009;338:a3037.

Hartas GA, Tsounias E, Gupta-Malhotra M. Approach to diagnosing congenital cardiac disorders. Crit Care Nurs Clin North Am 2009;21:27–36.

Jones RW, Baumer JH, Joseph MC, Shinebourne EA. Arterial oxygen tension and response to oxygen breathing in differential diagnosis of congenital heart disease in infancy. Arch Dis Child 1976;51:667–73.

Sadowski SL. Congenital cardiac disease in the newborn infant: past, present, and future. Crit Care Nurs Clin North Am 2009;21:37–48.

Sasidharan P. An approach to diagnosis and management of cyanosis and tachypnea in term infants. Pediatr Clin North Am 2004;51:999–1021.

Thangaratinam S, Daniels J, Ewer AK, Zamora J, Khan KS, et al. Accuracy of pulse oximetry in screening for congenital heart disease in asymptomatic newborns: a systematic review. Arch Dis Child Fetal Neonatal Ed 2007;92:F176–80.

Tingelstad J. Consultation with the specialist: nonrespiratory cyanosis. Pediatr Rev 1999;20:350–2.

Child with suspected CYANOTIC HEART DISEASE

(Cont'd from p 539)

(H)
- Echocardiogram or
- Immediate consultation with a pediatric cardiologist for potential transfer to tertiary care center

IV access and consider PGE_1 if unstable, severe cyanosis, absent femoral pulses, or ductal dependent lesion established by echo or suspected by screening/cardiology

Rheumatic Fever

Joshua A. Kailin, MD, and Michael S. Schaffer, MD

Rheumatic fever, which consists of delayed nonsuppurative sequelae of group A streptococcal (GAS) pharyngitis, is a diffuse inflammatory disease of the connective tissue involving the heart, joints, brain, blood vessels, and subcutaneous tissue. The term *acute rheumatic fever* (ARF) is a misnomer, for on occasion, the disease may not be acute, rheumatic, or febrile. Rheumatic fever is still the most common cause of heart disease in children worldwide. It causes 25% to 40% of all cardiovascular disease, including in tropical countries where it was once believed to be rare. Despite an apparent decline in incidence over time in the United States, rheumatic fever incidence rates remain relatively high in non-Western countries, particularly Eastern Europe, the Middle East, Asia, Australia, and New Zealand. In the United States, although the prevalence is low and still decreasing, rheumatic fever maintains its position as a leading cause of postnatally acquired heart disease in children. It has been estimated that 95% of the nearly 20 million cases of rheumatic heart disease (RHD) in the world and up to 500,000 deaths each year caused by ARF and RHD occur in developing countries.

ARF occurs most commonly in young school-age children (5–15 years old). No true differences in susceptibility according to sex, race, or ethnic group have been established. One typical feature of this disease process is a latent period between GAS pharyngitis and ARF varying from 7 to 35 days with an average of 18 days. The latent period may be 2 to 6 months in patients with Sydenham chorea (Table 1). The most popular theory of pathogenesis is that ARF results from some type of autoimmunity. The molecular mimicry between components of highly virulent strains of group A streptococcus, containing very large hyaluronate capsules and M-protein molecules with host tissues, may lead to a cross-reactive immune response, in which the immune system will damage both the streptococcus and certain tissues of the patient, especially the heart. Carditis is the most serious major manifestation of ARF. It is most common and severe in the young. It may cause acute heart failure or culminate in chronic valvar heart disease. The incidence rate of clinically evident carditis with ARF varies from 40% to 50%. Patients with carditis in the initial episode of ARF usually experience development of residual RHD. If RHD recurrences can be prevented, the long-term outcome is better.

The most effective preventive measures against rheumatic fever are socioeconomic and sanitary. Adequate housing and relief from crowding are important in prevention of outbreaks of streptococcal infection. The aim of primary prophylaxis is to prevent the initial attacks of rheumatic fever by identification and treatment of GAS pharyngitis. Secondary prophylaxis is the prevention of recurrences of rheumatic fever by continuous chemoprophylaxis. The most effective method has been a single intramuscular injection of 1.2 million units (600,000 units if <27 kg) benzathine penicillin every 3 to 4 weeks.

A. Ask about symptoms of a sore throat during the month (range, 1–5 weeks) before the onset of rheumatic fever symptoms. However, many patients have subclinical disease without any indication of a prior streptococcal infection. Ask about any potential recent exposures to family members with GAS pharyngitis. Ask about fever and painful, swollen joints. If they are present, determine the pattern of involvement. In rheumatic fever, patients get a migratory arthritis that usually presents 14 to 21 days after a GAS infection. The disease resolves after 4 to 7 days in the initial joints and then develops in new joints. ARF arthritis is migratory and transient, and affects mainly large joints, particularly the knees, ankles, elbows, and wrists. Polyarthritis occurs in about 75% of patients during the acute stage of the disease. Ask about the use of salicylates or other nonsteroidal anti-inflammatory drugs, which could mask arthritis. Ask about symptoms of congestive heart failure, such as increased sweating, poor feeding, cyanosis, shortness of breath, dyspnea, inability to sleep flat, edema, and exercise intolerance. Facial grimacing, odd movements, or unusual emotional outbursts suggest chorea. Chorea may also manifest as poor school performance secondary to handwriting difficulty and inability to concentrate.

B. On physical examination, the unequivocal signs of carditis in a patient with ARF are: (1) an organic heart murmur that is clearly mitral or aortic insufficiency, (2) pericardial friction rub or effusion, and (3) cardiac enlargement with or without heart failure. Unexplained tachycardia is also suggestive of inflamed myocardium. Congestive heart failure indicates significant myocarditis and occurs in 5% to 10% of first attacks, but it is more common as a manifestation of recurrence. Myocarditis in the absence of valvulitis is not likely to be rheumatic in origin. The mitral valve is the most common site of inflammation and is effected almost three times as frequently as the aortic valve. The murmur of mitral insufficiency is a holosystolic, apical blowing murmur that radiates to the axilla; the murmur of aortic insufficiency is heard in early diastole at the right upper sternal border. Also note any swollen or tender joints consistent with arthritis. Random, rapid, involuntary, purposeless, nonrhythmic movements (usually the face and upper extremities) indicate chorea. Another rare major ARF criterion is erythema marginatum, which is a fine, lacy, painless, nonpruritic erythematous rash found mainly over the trunk and inner surfaces of the arms and legs. Subcutaneous nodules that are movable, hard, round, painless swellings over bone prominences are also rarely seen.

C. A throat culture or rapid antigen detection test (RADT) is of uncertain practical value. Because there is usually a latent period of 2 to 3 weeks between pharyngitis and the appearance of ARF, a throat culture taken at the onset of ARF is frequently negative. A throat culture or RADT that is positive does not prove recent infection because children can be chronic streptococcal carriers. Only 80% of infected patients have an increased antistreptolysin O (ASO) titer. Request other streptococcal antibodies (e.g., anti-DNase B) for patients thought to have rheumatic

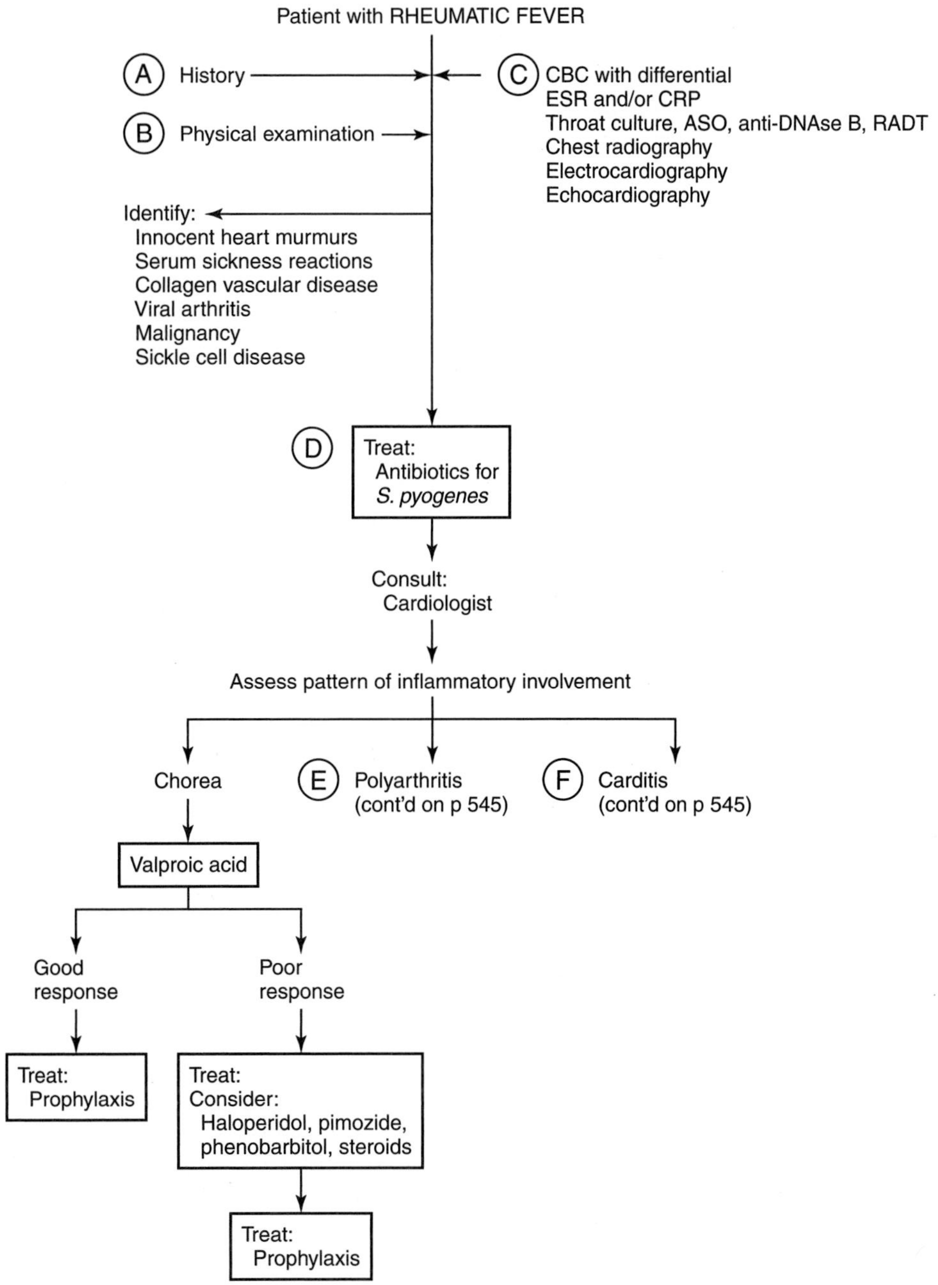
Patient with RHEUMATIC FEVER
(A) History
(B) Physical examination
(C) CBC with differential
ESR and/or CRP
Throat culture, ASO, anti-DNAse B, RADT
Chest radiography
Electrocardiography
Echocardiography
Identify:
Innocent heart murmurs
Serum sickness reactions
Collagen vascular disease
Viral arthritis
Malignancy
Sickle cell disease
(D) Treat:
Antibiotics for
S. pyogenes
Consult:
Cardiologist
Assess pattern of inflammatory involvement
Chorea
(E) Polyarthritis
(cont'd on p 545)
(F) Carditis
(cont'd on p 545)
Valproic acid
Good
response
Poor
response
Treat:
Prophylaxis
Treat:
Consider:
Haloperidol, pimozide,
phenobarbitol, steroids
Treat:
Prophylaxis

fever who have a normal ASO titer. Streptococcal antibodies may begin to decline after 2 months. Consider an ASO titer less than 250 Todd units normal, titers greater than 250 Todd units increased in adults, and titers greater than 333 Todd units increased in children. Increased titers are suggestive of an antecedent GAS pharyngeal infection. Erythrocyte sedimentation rate (ESR) and C-reactive protein (CRP) are not specific for rheumatic fever but are useful for determining inflammation (ESR usually >60 in ARF). Obtain a chest film to detect cardiac enlargement and pericardial effusion. Electrocardiographic changes include prolongation of the PR interval, flattened or inverted T waves caused by myocarditis, and elevation of the ST segment in pericarditis. In patients with suspected ARF presenting with chorea or polyarthritis but without a murmur, obtain an echocardiogram to evaluate for "subclinical" valvulitis and carditis.

D. Treat all patients with benzathine penicillin G to eradicate group A streptococcus. Subsequently, start a secondary prophylaxis program for prevention of recurrent ARF with intramuscular benzathine penicillin every 21 to 28 days, depending on the risk for recurrence. Oral alternatives such as penicillin V or sulfadiazine can be considered if intramuscular injections are poorly tolerated. Certain macrolides and azalides can also be used in penicillin-allergic patients as an alterative regimen. Prophylaxis is the most important aspect of disease management because recurrence for GAS infection can cause more severe carditis and valve injury. Secondary prophylaxis reduces the severity of RHD, is associated with regression of heart disease in approximately 50% to 70% of those with adequate adherence over a decade, and reduces RHD mortality.

Table 1. **Jones Criteria: Guidelines for the Diagnosis of an Initial Attack of Rheumatic Fever**

Requirements for Diagnosis	Criteria
Two major criteria *or* One major plus two minor criteria *plus* Evidence of previous GAS infection 1. History of (within last 45 days) a. Streptococcal sore throat b. Scarlet fever c. Positive throat culture or RADT 2. Raised ASO titer a. >333 units in children b. >250 units in adults 3. Anti-deoxyribonuclease B a. Normal values i. 1:60 units in preschool ii. 1:480 units in school-aged children iii. 1:340 in adults	**Major Criteria** Carditis Polyarthritis Chorea Erythema marginatum Subcutaneous nodules **Minor Criteria** Previous rheumatic fever Polyarthralgia (in absence of arthritis as a major criteria) ECG: prolonged PR interval Fever Increased ESR or CRP

ASO, antistreptolysin O; *CRP*, C-reactive protein; *ECG*, electrocardiogram; *ESR*, erythrocyte sedimentation rate; *GAS*, group A streptococcal; *RADT*, rapid antigen detection test.

E. Aspirin or naproxen is effective for arthritis and mild carditis. Arthritis of rheumatic fever characteristically heals without residual manifestations. Acetylsalicylic acid (ASA) is an analgesic and antipyretic, and generally causes dramatic improvement of the arthritis but has minimal impact on carditis. ASA is continued for 2 to 3 weeks or until inflammation subsides clinically or until all laboratory values are normal. After this, the dose is decreased gradually to avoid rebound inflammation. The dose of ASA is 60 to 100 mg/kg/day divided four times daily for 2 to 6 weeks. Serum ASA concentrations should be monitored with extended therapy (anti-inflammatory effect 150–300 μg/ml). The dose of naproxen ranges from 10 to 20 mg/kg/day.

F. Patients with moderate to severe carditis or severe arthritis with ARF should be hospitalized. It is important to limit exercise for 6 to 8 weeks.

G. For moderately to severely ill patients with carditis and congestive heart failure, prescribe a regimen of prednisone, 2 mg/kg/day, until the ESR normalizes, usually approximately 2 weeks. Taper prednisone over a 2- to 4-week period. Continue salicylates for a total treatment course of 12 weeks. Digoxin must be used with caution with ARF because inflamed myocardium can be hypersensitive to digoxin and toxicity with arrhythmias can occur. Consult a cardiologist before digoxin use.

H. Recommendations of the American Heart Association for the duration of prophylaxis are as follows: (1) ARF without carditis: duration of 5 years or until age 21 years, whichever is longer; (2) ARF with carditis but no residual heart disease and no valvar disease: 10 years or until 21 years of age, whichever is longer; (3) ARF with carditis and residual heart disease (persistent valve disease): at least 10 years since last episode and at least until age 40 years, sometimes lifelong prophylaxis.

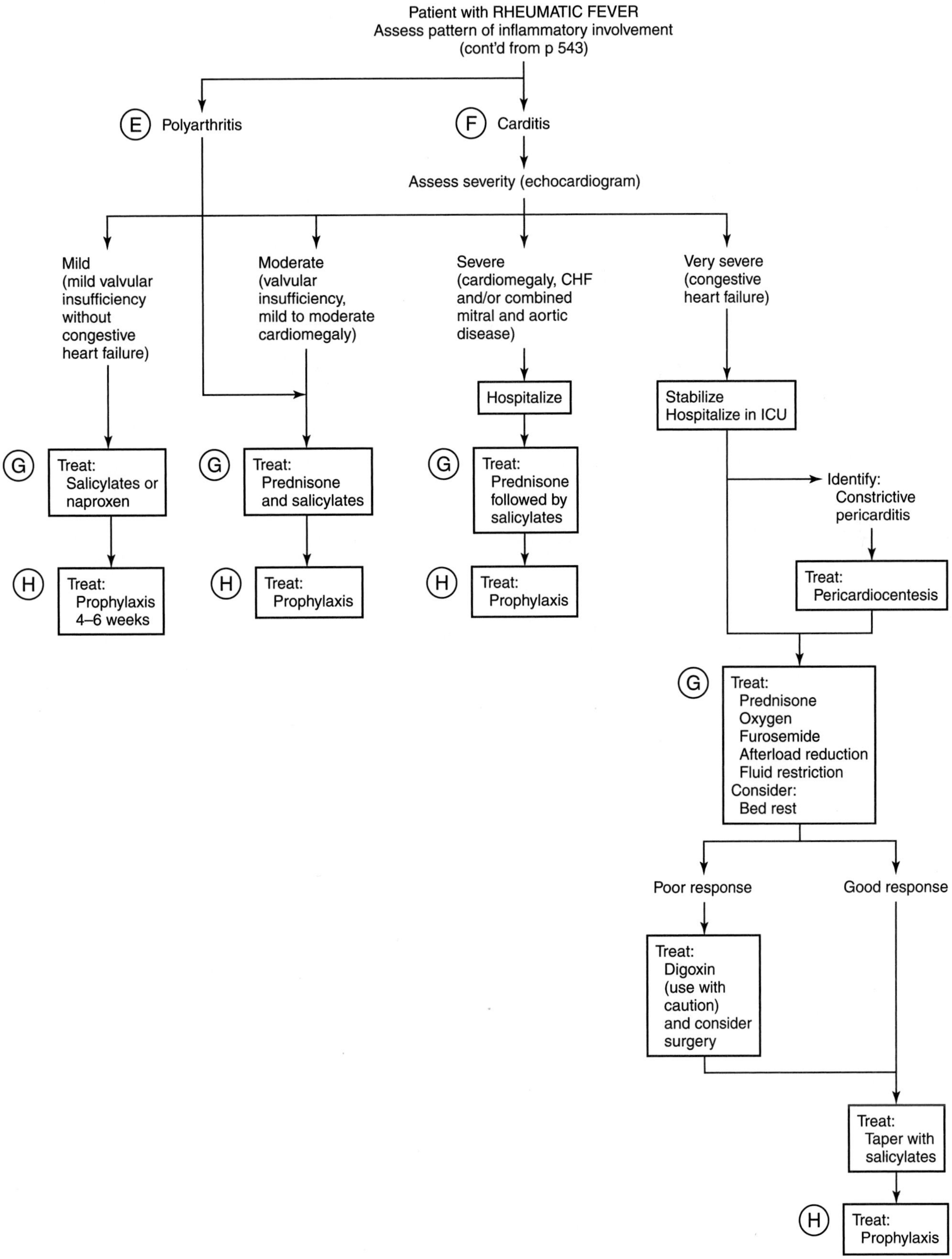
Patient with RHEUMATIC FEVER
Assess pattern of inflammatory involvement
(cont'd from p 543)
E
Polyarthritis
F
Carditis
Assess severity (echocardiogram)
Mild
(mild valvular insufficiency without congestive heart failure)
Moderate
(valvular insufficiency, mild to moderate cardiomegaly)
Severe
(cardiomegaly, CHF and/or combined mitral and aortic disease)
Very severe
(congestive heart failure)
Hospitalize
Stabilize
Hospitalize in ICU
Identify:
Constrictive pericarditis
Treat:
Pericardiocentesis
G
Treat:
Salicylates or naproxen
G
Treat:
Prednisone and salicylates
G
Treat:
Prednisone followed by salicylates
H
Treat:
Prophylaxis 4–6 weeks
H
Treat:
Prophylaxis
H
Treat:
Prophylaxis
G
Treat:
Prednisone
Oxygen
Furosemide
Afterload reduction
Fluid restriction
Consider:
Bed rest
Poor response
Good response
Treat:
Digoxin (use with caution) and consider surgery
Treat:
Taper with salicylates
H
Treat:
Prophylaxis

References

Atatoa-Carr P, Lennon D, Wilson N, et al. Rheumatic fever diagnosis, management, and secondary prevention: a New Zealand guideline. N Z Med J 2008;121:59–69.

Brundage JF, Gunzenhauser JD, Longfield JN, et al. Epidemiology and control of acute respiratory diseases with emphasis on group A beta-hemolytic streptococcus: a decade of U.S. Army experience. Pediatrics 1996;97(Pt 2):964–70.

Dajani A, Taubert K, Ferrieri P, et al. Treatment of acute streptococcal pharyngitis and prevention of rheumatic fever: a statement for health professionals. Committee on Rheumatic Fever, Endocarditis, and Kawasaki's Disease of the Council on Cardiovascular Disease in the Young, the American Heart Association. Pediatrics 1995;96 (Pt 1):758–64.

De Rosa G, Pardeo M, Stabile A, et al. Rheumatic heart disease in children: from clinical assessment to therapeutical management. Eur Rev Med Pharmacol Sci 2006;10:107–10.

El-Said GM, El-Refaee MM, Soroour KA, el-Said, HG. Rheumatic fever and rheumatic heart disease. In: Garson A Jr, Bricker JT, Fisher DJ, Neish SR, editors. The science and practice of pediatric cardiology. 2nd ed. Baltimore: Williams & Wilkins; 1998. p. 1691–1724.

Forster J. Rheumatic fever: keeping up with the Jones criteria. Contemp Pediatr 1993;10:51–60.

Gerber MA, Baltimore RS, Eaton CB, et al. Prevention of rheumatic fever and diagnosis and treatment of acute streptococcal pharyngitis: a scientific statement from the American Heart Association Rheumatic Fever, Endocarditis, and Kawasaki Disease in the Young, the Interdisciplinary Council on Functional Genomics and Translational Biology, and the Interdisiplinary Council on Quality of Care and Outcomes Research: endorsed by the American Academy of Pediatrics. Circulation 2009;119:1541–51.

Guilherme L, Kalil J, Cunningham M. Molecular mimicry in the autoimmune pathogenesis of rheumatic heart disease. Autoimmunity 2006;39:31–9.

Hashkes, PJ, Tauber T, Somekh E, et al. Naproxen as an alternative to aspirin for the treatment of arthritis of rheumatic fever: a randomized control trial. J Pediatr 2003;143:399–401.

Lennon D. Acute rheumatic fever. In: Feigen RD, Cherry JD, editors. Textbook of pediatric infectious diseases. 5th ed. Philadelphia: WB Saunders; 2004, p. 413–26.

Lennon D. Acute rheumatic fever in children: recognition and treatment. Pediatr Drugs 2004;6:363–73.

Lue HC, Wu MH, Wang JK, et al. Three- versus four-week administration of benzathine penicillin G: effects on incidence of streptococcal infections and recurrences of rheumatic fever. Pediatrics 1988;97 (Pt 2):984–8.

Stollerman GH. Rheumatic fever. Lancet 1997;349:934–42.

Stollerman GH. Rheumatic fever in the 21st century. Clin Infect Dis 2001;33:806–14.

Tibararwa KB, Volmink JA, Mayosi BM. Incidence of acute rheumatic fever in the world: a systematic review of population-based studies. Heart 2008;94:1534–40.

Veasy LG, Wiedmeier SE, Osmond FS, et al. Resurgence of acute rheumatic fever in the intermountain area of the United States. N Engl J Med 1987;316:421–7.

Working Group on Pediatric Acute Rheumatic Fever and Cardiology Chapter of Indian Academy of Pediatrics. Consensus Guidelines on Pediatric Acute Rheumatic Fever and Rheumatic Heart Disease. Indian Pediatr 2008;45:565–73.

Zangwill KM, Wald EM, Londino AV. Acute rheumatic fever in Western Pennsylvania: a persistent problem into the 1990s. J Pediatr 1991;118:561–3.

Children with Special Health Care Needs

Overview of Primary Care for the Child with Special Health Care Needs

Preventive Ambulatory Care of the Premature Infant

Medical Care of Children in Foster Care

Cerebral Palsy

Cleft Lip and Cleft Palate

Transitioning Young Adults with Special Health Care Needs to Adult Medical Care

Overview of Primary Care for the Child with Special Health Care Needs

David Fox, MD, Karen L. Kelminson, MD, and Ellen Roy Elias, MD

Advances in medical and surgical care have led to the long-term survival of children with chronic and often complex special medical issues. The Maternal and Child Health Bureau defines this population as "those (children) who have or are at increased risk for a chronic physical, developmental, behavioral or emotional condition and who also require health and related services of a type or amount beyond that required by children generally." As many as 13% of children in the United States are believed to have special health care needs, corresponding to greater than 9 million children nationwide. Many of these children with special health care needs (CSHCN) face developmental and behavioral, as well as medical, challenges.

A. Comprehensive Evaluation: Perform a comprehensive evaluation including a detailed history and physical examination that includes medical, surgical, and medication history. Diagnosis-specific issues are important to address, but common pediatric concerns must also be reviewed. Four specific areas often present problems for CSHCN:

1. Nutrition: Document growth parameters on age- and diagnosis-specific growth charts, when available. Ask about diet and feeding concerns that the family has about the child. Gagging or choking suggests the need for a swallow study to look for aspiration. Gastrointestinal symptoms must be explored, including vomiting and abnormal stooling patterns. Reflux and constipation occur frequently and often need therapy. Consult a nutrition specialist for concerns about significantly overweight or underweight children, or with help managing gastrostomy tube feedings.

2. Respiratory Status: Any use of supplemental oxygen or positive-pressure devices should be documented and the current management reviewed. Respiratory therapy or pulmonology consultation is often helpful. Upper airway concerns and tracheostomy management require the advice of ENT (ear, nose, and throat) specialists. All children with respiratory issues should be diligently immunized and offered immunoprophylaxis for respiratory syncytial virus when appropriate. Frequent respiratory illnesses requiring hospitalization should raise the concern of silent aspiration, reactive airway disease, or airway abnormalities.

(Continued on page 550)

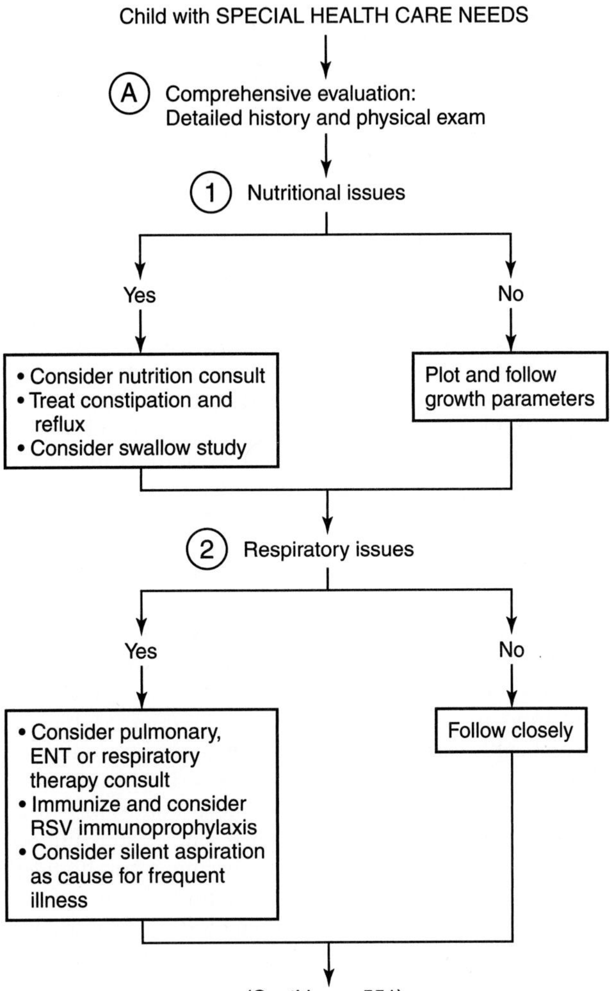
Child with SPECIAL HEALTH CARE NEEDS
A Comprehensive evaluation:
Detailed history and physical exam
1 Nutritional issues
Yes
No
• Consider nutrition consult
• Treat constipation and reflux
• Consider swallow study
Plot and follow growth parameters
2 Respiratory issues
Yes
No
• Consider pulmonary, ENT or respiratory therapy consult
• Immunize and consider RSV immunoprophylaxis
• Consider silent aspiration as cause for frequent illness
Follow closely

(Cont'd on p 551)

3. Sleep Issues: Ask routine questions about sleep patterns, sleep hygiene, and signs of abnormal sleep symptoms. Consider a sleep study to document obstructive breathing patterns that may benefit from surgical or medical intervention. For the child with significant neurologic impairment who does not respond to maximizing sleep hygiene and has no respiratory issues, sleep medications may be necessary.
4. Developmental Milestones: As with any pediatric patient, developmental assessment should be done at well-child visits. For the CSHCN, there needs to be a heightened awareness of developmental milestones and appropriate referral for any delays should be made. For children with significant physical challenges, rehabilitation medicine consultation is appropriate. The loss of language or motor milestones should prompt a genetic or metabolic consultation.

Allow sufficient time to review complex information: an hour for a new visit is appropriate, and increased time for follow-up visits may also be needed. Ask caregivers to send you a question list in advance of an appointment, so that you have time to research complex issues. Document the other health care providers who care for the child, including medical and surgical specialists, mental and behavioral health providers, and physical, speech, and occupational therapists. A medication list should be carefully reconciled at each visit. Document all home-care services to allow for efficient communication. Carefully document the child's diagnoses and maintain an updated problem list.

B. Family Support and Structure: Identify the family structure in which this child is living and discuss with the primary caregiver how the family has responded to the stress of a medically complex child. Parents of newborns with complex problems or those children with a severe acquired disability may express a grief reaction at the loss of their idealized child. Divorce and family discord are not uncommon sequelae of the stress of a child with special needs. Siblings of medically fragile children may suffer from a relative lack of attention or may express fears about the possibility of the death of their sibling. Provide the family with available resources for counseling and support that are culturally and medically appropriate.

C. Long-Term Planning: Discuss with the family the long-term plan they have for their child. Though providing a medical prognosis for the child in many cases is difficult, and perhaps unwise, discussing what the family wants for the future is invaluable. Frank discussions about the life-limiting nature of the child's underlying disease are often met with gratitude from the family that is grappling with such issues. Consider discussing the parent's feelings about the level of medical and technologic intervention with which they are comfortable and the appropriateness of an advance directive. Issues regarding finances and insurance need to be addressed with appropriate referral to financial counselors or social workers. In late adolescence and early adulthood, consider the relevance of discussing group homes, workshop settings, and other community-supported employment. The child should be included in these discussions to the extent possible and appropriate.

(Continued on page 552)

Child with SPECIAL HEALTH CARE NEEDS

(Cont'd from p 549)

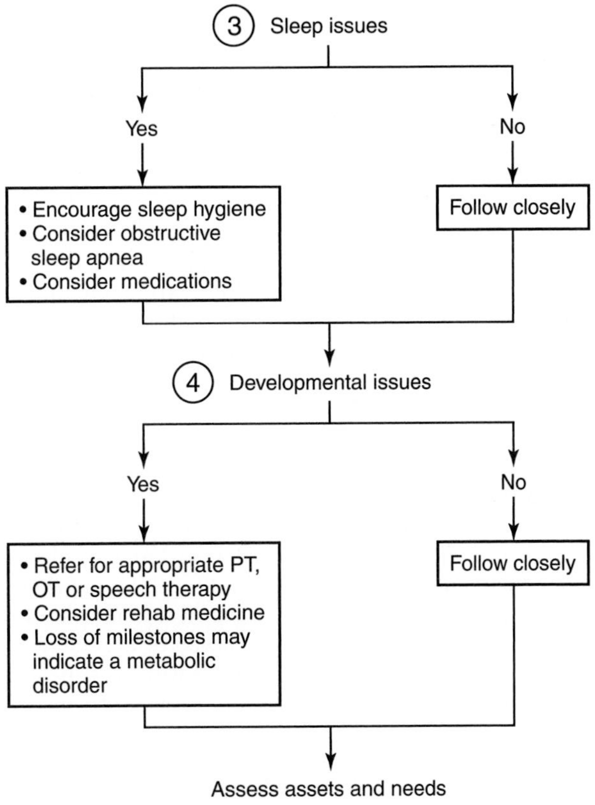
3 Sleep issues
Yes
No
• Encourage sleep hygiene
• Consider obstructive sleep apnea
• Consider medications
Follow closely
4 Developmental issues
Yes
No
• Refer for appropriate PT, OT or speech therapy
• Consider rehab medicine
• Loss of milestones may indicate a metabolic disorder
Follow closely
Assess assets and needs

(B) Family support and structure

i. Recognize the stress the family is under

(C) Long term planning

i. Discuss family's hopes for future

(Cont'd on p 553)

D. Education and Development: Review education issues and discuss the importance of early intervention services and their availability in the community. Speech therapy, hearing assistance devices, and sign language services can help ensure that communication is preserved. Services for visually impaired children are also crucial. Parents may desire to explore alternative, complementary, or nontraditional forms of therapy. Encourage those therapies that present no harm and are enjoyable to the family, and advise caution toward those that are invasive, expensive, and untested. In early childhood, present the options for preschool programs and begin planning for future school placement and performance. Public schools are required to develop an Individualized Educational Plan (IEP) for children to meet their academic needs, and this should be reviewed by the medical provider. Once the child is in school, assess the options for developing prevocational skills. During adolescence, discuss the appropriateness of school placement and adequate vocational training within the school curriculum.

E. Behavior and Mental Health: Address the behavioral and mental health issues of the child. Parents sometimes find it challenging to set appropriate limits with their child with disabilities out of a sense of guilt or sympathy for the child's situation. During early childhood (1–5 years of age), assess the child's behavior and develop a plan for behavioral management, socialization, and recreational skills. Mental health providers who have early childhood experience are in short supply and often have a heavy caseload. The primary care provider may be called on to do more screening, triaging, and comanaging of these challenging issues. In adolescence, ensure that the child and family have assistance in discussing psychosocial development, pubertal development, and sexuality in both girls and boys.

F. Provide a Medical Home: The medical home provides care that is accessible, continuous, comprehensive, family centered, coordinated, compassionate, and culturally competent. It encompasses well-child care and acute visits, together with the management of disease and chronic conditions. CSHCN and their families particularly benefit from primary care given in a medical home. These children require coordination of patient care (between health care professionals), case management, care plans, and help with care transitions. Families of these children should be included as members of the health care team to manage the child's health condition. The medical home improves effectiveness of care and health status for CSHCN and increases the likelihood that they will receive services such as mental health interventions, respite care, rehabilitation, and special education. Families of children who receive primary care in a medical home are often more satisfied, particularly with regard to family centeredness and timeliness of care, and also report that these services improve family functioning.

G. Implement a Care Plan: The health care plan begun at the initial visit should be reassessed and adjusted at each subsequent visit. The provider should encourage the participation of the family and other professionals involved in the patient's life when adjusting the care plan. This plan should include all pertinent medical, educational, and family-related issues important in the care of the patient. The goals of the care plan are to help the patient's caregivers prioritize needs and optimize the functional status of the child and family. The care plan should be flexible and accommodating to changes in the life of the child and family. The child's medical fragility and functional status, together with the level of family support necessary to maintain or improve family functioning, should be taken into consideration. At each visit, a written summary of critical information should be given to the family, and an advance directive should be prepared and/or updated if indicated.

H. Advocate for CSHCN: The primary care provider should be an active advocate for CSHCN. These children require advocacy in the medical setting, the education system, and at the local and state community levels. Families often require assistance with acquiring and maintaining health insurance. Support from the medical home should be provided when patients have difficulty accessing health services because of problems with their health insurance plans.

Providers can effectively advocate for improvement in the quality of medical care for CSHCN, for removal of barriers to beneficial services and programs, and for greater access to community-based services. Physicians can also advocate to improve the knowledge of health care professionals, families, and the public regarding CSHCN.

I. Monitor CSHCN: Providers can use the individual patient's health care plan to determine appropriate follow-up for the child. In general, all CSHCN should be evaluated at least every 6 months. Children with more complex problems, family dysfunction, or who are at high risk for deterioration should be seen at least every 1 to 2 months. Maintaining close communication with the family and other health care professionals involved in the patient's care helps ensure that the child's and family's needs are being adequately and efficiently provided.

References

American Academy of Pediatrics Policy Statement; Council on Children with Disabilities. Care Coordination in the Medical Home: Integrating health and related systems of care for children with special health care needs. Pediatrics 2005;116:1238–44.

Cooley CW. Redefining primary pediatric care for children with special health care needs: the primary care medical home. Curr Opin Pediatr 2004;16:689–92.

Homer CJ, Klatka K, Romm D, et al. A review of the evidence for the medical home for children with special health care needs. Pediatrics 2008;122:e922–37.

McAllister JW, Presler E, Cooley CW. Practice based care coordination: a medical home essential. Pediatrics 2007;120:e723–33.

Child with SPECIAL HEALTH CARE NEEDS

(Cont'd from p 551)

(D) Education and development

i. Discuss therapies and school progress

(E) Behavioral and mental health

i. Discuss behavior management and socialization

↓

Plan and coordinate

(F) Provide a medical home

i. Family-centered, coordinated care is the goal

(G) Implement a care plan

i. Consider advance directive

(H) Advocate for CSHCN

(I) Monitor CSHCN

i. More frequent visits are needed for CSHCN

Preventive Ambulatory Care of the Premature Infant

Adam Rosenberg, MD, and Edward Goldson, MD

Approximately 10% of newborns in the United States have birth weights of less than 2500 g. They make up a heterogeneous group; some have few problems, whereas others have many complications associated with their prematurity and low birth weight. With advances in obstetric and neonatal care, survival of infants less than 28 weeks' gestation and 1000 g has markedly improved. This group, however, has a considerable rate of long-term morbidities. In providing care to this group of children, two rules of thumb should be considered. First, the more immature and small the infant, the greater is the risk for complications. In addition, the greater the number of complications, the greater is the risk for an adverse medical or neurodevelopmental outcome. Second, any infant requiring neonatal intensive care is at increased risk for later medical, developmental, and behavioral difficulties, including late preterm infants (34–36 weeks gestational age).

A. Obtain a complete history and physical examination. If possible, it is helpful to visit the infant in the hospital before discharge, to discuss the infant's hospital course with the staff, to meet with the family, and to prepare for the infant's outpatient care. At the initial ambulatory clinic visit, review the discharge plans and identify ongoing issues that need to be addressed. Assess the family's psychosocial needs during the predischarge meeting, the initial clinic visit, and subsequent visits for ongoing care. Consult with mental health professionals and social workers. When appropriate, refer for services that cannot be provided by clinic personnel. Criteria for discharge include maintaining normal temperature in an open crib, adequate enteral intake with consistent weight gain, and absence of apnea and bradycardia spells requiring intervention.

B. Coordination of primary care and subspecialty services is central to caring for these children. Primary care services for the prematurely born child should be consistent with current American Academy of Pediatrics guidelines and include routine health maintenance, monitoring of growth and development, and provision of immunizations. Children should have their height, weight, and head circumference measured and their weight-to-length ratio or body mass index plotted at every well-child visit. Close monitoring of nutrition is essential in this group of children. For many, adequate nutrition for growth and development and good health is a problem. Many require administration of special convalescent formulas for premature infants (EnfaCare Lipil or Similac NeoSure, 22 calories/oz; in some cases, concentrated further to 24–26 calories/oz) or breast milk fortified with formula powder and the continued provision of high-calorie products after the first year of life. Collaboration with a dietitian is helpful in identifying and helping parents to meet the nutritional needs of their child. Because these infants are at high risk for developmental disturbances, close monitoring of all aspects of the infant's developmental progress is essential. The inclusion of occupational, physical, and speech-language therapists in the infant's routine care facilitates the identification of difficulties that would benefit from early intervention. Immunizations should be provided at the appropriate chronologic age, not age corrected for degree of prematurity. Preventive services also include the use of palivizumab (Synagis) for infants who meet the American Academy of Pediatrics criteria for administration. The criteria are based on the gestational age at birth, age at the onset of respiratory syncytial virus season, and whether the infant has chronic lung disease (CLD).

C. Children born prematurely are at high risk for developmental and behavioral difficulties. Early intervention with physical (PT), occupational (OT), and speech therapy can enhance outcome. Careful developmental screening should be done at 1 and 2 years of age. This should include a screen for findings consistent with autism spectrum disorder (ideally performed at 18 months of age). Consider periodic assessment and educational planning needs as children approach the preschool and school years. The early identification of learning difficulties can facilitate appropriate placement and access to necessary academic supports. During the school years, behavioral and attention problems may emerge. Consider financial issues, which include acquiring and maintaining health insurance and access to special services. A social worker or financial counselor can often be of considerable help.

(Continued on page 556)

Premature infant with PREVENTIVE AMBULATORY CARE

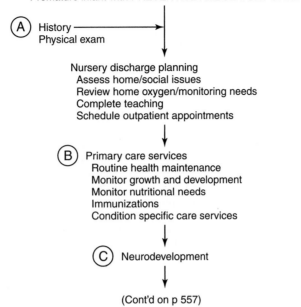

(A) History
Physical exam

Nursery discharge planning
- Assess home/social issues
- Review home oxygen/monitoring needs
- Complete teaching
- Schedule outpatient appointments

(B) Primary care services
- Routine health maintenance
- Monitor growth and development
- Monitor nutritional needs
- Immunizations
- Condition specific care services

(C) Neurodevelopment

(Cont'd on p 557)

D. Identify associated medical conditions and make appropriate referrals. Associated conditions are common among children born prematurely. It is essential to identify these as early as possible. Some of the problems include CLD (see sections E and F); cardiovascular sequelae; neurodevelopmental difficulties; gastroenterologic disturbances; otolaryngologic problems; ophthalmologic disorders, including retinopathy of prematurity, refractive errors, and strabismus; and endocrine disorders. Referral to the appropriate subspecialties and coordination of care fall under purview of the primary care physician. Systemic hypertension is a fairly uncommon complication of prematurity, but when present is usually related to high renin. Treat with captopril at a dose titrated between 0.1 and 0.5 mg/kg (maximum, 6 mg/kg/day) two to three times per day. The infants often outgrow this complication, so the medication can be weaned over time. Gastroesophageal reflux is relatively common during early infancy in former preterm infants. If not recognized and treated, it can lead to feeding aversions, failure to thrive, and recurrent aspiration. Medical treatment can include keeping the infant upright after feedings, thickening of feeds, use of ranitidine, 2 mg/kg twice a day, or lansoprazole, 1 to 1.5 mg/kg once or twice a day. Indications for surgical intervention (gastrostomy tube and fundoplication) include failure to thrive and exacerbation of pulmonary status because of recurrent aspiration episodes. Hypothyroidism is another fairly uncommon issue in premature infants, but some infants require thyroid hormone supplementation in the nursery. Most often, these infants do not have true primary hypothyroidism. Continue supplementation for a minimum of 2 years before withdrawal of therapy in consultation with an endocrinologist.

E. CLD is defined as a persistent oxygen requirement with an abnormal chest radiograph at 36 weeks postconceptual age. Associated symptoms include tachypnea, increased work of breathing, cough, audible wheeze, rhonchi or rales, and expiratory grunting. The incidence is greatest in infants of the lowest gestational age. A chest radiograph should be reviewed before hospital discharge, and pulse oximeter saturations should be assessed in room air and on supplemental oxygen. Targeted therapy includes diuretics (spironolactone-hydrochlorothiazide or furosemide at a dosage of 1–2 mg/kg/day for either), inhaled albuterol, and inhaled steroids.

F. Prevention of intercurrent viral infections is critical to the child with CLD. Avoidance of exposures, good hand hygiene, influenza vaccinations yearly, and monthly palivizumab injections to prevent severe respiratory syncytial virus infections are indicated. Rapid identification of intercurrent respiratory infections and reactive airways disease is important to allow early therapy with increased oxygen, use of inhaled bronchodilators, and possibly use of systemic corticosteroids. Any infant or child with recurrent wheezing episodes should be on an asthma controller medication.

G. The final dimension of the care of the prematurely born infant and the family is the implementation of a comprehensive care plan and monitoring of that plan. A family member will often serve as the care coordinator, although, on occasion, it is necessary to call on outside resources. Monitor the plan as part of the routine health maintenance visit. Consider periodic multidisciplinary conferences to ensure that the child is receiving the required services and to make adjustments as the child matures and his or her needs and the family's needs change.

References

American Academy of Pediatrics Section on Ophthalmology, American Academy of Ophthalmology and Association for Pediatric Ophthalmology and Strabismus. Screening examination of premature infants for retinopathy of prematurity. Pediatrics 2006;117:572.

Chyi LJ, Lee HC, Hintz SR, et al. School age outcomes of late preterm infants: special needs and challenges for infants born at 32-36 weeks gestation. J Pediatr 2008;153:25–31.

Eichenwald EC, Stark AR. Management and outcomes of very low birth weight. N Engl J Med 2008;358:1700–11.

Hack M, Taylor HG, Drotar D, et al. Chronic conditions, functional limitations, and special healthcare needs of school-aged children born with extremely-low-birth-weight in the 1990's. JAMA 2005;294:318–25.

Marlow N, Wolke D, Bracewell MA, Samara M. Neurologic and developmental disability at six years of age after extremely preterm birth. N Engl J Med 2005;352:9–19.

Moster D, Lie RT, Markestad T. Long-term medical and social consequences of preterm birth. N Engl J Med 2008;359:262–73.

Spittle AJ, Orten J, Doyle LW, Boyd R. Early developmental intervention programs post hospital discharge to prevent motor and cognitive impairments in preterm infants. Cochrane Database Syst Rev 2007;2:CD005495.

Stephens BE, Vohr BR. Neurodevelopmental outcome of the premature infant. Pediatr Clin North Am 2009;56:631–46.

Premature infant with PREVENTIVE AMBULATORY CARE
(Cont'd from p 555)

(D) Identify associated medical conditions

- (E) Chronic lung disease → Oxygen, diuretics, bronchodilators, inhaled steroids
  - (F) Prevention of intercurrent illnesses; Consider pulmonary consult
- Cardiac disease
  - Systemic hypertension → Consider echocardiogram, captopril
  - Pulmonary hypertension → Echocardiogram; Consider cardiology consult for a heart cath
- Neurologic conditions → EEG, consider MRI and neurology consult
  - Seizures
  - Hydrocephalus with or without shunt → CT scan or MRI, neurosurgery consult
  - Cerebral palsy → PT assessment; consider rehab consult for casting, botox, baclofen, orthopedic surgery, seating
- Development and behavior disorders
  - Gross and fine motor problems
  - Sensory integration
  - Speech/language
  - Behavior issues

  → Consult PT, OT, speech therapy; consider formal developmental evaluation; consider mental health input for behavior
- Ophthalmology
  - Retinopathy of prematurity (ROP)
  - Refractive errors
  - Strabismus

  → Consult ophthalmology; Follow ROP until retina is fully vascularized; then regular visits to assess refractive errors
- Gastroenterologic disorders
  - Gastroesophageal reflux → Medical therapy; consider pH impedance study, surgery referral
  - Short bowel syndrome → Use of elemental formula; ursodiol for cholestasis; fat soluble vitamins; nutrition and GI consultation
  - Feeding disorders; Gastrostomy feeds → Swallow study for aspiration; consult OT
- Endocrine disorders → Treat with levothyroxine until 2–3 years of age; consider endocrinology consult
  - Hypothyroidism
- Otolaryngologic disorders → Consult ENT and audiology
  - Recurrent ear infections
  - Sinusitis
  - Hearing loss
  - Tracheomalacia or airway stenosis

(G) Implement a care plan with follow up and monitoring

Medical Care of Children in Foster Care

Lora Melnicoe, MD, MPH

Nearly 500,000 children in the United States live in foster care, including foster homes, kinship placement, group homes, and residential treatment centers. Several studies have demonstrated that these children are at greatest risk for medical and developmental problems. Managing their health needs is complicated by the lack of medical and family history, their fragmentation of health care because of frequent and/or multiple changes in their living situation, difficulties in achieving follow-up care, and communication and consent barriers within the social work system. Ideally, each foster child obtains a medical home where medical, dental, and psychological services can be obtained.

A. Legal consent for treatment must be obtained before providing routine care. In general, social services has the authority to offer consent and provides foster parents with written documentation that authorizes routine medical treatment. If parental rights have not been terminated, biological parents need to give informed consent for invasive procedures.

Adolescents with the capacity to consent should be entitled to receive confidential services related to family planning, sexually transmitted infections, and substance abuse. Local and state statutes may have specifications regarding these issues, and foster care agencies may have varying policies, necessitating awareness of these policies in your community.

B. Commonly, foster parents are not able to provide medical information on a newly placed child. The social worker may have brief or cursory information regarding a child's current medical history, the past or family medical history, as well as developmental, educational, psychological, and dental histories. Often the parent is not cooperative in revealing or supplying health information, and medication and supplies, including eyeglasses, may be withheld. Older children are able to provide history regarding themselves and their siblings, but this information must be interpreted with caution. Foster parents should be carefully interviewed regarding their concerns and observations. Schools and state immunization registries can provide additional information, particularly regarding vaccination status. It is also important to obtain available information from medical records with the assistance of the case worker, who can sign consent for and request release of the medical records.

C. Initial Medical Screen: Ideally, an initial medical evaluation takes places within 48 to 72 hours of placement. The purpose of this visit is to identify any acute or contagious illness, evidence of abuse or neglect, chronic conditions requiring immediate treatment, and severe psychological or developmental concerns. This evaluation would include a review of any available medical information, nutritional screening and height and weight with percentiles, and complete bodily inspection and external genital examination. Assessment for any chronic conditions, pregnancy, and hygiene status is completed, and identification of priority areas for obtaining additional medical or developmental information.

D. Comprehensive Examination: Within 1 month of placement, a comprehensive medical assessment should occur, to review medical, developmental, educational, psychological, and dental information, to identify conditions that need treatment or further evaluation, and to develop a treatment plan. Federal social service statutes require that this visit is scheduled within 2 weeks of placement. Birth parents should be included at this appointment if appropriate and possible.

During this visit, a standard history, review of systems, and complete physical examination should be performed in a culturally competent environment. Older children and teens should be interviewed separately for part of the visit. Current child safety and response to the foster home should be assessed. Standardized developmental and mental health screens should be performed. Adolescents should be surveyed regarding their behavioral risk factors, and family planning and health education information should be provided as appropriate. Hearing and vision screens should be completed.

For children younger than 3 years who are at high risk for dental caries, fluoride varnish should be applied. Laboratory studies should include tuberculin skin test (TST), anemia and lead screening, and glucose, lipids, and liver function tests (LFTs) for obesity as indicated. Routine screening for sexually transmitted infections should be performed on sexually active teens.

Anticipatory guidance should include areas of particular concern among foster children, specifically sleep, hygiene, toileting, and mealtime behaviors; rules and limit-setting, aggressive or withdrawn behaviors, and building confidence and self-esteem; as well as the management of drug-exposed infants. Educational information should be provided as needed. At this time, subspecialty and mental health referrals are made as indicated. Foster families may need additional support through Women, Infants, and Children program referrals, provision of medical equipment and supplies including pull-ups, as well as in-home therapy services.

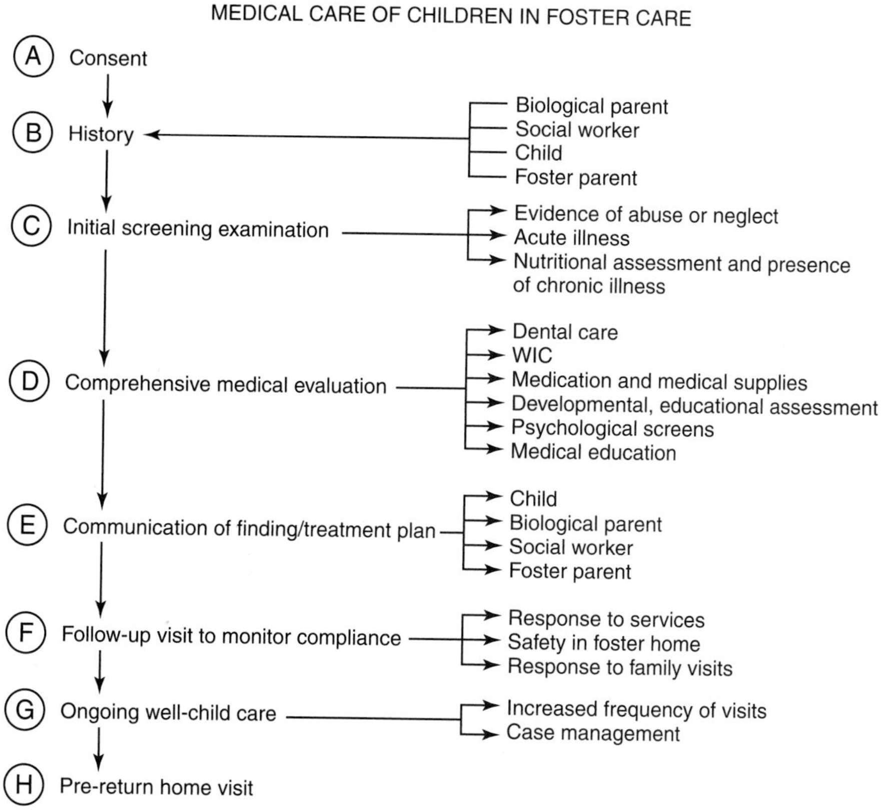
MEDICAL CARE OF CHILDREN IN FOSTER CARE
A Consent
B History
Biological parent
Social worker
Child
Foster parent
C Initial screening examination
Evidence of abuse or neglect
Acute illness
Nutritional assessment and presence of chronic illness
D Comprehensive medical evaluation
Dental care
WIC
Medication and medical supplies
Developmental, educational assessment
Psychological screens
Medical education
E Communication of finding/treatment plan
Child
Biological parent
Social worker
Foster parent
F Follow-up visit to monitor compliance
Response to services
Safety in foster home
Response to family visits
G Ongoing well-child care
Increased frequency of visits
Case management
H Pre-return home visit

E. Communication of Treatment Plan: Medical information and plans must be discussed with the foster parent, social worker, and foster child as appropriate. In some cases, the guardian ad litem, court personnel, foster care agency, or biological parents may need to be informed about relevant medical, behavioral, or developmental findings. This can be a challenging and time-consuming task for the medical provider, but is essential to ensure the successful completion of the treatment plan.

F. Follow-up Visit: A follow-up visit provides assurance that the recommended treatment plan is being carried out. Results of evaluations and referrals can be discussed, additional problems can be identified, and responses to treatment can be determined. It is imperative to document that acceptable weight gain has occurred; growth and developmental parameters should be closely monitored. Behavioral patterns related to feeding, sleeping, toileting, and communication and limit-setting can be discussed, and additional education can be provided to foster parents. Foster child safety and adjustment can be assessed, and older children and adolescents should be interviewed separately for a portion of the visit.

G. Ongoing Well-Child Care: Because of their complexity, children in out-of-home placement need to be seen at more frequent intervals than are recommended for other children. The AAP Task Force on Health Care for Children in Foster Care suggests monthly visits up to 6 months of age. After 2 years of age, well-child care should be scheduled every 6 months, to closely monitor growth, developmental, and psychosocial progress. Inspection for additional abuse or neglect can also be done at these visits. Ongoing case management is valuable to assure that medical, psychological, and developmental needs are being met.

H. Pre-return Home Visit: Before children return home from placement, it is useful to have a visit to clarify medical interventions that have occurred, update prescriptions and necessary medical supplies, and ensure that necessary therapy will continue after their return home. Ideally, the biological parent and possibly the guardian ad litem should attend the visit and have an opportunity to have their questions and concerns addressed. The social worker needs to be aware of needed treatment and follow-up visits, to ensure that the treatment plan is continued after the children return home.

References

AAP Task Force on Health Care for Children in Foster Care. Fostering health: health care for children and adolescents in foster care. 2nd ed. Elk Grove Village, IL: American Academy of Pediatrics; 2005.

Szilaggi M. Foster care. In: Parker S, Zuckerman B, Augustyn M, editors. Developmental and behavioral pediatrics. Philadelphia; Lippincott Williams & Wilkins; 2005. p. 401–4.

Cerebral Palsy

Susan D. Apkon, MD, and Jason T. Rhodes, MD

Cerebral palsy (CP) is a disorder of movement and posture that is caused by a nonprogressive injury to the developing brain. Cerebral palsy causes limitations in activity with motor impairments that are often accompanied by disturbances in sensation, perception, cognition, communication, and behavior. It is the most common physical disability affecting children, with an incidence of 2 to 3 per 1000 live births. The onset occurs prenatally, perinatally, or postnatally. The most common causative factors of CP are prenatal in timing and include infection, intrauterine stroke, and genetic malformations. Infants born before 32 weeks gestational age are at greater risk for development of CP. Classification of CP is based on body parts involved (hemiplegia, diplegia, and quadriplegia being most common) and movement patterns (spasticity, dystonia, choreoathetosis, or ataxia).

A. Obtain a complete history including prenatal, perinatal, and postnatal information. Determine medical history including growth and nutrition, medical complications, hospitalizations, medications, and allergies. Obtain developmental history including gross and fine motor and speech-language skills. The history should also include therapy interventions, functional and ambulatory status, and use of equipment and orthotics.

B. Perform a complete physical examination including weight, height, and head circumference (occipital-frontal circumference) at each visit. With the neurologic examination, assess tone and deep tendon reflexes, and note persistent primitive reflexes. Observe the child's skills, such as rolling, sitting, and walking, as well as hand use, communication, and play. In the musculoskeletal examination, evaluate range of motion in upper and lower extremities, the gait if the patient is ambulatory, and assess the hips and spine. Evaluate vision and hearing.

(Continued on page 562)

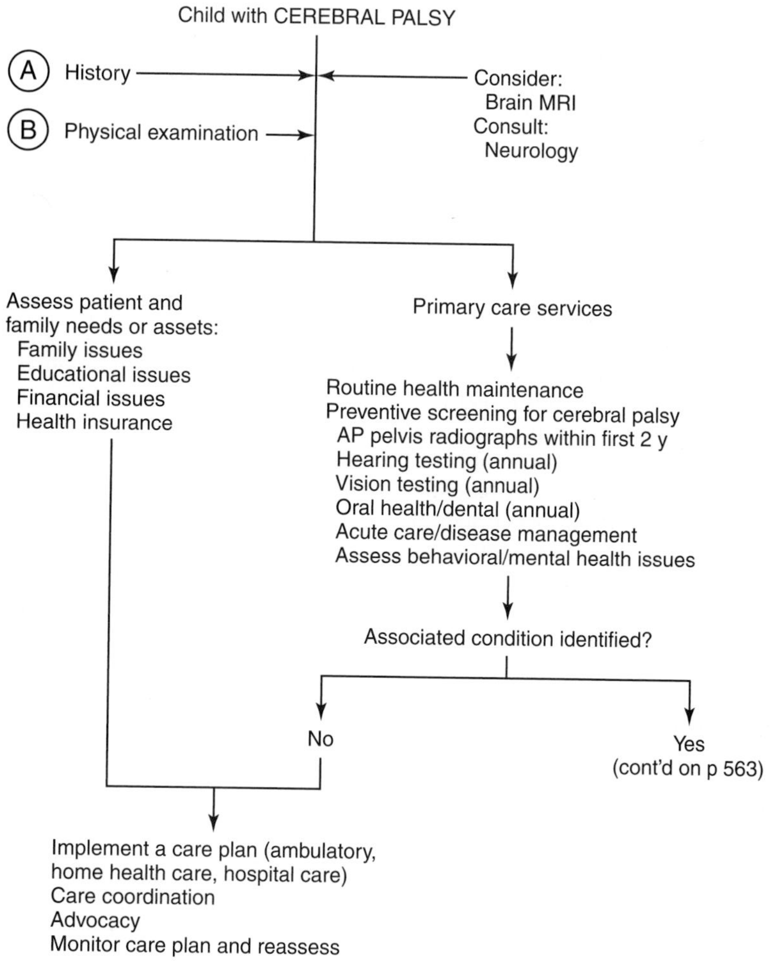
Child with CEREBRAL PALSY
A
History
B
Physical examination
Consider:
Brain MRI
Consult:
Neurology
Assess patient and family needs or assets:
Family issues
Educational issues
Financial issues
Health insurance
Primary care services
Routine health maintenance
Preventive screening for cerebral palsy
AP pelvis radiographs within first 2 y
Hearing testing (annual)
Vision testing (annual)
Oral health/dental (annual)
Acute care/disease management
Assess behavioral/mental health issues
Associated condition identified?
No
Yes
(cont'd on p 563)
Implement a care plan (ambulatory, home health care, hospital care)
Care coordination
Advocacy
Monitor care plan and reassess

C. Oral motor difficulties can affect nutritional status. Obtaining the child's weight at each visit is important to follow growth and general health. A history of choking or coughing during mealtime or frequent respiratory infections should prompt a referral to assess feeding and swallowing abilities. Based on results of the study, modification to diet may be made. Consider a gastrostomy tube for chronic malnutrition or severe aspiration.

D. Gastroesophageal reflux is a common problem for children with cerebral palsy. Consider dietary modifications. Medications such as H2 blockers and proton pump inhibitors may be necessary. Refer for surgical intervention if diet and medications are not effective.

E. Abnormalities in tone and movement can put children with cerebral palsy at risk for hip subluxation and/or dislocation, contractures of joints, and scoliosis. A baseline anterior-posterior (AP) radiograph of the pelvis should be obtained at 1 to 2 years of age and then repeated every 6 months to yearly depending on amount of subluxation and rate of progression. Refer to an orthopedic surgeon if evidence of subluxation is present. Scoliosis management should include radiographs at 2 to 3 years of age pending clinical findings and then monitoring if there is scoliosis found based on amount and rate of progression. With progression or curvature greater than 20 degrees, consult orthopedics for further management because brace treatment is not effective in CP and surgical management will possibly be needed. Generalized spasticity interfering with function, positioning, or comfort should be treated with medications, such as oral diazepam or baclofen. Use low doses initially to avoid sedating side effects. Intrathecal administration of baclofen is effective at reducing severe spasticity. Localized tone can be managed with nerve blocks using phenol or intramuscular injections of botulinum toxin. Common lower extremity muscles targeted include hip adductors, hamstrings, and gastrocnemius muscles. Spasticity in the upper extremity commonly affects the biceps, pronator, wrist and finger flexors, and thumb adductors. Contractures of joints may be managed with range-of-motion exercises, nerve and muscle blocks, or surgical intervention.

F. Early initiation of therapy services including physical, occupation, and speech therapy can facilitate acquisition of new skills and prevent complications that are secondary to the underlying pathologic process. Therapy can also assist families in interacting with, handling, and positioning their infants. As children become older, the therapy takes into account the child's age, cognitive ability, and level of functioning, with the overall goal of improving function, activity participation, and quality of life. Therapists can assist with ordering equipment including wheelchairs.

Reference

Olesek J, Davidson L. Cerebral palsy. In: Braddom RL, editor. Physical medicine and rehabilitation. 4th ed. Philadelphia: Elsevier; 2011. p. 1253–73.

Child with CEREBRAL PALSY
Associated condition identified?

↓

Yes
(cont'd from p 561)

Condition	Management	Consult
(C) Nutrition Feeding problems (p 548)	Consider swallow study	Consult: Feeding specialist Nutritionist
Growth problems (p 12)	Assess nutritional intake and exclude endocrine disorders	Consult: Nutritionist Endocrinologist
(D) Gastrointestinal Gastroesophageal reflux (p 584) Constipation (p 214)	Medical management Radiologic studies	Consult: Gastroenterology Surgery
(E) Musculoskeletal Hip dislocation	Radiologic studies AP pelvic films	Consult: Orthopedics
Scoliosis	Radiologic studies	Consult: Orthopedics
Spasticity/contractures	Consider: Durable medical equipment (wheelchair, car seat, bath seat) Diazepam, baclofen Physical and occupational therapy Neuromuscular block (phenol and/or botulinum toxin) Surgery	Consult: Rehabilitation medicine Orthopedics
Excessive secretions	Consider: Glycopyrrolate (Robinul) Scopolamine patch	Consult: ENT consult
Seizures (p 358)	Consider: Anti-epileptic drug level	Consult: Neurology consult
Gynecologic problems	Consider: Gynecology Adolescent medicine	
Behavioral and mental health problems (p 505)	Consider: Mental health professional	

↓

(F) Ancillary therapies
Speech, OT, PT, nutrition

Cleft Lip and Cleft Palate

Robert Brayden, MD, and Sondra Valdez, BSN

Cleft lip with or without cleft palate (CL ± P) and cleft palate only (CPO) are common malformations. The prevalence of CL ± P is approximately 1 in 1000 individuals. CPO occurs in 1 in 2500 individuals. Cleft lip results from the lack of fusion of the maxillary and nasomedial processes. The palate separates the naso-oral pharynx, impacting eustachian tube function, and plays a critical role in speech, as well as feeding. Numerous combinations and varying degrees of severity exist, ranging from unilateral cleft lip to bilateral cleft lip associated with or without clefting of the palate. Cleft palate results from incomplete or absence of the palatal shelves fusing. The extent of palatal clefting ranges from involvement of the entire length of the palate to something as minor as a bifid uvula with normal velopharyngeal functioning.

Women with a family history of cleft lip and palate or a history in their partner's family should be advised to begin taking 0.4 mg/day folic acid 3 months before conception to reduce the risk for recurrence in offspring.

Table 1. **Recurrence Risk**

Relationship to Index Case	CL ± P (%)	CPO (%)
Sibling (overall risk)	4.0	1.8
2 affected siblings	10.0	8.0
Sibling and one affected parent	10.0	
Anomaly		
Bilateral cleft lip and palate	5.7	
Unilateral cleft lip and palate	4.2	
Unilateral cleft lip	2.5	
General population	0.1	0.04

CL ± P, cleft lip with or without cleft palate; *CPO*, cleft palate only.

Table 2. **Acceptable Growth by Age of Child**

Age (months)	Weight Gain (g/day)
Birth to 3	20–30
3–6	15–20
6–9	10–15
9–12	6–11
12–18	5–8
18–25	3–7

A. The following elements of history are relevant to cleft lip or palate:

Prenatal history: parental ages and health status; gestation and duration; results of diagnostic procedures (ultrasonography, amniocentesis); complications (bleeding, high fever); fetal movement; and teratogen exposures (e.g., anticonvulsants, retinoids, alcohol and illegal drugs [cocaine, amphetamine]).

Family history: any cleft lip or palate in the first-degree or second-degree relatives (Table 1); other birth defects, developmental delays, or learning disabilities; genetic anomalies; multiple miscarriages or stillbirths.

Delivery history: gestational age at onset of labor; complications of labor; fetal presentation; mode of delivery; neonatal status and Apgar scores.

Birth history: newborn course (feeding, other obvious anomalies, complications) and physical growth (height, weight, head circumference) (Table 2).

Developmental history: early milestones, results of formal psychometric testing, and current therapies.

Medical history: general health; growth; illnesses; frequency of ear infections; surgical procedures; special studies, including brain imaging, echocardiography, abdominal ultrasonography; audiology, otolaryngology, plastic, dental, and ophthalmologic evaluation.

B. The physical examination of children with clefting concerns focuses on evidence of airway obstruction and/or the presence of Pierre Robin sequence (PRS). PRS results from a small mandible, which displaces the tongue, thus preventing the palatal shelves from fusing during embryologic development. PRS may result in respiratory obstruction from the posterior displacement of the tongue, sometimes requiring intubation at birth. Avoiding the supine position and placing these infants in the lateral or prone position will decrease the incidence of obstructive events. Feeding infants with PRS is often challenging and requires an upright or prone position. In addition, infants with PRS have an increased incidence of gastroesophageal reflux disease. Severely symptomatic children may require surgical intervention.

Cardiac anomalies are somewhat more likely to occur when a child has a cleft of the palate. A number of genetic syndromes are responsible for the structural components that result in the formation of the midline structures of the palate and heart muscle. A careful examination can detect whether a cardiac defect is present.

Facial characteristics may give further evidence to genetic abnormalities. A small but rounded face and a narrowness of the alae nasi are signs of 22q11.2 deletion or DiGeorge syndrome. The shape of the skull, the positioning of the eyes, and the eyelid openings may give evidence for the presence of syndromic associations with a cleft. Facial anomalies may also suggest amniotic band syndrome that can result in clefting.

Vertebral bodies are also midline structures and can, on occasion, be affected when clefting syndromes are present. Likewise, the penile shaft is more susceptible to hypospadias when a male has a cleft of the lip or palate.

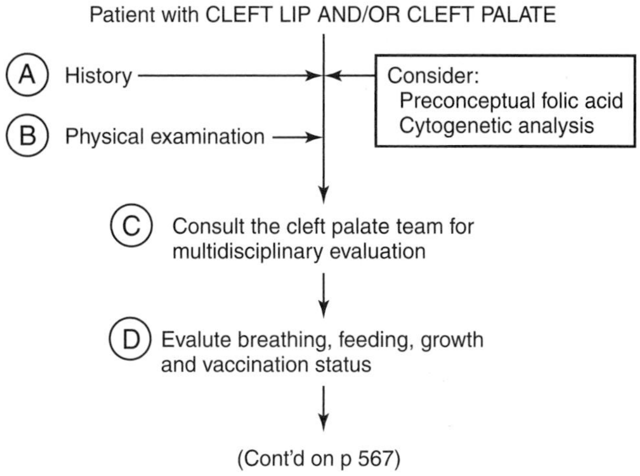
Patient with CLEFT LIP AND/OR CLEFT PALATE
A
History
B
Physical examination
Consider:
Preconceptual folic acid
Cytogenetic analysis
C
Consult the cleft palate team for multidisciplinary evaluation
D
Evalute breathing, feeding, growth and vaccination status
(Cont'd on p 567)

C. A multidisciplinary approach that integrates audiology, dentistry, genetics, orthodontics, otolaryngology, plastic surgery, primary care pediatrics, psychology, social work, and speech pathology is provided in many centers.

D. Primary care pediatricians and occupational therapists will review the approach to feeding with the family and will closely monitor the infant's weight gain and feeding difficulties. Problems such as coughing, choking, reflux through the nose, and extended feeding time lasting longer than 20 minutes should be addressed.

Some babies with particularly large palatal clefts may benefit from the early construction and placement of a palatal obturator prosthesis. This device provides an acrylic hard structure that, if accepted by the infant, can facilitate feeding.

For babies with cleft lip only, breast-feeding is usually possible. Babies with clefts of palatal structures rarely have successful breast-feeding. Babies with a cleft palate will usually need a specialized feeding system, such as the Haberman, Mead Johnson, or Pigeon bottle, and can receive pumped breast milk or formula.

Immunizations should be given at the usual times with one exception. The live virus vaccines replicate in the body and theoretically may interfere with wound healing because of the predilection to find sites of enhanced blood flow. An interval of 6 weeks either before or after live virus injected vaccines (MMR [mumps, measles, and rubella], varicella) and surgery is an ample separation.

E. Middle-ear effusions and hearing deficits should be closely monitored, especially early in life. Children with clefting of the palate and/or anomalies of the hearing apparatus, such as hemifacial microsomia or Goldenhar syndrome, should receive early and thorough evaluation of hearing and needed interventions to maximize hearing potential.

F. Surgical care may involve a plastic surgeon, otolaryngologist, and/or oral surgeon. Cleft lip malformations are usually closed at about 3 months of life. Repairing a bilateral cleft lip may require more than one operation. Cleft palate surgery is usually performed between 6 and 15 months of age. Good postoperative care is essential. Educate the parents carefully on proper incision care, diet restrictions (full liquid or soft diet), and guidelines for the safe use of arm restraints. When additional surgery is needed, there is usually a 4- to 6-month healing period between procedures. As the child grows, additional surgery may be indicated to improve palatal function. Indications for additional surgery include speech problems related to incomplete closure of the palate, airway obstruction, and breakdown of the initial repair.

G. Reflecting the influence of genetic, developmental, and environmental factors in its occurrence, CPO is more often syndromic and seen in association with other anomalies compared with CL ± P. However, both isolated and syndromic forms of each occur, and the general diagnostic approach is the same.

Decide initially whether structural anomalies are present (Table 3). Determining whether a cleft lip or palate is isolated versus syndromic is important. Cytogenetic testing is important for many children with clefts. Clefting may occur in chromosomal disorders (e.g., 22q11.2 deletion, trisomy 13, trisomy 18) or single-gene disorders (van der Woude syndrome, ectrodactyly-ectodermal dysplasia-clefting syndrome).

Individuals with 22q11.2 deletion syndrome have a range of findings that may include congenital heart disease, palatal abnormalities, characteristic facial features, and learning difficulties. Hypocalcemia and immune deficiency, although less common, are also seen. The severe end of the 22q11.2 deletion spectrum is known as DiGeorge syndrome.

Palatal clefts may be primary or secondary. Secondary clefting usually results from PRS. As described previously, PRS may be an isolated anomaly, or it may occur as part of a skeletal, muscular, connective tissue, or chromosomal syndrome. Stickler syndrome is a single-gene disorder that is sometimes associated with clefting of the palate based on a small mandible. Stickler syndrome is a disorder of collagen and also leads to hearing problems, vision disorders including early and severe myopia, and joint problems.

The risk rate for recurrence of CL ± P after one affected child is in the range of 4% (see Table 1). However, with a history of two affected first-degree relatives, the recurrence risk rate is about 10%. For isolated cleft palate, the recurrence risk rate after one affected child is 1.8%, increasing to 8% after two affected siblings.

H. Dental care should address problems that may be associated with clefts of the palate. An obturator may need to be fabricated to facilitate feeding. Nasal alveolar molding may be recommended; this presurgical appliance repositions the premaxilla and aligns the cleft edges, decreasing the number of surgeries required. The dentist also provides anticipatory guidance relating to missing or malformed teeth, crowding, spacing, and alveolar abnormalities. Children with clefts are at a greater risk for dental caries, and good oral hygiene should be promoted, starting when the first tooth erupts.

I. Speech therapy is important for the prevention and treatment of speech disorders. Therapy for clefting conditions most commonly is focused on expressive language and articulation skills and the development of a home-based parent–child program.

J. See the Child with Special Health Care Needs (p. 548) overview chapter for a discussion of family assets and needs, and behavioral and mental health services.

Table 3. **Common Genetic Anomalies Associated with Cleft Lip with or without Cleft Palate and Cleft Palate Only**

Genetic Anomalies	Clinical Description
Single-Gene Defects	
Stickler syndrome	Severe myopia, spondyloepiphyseal dysplasia
van der Woude syndrome	Lip pits, hypodontia
Ectrodactyly-ectodermal dysplasia-clefting (EEC) syndrome	Ectrodactyly, ectodermal dysplasia
Roberts syndrome	Microcephaly, hypomelia, hypotrichosis, facial hemangioma
Fryns syndrome	Diaphragmatic abnormalities, coarse face, digital hypoplasia
Oral-facial-digital	Oral frenula, hypoplasia of the alar cartilage, digital asymmetry
Chromosomal Anomalies	
22q11.2 deletion	Cardiac defects, velopharyngeal incompetence, dysmorphic facial features
Trisomy 13	Holoprosencephaly, polydactyly, cardiac defects, eye abnormalities
4p–syndrome	Hypertelorism, broad nose, microcephaly, low set ears

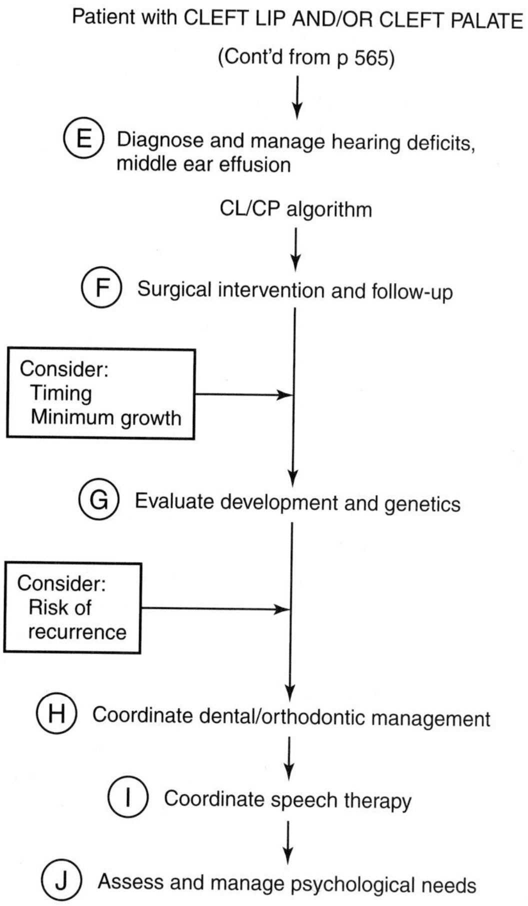
Patient with CLEFT LIP AND/OR CLEFT PALATE
(Cont'd from p 565)
E
Diagnose and manage hearing deficits, middle ear effusion
CL/CP algorithm
F
Surgical intervention and follow-up
Consider:
Timing
Minimum growth
G
Evaluate development and genetics
Consider:
Risk of recurrence
H
Coordinate dental/orthodontic management
I
Coordinate speech therapy
J
Assess and manage psychological needs

References

Jones KL, editor. Smith's recognizable patterns of human malformation. 6th ed. Philadelphia: WB Saunders; 2006.

Losee JE, Kirschner RE, editors. Comprehensive cleft care. New York: McGraw Hill; 2009.

Wilcox AJ, Lie RT, Solvoll K, et al. Folic acid supplements and risk of facial clefts: a national population based case-control study. BMJ 2007; 334:462. doi:10.1136/BMJ.39079.618287.OB.

Transitioning Young Adults with Special Health Care Needs to Adult Medical Care

Laura Pickler, MD, MPH

Children with complex medical and genetic conditions are living longer than was predicted in the past because of better treatments and overall care. Currently, greater than 90% of children born with special health care needs reach adulthood. According to 2000 nationwide census data, approximately 6% or 2.6 million children and youths age 5 to 15 years have a disability. Often, the success of excellent pediatric medicine results in young adults who require ongoing, sometimes intensive, medical supervision throughout their lives. Unfortunately, a significant proportion of youth lack access to a physician familiar with their condition and lack the ability to pay for necessary medical services. The challenges and failures of medical transition have been well documented and are available for review elsewhere.

Healthy People 2020 clearly established the goal that transition would be facilitated in all aspects of life to include health care. Having a source of medical care in the medical home model is the foundation on which all other aspects of adult life hinge, such as work and independent living. Medical transition does not necessarily require a change in the provider of health care but does encompass a shift in the scope of medical care regardless of where that care is provided.

GOALS OF TRANSITION

The ultimate goal of transition for a young adult from pediatric-focused care to adult-focused care is to facilitate high-quality medical care that meets the needs of the young adult from a biopsychosocial standpoint. The young adult must move from a patient giving assent to being an educated self-advocate and consumer of medical services. Medical providers need to be equipped to provide a medical home model of care where collaborative relationships between primary care providers and specialists are robust. This ideal model of care is difficult to achieve, even within programs intentionally organized to provide such resources to patients, their families, pediatricians, and adult medical providers. Successful transition requires a team approach using support services from a broad array of staff to ensure education, financing, case management, communication, and support through the process of transition. This task should not be underestimated in its scope and may take several years to accomplish. The algorithm summarizes decision points important in the transition process.

ROLE OF THE PEDIATRICIAN

The primary care pediatrician is frequently the person who identifies that transition is an issue needing to be addressed and decides how to proceed (plan A, A+, A++, B+, B++). A substantial burden for medical management and medical record assembly and transfer rests with the treating pediatrician. Ideally, the young adult has received comprehensive, coordinated care within the context of a medical home throughout childhood. Technology that is increasingly available may be able to facilitate organizing the medical record into a concise summary of major childhood medical events to serve as a bridge equipping the receiving adult provider to seamlessly take over medical management of ongoing problems. The pediatrician also serves as a leader in the transition process by setting the tone for the patient and the family, acknowledging the change in their relationship, supporting emotional bonds, and leading the process of developmentally appropriate intentional transition.

ROLE OF YOUNG ADULTS AND THEIR FAMILY MEMBERS

As more young adults have attempted transition to adult care, families have become increasingly vocal with regard to their needs in this process. The lack of well-coordinated processes to ensure safe and high-quality systems of care has been highlighted at the national level by family advocacy organizations and others. In the current economic and political landscape of health care, families must be willing to pilot strategies for transition, provide constructive feedback on what is and is not working, and allow youths to take more responsibility and eventually the lead in their own medical decisions. Families and youths as partners in the medical education process cannot be underestimated in their importance. Only through collaboration will the transition process improve for everyone involved.

ROLE OF THE ADULT PROVIDER

Adult medical providers have the role in assuming the care and management of these youths. Initially there may be comanagement with pediatric primary care and specialty providers while the patient is becoming established. Not insignificantly, the adult provider should assume a role in

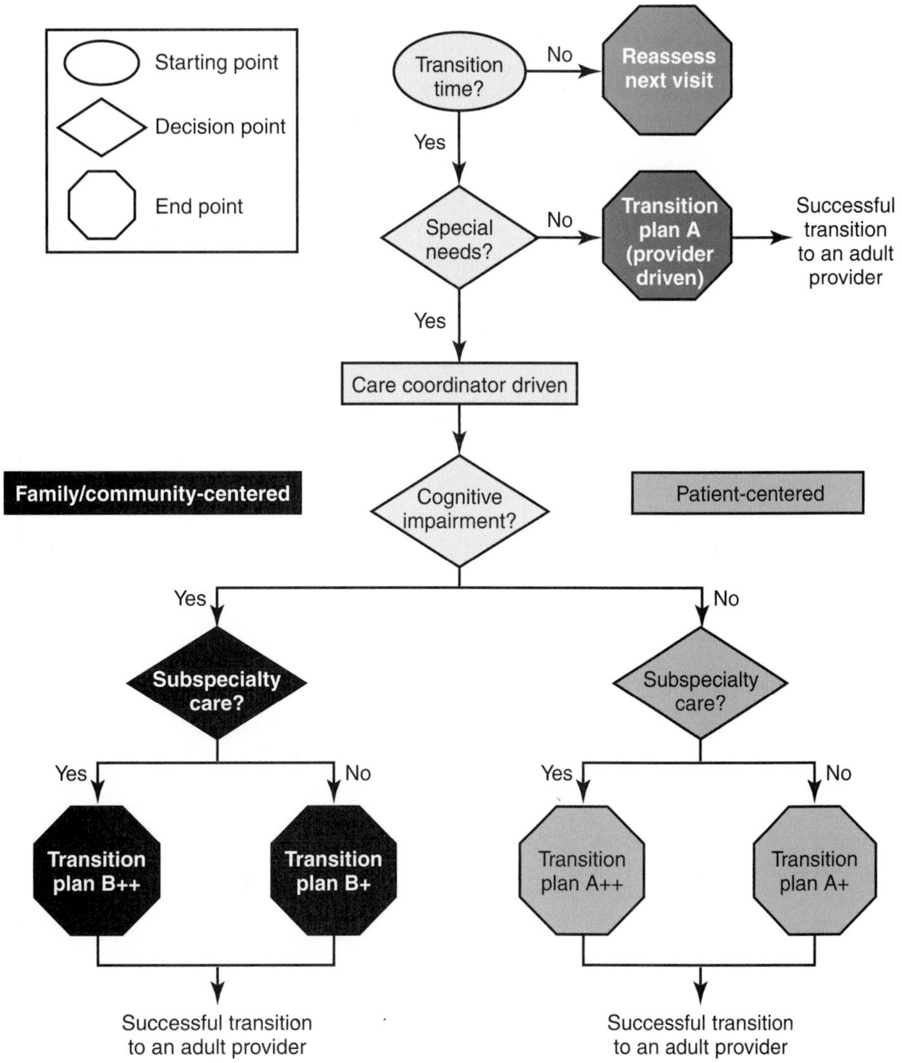
Starting point
Decision point
End point
Transition time?
No
Reassess next visit
Yes
Special needs?
No
Transition plan A (provider driven)
Successful transition to an adult provider
Yes
Care coordinator driven
Family/community-centered
Cognitive impairment?
Patient-centered
Yes
No
Subspecialty care?
Subspecialty care?
Yes
No
Yes
No
Transition plan B++
Transition plan B+
Transition plan A++
Transition plan A+
Successful transition to an adult provider
Successful transition to an adult provider

supporting the young adult and his or her family in finding a new balance in the adult medical setting. The continued involvement of the family should be expected and encouraged during this transitioning period. In addition, working with the family and others to assure adequate health care financing for these youths is a major goal of transition.

RESOURCES

Excellent resources are readily available at no or low cost to aid in the transition process. Although this section is focused on youths with special health care needs, transition for all young adults should be a goal. The young adult with complex medical needs is at greater risk during this time than typically developed youths with minimal health care needs. The transition process in and of itself may be a risk factor for adverse health outcomes with high-risk youths, even youths perceived to be medically stable. Checklists may prove helpful in starting the transition discussion. Development of short-term goals can help move young adults toward greater independence. Readiness to transfer responsibility of medical management to an adult provider also may be facilitated by use of a checklist tool in busy practices. A sampling of Web-based resources includes:

- Healthy and Ready to Work: www.hrtw.org
- Family Voices: www.familyvoices.org
- El Grupo Vida: www.elgrupovida.org
- American Academy of Pediatrics, National Center for Medical Home Implementation: www.medicalhomeinfo.org
- It's Time to Transition Workbook: www.cdphe.state.co.us/ps/hcp/transition/workbook.pdf

Transition is a challenging process but may be navigated successfully using a team approach within the medical home model of care.

References

American Academy of Pediatrics. A consensus statement on health care transitions for young adults with special health care needs. Pediatrics 2002;110:1304–6.

Annunziato RA, Emre S, Shneider B, et al. Adherence and medical outcomes in pediatric liver transplant recipients who transition to adult services. Pediatr Transplant 2007;11:578–81.

Newacheck PW, Strickland B, Shonkoff JP. An epidemiologic profile of children with special health care needs. Pediatrics 1998;102:117–23.

Okumura MJ, Heisler M, Davis MM, et al. Comfort of general internists and general pediatricians in providing care for young adults with chronic illnesses of childhood. J Gen Intern Med 2008;23: 1621–7.

Peter NG, Forke CM, Ginsburg KR, Schwarz DF. Transition from pediatric to adult care: internists' perspectives. Pediatrics 2009;123: 417–23.

U.S. Department of Health and Human Services. Healthy people 2020: understanding and improving health, 2nd ed. Washington, DC: U.S. Government Printing Office; 2010.

Dermatology

Acne

Arelis Burgos-Zavoda, MD, and Joanna M. Burch, MD

Acne vulgaris is the most common skin problem in the United States, affecting nearly 80% to 85% of individuals between 11 and 30 years of age. The skin lesions in acne are initiated by hormonal changes of puberty that stimulate increased sebum production and hyperkeratinization of the pilosebaceous duct. The hyperkeratinization and excess sebum production lead to obstruction of the follicular opening (the pore clogs). During puberty, the hair follicle becomes colonized by bacteria (*Propionibacterium acnes*). The combination of these changes can in some lesions initiate an inflammatory response. These lesions are red clinically. If there is rupture of the follicular wall, inflammatory nodules result. Inflammatory acne presents with raised red papules, pustules, nodules, or cystic lesions. Noninflammatory acne includes open comedones (blackheads) and closed comedones (whiteheads).

A. Acne severity can be objectively classified using several scales, for example, mild (6–20 lesions), moderate (21–50 lesions), or severe (>50 lesions). Untreated inflammatory acne or nodulocystic acne can cause dyspigmentation or permanent scarring.

B. Skin Care: Educate the patient about proper washing with mild soap and avoiding excessive scrubbing. Look for oil-free or noncomedogenic cosmetics and lubricants. Oil-free or water-based moisturizers may help the skin dryness and irritation that can result from acne treatment. Diet usually does not affect acne.

C. Topical Treatments (Retinoids): Retinoids prevent hyperkeratinization and blockage of the pore. They are the most effective keratolytic agents. They have also been shown in several studies to have anti-inflammatory and antibacterial properties. The first retinoid brought to market was tretinoin (Retin-A), available in gel (0.01% and 0.025%), cream (0.025%, 0.05%, and 0.1%), and microgel (0.04% and 0.1%). Adapalene, available as a cream (0.1%) or gel (0.1% and 0.3%), is a synthetic retinoid that has been shown to be less irritating that tretinoin in several studies. Another topical retinoid product tazarotene (Tazorac), available in a cream (0.1%) and gel (0.1%), is one of the most effective retinoids, but often the most irritating. In general, all retinoids can be drying and irritating to the skin. These products should be applied to the face in the evening. A useful analogy for the patient is to use a "pea-sized" amount of product for a full face application, avoiding areas around the eyes, nose, and mouth. It is important to use a sunscreen (SPF 15 or higher) while outdoors. Use of retinoids can seem to worsen acne initially because of irritation, redness, and peeling. Another useful strategy to decrease the incidence of irritation is to have the patient begin therapy 3 nights a week, increasing as tolerated over a few weeks to nightly application. In patients with sensitive skin, adapalene is a good choice in the treatment of acne vulgaris with less adverse effects and high efficacy. A 12-week course is required to evaluate response. More severe or resistant acne cases can be treated with a retinoid in the evening and benzoyl peroxide (BPO) or a topical antibiotic during the day.

D. Topical Treatments (Nonretinoid):

1. BPO has antibacterial action, reduces free fatty acid concentrations, and has comedolytic activity. Use a 5% gel; it is as effective as 10% gel but less irritating. Although the liquid and cream forms are less irritating, they are much less effective. BPO washes and cleansers are useful in covering large areas such as the back and chest. BPO products may bleach colored clothing or linens. More recently, combination products containing both BPO and topical clindamycin are available, and these agents have been shown in several studies to be more effective than either ingredient used alone.
2. Azelaic acid 15% and 20% cream has mild antibacterial and comedolytic activity. It is effective for mild acne in darker skinned patients because it can lighten postinflammatory hyperpigmentation. Start with daily application and increase to twice daily if needed. A thin layer should be applied to the entire face when it is completely dry, avoiding the areas around the eyes and mouth. The layer is left on all day.
3. Topical antibiotics like erythromycin 2% gel and clindamycin 1% gel, solution, lotion, and pledgets should only be used on inflammatory acne in combination with a product with comedolytic activity. Many over-the-counter "acne" products contain some BPO, salicylic acid, and α-hydroxy acid (AHA). These ingredients may contribute to the dryness and peeling if combined with prescription therapy. If adverse effects from topical treatment persist, consider alternate-day application. Failure to improve after 12 weeks is an indication for additional therapy.

E. Topical antibiotics should be used only in combination with a keratolytic agent for mild-to-moderate inflammatory acne. Antibiotics should never be used alone for acne.

F. Treat moderate-to-severe inflammatory acne with oral tetracycline, minocycline, or doxycycline for 3 to 6 months (Table 1). Erythromycin is not an appropriate first-line choice for acne unless the tetracycline class of antibiotics is contraindicated. A topical keratolytic therapy should always be combined with an oral antibiotic. In 3 to 6 months, if the patient is improved, try to wean the dose to once a day for 2 to 3 months, then discontinue.

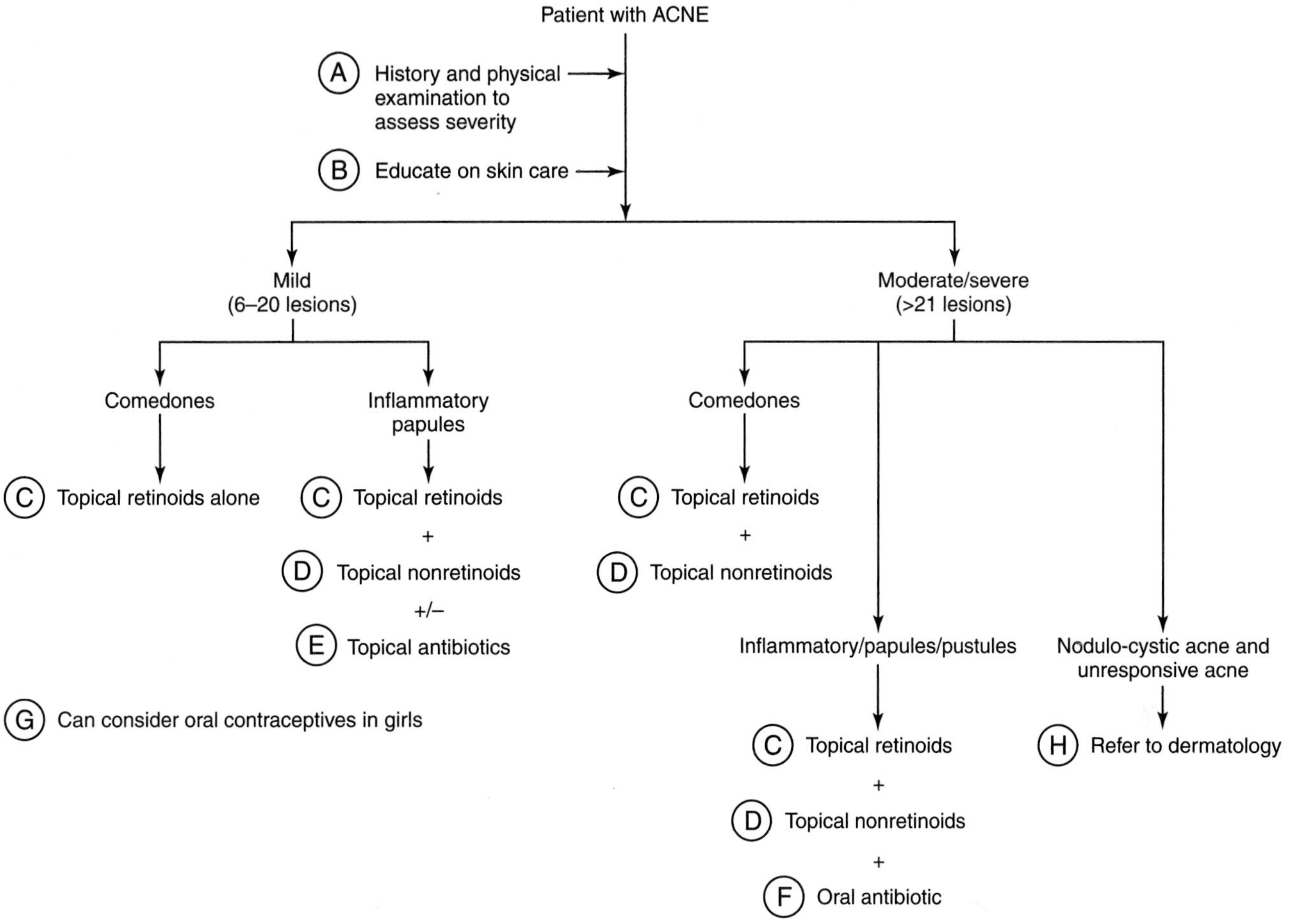
Patient with ACNE
A History and physical examination to assess severity
B Educate on skin care
Mild (6–20 lesions)
Moderate/severe (>21 lesions)
Comedones
Inflammatory papules
Comedones
C Topical retinoids alone
C Topical retinoids
+
D Topical nonretinoids
+/–
E Topical antibiotics
C Topical retinoids
+
D Topical nonretinoids
Inflammatory/papules/pustules
Nodulo-cystic acne and unresponsive acne
G Can consider oral contraceptives in girls
C Topical retinoids
+
D Topical nonretinoids
+
F Oral antibiotic
H Refer to dermatology

Table 1. **Oral Antibiotics Used in the Treatment of Acne in Adolescents**

Drug	Dosage	Product Availability
Erythromycin	500 mg bid PO	Tablets: 250, 500 mg
Tetracycline	500 mg bid PO	Tablets: 250, 500 mg
Minocycline	50–100 mg bid PO	Tablets: 50, 100 mg
Doxycycline	50–100 mg bid PO	Tablets: 50, 100 mg

Doxycycline and minocycline should be given with food, whereas tetracycline should be given on an empty stomach. Doxycycline is the most photosensitizing. Avoid tetracycline-class antibiotics in pregnancy or in children younger than 8 years. After discontinuation of oral or topical antibiotic therapy, maintenance therapy with a retinoid should be continued. If this is not done, it is likely that the primary process will restart and acne vulgaris will recur.

G. Oral contraceptives have been shown to be effective in the treatment of acne vulgaris in female individuals. Ortho Tri-Cyclen, Estrostep, and Yaz are FDA approved for the treatment of acne vulgaris.

H. Consider referral to a dermatologist for isotretinoin (Accutane) treatment of patients who have cystic acne with scarring that fails to respond to topical therapy plus oral antibiotics. Isotretinoin should not be used by pregnant or nursing mothers (causes severe birth defects) and should be used with caution by sexually active women and girls (only when an acceptable contraceptive method is being used). Adverse effects include cheilitis, dry skin, epistaxis, conjunctivitis, arthralgias, headache, fatigue, photosensitivity, hepatitis, depression, and elevation of triglycerides. Monitor pregnancy status, fasting triglyceride levels, cholesterol level, complete blood count, and liver function test results every 4 weeks.

References

Fitzpatrick JE, Morelli JG, Burch JM. Dermatology secrets. 3rd ed. St. Louis, MO: Mosby; 2007.

Hayashi N, Akamatsu H, Kawashima M; Acne Study Group. Establishment of grading criteria for acne severity. J Dermatol 2008;35(5):255–60.

Iraji F, Sadeghinia A, Shahmoradi Z, et al. Efficacy of topical azelaic acid gel in the treatment of mild-moderate acne vulgaris. Indian J Dermatol Venereol Leprol 2007;73(2):94–6.

Paller AS, Mancini AJ. Hurwitz clinical pediatric dermatology. 3rd ed. New York: Elsevier; 2006.

Piskin S, Uzunali E. A review of the use of adapalene for the treatment of acne vulgaris. Ther Clin Risk Manag 2007;3(4):621–4.

Thiboutot DM. Overview of acne and its treatment. Cutis 2008; 81(1 Suppl):3–7.

Thielitz A, Gollnick H. Topical retinoids in acne vulgaris: update on efficacy and safety. Am J Clin Dermatol 2008;9(6):369–81.

Weston WL, Lane AT, Morelli JG. A color textbook of pediatric dermatology. 4th ed. St. Louis, MO: Mosby; 2007.

Vascular Birthmarks

Arelis Burgos-Zavoda, MD, Joseph Morelli, MD, and Joanna M. Burch, MD

Vascular birthmarks are the most common type of cutaneous birth defect. They should be classified as either hemangiomas or vascular malformations. Vascular malformations are defined by the predominant vessel type within the birthmark.

A. Hemangiomas, the most common tumor of childhood, are benign tumors of capillary endothelium. Hemangiomas should not be described as capillary or cavernous; all hemangiomas are capillary, and the terms *superficial, deep,* and *mixed* should be used. Some 20% are present at birth; the rest arise during the first 8 weeks of life. Hemangiomas have a predictable natural history. They grow rapidly for the first year of life, especially during the first 6 months. During the second year of life, growth stops and involution begins. Regression takes place slowly for years; 50% are maximally regressed by age 5 years, and 90% are maximally regressed by age 9 years. Regression does not define return of the skin to normal. Most hemangiomas are not associated with complications and do not require treatment. Any facial or diaper area hemangioma should be treated, as should those causing high-output cardiac failure. If there is a question whether treatment of a hemangioma is necessary, referral should be made to a pediatric dermatologist as early as possible. Treatment options include vascular pulsed dye laser, oral glucocorticosteroids, and interferon alfa-2a. There is new, case-reported evidence that propranolol is effective in speeding the involution of large, complicated hemangiomas. This treatment should be monitored for adverse effects. Larger studies are needed.

B. Capillary malformations (port-wine stains) are the most common vascular malformation. They occur in 3 of 1000 births. Port-wine stains, always present at birth, are usually flat and light pink at birth and become progressively darker and thicker with age. Port-wine stains covering a large portion of the face including the first division of the trigeminal nerve can be associated with Sturge–Weber syndrome (SWS). SWS is the association of a facial port-wine stain with central nervous system (seizures, mental retardation, hemiplegia) and ophthalmologic (glaucoma) abnormalities. All port-wine stains have the potential to lead to overgrowth of the underlying skin and subcutaneous tissue. Overgrowth of an extremity covered by a port-wine stain is called *Klippel-Trénaunay syndrome.* Treatment of choice for port-wine stains is the vascular pulsed dye laser. There is considerable evidence warranting the beginning of laser treatments as soon after birth as possible.

C. Other vascular malformations, including lymphangiomas, should be defined by the predominant vessel within the lesion. These vascular malformations are much less common than port-wine stains. They are all difficult to treat and are best managed with the input of a specialized vascular malformation clinic.

References

Boye E, Jinnin M, Olsen BR. Infantile hemangioma: challenges, new insights, and therapeutic promise. J Craniofac Surg 2009;20 (Suppl 1):678–84.

Ch'ng S, Tan ST. Facial port-wine stains—clinical stratification and risks of neuro-ocular involvement. J Plast Reconstr Aesthet Surg 2008;61(8):889–93.

Léauté-Labrèze C, Dumas de la Roque E, Hubiche T, et al. Propranolol for severe hemangiomas of infancy. N Engl J Med 2008;358:2649–51.

O'Regan GM, Watson R, Orr D, et al. Management of vascular birthmarks: review of a multidisciplinary clinic. Ir Med J 2007;100(4): 425–7.

Siegfried EC, Keenan WJ, Al-Jureidini S. More on propranolol for hemangiomas of infancy. N Engl J Med 2008;359(26):2846.

Stier MF, Glick SA, Hirsch RJ. Laser treatment of pediatric vascular lesions: port wine stains and hemangiomas. J Am Acad Dermatol 2008;58(2):261–85.

Weston WL, Lane AT, Morelli JG. A color textbook of pediatric dermatology. 4th ed. St. Louis, MO: Mosby; 2007.

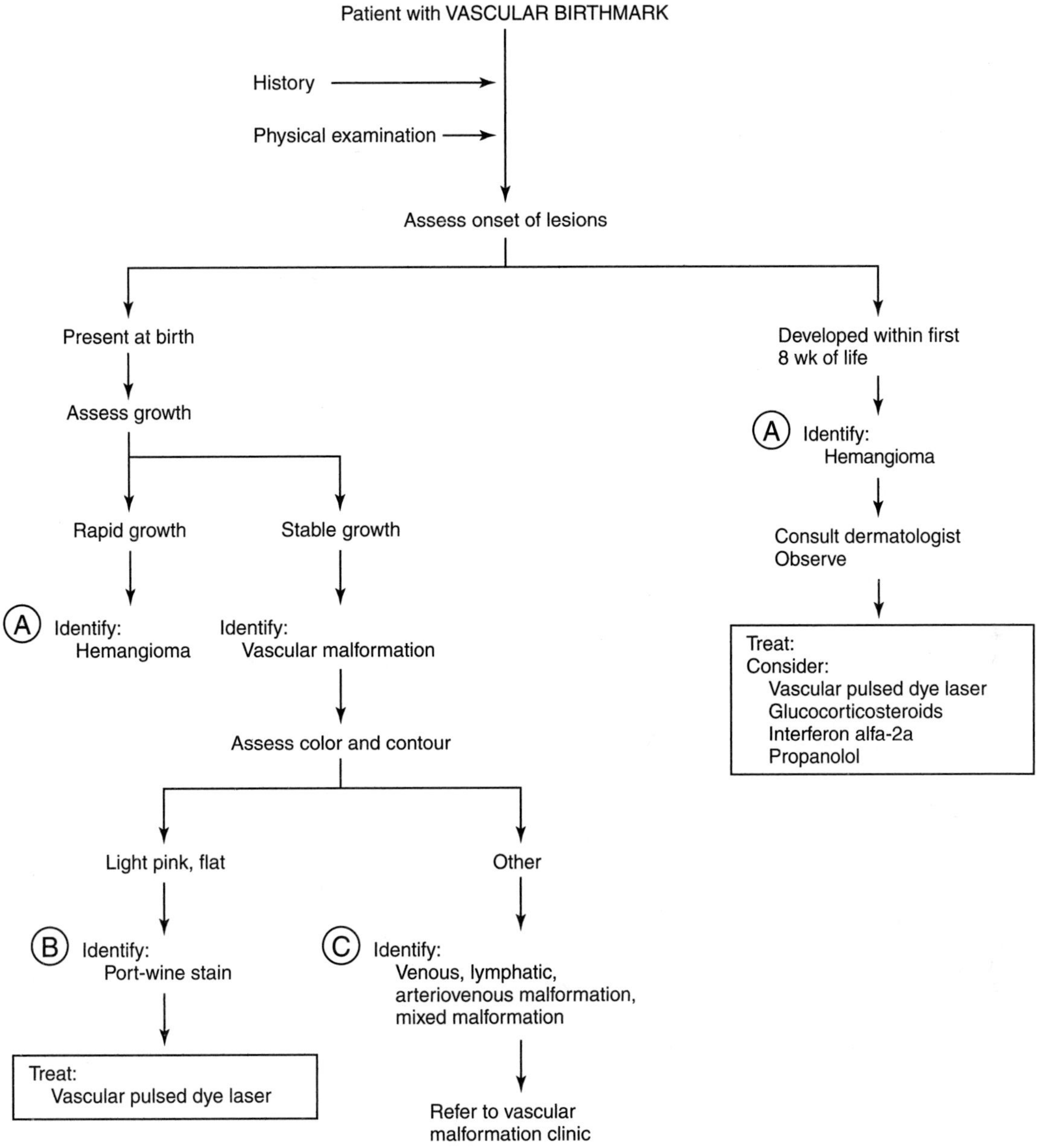
Patient with VASCULAR BIRTHMARK
History
Physical examination
Assess onset of lesions
Present at birth
Assess growth
Rapid growth
Stable growth
(A) Identify:
Hemangioma
Identify:
Vascular malformation
Assess color and contour
Light pink, flat
Other
(B) Identify:
Port-wine stain
Treat:
Vascular pulsed dye laser
(C) Identify:
Venous, lymphatic, arteriovenous malformation, mixed malformation
Refer to vascular malformation clinic
Developed within first 8 wk of life
(A) Identify:
Hemangioma
Consult dermatologist
Observe
Treat:
Consider:
Vascular pulsed dye laser
Glucocorticosteroids
Interferon alfa-2a
Propanolol

GASTROENTEROLOGIC DISORDERS

Inflammatory Bowel Diseases: Crohn Disease and Ulcerative Colitis

Samantha A. Woodruff, MD, and Edward J. Hoffenberg, MD

Inflammatory bowel diseases (IBDs) include Crohn disease and ulcerative colitis. Both appear to be precipitated by infection or environmental triggers in a genetically susceptible host. Involvement in Crohn disease is variable and can affect all areas of the gastrointestinal tract from the mouth to the anus. The inflammation of the intestines may be continuous or segmental, leaving normal "skip areas" between involved intestine. The inflammation is transmural, which predisposes to fistula formation. The disease can be categorized by the pattern of involvement: ileocolitis (52%), diffuse small intestine (20%), ileitis (19%), and colitis (9%). In ulcerative colitis, the inflammation may affect the entire colon (pancolitis) or just the distal colon. Over time, the process can extend from the distal colon to involve the entire colon. Patients with pancolitis have more severe disease, a greater incidence of extraintestinal manifestations, and an increased risk for toxic megacolon and cancer. After about 7 years of pancolitis, the risk for colon cancer increases significantly so that surveillance, which is imperfect, or colectomy should be considered to prevent colon cancer. The distinction between ulcerative colitis and Crohn disease may be "indeterminate" in 10% to 20% of patients with colitis. Patients most often have diarrhea, bloody stools, tenesmus, and abdominal pain and anemia. Presentation in Crohn disease is sometimes more subtle with growth and pubertal delay, abscess, intestinal stricture, or perianal disease including chronic fissure, or a fistula. Common extraintestinal manifestations, which may precede overt IBD, include oral aphthoid ulcers, anemia, arthritis, skin manifestations of erythema nodosa or pyoderma gangrenosum, and liver disease, most commonly sclerosing cholangitis or autoimmune hepatitis. Sclerosing cholangitis is a risk factor for development of cancer of the bile ducts (cholangiocarcinoma). The clinical, radiographic, endoscopic, and histologic findings reflect the involvement and severity of inflammation (Table 1). The goal of management is to induce a rapid clinical response and prolonged remission and also address nutrition and growth problems.

Table 1. **Degrees of Illness in Patients with Crohn Disease or Ulcerative Colitis**

Moderate: Mild systemic signs such as fever, anemia, weight loss, while tolerating oral fluids and nutrition
Severe: Severe anemia, severe hypoalbuminemia, marked malnutrition, dehydration or electrolyte disturbance *or*
Inability to tolerate oral feedings because of abdominal pain, vomiting, or intermittent partial intestinal obstruction
Very Severe: Sepsis, toxic megacolon, shock, or severe hemorrhage *or*
Complication requiring surgery

A. In the patient's history, ask about the onset and frequency of stools, including nocturnal stools; visible blood in the stools; and symptoms of urgency, cramping, and abdominal pain. Ask about nausea, vomiting, fullness, oral ulcers or stomatitis, and perianal pain (ulcers, fissures, abscess, and fistula). Right lower quadrant crampy abdominal pain may mimic appendicitis. Severe anorexia and protracted vomiting suggest intestinal obstruction related to edema or stricture, but also consider an alternative cause of an obstruction from a mass or tumor (lymphoma). With ulcerative colitis, the duration of symptoms before the patient seeks medical attention is often short (days to weeks). Recognize that ulcerative colitis may occur soon after an infectious colitis with symptoms similar to recurrent infection. Crohn disease may have a more insidious onset with longer duration of symptoms, malaise, and weight loss before seeking medical attention. Ask about systemic extraintestinal symptoms, such as fatigue, poor weight gain or weight loss, fever, arthritis or arthralgia, delayed growth and sexual development, eye pain or vision difficulty (conjunctivitis, uveitis, iritis, episcleritis), flank pain (renal stones), jaundice, pruritus, and rashes (pyoderma gangrenosum, erythema nodosa).

B. In the physical examination, document the pattern of growth (weight and height) and sexual maturation or pubertal development. Assess for signs of chronic malnutrition and hypoalbuminemia (muscle wasting, peripheral edema, clubbing of the fingers and toes) and signs of vitamin deficiency. Assess for abdominal distention, focal or diffuse tenderness, and bowel sounds. Suspect toxic megacolon in a toxic-appearing patient with abdominal distention and peritoneal signs with or without shock. The more severe the presenting symptoms, the greater the consideration for toxic megacolon. Bowel wall edema, especially in the right lower quadrant, may present as an abdominal mass. Note perianal findings (ulcers, skin tags, fissures, abscess, and fistula) that suggest Crohn disease. Note extraintestinal manifestations, such as oral ulcers or stomatitis, fever, anemia (pallor, tachycardia, hypotension), arthritis, ophthalmologic disorders (uveitis, iritis, episcleritis), jaundice (hepatitis, sclerosing cholangitis), and dermatologic findings (pyoderma gangrenosum, erythema nodosa).

C. Laboratory studies are useful in excluding alternative diagnoses (such as infection) and in assessing the severity of the disease, degree of blood loss, nutritional status, and extraintestinal involvement. Screening blood work should include a complete blood count (CBC), C-reactive protein (CRP), erythrocyte sedimentation rate (ESR), basic metabolic panel, and liver

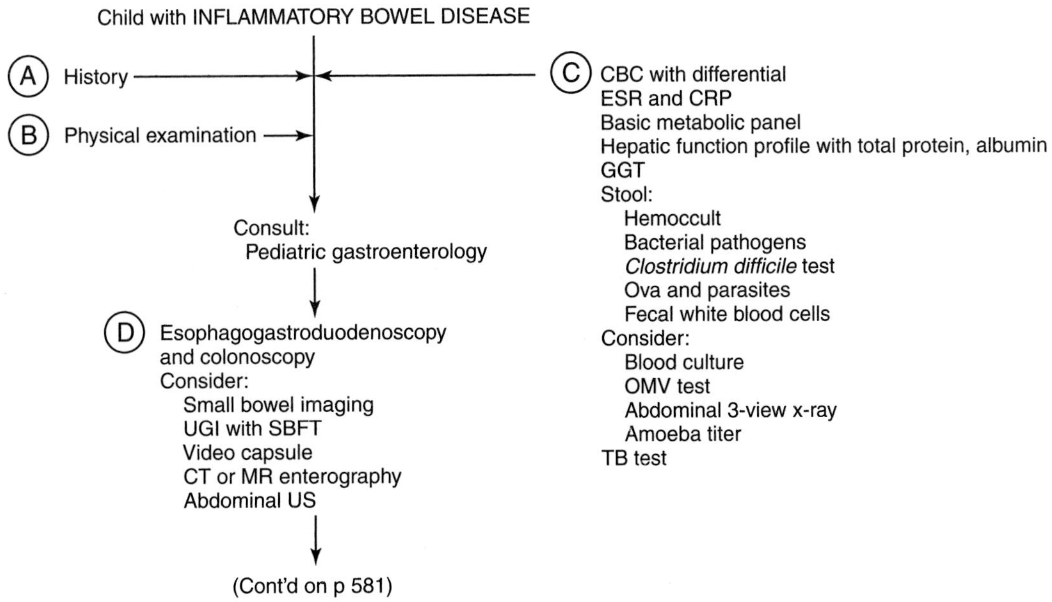
Child with INFLAMMATORY BOWEL DISEASE
A History
B Physical examination
C CBC with differential
ESR and CRP
Basic metabolic panel
Hepatic function profile with total protein, albumin
GGT
Stool:
Hemoccult
Bacterial pathogens
Clostridium difficile test
Ova and parasites
Fecal white blood cells
Consider:
Blood culture
OMV test
Abdominal 3-view x-ray
Amoeba titer
TB test
Consult:
Pediatric gastroenterology
D Esophagogastroduodenoscopy
and colonoscopy
Consider:
Small bowel imaging
UGI with SBFT
Video capsule
CT or MR enterography
Abdominal US
(Cont'd on p 581)

function tests with gamma-glutamyl transferase (GGT). Chronic intestinal losses of blood and protein may lead to hypochromic microcytic anemia and hypoalbuminemia. Diarrhea may lead to electrolyte abnormalities. Hepatitis and sclerosing cholangitis, present in up to 10% of patients (more commonly, ulcerative colitis), are associated with increased liver function tests, with GGT being the most sensitive screening test. Bacterial colitis including *Clostridium difficile* and viral colitis may mimic IBD and should be ruled out with stool studies. Testing for tuberculosis (TB) should be performed. Identify infections with *Entamoeba histolytica* with amoeba titers in low prevalence populations or stool staining in higher prevalence areas. Anti-*Saccharomyces cerevisiae* antibody (ASCA) may be positive in approximately 60% to 70% of children with Crohn disease. However, ASCA and anti-neutrophil cytoplasmic antibody (p-ANCA) serologic markers are not accurate enough for use in differentiating IBD from infectious colitis or other mimics of IBD. Serologic testing may be useful in guiding management of the 20% of patients who have indeterminate IBD. Specialized stool testing with fecal lactoferrin and calprotectin (neutrophil-derived proteins) may be useful in the monitoring of IBD, although normal values in children have not been verified. When assessing a patient for flare, infectious colitis, including cytomegalovirus (CMV) and *C. difficile,* should be considered before starting treatment with anti-inflammatory agents.

D. If toxic megacolon is suspected or the patient has signs of significant obstruction, blood loss, or shock, first order three-view radiographs of the abdomen and consult a surgeon. Avoid doing further radiologic studies and colonoscopy until the patient is stable. If the patient is stable and not toxic, consider repeating upper endoscopy and colonoscopy to assess the extent and severity of disease and to exclude infectious causes of the colitis. In Crohn disease, colonoscopy may show colitis or linear ulcerations separated by normal mucosa (skip areas) or pancolonic involvement. Characteristic findings of Crohn disease include thickened mucosa, ulcerations, pseudopolypoid formation with cobblestoning, and stenotic areas with proximal dilatation. There may be upper tract involvement with esophagitis, gastritis, or duodenitis as well. Biopsy findings include acute and chronic inflammation and, in about 25% of cases of Crohn disease, noncaseating granulomas. To assess and stage small-bowel involvement, obtain imaging test with one of the following: upper gastrointestinal series with small-bowel follow-through, video capsule endoscopy, computed tomographic (CT) enterography, or magnetic resonance (MR) enterography. Consider obtaining an abdominal ultrasound examination or computed tomographic scan with contrast enhancement when signs of an abscess, mass, or appendicitis are present.

In ulcerative colitis, there is generally a symmetric and continuous involvement of the colon with a sharp demarcation between involved and normal colon. Typical findings include erythema, friability, and aphthous ulcers. Mild terminal ileal abnormalities can occur with the pancolitis of ulcerative colitis and do not always indicate Crohn disease. Upper intestinal endoscopy with biopsy should be performed to help distinguish Crohn disease of the upper gastrointestinal tract from peptic ulcer disease or eosinophilic gastroenteropathy. However, upper endoscopy may reveal mild gastroduodenitis in up to 30% of patients with ulcerative colitis and should not be interpreted as evidence of Crohn disease. Colonic biopsy findings include acute and chronic inflammation. After the colonoscopy, obtain an upper gastrointestinal series with small-bowel follow-through to assess or stage upper gastrointestinal tract involvement by Crohn disease.

E. Therapy is based on both severity (see Table 1) and location of disease. Local therapy (suppositories and enemas) may be sufficient for left-sided disease distal to the splenic flexure. Pancolitis requires systemic therapy to induce a rapid clinical response and remission. In patients with severe and very severe illness, initial therapy may require fluid resuscitation, correction of anemia, and normalization of electrolyte imbalance. When the colitis is severe and associated with marked pain or bleeding, provide bowel rest by restricting to nothing by mouth and consider nasogastric decompression if significant cramping or vomiting. Attention to nutrition is important to promote healing as well as growth. Involvement of the gastrointestinal tract, especially the small bowel in Crohn disease, leads to impaired absorption of nutrients as well as to increased losses (i.e., calories, protein, iron). Calorie requirements may be up to 140% of baseline needs. Often, vitamin (B_{12}, folate), mineral (calcium, magnesium), and metal (zinc, copper, iron) supplementations are required. Methods to provide adequate nutrition include high-calorie liquid or elemental supplements, nasogastric feedings, and, rarely, parenteral nutrition. If significant nutritional rehabilitation is required, monitor for refeeding syndrome. Lactose intolerance, secondary to small-bowel involvement, may mimic Crohn disease and may be documented by a lactose breath test. Treatment is by avoidance of lactose-containing foods or use of lactase supplements. A low-residue diet may improve cramping and diarrhea.

F. For mild disease, oral preparations designed to deliver salicylates directly to the colon may be sufficient therapy (Table 2) to induce and maintain remission. Sulfasalazine, a salicylate attached to a sulfa carrier, is released in the colon, where it acts locally and is effective in both Crohn colitis and ulcerative colitis. Because sulfasalazine inhibits absorption of folate, supplementation with 1 mg/day is recommended. Mesalamine oral and rectal preparations also deliver salicylate to the colon, are equally effective in treating colitis, and should be used in those with sulfa allergies or intolerance to sulfasalazine. Mesalamine preparations come with different delivery systems for release in the small bowel as well as colon (Asacol has a pH-sensitive resin and is released in the distal ileum and colon, whereas Pentasa microspheres are released in jejunum, ileum, and colon). Folate supplementation is not needed when these preparations are used. For isolated proctitis, local therapy with salicylate suppositories or corticosteroid enemas may avoid adverse effects of systemic treatments. Adverse effects include headache, nausea, abdominal pain, and rashes. Rare complications from therapy are serum sickness reactions, hemolytic anemia, aplastic anemia, and pancreatitis.

G. Perianal lesions suggest Crohn disease and are treated with warm soaks, antibiotics such as metronidazole (15–30 mg/kg/day) or ciprofloxacin, immunomodulators such as 6-mercaptopurine or azathioprine (Imuran), and anti–tumor necrosis factor-α (anti–TNF-α) agents. Long-term therapy with metronidazole may lead to peripheral neuropathy. Anti–TNF-α therapy combined with immunomodulators has been associated with rare hepatosplenic T-cell lymphoma.

H. In moderate or severe IBD (systemic involvement), corticosteroids may be needed to induce a rapid clinical response, and there is systemic involvement. Anemia and iron deficiency are common. Immunize against varicella if there is not a definite history of prior disease. For severe and very severe illness, treat with intravenous methylprednisolone or oral prednisone (1 mg/kg/day up to 60 mg daily) until clinical improvement (usually 1–2 weeks). In very severe patients, intravenous therapy may be required, as well as intravenous nutritional rehabilitation. Consider secure intravenous (IV) access for prolonged therapy.

I. Indications for surgery include failure of medical management, toxic megacolon, severe hemorrhage, abscess, perforation, obstruction or stricture, growth failure, intractable pain, prevention of malignancy, and long-term corticosteroid use. In children with ulcerative colitis, consider colectomy for prevention of colon cancer after 7 years of pancolitis or persistent symptoms despite maximum medical management. In Crohn disease, surgery is not curative, so it is usually reserved for those with persistent symptoms, a small focus of intestinal disease, or the earlier surgical complications.

J. Once a response has been obtained, begin tapering corticosteroids by 10-mg weekly until at 20 mg/day. Then gradually taper by 5 mg/wk. If no response within a few days, consider surgical consult. Patients with moderate-to-severe IBD who are steroid responsive may benefit from an immunomodulator, such as 6-mercaptopurine, azathioprine, or methotrexate. These medications should be considered early in course of therapy for best chance to maintain remission and discontinue corticosteroids. Complications of immunomodulators include leukopenia, nausea, acute pancreatitis, hepatotoxicity, and shingles. Steroid-dependent or resistant and fistulizing Crohn disease patients may benefit from the use of anti–TNF-α agents, such as infliximab or adalimumab. Consider use of anti–TNF-α agents as first-line therapy in moderate-to-severe IBD, or after minimal response to 3 to 7 days of IV corticosteroids. Consider maintenance therapy until growth and sexual maturation are complete. For steroid-dependent or steroid-resistant ulcerative colitis, consider a colectomy or alternative therapies such as infliximab, tacrolimus, or cyclosporine. Also consider assessing bone mineral density.

K. Maintenance nutritional support provides adequate calorie intake for growth and replenishes deficiencies. Iron supplementation is common. A low-residue diet may reduce diarrhea and crampy abdominal pain. An elemental diet can be used to induce remission in Crohn disease, but is not effective in ulcerative colitis.

(Continued on page 582)

Child with INFLAMMATORY BOWEL DISEASE

(Cont'd from p 579)

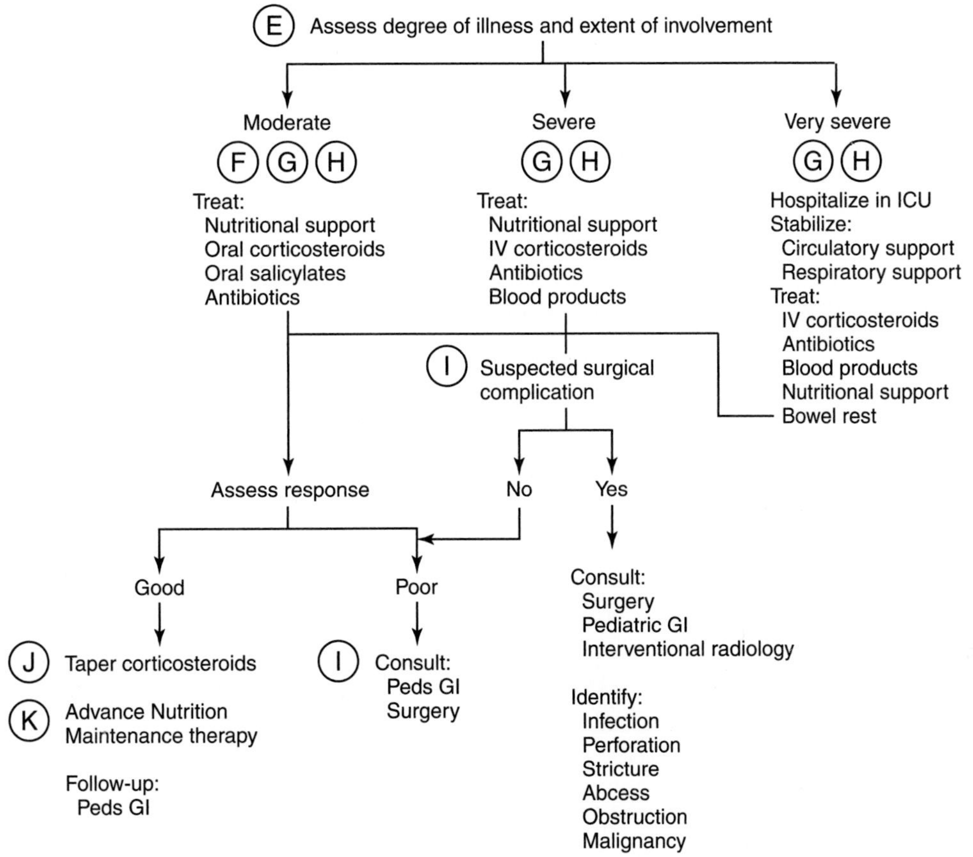
E Assess degree of illness and extent of involvement
Moderate
F G H
Treat:
Nutritional support
Oral corticosteroids
Oral salicylates
Antibiotics
Severe
G H
Treat:
Nutritional support
IV corticosteroids
Antibiotics
Blood products
Very severe
G H
Hospitalize in ICU
Stabilize:
Circulatory support
Respiratory support
Treat:
IV corticosteroids
Antibiotics
Blood products
Nutritional support
Bowel rest
I Suspected surgical complication
No
Yes
Assess response
Good
Poor
J Taper corticosteroids
K Advance Nutrition
Maintenance therapy
Follow-up:
Peds GI
I Consult:
Peds GI
Surgery
Consult:
Surgery
Pediatric GI
Interventional radiology
Identify:
Infection
Perforation
Stricture
Abcess
Obstruction
Malignancy

Table 2. **Medical Therapy for Crohn Disease or Ulcerative Colitis**

Medication	Dosage	Product Availability
Salicylate Derivatives		
Sulfasalazine (release in colon only)	25–75 mg/kg/day in 2–4 divided doses	500-mg tablets
Mesalamine	1–4.8 g/day in 1–4 divided doses	Multiple strengths
Multiple formulations: slow release, colon only, ileum and colon, or throughout small and large intestine		
5-ASA salicylate suppository	1–2 times a day per rectum	1-g suppository
Mesalamine enema	1–2 times a day per rectum	4 g/60 ml
Corticosteroids		
Prednisone, methylprednisolone	1 mg/kg/day to maximum of 60 mg	Multiple strengths Suspension: 5 and 15 mg/5 ml
Hydrocortisone enema	Apply per rectum 1–2 times a day	100 mg/60 ml
Immunosuppressives		
Azathioprine	1–2.5 mg/kg/day	50-mg tablet
6-Mercaptopurine	1–1.5 mg/kg/day	50-mg tablet
Methotrexate	10–20 mg/m²/wk (maximum: 25 mg) PO, SC, or IM	2.5-mg tablet
Anti–TNF-α		
Infliximab	5–10 mg/kg IV infusion: Induction: 0, 2, 6 weeks Maintenance: q8wk	100-mg vials
Antibiotics		
Metronidazole	15–30 mg/kg/day divided tid	250, 500 mg
Ciprofloxacin	20–30 mg/kg/day divided bid maximum: 1.5 g	100, 250, 500, 750 mg Suspension: 50, 100 mg/ml

IM, intramuscularly; *IV*, intravenously; *PO*, orally; *SC*, subcutaneously; *TNF*, tumor necrosis factor.

References

Mackey AC, Green L, Liang L, et al. Hepatosplenic T cell lymphoma associated with infliximab use in young patients treated for inflammatory bowel disease. J Pediatr Gastroenterol Nutr 2007;44:265–7.

Markowitz J. Current treatment of inflammatory bowel disease in children. Dig Liver Dis 2008;40:16–21.

NASPGHAN/CCFA Working Group. Differentiating ulcerative colitis from Crohn disease in children and young adults: report of a working group of the North American Society for Pediatric Gastroenterology, Hepatology and Nutrition and the Crohn's and Colitis Foundation of America. J Pediatr Gastroenterol Nutr 2007;44:653–74.

Rufo AB, Bousvaros A. Challenges and progress in pediatric inflammatory bowel disease. Curr Opin Gastroenterol 2007;23:406–12.

Rufo AB, Bousvaros A. Current therapy of inflammatory bowel disease in children. Pediatr Drugs 2006;8(5):279–302.

Wong A, Bass D. Laboratory evaluation of inflammatory bowel disease. Curr Opin Pediatr 2008;20:566–70.

Gastroesophageal Reflux

Judith A. O'Connor, MD

Gastroesophageal reflux (GER) is the passage of gastric contents into the esophagus through the lower esophageal sphincter, and gastroesophageal reflux disease (GERD) is defined as symptoms or complications of GER. The reasons for reflux include transient relaxation of the lower esophageal sphincter, increased intragastric pressure, and decreased basal lower esophageal sphincter tone. Clinical consequences depend on the frequency and acidity of reflux, esophageal clearance mechanisms, esophageal mucosal barrier, visceral hypersensitivity, and airway responsiveness. Clinical manifestations of GERD in children include vomiting, poor weight gain, dysphagia, abdominal or substernal pain, esophagitis, and respiratory disorders. When severe, GERD can result in failure to thrive, erosive esophagitis or esophageal strictures, aspiration pneumonia, asthma, and apnea.

A. In the patient's history, ask about the onset, frequency, and severity (quantity, degree of forcefulness, presence of bile or blood) of the vomiting. Determine the type of formula, manner of preparation, quantity ingested, and feeding position and technique. Establish the time of vomiting in relation to the feeding. Spitting up or regurgitation of small amounts of formula during or soon after feeding suggests an improper feeding technique, such as bottle propping, or overfeeding. Note associated symptoms, such as fever, cough, coryza, respiratory distress, diarrhea, altered mental status, seizures, and failure to thrive. Inquire about perinatal deaths in the family that suggest inborn errors of metabolism or adrenal insufficiency (Table 1).

B. In the physical examination, assess hydration and circulatory status by determining blood pressure, pulse, respiratory rate, capillary refill, skin color and turgor, tears, fullness of the fontanelle, and urine output. Plot the infant's height, weight, and head circumference on a growth grid to identify failure to thrive or rapid head growth. Assess mental status. Note any acute otitis media, irritability, lethargy, jaundice, hepatosplenomegaly, seizures, or focal neurologic signs. Observe a feeding and note the peristaltic waves. Palpation of an abdominal mass (olive) in an infant suggests pyloric stenosis (Table 2).

C. Consider lifestyle changes to include diet modification and positioning. In the infant, a strong family history of atopy is suggestive of cow's milk protein intolerance. In cases of mild GER with good weight gain, try 1 to 2 weeks of a hypoallergenic formula. If the vomiting fails to resolve, add cereal to the formula (2–3 teaspoons per ounce of formula) to reduce the number of vomiting episodes. In cases with moderate GER and poor weight gain, increase the caloric density of the formula and consider feeding smaller volumes of formula given more frequently to reduce gastric distention. When adequate growth is still not achieved, especially in infants with neurologic impairment, consider continuous nasogastric or nasoduodenal feedings in an attempt to avoid surgery. GER is significantly less common in the prone position; however, increased risk for SIDS outweighs the potential benefits of prone sleeping. If necessary, attempt to position the infant's body prone at a 30-degree incline throughout most of the day when the infant is awake. This can best be accomplished when the infant straddles a padded post or uses a GER harness.

In children and adolescents, diet modification should include avoidance of caffeine, chocolate, and spicy foods. Counsel to avoid obesity (or weight reduction), exposure to tobacco smoke, and alcohol. Prone sleeping position with head elevated is the position of choice in children and adolescents.

D. Consider acid-suppressant therapy to decrease the quantity of gastric acid. Antisecretory agents include H2 receptor antagonists (H2RA) and proton pump inhibitors (PPIs). PPIs produce greater acid suppression and have a longer duration of action. Although used frequently, currently, no PPIs are approved for patients younger than 1 year. Published studies use 0.5 to 1.0 mg/kg dose (Table 3). In adults, a step-down approach using a greater dose of PPI to achieve improvement, followed a standard dose of PPI and then H2RA to maintain improvement, has been shown to be cost-effective and is now advocated. Duration is variable, but is usually 3 months, if improvement occurs, with attempts to discontinue thereafter.

E. Obtain an upper gastrointestinal (GI) series when growth deficiency is present and an anatomic abnormality is suspected. Barium studies will fail to identify about 40% of patients with esophagitis secondary to reflux. False-negative studies result from the relatively brief duration of the study and false-positive studies occur because of the occurrence of physiologic reflux. Thus, an upper GI series does not reliably determine the presence or absence of GER. Anatomic conditions that occur with vomiting during infancy include esophageal stricture or web, duodenal web, hiatal hernia, diaphragmatic hernia, pyloric stenosis, antral web, intestinal obstruction, annular pancreas, malrotation, and volvulus.

F. Esophageal pH and impedance-pH monitoring are the most sensitive methods of confirming reflux and correlating reflux with symptoms. pH monitoring measures the frequency and duration of acid reflux. It is useful in diagnosing acid reflux and assessing the adequacy of treatment with acid suppression when symptoms persist. Limitations include the inability to detect nonacid reflux. Impedance-pH monitoring detects all reflux events and characterizes the reflux as acid, nonacid, or weakly acid, and thus can correlate these events with individual symptoms. Both are placed into the distal esophagus and require continuous monitoring for 12 to 24 hours.

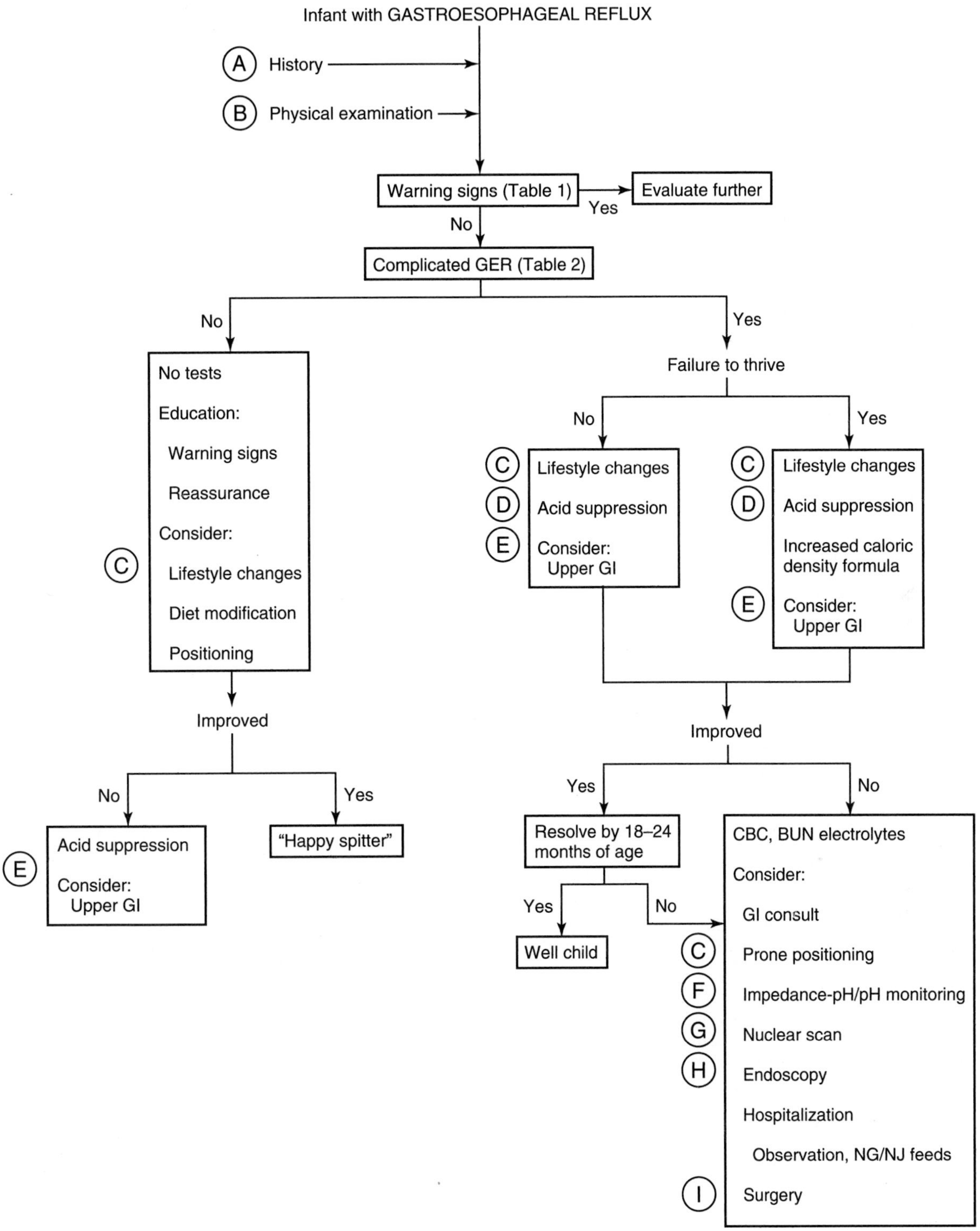

Infant with GASTROESOPHAGEAL REFLUX
A History
B Physical examination
Warning signs (Table 1)
Yes
Evaluate further
No
Complicated GER (Table 2)
No
Yes
No tests
Education:
Warning signs
Reassurance
Consider:
C Lifestyle changes
Diet modification
Positioning
Improved
No
Yes
E Acid suppression
Consider:
Upper GI
"Happy spitter"
Failure to thrive
No
Yes
C Lifestyle changes
D Acid suppression
E Consider:
Upper GI
C Lifestyle changes
D Acid suppression
Increased caloric density formula
E Consider:
Upper GI
Improved
Yes
No
Resolve by 18–24 months of age
Yes
No
Well child
CBC, BUN electrolytes
Consider:
GI consult
C Prone positioning
F Impedance-pH/pH monitoring
G Nuclear scan
H Endoscopy
Hospitalization
Observation, NG/NJ feeds
I Surgery

G. A nuclear scan after a feeding with technetium Tc 99m may be useful in identifying pulmonary aspiration and is helpful in assessing the rate of gastric emptying.

H. Endoscopy will assess the extent and severity of esophagitis and identify any bleeding or strictures. It can also identify other conditions, such as peptic ulcer disease, *Helicobacter pylori* gastritis, eosinophilic, infectious or caustic esophagitis, and Crohn disease. Esophageal biopsy is indicated to exclude causes of esophagitis other than GER.

I. Consider surgery (Nissen fundoplication) if growth failure and severe symptoms persist, if an esophageal stricture develops, or when unable to wean off medications.

Table 1. Warning Signs of Vomiting

Bilious vomiting (hematemesis/ hematochezia)	Gastrointestinal bleeding
Onset of vomiting after 6 months of life	Fever
Lethargy	Hepatosplenomegaly
Bulging fontanelle	Macro/microcephaly
Seizures	Abdominal tenderness/distention
Chromosomal disorders	Other chronic disorders

Table 2. Complications of Gastroesophageal Reflux

Symptoms	Findings
Recurrent vomiting	Esophagitis
Failure to thrive	Esophageal stricture
Irritability	Barrett esophagitis
Regurgitation	Anemia
Heartburn, chest or abdominal pain	Hypoproteinemia
Hematemesis	Recurrent pneumonia
Dysphagia	Refractory asthma
Abnormal posturing (Sandifer syndrome)	Laryngitis
Respiratory symptoms	
Apnea	
Hoarseness	
Wheezing/stridor	
Cough	

Table 3. Medications Demonstrated to Be Effective in Pediatric Gastroesophageal Reflux Disease

Medication	Standard Recommended Dosage
Histamine$_2$ Receptor Antagonists	
Cimetidine	40 mg/kg/day, divided q6–8h (Adult dose: 800–1200 mg/dose, 2 or 3 times a day)
Nizatidine	10 mg/kg/day, divided q12h (Adult dose: 150 mg twice daily or 300 mg every hour of sleep)
Ranitidine	5–10 mg/kg/day, divided q8h (Adult dose: 300 mg twice daily)
Famotidine	1 mg/kg/day, divided q12h (Adult dose: 20 mg twice daily)
Proton Pump Inhibitors	
Omeprazole	1–18 years: 5–<10 kg; 5 mg daily 10–<20 kg; 10 mg daily >20 kg; 20 mg daily (Adult dose: 20 mg daily, esophagitis, 40 mg daily, ulcer disease)
Lansoprazole	
Erosive esophagitis	1–11 years of age: <30 kg: 15 mg daily >30 kg: 30 mg daily 12–18 years of age: 30 mg daily (adult dose)
Nonerosive esophagitis	1–18 years of age: 15 mg daily (adult dose)
Pantoprazole	No pediatric dose, 40 mg daily (adult dose)
Rabeprazole	No pediatric dose, 20 mg daily (adult dose)

References

Fiedorek S, Tolia V, Gold BD, et al. Efficacy and safety of lansoprazole in adolescents with symptomatic erosive and non-erosive gastroesophageal reflux disease. J Pediatr Gastroenterol Nutr 2005;40:319.

Gremse D, Winter H, Tolia V, et al. Pharmacokinetics and pharmacodynamics of Lansoprazole in children with gastroesophageal reflux disease. J Pediatr Gastroenterol Nutr 2002;35:S319.

Gunasekaran TS, Hassall EG. Efficacy and safety of omeprazole for severe gastroesophageal reflux in children. J Pediatr 1993;123:148.

Lee WS, Beattie RM, Meadows N, et al. Gastroesophageal reflux: clinical profiles and outcomes. J Paediatr Child Health 1999;35:568–71.

Nelson SP, Chen EH, Synian OM, Christoffel KK. Prevalence of symptoms of gastroesophageal reflux during childhood—a pediatric practice-based survey. Pediatric Practice Research Group. Arch Pediatr Adolesc Med 2000;154:150–4.

Vandenplas Y. Gastroesophageal reflux in pediatric gastrointestinal and liver disease. In: Wyllie R, Hyams J, editors. Pediatric gastrointestinal and liver disease. 3rd ed. Philadelphia: Saunders Elsevier; 2006. p. 305.

Vandenplas YM, Rudolph CM, DiLorenzo C, et al. Pediatric gastroesophageal reflux clinical practice guidelines: joint recommendations of the North American Society of Pediatric Gastroenterology, Hepatology and Nutrition and the European Society of Pediatric Gastroenterology, Hepatology and Nutrition. J Pediatr Gastroenterol Nutr 2009;49:498.

Zang W, Kukilka M, Witt G, et al. Age-dependent pharmacokinetics of Lansoprazole in neonates and infants. Paediatr Drugs 2008;10:265.

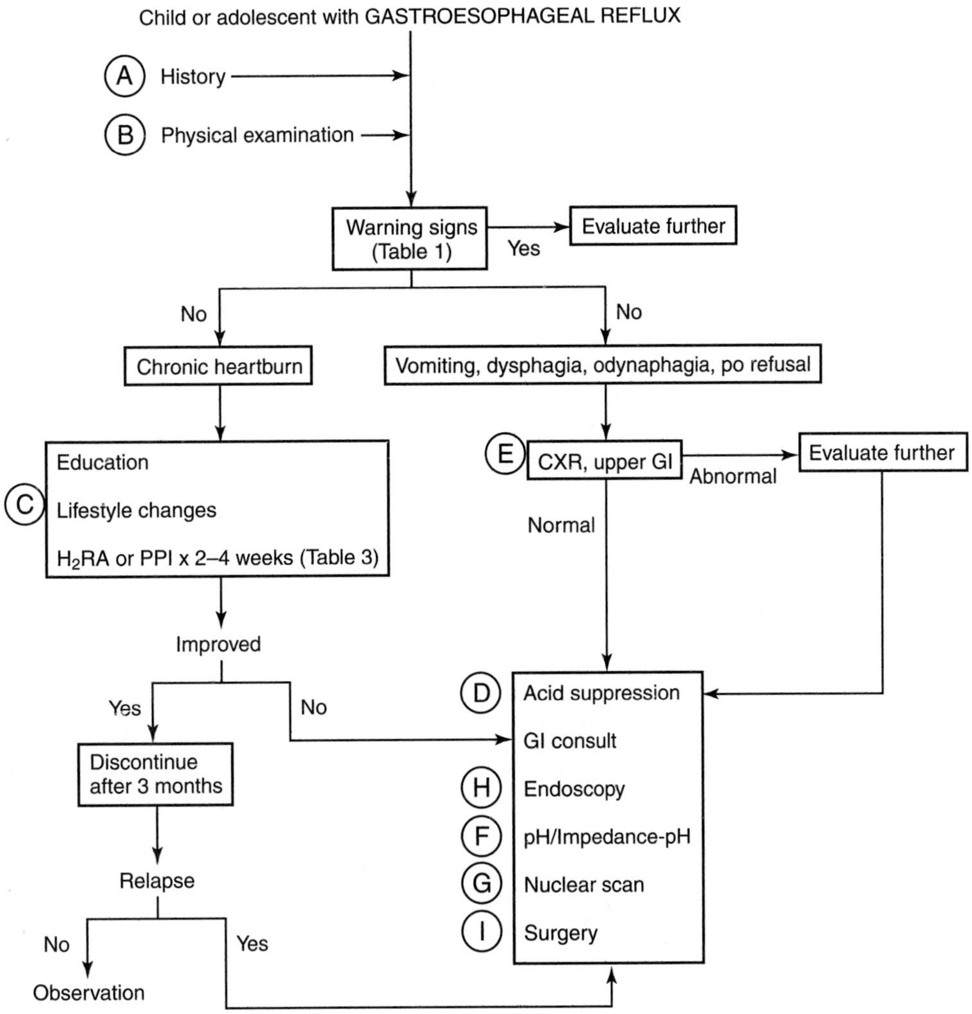
Child or adolescent with GASTROESOPHAGEAL REFLUX
A
History
B
Physical examination
Warning signs (Table 1)
Yes
Evaluate further
No
No
Chronic heartburn
Vomiting, dysphagia, odynaphagia, po refusal
Education
C
Lifestyle changes
H2RA or PPI x 2–4 weeks (Table 3)
E
CXR, upper GI
Abnormal
Evaluate further
Normal
Improved
Yes
No
Discontinue after 3 months
Relapse
No
Yes
Observation
D
Acid suppression
GI consult
H
Endoscopy
F
pH/Impedance-pH
G
Nuclear scan
I
Surgery

Infectious Hepatitis

Brandy Lu, MD, and Cara L. Mack, MD

Hepatitis A, caused by the single-stranded RNA hepatitis A virus (HAV), is transmitted fecal-orally and the incubation period is 15 to 50 days. Diagnosis is confirmed with the presence of anti-HAV immunoglobulin M (IgM) antibody in serum. There is no carrier state or chronic infection. A vaccine is available and routine immunization is recommended for all children starting at 1 year of age.

Hepatitis B, caused by the double-stranded DNA hepatitis B virus (HBV), can be transmitted vertically, parenterally, or sexually. The incubation period is 50 to 180 days, and there is a carrier state and chronic infection. A carrier state is a persistent infection without biochemical or clinical signs of ongoing hepatic injury, and carriers are infectious. Perinatal transmission rates vary from 20% to 90% depending on maternal hepatitis B surface antigen (HBsAg) titer and hepatitis B e antigen (HBeAg) status. The development of chronic disease varies based on age, where infected infants have a 90% chance of development of chronic disease, children between 1 and 5 years have a 30% chance, and children older than 5 years have a 6% chance. Diagnostic tests include HBsAg, HBeAg, anti-HBe, anti-HBs, and HBV DNA. Infants younger than 6 months can have false-positive HBV DNA and antibodies because of placenta passage. Positive HBsAg represents infection, and positive HBeAg represents high infectivity.

Chronic active hepatitis is associated with persistence of HBsAg more than 6 months, HBV DNA greater than 10^5 copies/ml, and increased alanine transaminase (ALT) and aspartate transaminase (AST) levels. HBV carrier is associated with the presence of HBsAg and normal ALT/AST levels. Of the neonates who become chronic carriers, many will develop an "immune-tolerant" phase, represented by a normal ALT/AST despite high HBV DNA levels and persistent HBeAg. The development of anti-HBs is rare but represents protective immunity. A vaccine and serum immunoglobulin is available, and routine immunization is recommended for all children.

Hepatitis C, caused by the single-stranded RNA hepatitis C virus (HCV), is transmitted vertically, parenterally, or sexually. The incubation period is 30 to 150 days, and there is a carrier state and chronic infection. Perinatal transmission rates are 5% and increase to 15% if the mother is coinfected with human immunodeficiency virus (HIV). Chronic infection will develop in 60% to 80% of exposed children. Diagnostic tests include anti-HCV antibodies for children older than 18 months and a positive HCV RNA polymerase chain reaction (PCR) test at 3 and 12 months of age.

Hepatitis D is caused by a defective RNA hepatitis D virus (HDV) that cannot replicate without a coexisting infection with hepatitis B. The incubation period is 20 to 90 days, and there is a carrier state and chronic infection. Coinfection with hepatitis D is more severe than hepatitis B alone and can progress more rapidly to liver failure and cirrhosis. The diagnostic test is anti-HDV antibody.

Hepatitis E, caused by the single-stranded RNA hepatitis E virus (HEV), is transmitted fecal-orally, and the incubation period is 15 to 40 days. There is no carrier state or chronic infection. Infection can be very severe in pregnant women, with 20% mortality rate. The diagnostic test is anti-HEV antibody. The characteristics and terminology of associated antigens and antibodies for hepatitis viruses are reviewed in Table 1.

A. In the patient's history, ask about any fever, anorexia, malaise, vomiting, abdominal pain, jaundice, dark urine, bleeding, or clay-colored stools. Ask whether there has been travel outside the United States, blood product transfusions, or exposure to jaundiced individuals. Inquire as to whether other family members have a history of viral hepatitis, and if so, their treatment and immunization history.

B. In the physical examination, note any jaundice, hepatomegaly, splenomegaly, or abdominal mass. Consider infectious mononucleosis (Epstein–Barr virus [EBV]) when exudative tonsillitis, lymphadenopathy, or splenomegaly is present.

C. Hepatitis is due to hepatocyte membrane disruption and is defined as two times the upper limit of normal of levels of the serum transaminases (ALT and AST). Other causes of infectious hepatitis (besides hepatitis A–E) include viral infections ([EBV], cytomegalovirus [CMV]), herpes simplex virus, influenza, varicella virus, adenovirus, echovirus, coxsackievirus, enterovirus, parvovirus, rubella, arbovirus), bacterial infections (mycoplasma, brucellosis, tularemia, leptospirosis, syphilis, gonorrhea, chlamydia), and parasitic infections (cryptosporidium, malaria, amoeba). Screen for these infections based on history. The "monospot" test has a high false-negative rate in children younger than 4 years and in early disease; therefore, it should not be used solely to diagnosis EBV infection.

Pediatric acute liver failure is defined as: (1) children with no known evidence of chronic liver disease, (2) biochemical evidence of acute liver injury, and (3) hepatic-based coagulopathy defined as an international normalized ratio (INR) $\geq$1.5 not corrected by vitamin K in the presence of clinical hepatic encephalopathy or an INR $\geq$2.0 regardless of the presence or absence of encephalopathy. Patients in liver failure should be transferred to a pediatric tertiary care center with consultation from a pediatric gastroenterology specialist.

(Continued on page 590)

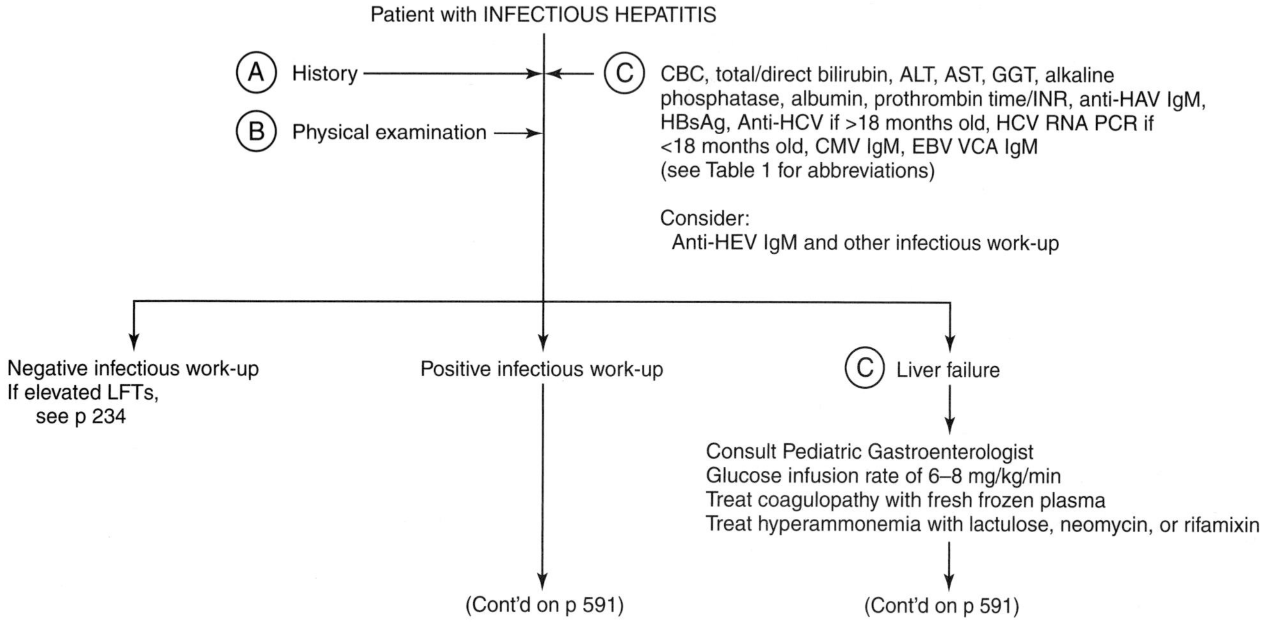
Patient with INFECTIOUS HEPATITIS
(A) History
(B) Physical examination
(C) CBC, total/direct bilirubin, ALT, AST, GGT, alkaline phosphatase, albumin, prothrombin time/INR, anti-HAV IgM, HBsAg, Anti-HCV if >18 months old, HCV RNA PCR if <18 months old, CMV IgM, EBV VCA IgM (see Table 1 for abbreviations)
Consider: Anti-HEV IgM and other infectious work-up
Negative infectious work-up If elevated LFTs, see p 234
Positive infectious work-up
(C) Liver failure
Consult Pediatric Gastroenterologist
Glucose infusion rate of 6–8 mg/kg/min
Treat coagulopathy with fresh frozen plasma
Treat hyperammonemia with lactulose, neomycin, or rifamixin
(Cont'd on p 591)
(Cont'd on p 591)

Table 1. **The Hepatitis Viruses: Characteristics and Terminology of Associated Antigens and Antibodies**

Serologic Markers of HAV		
Anti-HAV IgM	Antibody (IgM subclass) directed against HAV	Indicates current or recent infection
Anti-HAV IgG	Antibody (IgG subclass) directed against HAV	Indicates previous HAV infection/vaccine Protective immunity
Serologic Markers of HBV		
HBsAg	Hepatitis B surface antigen; found on the surface of the intact virus and in serum as free particles	Indicates infection with HBV
HBcAg	Hepatitis B core antigen; found within the core of the intact virus	Detectable in liver tissue only
HBeAg	Hepatitis B e antigen; soluble antigen produced during self-cleavage of HBcAg	Indicates active HBV infection Signifies high infectivity
HBV DNA	DNA of HBV	Indicates active HBV replication
Anti-HBs IgG	Antibody (IgG subclass) to HBsAg	Indicates protective immunity from previous infection/vaccine
Anti-HBc IgM	Antibody (IgM subclass) to HBcAg	Indicates early infection
Anti-HBc IgG	Antibody (IgG subclass) to HBcAg	Indicates infection
Anti-HBe	Antibody to HBeAg	Indicates resolution of replication
Serologic Markers of HCV		
Anti-HCV	Antibody to HCV	Indicates exposure to HCV; not protective
HCV RNA	RNA (PCR) of HCV	Indicates HCV infection
Serologic Markers of HDV		
HDVAg	Hepatitis D antigen	Indicates HDV infection
Anti-HDV	Antibody (IgM/IgG subclass) to HDV	Indicates exposure to HDV
HDV RNA	RNA of HDV	Indicates HDV replication
Serologic Markers of HEV		
HEVAg	Antigen associated with HEV	Stool test, indicates recent infection
HEV RNA	RNA of HEV	Indicates early HEV infection
Anti-HEV	Antibody (IgM subclass) to HEV	Indicates early exposure to HEV
Serologic Markers of EBV		
Anti-EBV VCA IgM	Antibody (IgM subclass) to VCA of EBV	Indicates early infection
Anti-EBV VCA IgG	Antibody (IgG subclass) to VCA of EBV	Indicates past infection
Anti-EBNA IgG	Antibody (IgG subclass) to EBV nuclear antigen	Present after acute infection has cleared
Anti-EA IgG	Antibody (IgG subclass) to EBV early antigen	Indicates early infection
Serologic Markers of CMV		
Anti-CMV IgM	Antibody (IgM subclass) to CMV	Indicates early infection
Anti-CMV IgG	Antibody (IgG subclass) to CMV	Indicates past infection

CMV, cytomegalovirus; *EA*, early antigen; *EBNA*, EBV nuclear antigen; *EBV*, Ebstein–Barr Virus; *HAV*, hepatitis A virus; *HBcAg*, hepatitis B core antigen; *HBeAg*, hepatitis B e antigen; *HBsAg*, hepatitis B surface antigen; *HBV*, hepatitis B virus; *HCV*, hepatitis C virus; *HDV*, hepatitis D virus; *HEV*, hepatitis E virus; *PCR*, polymerase chain reaction; *VCA*, viral capsid antigen.

Modified from Hochman JA, Balistreri WF. Acute and chronic viral hepatitis. In: Suchy FJ, Sokol RJ, Balistreri WF, editors. Liver disease in children. Cambridge, NY: Cambridge University Press; 2007. p. 370.

D. In hepatitis A, only 30% of infants and preschool-age children exhibit symptoms, whereas older children will present with fever, abdominal pain, emesis, diarrhea, and jaundice. Hepatitis A is typically characterized by clinical improvement with the onset of jaundice and a normalization of bilirubin and transaminases within 4 to 6 weeks. Slight increase of unconjugated bilirubin and serum transaminase levels may persist for up to 2 months. Immunoglobulin should only be administered to close contacts (e.g., household members) within 2 weeks of exposure. Offer the hepatitis A vaccine to all contacts.

E. When an individual is exposed to a person with acute hepatitis B, treat with hepatitis B immunoglobulin within 2 weeks of exposure if not previously vaccinated and begin the vaccination series. Prevent perinatal transmission by giving newborns hepatitis B vaccine and 0.5 ml hepatitis B immunoglobulin at birth. Chronic hepatitis B rarely presents with clinical symptoms; however, once chronic disease is established, it is important to screen for hepatocellular carcinoma with an annual α-fetoprotein (AFP) serum level and a liver ultrasound every other year. The majority of children with perinatal acquisition of hepatitis B are asymptomatic with positive HBsAg and HBeAg and negative anti-HBs and anti-HBe. When signs of inflammation (ALT more than two times the upper limit of normal) persist beyond 6 months, referral to a pediatric gastroenterologist is indicated. Treatment of chronic hepatitis B with α-interferon or lamivudine is effective in only about 30% of patients. α-interferon is associated with adverse effects and lamivudine with the inevitable development of viral resistance. Approximately 0.6% of children will spontaneously clear their hepatitis B infection per year, so treatment is often reserved until children are older.

F. Hepatitis C infection is usually asymptomatic in childhood, but infection can rarely progress to cirrhosis or develop into hepatocellular carcinoma. When chronic disease has been established, screen for hepatocellular carcinoma with yearly AFP levels and every other year liver ultrasounds. When signs of inflammation (ALT more than two times the upper limit of normal) persist beyond 6 months, referral to a pediatric gastroenterologist is indicated. Potential therapies for chronic hepatitis C include combination pegylated α-interferon and ribavirin.

References

Hsu EH, Murrary KF. Hepatitis B and C in children. Nat Clin Pract Gastroenterol Hepatol 2008;5:311–20.

Narkewicz MR, Cabrera R, Gonzalez-Peralta RP. The "C" of viral hepatitis in children. Semin Liver Dis 2007;3:295–311.

Slowik MK, Jhaveri R. Hepatitis B and C viruses in infants and young children. Semin Pediatr Infect Dis 2005;16:296–305.

Suchy FJ, Sokol RJ, Balistreri WF, editors. Liver diseases in children. 3rd ed. Cambridge, NY: Cambridge University Press; 2007.

Patient with INFECTIOUS HEPATITIS

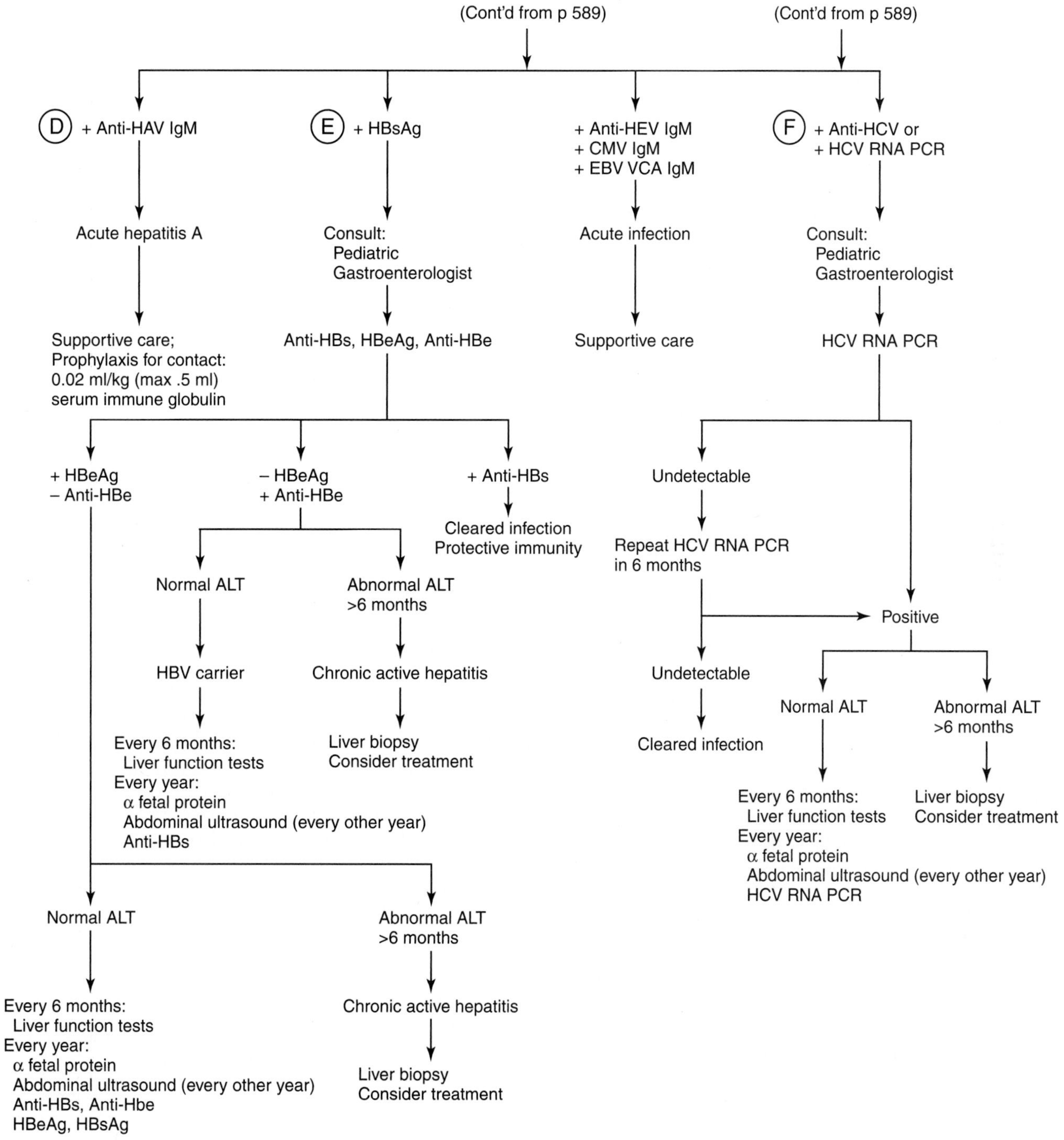

(Cont'd from p 589)
(Cont'd from p 589)
D + Anti-HAV IgM
E + HBsAg
+ Anti-HEV IgM
+ CMV IgM
+ EBV VCA IgM
F + Anti-HCV or
+ HCV RNA PCR
Acute hepatitis A
Consult: Pediatric Gastroenterologist
Acute infection
Consult: Pediatric Gastroenterologist
Supportive care; Prophylaxis for contact: 0.02 ml/kg (max .5 ml) serum immune globulin
Anti-HBs, HBeAg, Anti-HBe
Supportive care
HCV RNA PCR
+ HBeAg
– Anti-HBe
– HBeAg
+ Anti-HBe
+ Anti-HBs
Cleared infection
Protective immunity
Undetectable
Repeat HCV RNA PCR in 6 months
Normal ALT
Abnormal ALT >6 months
Positive
HBV carrier
Chronic active hepatitis
Undetectable
Normal ALT
Abnormal ALT >6 months
Cleared infection
Every 6 months:
Liver function tests
Every year:
α fetal protein
Abdominal ultrasound (every other year)
Anti-HBs
Liver biopsy
Consider treatment
Every 6 months:
Liver function tests
Every year:
α fetal protein
Abdominal ultrasound (every other year)
HCV RNA PCR
Liver biopsy
Consider treatment
Normal ALT
Abnormal ALT >6 months
Chronic active hepatitis
Every 6 months:
Liver function tests
Every year:
α fetal protein
Abdominal ultrasound (every other year)
Anti-HBs, Anti-Hbe
HBeAg, HBsAg
Liver biopsy
Consider treatment

Acute Pancreatitis

Henry R. Thompson, MD

Acute pancreatitis is inflammation of the pancreas with activation of pancreatic enzymes within the organ. This leads to tissue destruction. Patients classically present with pain (94%), vomiting (64%), and fever (33%). This is a relatively uncommon diagnosis in childhood and is often missed. Diagnosis is based on clinical symptoms, a three times increase in pancreatic enzymes, and radiologic evaluation. Causes of pancreatitis range from idiopathic (27%), systemic disease (23%), biliary tract disease (21%), and trauma (16%). Causative factors include medications (sulfasalazine, azathioprine, and valproic acid), infections (viral), or systemic disorder (cystic fibrosis, hemolytic uremic syndrome, diabetes mellitus, and Kawasaki disease).

Table 1. **Severity of Illness in Pancreatitis**

Severe	Very Severe
Severe abdominal pain with nausea and vomiting *and* Increased serum amylase or lipase	Signs of shock *or* Disseminated intravascular coagulation *or* Severe respiratory distress/impending respiratory failure *or* Signs of pancreatic necrosis *or* Signs of peritonitis

A. In the patient's history, ask about acute abdominal pain in left upper quadrant (LUQ) that radiates to the back or right upper quadrant (RUQ) and is associated with nausea and vomiting. This may be with or without fever.

B. In the physical examination, note abdominal distention with or without peritoneal signs, and ascites. There may be signs of an ileus with absent bowel sounds. Discoloration around the umbilicus or flank suggests pancreatic necrosis (Cullen sign). Note signs of respiratory distress associated with pleural effusions or pneumonitis. Assess circulatory status and peripheral perfusion to identify intravascular volume loss secondary to third spacing. Note purpura or bleeding that suggests disseminated intravascular coagulation.

C. Laboratory findings of pancreatitis include increases in serum amylase and lipase levels. Comprehensive metabolic panel including liver function test results may be abnormal when choledocholithiasis or hepatitis is present. Glucose may be increased and calcium decreased with severe disease. The white blood cell (WBC) count is often increased (10,000–25,000 K/μl).

D. Assess degree of illness (Table 1). For mild degree of illness, observe the patient. Provide hydration and symptomatic treatment. Start with a clear or low-fat diet. For severe pain, patient should be hospitalized. For very severe illness that may include respiratory distress and shock, admit to the intensive care unit (ICU).

E. Provide fluid resuscitation intravenously and correct electrolyte abnormalities. Control pain with narcotics. Prevent stress ulcer with a proton pump inhibitor (1–3 mg/kg IV every 24 hours) or use an H2 receptor antagonist (ranitidine 1 mg/kg intravenously [IV] every 8 hours).

F. Consider evaluation with ultrasound or abdominal computed tomography (CT) if increased liver function tests or physical examination findings of shock or peritonitis. In severe cases, treat with Octreotide (1–10 μg/kg/day IV divided every 12 hours). In severe cases, use nasogastric decompression.

G. Follow up by re-evaluation over 24 to 72 hours. If improved with decreased amylase and lipase, consider feeds. If not improved clinically and with increased amylase and lipase, consider repeat ultrasound or CT and consider nasojejunal feeds or total parenteral nutrition.

References

Benifla M, Weizman Z. Acute pancreatitis in childhood: analysis of literature. J Clin Gastroenterol 2003;37:169–72.

Chen CF, Kong MS, Lai MW, Wing CJ. Acute pancreatitis in children: a 10-year experience in a medical center. Acta Paediatr Taiwan 2006;47(4):192–6.

Lowe ME, Greer JB. Pancreatitis in children and adolescents. Curr Gastroenterol Rep 2008;10(2):128–35.

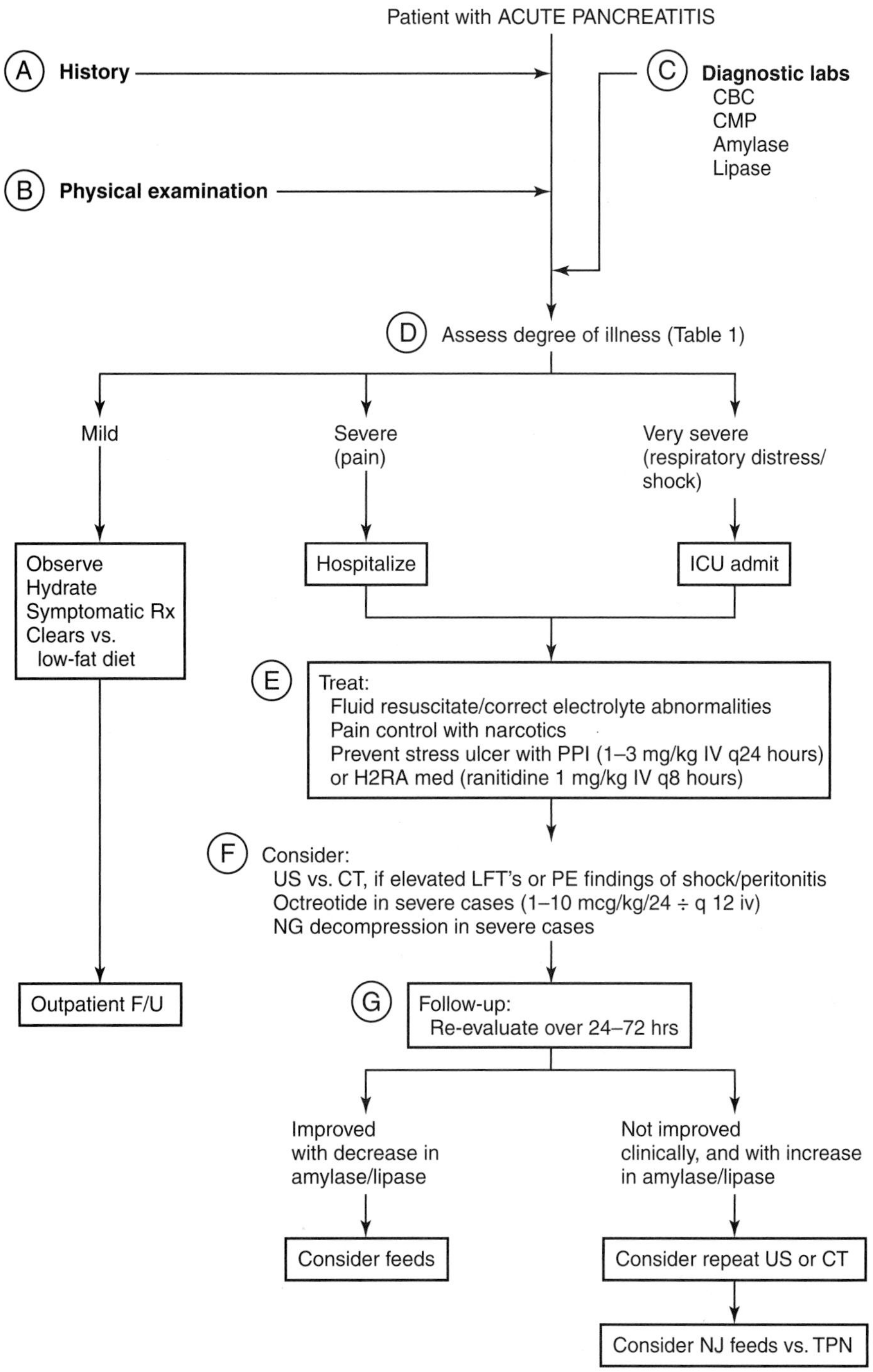
Patient with ACUTE PANCREATITIS
A History
B Physical examination
C Diagnostic labs
CBC
CMP
Amylase
Lipase
D Assess degree of illness (Table 1)
Mild
Severe (pain)
Very severe (respiratory distress/ shock)
Observe
Hydrate
Symptomatic Rx
Clears vs. low-fat diet
Hospitalize
ICU admit
E Treat:
Fluid resuscitate/correct electrolyte abnormalities
Pain control with narcotics
Prevent stress ulcer with PPI (1–3 mg/kg IV q24 hours)
or H2RA med (ranitidine 1 mg/kg IV q8 hours)
F Consider:
US vs. CT, if elevated LFT's or PE findings of shock/peritonitis
Octreotide in severe cases (1–10 mcg/kg/24 ÷ q 12 iv)
NG decompression in severe cases
Outpatient F/U
G Follow-up:
Re-evaluate over 24–72 hrs
Improved with decrease in amylase/lipase
Not improved clinically, and with increase in amylase/lipase
Consider feeds
Consider repeat US or CT
Consider NJ feeds vs. TPN

Hematologic Disorders

Hemolytic Anemia

Microcytic Anemia

Normocytic and Macrocytic Anemia

Bleeding Disorders

Venous Thromboembolism

Fever or Acute Illness in a Child with Sickle Cell Disease

Thrombocytopenia

Neutropenia

Hemolytic Anemia

Julie D. Zimbelman, MD

A. Hemolytic anemia is defined by a reduction in red blood cell survival. In the history, key presenting features to assess include headache, dizziness, syncope, fever, chills, abdominal pain and/or distention, back pain, tea-colored/cola-colored urine, jaundice (current or history of neonatal or recurrent jaundice, and history of gallstones. It is important to note the presence of any systemic symptoms such as arthritis, rash, mouth ulcers, thrombosis or thyroid disease (autoimmune), infection (Epstein–Barr virus, mycoplasma), or autoimmune hemolytic anemia. The patient's ethnicity may suggest thalassemia/hemoglobinopathy, G6PD (glucose 6-phosphate dehydrogenase) deficiency, or sickle cell disease. Neonatal history of Rh/ABO disease and family history of jaundice, gallstones, splenectomy, or hemolytic anemia is important to note.

B. In the physical examination, assess vital signs and perfusion. Growth parameters to include height and weight as growth retardation suggests longstanding anemia or diseases associated with autoimmune hemolysis. Look for jaundice/pallor, splenomegaly (autoimmune hemolytic anemia, sickle cell disease, spherocytosis, or other red blood cell membrane abnormality), petechiae/bruising (associated thrombocytopenia, disseminated intravascular coagulation [DIC], hemolytic uremic syndrome, autoimmune, malignancy), and presence of arthritis or rash (collagen vascular disease).

C. Laboratory evaluation should include a complete blood cell count (CBC) and reticulocyte count. The reticulocyte count is generally increased unless a patient has an aplastic crisis. A comprehensive metabolic panel and lactate dehydrogenase (LDH) should be performed to evaluate for hemolysis and hemolytic uremic syndrome (HUS). The indirect bilirubin, aspartate aminotransferase (AST) and LDH may be elevated in hemolysis. An elevated creatinine in addition is concerning for HUS. Any abnormal hemoglobin at birth from newborn screen results should be noted.

D. Obtain a Coombs test (direct, indirect, complement).

E. Discern the thermal amplitude (warm vs. cold) and antigen specificity of the antibody. The thermal amplitude is the temperature at which the antibody reacts maximally with the antigen on the red cell. It is warm reacting if that temperature is 37° C and cold reacting if that temperature is less. Consider a Donath–Landsteiner antibody. Obtain a partial thromboplastin time (PTT) and antinuclear antibody (ANA) if autoimmune to evaluate for other antibodies. Evaluate for infection if symptoms are suggestive (Epstein–Barr virus, mycoplasma). Review the peripheral blood smear. Haptoglobin is usually low in hemolytic anemia, is unreliable in newborns, and is an acute phase reactant so may be falsely elevated. A urinalysis is helpful to assess for evidence for increased urobilinogen (extravascular hemolysis) and hemoglobinuria (intravascular hemolysis).

F. Morphology with elliptocytes/spherocytes can occur as a result of nonhereditary causes, so it is difficult to state with certainty in acute hemolytic crisis whether the spherocytes are a cause or an effect of hemolytic disease. A review of the parental blood smears may be helpful. Hereditary spherocytosis and elliptocytosis are usually autosomal dominant.

G. Target cells may be seen in liver disease and hemoglobinopathy. A sickly solubility test (e.g., sickle preparation) confirms the presence of sickle hemoglobin, but the result is negative in infants with sickle disease owing to high levels of fetal hemoglobin. Older children with sickle cell trait have a positive sickle solubility test result but do not have hemolysis, anemia, or an abnormal blood smear. Obtain a hemoglobin electrophoresis to investigate the possibility of a hemoglobinopathy.

H. Red cell fragmentation with helmet cells is suggestive of microangiopathic hemolytic process such as disseminated intravascular coagulation (DIC) or HUS.

I. Red cell morphology may not suggest a specific diagnosis. G6PD and pyruvate kinase deficiencies are the most common inherited defects of red cell metabolism. Unstable hemoglobins usually show autosomal dominance inheritance because heterozygotes are affected. Oxidant-mediated hemolysis may be induced by infection or oxidant medications in patients with G6PD deficiency or with some unstable hemoglobinopathies; in such cases, there may be blister cells or bite cells on the peripheral blood smear, and a Heinz body preparation may be positive. Consideration of other causative factors includes other red cell enzyme assays, and flow cytometry for paroxysmal nocturnal hemoglobinuria (PNH).

Treatment considerations include supportive care and transfusion if necessary. If autoimmune, may be unable to find in vitro cross-match compatible blood. Donor erythrocytes with the least agglutination with patient's sample should be transfused and red cells should be washed before transfusion. Consider warming the blood *with appropriate blood bank protocols* in cold autoimmune hemolytic anemia. (Do *not* warm the blood in an uncontrolled fashion.) In vivo cross match with transfusion of small volume of blood and concomitant use of high-dose corticosteroids. Consider steroids in autoimmune disease and try to control the underlying diagnosis (e.g., autoimmune disease, infection). Close monitoring is indicated (laboratory tests, physical examination). In autoimmune hemolytic anemia, may need a hemoglobin evaluation every 4 hours. Consider folic acid administration and consultation with a hematologist.

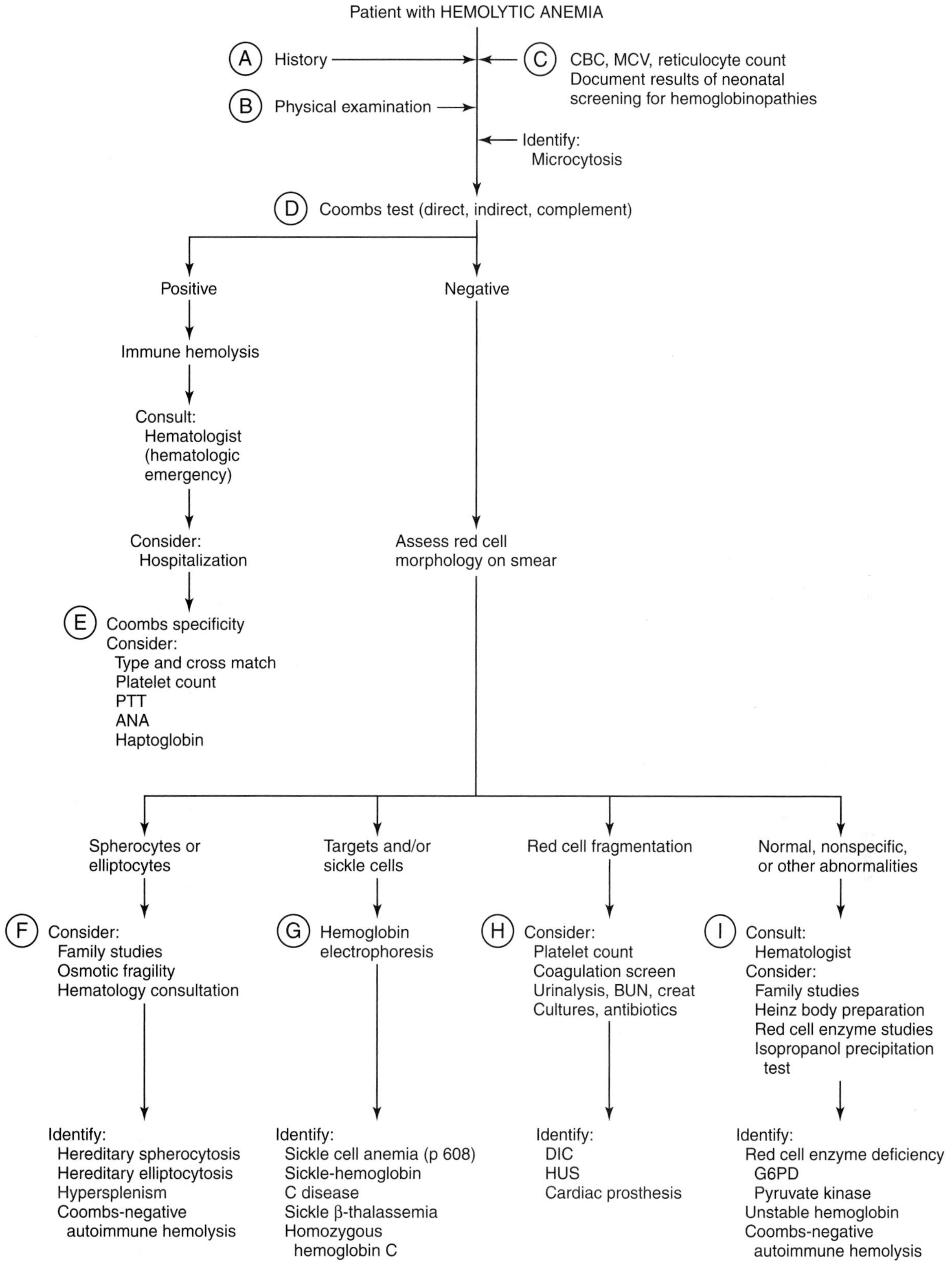
Patient with HEMOLYTIC ANEMIA
A
History
B
Physical examination
C
CBC, MCV, reticulocyte count
Document results of neonatal screening for hemoglobinopathies
Identify:
Microcytosis
D
Coombs test (direct, indirect, complement)
Positive
Negative
Immune hemolysis
Consult:
Hematologist (hematologic emergency)
Consider:
Hospitalization
E
Coombs specificity
Consider:
Type and cross match
Platelet count
PTT
ANA
Haptoglobin
Assess red cell morphology on smear
Spherocytes or elliptocytes
Targets and/or sickle cells
Red cell fragmentation
Normal, nonspecific, or other abnormalities
F
Consider:
Family studies
Osmotic fragility
Hematology consultation
G
Hemoglobin electrophoresis
H
Consider:
Platelet count
Coagulation screen
Urinalysis, BUN, creat
Cultures, antibiotics
I
Consult:
Hematologist
Consider:
Family studies
Heinz body preparation
Red cell enzyme studies
Isopropanol precipitation test
Identify:
Hereditary spherocytosis
Hereditary elliptocytosis
Hypersplenism
Coombs-negative autoimmune hemolysis
Identify:
Sickle cell anemia (p 608)
Sickle-hemoglobin C disease
Sickle β-thalassemia
Homozygous hemoglobin C
Identify:
DIC
HUS
Cardiac prosthesis
Identify:
Red cell enzyme deficiency
G6PD
Pyruvate kinase
Unstable hemoglobin
Coombs-negative autoimmune hemolysis

References

Bain BJ. Diagnosis from the blood smear. N Engl J Med 2005;353: 499–500.

Lanzkowsky P. Hemolytic anemia. In: Lanzkowsky P, editor. Manual of pediatric hematology and oncology. 4th ed. New York: Elsevier; 2005. p. 136–98.

Rosse WF, Hillmen P, Schreiber AD. Immune mediated hemolytic anemia. Hematology Am Soc Hematol Educ Program 2004; 48–62.

Microcytic Anemia

Julie D. Zimbelman, MD

A. The differential diagnosis of microcytic anemia includes iron deficiency, α- or β-thalassemia, hemoglobinopathy, lead poisoning, chronic inflammation, copper deficiency, and atransferrinemia. Presenting features to assess include bleeding, pallor, jaundice, and symptoms of chronic disease/inflammation (fever, pain). History should include a dietary history for symptoms of pica, ethnicity (thalassemia, hemoglobinopathy), history of jaundice or splenomegaly, and family history of jaundice. Age of patient is important because iron deficiency is common in children 6 to 36 months old and in adolescent girls who are menstruating and have suboptimal diets. Growth history and lead exposure are important.

B. Physical examination includes vital signs, cardiovascular status (syncope, shortness of breath, decrease in exercise tolerance), growth (delayed growth with chronic disease), jaundice, splenomegaly, frontal bossing (thalassemia), and signs of systemic disease (infection, collagen vascular disease, malignancy).

C. Laboratory evaluation should include complete blood cell count (CBC) and reticulocyte count (note normal values for age). Pay attention to erythrocyte indices because erythrocyte count is usually increased in thalassemia, though this is not a reliable parameter in children up to 48 months old, and the mean cell volume (MCV)/red blood cell (RBC) ratio less than 13 favors thalassemia. The RBC distribution width (RDW) is generally increased in iron deficiency but not with thalassemia trait. Note normal values vary with age. Review peripheral blood smear.

D. Treatment for iron deficiency consists of elemental iron 4 to 6 mg/kg/24 hours divided two to three times daily. Elemental iron is best absorbed with vitamin C. Response to treatment should be verified within 1 to 2 weeks after initiation of iron. Limit cow's milk to 24 ounces per day or less.

E. In moderately severe microcytic anemia, the diagnosis of iron deficiency should only be made with a history of an iron poor diet (ages 6 to 36 months) or explained blood loss without a history and physical exam suggesting another cause.

F. In severe microcytic anemia consult hematology. Consider hospitalization.

G. A reticulocytosis should be seen within several days of initiating iron therapy, and the hemoglobin should begin to increase within the first week. If this is not the case, consider ongoing iron loss, poor compliance, or other contributing cause for the anemia. Depending on age, consider further evaluation for iron deficiency. Consider a hematology consult if not readily corrected or if thalassemia or hemoglobinopathy is identified. Correction of underlying disease in chronic inflammation is helpful in correcting anemia.

H. The peripheral smear may reflect hypochromia (iron deficiency), target cells (thalassemia), or basophilic stippling (unstable hemoglobin, thalassemia, lead poisoning). Additional studies include free erythrocyte porphyrin (FEP), ferritin, total iron binding capacity (TIBC), serum iron, and lead level. The serum ferritin is typically low in iron deficiency (low serum iron) but high in anemia of chronic inflammation (low serum iron). The serum ferritin may be falsely normal or elevated in acute illness. TIBC is usually elevated in iron deficiency and normal or low in anemia of chronic inflammation. Quantitative hemoglobin electrophoresis shows an elevated A2 or F (fetal) in β-thalassemia, a hemoglobin S greater than hemoglobin A in sickle β-thalassemia and hemoglobin C or E in hemoglobin C or E disorders. It is usually normal in α-thalassemia trait except in the newborn when Bart's hemoglobin is present.

I. Lead poisoning has been associated with microcytic anemia but most of the anemia associated with lead poisoning is due to coexistent iron deficiency. It is important to evaluate for lead poisoning.

J. Iron therapy should be continued until iron stores are replenished. The possibility of blood loss should be thoroughly investigated when iron deficiency occurs in children older than 3 years or in younger children with adequate dietary iron.

References

Aslan D, Altay C. Incidence of high erythrocyte counts in infants and young children with iron deficiency anemia: re-evaluation of an old parameter. J Ped Hem-Onc 2003;25:303–6.

Barkin, R, Rosen, P. Anemia. In: Emergency Pediatrics: A Guide to Ambulatory Care. 6th ed. Philadelphia: Mosby; 2003. p. 212–6.

Jain, S, Kamat, D. Evaluation of microcytic anemia. Clin Pediatr (Phila) 2009;48:7–12.

Lanzkowsky, P. Iron-Deficiency Anemia. In: Lanzkowsky P, editor. Manual of Pediatric Hematology and Oncology. 4th ed. New York: Elsevier; 2005. p. 31–46.

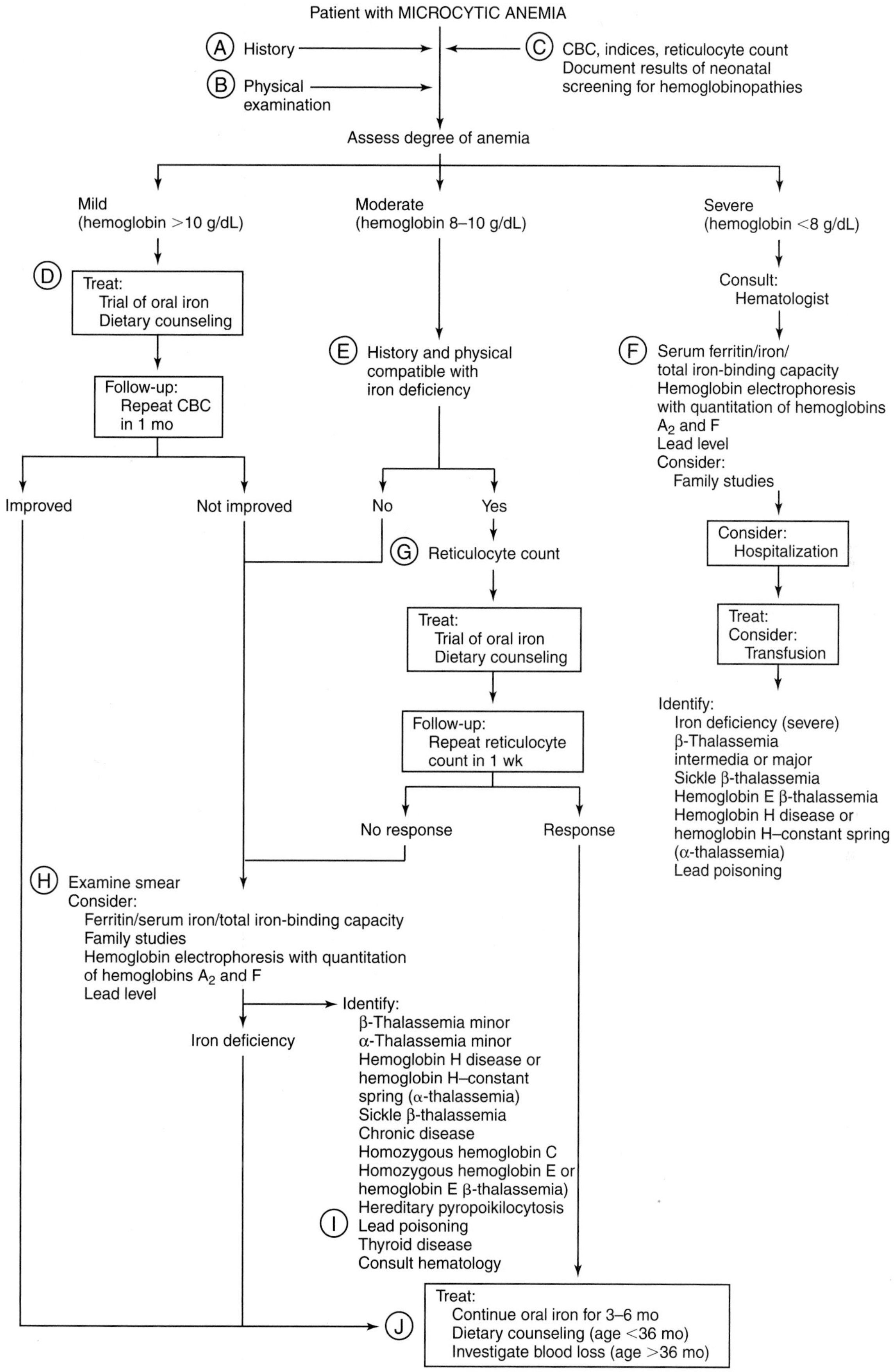
Patient with MICROCYTIC ANEMIA
(A) History
(B) Physical examination
(C) CBC, indices, reticulocyte count
Document results of neonatal screening for hemoglobinopathies
Assess degree of anemia
Mild (hemoglobin >10 g/dL)
Moderate (hemoglobin 8–10 g/dL)
Severe (hemoglobin <8 g/dL)
(D) Treat:
Trial of oral iron
Dietary counseling
Follow-up:
Repeat CBC in 1 mo
Improved
Not improved
(E) History and physical compatible with iron deficiency
No
Yes
(G) Reticulocyte count
Treat:
Trial of oral iron
Dietary counseling
Follow-up:
Repeat reticulocyte count in 1 wk
No response
Response
Consult:
Hematologist
(F) Serum ferritin/iron/total iron-binding capacity
Hemoglobin electrophoresis with quantitation of hemoglobins A2 and F
Lead level
Consider:
Family studies
Consider:
Hospitalization
Treat:
Consider:
Transfusion
Identify:
Iron deficiency (severe)
β-Thalassemia intermedia or major
Sickle β-thalassemia
Hemoglobin E β-thalassemia
Hemoglobin H disease or hemoglobin H–constant spring (α-thalassemia)
Lead poisoning
(H) Examine smear
Consider:
Ferritin/serum iron/total iron-binding capacity
Family studies
Hemoglobin electrophoresis with quantitation of hemoglobins A2 and F
Lead level
Iron deficiency
Identify:
β-Thalassemia minor
α-Thalassemia minor
Hemoglobin H disease or hemoglobin H–constant spring (α-thalassemia)
Sickle β-thalassemia
Chronic disease
Homozygous hemoglobin C
Homozygous hemoglobin E or hemoglobin E β-thalassemia)
Hereditary pyropoikilocytosis
(I) Lead poisoning
Thyroid disease
Consult hematology
(J) Treat:
Continue oral iron for 3–6 mo
Dietary counseling (age <36 mo)
Investigate blood loss (age >36 mo)

Normocytic and Macrocytic Anemia

Julie D. Zimbelman, MD

A. Key presenting features of normocytic and macrocytic anemia to assess include presence of fatigue, pallor, and jaundice (hemolysis). Fever that is persistent or recurrent may indicate infection, malignancy, or collagen vascular disease. Note pain (juvenile rheumatoid arthritis, leukemia, or other malignancy), diarrhea (malabsorption, hemolytic uremic syndrome), bleeding (acute blood loss, low platelets), and bruising (low platelets). A medication history is important because some medications can cause anemia (i.e., antimetabolites, anticonvulsants). The dietary history may suggest vitamin B_{12} or folate deficiency. Obtain a family history for history of anemia, jaundice, splenomegaly, or gallstones. The patient's growth history or short stature should be documented (hypothyroidism, chronic anemia, Fanconi, Diamond–Blackfan). Microcephaly or congenital anomalies may indicate Fanconi anemia. Systemic abnormalities suggestive of chronic disease include hypertension, edema, petechiae/bruising, jaundice, lymphadenopathy, joint heat or swelling, and splenomegaly.

B. Physical examination components include vital signs, perfusion, and growth history to include height, weight, and head circumference. Dysmorphism may indicate Down syndrome (macrocytosis) or Fanconi anemia (macrocytosis). Skin jaundice (liver disease, hemolysis), bruising/petechiae (leukemia, hemolytic uremic syndrome, aplastic anemia), lymphadenopathy (juvenile rheumatoid arthritis, leukemia/lymphoma), joint heat or swelling (juvenile rheumatoid arthritis), splenomegaly (leukemia/lymphoma, hereditary spherocytosis or other red blood cell membrane defect, liver disease, hypersplenism, sickle syndromes), and evidence for infection (fever/pain) should be assessed.

C. Laboratory evaluation should include complete blood cell count (CBC) and reticulocyte count (red blood cell indices; note normal red blood cell indices for age). In macrocytic anemia, additional studies include vitamin B_{12} level, folate level, consideration of B_{12} absorption studies, consideration of bone marrow evaluation (myelodysplasia, Blackfan–Diamond anemia). Consider evaluation for Fanconi anemia (chromosomal fragility studies) and hemoglobin electrophoresis. Normocytic anemia should include a comprehensive metabolic panel (liver disease, renal disease, other [e.g., hypoalbuminemia in primary gastrointestinal diseases]), consideration of bone marrow evaluation (malignancy, sideroblastic anemia, dyserythropoietic anemia) and other studies related to symptoms such collagen vascular disease studies (antinuclear antibody [ANA], complement), infectious evaluation (serologies [e.g., human immunodeficiency virus]), imaging (pneumonia, deep abscess, osteomyelitis), thyroid studies, tissue biopsy of abnormality (e.g., lymph node), and suspected hemolytic anemia (see Hemolytic Anemia chapter, p. 596).

D. The reticulocyte count helps differentiate anemias caused by increased peripheral red blood cell destruction from those caused by underproduction. A low or "normal" reticulocyte count in the face of significant anemia is inappropriate and suggests bone marrow failure. However, a low reticulocyte count does not exclude hemolysis; hemolytic anemias sometimes present with aplastic crisis.

E. Review of the peripheral blood smear is important and helpful. Red cell morphology may show anisocytosis or poikilocytosis, tear drops, polychromasia (hemolysis, recent blood loss or recovery from marrow suppression). Hypersegmented neutrophils are associated with megaloblastic anemia. Sickle forms, red cell fragmentation (disseminated intravascular coagulation, hemolytic uremic syndrome) or spherocytes (hereditary spherocytosis, autoimmune hemolytic anemia) suggest hemolysis.

F. Attention to other cytopenias, including platelet and neutrophil counts is important. If neutropenia or a decreased platelet count is also present, consider malignancy, dysplasia or aplasia.

G. Consult hematology prior to performing a marrow evaluation to ensure all necessary studies are included (flow cytometry, cytogenetics).

H. Pure red blood cell aplasia of unknown origin often requires a bone marrow examination. However, if the history, physical examination, and laboratory results are all consistent with transient erythroblastopenia of childhood (TEC), then bone marrow examination may be deferred and the child observed closely with at least weekly examinations and complete blood counts.

References

Abshire TC. The anemia of inflammation, a common cause of childhood anemia. Pediatr Clin North Am 1996;43:623–37.

Bain BJ. Diagnosis from the blood smear. N Engl J Med 2005;353: 498–507.

Coyer SM. Anemia: diagnosis and management. J Pediatr Hematol Oncol 2005;19:380–5.

Lanzkowsky P. Classification and diagnosis of anemia during childhood. In: Lanzkowsky P, editor. Manual of Pediatric Hematology and Oncology. 4th ed. New York: Elsevier; 2005. p. 1–11.

Rossbach HC. The role of four: a systematic approach to diagnosis of common pediatric hematologic and oncologic disorders. Fetal Pediatr Pathol 2005;24:277–296.

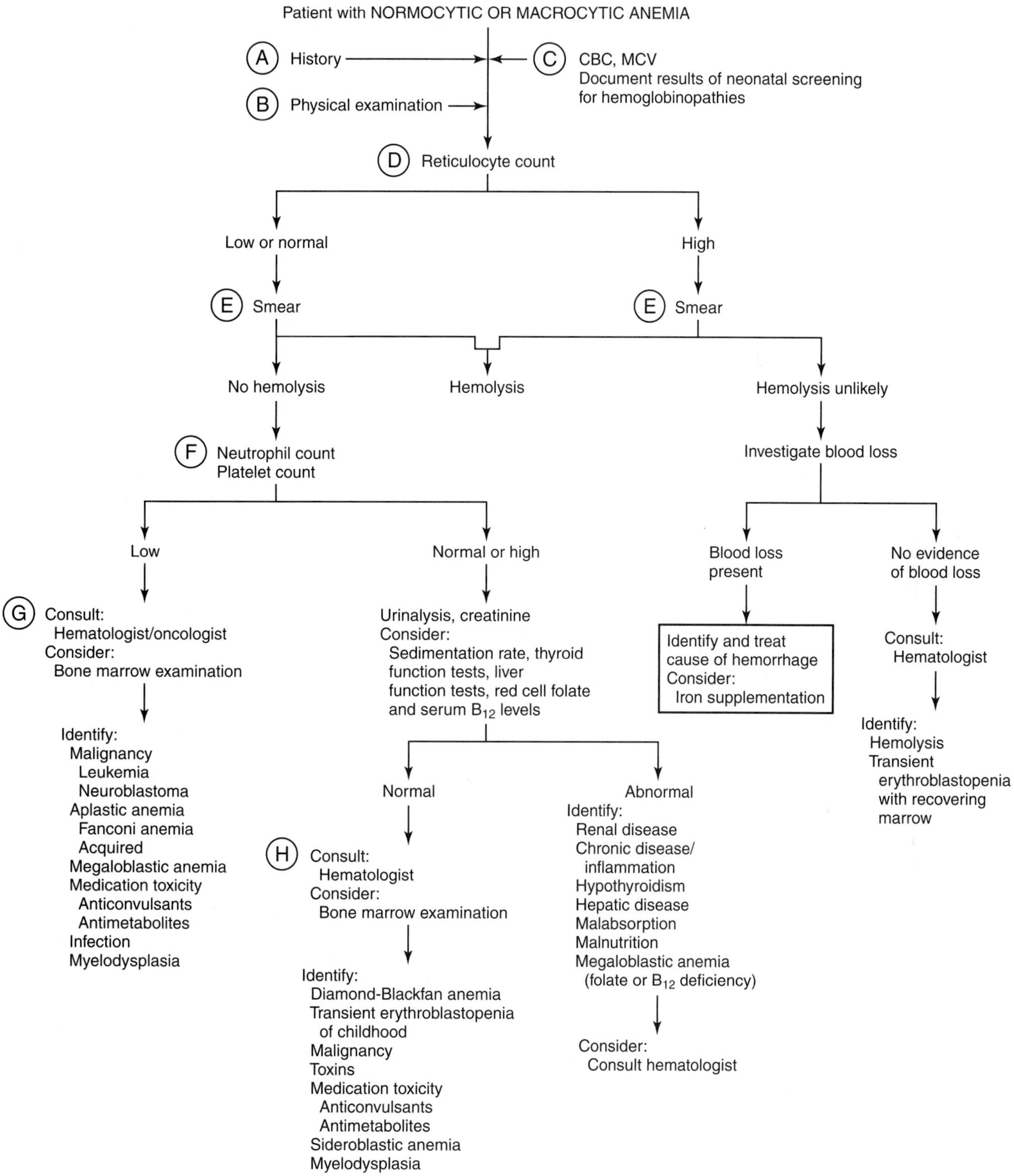
Patient with NORMOCYTIC OR MACROCYTIC ANEMIA
(A) History
(B) Physical examination
(C) CBC, MCV
Document results of neonatal screening for hemoglobinopathies
(D) Reticulocyte count
Low or normal
High
(E) Smear
(E) Smear
No hemolysis
Hemolysis
Hemolysis unlikely
(F) Neutrophil count
Platelet count
Investigate blood loss
Low
Normal or high
Blood loss present
No evidence of blood loss
(G) Consult:
Hematologist/oncologist
Consider:
Bone marrow examination
Urinalysis, creatinine
Consider:
Sedimentation rate, thyroid function tests, liver function tests, red cell folate and serum B_{12} levels
Identify and treat cause of hemorrhage
Consider:
Iron supplementation
Consult:
Hematologist
Identify:
Malignancy
Leukemia
Neuroblastoma
Aplastic anemia
Fanconi anemia
Acquired
Megaloblastic anemia
Medication toxicity
Anticonvulsants
Antimetabolites
Infection
Myelodysplasia
Normal
Abnormal
Identify:
Hemolysis
Transient erythroblastopenia with recovering marrow
(H) Consult:
Hematologist
Consider:
Bone marrow examination
Identify:
Renal disease
Chronic disease/inflammation
Hypothyroidism
Hepatic disease
Malabsorption
Malnutrition
Megaloblastic anemia (folate or B_{12} deficiency)
Identify:
Diamond-Blackfan anemia
Transient erythroblastopenia of childhood
Malignancy
Toxins
Medication toxicity
Anticonvulsants
Antimetabolites
Sideroblastic anemia
Myelodysplasia
Consider:
Consult hematologist

Bleeding Disorders

Mindy L. Grunzke, MD, and Neil A. Goldenberg, MD, PhD

Bleeding of recent onset in an ill child is often an acquired phenomenon, caused by, for example, platelet inhibition by medicines or consumption coagulopathy (e.g., disseminated intravascular coagulation [DIC]) in severe infection. However, recurrent bleeding in an otherwise healthy child who takes no medications or herbal preparations is concerning for a congenital bleeding disorder. Congenital bleeding disorders range from relatively common (e.g., von Willebrand disease [vWD]: estimated prevalence of 1% in the United States), to less common (e.g., hemophilia A: incidence of 1 in 5000 male births per year), to very rare (factor XIII deficiency: estimated prevalence of 1 in 2 million). Although severe congenital disorders are relatively infrequent in the population, their prompt diagnosis can avoid catastrophic consequences.

A. History: A detailed history is essential for a bleeding evaluation. A thorough bleeding history defines the level of clinical suspicion for bleeding disorder, which, in turn, influences the type and extent of diagnostic laboratory evaluation. History should note sex, age at onset, clinical presentation, all medications (especially platelet inhibitors and warfarin), past/present medical diagnoses (with particular attention to hepatic synthetic dysfunction, renal insufficiency, malabsorption, or connective tissue disorders as possible causes of, or contributors to, bleeding manifestations), family medical history (with emphasis on bleeding histories), and a complete review of symptoms. Pertinent details on clinical presentation and personal history of bleeding include mode of onset (spontaneous vs. trauma induced), location/distribution, duration, and response to intervention. Specific questioning should be undertaken regarding prior hemostatic challenges, including fractures, other traumatic injuries, surgeries, other invasive procedures (e.g., circumcision in male patients), and dental extractions. Mucosal bleeding (epistaxis, gum bleeding, menorrhagia) and easy bruising may indicate a disorder of primary hemostasis (including vWD, thrombocytopenia, and platelet dysfunction). Bleeding into soft tissues (e.g., muscle) or joints is suggestive of a secondary hemostatic defect (i.e., coagulation factor deficiencies, such as hemophilia A or B or deficiency/dysfunction of fibrinogen). Hemorrhagic stroke at birth in a term infant or delayed/protracted bleeding from the umbilical stump may be presentations of factor XIII deficiency or a primary defect in fibrinolysis. Mild bleeding disorders may be present in the absence of substantial bleeding history, particularly among children for whom there has been no history of surgery or trauma. By contrast, spontaneous bleeding that requires medical attention is highly suspicious for a severe underlying bleeding disorder.

B. Physical Examination: A complete physical examination evaluates for signs of systemic disorders (e.g., lymphadenopathy, hepatosplenomegaly, rash). Examination should note the presence, location, and characteristics of any ecchymoses or petechiae. Areas of ecchymoses, in particular, should be palpated for evidence of hematoma. Joints should be examined for any tenderness, swelling, or limitation in range of motion that may indicate hemarthrosis. Although these positive findings are helpful, a normal examination at the time of evaluation does not rule out an underlying bleeding disorder.

C. Diagnostic Evaluation: Always consider nonaccidental trauma. Radiologic imaging may be warranted in areas of bony tenderness/deformity or extensive ecchymosis/hematoma (particularly in the head, neck, and thorax).

Properly obtained laboratory blood samples are important in determining the causes of bleeding. Samples for coagulation testing should ideally be drawn via clean peripheral venipuncture to avoid spurious results.

First-stage diagnostic testing includes a complete blood cell count (CBC), review of the peripheral blood smear, prothrombin time (PT), activated partial thromboplastin time (aPTT), fibrinogen "level" (i.e., clotting activity), and thrombin time (TT). If the history includes mucocutaneous bleeding, first-stage testing should also include platelet function assessment by Platelet Function Analyzer-100 (PFA-100) or standardized bleeding time. The CBC assesses platelet number and may suggest iron-deficiency anemia in the setting of chronic/significant blood loss. Pancytopenia may indicate underlying malignancy or bone marrow failure. The PT interrogates the extrinsic and common pathways of the coagulation cascade (including tissue factor and factors VII, X, V, II, and fibrinogen) and is sensitive to vitamin K deficiency (therefore warfarin therapy) and high concentrations of heparin. The aPTT tests the intrinsic and common coagulation pathways (including factors XI, IX, VIII, X, V, II, and fibrinogen). The aPTT is quite sensitive to heparin, as well as to lupus anticoagulant antibodies (which are not infrequent among children with recent infection/inflammatory illness, and also are common in children with thrombosis). In addition, the aPTT detects high-molecular-weight kininogen, prekallikrein, and factor XII, which comprise the "contact" factor pathway, wherein deficiencies do not cause a bleeding diathesis. The TT is sensitive to dysfunctional fibrinogen (also to heparin and to the effects of fibrin split products) and supports the fibrinogen clotting assay in the assessment of fibrinogen. The PFA-100 is sensitive to aspirin and other cyclo-oxygenase-1 inhibitors (e.g., nonsteroidal anti-inflammatory agents such as ibuprofen), as well

BLEEDING ALGORITHM

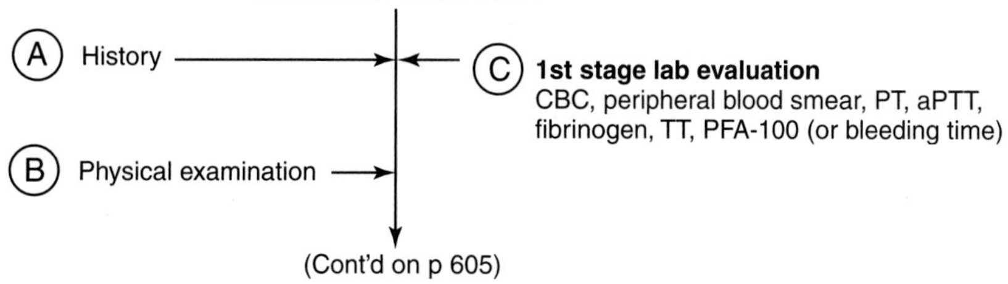
A History
B Physical examination
C 1st stage lab evaluation
CBC, peripheral blood smear, PT, aPTT, fibrinogen, TT, PFA-100 (or bleeding time)
(Cont'd on p 605)

as to some congenital platelet function disorders (e.g., Glanzmann thrombasthenia); however, it does not reliably evaluate platelet function in the setting of anemia or thrombocytopenia. It is prolonged in many patients with vWD and has largely replaced the bleeding time in most clinical settings. The bleeding time is sensitive to both primary and secondary hemostatic defects, and may also be prolonged in connective tissue disorders.

D. Disorders of primary hemostasis typically include mucocutaneous bleeding. In patients with mucocutaneous bleeding, platelet number, morphology, and function are particularly important to assess. Investigate thrombocytopenia if present. Thrombocytopenia with large platelets may indicate immune-mediated causes (e.g., idiopathic thrombocytopenic purpura [ITP]) or rare congenital macrothrombocytopenias (e.g., Bernard–Soulier syndrome). Acute leukemia, bone marrow failure, and drug-related thrombocytopenia are typically associated with normal-sized platelets. Small platelets are seen in Wiskott–Aldrich syndrome. Absence of α granules in gray platelet syndrome results in a ghost-like or gray appearance of platelets on Romanowsky stain of the peripheral blood smear. Platelet function was classically assessed with the bleeding time; PFA-100 is often used now instead. Nevertheless, platelet aggregation studies remain the gold standard in assessing platelet function defects, despite technical limitations and suboptimal reproducibility. Platelet aggregation testing is particularly useful for further evaluation of mucocutaneous bleeding when first-stage testing is normal or when the PFA-100 collagen/ADP (adenosine diphosphate) closure time is prolonged but testing for vWD is normal. vWD is among the most common of inherited bleeding disorders; evaluation includes von Willebrand factor (vWF) antigen, vWF activity (both by Ristocetin cofactor assay and collagen binding assay), and factor VIII activity (in addition to first-stage tests). Confirmatory testing for vWD involves repeat testing on a separate venipuncture specimen, with the addition of vWF multimeric assay.

E. Disorders of secondary hemostasis typically include joint/soft-tissue bleeding. In patients with joint or soft-tissue bleeding, the PT, aPTT, fibrinogen, and TT are particularly important to assess. Consider the possibilities of absent/low fibrinogen (afibrinogenemia/hypofibrinogenemia) and heparin contamination when PT, aPTT, and TT are all prolonged. Dual PT and aPTT prolongation with a normal TT may suggest a deficiency of factors V, X, or prothrombin; vitamin K deficiency (supported by low activities of factors II (prothrombin), VII, IX, and X that correct after vitamin K supplementation); or hepatic synthetic dysfunction (supported by low albumin levels and biochemical indices of hepatic injury). If the PT or aPTT is prolonged, assess for factor deficiencies, specific factor inhibitors, and lupus-type inhibitors (i.e., lupus anticoagulants) by mixing study (1:1 ratio of patient plasma/pooled normal plasma); normalization of the PT or aPTT suggests a factor deficiency, whereas noncorrection suggests the presence of an inhibitor. An inhibitor is also suggested by increase in factor activity with serial dilution of plasma. Perform the individual factor assays as indicated to confirm the diagnosis of specific factor deficiencies/inhibitors. If the PT, aPTT, and TT are all normal, consider more rare diagnoses including disorders of fibrinolysis, factor XIII deficiency, or vascular injury.

F. When PT, aPTT, and TT are all prolonged in the presence of thrombocytopenia, consider DIC.

G. Other causes of bleeding also need to be considered. The euglobulin lysis time (ELT) evaluates clot lysis and is sensitive to disorders such as plasminogen activator inhibitor-1 (PAI-1) deficiency, in which traumatic bleeding results from excessive fibrinolysis. Factor XIII urea clot solubility assay evaluates for impaired fibrin cross-linking caused by factor XIII deficiency, which is not detected by the PT or aPTT. Vasculitis and vascular anomalies may also cause bleeding, often in association with thrombocytopenia or consumption coagulopathy; however, bleeding may have a uniquely anatomic cause. Connective tissue diseases, particularly collagen defects, often have normal coagulation testing and may occasionally have physical findings (e.g., joint hyperextensibility in Ehlers–Danlos syndrome).

Treatment: Treatment strategies depend on diagnosis. Consultation with pediatric hematology is warranted. Therapeutic approach should also address any comorbid conditions that may contribute to the bleeding symptoms and limit any medications that impair platelet function.

For disorders of primary hemostasis caused by defective platelet function, platelet transfusion is the mainstay of therapy for clinically significant hemorrhage. 1-Deamino-8-D-arginine vasopressin (DDAVP) may be effective in select circumstances. ε-Aminocaproic acid (EACA) is often effective as an adjunctive therapy or in the setting of minor bleeding episodes. For vWD, depending on the type and severity of the defect (and of the bleeding episode, in type 1 vWD), agents may include DDAVP, EACA, or highly purified, viral-inactivated, plasma-derived concentrate of factor VIII/vWF complex. Oral contraceptive pills may be useful for menorrhagia.

With regard to secondary hemostatic defects, single-factor replacement is available as either recombinant or highly purified, viral-inactivated, plasma-derived concentrates of factor VIII or IX for hemophilia A and B, respectively. The presence of a high-titer factor VIII–inhibitory antibody in hemophilia A requires treatment with a bypassing agent such as recombinant activated factor VII or a prothrombin complex concentrate for the management of acute bleeding episodes. Recombinant activated factor VII is also used for factor VII deficiency. In afibrinogenemia/hypofibrinogenemia, fibrinogen concentrate is preferred; alternatively, cryoprecipitate is indicated. Fresh frozen plasma (FFP) is used for factor XI and plasminogen deficiencies. In DIC, treatment is focused on the underlying condition, and supportive care includes replacement of consumed coagulation components via platelet transfusions, FFP, and cryoprecipitate, as needed for bleeding. Heparin is sometimes also used to attenuate coagulation activation in DIC. Bleeding caused by antibody-mediated inhibition of specific coagulation factors is rare in children; corticosteroids may be useful in this scenario.

Bleeding in factor XIII deficiency is managed with cryoprecipitate. Defects of excessive fibrinolytic function may be treated with antifibrinolytic agents, such as EACA or tranexamic acid.

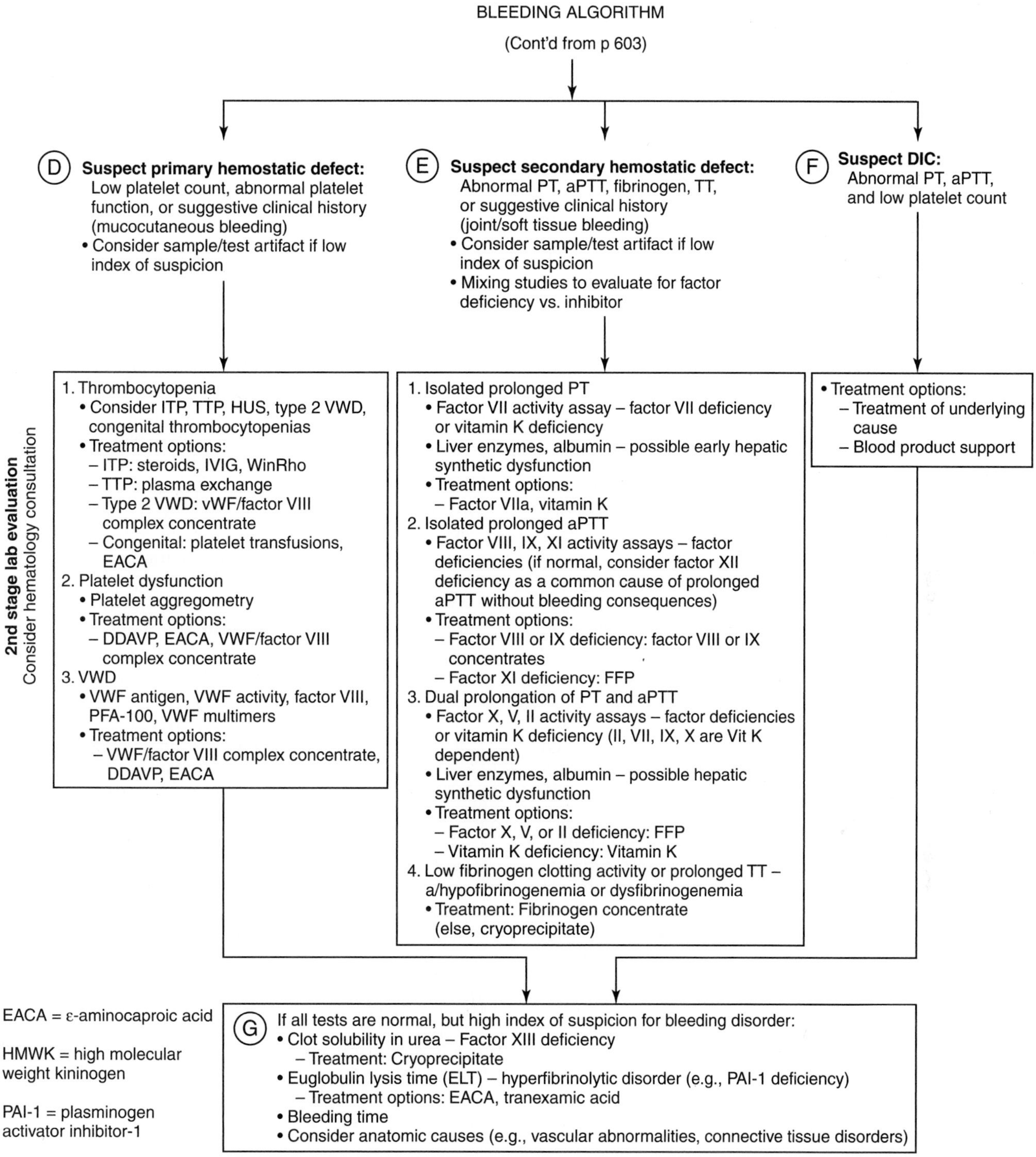
BLEEDING ALGORITHM
(Cont'd from p 603)
D Suspect primary hemostatic defect:
Low platelet count, abnormal platelet function, or suggestive clinical history (mucocutaneous bleeding)
• Consider sample/test artifact if low index of suspicion
E Suspect secondary hemostatic defect:
Abnormal PT, aPTT, fibrinogen, TT, or suggestive clinical history (joint/soft tissue bleeding)
• Consider sample/test artifact if low index of suspicion
• Mixing studies to evaluate for factor deficiency vs. inhibitor
F Suspect DIC:
Abnormal PT, aPTT, and low platelet count
2nd stage lab evaluation
Consider hematology consultation
1. Thrombocytopenia
• Consider ITP, TTP, HUS, type 2 VWD, congenital thrombocytopenias
• Treatment options:
– ITP: steroids, IVIG, WinRho
– TTP: plasma exchange
– Type 2 VWD: vWF/factor VIII complex concentrate
– Congenital: platelet transfusions, EACA
2. Platelet dysfunction
• Platelet aggregometry
• Treatment options:
– DDAVP, EACA, VWF/factor VIII complex concentrate
3. VWD
• VWF antigen, VWF activity, factor VIII, PFA-100, VWF multimers
• Treatment options:
– VWF/factor VIII complex concentrate, DDAVP, EACA
1. Isolated prolonged PT
• Factor VII activity assay – factor VII deficiency or vitamin K deficiency
• Liver enzymes, albumin – possible early hepatic synthetic dysfunction
• Treatment options:
– Factor VIIa, vitamin K
2. Isolated prolonged aPTT
• Factor VIII, IX, XI activity assays – factor deficiencies (if normal, consider factor XII deficiency as a common cause of prolonged aPTT without bleeding consequences)
• Treatment options:
– Factor VIII or IX deficiency: factor VIII or IX concentrates
– Factor XI deficiency: FFP
3. Dual prolongation of PT and aPTT
• Factor X, V, II activity assays – factor deficiencies or vitamin K deficiency (II, VII, IX, X are Vit K dependent)
• Liver enzymes, albumin – possible hepatic synthetic dysfunction
• Treatment options:
– Factor X, V, or II deficiency: FFP
– Vitamin K deficiency: Vitamin K
4. Low fibrinogen clotting activity or prolonged TT – a/hypofibrinogenemia or dysfibrinogenemia
• Treatment: Fibrinogen concentrate (else, cryoprecipitate)
• Treatment options:
– Treatment of underlying cause
– Blood product support
G If all tests are normal, but high index of suspicion for bleeding disorder:
• Clot solubility in urea – Factor XIII deficiency
– Treatment: Cryoprecipitate
• Euglobulin lysis time (ELT) – hyperfibrinolytic disorder (e.g., PAI-1 deficiency)
– Treatment options: EACA, tranexamic acid
• Bleeding time
• Consider anatomic causes (e.g., vascular abnormalities, connective tissue disorders)
EACA = ε-aminocaproic acid
HMWK = high molecular weight kininogen
PAI-1 = plasminogen activator inhibitor-1

References

Goldenberg NA, Manco-Johnson MJ. Pediatric hemostasis and use of plasma components. Best Pract Res Clin Haematol 2006;19: 143–55.

Rajpurkar M, Lusher JM. Clinical and laboratory approach to the patient with bleeding. In: Orkin SH, Nathan DG, Ginsburg D, et al, editors. Nathan and Oski's hematology of infancy and childhood. 7th ed. Philadelphia: Saunders; 2009. p. 1449–61.

Venous Thromboembolism

Mindy L. Grunzke, MD, and Neil A. Goldenberg, MD, PhD

The incidence rate of venous thromboembolism (VTE) in children is bimodal, with peak rates in the neonatal period and adolescence. The overall incidence rate of VTE is 0.49 per 10,000 per year in the United States. Remember the Virchow triad (venous stasis, endothelial damage, and hypercoagulable state) when considering the pathogenesis of VTE. In children, more than 90% of VTEs are associated with an identified clinical triggering event or condition (compared with 60% in adults). Furthermore, more than 50% of deep vein thromboses (DVTs) in children and more than 80% in neonates occur in association with indwelling central venous catheters.

A. History: Determine the onset and location of symptoms, surrounding events (trauma), associated risk factors, and detailed family history of thrombophilia traits, early-onset (i.e., before age 55 years) VTE, stroke, or myocardial infarction, or recurrent fetal loss. Clinical risk factors for VTE include central venous access, trauma, surgery, immobilization, pregnancy, exogenous estrogen (oral contraceptives), infection, malignancy, or other systemic disorders such as collagen vascular disease, renal disease, or inflammatory bowel disease. Symptoms may include painful limb swelling (extremity DVTs), sudden-onset shortness of breath or pleuritic chest pain (pulmonary embolism [PE]), severe, persistent headache, or blurred vision (cerebral sinovenous thrombosis [CSVT]), among others.

B. Physical Examination: Signs are often subtle in children. Examine limbs for tenderness, swelling, discoloration, palpable cord in popliteal fossa, Homans' sign (calf pain on forced ankle dorsiflexion, which may indicate DVT; however, this sign is neither sensitive nor specific), and signs of chronic venous insufficiency such as edema, dilated superficial collateral veins, venous stasis dermatitis, or skin ulceration. Upper extremity or neck thromboses may also cause neck/facial swelling and/or bilateral periorbital edema, particularly when the superior vena cava is occluded (superior vena cava syndrome). Tachypnea, hypoxia, a loud second heart sound, and/or signs of right-heart failure (hepatomegaly, peripheral edema) may be found in PE, particularly with proximal or extensive involvement of the pulmonary arterial tree. Neurologic signs (cranial nerve palsy, papilledema) may indicate CSVT, whereas the triad of flank mass, hematuria, and thrombocytopenia is associated with renal vein thrombosis.

DIAGNOSIS

C. Appropriate radiologic imaging is required to confirm the presence of a thrombus and to define its extent and occlusiveness. Venography is the historical gold standard diagnostic modality, but it is invasive. Lower extremity DVT is effectively imaged via compression ultrasound with Doppler; computed tomography (CT) or magnetic resonance imaging (MRI) with venography (CTV or MRV) is sometimes required for proximal visualization of the involved pelvic, abdominal, or thoracic vasculature. For upper extremity DVT, echo may be useful centrally in combination with ultrasound peripherally; however, venography is sometimes required for definitive diagnosis in noncompressible areas. PE requires spiral computed tomographic angiogram (CTA) and/or ventilation/perfusion scan for diagnosis; at many pediatric tertiary care centers, expertise is greatest with spiral CTA. CSVT may be disclosed by CTV or MRV. For serial imaging, CT should be avoided if possible given the radiation exposure with this modality.

D. With regard to laboratory evaluation, a complete blood cell count (CBC), disseminated intravascular coagulation (DIC) panel (prothrombin time [PT], activated partial thromboplastin time (aPTT), fibrinogen, and D-dimer), and a comprehensive thrombophilia panel are recommended to define the extent of underlying thrombophilia and appropriate treatment options. Thrombophilia states include anticoagulant deficiency or resistance states (deficiency of protein C, protein S, or antithrombin; presence of the factor V Leiden polymorphism); excess procoagulant states (elevated factor VIII; presence of the prothrombin G20210A mutation); and mediators of hypercoagulability or endothelial damage (elevated lipoprotein[a], hyperhomocysteinemia; or the presence of antiphospholipid antibodies such as the lupus anticoagulant [often measured by dilute Russell viper venom time] and IgG or IgM anticardiolipin or anti–β2-glycoprotein-1 antibodies).

TREATMENT

Consultation with pediatric hematology is warranted. Identified clinical triggers for thrombosis should be mitigated, if possible (e.g., discontinuing estrogen-containing oral contraceptives, treating underlying infectious diseases or inflammatory conditions).

Conventional treatment for a first thrombotic event involves acute anticoagulation with a heparin-based agent (unfractionated heparin [UFH] or low-molecular-weight heparin [LMWH]) for approximately 1 week, followed by subacute/extended anticoagulation with LMWH or warfarin. Anticoagulation is given to reduce the risk for thrombus progression or embolism; thrombus regression is believed to rely on intrinsic fibrinolytic mechanisms to dissolve thrombosis over time. Duration of anticoagulation is risk stratified, currently based largely on adult evidence: For VTE associated with a risk factor that has resolved, recommended duration is 3 to 6 months

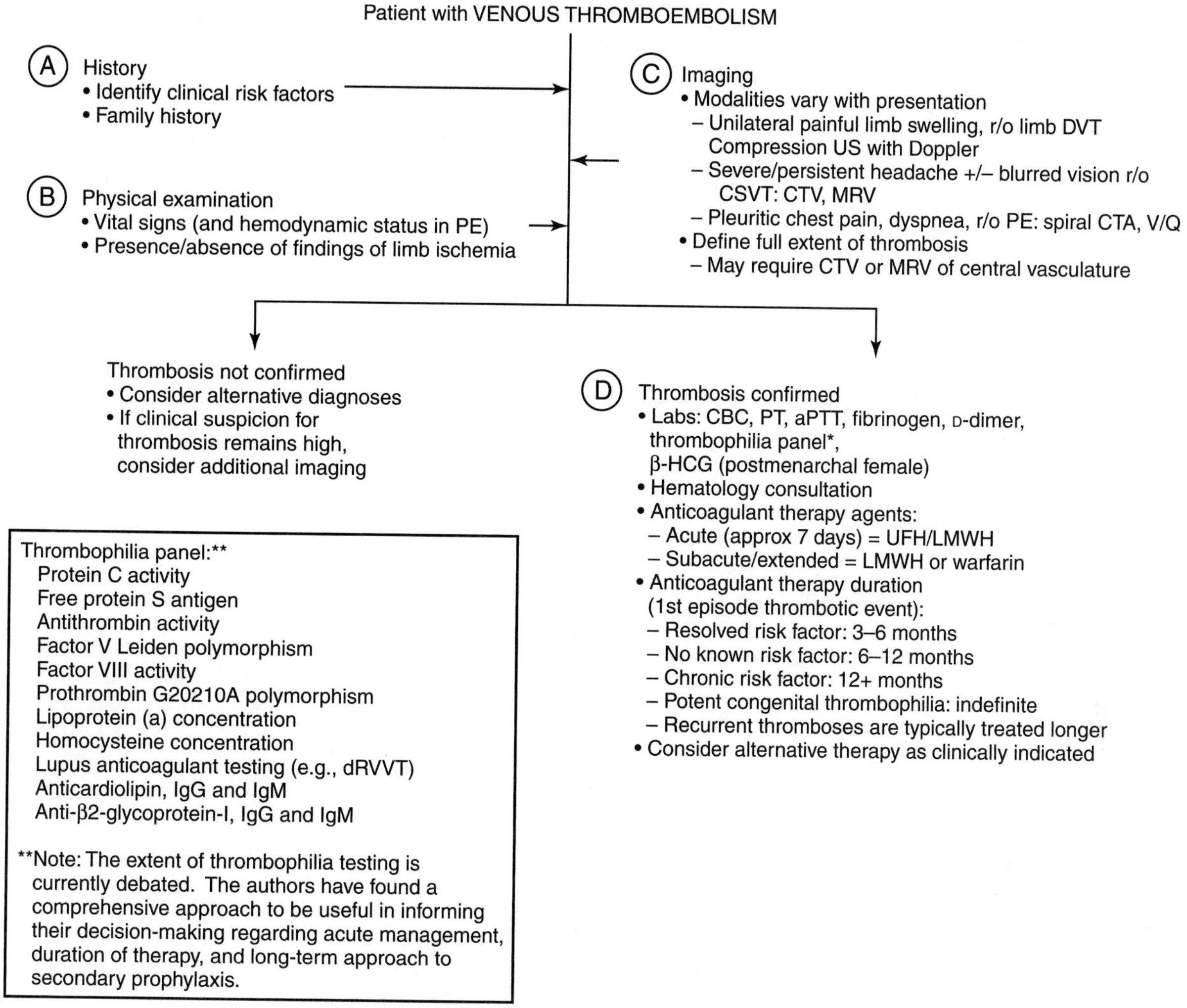
Patient with VENOUS THROMBOEMBOLISM
A History
• Identify clinical risk factors
• Family history
B Physical examination
• Vital signs (and hemodynamic status in PE)
• Presence/absence of findings of limb ischemia
C Imaging
• Modalities vary with presentation
– Unilateral painful limb swelling, r/o limb DVT Compression US with Doppler
– Severe/persistent headache +/– blurred vision r/o CSVT: CTV, MRV
– Pleuritic chest pain, dyspnea, r/o PE: spiral CTA, V/Q
• Define full extent of thrombosis
– May require CTV or MRV of central vasculature
Thrombosis not confirmed
• Consider alternative diagnoses
• If clinical suspicion for thrombosis remains high, consider additional imaging
D Thrombosis confirmed
• Labs: CBC, PT, aPTT, fibrinogen, D-dimer, thrombophilia panel*, β-HCG (postmenarchal female)
• Hematology consultation
• Anticoagulant therapy agents:
– Acute (approx 7 days) = UFH/LMWH
– Subacute/extended = LMWH or warfarin
• Anticoagulant therapy duration (1st episode thrombotic event):
– Resolved risk factor: 3–6 months
– No known risk factor: 6–12 months
– Chronic risk factor: 12+ months
– Potent congenital thrombophilia: indefinite
– Recurrent thromboses are typically treated longer
• Consider alternative therapy as clinically indicated
Thrombophilia panel:**
Protein C activity
Free protein S antigen
Antithrombin activity
Factor V Leiden polymorphism
Factor VIII activity
Prothrombin G20210A polymorphism
Lipoprotein (a) concentration
Homocysteine concentration
Lupus anticoagulant testing (e.g., dRVVT)
Anticardiolipin, IgG and IgM
Anti-β2-glycoprotein-I, IgG and IgM
**Note: The extent of thrombophilia testing is currently debated. The authors have found a comprehensive approach to be useful in informing their decision-making regarding acute management, duration of therapy, and long-term approach to secondary prophylaxis.

(3 months is most often used); for idiopathic VTE, suggested duration is 6 to 12 months; for VTE occurring in the setting of a chronic prothrombotic risk factor, recommended duration is 12 months at minimum. In each of the aforementioned categories, a longer duration of anticoagulation for acute VTE is recommended in patients who have had a previous thrombotic event. Indefinite treatment is often warranted in the setting of potent congenital thrombophilia (e.g., severe protein C deficiency). In antiphospholipid antibody syndrome, treatment duration is unclear and often individualized. Anticoagulant dosing and monitoring recommendations have been previously published by Monagle and colleagues. Heparin-based therapy is ideally monitored by anti–factor Xa activity level, whereas warfarin is monitored via the international normalized ratio (calculated from the measured PT).

Alternative treatment approaches to conventional anticoagulation may be warranted in select cases. These include systemic or local pharmacologic thrombolysis, with or without interventional mechanical thrombolysis (e.g., in the setting of occlusive DVT with evidence of or high risk for end-organ or tissue damage); direct thrombin inhibitors (e.g., in heparin-induced thrombocytopenia); and replacement of clinically significant deficiencies of native anticoagulants (e.g., protein C, antithrombin).

References

Monagle P, Chalmers E, Chan A, et al; American College of Chest Physicians. Antithrombotic therapy in neonates and children: American College of Chest Physicians Evidence-Based Clinical Practice Guidelines (8th edition). Chest 2008;133(6 Suppl): 887S–968S.

Pipe SW, Goldenberg NA. Acquired disorders of hemostasis. In: Orkin SH, Nathan DG, Ginsburg D, et al, editors. Nathan and Oski's hematology of infancy and childhood. 7th ed. Philadelphia: Saunders; 2009. p. 1591–1620.

Fever or Acute Illness in a Child with Sickle Cell Disease

Julie A. Panepinto, MD

Sickle cell disease is an autosomal recessive disease that results from a substitution of valine for glutamic acid in the sixth position of the β-globin chain of hemoglobin. This results in abnormal hemoglobin and causes the red blood cells to become sickle shaped and lead to vaso-occlusive complications that are common in sickle cell disease. The diagnosis is usually made at birth in the United States through newborn screening and occurs in approximately 1 in 400 African American births.

A. In the patient's history, review prior sickle cell disease complications, as well as the details of the acute illness. Triage all patients with fever (temperature >38.5° C) for rapid history and physical assessment. Draw a blood sample for complete blood cell count (CBC), reticulocyte count, and blood culture, and give parenteral antibiotics immediately (see section C). Obtain a chest radiograph to evaluate the patient with fever for an infiltrate. Inquire specifically about fever, pain, chest pain, cough, shortness of breath, and neurologic symptoms. Ask whether pain is similar or dissimilar to previous sickle pains. Determine from the patient or from medical records the precise diagnosis (homozygous sickle cell anemia, sickle cell–hemoglobin C disease, sickle β+- or β0-thalassemia), as well as the patient's baseline values for hemoglobin, hematocrit, platelet count, and reticulocyte count.

B. Perform a complete physical examination; search for foci of infection. Note fever (infection such as bacteremia or osteomyelitis, infarction, or acute chest syndrome), tachypnea (acute chest syndrome, asthma, sepsis, splenic sequestration, or aplastic crisis), or tachycardia or hypotension (splenic sequestration, severe infection). Extreme pallor suggests splenic sequestration or aplastic crisis. Significant splenomegaly (size larger than baseline examination) suggests splenic sequestration. Note any neurologic abnormalities (stroke, meningitis), right upper quadrant abdominal tenderness (biliary colic secondary to cholelithiasis, vaso-occlusive crisis), knee or hip pain (aseptic necrosis of the femoral head), any persistent focal bone pain (infarction or osteomyelitis) or priapism (Table 1).

C. Assess the risk for infection. Because functional asplenia develops at an early age, infants and children with sickle cell disease commonly acquire bacterial sepsis and meningitis. Patients with a temperature greater than 38.5° C (with or without a focus of infection) or with unexplained lethargy or diarrhea may have overwhelming sepsis (*Streptococcus pneumoniae* is the most common organism). Immediately obtain blood and other culture specimens, and begin broad-spectrum parenteral antibiotics (e.g., cefuroxime, cefotaxime, or ceftriaxone). Because of the prevalence of resistant organisms, vancomycin should be added for severe illness or proven or suspected central nervous system infection. Perform a lumbar puncture for patients with meningismus or young children with excessive lethargy or toxicity.

D. Consider the possibility of an illness unrelated to sickle cell disease (e.g., appendicitis presenting with abdominal pain). Acute splenic enlargement with a hematocrit less than the baseline value or signs of intravascular volume depletion indicate splenic sequestration. A hematocrit less than the baseline value in association with a very low reticulocyte count suggests an aplastic crisis. A decreased (from baseline) platelet count may indicate sepsis, splenic sequestration, or acute chest syndrome. More than one acute complication may be present simultaneously.

(Continued on page 610)

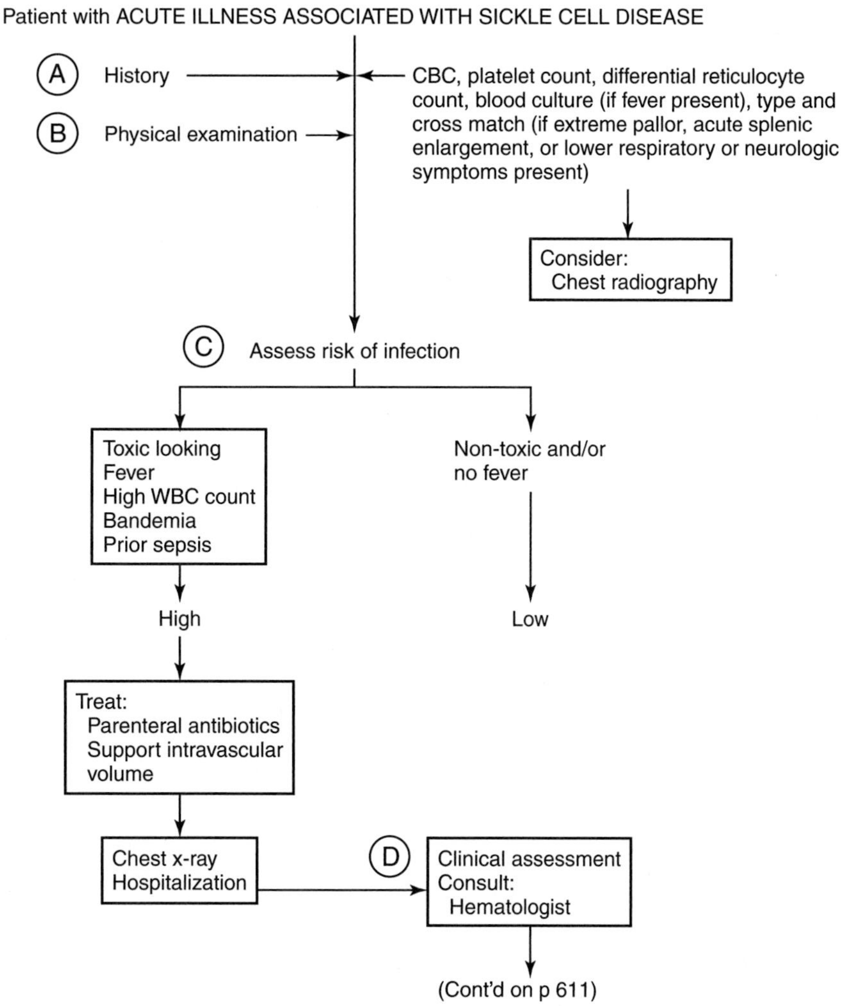
Patient with ACUTE ILLNESS ASSOCIATED WITH SICKLE CELL DISEASE
A
History
B
Physical examination
CBC, platelet count, differential reticulocyte count, blood culture (if fever present), type and cross match (if extreme pallor, acute splenic enlargement, or lower respiratory or neurologic symptoms present)
Consider:
Chest radiography
C
Assess risk of infection
Toxic looking
Fever
High WBC count
Bandemia
Prior sepsis
Non-toxic and/or no fever
High
Low
Treat:
Parenteral antibiotics
Support intravascular volume
Chest x-ray
Hospitalization
D
Clinical assessment
Consult:
Hematologist
(Cont'd on p 611)

Table 1. **Degree of Illness in Sickle Cell Patients with an Acute Illness**

Mild	Moderate	Severe	Very Severe
Vaso-occlusive painful event: responsive to oral pain medications	Vaso-occlusive painful event: requires parental analgesics	Vaso-occlusive painful event: requires parental analgesics	Vaso-occlusive painful event: requires parental analgesics
Fever: nontoxic, white blood cell count <25,000/μl, no infiltrate on chest radiograph	Fever: osteomyelitis, bacteremia	Fever: osteomyelitis, bacteremia	Fever: sepsis
	Priapism: resolves spontaneously without intervention	Priapism: requires intervention for resolution	Priapism: prolonged and/or refractory to intervention
		Acute chest syndrome without respiratory distress	Acute chest syndrome with respiratory distress
	Aplastic crisis, asymptomatic	Aplastic crisis with severe anemia and symptoms of severe anemia	
		Splenic sequestration without signs of shock yet	Splenic sequestration with shock
		Cerebrovascular accident	

E. A vaso-occlusive complication secondary to ischemia may occur in any part of the body. Treatment includes hydration with maintenance fluids (sickle cell patients have hyposthenuria, but avoid excessive hydration, which may precipitate or exacerbate acute chest syndrome), oxygen for hypoxemia if it is present, and adequate analgesia (oral analgesics or intravenous medications such as morphine or hydromorphone for severe pain). Nonsteroidal anti-inflammatory analgesics (e.g., ibuprofen, ketorolac) may also be useful in some cases. Do not use repeated doses of meperidine because it has the potential to induce seizures. Indications for hospitalization for pain include the inability to maintain hydration orally, the failure of oral analgesics to relieve pain adequately, and the presence of a coexistent complication, such as acute chest syndrome, splenic sequestration, or stroke. It is sometimes difficult to differentiate vaso-occlusive abdominal pain from cholecystitis. Imaging studies, surgical consultation, and liver function tests may be helpful. Consider the possibility of acute osteomyelitis *(Staphylococcus aureus, Salmonella)* in patients thought to have bone infarctions, but infarction is far more common. The term *acute chest syndrome* defines any acute illness with a new pulmonary infiltrate. Causes of acute chest syndrome, such as bone marrow fat embolism and pulmonary infarction, are difficult to differentiate from bacterial pneumonia *(S. pneumoniae, Haemophilus influenzae, S. aureus, Mycoplasma, Chlamydia);* thus, broad-spectrum antibiotic coverage that includes a macrolide should be provided if fever is present. A cerebrovascular accident is an indication for an immediate simple red blood cell transfusion, followed by an exchange transfusion and subsequent chronic transfusions to decrease the amount of sickle hemoglobin. Boys with prolonged priapism should receive a simple red blood cell transfusion, analgesics, intravenous fluids, and be seen by a urologist for possible surgical intervention such as penile aspiration and irrigation.

F. Aplastic crises are typically caused by parvovirus B19 and represent a transient inability of erythropoiesis to keep pace with chronic hemolysis. The rapidly declining hemoglobin level may result in congestive heart failure; red blood cell transfusions are sometimes needed to support the patient until adequate red blood cell production resumes. Use droplet isolation to protect immunodeficient patients and pregnant health care providers.

G. Splenic sequestration can be a life-threatening emergency requiring urgent red blood cell transfusions to maintain intravascular volume. Such episodes, often triggered by infection, tend to recur.

H. Sickle cell patients with a hemoglobin level less than 10 g/dl who require general anesthesia for surgical procedures are generally transfused before surgery to reduce the risk for perioperative sickling complications.

References

Cage CS. Sickle cell disease. Hematol Oncol Clin North Am 2005;19:771–987.

Field JJ, Knight-Perry JE, Debaun MR. Acute pain in children and adults with sickle cell disease: management in the absence of evidence-based guidelines. Curr Opin Hematol 2009;16:173–8.

National Institutes of Health, National Heart, Lung, and Blood Institute. The management of sickle cell disease. 4th ed. Bethesda, MD: National Institutes of Health; 2002.

Vichinsky EP, Haberkern CM, Neumayr L, et al. A comparison of conservative and aggressive transfusion regimens in the perioperative management of sickle cell disease. N Engl J Med 1995; 333:206.

Vichinsky EP, Neumayr L, Earles AN, et al. Causes and outcomes of the acute chest syndrome in sickle cell disease. N Engl J Med 2000; 342:1855.

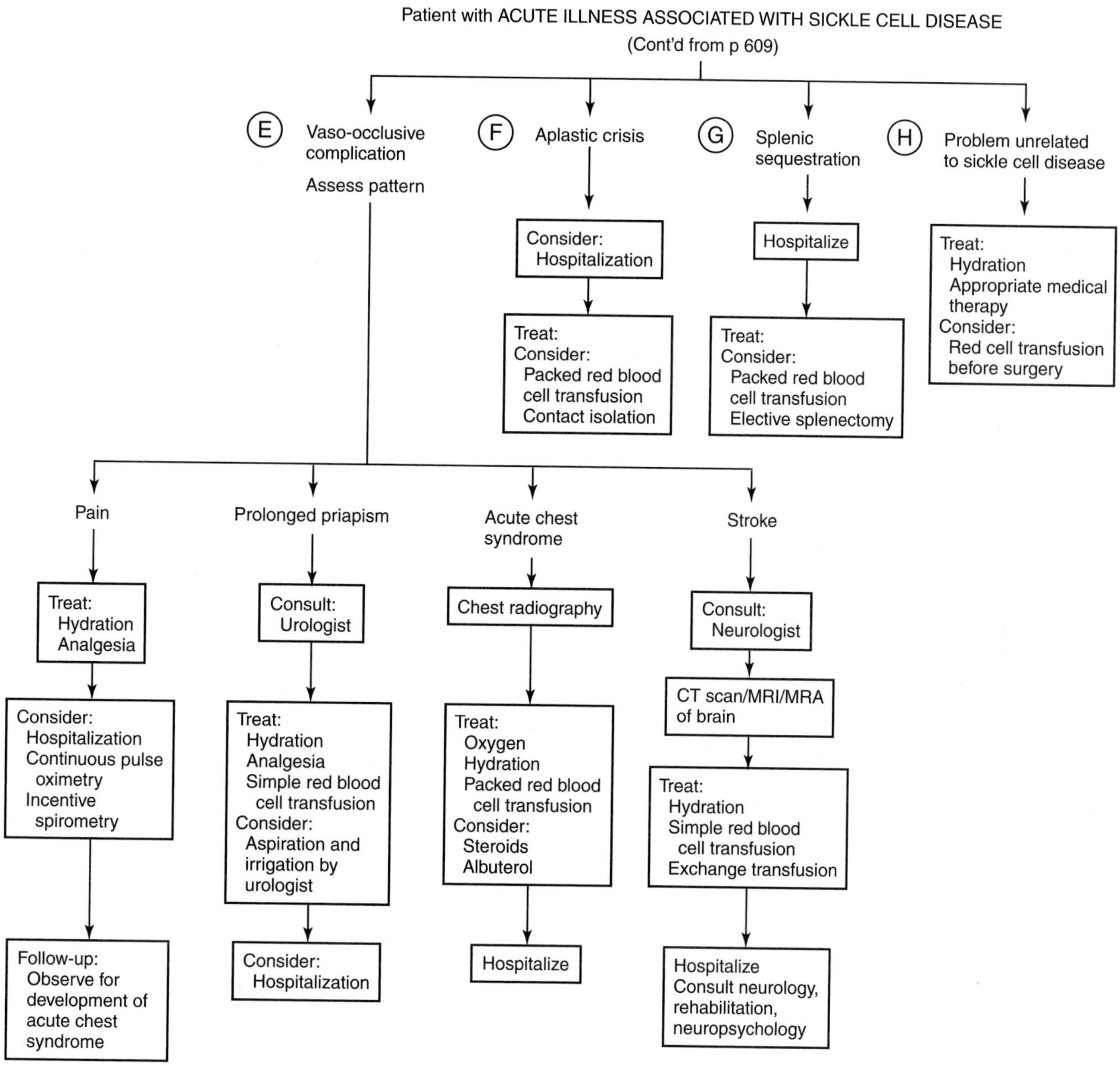
Patient with ACUTE ILLNESS ASSOCIATED WITH SICKLE CELL DISEASE
(Cont'd from p 609)
E Vaso-occlusive complication
Assess pattern
F Aplastic crisis
G Splenic sequestration
H Problem unrelated to sickle cell disease
Consider: Hospitalization
Treat: Consider: Packed red blood cell transfusion Contact isolation
Hospitalize
Treat: Consider: Packed red blood cell transfusion Elective splenectomy
Treat: Hydration Appropriate medical therapy Consider: Red cell transfusion before surgery
Pain
Prolonged priapism
Acute chest syndrome
Stroke
Treat: Hydration Analgesia
Consult: Urologist
Chest radiography
Consult: Neurologist
CT scan/MRI/MRA of brain
Consider: Hospitalization Continuous pulse oximetry Incentive spirometry
Treat: Hydration Analgesia Simple red blood cell transfusion Consider: Aspiration and irrigation by urologist
Treat: Oxygen Hydration Packed red blood cell transfusion Consider: Steroids Albuterol
Treat: Hydration Simple red blood cell transfusion Exchange transfusion
Follow-up: Observe for development of acute chest syndrome
Consider: Hospitalization
Hospitalize
Hospitalize Consult neurology, rehabilitation, neuropsychology

Thrombocytopenia

Julie A. Panepinto, MD

Thrombocytopenia is a lower than normal number of platelets. Usually, platelet counts are between 150,000 and 500,000/μl blood in children but may be higher in infants. Thrombocytopenia is most likely to be secondary to an autoimmune process and rarely is due to a congenital disease.

A. In the patient's history, ask about the type and duration of bruising, bleeding, or petechiae. Note recent illnesses, such as diarrhea (hemolytic-uremic syndrome [HUS]), neurologic symptoms (thrombotic thrombocytopenic purpura [TTP]), and sore throat (infectious mononucleosis, acute poststreptococcal glomerulonephritis). Document associated symptoms, such as fever (infection, leukemia or other malignancy, autoimmune disease), limp, and limb pain (leukemia, autoimmune disease). Note any medications (platelet-antibody effects). Obtain a family history of bleeding disorders. Assess risk for human immunodeficiency virus (HIV) infection or other immunodeficiency disorder.

B. In the physical examination, note fever and assess the degree of illness. Acutely ill and toxic-appearing children with thrombocytopenia require expeditious evaluation (disseminated intravascular coagulation [DIC], sepsis, HUS, TTP, severe hemorrhage). Note the extent and type of manifestations of bleeding. Short stature, microcephaly, skeletal anomalies, hyperpigmentation, hypogenitalism (Fanconi anemia), absent radii with normal thumbs (thrombocytopenia with absent radii), and chronic eczema and recurrent infections in a boy (Wiskott–Aldrich syndrome) are all clues to congenital thrombocytopenia. Splenomegaly or generalized lymphadenopathy suggests leukemia, malignant neoplasia, infection such as with HIV or infectious mononucleosis, a storage disease, or hypersplenism. Children with idiopathic thrombocytopenic purpura (ITP) do not have jaundice or hepatosplenomegaly. Arthritis, mouth ulcers, or a characteristic rash may suggest an autoimmune disease.

C. Order a complete blood cell count (CBC) with differential and platelet count. The finding of anemia or neutropenia (absolute neutrophil count $<1500/mm^3$) in association with thrombocytopenia helps direct the subsequent workup. Whereas neutropenia may occur with infection, its association with significant thrombocytopenia also suggests bone marrow failure. Anemia suggests bone marrow failure, intravascular hemolysis, autoimmune disease, HIV infection, or blood loss secondary to thrombocytopenic bleeding.

D. Review the peripheral blood smear. Red blood cell fragmentation suggests intravascular hemolysis. Spherocytes (autoimmune hemolysis) or macrocytes (bone marrow failure, Fanconi anemia, or brisk reticulocytosis) are also helpful clues. Note platelet size and morphology and homogeneity of the platelets. Boys with Wiskott–Aldrich syndrome have tiny platelets; large platelets suggest rapid platelet turnover, as seen in ITP, or a congenital thrombocytopenia, such as Bernard–Soulier syndrome, or MYH9-related disease, such as May–Hegglin anomaly. Type 2b von Willebrand disease is associated with thrombocytopenia.

(Continued on page 614)

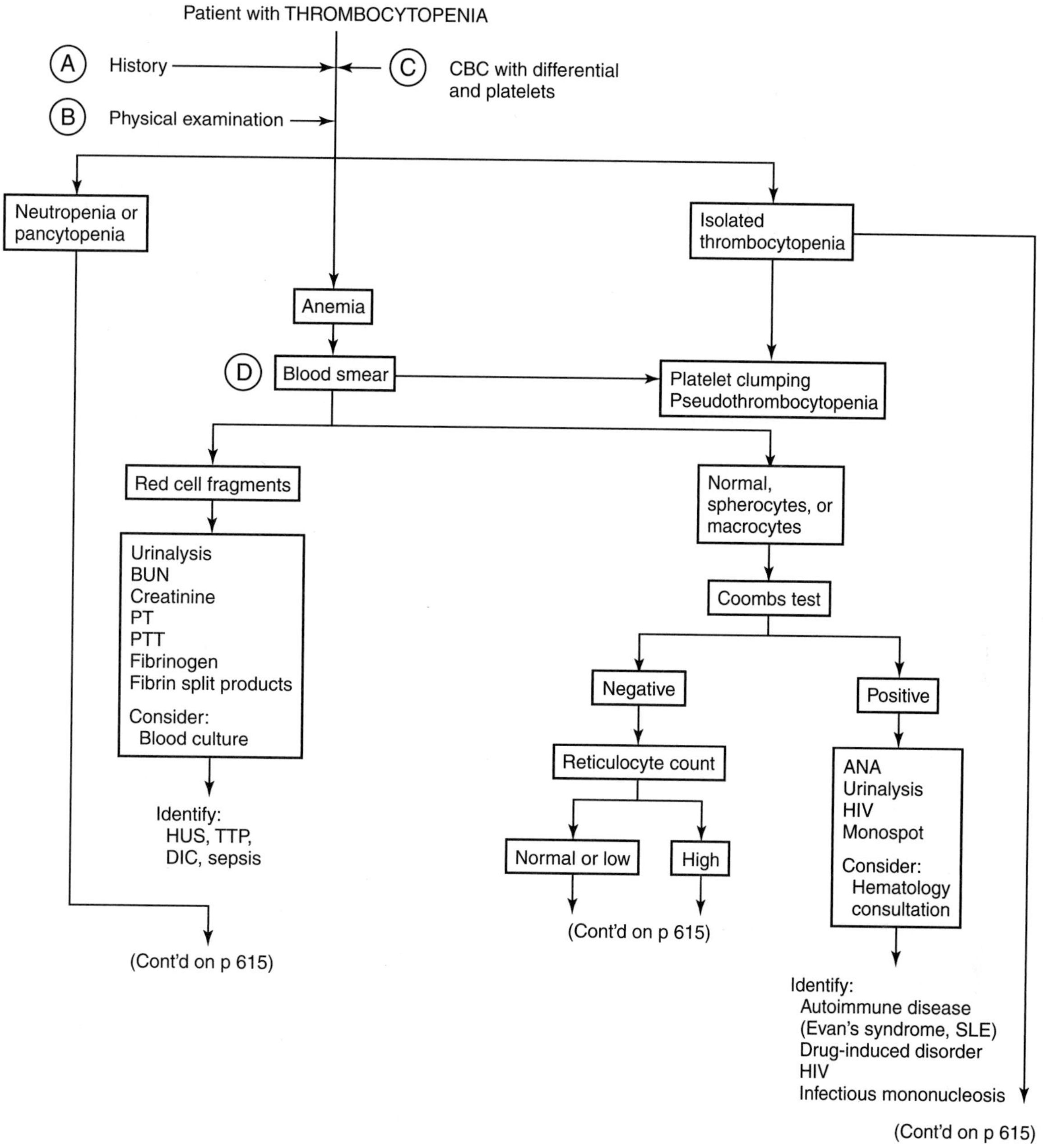
Patient with THROMBOCYTOPENIA
A History
B Physical examination
C CBC with differential and platelets
Neutropenia or pancytopenia
Anemia
Isolated thrombocytopenia
D Blood smear
Platelet clumping Pseudothrombocytopenia
Red cell fragments
Normal, spherocytes, or macrocytes
Urinalysis
BUN
Creatinine
PT
PTT
Fibrinogen
Fibrin split products
Consider:
Blood culture
Coombs test
Negative
Positive
Reticulocyte count
ANA
Urinalysis
HIV
Monospot
Consider:
Hematology consultation
Identify:
HUS, TTP,
DIC, sepsis
Normal or low
High
(Cont'd on p 615)
(Cont'd on p 615)
Identify:
Autoimmune disease
(Evan's syndrome, SLE)
Drug-induced disorder
HIV
Infectious mononucleosis
(Cont'd on p 615)

E. Consult a hematologist before performing a bone marrow examination to avoid omitting important special studies (biopsy, chromosomes, lymphoid markers). The absence of lymphadenopathy, organomegaly, and leukemic blasts on the blood smear does not exclude leukemia.

F. ITP is the most common cause of acute thrombocytopenia in an otherwise well child. In addition, in an otherwise healthy neonate, alloimmune thrombocytopenia should be considered. However, other diagnostic possibilities must always be entertained as the cause of the thrombocytopenia. A positive antinuclear antibody (ANA) or Coombs test result indicates other autoantibodies and suggests an underlying autoimmune disease such as systemic lupus erythematosus (SLE). The decision to perform a bone marrow examination may be individualized. Children without significant clinical bleeding are observed with serial CBCs and platelet counts. When the platelet count normalizes, further counts are not needed. Recurrence is rare.

G. Because splenomegaly and lymphadenopathy are unusual in children with ITP, these findings in a child with significant thrombocytopenia (lacking a clear alternative explanation, such as long-standing splenomegaly with portal hypertension suggesting hypersplenism or test results indicating HIV infection) dictate an early bone marrow examination.

References

Cines DB, Bussel JR, McMillan RB, Zehnder JL. Congenital and acquired thrombocytopenia. In: Hematology 2004: education program book. Washington, DC: American Society of Hematology; 2004. p. 390–406.

Veneri D, Franchini M, Randon F, et al. Thrombocytopenias: a clinical point of view. Blood Transfus 2009;7:75–85.

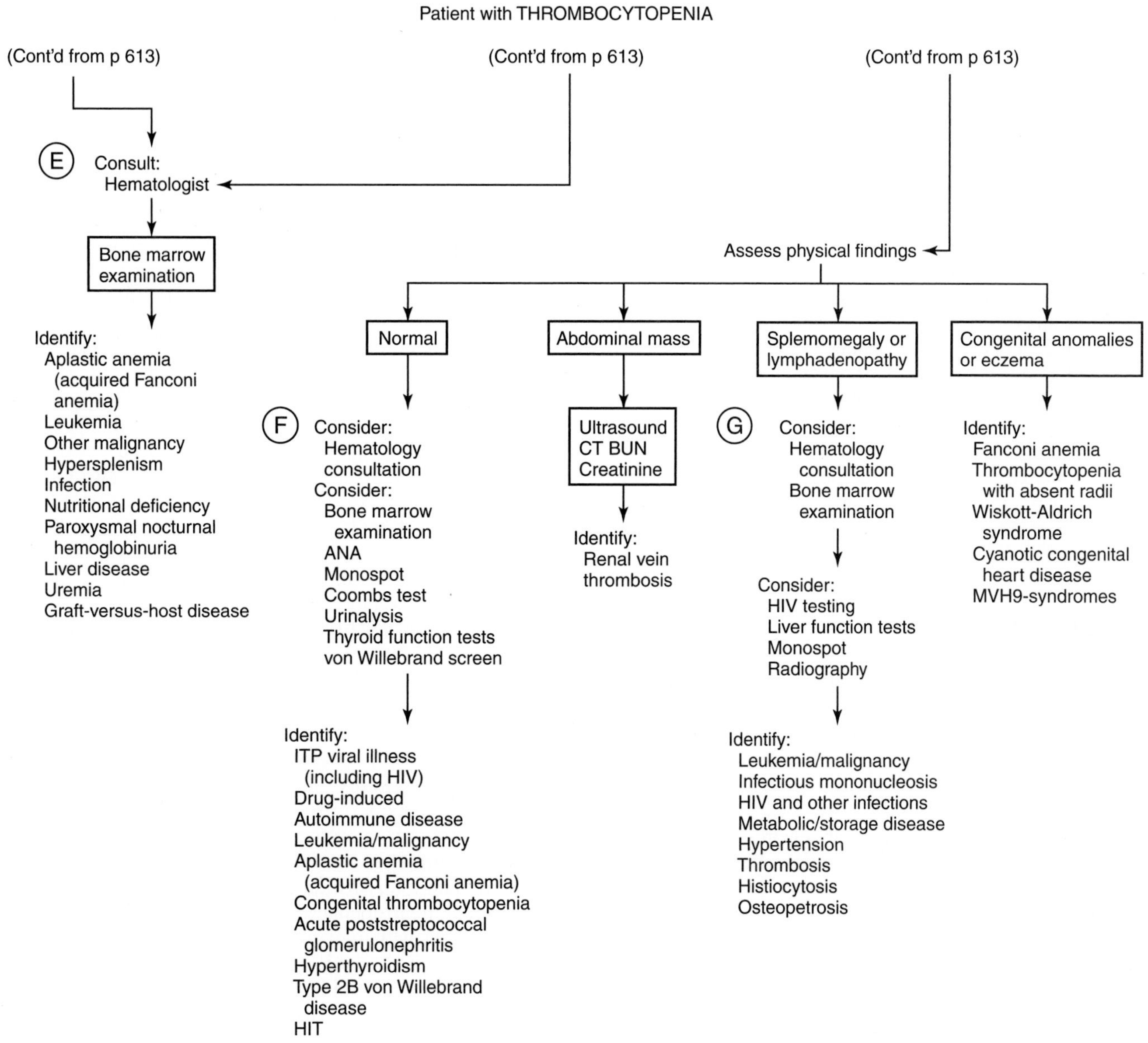
Patient with THROMBOCYTOPENIA
(Cont'd from p 613)
(Cont'd from p 613)
(Cont'd from p 613)
E
Consult: Hematologist
Bone marrow examination
Identify:
Aplastic anemia (acquired Fanconi anemia)
Leukemia
Other malignancy
Hypersplenism
Infection
Nutritional deficiency
Paroxysmal nocturnal hemoglobinuria
Liver disease
Uremia
Graft-versus-host disease
Assess physical findings
Normal
Abdominal mass
Splemomegaly or lymphadenopathy
Congenital anomalies or eczema
F
Consider:
Hematology consultation
Consider:
Bone marrow examination
ANA
Monospot
Coombs test
Urinalysis
Thyroid function tests
von Willebrand screen
Identify:
ITP viral illness (including HIV)
Drug-induced
Autoimmune disease
Leukemia/malignancy
Aplastic anemia (acquired Fanconi anemia)
Congenital thrombocytopenia
Acute poststreptococcal glomerulonephritis
Hyperthyroidism
Type 2B von Willebrand disease
HIT
Ultrasound
CT BUN
Creatinine
Identify:
Renal vein thrombosis
G
Consider:
Hematology consultation
Bone marrow examination
Consider:
HIV testing
Liver function tests
Monospot
Radiography
Identify:
Leukemia/malignancy
Infectious mononucleosis
HIV and other infections
Metabolic/storage disease
Hypertension
Thrombosis
Histiocytosis
Osteopetrosis
Identify:
Fanconi anemia
Thrombocytopenia with absent radii
Wiskott-Aldrich syndrome
Cyanotic congenital heart disease
MVH9-syndromes

Neutropenia

Ann-Christine Nyquist, MD, MSPH, Rachelle Nuss, MD,
and Peter A. Lane, MD

DEFINITION

Neutropenia is an absolute decrease in the number of circulating neutrophils in the blood. The absolute neutrophil count is determined by multiplying the total white blood cell count by the percentage of neutrophils plus bands. Neutropenia is mild if the absolute neutrophil count is between 1000 and 1500/μL^3, moderate if it is between 500 and 1000/μL^3, and severe if it is less than 500/μL^3. For children 2 weeks to 1 year of age, the lower limit of normal is 1000/μL^3 rather than 1500/μL^3. In general, the severity of neutropenia correlates with risk for bacterial infection. The most common bacterial and fungal infections are cellulitis, skin abscesses, pneumonia, and septicemia.

CAUSATIVE FACTORS

Most cases of childhood neutropenia are self-limited and associated with a viral illness or drug therapy. Influenza, hepatitis, rubella, adenovirus, enterovirus, measles (rubeola), mumps, Epstein–Barr virus, and cytomegalovirus have been associated with neutropenia.

A. In the patient's history, ask about previous and current infections; include bacterial and viral infections. A family history of recurrent infection or unexplained childhood deaths suggests a congenitally acquired immunodeficiency. Risk factors for human immunodeficiency virus infection should be determined, but all patients should have HIV antibody testing. Fever, weight loss, and bone pain suggest leukemia. Similar symptoms and rash may indicate collagen vascular disease.

B. In the physical examination, note the nutritional status of the child; marasmus and vitamin B_{12}, folate, and copper deficiencies are associated with neutropenia. Fanconi anemia, osteopetrosis, dyskeratosis congenita, and aminoacidurias may have physical stigmata and may also have associated neutropenia. Children with neutropenia may be at risk for pyogenic bacterial infection with endogenous skin flora such as *Staphylococcus aureus* and gram-negative rods (especially *Pseudomonas aeruginosa*). The skin should be examined for signs of cellulitis or abscess formation. Note gingivostomatitis, perirectal cellulitis, otitis media, and signs of pneumonia and septicemia. Lymphadenopathy, hepatomegaly, or splenomegaly suggests an underlying malignant disease or immunodeficiency. Arthritis suggests a collagen vascular disease.

C. A moderately or severely ill child has one or more of the following findings: (1) abnormal nutrition, growth, and development; (2) severe, chronic, or recurrent infection; (3) unexplained hepatosplenomegaly or lymphadenopathy; (4) signs of collagen vascular disease; (5) immature white blood cells, anemia, or thrombocytopenia; or (6) a family history of neutropenia or recurrent infection.

D. If the child remains well, another complete blood cell count (CBC) can be obtained in 6 to 8 weeks. If in the interim the child has signs of moderate or severe illness, a CBC should be obtained sooner. A normal neutrophil count during a febrile illness suggests a benign cause of the neutropenia.

E. Otherwise healthy children with isolated, transient neutropenia discovered during a minor acute illness or routine preoperative screening are at little risk for serious infectious complications. Once a normal count is obtained, no further counts are indicated.

F. Chronic neutropenia may be benign, cyclic, severe, or associated with metabolic or immune diseases. In an otherwise well child, obtaining biweekly blood counts for 4 to 6 weeks is indicated to determine whether cyclic neutropenia occurs. Most individuals with cyclic neutropenia become neutropenic every 12 to 21 days, and the count remains low for 3 to 10 days, during which time they may have fever, stomatitis, pharyngitis, and cervical adenopathy. If this 4- to 6-week evaluation does not reveal cycling or the child's condition becomes worrisome, consult a hematologist to exclude a more serious cause of the neutropenia. Children with severe congenital neutropenia generally respond to treatment with granulocyte colony-stimulating factor.

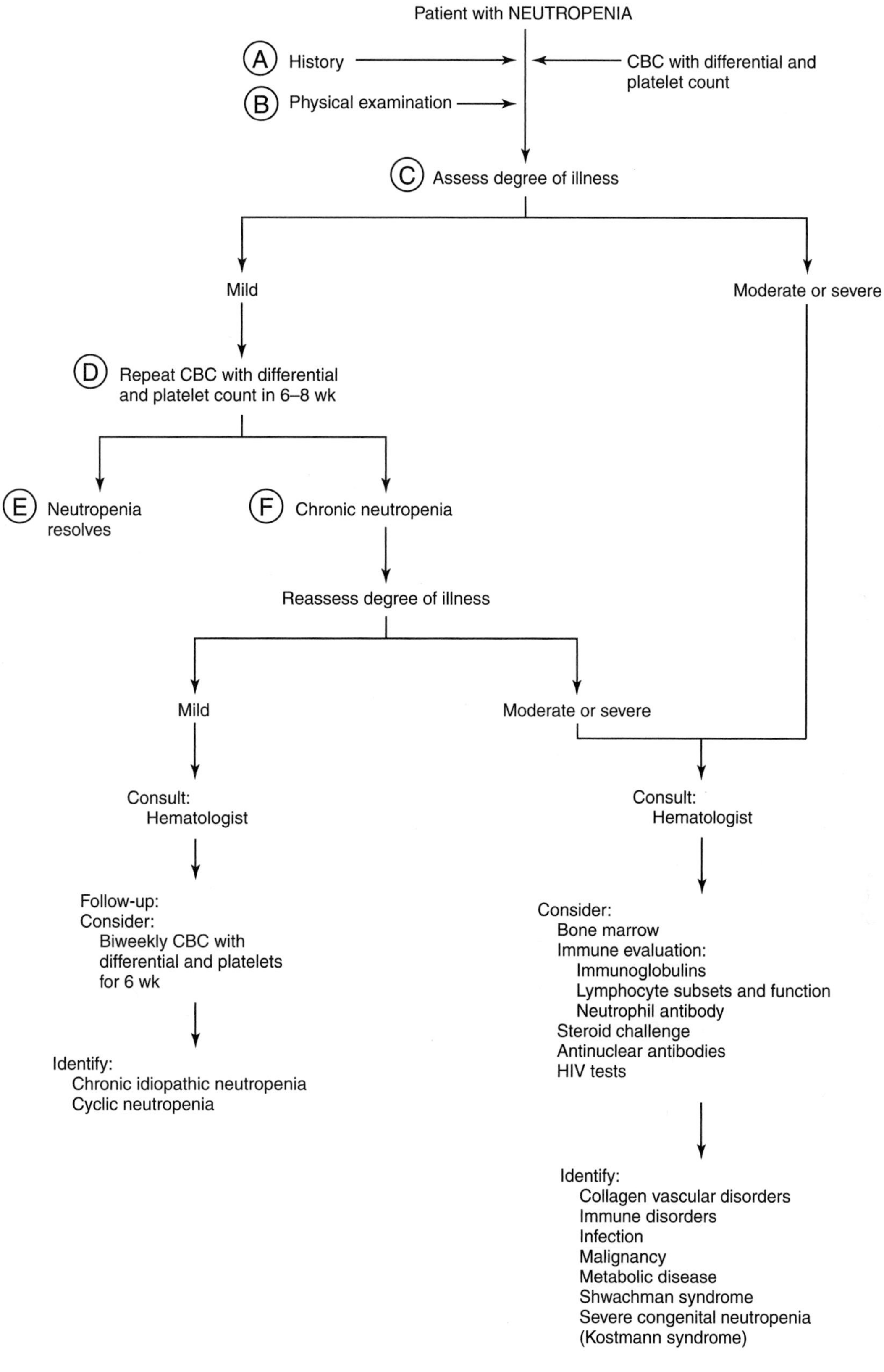
Patient with NEUTROPENIA
(A) History
(B) Physical examination
CBC with differential and platelet count
(C) Assess degree of illness
Mild
Moderate or severe
(D) Repeat CBC with differential and platelet count in 6–8 wk
(E) Neutropenia resolves
(F) Chronic neutropenia
Reassess degree of illness
Mild
Moderate or severe
Consult: Hematologist
Consult: Hematologist
Follow-up:
Consider:
Biweekly CBC with differential and platelets for 6 wk
Identify:
Chronic idiopathic neutropenia
Cyclic neutropenia
Consider:
Bone marrow
Immune evaluation:
Immunoglobulins
Lymphocyte subsets and function
Neutrophil antibody
Steroid challenge
Antinuclear antibodies
HIV tests
Identify:
Collagen vascular disorders
Immune disorders
Infection
Malignancy
Metabolic disease
Shwachman syndrome
Severe congenital neutropenia (Kostmann syndrome)

References

Bernini JC. Diagnosis and management of chronic neutropenia during childhood. Pediatr Clin North Am 1996;43:773.

Boztug K. Congenital neutropenia syndromes. Immunol Allergy Clin North Am 2008;28:259.

Infectious Diseases

Human Immunodeficiency Virus Infection

Elizabeth J. McFarland, MD

Human immunodeficiency virus (HIV) is a cytopathic human retrovirus that primarily infects $CD4^+$ helper T lymphocytes, leading to the loss in number and function of these and other cells critical to the immune system. HIV is transmitted by percutaneous or mucous membrane exposure to blood, semen, cervical secretions, and human milk. Infants are infected by maternal transmission. Older children and adolescents are infected through sexual transmission and injecting drug use. Progression of HIV infection leads to acquired immune deficiency syndrome (AIDS). HIV infection is diagnosed by blood tests to detect HIV-specific antibody or viral nucleic acid. An AIDS diagnosis is determined by the occurrence of specific opportunistic infections or specific malignancies. For adolescents and adults older than 13 years, severe immunosuppression with a CD4 T-lymphocyte count less than 200 cells/mm^3 or percentage of less than 14 also meets criteria for an AIDS diagnosis. Table 1 lists the AIDS-defining conditions.

A. Consider HIV in children with signs and symptoms suggesting immunodeficiency or chronic disease. Diagnosis of an AIDS-defining condition (see Table 1) should prompt HIV testing if another specific reason for immunodeficiency is not known. The presence of diagnoses listed in Table 2 would be an indication to consider HIV testing. In the history, inquire about symptoms of early disease, such as frequent upper or lower respiratory infections, sinusitis, otitis media, chronic cough or wheezing, recurrent/chronic parotitis, rashes, eczema, extensive warts, recurrent fevers, and night sweats. Failure to thrive and developmental delay are common, particularly during the first years of life. Ask about evidence of more advanced disease: recurrent invasive bacterial infections (bacteremia, pneumonia, urinary tract infections), recurrent shingles (herpes zoster), *Candida* infections (mucous membranes, skin, and nails), chronic diarrhea, and hepatitis. Consider organ-specific disease, particularly congestive heart failure secondary to cardiomyopathy; edema, hematuria, or proteinuria caused by nephropathy; and bruising caused by thrombocytopenia. Adolescents are at risk for HIV infection through sexual activity without barrier protection and parenteral exposure (unclean needles). Acute infection is frequently (40%–90%) associated with acute retroviral syndrome with typical viral syndrome symptoms of fever, sore throat, myalgia, arthralgias, headache, diarrhea, nausea, and vomiting. Features that are more particular to acute HIV may include lymphadenopathy, rash, oral ulcers, weight loss, aseptic meningitis, and thrush. A sizable proportion of individuals with acute HIV infection will seek medical care for their illness, but diagnosis is made only if the provider has a high index of suspicion. Infants born to HIV-infected women have a 13% to 39% risk for HIV infection if there is no intervention. If the woman and infant receive effective antiretroviral prophylaxis, in conjunction with scheduled C-section when indicated, the risk for mother-to-child transmission is less than 1%. The Centers for Disease Control and Prevention recommends routine HIV testing with right of refusal for all pregnant women irrespective of known risk factors. Women who do not have documented HIV test results at the time of labor and delivery should be offered rapid HIV testing and antiretroviral prophylaxis provided to the woman and infant if the result is positive, pending confirmation. Infected infants rarely have symptoms in the newborn period. All HIV-exposed infants require sequential diagnostic testing to determine their infection status.

B. For infected infants, the findings of physical examination are usually normal in the first weeks to months of life. Hepatosplenomegaly or lymphadenopathy may rarely be observed in the newborn period. Without treatment, 30% of infants will develop signs during the first year of life. Look for failure to thrive and developmental delay or loss of milestones. In the central nervous system, signs include increased tone, spasticity, encephalopathy (irritability, apathetic, weak, disoriented), and microcephaly. Identify cardiomyopathy (gallop rhythm, tachypnea, tachycardia, lung crackles, hepatomegaly, and decreased peripheral pulses) and pneumonia (tachypnea, retractions, grunting, lung crackles). Children identified after infancy may have adenopathy, splenomegaly, hepatomegaly, salivary gland enlargement (parotitis), wheezing (caused by lymphocytic interstitial pneumonia), failure to thrive, wasting, and signs of nephropathy (proteinuria, hypertension). Recurrent invasive bacterial infections include pneumonia, bone or joint infection (painful limb, joint swelling, limitation of motion), and meningitis (lethargy, altered mental status, meningismus). Also look for *Candida* rashes, extensive warts and molluscum, vesicular lesions of herpes zoster, petechiae, and purpura. Acute retroviral syndrome presents with fever, lymphadenopathy, pharyngitis, macular-papular rash, oral ulcers, hepatosplenomegaly, white oral plaques (thrush), aseptic meningitis (photophobia, meningismus), and other neurologic manifestations (facial palsy, peripheral neuropathy, brachial neuritis, cognitive impairment or psychosis).

C1. HIV antibody testing is the standard for diagnosis in patients older than 18 months (after placentally transferred maternal antibodies are no longer detectable) with symptoms of established HIV infection. The two-part test is performed by an initial enzyme-linked immunosorbent assay (ELISA) or one of several rapid antibody tests. These ELISA and rapid

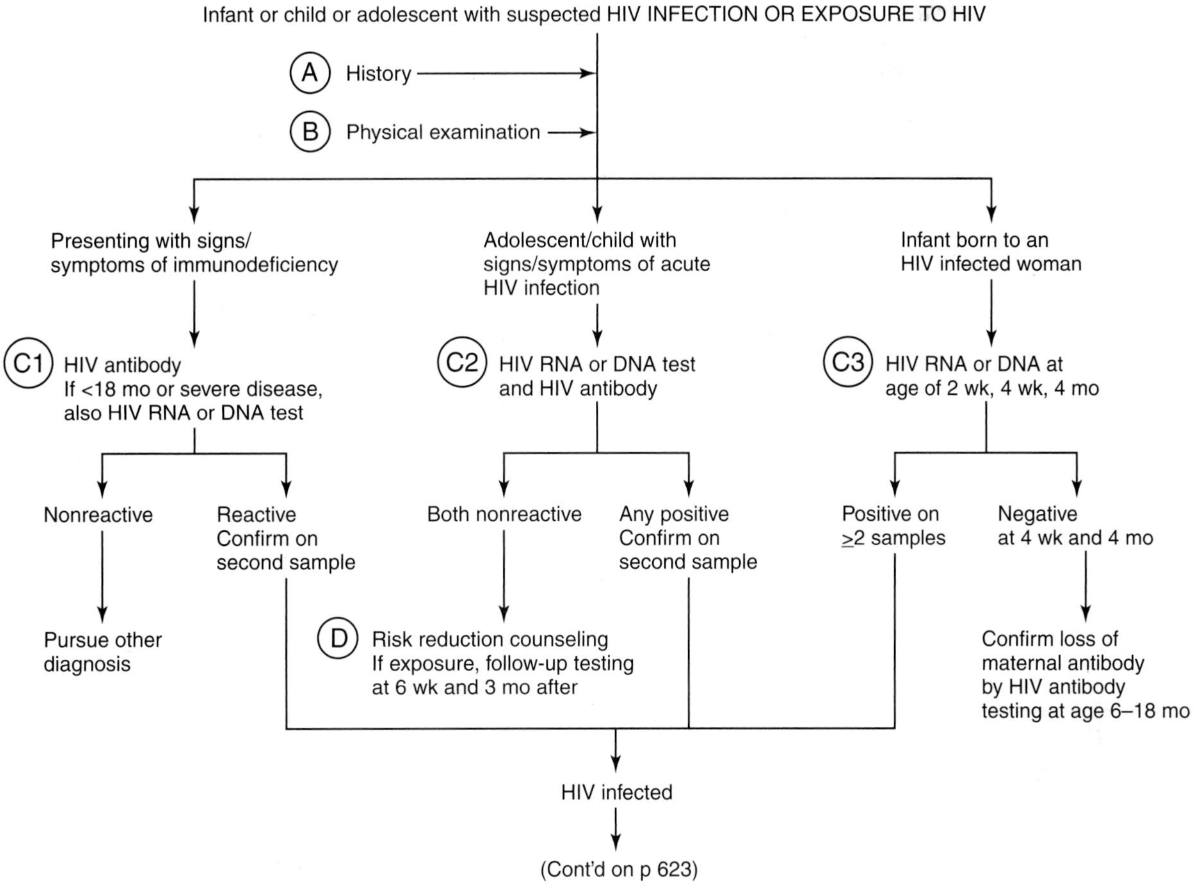

Infant or child or adolescent with suspected HIV INFECTION OR EXPOSURE TO HIV
A History
B Physical examination
Presenting with signs/ symptoms of immunodeficiency
Adolescent/child with signs/symptoms of acute HIV infection
Infant born to an HIV infected woman
C1 HIV antibody If <18 mo or severe disease, also HIV RNA or DNA test
C2 HIV RNA or DNA test and HIV antibody
C3 HIV RNA or DNA at age of 2 wk, 4 wk, 4 mo
Nonreactive
Reactive Confirm on second sample
Both nonreactive
Any positive Confirm on second sample
Positive on ≥2 samples
Negative at 4 wk and 4 mo
Pursue other diagnosis
D Risk reduction counseling If exposure, follow-up testing at 6 wk and 3 mo after
Confirm loss of maternal antibody by HIV antibody testing at age 6–18 mo
HIV infected
(Cont'd on p 623)

assays are highly sensitive, and false-positive results occur rarely. Therefore, a positive initial result must be confirmed with an alternative assay, usually a Western blot, to detect antibody to specific HIV proteins. A second separate specimen should be obtained to preclude the possibility of laboratory error or contamination before a final diagnosis of infection. Nucleic acid testing to identify HIV DNA in blood cells or HIV RNA in plasma is used to assist in diagnosis of HIV infection during acute infection or in the infant born to an HIV-infected woman. Patients with very advanced disease may lack specific antibody production, in which case testing for viral nucleic acid may be necessary to make the diagnosis.

C2. If acute infection is suspected, both HIV nucleic acid and antibody testing are needed to determine whether the infection is acute. In the first weeks to months after infection, HIV antibody by ELISA and Western blots may be negative or indeterminant. However, HIV nucleic acid testing will be positive by 2 to 3 weeks after exposure. HIV antibody test results are positive in most people by 6 weeks after infection and in virtually all by 3 months.

C3. Diagnosis in HIV-exposed infants is complicated by placental transfer of maternal antibodies against HIV, which may persist as long as 18 months; therefore, HIV antibody tests indicate exposure but are not diagnostic of infection. However, HIV nucleic acids are demonstrated in almost all infants by 2 to 4 weeks of age and in essentially all by 1 to 4 months of age. Viral nucleic acid testing is performed at birth (optional) and age 2, 4, and 16 weeks. Criteria for early diagnosis of infection or exclusion of infection are shown in Table 3. Most experts recommend that infants with negative virologic tests have HIV antibody testing at age 6 to 18 months to confirm absence of infection after loss of maternal antibody (seroreverter).

D. Discussion of negative results of HIV diagnostic testing provides an excellent opportunity for counseling adolescents about reducing their risk for HIV infection. Typically, this includes an open discussion of safer sexual practices and a demonstration of the use of condoms. If there has been a specific exposure, repeat HIV antibody testing after 6 weeks and 3 months is indicated to confirm absence of infection.

Table 1. **Centers for Disease Control and Prevention Surveillance Case Definition of Acquired Immune Deficiency Syndrome: Diagnoses Indicative of Acquired Immune Deficiency Syndrome in Children, Adolescents, and Adults**

All Ages
Candidiasis, esophageal or pulmonary
Coccidioidomycosis, disseminated
Cryptococcosis, extrapulmonary
Cryptosporidiosis or isosporiasis with diarrhea persisting >1 month
Cytomegalovirus disease with onset at age >1 month (at site other than liver, spleen, nodes)
Encephalopathy
Herpes simplex virus: oral lesion persisting >1 month, or bronchitis, pneumonitis, esophagitis at age >1 month
Histoplasmosis, disseminated or extrapulmonary
Kaposi sarcoma
Lymphoma (Burkitt; immunoblastic, or primary, of brain)
Mycobacterium tuberculosis, disseminated or extrapulmonary
Mycobacterium infection, other species, disseminated
Pneumocystis jiroveci pneumonia
Progressive multifocal leukoencephalopathy
Salmonella (nontyphoid) septicemia, recurrent
Toxoplasmosis of the brain with onset at age >1 month
Wasting syndrome
Age <13 years
Serious bacterial infections, multiple or recurrent (two within 2-year period)
Age >13 years
Cervical cancer, invasive
Mycobacterium tuberculosis, pulmonary
Pneumonia, recurrent

Adapted from Centers for Disease Control and Prevention. 1994 revised classification system for human immunodeficiency virus infection in children less than 13 years of age. MMWR Recomm Rep 1994;43(RR-12):8; and Centers for Disease Control and Prevention. Revised surveillance case definitions for HIV infection among adults, adolescents, and children aged <18 months and for HIV infection and AIDS among children 18 months to <13 years—United States, 2008. MMWR 2008; 57(RR-10):9.

E. Assess the degree and risk for disease progression using $CD4^+$ T-lymphocyte count and percentage (Table 4), clinical classification (see Tables 1 and 2), and quantitative plasma HIV RNA. CD4 T-lymphocyte count in healthy infants and young children (age <5 years) are greater than in adults; therefore, age-adjusted counts must be used. Low CD4 T-lymphocyte parameters predict a greater risk for HIV morbidity and mortality. Greater HIV RNA levels are associated with increased rate of CD4 T-cell decline and, in children, also predict HIV morbidity and mortality independent of CD4 T-cell parameters. Assess organ system dysfunction with laboratory tests for anemia, neutropenia, thrombocytopenia, hepatitis, and nephropathy. Serum immunoglobulin G (IgG), IgM, and IgA are often increased but may decline below normal with disease progression. Evaluate for common coinfections including hepatitis B and C viruses. Determine the risk for reactivation of latent infections with skin testing for *Mycobacterium tuberculosis* (5-mm induration is positive), serology for toxoplasmosis, cytomegalovirus, varicella zoster virus, and testing for sexually transmitted infections for behaviorally infected adolescents.

F. Patients with severe immunosuppression based on specific CD4 T-lymphocyte cutoffs should initiate prophylaxis for selected opportunistic infections once active infection is excluded (Table 5). As for all children, ingestion of raw meat, eggs, seafood, and soil should be avoided, and careful hand washing should follow contact with animals, especially reptiles or animals with diarrhea.

G. Begin education, counseling, and motivational interviewing to prepare patients to adhere to lifelong therapy because essentially all patients will eventually require antiretroviral treatment. Individuals must have high rates of adherence to treatment to prevent induction of resistant virus.

H. HIV treatment management (deciding when to initiate HIV-specific treatment, selecting antiretroviral drugs, monitoring efficacy and toxicity, selecting second-line therapy for treatment failure) is complex. HIV expert consultation is recommended for all patients and is associated with better outcomes. Timing for initiation of antiretroviral treatment is currently based on patient age, clinical stage, age-adjusted CD4 T-lymphocyte parameters, and plasma HIV RNA (see Table 6 for 2010 recommendations). Published guidelines on antiretroviral treatment can be found online (http://aidsinfo.nih.gov). These guidelines are updated regularly, so current references should be consulted.

I. Standard treatment for HIV is a combination of three antiretroviral drugs with at least two having different mechanisms of action. Combination treatment is required to achieve potent viral suppression and to prevent outgrowth of virus resistant to the drugs. The initial regimen will include two nucleoside reverse transcriptase inhibitors (NRTI) plus either a non-nucleoside reverse transcriptase inhibitor (NNRTI) or a protease inhibitor (PI). Currently, seven NRTIs, four NNRTIs, and nine PIs have FDA approval; many have approved pediatric dosing and formulations (Table 7). For patients who need subsequent regimens after treatment failure, drugs with other mechanisms of action (inhibition of virus entry to the cell; inhibition of viral nucleic acid integration) have been developed; pediatric studies of safety and dosing for these drugs are under way. The goal of treatment is consistent suppression of plasma virus below the limit of detection. Plasma HIV RNA is measured at 4 to 8 weeks after starting a regimen, and then both HIV RNA and CD4 T-cell parameters are tested every 3 to 4 months. Treatment failure is defined as plasma HIV RNA copies/ml that have not decreased by at least 1 og_{10} at 8 to 12 weeks or are more than 400 cp/ml at 6 months after starting treatment. Patients with treatment failure are evaluated for problems with adherence to treatment, pharmacokinetics, and viral resistance. An alternative treatment regimen is determined based on findings of the evaluation.

J. Antiretroviral treatment may result in drug toxicity. The adverse effects that are either common and dose limiting or rare but severe for particular drugs or classes of drugs are listed in Table 7.

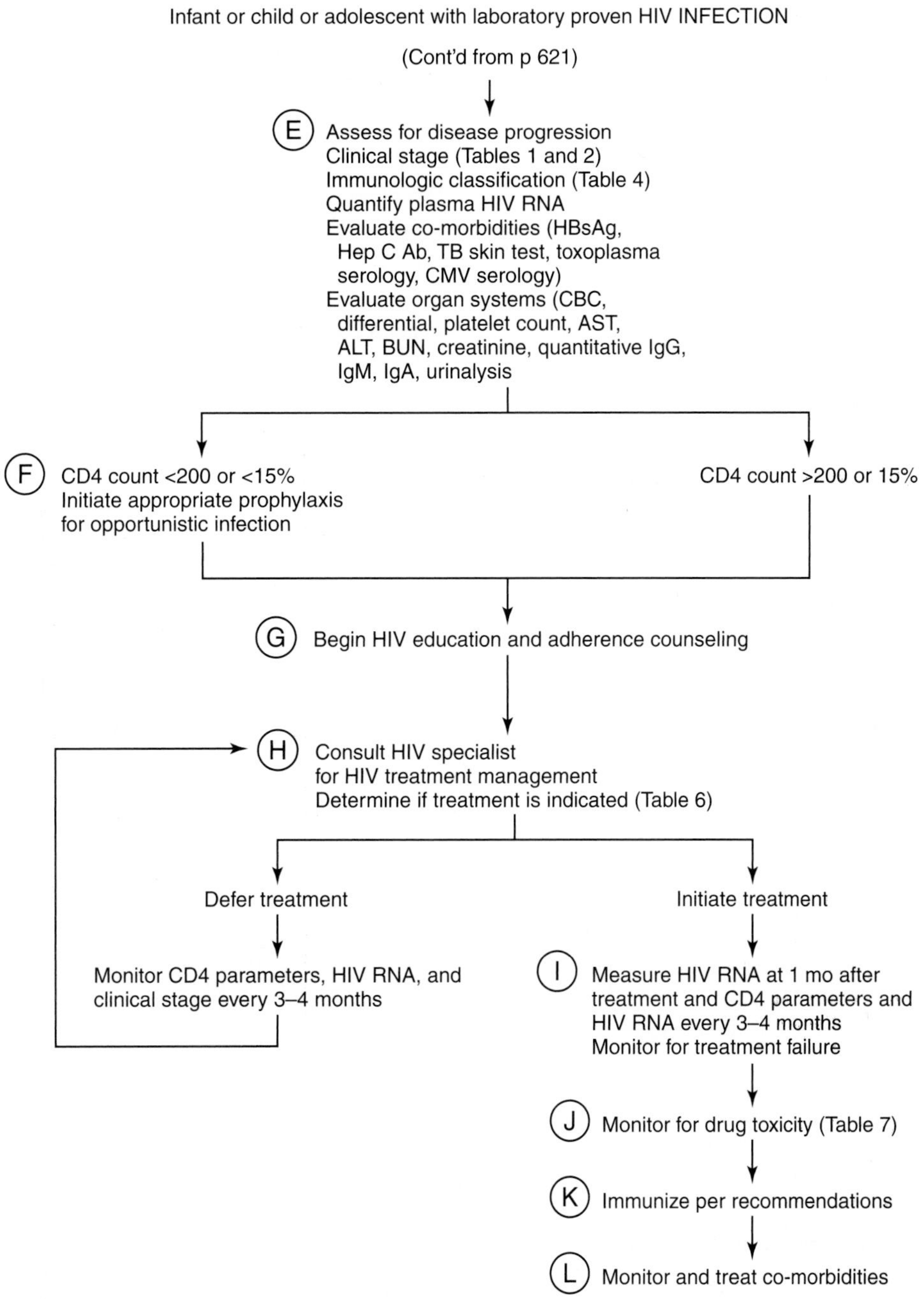
Infant or child or adolescent with laboratory proven HIV INFECTION
(Cont'd from p 621)
E
Assess for disease progression
Clinical stage (Tables 1 and 2)
Immunologic classification (Table 4)
Quantify plasma HIV RNA
Evaluate co-morbidities (HBsAg, Hep C Ab, TB skin test, toxoplasma serology, CMV serology)
Evaluate organ systems (CBC, differential, platelet count, AST, ALT, BUN, creatinine, quantitative IgG, IgM, IgA, urinalysis
F
CD4 count <200 or <15%
Initiate appropriate prophylaxis for opportunistic infection
CD4 count >200 or 15%
G
Begin HIV education and adherence counseling
H
Consult HIV specialist for HIV treatment management
Determine if treatment is indicated (Table 6)
Defer treatment
Initiate treatment
Monitor CD4 parameters, HIV RNA, and clinical stage every 3–4 months
I
Measure HIV RNA at 1 mo after treatment and CD4 parameters and HIV RNA every 3–4 months
Monitor for treatment failure
J
Monitor for drug toxicity (Table 7)
K
Immunize per recommendations
L
Monitor and treat co-morbidities

K. Immunization for HIV-infected children should include hepatitis B, diphtheria-tetanus-acellular pertussis, inactivated polio, *Haemophilus influenzae* type b, and conjugated pneumococcal vaccine given on the standard schedule. In general, live virus vaccines should be avoided; however, two doses of MMR (measles, mumps, and rubella) and VZV (varicella zoster virus) vaccines are recommended for children who are not CDC stage C or immune category 3. Pneumovax after age 2 years and a second dose after 3 to 5 years, as well as annual influenza vaccines, are recommended. Responses to vaccines are improved when administered after starting effective antiretroviral treatment, when plasma HIV RNA is low and CD4 T-lymphocyte numbers have recovered.

L. Monitor and treat comorbid conditions. Rates of mental health disorders (attention-deficit disorder, depression, behavioral disorders) occur at a high rate among children and adolescents infected and affected with HIV. Dietary counseling is provided to reduce the risk for metabolic disorders associated with HIV and/or antiretroviral treatment (hypertriglyceridemia, abnormal cholesterol, glucose intolerance, low bone mineralization), as well as failure to thrive or wasting with advanced HIV disease. Children with HIV, even on antiretroviral treatment, remain at greater risk for invasive bacterial infections, herpes zoster, nephropathy, progressive cervical cancer, and certain other malignancies.

Table 2. **Centers for Disease Control and Prevention Clinical Categories of Children with Human Immunodeficiency Virus Infection**

Category N: Not Symptomatic

No signs or symptoms or only one of the conditions listed in category A

Category A: Mildly Symptomatic

Having two or more of the following conditions and none of those listed in category B:
- Lymphadenopathy
- Hepatomegaly
- Splenomegaly
- Dermatitis
- Parotitis
- Recurrent or persistent upper respiratory infection, sinusitis, or otitis media

Category B: Moderately Symptomatic

Having symptoms attributed to human immunodeficiency virus infection other than those in category A or C

Examples:
- Anemia, neutropenia, thrombocytopenia
- Bacterial meningitis, pneumonia, sepsis (single episode)
- Candidiasis, oropharyngeal, persisting >2 months
- Cardiomyopathy
- Cytomegalovirus infection with onset at age <1 month
- Diarrhea, recurrent or chronic
- Hepatitis
- Herpes simplex virus recurrent stomatitis (more than two episodes in 1-year period) or bronchitis, pneumonitis, esophagitis with onset at age <1 month
- Herpes zoster, two or more episodes or more than one dermatome
- Leiomyosarcoma
- Lymphoid interstitial pneumonia
- Nephropathy
- Nocardiosis
- Fever lasting >1 month
- Toxoplasmosis with onset at age <1 month
- Varicella, complicated

Category C: Severely Symptomatic

Children with any acquired immune deficiency syndrome–defining condition (see Table 1)

Adapted from Centers for Disease Control and Prevention. 1994 revised classification system for human immunodeficiency virus infection in children less than 13 years of age. MMWR Recomm Rep 1994;43(RR-12):8.

Table 3. **Criteria for Human Immunodeficiency Virus Diagnosis for Infant Born to Human Immunodeficiency Virus–Infected Woman**

Children Younger than 18 Months and Born to an HIV-Infected Mother

Definitively Infected

Positive results on two separate determinations on blood or tissue (excluding cord blood) for one or more of the following HIV detection tests: HIV nucleic acid detection (DNA or RNA); p24 antigen test with neutralization (age≥1 month); HIV isolation by culture

Definitively Uninfected

At least two negative HIV nucleic acid (DNA or RNA) detection tests from separate specimens, both obtained at age >1 month and one obtained at age >4 months

or

At least two negative HIV antibody tests from separate specimens obtained at age >6 months

and

No other laboratory (prior positive nucleic acid tests) or clinical evidence of HIV infection/AIDS (see Table 1)

Presumptively Uninfected

Two negative HIV nucleic acid detection (DNA or RNA) tests from separate specimens, both obtained at age >2 weeks and one obtained at age >4 weeks

or

One negative HIV nucleic acid detection test obtained at age >8 weeks

or

One negative HIV antibody test obtained at age >6 months

and

No other laboratory (prior positive nucleic acid tests) or clinical evidence of HIV infection/AIDS (see Table 1)

AIDS, acquired immune deficiency syndrome; *HIV*, human immunodeficiency virus.

Adapted from Centers for Disease Control and Prevention. Revised surveillance case definitions for HIV infection among adults, adolescents, and children aged <18 months and for HIV infection and AIDS among children aged 18 months to <13 years—United States, 2008. MMWR Recomm Rep 2008;57(RR-10):1-9.

Table 4. **Immunologic Categories Based on Age-Specific CD4 Lymphocyte Counts and Percentages of Total Lymphocytes**

	Age of Child		
Immunologic Category	**<12 months**	**1–5 years**	**6–12 years**
1. No evidence of suppression	≥1500 cells/μl (≥25%)	≥1000 cells/μl (≥25%)	≥500 cells/μl (≥25%)
2. Evidence of moderate suppression	750–1499 cells/μl (15%–24%)	500–999 cells/μl (15%–24%)	200–499 cells/μl (15%–24%)
3. Evidence of severe suppression	<750 cells/μl (<15%)	<500 cells/μl (<15%)	<200 cells/μl (<15%)

Adapted from Centers for Disease Control and Prevention. 1994 revised classification system for human immunodeficiency virus infection in children less than 13 years of age. MMWR Recomm Rep 1994;43(RR-12):4.

Table 5. **Prophylaxis to Prevent the First Episode of Selected Opportunistic Pathogens**

Pathogen	Indication	First Choice Preventative Regimen
Pneumocystis pneumonia	HIV indeterminant age <12 months* HIV-infected age: <12 months with any CD4 count 1–5 years with CD4 <500 cells/μl or <15% >6 years with CD4 <200 cells/μl or <15%	TMP-SMX, 150/750 mg/m² body surface area per day (maximum: 320/1600 mg) orally divided into two doses daily and administered three times weekly on consecutive or alternate days or undivided single doses three times weekly on consecutive days†
Mycobacterium avium complex	HIV-infected age: <1 year with CD4 <750 cells/μl 1–2 years with CD4 <500 cells/μl 2–5 years with CD4 <75 cells/μl >6 years with CD4 <50 cells/μl	Clarithromycin, 7.5 mg/kg (maximum: 500 mg) orally two times daily or azithromycin 20 mg/kg (maximum: 1200 mg) orally weekly†
Toxoplasmosis gondii	HIV-infected with IgG antibody to *Toxoplasma* <6 years with CD4 <15% >6 years with CD4 <100 cells/μl	TMP-SMX 150/750 mg/m² body surface area daily orally in two divided doses†

TMP-SMX=Trimethoprim-sulfamethoxazole

*Prophylaxis not indicated for exposed infants with testing consistent with presumed uninfected.

†Alternative treatments found in Centers for Disease Control and Prevention. Guidelines for the prevention and treatment of opportunistic infections among HIV-exposed and HIV-infected children. MMWR Recomm Rep 2009;58(RR-11):1-168.

Adapted from Centers for Disease Control and Prevention. Guidelines for the prevention and treatment of opportunistic infections among HIV-exposed and HIV-infected children. MMWR Recomm Rep 2009;58(RR-11):127, <http://www.aidsinfo.nih.gov/>;[accessed 05.05.2011].

Table 6. **Guidelines for Indications to Start Antiretroviral Therapy for Human Immunodeficiency Virus–Infected Children**

Age	Criteria	Recommendation
<12 months	Regardless of clinical symptoms, immune status, or viral load	Treat
1 to <5 years	Clinical category B or C	Treat
	CD4 <25%	Treat
	Clinical category A or N and CD4 ≥25% with:	
	• HIV RNA >100,000 cp/ml	Treat
	• HIV RNA <100,000 cp/ml	Consider or defer, re-evaluate every 3–4 months
>5 to <13 years	Clinical category B or C	Treat
	CD4 <350 cells/m³	Treat
	Clinical category A or N and CD4 ≥350 cells/mmm with:	
	• HIV RNA ≥100,000 cp/ml	Treat
	• HIV RNA <100,000 cp/ml	Consider or defer, re-evaluate every 3–4 months
>13 years	AIDS-defining illness or HIV-associated nephropathy, HBV coinfection when treatment of HBV is indicated	Treat
	CD4 <350 cells/m³	Treat
	CD4 350–500 cells/m³	Recommended*
	CD4 >500 cells/m³	Consider

*The advisory panel was divided on the strength of this recommendation: 55% voted for strong recommendations, and 45% voted for moderate recommendation.

AIDS, acquired immune deficiency syndrome; *HBV*, hepatitis B virus; *HIV*, human immunodeficiency virus.

Adapted from Panel on Antiretroviral Therapy and Medical Management of HIV-infected Children. Guidelines for the use of antiretroviral agents in pediatric HIV infection. <http://aidsinfo.nih.gov/contentFiles/PediatricGuidelines.pdf>; [accessed 05.05.10] ; and Panel on Antiretroviral Guidelines for Adults and Adolescents. Guidelines for the use of antiretroviral agents in HIV-1-infected adults and adolescents. Department of Health and Human Services. <http://www.Aidsinfo.nih.gov/ContentFiles/AdultandAdolescentGL.pdf>; 2011 [accessed 05.05.10], p. 22.

Table 7. **Antiretroviral Medications for Human Immunodeficiency Virus Infection and Associated Adverse Effects**

Drug Name*	Adverse Effects†
Nucleoside Reverse Transcriptase Inhibitor Class (NRTI)	
Abacavir (ABC)	Hypersensitivity reaction (can be fatal), do not rechallenge
Didanosine (ddI)	Pancreatitis, peripheral neuropathy
Emtricitabine (FTC)	Minimal toxicity
Lamivudine (3TC)	Minimal toxicity
Stavudine (d4T)	Lipodystrophy, peripheral neuropathy
Tenofovir (TDF)‡	Bone demineralization, renal insufficiency (rare)
Zidovudine (ZDV)	Anemia, neutropenia, myopathy
All in class	Lactic acidosis (rare but potentially fatal)
Nonnucleoside Reverse Transcriptase Inhibitor Class (NNRTI)§	
Delavirdine (DLV)‡	Increased transaminases
Efavirenz (EFV)	Central nervous system symptoms, concern for teratogenicity in first trimester
Etravirine (ERV)‡	Nausea, rash
Nevirapine (NVP)	Rash, hepatitis (may be associated with hypersensitivity)
All in class	Rash (rarely Stevens–Johnson syndrome)
Protease Inhibitor Class (PI)§	
All in class	Gastrointestinal (GI) intolerance, transaminase increase, dyslipidemia, lipodystrophy, risk for bleeding in patients with hemophilia
Atazanavir (ATV)¶	Elevated indirect bilirubin, atrio-ventricular heart block
Darunavir (DRV)¶	Rash (cross-reaction with sulfonamides)
Fosamprenavir (FPV)¶	Rash, oral paresthesia, increased creatinine kinase
Indinavir (IDV)‡	Nephrolithiasis, elevated indirect bilirubin
Lopinavir/ritonavir (LPV/r)	GI intolerance
Nelfinavir (NFV)	Diarrhea
Ritonavir (RTV)	Circumoral paraesthesias, GI intolerance
Saquinavir hard gel (SQV)‡¶	GI intolerance
Tipranavir (TPV)¶	Rash (cross-reaction with sulfonamides), possible association with intracranial hemorrhage
Integrase Inhibitor Class	
Raltegravir (RAL)‡	GI intolerance, headache, increased creatinine kinase level, myopathy
Entry Inhibitors Class	
Enfuvirtide (T-20)	Injection-site reactions, increase rate of bacterial pneumonia, hypersensitivity
Maraviroc (MVC)‡§	Cough, fever, upper respiratory infections, dizziness, hepatic toxicity, cardiac events

*Several of the individual drugs are available as fixed drug combinations at dose appropriate for adults and older adolescents. Adverse effects are those of the individual components.

†Adverse effects listed are either common and dose limiting or rare but severe. The frequency of the events among treated children has not always been determined. Additional adverse events may occur.

‡No pediatric formulation or dosing recommendations.

§The PIs and NNRTIs are metabolized by the cytochrome P450 system. Potentially significant drug interactions with multiple agents are possible. See the product label for contraindicated concurrent medication dose adjustments.

¶Usually given with low-dose ritonavir to take advantage of drug interaction that will boost pharmacokinetics parameters of the primary PI.

Adapted from Panel on Antiretroviral Therapy and Medical Management of HIV-infected Children. Guidelines for the use of antiretroviral agents in pediatric HIV infection. <www.aidsinfo.nih.gov>; [accessed 05.05.10].

References

American Academy of Pediatrics Committee on Pediatric AIDS. HIV testing and prophylaxis to prevent mother-to-child transmission in the United States. Pediatrics 2009;122:1127–34.

Centers for Disease Control and Prevention. Guidelines for the prevention and treatment of opportunistic infections among HIV-exposed and HIV-infected children. MMWR Recomm Rep 2009;58(RR-11):1–168.

Centers for Disease Control and Prevention. Revised surveillance case definitions for HIV infection among adults, adolescents, and children aged <18 months and for HIV infection and AIDS among children aged 18 months to <13 Years—United States, 2008. MMWR Recomm Rep 2008;57(RR-10):1–9.

Centers for Disease Control and Prevention. 1994 revised classification system for human immunodeficiency virus infection in children less than 13 years of age. MMWR Recomm Rep 1994;43(RR-12):1.

Giaquinto C, Morelli E, Fregonese F, et al. Current and future antiretroviral treatment options in paediatric HIV infection. Clin Drug Invest 2008;28:375–97.

Havens PL, Mofenson LM, Committee on Pediatric AIDS. Evaluation and management of the infant exposed to HIV-1 in the United States. Pediatrics 2009;123:175–87.

Panel on Antiretroviral Guidelines for Adults and Adolescents. Guidelines for the use of antiretroviral agents in HIV-1-infected adults and adolescents. Department of Health and Human Services. <http://Aidsinfo.nih.gov/ContentFiles/AdultandAdolescentGL.pdf>; 2011 [accessed 05.05.10], p. 34.

Reisner SL, Mimiaga MJ, Skeer M, et al. A review of HIV antiretroviral adherence and intervention studies among HIV-infected youth. Top HIV Med 2009;17:14–25.

Panel on Antiretroviral Therapy and Medical Management of HIV-Infected Children: Guidelines for the use of antiretroviral agents in pediatric HIV infection. <http://aidsinfo.nih.gov/ContentFiles/PediatricGuidelines.pdf>; 2010 [accessed 05.05.10], p. 1–219.

Zetola NM, Pilcher CD. Diagnosis and management of acute HIV infection. Infect Dis Clin North Am 2007;21:19.

Kawasaki Disease

Marsha S. Anderson, MD, and Mary P. Glodé, MD

Kawasaki disease, a self-limited acute febrile illness caused by a systemic vasculitis, is the leading cause of pediatric acquired heart disease in the United States. Kawasaki disease is a clinical diagnosis, and no confirmatory laboratory test is available. Kawasaki disease is characterized by fever for at least 4 days with four of the following five signs in the absence of another compatible known disease or infection: (1) bilateral nonexudative, conjunctival injection; (2) oral changes including chapped, dry, red, and/or fissured lips, diffuse injection of the oral mucosa and pharynx, or strawberry tongue; (3) changes of peripheral extremities, such as edema, erythema, or induration of hands and feet; (4) polymorphous erythematous rash (usually morbilliform, maculopapular, scarlatiniform, or erythema multiforme-like); and (5) lymphadenopathy, often cervical, with enlargement of a node to more than 1.5 cm in diameter. Patients with fever for more than 5 days and fewer than four diagnostic features can be diagnosed as having Kawasaki disease when coronary artery disease is detected by echocardiogram or coronary angiography. Presumptive diagnosis of Kawasaki disease and initiation of therapy do not require waiting for 4 to 5 days of fever. Additional findings that may be observed include irritability, arthritis or arthralgia, vomiting, diarrhea, abdominal pain, hepatitis, obstructive jaundice, hydrops of the gallbladder, aseptic meningitis, urethritis, and cardiac disease. Most children have at least some desquamation of the palms and soles 10 to 20 days after onset of fever. Some children do not experience development of four or more of the major clinical signs described earlier, and this has been termed *incomplete Kawasaki disease.* Evaluation of these children is complicated, and a diagnostic algorithm has been developed to aid in the evaluation of children with suspected Kawasaki disease (see Newburger JW 2004).

The median age of onset of Kawasaki disease is 2 years; most patients are younger than 5 years. Infants younger than 6 months who have Kawasaki disease may not meet the case definition. These patients appear to be at increased risk for severe disease and coronary artery aneurysms.

A. A complete history is essential to help sort through the possibilities on the differential diagnosis. Include the following in the history: recent medications or immunizations (drug reaction, Stevens–Johnson syndrome, MMR [measles, mumps, and rubella] reaction), recent travel (measles, tick-borne illness), recent animal exposure (leptospirosis), ill contacts (viral illness, especially adenovirus), joint swelling or pain (juvenile idiopathic arthritis, other collagen vascular disease). Laboratory evaluation may show leukocytosis, thrombocytosis (approximately 2–3 weeks after onset), high sedimentation rate, high C-reactive protein, high transaminases, low albumin, and sterile pyuria. Identify *Streptococcus pyogenes* pharyngitis. Other laboratory studies to consider in the evaluation depending on the clinical presentation include lumbar puncture, sinus computed tomographic (CT) scan, chest radiograph, urine culture, anti-DNAse B, and anti-streptolysin antibody.

B. Tachycardia out of proportion to the level of fever is seen in many patients with Kawasaki disease and may reflect underlying myocarditis. A gallop may also be present. Patients with very severe illness may have unstable vital signs (hypotension and shock), myocarditis, or signs of congestive heart failure, and may need intensive care management. Consultation with someone with experience in treating Kawasaki disease is recommended for all cases if possible.

(Continued on page 630)

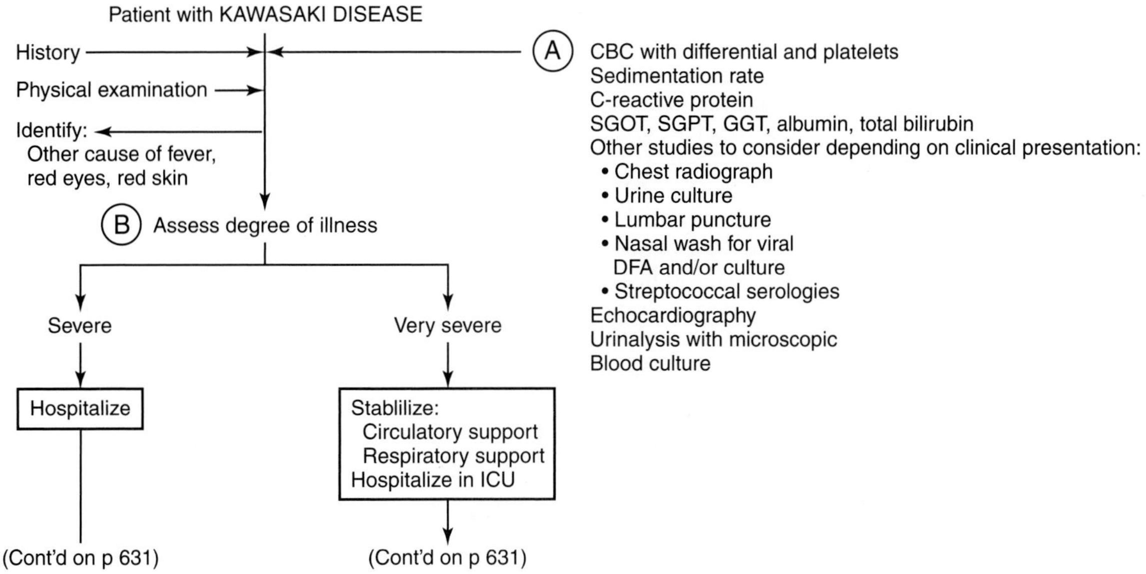
Patient with KAWASAKI DISEASE
History
Physical examination
Identify:
Other cause of fever, red eyes, red skin
(A) CBC with differential and platelets
Sedimentation rate
C-reactive protein
SGOT, SGPT, GGT, albumin, total bilirubin
Other studies to consider depending on clinical presentation:
• Chest radiograph
• Urine culture
• Lumbar puncture
• Nasal wash for viral DFA and/or culture
• Streptococcal serologies
Echocardiography
Urinalysis with microscopic
Blood culture
(B) Assess degree of illness
Severe
Very severe
Hospitalize
Stablilize:
Circulatory support
Respiratory support
Hospitalize in ICU
(Cont'd on p 631)
(Cont'd on p 631)

C. As soon as the diagnosis is established, treat with intravenous immunoglobulin (IVIG; 2 g/kg) given over 10 to 12 hours as a single dose. Studies have shown IVIG given in the first 10 days of illness substantially decreases risk for development of coronary artery lesions. No studies have evaluated risk reduction using IVIG after the 10th day of illness, but it is still recommended as treatment if the patient is symptomatic and/or has signs of ongoing inflammation. The most common adverse effects of IVIG include fever, chills, and headaches. A hemolytic reaction or anaphylaxis is rare. Immunoglobulin preparations have been screened for hepatitis and human immunodeficiency viruses. MMR and varicella vaccines should not be given within 11 months of treatment with IVIG (patients may not develop good immune responses because IVIG contains antibody to these antigens).

D. At the time of diagnosis and treatment with IVIG, high-dose oral aspirin (80–100 mg/kg/day in four divided doses) should be initiated and continued until the patient has been afebrile for 3 to 5 days. At this point, the dose and frequency of the aspirin can be reduced to 3 to 5 mg/kg/day given orally once a day. Signs of aspirin toxicity are only occasionally seen at high doses, but be alert for the signs such as vomiting, hyperpnea, lethargy, and liver function alterations. In patients without development of coronary artery abnormalities, low-dose aspirin is continued until the 6- to 8-week follow-up echocardiogram has been obtained and has been declared normal. In patients with coronary artery findings, the decision on when to stop the aspirin will be made by the cardiologist (some patients take aspirin indefinitely). Use of aspirin during varicella or influenza infections has been associated with Reye syndrome. Therefore, it is important that the patient and family receive influenza vaccines before discharge (seasonally) if they have not previously received them this season. The patient should receive trivalent inactivated (injectable) influenza vaccine; the live attenuated vaccine (intranasal) is contraindicated in patients taking aspirin. If the patient receiving aspirin is exposed or has symptoms of varicella infection or influenza, the aspirin should be stopped immediately and the cardiologist contacted for advice on an alternative agent to use. Dipyridamole is one such alternative antiplatelet drug, but there are others, and cardiologists may have personal preferences or recommendations based on the presence or absence of coronary artery disease.

E. Cardiac complications include pericardial effusion, myocarditis with arrhythmias or congestive heart failure, coronary artery aneurysms, late coronary artery occlusion with myocardial infarction, acute and chronic valvulitis, and aneurysms of the aorta and other noncoronary arteries. Patients who experience development of giant coronary aneurysms (≥8 mm) are at high risk for myocardial ischemia/infarction. Deaths are most frequent between days 20 and 40 of the illness. A small number of patients continue to have fever and lack of resolution of signs and symptoms after treatment with IVIG. Patients who do not become afebrile within 36 hours after the immunoglobulin infusion finishes are termed *IVIG resistant.* These patients need to be treated either with a second dose of IVIG or with one of the newer agents under study. Consultation with an expert on Kawasaki disease is recommended.

References

Anderson MS, Todd JK, Glode MP. Delayed diagnosis of Kawasaki syndrome: an analysis of the problem. Pediatrics 2005;115(4): e428–33.

Bradley DJ, Glode MP. Kawasaki disease: the mystery continues. West J Med 1998;168:23.

Burns JC, Best BM, Mejias A, et al. Infliximab treatment of intravenous immunoglobulin–resistant Kawasaki disease. J Pediatr 2008;153:833–8.

Burns JC, Glode MP. Kawasaki syndrome. Lancet 2004;364:533.

Burns JC, Shike S, Gordon JB, et al. Sequelae of Kawasaki disease in adolescents and young adults. J Am Coll Cardiol 1996;28:253.

Chang FY, Hwang B, Chen SJ, et al. Characteristics of Kawasaki disease in infants younger than six months of age. Pediatr Infect Dis J 2006; 25:241–4.

Dhillon R, Clarkson P, Donald AE, et al. Endothelial dysfunction late after Kawasaki disease. Circulation 1996;94:2103.

Dominguez SR, Friedman K, Seewald R, et al. Kawasaki disease in a pediatric intensive care unit: a case-control study. Pediatrics 2008; 122:e786.

Melish ME. Kawasaki syndrome. In: Krugman S, Katz SL, Gershon AE, Wilfert C, editors. Infectious diseases of children. 9th ed. St. Louis, MO: Mosby; 1992. p. 211.

Newburger JW, Takahashi M, Beiser AS, et al. A single intravenous infusion of gamma globulin as compared with four infusions in the treatment of acute Kawasaki syndrome. N Engl J Med 1991; 324:1633.

Newburger JW, Takahashi M, Burns JC, et al. The treatment of Kawasaki syndrome with intravenous gamma globulin. N Engl J Med 1986;315:341.

Newburger JW, Takahashi M, Gerber MA, et al. Diagnosis, treatment, and long term management of Kawasaki disease, a statement for health professionals from the Committee on Rheumatic Fever, Endocarditis and Kawasaki Disease, Council on Cardiovascular Disease in the Young, American Heart Association. Circulation 2004;110:2747.

Senzaki H. Long-term outcome of Kawasaki disease. Circulation 2008;118:2763–72.

Sundel RP, Burns JC, Baker A, et al. Gamma globulin re-treatment in Kawasaki disease. J Pediatr 1993;123:657.

Tremoulet AH, Best BM, Song S, et al. Resistance to intravenous immunoglobulin in children with Kawasaki disease. J Pediatr 2008;153(1):117–21.

Wright DA, Newburger JW, Baker A, Sundel RP. Treatment of immune globulin–resistant Kawasaki disease with pulsed doses of corticosteroids. J Pediatr 1996;128:146.

Patient with KAWASAKI DISEASE

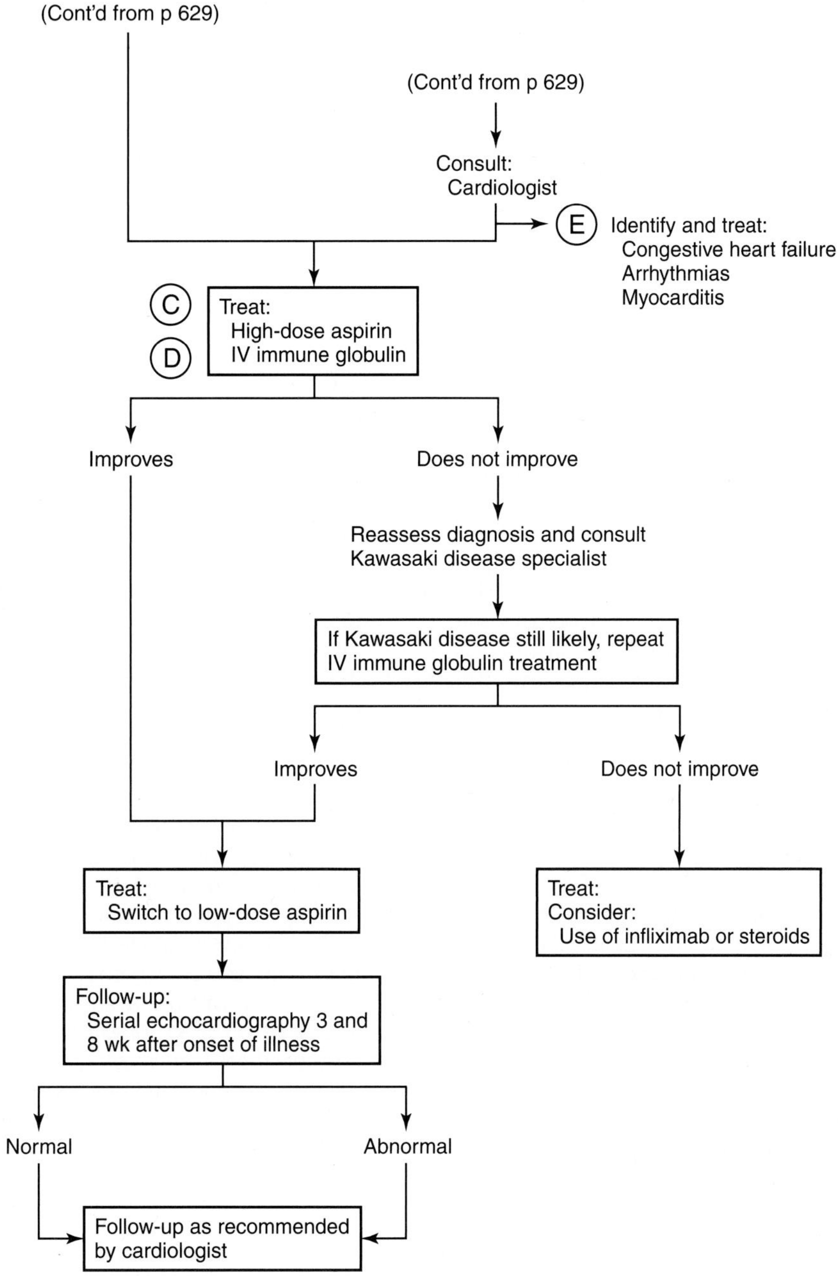
(Cont'd from p 629)
(Cont'd from p 629)
Consult:
Cardiologist
E
Identify and treat:
Congestive heart failure
Arrhythmias
Myocarditis
C
D
Treat:
High-dose aspirin
IV immune globulin
Improves
Does not improve
Reassess diagnosis and consult Kawasaki disease specialist
If Kawasaki disease still likely, repeat IV immune globulin treatment
Improves
Does not improve
Treat:
Switch to low-dose aspirin
Treat:
Consider:
Use of infliximab or steroids
Follow-up:
Serial echocardiography 3 and 8 wk after onset of illness
Normal
Abnormal
Follow-up as recommended by cardiologist

Lyme Disease

Julie-Ann Crewalk, MD, and Roberta L. DeBiasi, MD

Lyme disease is a multisystem inflammatory disorder caused by infection with the spirochete, *Borrelia burgdorferi*. The disease is transmitted by the bite of an *Ixodes* tick (*I. scapularis* or *I. pacificus*, *I. rincinus* in Europe, *I. persulacatus* in Asia). Transmission has been confirmed on at least three continents. Inoculation from the *Ixodes* tick may lead to isolated Lyme disease, as well as possible coinfection with *Anaplasma phaygocytophilium* or *Babesia microti*.

A. History: When obtaining the patient's history, ask about potential exposure to ticks and recognized tick bites, as well as rashes or an influenza-like illness (without respiratory symptoms). Ticks are found not only in wooded areas, but also in grasses, shrubs, and bushes surrounding the yard. Generalized symptoms of fever, malaise, fatigue, conjunctivitis, sore throat, arthralgias, nausea, vomiting, stiff neck, and headache are often noted in early Lyme disease and may accompany the initial rash.

B. Physical Examination: Be observant for skin lesions. When erythema migrans rash is present (approximately 50% of cases), it initially manifests 1 to 32 days after the tick bite. This skin lesion begins as an erythematous papule and expands circumferentially to a large circular or oval erythematous lesion, with our without partial central clearing ("bull's-eye" lesion), that may reach a diameter of 60 cm. The lesion may resemble cellulitis, the center may vesiculate or ulcerate, and secondary lesions may develop. The lesion is typically present for approximately 4 to 6 weeks. Additional physical signs that may be present include lymphadenopathy, mild meningismus, ocular findings (conjunctivitis, iritis, keratitis), bradycardia, splenomegaly, arthritis, and less commonly, hepatomegaly (anicteric hepatitis) or testicular swelling.

C. Assess the Pattern of Disease: Lyme disease has early- and late-stage manifestations. Early localized disease is often limited to isolated erythema migrans rash, with or without fever, headache, and/or myalgia. Early disseminated disease occurs in about 15% of patients, most commonly manifesting as multiple erythema migrans lesions, with or without fever, headache, myalgia, and/or meningismus. Secondary erythema migrans lesions develop within several weeks of infection, consisting of smaller annular lesions in comparison with the initial primary lesion. Other potential manifestations of early disseminated disease include central nervous system abnormalities (aseptic meningitis, facial nerve palsy, radiculopathy, cerebellar ataxia, transverse myelitis) or rarely cardiac abnormalities (heart block or myocarditis). Late disease presents months after initial infection, usually as recurrent arthritis of the large joints, such as the knees, and rarely as neurologic disease (encephalitis, polyneuritis).

D. Serologic Testing: Early localized disease is primarily a clinical diagnosis. Serologic testing is commonly negative during early localized disease, as a minimum of 3 to 4 weeks are required to develop a reliably detectable serologic response. Serologic testing for Lyme disease is indicated for suspected early disseminated and late Lyme disease. A two-step testing approach is recommended, consisting of an initial quantitative screening test (EIA or IFA) for serum antibodies (sensitive but not specific). Equivocal or positive results should be followed by confirmatory testing by Western immunoblot IgG and IgM (specific but potentially overly sensitive in absence of screening ELISA).

(Continued on page 634)

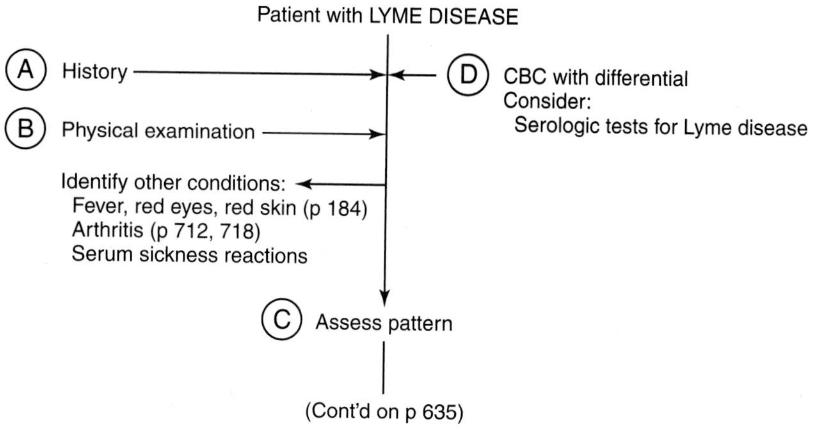
Patient with LYME DISEASE
(A) History
(B) Physical examination
Identify other conditions:
Fever, red eyes, red skin (p 184)
Arthritis (p 712, 718)
Serum sickness reactions
(D) CBC with differential
Consider:
Serologic tests for Lyme disease
(C) Assess pattern
(Cont'd on p 635)

E. Localized Erythema Migrans: Treatment of early localized and disseminated disease effectively prevents progression to manifestations of late disease. All symptoms and signs should resolve promptly during treatment of early disease.

F. Cardiac manifestations of early disseminated disease usually develop 3 to 21 weeks after the bite, most commonly as various stages of atrioventricular block, but also as myocarditis and left ventricular dysfunction. Carditis is rare in children.

G. Neurologic manifestations can be present initially but more often develop 4 to 6 weeks after the tick bite. The most frequent manifestations are meningitis and cranial nerve palsies, as well as peripheral radiculoneuropathies. Less common are transverse myelitis, Guillain-Barré syndrome, cerebellar ataxia, encephalitis, and pseudotumor cerebri (seen primarily in children). Neuro-ophthalmologic findings can include neuroretinitis and optic neuritis. Neurologic abnormalities may progress in untreated patients during months to years into chronic syndromes. Bell's palsy is the most common cranial neuropathy and can occur either as an isolated neurologic manifestation or in conjunction with aseptic meningitis.

H. Arthritis usually develops months after the tick bite. The pattern of joint involvement may be variable and can be monoarticular, oligoarticular, migratory, or additive. Monoarticular or pauciarticular involvement of the knee is the most common presentation. Other joints may include shoulder, elbow, temporomandibular joint, ankle, wrist, and hip. Joints are characteristically warm and swollen, but rarely erythematous. Waxing and waning symptoms are common. Without treatment, the arthritis usually lasts several weeks, often remits and recurs, and can become debilitating.

(Continued on page 636)

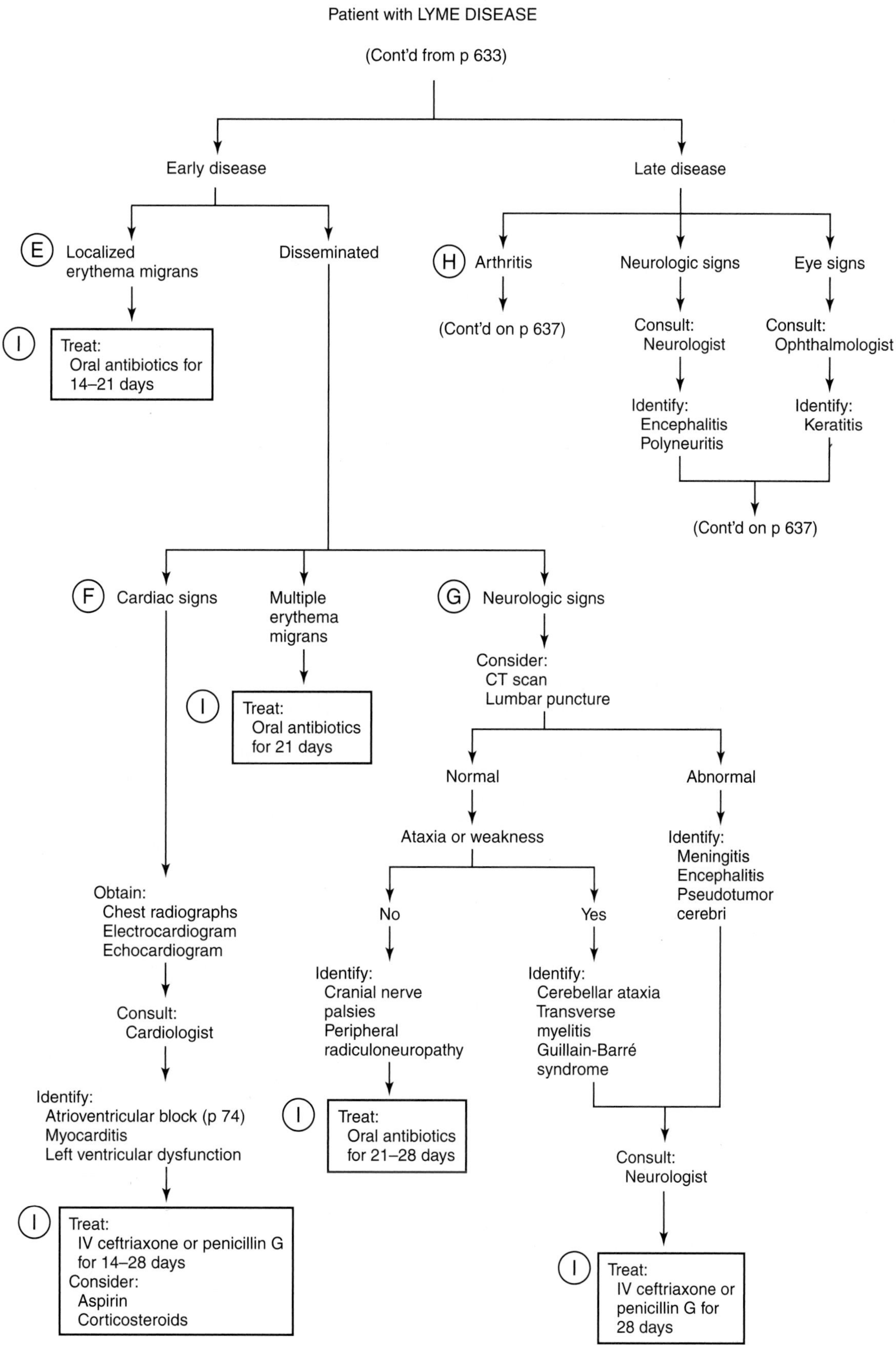
Patient with LYME DISEASE
(Cont'd from p 633)
Early disease
Late disease
E Localized erythema migrans
I Treat: Oral antibiotics for 14–21 days
Disseminated
H Arthritis
(Cont'd on p 637)
Neurologic signs
Consult: Neurologist
Identify: Encephalitis Polyneuritis
Eye signs
Consult: Ophthalmologist
Identify: Keratitis
(Cont'd on p 637)
F Cardiac signs
Obtain: Chest radiographs Electrocardiogram Echocardiogram
Consult: Cardiologist
Identify: Atrioventricular block (p 74) Myocarditis Left ventricular dysfunction
I Treat: IV ceftriaxone or penicillin G for 14–28 days Consider: Aspirin Corticosteroids
Multiple erythema migrans
I Treat: Oral antibiotics for 21 days
G Neurologic signs
Consider: CT scan Lumbar puncture
Normal
Ataxia or weakness
No
Identify: Cranial nerve palsies Peripheral radiculoneuropathy
I Treat: Oral antibiotics for 21–28 days
Yes
Identify: Cerebellar ataxia Transverse myelitis Guillain-Barré syndrome
Abnormal
Identify: Meningitis Encephalitis Pseudotumor cerebri
Consult: Neurologist
I Treat: IV ceftriaxone or penicillin G for 28 days

Table 1. **Drugs Used in the Treatment of Lyme Disease**

Drugs/Antibiotics	Dosage	Duration
Amoxicillin	50 mg/kg/day PO divided tid (maximum: 500 mg per dose)	
Cefuroxime axetil	30 mg/kg/day PO divided bid (maximum 1 gm per day)	Early localized: 21 days Early disseminated: Multiple EM: 21 days Facial Palsy: 21–28 days Late arthritis: 28 days
Doxycycline	≥8 years of age: 100 mg per dose bid <8 years of age: 4 mg/kg/day PO divided bid (maximum: 100 mg per dose)	Early localized: 14–21 days Early disseminated: 21–28 days
Ceftriaxone	75–100 mg/kg/day IV once daily (maximum: 2 g per day)	
Cefotaxime	150 mg/kg/day IV divided every 8 hrs (maximum: 2 g per dose)	Early (carditis/meningitis): 14–28 days
Penicillin G	300,000 U/kg/day IV divided every 4 hrs (maximum: 20 million units per day)	Late (persistent arthritis, encephalitis): 14–28 days
°Erythromycin ethyl succinate	50 mg/kg/day PO divided q6h (maximum: 500 mg per dose)	Early localized: 14–21 days
°Azithromycin	10 mg/kg/day PO once daily (maximum: 500 mg per dose)	Early localized: 7–10 days

°Not first line treatment due to lower response rate.
IV, intravenously; *PO*, orally.

I. Treatment:

1. Early localized disease (erythema migrans, arthralgias, headaches, and other early manifestations) should be treated with oral doxycycline or tetracycline (for children ≥8 years old) or amoxicillin (for children <8 years old) for 14 to 21 days. Cefuroxime is an acceptable alternative for patients allergic to amoxicillin (Table 1). The macrolides are not recommended as first-line therapy because they were found to be less effective than other antimicrobials. First-generation cephalosporins should not be used for treatment.

2. Treatment of patients with early disseminated disease is based on the presenting clinical manifestation:

a. Multiple erythema migrans can be treated with the same oral regimens as described above, but for 21 days.

b. Patients with isolated facial nerve palsy (in absence of aseptic meningitis) can be treated orally for 21 to 28 days. Treatment prevents progression of neurologic disease; however, it will not affect time or likelihood of resolution of the cranial nerve palsy. Steroids are not indicated for treatment of Bell's palsy caused by Lyme disease. Intravenous antimicrobial therapy is indicated for treatment of aseptic meningitis and other neurologic manifestations of Lyme disease.

c. Carditis should be treated with intravenous ceftriaxone or penicillin G for 14 to 28 days.

3. Late disease:

a. Patients with arthritis in absence of neurologic disease can be treated orally for 28 days. One third of patients with arthritis will have persistent symptoms/signs at conclusion of therapy that almost always resolves within an additional month. However, some patients may require a second course of oral therapy. Refractory or recurrent arthritis should be treated with intravenous therapy. NSAID treatment in conjunction with antimicrobial therapy is often utilized.

b. Treatment of neurologic disease (with exception of isolated cranial nerve palsy), should be completed with intravenous ceftriaxone or penicillin G for 21 to 28 days.

c. Although unusual in the pediatric population, a small subset of patients may report ongoing symptoms including headache, fatigue, and myalgia persisting longer than 6 months after completion of standard therapy for any stage of Lyme disease. This entity, termed *post-Lyme syndrome,* is an area of active study but does not represent active or chronic infection. Prolonged antimicrobial therapy is not indicated in these patients. Advise all patients to take appropriate precautions for preventing subsequent tick bites, such as protective clothing, use of insect repellents, and daily inspection for attached ticks.

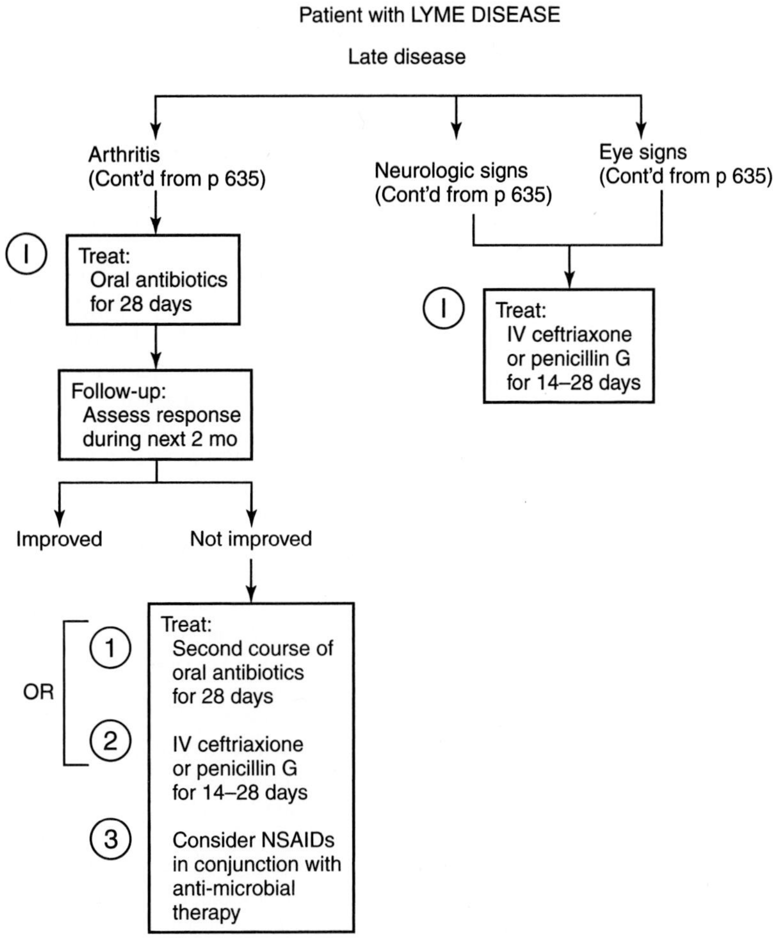
Patient with LYME DISEASE
Late disease
Arthritis
(Cont'd from p 635)
Neurologic signs
(Cont'd from p 635)
Eye signs
(Cont'd from p 635)
I
Treat:
Oral antibiotics
for 28 days
I
Treat:
IV ceftriaxone
or penicillin G
for 14–28 days
Follow-up:
Assess response
during next 2 mo
Improved
Not improved
OR
1
2
3
Treat:
Second course of
oral antibiotics
for 28 days
IV ceftriaxione
or penicillin G
for 14–28 days
Consider NSAIDs
in conjunction with
anti-microbial
therapy

References

American Academy of Pediatrics. Lyme disease. In: Pickering LK, Baker CJ, Long SS, et al, editors. Red Book: 2006 report of the committee on infectious diseases. 28th ed. Elk Grove Village, IL: American Academy of Pediatrics; 2009. p. 430–7.

Baltimore RS, Shapiro ED. Lyme disease. Pediatr Rev 1994;15:167.

Christy C, Siegel DM. Lyme disease—what it is, what it isn't. Contemp Pediatr 1995;12:64.

Eppes SC, Nelson DK, Lewis LL, Klein JE. Characterization of Lyme meningitis and comparison with viral meningitis in children. Pediatrics 1999;103:957–60.

Rothermel H, Hedges TR, Steere AC. Optic neuropathy in children with Lyme disease. Pediatrics 2001;108:477–81.

Steere AC. Lyme disease. N Engl J Med 2001;345(2):115–25.

Wormser GP, Dattwyler RJ, Shapiro ED, et al. The clinical assessment, treatment, and prevention of lyme disease, human granulocytic anaplasmosis, and babesiosis: clinical practice guidelines by the Infectious Diseases Society of America. Clin Infect Dis 2006;43:1089–1134.

Meningitis

Donna Curtis, MD, MPH, and Ann-Christine Nyquist, MD, MSPH

Meningitis is an inflammation of the meninges, the membranes that surround the brain and spinal cord. Related conditions include encephalitis, inflammation of the brain, and meningoencephalitis, which is inflammation of both the meninges and the brain.

Infectious causes of meningitis include viruses and bacteria, and fungi and parasites (rare causes of meningitis). The epidemiology of meningitis depends on many things, but the age of the patient and the time of year often dictate treatment decisions before a pathogen is known. For the purposes of this chapter, epidemiology, diagnosis, and management are discussed in the context of developed countries. Among viruses, enteroviruses and herpes simplex virus (HSV) are the most common causes of viral meningitis in infants. In older children, enteroviruses continue to dominate, other viruses include HSV, arboviruses, influenza, Epstein–Barr virus, and human immunodeficiency virus. The most common causes of bacterial meningitis also vary by age of the child. Among infants, newborn to 4 to 6 weeks, group B streptococcus and Enterobacteriaceae, particularly *Escherichia coli,* are the most common causes of bacterial meningitis. The pathogens in this age group reflect exposure to vaginal and perineal flora of the mother. There is no definite time period distinguishing causes of bacterial meningitis in various age ranges, but after about 1 month of age, *Streptococcus pneumoniae* and *Neisseria meningitidis* become more common, and they are the predominant organisms after approximately 3 months of age. Other bacteria to consider based on maternal history, exposures, and immune status include, but are not limited to, *Listeria monocytogenes,* enterococci, *Staphylococcus aureus, Citrobacter, Salmonella, Haemophilus influenzae* (type a, nontypeable, type b), *Mycoplasma, Mycobacterium tuberculosis, Streptococcus anginosus,* and anaerobes. The frequency of *H. influenzae* type b infection has decreased dramatically with immunization; however, in areas of the world where conjugate *H. influenzae* type b vaccine is not administered, this organism remains a common cause of meningitis. Invasive *H. influenzae* type a infections are reported as a rare cause of meningitis. As the use of conjugate pneumococcal vaccine increases, the frequency of pneumococcal meningitis will decrease and the relative proportion of meningococcal meningitis will increase. In Lyme-endemic areas, Lyme meningitis should also be considered. Fungal meningitis is rare and is typically restricted to particular patient groups. For example, cryptococcal meningitis should be considered in patients with human immunodeficiency virus (HIV) or other immunodeficiency, and Candidal meningitis can occur in premature infants in neonatal intensive care units (NICUs), patients with ventricular shunts, or immunodeficient patients. Parasitic meningitis is also rare but can include amoebic meningitis in patients who are immunocompromised or with exposure to freshwater.

Morbidity and mortality for bacterial meningitis depends on the age of the patient and the bacteria, but can be significant. The mortality rate for bacterial meningitis is 10% to 20% in the neonatal period and 3% to 10% in infants and children. Morbidity includes sensorineural hearing loss (most common sequelae), intellectual delay, obstructive hydrocephalus, or seizure disorder. Viral meningitis generally has much less morbidity and mortality; however, notable exceptions include herpes simplex meningoencephalitis, neonatal enteroviral sepsis, influenza necrotizing encephalitis, and enterovirus 71 meningoencephalitis.

A. The patient's history should include details of fever, irritability, and other new symptoms noted by the caregiver. Look for alterations in the mental status and normal level of activity, including playfulness, irritability, feeding and sleeping patterns, responsiveness, and seizures. A full review of systems should be elicited with particular attention to recent respiratory symptoms (cough, congestion, coryza, sore throat, earache, fast or difficult breathing, chest indrawing [retractions]), treatment with antibiotics, and gastrointestinal symptoms (vomiting, diarrhea, abdominal distention, abdominal pain, blood in stools). Pertinent aspects of history include maternal prenatal labs and group B streptococcus status for infants, any known sick contacts, vaccination history, underlying medical conditions (especially exposure to HIV, other known immunodeficiency or immunosuppressive medications, sickle cell disease, heart disease with single-ventricle physiology), contact with animals, travel history, family history of immune disorders, and any indwelling foreign bodies (ventricular shunt, central venous catheters).

B. A complete physical examination should be performed with particular attention to mental status, neurologic examination, and cardiovascular examination. The neurologic examination should evaluate for nuchal rigidity, including Brudzinski and Kernig signs, a bulging fontanelle in infants, papilledema, and focal neurologic signs such as cranial nerve abnormalities (3, 4, and 6 can indicate increased intracranial pressure), weakness, or asymmetric reflexes. In Brudzinski sign, the knees flex in response to rapid flexion of the neck. Kernig sign is resistance to extension of the leg when the hips are flexed. In infants with a fontanelle, the baseline head circumference should be measured and the fontanelle width can also be measured and followed daily to monitor for development of complications such as subdural effusion or hydrocephalus. Cardiovascular examination should concentrate on signs of shock such as tachycardia, low blood pressure, delayed capillary refill, or weak pulses. Other notable findings could include respiratory distress, seizures, petechiae and/or purpura, other skin rash, and bone or joint infections.

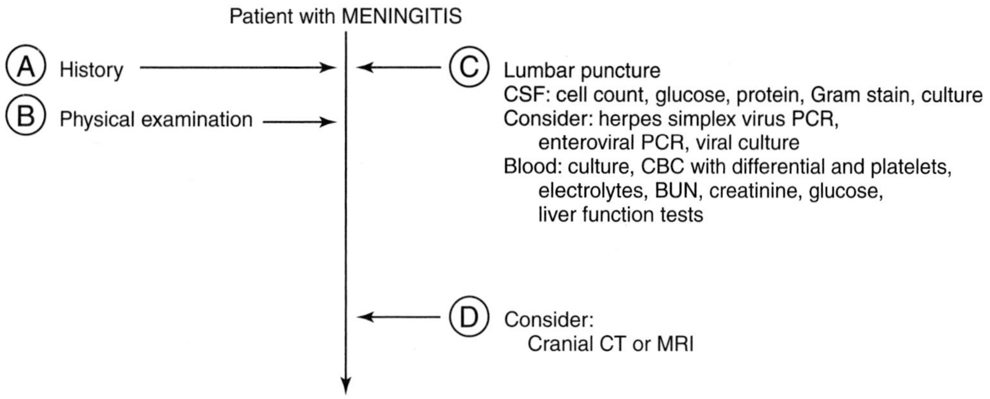
Patient with MENINGITIS
A History
B Physical examination
C Lumbar puncture
CSF: cell count, glucose, protein, Gram stain, culture
Consider: herpes simplex virus PCR, enteroviral PCR, viral culture
Blood: culture, CBC with differential and platelets, electrolytes, BUN, creatinine, glucose, liver function tests
D Consider: Cranial CT or MRI

(Cont'd on p 641)

C. The diagnosis of meningitis is based on signs of inflammation in the cerebrospinal fluid (CSF); therefore, a lumbar puncture (LP) should be performed unless clinically contraindicated. Contraindications to performing a LP include: concern for increased intracranial pressure (refer to section D) or respiratory or cardiovascular instability. Antibiotics should not be delayed if a LP is not performed before stabilization or further testing. CSF should be sent for cell count, glucose, protein, bacterial culture, and possibly for viral studies based on clinical presentation. Common CSF viral studies include HSV polymerase chain reaction (PCR) and enterovirus PCR. Other studies may be sent on the CSF based on history and physical, for example, mycobacterial culture, fungal culture, West Nile virus IgG/IgM, viral culture, and cryptococcal antigen. CSF laboratory parameters can vary based on age. After the neonatal period, a normal CSF should have no more than 10 white blood cells (WBCs) per cubic millimeter, a glucose level greater than 50% of the serum concentration, a protein level less than 45 mg/dl, and a negative Gram stain. Sterilization of the CSF can occur within 1 hour of parenteral administration of antibiotics for meningococcal infection and within 4 hours for pneumococcal infection. CSF cell counts greater than $500/mm^3$ are suggestive but not diagnostic of bacterial infection because 45% of patients with enteroviral meningitis have CSF counts greater than $500/mm^3$. A majority of patients with enteroviral meningitis also demonstrate polymorphonuclear leukocyte predominance in the CSF. CSF parameters can also be normal early on in infection, so treatment should be initiated if there is a clinical suspicion of meningitis even with normal CSF cell count and chemistries. In this case, if culture or PCRs are negative, the LP can be repeated in 24 to 48 hours. There is no definite cutoff for WBCs to distinguish between viral and bacterial meningitis; however, in general, the higher the WBCs, the more likely the cause is bacterial. Additional studies that can aid in diagnosis of meningitis include throat and rectal PCRs for enterovirus, surface cultures (or PCRs) for HSV, and serum PCR for viruses. Other laboratory abnormalities may include disseminated intravascular coagulation (seen with disseminated HSV, neonatal enterovirus, bacteremia suggesting pneumococcal or meningococcal infection), elevated liver function tests (HSV or neonatal enterovirus), and hyponatremia (syndrome of inappropriate antidiuretic hormone secretion [SIADH] from bacterial meningitis).

D. When there is clinical concern for increased intracranial pressure (papilledema, bulging fontanelle, cardiovascular instability), a computed tomography (CT) scan or magnetic resonance imaging (MRI) of the head should be obtained before performing a LP. Performing either imaging test with contrast will allow visualization of abscess, and on an MRI, inflammation of the meninges or brain will occur with meningitis, encephalitis, or both. Findings of temporal lobe involvement in patients with seizures suggest herpes central nervous system infection.

E. Assess the degree of illness. Very severely ill patients have signs of severe dehydration, shock, respiratory distress, disseminated intravascular coagulation, electrolyte abnormalities, hypoglycemia, markedly altered mental status, prolonged seizures, or focal neurologic signs.

F. For the initial 24 to 48 hours, patients with bacterial meningitis should be monitored for hemodynamic stability, neurologic status, urine output, electrolyte levels, glucose concentration, and calcium concentration. Maintain the patient's hydration in the normal range. Correct significant dehydration and avoid overhydration.

G. Initial empiric antibiotic therapy is typically based on the age of the patient (Table 1). Neonates to approximately 4 to 6 weeks should be started on ampicillin and cefotaxime or an aminoglycoside (typically gentamicin). The ampicillin will cover group B streptococcus, listeria, and enterococci. Doses should be maximized for the age and weight. If gentamicin is used, levels should be followed closely to avoid additional potential effects on hearing or renal function. Infants in the NICU or any infant with a central line should be treated with vancomycin given the risk for central line infection. Older infants (i.e., >4–6 weeks) should be empirically started on vancomycin and cefotaxime (or ceftriaxone). The switch to vancomycin is based on the risk for resistant *Streptococcus pneumoniae.* If a resistant pneumococcus is isolated, or if there is no clinical improvement in 24 to 48 hours, adding rifampin (20 mg/kg per day in two doses) is indicated. Vancomycin levels should be followed closely to ensure adequate serum concentrations and monitor for toxicity. Serum creatinine should be followed closely for either vancomycin or gentamicin to monitor for renal toxicity. Acyclovir should be added to the empiric treatment regimen if there is any clinical concern for HSV meningitis. Once a pathogen has been identified, the antibiotic regimen should be tailored to the recommended treatment regimen for that pathogen. Treatment duration is typically pathogen specific and can change based on whether there are any clinical complications. In general, for a non-complicated meningitis treat gram-negative enterics for 21 days, group B streptococcus for 14 to 21 days, *S. pneumoniae* for 10 to 14 days, *H. influenzae* for 7 to 10 days, and *N. meningitidis* for 7 days.

H. Begin therapy with acyclovir when herpes infection is suspected or identified. Under 6 months of age, a dosage of 20 mg/kg intravenously (IV) every 8 hours can be used. After 6 months of age, the standard dosage of 10 mg/kg IV every 8 hours (or better, 1500 mg/m^2 per 24 hours divided every 8 hours) should be used. In certain severe infections, the 20 mg/kg IV every 8 hours dosage is used for older children. Ensure the adult maximum dosage is not exceeded. Typical length of treatment for HSV meningitis/encephalitis is 21 days IV.

I. Neurologic sequelae of bacterial meningitis is related to the inflammation of the body's immune response to the pathogen. Many studies have tried to evaluate the effects of steroids on neurologic outcomes; and although results are mixed, many experts recommend using steroids in addition to antibiotics concurrently with the antibiotics or very soon after. The potential benefits include decreased sensorineural hearing loss and improvement in other neurologic sequelae. This has been shown in *Haemophilus* type b meningitis, and there is some data for *Streptococcus pneumoniae* meningitis in adults. The concern for using dexamethasone is based on decreased CSF concentrations of vancomycin and other medications caused by decreased inflammation of the meninges, because the inflammation of the meninges allows for better passage of antibiotics across the blood–brain barrier. Another concern is that the anti-inflammatory effects may mask clinical conditions that fail to respond to standard empiric antibiotics such as resistant *Streptococcus pneumoniae,* mycobacteria, or fungal infections. Of note, it is not uncommon for the patient to have another fever once the dexamethasone is stopped; however, this does not necessarily represent treatment failure and the patient must be evaluated clinically. The recommended dosage for dexamethasone is 0.15 mg/kg IV every 6 hours for 4 days.

(Continued on page 642)

Table 1. **Therapy for Meningitis**

Drug	IV Dose
Acyclovir	1500 mg/m^2/24 hr (30 mg/kg 24 hr) divided every 8h
Ampicillin sodium	50–75 mg/kg every 6h
Cefotaxime (Claforan)	50–75 mg/kg every 6h
Ceftriaxone (Rocephin)	100 mg/kg daily
Dexamethasone	0.15 mg/kg every 6h IV × 4 days
Gentamicin	2.5 mg/kg every 8h (infants <7 days, every 12h)
Vancomycin (Vancocin)	15 mg/kg every 6h (infants >30 days) 15 mg/kg every 8h (infants 7–30 days) 15 mg/kg every 12h (infants <7 days)

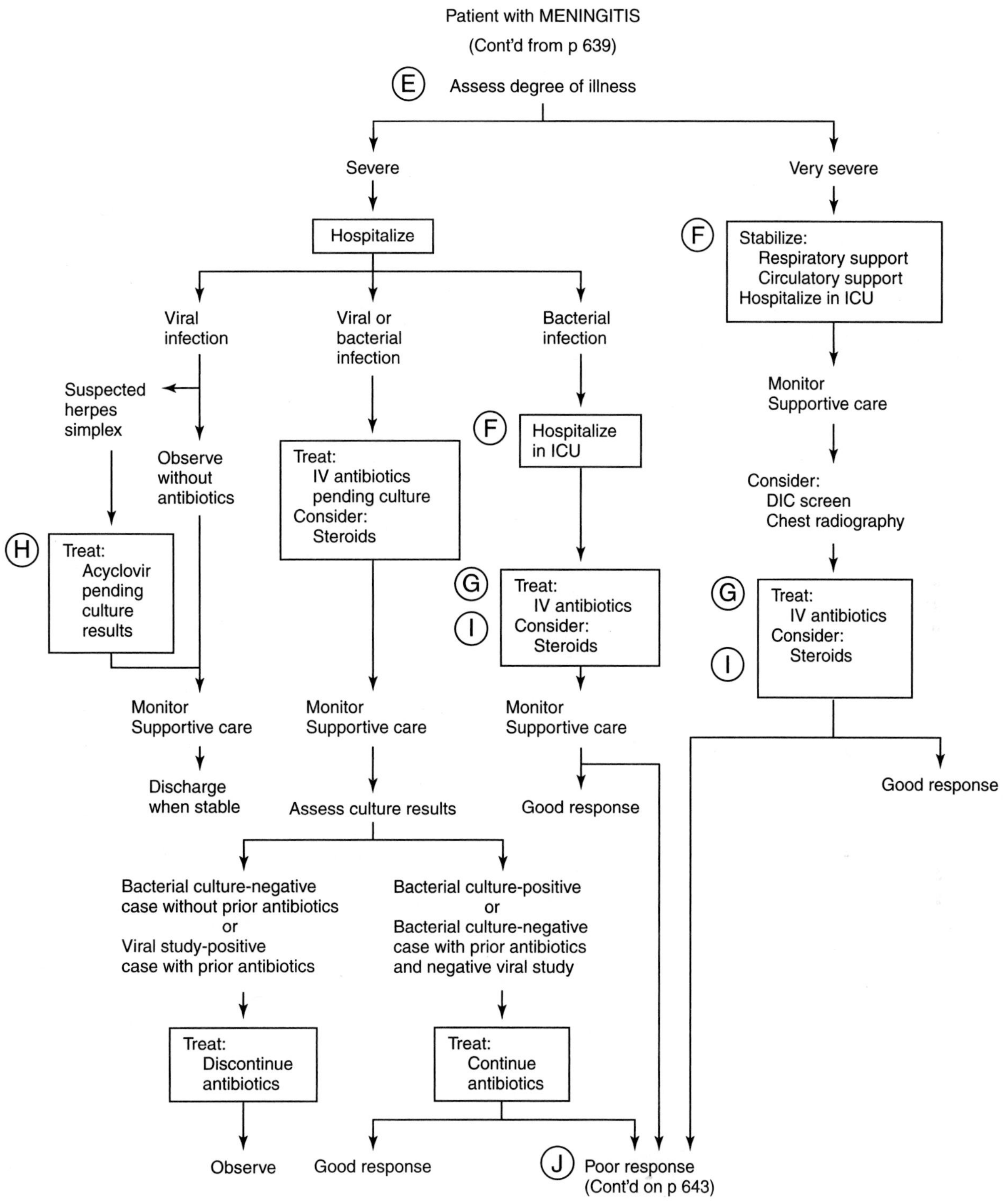

Patient with MENINGITIS
(Cont'd from p 639)
E Assess degree of illness
Severe
Very severe
Hospitalize
F Stabilize: Respiratory support Circulatory support Hospitalize in ICU
Viral infection
Viral or bacterial infection
Bacterial infection
Suspected herpes simplex
Observe without antibiotics
Treat: IV antibiotics pending culture Consider: Steroids
F Hospitalize in ICU
Monitor Supportive care
Consider: DIC screen Chest radiography
H Treat: Acyclovir pending culture results
G I Treat: IV antibiotics Consider: Steroids
G I Treat: IV antibiotics Consider: Steroids
Monitor Supportive care
Monitor Supportive care
Monitor Supportive care
Good response
Discharge when stable
Assess culture results
Good response
Bacterial culture-negative case without prior antibiotics or Viral study-positive case with prior antibiotics
Bacterial culture-positive or Bacterial culture-negative case with prior antibiotics and negative viral study
Treat: Discontinue antibiotics
Treat: Continue antibiotics
Observe
Good response
J Poor response (Cont'd on p 643)

J. Patients should improve within 24 to 48 hours after initiation of antibiotic therapy. Indications of a poor response include persistent opisthotonos, seizures, coma or altered mental status, and signs suggesting central nervous system complication (focal neurologic signs, enlarging head circumference, ataxia, persistent seizures, prolonged coma, altered mental status). Patients can have prolonged fevers, particularly with *Haemophilus influenzae* meningitis (10%–15%); however, other causes of prolonged fevers such as phlebitis, soft-tissue infection, urinary tract infection, and bone joint infection must be evaluated. Drug fever must be considered.

K. Consider repeating LP in 24 to 36 hours to document an adequate therapeutic response in all neonates, infections with nonsusceptible *S. pneumoniae* and gram-negative enteric bacilli, immunocompromised patients, recurrent meningitis, and failure to respond to therapy. Routine LP at the end of therapy is unnecessary; however, consider repeating LP in the patient with persistent fever. A repeat LP is also often recommended in neonates with gram-negative bacilli. The repeat LP will document end-of-therapy CSF parameters in the event that the infant returns for treatment and requires a repeat LP.

L. Signs of central nervous system complications include focal neurologic findings, prolonged seizures, persistent alterations in mental status, enlarging head circumferences, and ataxia. A CT or MRI scan will identify significant central nervous system disease: subdural effusion or empyema, cerebral edema, cerebral abscess, cerebral infarction, or hydrocephalus. Small subdural effusions are common and should not be drained. Aspirate an effusion or empyema if it is large and associated with ventricular displacement, focal neurologic signs, signs of increased intracranial pressure, or deterioration in the patient's condition. Patients with meningitis should have a hearing screen and be followed closely for developmental abnormalities.

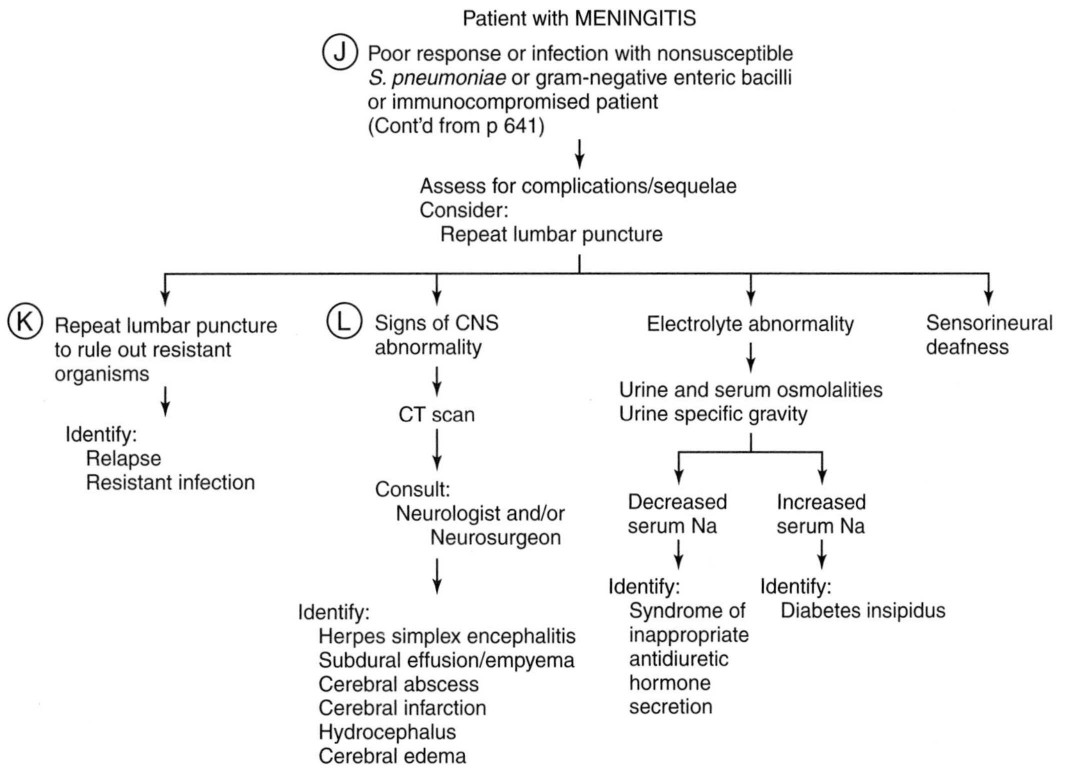
Patient with MENINGITIS
J
Poor response or infection with nonsusceptible *S. pneumoniae* or gram-negative enteric bacilli or immunocompromised patient
(Cont'd from p 641)
Assess for complications/sequelae
Consider:
Repeat lumbar puncture
K
Repeat lumbar puncture to rule out resistant organisms
Identify:
Relapse
Resistant infection
L
Signs of CNS abnormality
CT scan
Consult:
Neurologist and/or
Neurosurgeon
Identify:
Herpes simplex encephalitis
Subdural effusion/empyema
Cerebral abscess
Cerebral infarction
Hydrocephalus
Cerebral edema
Electrolyte abnormality
Urine and serum osmolalities
Urine specific gravity
Decreased serum Na
Identify:
Syndrome of inappropriate antidiuretic hormone secretion
Increased serum Na
Identify:
Diabetes insipidus
Sensorineural deafness

References

Arditi M, Mason EO Jr, Bradley JS, et al. Three-year multicenter surveillance of pneumococcal meningitis in children: clinical characteristics and outcome related to penicillin susceptibility and dexamethasone use. Pediatrics 1998;102:1087–97.

Bonadio WA. The cerebrospinal fluid: physiologic aspects and alterations associated with bacterial meningitis. Pediatr Infect Dis J 1992;11:423.

Bradley JS. Dexamethasone therapy in meningitis: potentially misleading antiinflammatory effects in central nervous system infections. Pediatr Infect Dis J 1994;13:823.

Brouwer MC, McIntyre P, de Gans J, Prasad K, van de Beek D. Corticosteroids for acute bacterial meningitis. Cochrane Database Syst Rev 2010;(9):CD004405.

Chavez-Bueno S, McCracken GH. Bacterial Meningitis in Children. Pediatr Clin N Am 2005;52:795.

Dodge PR. Neurological sequelae of acute bacterial meningitis. Pediatr Ann 1994;23:101.

Durbin WJ. Pneumococcal Infections. Pediatr Rev 2004;25:418.

Feigin RD. Use of Corticosteroids in Bacterial Meningitis. Pediatr Infect Dis J 2004;23:355.

Greenwood BM. Corticosteroids for acute bacterial meningitis. N Engl J Med 2007;357:2507.

Grimwood K, Anderson VA, Bond L, et al. Adverse outcomes of bacterial meningitis in school-age survivors. Pediatrics 1995;95:646.

Kanegaye JT, Soliemanzadeh P, Bradley JS. Lumbar puncture in pediatric bacterial meningitis: defining the time interval for the recovery of cerebrospinal fluid pathogens after parenteral antibiotic pretreatment. Pediatrics 2001;108:1169–74.

Kim KS. Acute bacterial meningitis in infants and children. Lancet Infect Dis 2010;10:32.

Lee BE, Davies HD. Aseptic meningitis. Curr Opin Infect Dis 20:272.

Mann K, Jackson MA. Meningitis. Pediatr Rev 2008;29;417.

Negrini B, Kelleher KJ, Wald ER. Cerebrospinal fluid findings in aseptic versus bacterial meningitis. Pediatrics 2000;105:316–9.

Odio CM, Faingezicht I, Paris M, et al. The beneficial effects of early dexamethasone administration on infants and children with bacterial meningitis. N Engl J Med 1991;324:1525.

Sáez-Llorens X, McCracken GH. Bacterial meningitis in children. Lancet 2003;361:2139.

Snedeker JD, Kaplan SL, Dodge PR, et al. Subdural effusion and its relationship with neurologic sequelae of bacterial meningitis in infancy: a prospective study. Pediatrics 1990;86:163.

van de Beek D, de Gans J, Tunkel AR, Wijdicks EF. Community-acquired bacterial meningitis in adults. N Engl J Med 2006;354:44.

van Rossum AMC, Wulkan RW, Oudesluys-Murphy AM. Procalcitonin as an early marker of infection in neonates and children. Lancet Infect Dis 2004;4:620.

Wald ER, Kaplan SL, Mason EO, et al. Dexamethasone therapy for children with bacterial meningitis. Meningitis Study Group. Pediatrics 1995;95:21–8.

Waler JA, Rathore MH. Outpatient management of pediatric bacterial meningitis. Pediatr Infect Dis J 1995;14:89.

Yogev R, Guzman-Cottrill J. Bacterial Meningitis in Children: Critical Review of Current Concepts. Drugs 2005;65(8):1097.

INTERNATIONAL PEDIATRICS

Common Illness after International Travel

Roopal Patel, MD, DTMH, and Judith C. Shlay, MD, MSPH

Each year, more than 50 million people from the industrialized countries visit the developing world, including more than 2 million children. Up to 8% of returning travelers are ill enough to seek medical care while either abroad or on returning home.

A. When a child presents with a medical condition, it is important to know the areas where the family has traveled, because the differential diagnosis will vary depending on the location(s) visited. Using information from the GeoSentinel surveillance network, a system of specialized travel and tropical medicine clinics on six continents, region-specific diagnoses have been elucidated. In addition, it is important to determine details of the child's travels: exposure to freshwater, contact with animals, mingling with local people, and receipt of travel immunizations and malaria chemoprophylaxis.

When a traveler presents with a medical condition, the evaluation should focus on the following questions:

- What infections are possible given the places visited?
- Which of these infections is more probable given the patient's clinical findings?
- Which of these infections is life-threatening, treatable, or transmissible?

The three most common symptoms reported after travel are diarrhea, fever (with or without systemic illness), and dermatologic conditions.

DIARRHEA

B. Traveler's diarrhea (TD), the sudden onset of three or more unformed stools in 24 hours, is a common complaint during or shortly after travel to a developing country. TD is usually acquired from drinking contaminated water and ingesting contaminated food, specifically through exposure to unboiled water or raw foods, but exposure history may be limited. Determine duration of symptoms, severity of symptoms, and whether diarrhea is associated with fever, vomiting, or blood in stools. Assess fluid intake and output. Most TD is self-limited, but persistent symptoms can occur in a small percentage of travelers. Diarrhea with onset more than 1 month after travel is unlikely to be due to exposure during travel.

Physical examination should include assessment of hydrations status, especially in infants and young children, with appropriate fluid administration if necessary (see p. 220).

C. Acute TD is defined as lasting less than 2 weeks; infectious agents are the predominant cause. Worldwide, enterotoxigenic *Escherichia coli*, which causes a secretory diarrhea, is the most common bacterial pathogen isolated. *Campylobacter jejuni*, *Salmonella* spp., *Shigella* spp., and enteroinvasive *E. coli* are less common causes of TD but are invasive pathogens that can cause more severe disease. Fever, bloody stools, or leukocytes seen on stool microscopy indicate probable invasive inflammatory enteropathy; however, a secretory diarrhea may predominate early in the course of illness. Viral pathogens such as rotavirus, which can cause significant morbidity in children, calicivirus (Norwalk and Norwalk-like viruses), and enteroviruses account for 5% to 10% of acute TD.

D. Persistent diarrhea is present if symptoms persist for longer than 2 weeks. *Giardia lamblia* is the most commonly identified intestinal parasite and presents with acute, watery diarrhea with abdominal pain and in protracted courses with foul-smelling stools and flatulence. Other enteric protozoa include *Entamoeba histolytica*, *Cryptosporidium parvum*, and *Cyclospora cayetanensis*. *E. histolytica*, although a rarer cause of persistent diarrhea, can cause severe invasive disease that can be complicated by liver abscess. Parasitic infections are more common in long-term travelers. Some travelers with prolonged diarrhea will no longer have an infectious cause but will have developed a postinfectious irritable bowel syndrome or a malabsorption syndrome.

E. A pathogen is identified in only 40% to 60% of patients with TD, and culture may not be necessary in mild, acute, secretory diarrhea. Collect a stool specimen for culture for enteric pathogens and microscopic examination for ova and parasites and leukocytes if there is evidence of invasive diarrhea, for persistent diarrhea, if the diarrhea was unresponsive to empirical therapy, or if the patient is immunocompromised. Antigen detection assays for *Giardia* are available.

F. Acute, noninflammatory mild diarrhea can be treated empirically with fluids and antibiotic administration. Widespread antibiotic resistance has developed among many enteric pathogens; therefore, antibiotics that are no longer recommended are the sulfonamides, neomycin, ampicillin, doxycycline, tetracycline, trimethoprim alone, and trimethoprim-sulfamethoxazole. Azithromycin is considered the first-line antibiotic therapy in children and will cover TD acquired in all destinations, including potential fluoroquinolone-resistant *Campylobacter* found in Southeast Asia. Duration of treatment is usually 3 days for acute diarrhea. Fluoroquinolones are first line in adults. Although there is some concern that fluoroquinolones, such as ciprofloxacin, are associated with transient musculoskeletal adverse effects in children, increasing evidence supports the pediatric use

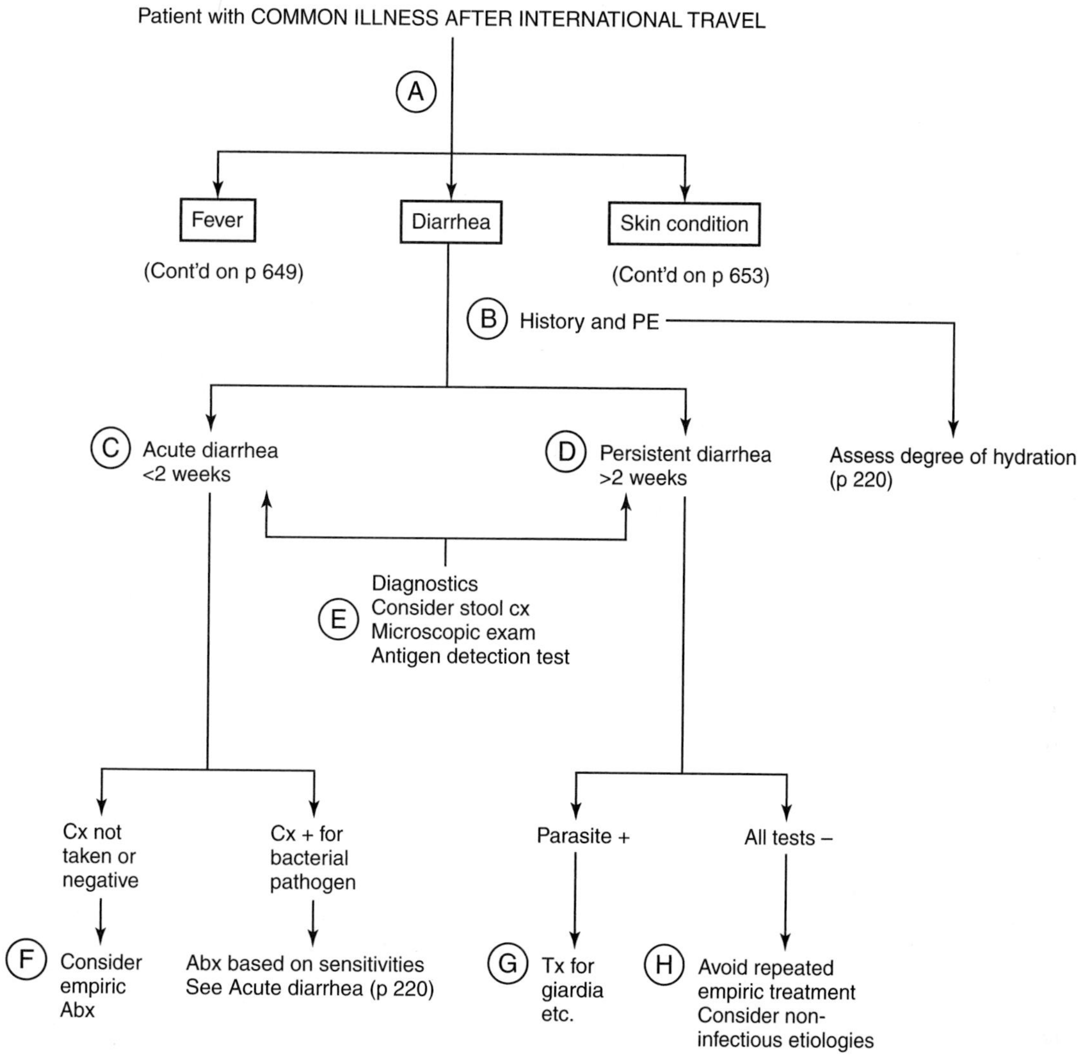
Patient with COMMON ILLNESS AFTER INTERNATIONAL TRAVEL
A
Fever
(Cont'd on p 649)
Diarrhea
Skin condition
(Cont'd on p 653)
B History and PE
C Acute diarrhea <2 weeks
D Persistent diarrhea >2 weeks
Assess degree of hydration (p 220)
E Diagnostics
Consider stool cx
Microscopic exam
Antigen detection test
Cx not taken or negative
Cx + for bacterial pathogen
Parasite +
All tests –
F Consider empiric Abx
Abx based on sensitivities
See Acute diarrhea (p 220)
G Tx for giardia etc.
H Avoid repeated empiric treatment
Consider non-infectious etiologies

of ciprofloxacin, particularly for short-course treatment. Rifaximin, a semisynthetic antibiotic, is an alternative for afebrile, nondysenteric TD and is approved for children older than 12 for the treatment of toxigenic *E. coli*. Antimotility agents, although effective in adults with TD, are not recommended in children younger than 2 years and should be used with caution in children between 2 and 12 years of age.

G. Metronidazole (5- to 10-day course) or tinidazole (single dose) are the drugs of choice for *Giardia*. Furazolidone and quinacrine are alternatives available outside of the United States. Treatment for symptomatic *E. histolytica* includes metronidazole or tinidazole, followed by a luminal amebicide such as iodoquinol and paromomycin.

H. Even if infectious causes for persistent diarrhea are not found, a single course of empiric treatment with azithromycin and/or metronidazole is warranted. Avoid repeated courses of empiric treatment. Dietary changes, include limiting lactose and fructose, may alleviate symptoms. Consider evaluation for noninfectious causes including postinfectious malabsorption, irritable bowel syndrome, and, if bloody stools are present, inflammatory bowel disease. Persistent diarrhea is often self-limited and will resolve over time.

FEVER

I. A febrile illness, with or without systemic symptoms, is a frequent presentation in a patient who has recently traveled internationally. Although potentially serious tropical infections such as malaria and dengue need prompt diagnosis and treatment, clinicians should not overlook common childhood illnesses including acute viral or bacterial infections.

Elicitation of travel history will help to narrow the differential diagnosis of fever. For example, malaria is the most frequently reported cause of fever in travelers returning from sub-Saharan Africa, whereas dengue is more commonly reported after travel to Southeast Asia. A careful review of the duration of travel, timing of symptom(s) onset related to dates of travel, and known incubation periods of key infectious diseases may help rule out certain causative factors. Exposure history, such as insect bites, whether the patient was visiting friends and family, or ingestion of raw foods may provide further clues to the cause of the febrile illness.

Perform a complete physical examination with a specific focus on vital signs, appearance (toxic or non-toxic), weight loss, pallor, rashes, including insect bites, and eschars, abdominal tenderness, hepatosplenomegaly, and lymphadenopathy.

Preliminary laboratory tests should identify the more common and potentially serious and treatable infections. Thick and thin smears should always be collected for immediate malaria testing. Blood cultures should also be sent, although empiric antibiotics may be needed before availability of results if the patient is very ill or clinical suspicion for a specific bacterial infection is high. Results of the complete blood cell count may help support preliminary diagnosis while other test results are pending.

(Continued on page 650)

Patient with COMMON ILLNESS AFTER INTERNATIONAL TRAVEL

(Cont'd from p 647)

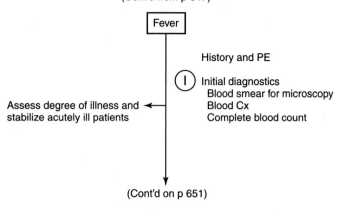

Fever

History and PE

(I) Initial diagnostics
- Blood smear for microscopy
- Blood Cx
- Complete blood count

→ Assess degree of illness and stabilize acutely ill patients

(Cont'd on p 651)

J. Malaria infections in humans are primarily caused by four *Plasmodium* species (*P. falciparum, P. vivax, P. malariae,* and *P. ovale*). The parasite is transmitted by an infective female *Anopheles* mosquito and transmission occurs worldwide in developing countries. Malaria in travelers, especially caused by *P. falciparum,* can cause severe and life-threatening disease, which can be prevented by appropriate chemoprophylaxis and prompt recognition by clinicians on return from travel. However, even with proper preventative measures, malaria can occur and a history of chemoprophylaxis should not exclude an evaluation for malaria. There are approximately 1500 imported cases reported annually in the United States, of which about two thirds are due to *P. falciparum* and one third due to *P. vivax*.

Most travelers (95%) become symptomatic within 30 days after return from travel. The incubation period depends on the species of *Plasmodium* and can be as short as 6 days, or for cases of *P. vivax* and *P. ovale,* up to years after the exposure. Fever is the predominant symptom, but sweats, rigors, gastrointestinal symptoms, headache, and/or malaise are often present. Early symptoms in children may mimic other common pediatric febrile illnesses, which may lead to a delay in diagnosis and treatment. Severe malaria presents with seizures, coma, renal failure, shock, or respiratory distress.

The gold standard for malaria diagnosis is the microscopic examination for parasites of thick and thin blood smears. The thick smear can detect even low levels of parasite, whereas the thin smear is used for species determination and parasitemia quantification. If the smears are negative, repeat blood smears should be taken 12 to 24 hours later. Three sets of negative smears taken 12 to 24 hours apart effectively exclude malaria as the cause of the fever. Supporting laboratory findings include thrombocytopenia without leukocytosis and, in cases of *P. falciparum,* increase of bilirubin and aminotransferases.

Patients with severe malaria, malaria caused by *P. falciparum,* or an unidentified species should be admitted to the hospital for initial treatment and monitoring of complications. *P. falciparum* resistance to chloroquine is widespread and increasing for *P. vivax;* therefore, treatment will depend on the drug susceptibility of the infecting parasites as determined by the geographic area where the infection was acquired (Table 1). Severe malaria should be treated with parenteral antimalarial therapy, and exchange transfusion should be strongly considered if the parasite density is more than 10% or if complications such as cerebral malaria, acute respiratory distress syndrome, or renal insufficiency exist.

K. Typhoid fever is a potentially severe, systemic illness caused by the bacterium *Salmonella enterica.* Travelers to endemic areas, including South Asia, Central and South America, Africa, and the Caribbean are exposed to the bacteria by the ingestion of contaminated food and beverages. Although immunization for typhoid fever is recommended for travelers, demonstrated effectiveness ranges from 50% to 80% for both oral Ty21a and intramuscular Vi capsular polysaccharide vaccines.

Incubation period is usually 7 to 14 (range, 3–60) days. Fever and malaise present early, followed by headache, abdominal pain, and diarrhea (more common in children, whereas constipation is more typical in adults). The fever increases in the second week of illness and "rose spots," a blanching erythematous maculopapular rash, can occur, but are reported in only 5% to 30% of cases. Other physical findings include a relative bradycardia, hepatosplenomegaly, and splenomegaly. Mental status changes can also occur. Severe typhoid with complications, which occur in 10% to 15% of cases, includes gastrointestinal bleeding, perforation, and typhoid encephalopathy accompanied by shock. Young children may present with a mild, febrile disease with sustained or intermittent bacteremia.

Isolation of *Salmonella typhi* from blood is diagnostic, with the highest sensitivity (60%–80%) in the first week of the disease. Multidrug-resistant isolates are common, especially in travelers returning from South Asia. Antibiotic choice should be based on severity of disease and susceptibility of the organism, but possible first-line options include third-generation cephalosporin, azithromycin, or a fluoroquinolone. Retreatment may be required if relapse of enteric fever occurs (up to 10% of patients).

L. The probable incubation period of the illness and travel destinations should be considered to focus the differential if initial tests are negative and suspicion for more common diseases is low (Table 2). Associated findings, such as hemorrhage, respiratory symptoms, eosinophilia, or rash, may also help narrow the differential. Further diagnostics, especially specific serologic assays, should be undertaken, and consultation with a travel medicine specialist may be warranted. Exotic travel-related diagnoses such as Ebola virus, rabies, Japanese encephalitis, plague, tularemia, yellow fever, among others, are quite rare; none of these infections is found in 17,353 returning travelers studied in 2006 from the GeoSentinel Surveillance.

M. *Dengue,* an arboviral infection that is transmitted by the *Aedes aegypti* mosquito, is seen most commonly in travelers from Asia and the Americas, with only a small proportion from Africa. After a typical incubation period of 4 to 7 days (range, 3–14 days), patients may experience a range of symptoms from a mild acute febrile illness to dengue hemorrhagic fever (DHF) or shock syndrome. DHF and dengue shock syndrome are not common among travelers because they occur primarily in patients who had a prior infection by a different dengue serotype. Dengue presents more classically in older children with sudden-onset fever, headache, retro-orbital pain, and myalgias, and in 50% of patients, a macular or maculopapular rash that appears at the end of the fever. Infants and young children may present with an undifferentiated fever, with or without the rash. Laboratory findings include thrombocytopenia, leukopenia with lymphopenia, mild-to-moderate increases in hepatic aminotransferases, and hyponatremia.

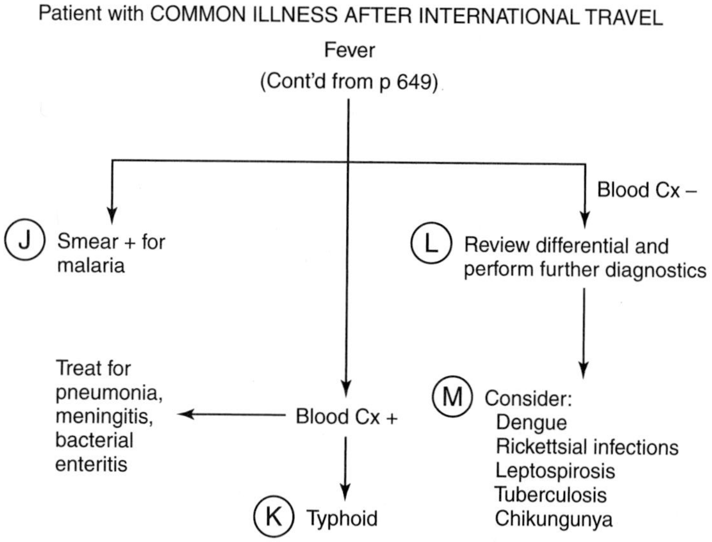
Patient with COMMON ILLNESS AFTER INTERNATIONAL TRAVEL
Fever
(Cont'd from p 649)
Blood Cx –
J
Smear + for malaria
L
Review differential and perform further diagnostics
Treat for pneumonia, meningitis, bacterial enteritis
Blood Cx +
M
Consider:
Dengue
Rickettsial infections
Leptospirosis
Tuberculosis
Chikungunya
K
Typhoid

Diagnosis of dengue is mainly clinical but can be confirmed by a fourfold increase in serum antibody in acute and convalescent serum. Diagnosis by viral culture or polymerase chain reaction tests is possible but limited by the sensitivity of the test.

Treatment is supportive and symptomatic because no specific therapeutic agents exist for dengue. For mild dengue, use antipyretics, bed rest, and fluid replacement. DHF may be heralded by decreasing platelet counts, especially at time of defervescence, and platelet counts should be monitored. Fresh frozen plasma should be administered if signs of disseminated intravascular coagulation are present, and prompt administration of intravenous fluids is indicated for DHF and signs of shock.

Rickettsial infections such as African tick typhus *(Rickettsia africae),* scrub typhus *(Orientia tsutsugamushi),* and Mediterranean tick typhus *(R. conorii),* are transmitted by arthropods and are more common after exposures to grassy areas such as on safari in sub-Saharan Africa. Symptoms of fever, headache, and myalgia are acute after an incubation period of 7 to 10 days (range, 3–21 days), and on physical examination a painless eschar at the inoculation site helps support the diagnosis. Other signs include rash, thrombocytopenia, leucopenia, and lymphadenopathy. Treatment should be given based on clinical suspicion while serologic confirmation of diagnosis is pending. Tetracyclines are the drug of choice even for children younger than 8 years, because effective treatment outweighs minimal risk for dental staining from one course of treatment.

Reports of *leptospirosis,* caused by growth in ecotourism and adventure sports, have increased in returning travelers and should be considered in older children with a history of exposure to freshwater (swimming, rafting, hiking). Symptoms include fever, headache, myalgia, and rash. Conjunctival suffusion occurs in less than half of the cases, and severe disease with jaundice and renal dysfunction (Weil syndrome), hemorrhagic pneumonitis, or circulatory collapse occurs in approximately 10% of patients. Diagnosis is made by isolation of spirochetes from blood or urine (low sensitivity) or by serologic diagnosis. The treatment of choice for hospitalized patients is intravenous penicillin. For milder disease, doxycycline can be used in children older than 8 years and ceftriaxone in younger patients.

Tuberculosis should be considered in pediatric patients who present with fever lasting longer than 2 weeks, in whom symptoms commence more than 2 weeks (up to months) after travel, patients with central nervous system findings, and especially, if patient had exposure to friends or family rather than short-term tourist destinations. A tuberculin skin test should be placed and radiographs considered (see p. 664).

Chikungunya virus, transmitted by the *Aedes* mosquito, is endemic to areas of Africa and Asia. The illness presents with acute onset of joint pain, followed by myalgia, fever, and rash with recovery usually within weeks. Clinical diagnosis is made first because confirmation requires demonstrating increase in antibodies using acute and convalescent serum. Chikungunya can present similarly to dengue; however, chikungunya infections are shorter in duration, and include a terminal maculopapular rash, arthralgia or arthritis, and conjunctival involvement. Hemorrhagic phenomena rarely occur with chikungunya infections. Treatment is supportive with antipyretics, analgesics, and fluids.

DERMATOLOGIC CONDITIONS

N. Skin conditions are common among persons who recently traveled. Most patients report that the skin lesions began while abroad. In the history, determine the duration of symptoms, relation to travel period, and possible exposures such as to freshwater or seawater, animals, or bites by insects or arthropods. The location of the lesions, their pattern (maculopapular, nodular, ulcerative, or linear), and the presence or absence of associated symptoms (such as pain, pruritus, fever, or other systemic symptoms) are useful in establishing the diagnosis. With symptoms of fever and rash, consider chikungunya virus, dengue, and rickettsial infections (see earlier). When the skin condition is the predominant presenting symptom, characterize on physical examination whether it is papular, nodular, an ulcer, or linear in nature. The most common dermatologic disorders reported by the GeoSentinel network included cutaneous larva migrans (9.8%), insect bites (8.2%), skin abscesses (7.7%), superinfected insect bites (6.8%), and allergic rash (5.5%). Other infections include dengue (3.4%) and leishmaniasis (3.3%).

O. Pruritic papules:

- *Insect bites* (bedbugs, fleas, scabies) generally occur in clusters or linear distributions. Bedbugs and fleas usually require only symptomatic therapy. For scabies, first-line treatment is either topical permethrin 5% cream or oral ivermectin. Close contacts need to be treated, and clothing and linen should be washed and dried or bagged for several days.
- *Seabather's eruption* is confined to skin covered by a bathing suit and associated with saltwater exposure. It is caused by larval forms of sea anemones and jellyfish. Treatment is usually with topical antihistamines and corticosteroids.
- *Cercarial* or *Schistosomal dermatitis* affects exposed skin and is caused by penetration of the skin by schistosomal cercariae in freshwater, resulting in an intense inflammatory response that is more rapid and severe if repeat exposures occur. Lesions usually resolve within a week. Treatment is symptomatic.
- *"Hot tub" folliculitis* is a diffuse folliculitis caused by *Pseudomonas aeruginosa* that contaminates swimming pools, hot tubs, whirlpools, or water slides. An itchy maculopapular eruption develops within 48 hours of exposure, especially in areas covered by bathing garments. Treatment is symptomatic.

P. Subcutaneous swelling and nodules:

- Common causes of fixed, painful subcutaneous swelling include myiasis, tungiasis, and furuncles. *Myiasis* is the invasion of the skin by the larvae of Diptera (flies) including the tumbu fly in Africa and the botfly in Latin America. Lesions resemble boils but have a central opening through which serosanguineous material oozes and where the larvae may emerge. Removal of the larvae is curative. *Tungiasis* (i.e., jiggers) develops after a female sand fly invades the skin, often around the toenail or soles of the feet, and is seen in travelers returning from Africa, South America, or India. Treatment is removal of the flea.
- Many parasites and other pathogens can cause nodules. Examples include echinococcosis, dirofilariasis, cysticercosis, coenurosis, and toxocariasis. Most occur in long-term travelers or immigrants and are rare in short-term travelers. Biopsy of accessible nodules is needed for diagnosis. Treatment is directed to the type of organism identified.

Q. Ulcers:

- *Ecthyma* (pyoderma) is the most frequent ulcer among travelers. It is a shallow, painful, purulent ulcer that results from skin trauma or bites that become secondarily infected, usually with *Staphylococcus aureus* or group A streptococci. Treatment consists of wound care and provision of antibiotics directed at the potential organisms.
- *Cutaneous leishmaniasis* presents with painless ulcers that typically enlarge slowly with a granulomatous or crusted base and raised margins. Leishmaniasis is spread by the bite of a female sandfly; it is diagnosed by finding amastigotes in tissue or on smears. Other manifestations include mucocutaneous and visceral, reflecting the tissue location of the infected macrophage. The drug of choice is either sodium stibogluconate or meglumine antimonate. Alternatives include pentamidine or paromomycins. Treatment duration may vary based on symptoms, host immune status, species, and the area of the world where the infection was acquired.

R. Linear and migratory lesions:

- *Cutaneous larva migrans* is the most frequent serpiginous lesion among travelers. It results from migration of animal hookworms in superficial tissues and is due to contact with contaminated soil/sand with dog/cat feces. It is most common on the foot or buttock. Indications for treatment are to relieve cutaneous symptoms and to prevent bacterial superinfections. Options include thiabendazole (topical), ivermectin (systemic), or albendazole (systemic). Antihistamines can be helpful in controlling pruritus.

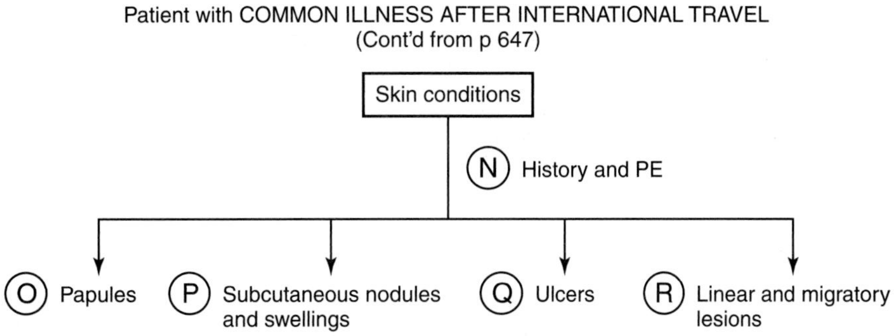
Patient with COMMON ILLNESS AFTER INTERNATIONAL TRAVEL
(Cont'd from p 647)
Skin conditions
(N) History and PE
(O) Papules
(P) Subcutaneous nodules and swellings
(Q) Ulcers
(R) Linear and migratory lesions

Table 1. **Pediatric Treatment Regimens for Uncomplicated and Severe Malaria**

Drug Options	Pediatric Dosage
Treatment for *Plasmodium falciparum* Acquired in Chloroquine-Resistant Areas or Species not Known—Uncomplicated Malaria	
Quinine sulfate + clindamycin (<8 years) or doxycycline, tetracycline (>8 years) (all oral) *or*	Quinine: 8.3-mg base/kg (= 10 mg salt/kg) orally (not to exceed the adult dose of 650 mg) three times daily for 3 days (infections acquired outside Southeast Asia) to 7 days (infections acquired in Southeast Asia) Clindamycin: 20-mg base/kg/day divided three times daily for 7 days Doxycycline: 2.2 mg/kg orally (not to exceed the adult dose of 100 mg) every 12 hours for 7 days Tetracycline: 25 mg/kg/day orally (not to exceed the adult dose of 250 mg) divided four times daily for 7 days
Artemether-lumefantrine (oral) *or*	1 tablet = 20 mg artemether and 120 mg lumefantrine A 3-day treatment schedule with a total of six oral doses is recommended for both adult and pediatric patients based on weight; the patient should receive the initial dose, followed by the second dose 8 hours later, then 1 dose PO bid for the following 2 days 5–<15 kg: 1 tablet per dose 15–<25 kg: 2 tablets per dose 25–<35 kg: 3 tablets per dose ≥35 kg: 4 tablets per dose
Atovaquone-Proguanil (oral) *or*	Pediatric tablet = 62.5 mg atovaquone/25 mg proguanil Adult tablet = 250 mg atovaquone/100 mg proguanil 5–8 kg: 2 pediatric tablets per day for 3 days >8–10 kg: 3 pediatric tablets per day for 3 days >10–20 kg: 1 adult tablet per day for 3 days >20–30 kg: 2 adult tablets per day for 3 days >30–40 kg: 3 adult tablets per day for 3 days >40 kg: 4 adult tablets per day for 3 days
Mefloquine (oral) *or*	13.7-mg base/kg (= 15 mg salt/kg) as initial dose, followed by 9.1-mg base/kg (= 10 mg salt/kg) given 6–12 hours after initial dose Total dose = 25 mg salt/kg (not to exceed the adult dose of 1250 mg salt)
Treatment for *P. falciparum* Acquired in Chloroquine-Sensitive Areas—Uncomplicated Malaria	
Chloroquine phosphate (oral)	10-mg base/kg immediately, followed by 5-mg base/kg at 6, 24, and 48 hours Total dose: 25-mg base/kg (not to exceed the adult dose of 1500-mg base)
Hydroxychloroquine sulfate (oral)	10-mg base/kg immediately, followed by 5-mg base/kg at 6, 24, and 48 h Total dose: 25-mg base/kg (not to exceed the adult dose of 1550-mg base)
Treatment of *P. vivax* Acquired in Chloroquine-Resistant Areas (See Later for Prevention of Relapse after Treatment)	
Atovaquone-Proguanil	As above
Oral quinine sulfate + doxycycline, tetracycline (>8 years)	As above
Mefloquine	As above
Treatment of all Plasmodium Other Than Chloroquine-Resistant *P. Falciparum* and *P. Vivax*	
Chloroquine phosphate	As above
Hydroxychloroquine	As above
Prevention of Relapse After Treatment for *P. Vivax and P. Ovale*	
Primaquine (if not G6PD deficient)	0.5-mg base/kg orally (not to exceed the adult dose of 30-mg base) per day for 14 days

Continued

Table 1. **Pediatric Treatment Regimens for Uncomplicated and Severe Malaria—cont'd**

Drug Options	Pediatric Dosage
Severe Malaria or Unable to Take Oral Medications	
Intravenous quinidine gluconate plus clindamycin (<8 years) or doxycycline, tetracycline (>8 years)	Quinidine: 6.25-mg base/kg (= 10 mg salt/kg) loading dose IV over 1–2 hours, then 0.0125-mg base/kg/min (= 0.02 mg salt/kg/min) continuous infusion for at least 24 hours Alternative regimen exist (see package insert) Once parasite density <1% and patient can take oral medication, complete treatment with oral quinine, dose as above Clindamycin: 10-mg base/kg loading dose IV followed by 5-mg base/kg IV every 8 h; switch to oral clindamycin as soon as patient can take oral medication; treatment course is 7 days Doxycycline: IV only if patient is not able to take oral medication; for children <45 kg, give 2.2 mg/kg IV every 12 hours and then switch to oral doxycycline as soon as patient can take oral medication; for children >45 kg, start with 100 mg IV every 12 hours; treatment course is 7 days Tetracycline: IV dose same as oral, use until able to take oral medications Investigational new drug (contact CDC for information): artesunate followed by one of the following: atovaquone-proguanil, doxycycline (clindamycin in pregnant women), or mefloquine

CDC, Centers for Disease Control and Prevention; *G6PD,* glucose 6-phosphate dehydrogenase; *IV,* intravenously; *PO,* orally.

Table 2. **Incubation Period of Infections That May Cause Fever in Pediatric Travelers**

Incubation Period	Diseases
<14 days	Malaria, dengue, typhoid, chikungunya, rickettsial infections, leptospirosis, salmonellosis, shigellosis, acute hepatitis, influenza, yellow fever,* East African trypanosomiasis, meningococcemia, enteroviruses, rabies,* bacterial and viral pneumonia, parvovirus B19, acute histoplasmosis,* acute coccidioidomycosis,* measles, varicella, arboviral encephalitis, bacterial or viral meningitis, acute human immunodeficiency virus infection,* viral hemorrhagic infections*
14 days to 6 weeks	Malaria, typhoid, tuberculosis, acute schistosomiasis, hepatitis A, hepatitis E,* amebic liver abscess, leptospirosis
>6 weeks	Malaria, tuberculosis, visceral leishmaniasis,* lymphatic filariasis, onchocerciasis, schistosomiasis, amebic liver abscess, rabies,* African trypanosomiasis, typhoid fever

*Rare causes in pediatric travelers.

References

Centers for Disease Control and Prevention. Health information for international travel 2008. Atlanta, GA: U.S. Department of Health and Human Service, Public Health Service; 2007.

Freedman DO. Clinical practice. Malaria prevention in short-term travelers. N Engl J Med 2008;359(6):603–12.

Freedman DO, Weld LH, Kozarsky PE, et al. Spectrum of disease and relation to place of exposure among ill returned travelers. N Engl J Med 2006;354(2):119–30.

Greenwood Z, Black J, Weld L, et al. Gastrointestinal infection among international travelers globally. J Travel Med 2008;15(4):221–8.

Griffith KS, Lewis LS, Mali S, Parise ME. Treatment of malaria in the United States: a systematic review. JAMA 2007;297(20):2264–77.

Hill DR, Ericsson CD, Pearson RD, et al. The practice of travel medicine: guidelines by the Infectious Diseases Society of America. Clin Infect Dis 2006;43:1499–1539.

Parry CM, Hien TT, Dougan G, et al. Typhoid fever. N Engl J Med 2002;347(22):1770–82.

Ryan ET, Wilson ME, Kain KC. Illness after international travel. N Engl J Med 2002;347(7):505–16.

Sethuraman U, Kamat D. Management of child with fever after international travel. Clin Pediatr 2007;46:222–7.

Taylor DN, Connor BA, Shlim DR. Chronic diarrhea in the returned traveler. Med Clin North Am 1999;83(4):1033–52. p. vii.

Thielman NM, Guerrant RL. Clinical practice: Acute infectious diarrhea. N Engl J Med 2004;350(1):38–47.

Wilder-Smith A, Schwartz E. Dengue in travelers. N Engl J Med 2005;353(9):924–32.

Management of Common Illnesses in Developing Countries at First-Level Health Facilities

Roopal Patel, MD, DTMH, and Eric A. F. Simoes, MBBS, DCH, MD

According to the World Health Organization (WHO) and UNICEF, almost 10 million deaths per year occur in children younger than 5 years, mostly in developing countries. One third of the deaths occur during the first month of life mainly because of prematurity and low birth weight, neonatal infections (sepsis and pneumonia), birth asphyxia, and birth trauma. After the neonatal period, the most common causes of death are pneumonia (19%), diarrhea (17%), malaria (8%), and measles (4%). Human immunodeficiency virus/acquired immune deficiency syndrome (HIV/AIDS) accounts for only 3% of deaths overall but may be an underlying condition leading to other causes of death, and prevalence in children varies by region across resource-limited settings. Malnutrition is an underlying factor in 35% to 50% of deaths. Poverty, unsafe water, poor sanitation, and limited access to medical care contribute to high rates of death in young children in developing countries. Effective prevention and treatment strategies such as vaccines, antibiotics, and oral rehydration exist for the most common illnesses seen in developing countries. However, the fundamental challenge is to deliver these services in the context of poverty, limited access to medical care, and the underdeveloped medical infrastructure seen in many developing countries.

The Integrated Management of Childhood Illness (IMCI) is a strategy developed in the 1990s by WHO and other institutions to provide evidence-based and effective prevention and treatment measures for the most common childhood illnesses in resource-limited settings. In developing countries, patients often seek initial medical care at first-level health facilities such as health posts or health centers. Primary health facilities are usually staffed by health care workers with limited medical training. IMCI guidelines therefore rely on simple clinical symptoms and signs to allow the health worker to assess a child's symptoms, classify the illness, and guide management, including determining which children need referral to higher levels of care. IMCI focuses on pneumonia, diarrhea, malaria, measles, malnutrition, immunization, and treatment of the infant younger than 60 days. Since the 1990s, several revisions have been made to the IMCI guidelines based on research and field tests, including recommendations for use in high HIV transmission settings, inclusion of dengue, care for child development, and a new guideline for the young infant that extends from birth to 60 days of age. This chapter uses the IMCI approach to outline the management of the most common illnesses in children younger than 5, excluding the first 60 days of age, at primary level health facilities.

A. Important first steps in the assessment of a sick child at the first-level health facility begin with an assessment for general danger signs to determine whether immediate referral to a higher level of care is needed. The health worker should inquire about seizures, determine whether the child is lethargic or unconscious, if they vomit everything, and whether they are able to drink. These findings are indicative of very severe disease such as cerebral or other forms of severe malaria, severe hypoxemic pneumonia, meningitis, severe dehydration, or shock caused by other serious illnesses (e.g., sepsis and dengue shock syndrome). A child with one or more of these signs should be considered seriously ill, and after the administration of prereferral treatment, referred urgently to a higher level of care for further evaluation, diagnosis, and treatment.

(Continued on page 658)

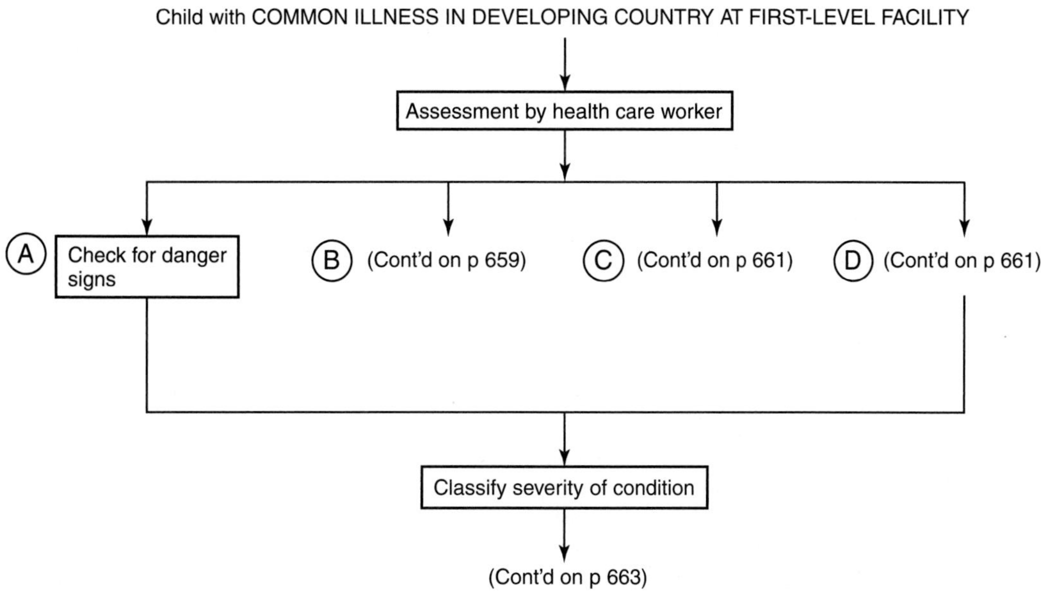
Child with COMMON ILLNESS IN DEVELOPING COUNTRY AT FIRST-LEVEL FACILITY
Assessment by health care worker
A
Check for danger signs
B
(Cont'd on p 659)
C
(Cont'd on p 661)
D
(Cont'd on p 661)
Classify severity of condition
(Cont'd on p 663)

B. Next, the health worker asks the caretaker about the presence of four main presenting symptoms: cough or difficulty breathing, diarrhea, fever, and ear problems. For each symptom, the IMCI algorithm uses a limited number of clinical signs, based on evidence of their sensitivity and specificity, to detect and then classify the severity of disease. Every child (even those with general danger signs) is assessed for the presence or absence of these symptoms.

Pneumonia, or acute lower respiratory tract infection, is the single most important cause of mortality in children younger than 5 years in developing countries. A child with cough or difficulty breathing should be evaluated for: (1) respiratory rate, (2) lower chest wall in-drawing, and (3) stridor. Increases to greater than age-specific respiratory rates have been shown to have a good sensitivity and specificity for detecting pneumonia in children. For infants 2 to 11 months of age, fast breathing is defined as 50 or more breaths per minute, and for 1 to 5 years of age, it is more than 40 breaths per minute. Lower chest wall in-drawing, noted in the absence of agitation, nose blockage, or active breastfeeding, indicates severe pneumonia. The presence of stridor, a sign of upper airway obstruction such as croup, requires urgent referral. Infants and children are classified as having severe pneumonia or very severe disease (danger signs, lower chest wall in-drawing, stridor), pneumonia (fast breathing alone), or upper respiratory tract infections (cough or difficult breathing without significant findings). Although several pathogens may cause pneumonia, the best evidence suggests that respiratory syncytial virus, *Haemophilus influenzae* type b (Hib), and *Streptococcus pneumoniae* are the leading causes in developing countries. Pulmonary tuberculosis (TB) presenting as pneumonia is increasingly common in young children in areas of high HIV transmission. Overlap of TB and pneumonia symptoms may initially lead to antibiotic treatment for cases of pulmonary TB, but health workers should be trained to refer patients who return without response to treatment, with chronic cough, or other signs of worsening.

A sick child with watery or bloody *diarrhea* is assessed to identify acute watery diarrhea, dysentery (bloody diarrhea), or persistent diarrhea (>14 days), and to classify hydration status. Bacterial pathogens are more common than viral pathogens in developing countries. The most common bacterial causes of diarrhea are *Escherichia coli, Shigella* spp., *Campylobacter* spp., *Salmonella,* and *Vibrio* spp. In countries where mortality caused by diarrhea is decreasing, viral pathogens such as rotavirus and noroviruses may have increased importance as causative agents of diarrhea. Parasitic causative agents, such as *Giardia lamblia, Cryptosporidium parvum, Cyclospora cayetanensis,* and, rarely in this age group, *Entamoeba histolytica,* are less common than bacterial and viral agents in developing countries. However, the former three are increasingly being recognized as important causes of diarrhea and persistent diarrhea in HIV-positive infants and children. Persistent diarrhea accounts for 10% to 15% of all diarrhea cases seen at first-level facilities, but accounts for up to 50% of deaths caused by diarrhea.

Table 1. **Classification of Dehydration Based on Clinical Signs**

Degree of Dehydration	Findings
Severe dehydration	Two of the following signs: Lethargic or unconscious Sunken eyes Not able to drink or drinks poorly (weak and requires help) Skin pinch test is very slow (>2 seconds)
Some dehydration	Two of the following signs: Restless or irritable Sunken eyes Drinks eagerly, thirsty Skin pinch test is slow (<2 seconds, skin stays up even briefly after pinch)
No dehydration	Not enough signs to classify as severe or some dehydration

Health care workers should ask how long the diarrhea has lasted and if there is blood in the stool. Assessment for dehydration should include the degree of lethargy or restlessness, sunken eyes, reaction when offered a drink, and elasticity of skin. There may be overlap of findings that are actually caused by severe malnutrition rather than diarrhea (sunken eyes). The degree of dehydration (Table 1) and classification of acute, persistent, or bloody diarrhea will then determine the treatment.

Fever is often the main reason a child presents to the health facility. A fever may be caused by a minor viral illness or an upper respiratory infection, but of immediate concern is the need to identify children with potentially life-threatening conditions, such as malaria, measles, meningitis/sepsis, or dengue. The guidelines use a temperature greater than 37.5° C axillary or 38° C rectal to define a fever; in the absence of a thermometer, feeling "hot" by history or examination is acceptable to enter into the algorithm. The duration of fever should also be determined. To identify other possible conditions, a child with fever should also be assessed for a stiff neck, upper respiratory tract symptoms, rash or history of rash, and other accompanying symptoms.

Malaria transmission is widespread in tropical and some subtropical countries, and causes an estimated 250 to 500 million cases each year. Four species of *Plasmodium* cause human malaria (*P. falciparum, P. vivax, P. malariae,* and *P. ovale*); *P. falciparum* predominates in Africa (except North Africa), and *P. vivax* is more often found in Central America, Asia, and North Africa. Uncomplicated malaria usually presents with fever, sweats, rigors, gastrointestinal symptoms, headache, and/or malaise. Early symptoms in children may mimic other common pediatric febrile illnesses, and severe malaria may commence with fever but then quickly lead to respiratory distress, shock, impaired consciousness, and/or seizures. The gold standard for diagnosis is microscopic detection of parasites on a stained peripheral blood smear. The availability of rapid diagnostic tests for malaria, decreasing malaria transmission, and

Child with COMMON ILLNESS IN DEVELOPING COUNTRY AT FIRST-LEVEL FACILITY

(Cont'd from p 657)

(B) Main symptoms:
- Cough/difficulty breathing
- Diarrhea
- Fever
- Ear problems

increasing resistance of antimalarials with the need to use more expensive drugs such as Artemisinin-based combination treatments has led to a shift away from presumptive treatment for malaria. WHO now recommends prompt parasitologic confirmation of malaria infection before treatment. As a result, developing countries are expanding the use of rapid diagnostic tests and microscopy at primary health facilities. Treatment based solely on clinical suspicion should be reserved for settings where diagnostics are not available.

The classification of fever includes severe febrile disease, defined as fever in combination with any danger sign or stiff neck; urgent referral with pretreatment is required. These children may have severe malaria, severe pneumonia, or other life-threatening infections such as bacterial sepsis or meningitis. *S. pneumoniae,* Hib, and meningococcus are the leading causes of meningitis and serious bacterial infections in the developing world; however, the burden of these infections is expected to decrease with the anticipated increased coverage of Hib and pneumococcal vaccines in developing countries. *Salmonella typhi* and *Staphylococcus aureus* are also important pathogens that cause meningitis or sepsis, especially in high HIV prevalence settings.

According to WHO estimates, there are 30 million cases of *measles* annually. Measles is an acute, viral illness characterized initially by fever, cough, coryza, conjunctivitis, and pinpoint blue and white spots in the buccal mucosa called *Koplik spots.* An erythematous rash then appears that typically starts at the hairline and forehead, then moves downward to involve the rest of the body. Other symptoms include anorexia, stomatitis, and generalized lymphadenopathy. Measles virus has a prolonged immunomodulatory effect (decreases both T and B lymphocytes), predisposing patients to secondary viral and bacterial infections, as well as reactivation of TB. Complications of measles can be severe and include otitis media, pneumonia, croup, diarrhea, and xerophthalmia, which can rapidly progress to keratomalacia, especially in the context of vitamin A deficiency. Complications can occur up to 3 months after the initial illness. Vitamin A deficiency is a major public health problem in Africa and South East Asia and is a significant cause of preventable blindness in children and a risk factor for severe measles. Administration of vitamin A as part of the treatment of measles has been associated with improved outcomes in children in developing countries. An effective measles vaccine is available as part of routine global immunization programs for children, and there have been recent efforts to improve vaccination coverage in young children in developing countries. According to IMCI, severe measles is fever and rash in addition to runny nose, conjunctivitis, or cough, and with any danger sign, severe stomatitis, or eye ulceration. A child with less severe measles, no danger signs, and only minor eye and mouth complications does not require urgent referral.

The next step in the IMCI algorithm is to assess for *ear problems*. Ear problems, such as chronic ear infections, are potentially preventable causes of deafness in developing countries. Furthermore, an ear infection could be a complication of measles and chronic ear drainage may be an indication of underlying HIV disease in areas of high transmission. If otoscopy is not available, the assessment includes determination of whether there is a history of ear pain or ear drainage and examining the child for signs of mastoiditis, specifically for tenderness and swelling behind the ear. The health care worker should distinguish mastoiditis, which would need referral, from acute and chronic ear infections, which may be managed in the outpatient setting.

C. After assessing danger signs and the four main symptoms (cough or difficult breathing, diarrhea, fever, and ear problems), *nutritional status* is assessed for all children. All children younger than 2 years have their feeding assessed and any feeding problems remedied. Malnutrition in developing countries is most often due to inadequate diet and affects an estimated 55 million children. Poverty, food insecurity and conflict, poor sanitation, maternal undernutrition, and chronic infections all contribute to malnutrition. Among children in developing countries throughout the world, repeated episodes of infection, together with mild but continued deficits in dietary intake, result in a process of suboptimal growth. The usual outcome of this process is that the child becomes stunted, and has height and consequently also weight below that of adequately nourished children of the same age. Stunting generally begins in infancy and develops in the first 2 years of life; after this age, stunting reflects past malnutrition. Therefore, although a nutrition intervention such as a program of sustained supplementation can improve linear growth among the very young, it will have little effect for children older than 2 to 3 years. By contrast, infections, such as dysentery or persistent diarrhea, and acute severe food deprivation generally result in wasting, a condition some authors call *acute malnutrition*. This form of malnutrition can be seen as an acute disease, which develops relatively rapidly, and may respond well to acute treatment. Severe acute malnutrition can be seen as a medical emergency because the immediate mortality is high.

The conventional assessment of nutritional status depends on the interpretation of several indicators (weight-for-age, height-for-age, and weight-for-height, collectively called *anthropometry*). Because IMCI is designed for use in settings where length boards are not generally available, indicators that do not require the measurement of length or height are used. The clinical assessment for malnutrition also includes examination for signs of severe physical wasting, seen often in the extremities, buttocks and rib cage, and edema of feet. Pallor of the palms is a nonspecific measure of anemia.

For severe malnutrition, IMCI uses edema of both feet to diagnose kwashiorkor and visible severe wasting to diagnose marasmus, both detected by visual inspection by a trained observer. These indicators are associated with an increased short-term risk for death, and intervention has been shown to avert some of these deaths. For these children, urgent referral to the hospital is needed.

For moderate acute malnutrition, the usual indicator is low weight-for-height. Because height or length measurements will not be available in most settings, ICMI uses very low weight-for-age as the indicator for protein-energy malnutrition. These children need a careful feeding assessment, and any feeding problems need to be remedied by nutritional counseling. These very low weight-for-age children have their weight gain monitored in a follow-up visit.

Severely malnourished children should also be assessed for HIV infection and accompanying serious bacterial infection, which can occur in up to 60% of cases. Anemia may be a result of malnutrition, iron deficiency, chronic infections including intestinal parasites, or malaria. In areas endemic with hookworm, ascaris, or other intestinal parasites, routine, presumptive administration of mebendazole is often recommended.

For all children, the immunization status should then be reviewed. In most cases, vaccination updates can be given at the same health care visit. Obvious exceptions may include those requiring immediate referral for serious conditions.

D. Depending on the burden of other infectious diseases in a country, the health care worker may need to consider other diagnoses. For example, an estimated 2.3 million children are living with *HIV/AIDS* worldwide, most in developing countries, particularly sub-Saharan Africa. More than half of children with HIV/AIDS who are not started on antiretroviral therapy die before 2 years of age from opportunistic infections and common diseases targeted by IMCI. Therefore, IMCI guidelines have been tailored for areas of high HIV transmission to include an assessment aimed at identification of HIV-exposed or HIV-infected children. If the results of the initial assessment identify a child with possible pneumonia, persistent diarrhea, chronic ear discharge, malnutrition, or if the mother is known to be HIV positive, then the health care workers should assess for other signs of HIV infection such as persistent skin and mouth conditions, oral thrush, generalized lymphadenopathy, or history of repeated infections such as pneumonia or diarrhea that were not responsive to standard treatment. TB and *Pneumocystis carinii,* infections found in children with moderate and severe HIV disease, may initially be confused with bacterial pneumonia; however, severity or recurrence of symptoms should prompt referral for further evaluation. Children with suspected HIV infection should be referred to appropriate facilities for further care, including counseling and testing, if HIV services are not available at the primary care level.

Dengue, an arboviral infection that is transmitted by the *Aedes aegypti* mosquito, is not included in the standard IMCI guidelines but is a potentially serious cause of childhood fever and rash in areas such as tropical Asia, Latin America, and the Caribbean. There are four serotypes of the virus that cause infection, and the risk for severe disease is greatly increased during secondary infections, in part because immunity is serotype specific. Primary infection, which is often asymptomatic or a mild febrile illness, occurs more commonly in children younger than 5; severe forms of dengue such as dengue hemorrhagic fever and dengue shock syndrome may occur in older children who are not covered under IMCI guidelines. Major signs with highest sensitivity and specificity for severe dengue requiring urgent referral are shock, altered sensorium, and bleeding. Some countries with endemic dengue have also instituted separate algorithms for the diagnosis and management of dengue to cover all at-risk age groups.

(Continued on page 662)

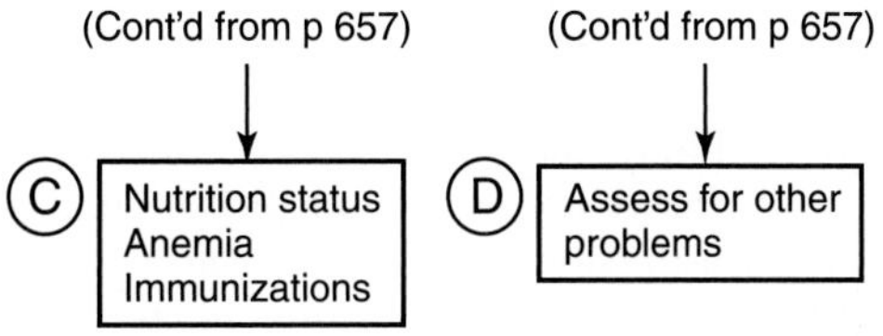
(Cont'd from p 657)
(Cont'd from p 657)
C
Nutrition status
Anemia
Immunizations
D
Assess for other
problems

E. Children with severe disease with or without danger signs should be referred to secondary or tertiary levels of care where a specific diagnosis can be made and appropriate treatment given. Prereferral treatment for specific conditions is warranted because delays in reaching referral facilities may lead to increased morbidity and mortality of disease (Table 2). For example, for severe febrile illness in areas of high malaria transmission, IMCI guidelines recommend giving a dose of injectable quinine. Artemisinins act more rapidly than other classes of antimalarial drugs to clear parasites, and national treatment guidelines may recommend injectable artemether or rectal artesunate as preferred alternatives to quinine. Antibiotics are also recommended because at the primary health level, serious bacterial infection cannot be differentiated from severe malaria. Intramuscular administration of ampicillin and gentamicin, chloramphenicol, or ceftriaxone should be given, which provide appropriate coverage for the most common causes of serious bacterial infections. Antibiotic administration is also warranted in the case of referral of severe measles because of the risk for bacterial superinfection. In most settings, district and referral hospitals have diagnostic capabilities to confirm a diagnosis and provide directed rather than presumptive treatment.

F. Treatment for less severe conditions is given on an outpatient basis and should also include clear follow-up instructions. For pneumonia, oral amoxicillin or cotrimoxazole for 5 days offers appropriate coverage for *S. pneumoniae* or *H. influenzae.* However, if a cough is present for more than 3 weeks or if there is recurrent wheezing, the patient should be referred for assessment of possible TB or asthma.

Antibiotics are not routinely used for acute or persistent diarrhea; however, ciprofloxacin is given in cases of dysentery, specifically targeting *Shigella*. Management of diarrhea includes addressing dehydration with oral rehydration solutions and encouraging continued feeding and breast-feeding. IMCI guidelines include specific rehydration instructions depending on weight and degree of response to rehydration.

In the face of increasing resistance, Artemisinin-based combination treatments are recommended as first-line agents for uncomplicated malaria. In settings without diagnostics to confirm malaria in suspected fever cases, antimalarials should only be given for fever in the absence of other symptoms such as upper respiratory tract symptoms, measles, or other obvious cause of fever.

Measles without severe complications should be treated with vitamin A, and if eye findings are present, with tetracycline eye ointment. Gentian violet may also be applied to stomatitis.

Acute ear infections can be managed in the outpatient setting with oral antibiotics (usually same as used for pneumonia) and drainage from chronic ear infections can be cleaned, although antibiotics are not recommended in this setting.

Moderate malnutrition can be effectively managed in the outpatient setting with the use of nutrient-rich supplemental foods. Home-based treatment with ready-to-use therapeutic food has been show to be effective even in cases of stabilized severe malnutrition.

Anemia may be treated with iron, mebendazole if the child is older than 1 year and has not received treatment within 6 months, and an antimalarial in high transmission areas may be considered. Response to treatment should be assessed in regular follow-up and the child referred if the pallor does not resolve within 2 months.

G. Home management is appropriate for mild illnesses such as upper respiratory infections, mild diarrhea without dehydration, or simple measles, after vitamin A administration. Successful home treatment depends on how well the caretaker understands the instructions given by the health care worker, and IMCI training includes modules on giving appropriate treatment advice.

H. Counseling of caretakers is an essential component contributing to the effectiveness of the IMCI strategy. For any ill child who is sent home, counseling about appropriate feeding and rehydration during illness and for follow-up care should be given. In practice, the following tasks are performed: (1) assessing the child's feeding; (2) identifying feeding problems; (3) counseling the mother about feeding problems; (4) advising the mother to increase fluid during illness; and (5) advising the mother when to return for follow-up visits, when to return immediately for further care, and when to return for immunizations.

Health workers also provide counseling about disease prevention, nutrition, and immunizations. The impact of the nutrition counseling component of IMCI has been studied in randomized, controlled trials and has been shown to result in improved weight gain in children contributing to the prevention of malnutrition. IMCI counseling also contains a holistic approach to disease prevention and emphasizes counseling mothers about their own health.

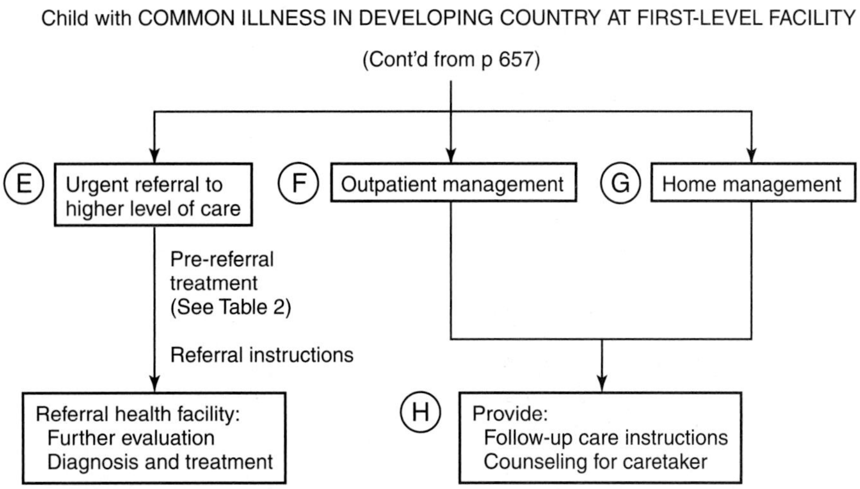
Child with COMMON ILLNESS IN DEVELOPING COUNTRY AT FIRST-LEVEL FACILITY
(Cont'd from p 657)
E
Urgent referral to higher level of care
F
Outpatient management
G
Home management
Pre-referral treatment (See Table 2)
Referral instructions
Referral health facility: Further evaluation Diagnosis and treatment
H
Provide: Follow-up care instructions Counseling for caretaker

Table 2. **Conditions Requiring Urgent Referral with Recommended Prereferral Treatment**

Classification of Illness	Prereferral Treatment
For all children before referral: Prevent low blood sugar by giving breast milk or sugar water.	
Seizure	Administer diazepam rectally, repeat dose if seizure continues
	Oxygen
Severe pneumonia or very severe disease	First dose of appropriate antibiotic
	Recommendations: ampicillin and gentamicin (IM)
	Chloramphenicol (IM)
	Ceftriaxone (IM)
	If able to take oral medications, can consider cotrimoxazole, amoxicillin
Severe febrile illness	First dose of intramuscular quinine or artemether
	First dose of antibiotics (as above)
	Antipyretic
Severe complicated measles	First dose of antibiotics (as above)
	Vitamin A
	Tetracycline eye ointment for eye findings
Severe dehydration	If facility can give intravenous fluid, start Ringer lactate solution (normal saline if not available); otherwise, refer as soon as possible
	ORS as soon as patient able to drink
	If delays in referral anticipated, consider nasogastric tube for ORS administration
Severe persistent diarrhea	Treat dehydration if present before referral
Mastoiditis	First dose of antibiotics (as above)
Severe malnutrition	First dose of antibiotics (as above) if signs of severe febrile disease also present
	Vitamin A

IM, intramuscularly; *ORS,* oral rehydration solution.

References

Black RE, Allen LH, Bhutta ZA, et al. Maternal and child undernutrition: global and regional exposures and health consequences. Lancet 2008;371(9608):243–60.

Black RE, Morris SS, Bryce J. Where and why are 10 million children dying every year? Lancet 2003;361:2226–34.

Boschi-Pinto C, Velebit L, Shibuya K. Estimating child mortality due to diarrhea in developing countries. Bull World Health Organ 2008;86:710–17.

Crawley J, Nahlen B. Prevention and treatment of malaria in young African children. Semin Pediatr Infect Dis 2004;15:169–80.

Gove S. Integrated management of childhood illness by outpatient health workers: technical basis and overview. Bull World Health Organ 1997;75:7–24.

Hoekstra EJ, McFarland JW, Shaw C, Salama P. Reducing measles mortality, reducing child mortality. Lancet 2006;368(9541):1050–2.

Manary MJ, Sandige HL. Management of acute moderate and severe childhood malnutrition. BMJ 2008;337:a2180.

Podewils LJ, Mintz ED, Nataro JP, Parashar UD. Acute, infectious diarrhea among children in developing countries. Semin Pediatr Infect Dis 2004;15(3):155–68.

Santos I, Victora CG, Martines J, et al. Nutrition counseling increases weight gain among Brazilian children. J Nutr 2001;131:2866–73.

Simoes EA, Desta T, Tessema T, et al. Performance of health workers after training in integrated management of childhood illness in Gondar, Ethiopia. Bull World Health Organ 1997;75:43–53.

Williams BG, Gouws E, Boschi-Pinto C, et al. Estimates of world-wide distribution of child deaths from acute respiratory infections. Lancet Infect Dis 2002;2:25–32.

World Health Organization, Department of Child and Adolescent Health and Development. Dengue, dengue haemorrhagic fever and dengue shock syndrome in the context of the integrated management of childhood illness. Geneva, Switzerland: World Health Organization; 2005.<http://whqlibdoc.who.int/hq/2005/WHO_FCH_CAH_05.13_eng.pdf>; 2005 [accessed 29.04.11].

World Health Organization, Department of Child and Adolescent Health and Development. Integrated management of childhood illness. WHO recommendations on the management of diarrhoea and pneumonia in HIV-infected infants and children. Geneva, Switzerland: World Health Organization; 2009. <http://whqlibdoc.who.int/publications/2010/9789241548083_eng.pdf>; 2009 [accessed 29.04.11].

Yehuda B, Fernando S. Integrated management of childhood illness: an emphasis on the management of infectious diseases. Semin Pediatr Infect Dis 2006;17:80–98.

Tuberculosis

John W. Ogle, MD

Tuberculosis (TB) is a disease caused by *Mycobacterium tuberculosis* and other closely related mycobacterial species (*M. bovis, M. africanum*). *M. tuberculosis* produces either latent infection or active tuberculous disease. Latent infection is the presence of a positive skin test with no sign or symptom of active TB and a normal chest radiograph. Active TB can involve almost any organ system but most commonly infects the lungs, pleura, central nervous system, lymphatic system, kidneys, bladder, bones, and joints.

A. Ask about exposures to active TB and any risk factors for development of active TB. In childhood TB, the disease is usually contracted from an adult with active TB. Detail any close contact with persons at high risk for TB, including foreign-born persons from high-prevalence areas, the homeless, the incarcerated, human immunodeficiency virus (HIV)–positive individuals, intravenous drug users, nursing home residents, and the medically underserved. Risk factors for progression of infection to active TB include young age (<4 years), recent infection with TB (<2 years), HIV infection, diabetes mellitus, prolonged corticosteroid therapy, other immunosuppressive therapy, leukemia, lymphoma, other cancers, end-stage renal disease, chronic malabsorption syndromes, and low body weight (10% or more less than ideal).

Symptoms of pulmonary TB include a prolonged or productive cough, hemoptysis, and chest pain. Symptoms of TB meningitis include changes in mental status, irritability, difficulty feeding, decreased responsiveness, and seizures. Systemic symptoms of active TB include fever, chills, night sweats, weight loss, and easy fatigability. Many children with active TB have subtle symptoms or are asymptomatic.

B. TB is often a slowly progressive disease, and many children with active TB have normal examinations. On physical examination, look, listen, and feel for findings that suggest meningitis (irritability, lethargy, unresponsiveness, full fontanelle, nuchal rigidity, presence of Kernig and Brudzinski signs) or pneumonia (tachypnea, retractions, nasal flaring, crackles). Examine for signs of adenitis or soft-tissue abscess (swelling, redness, or induration) or bone or joint infection (refusal to use limb, swollen joint, limitation of joint motion).

C. The Mantoux method of tuberculin skin testing (referred to as PPD or TST) is the preferred method of testing for TB infection in children. A PPD test can be performed during the same visit that immunizations are given, and a previous immunization with bacille Calmette–Guérin (BCG) is not a contraindication to placement of a PPD. The test involves the intradermal administration of 0.1 ml of 5 tuberculin units of purified protein derivative on the volar surface of the forearm to produce a wheal 6 to 10 mm in diameter. The test should be read at 48 to 72 hours, measuring only the induration in millimeters. Measure with a ruler perpendicular to the long axis of the arm. A skin test response is typically positive 2 to 12 weeks after infection. Table 1 details interpretation of the skin test. Results are interpreted regardless of prior BCG vaccination.

Measurement of γ-interferon released from white blood cells stimulated by *M. tuberculosis* antigens forms the basis of a new diagnostic test for TB. In adult patients, these tests have equal sensitivity and greater specificity than Mantoux testing. These tests are not yet FDA approved in children.

D. Children who are PPD positive with a normal chest radiograph, with no symptoms or signs of active TB, have latent TB infection. Treat with isoniazid, 10 to 15 mg/kg/day, for 9 months. Breast-fed and malnourished children warrant supplemental vitamin B_6 (Pyridoxine) therapy, 1 to 2 mg/kg/day (25 mg maximum), to prevent peripheral neuropathy. Treat children younger than 4 years with close exposure to a case of active TB with isoniazid, even if the child is PPD negative and the chest radiograph is normal, for 10 to 12 weeks after the last exposure; then repeat the PPD test. A newborn exposed to TB should have a chest radiograph, a PPD test; consider a lumbar puncture. If findings of TB are not present, treat with isoniazid for 3 to 4 months; then repeat the PPD test. Some experts treat these neonates with 9 months of isoniazid. If the contact case has isoniazid-resistant, rifampin-sensitive TB, treat with rifampin. Treatment of latent TB infection provides substantial protection against development of subsequent active TB.

E. The diagnostic tests for active TB are directed at confirming the diagnosis, obtaining a specimen for culture and sensitivities, and detailing the extent of disease. Always obtain a chest radiograph, even in those without pulmonary symptoms. A culture is important to confirm the diagnosis of TB and to guide TB therapy. Specimens can be obtained from sputum, early-morning gastric aspirates (useful in infants and young children who cannot produce sputum), bronchoalveolar lavage fluid, pleural fluid, pus, urine, cerebrospinal fluid, or a biopsy specimen. TB in children can be confirmed microbiologically in only 30% to 40% of cases. The decision to hospitalize a child for diagnostic testing balances the risks and costs of obtaining specimens along with the seriousness of the disease and the likelihood of alternate diagnoses.

F. The treatment of active TB is complicated by the long duration of therapy, difficulties with compliance of patients, emergence of multidrug resistance, and coexisting diseases such as HIV infection. Therapy of active TB is directly observed therapy with isoniazid, rifampin, and pyrazinamide. Those patients with both HIV infection and TB should ideally be treated by experts in both HIV and TB care. For all patients, if the TB strain is resistant to any of the first-line TB drugs, or if the patient remains symptomatic after 3 months, consult a TB medical expert. Because we cannot test visual acuity

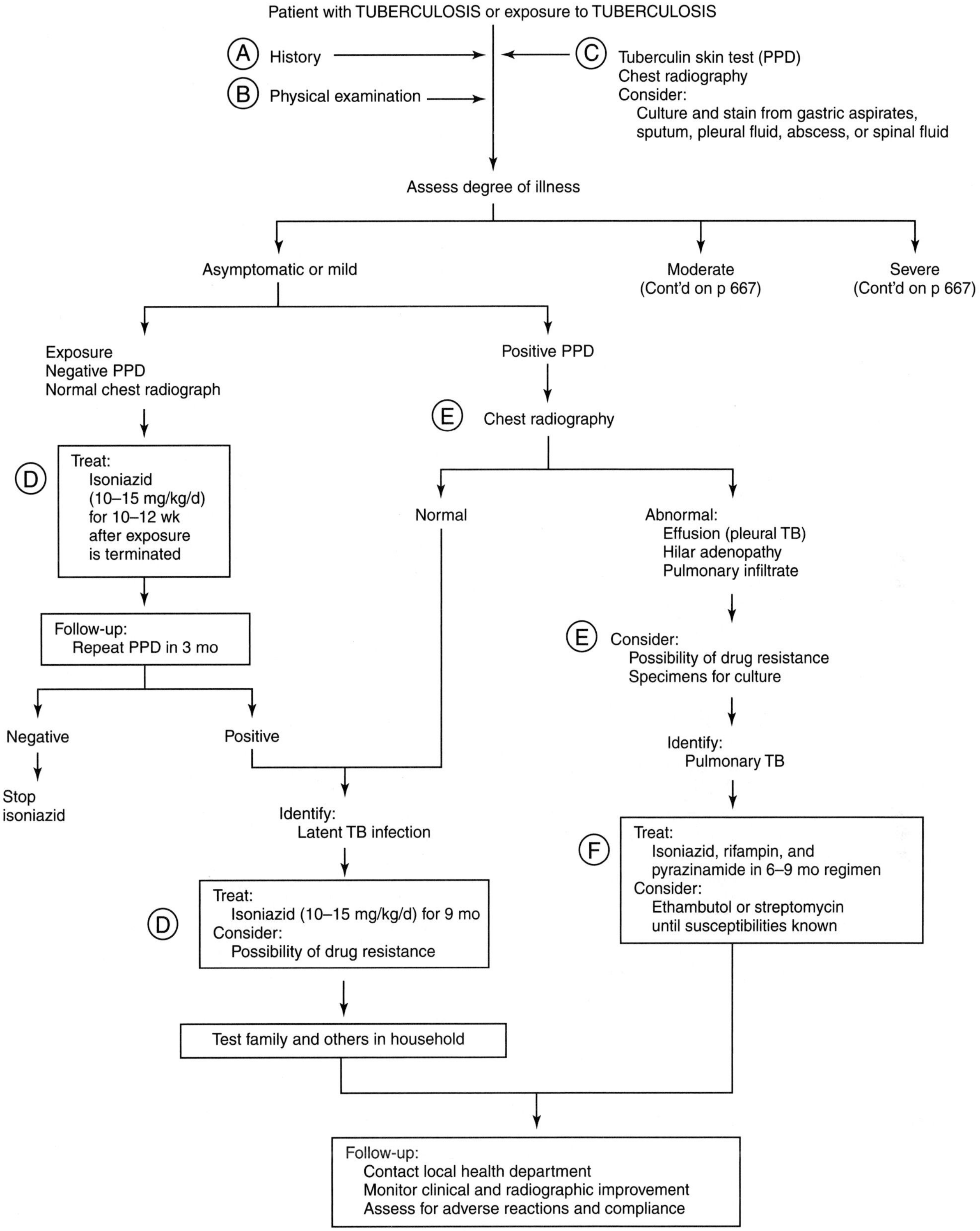
Patient with TUBERCULOSIS or exposure to TUBERCULOSIS
(A) History
(B) Physical examination
(C) Tuberculin skin test (PPD)
Chest radiography
Consider:
Culture and stain from gastric aspirates, sputum, pleural fluid, abscess, or spinal fluid
Assess degree of illness
Asymptomatic or mild
Moderate (Cont'd on p 667)
Severe (Cont'd on p 667)
Exposure
Negative PPD
Normal chest radiograph
(D) Treat:
Isoniazid (10–15 mg/kg/d) for 10–12 wk after exposure is terminated
Follow-up:
Repeat PPD in 3 mo
Negative
Stop isoniazid
Positive
Positive PPD
(E) Chest radiography
Normal
Abnormal:
Effusion (pleural TB)
Hilar adenopathy
Pulmonary infiltrate
(E) Consider:
Possibility of drug resistance
Specimens for culture
Identify:
Pulmonary TB
Identify:
Latent TB infection
(D) Treat:
Isoniazid (10–15 mg/kg/d) for 9 mo
Consider:
Possibility of drug resistance
(F) Treat:
Isoniazid, rifampin, and pyrazinamide in 6–9 mo regimen
Consider:
Ethambutol or streptomycin until susceptibilities known
Test family and others in household
Follow-up:
Contact local health department
Monitor clinical and radiographic improvement
Assess for adverse reactions and compliance

in young children, ethambutol has been avoided in the past. Because there is no evidence that ethambutol in the doses used causes visual problems in young children, many experts use ethambutol in young children when four-drug therapy is indicated.

Children with latent TB and most children with active TB are not contagious. Children with cavitary TB, laryngeal TB, intubated patients, patients with positive smears for acid fast bacilli, and some immune-suppressed patients may pose contagious risk.

Table 1. **Definitions of Positive Tuberculin Skin Test: Results in Infants, Children, and Adolescents**

Induration ≥5 mm

Children in close contact with known or suspected contagious people with tuberculosis disease
Children suspected to have tuberculosis disease:
- Findings on chest radiograph consistent with active or previous tuberculosis disease
- Clinical evidence of tuberculosis disease*

Children receiving immunosuppressive therapy† or with immunosuppressive conditions, including HIV infection

Induration ≥10 mm

Children at increased risk for disseminated tuberculosis disease:
- Children younger than 4 years
- Children with other medical conditions, including Hodgkin disease, lymphoma, diabetes mellitus, chronic renal failure, or malnutrition

Children with increased exposure to tuberculosis disease:
- Children born in high-prevalence regions of the world
- Children frequently exposed to adults who are HIV infected, homeless, users of illicit drugs, residents of nursing homes, incarcerated or institutionalized, or migrant farm workers
- Children who travel to high-prevalence regions of the world

Induration ≥15 mm

Children 4 years of age or older without any risk factors

These definitions apply regardless of previous bacilli Calmette–Guérin (BCG) immunization; erythema at tuberculin skin test (TST) site does not indicate a positive test result. Tests should be read at 48 to 72 hours after placement.
*Evidence by physical examination or laboratory assessment that would include tuberculosis in the working differential diagnosis (e.g., meningitis).
†Including immunosuppressive doses of corticosteroids.
HIV, human immunodeficiency virus.
From American Academy of Pediatrics. Tuberculosis. In: Pickering LK, editor. Red book: 2009 report of the committee on infectious diseases. 28th ed. Elk Grove Village, IL: American Academy of Pediatrics; 2009. p. 681. By permission.

G. Consider the use of corticosteroids for 6 to 8 weeks when there is severe morbidity from inflammation. Corticosteroids are indicated for children with tuberculous meningitis because steroids have been shown to lower mortality and long-term neurologic sequelae. Indications in addition to meningitis may include pleural and pericardial effusions, severe miliary disease, and intrinsic or extrinsic bronchial obstruction and atelectasis.

H. Tuberculous meningitis has a high mortality rate and is associated with severe neurologic sequelae in survivors. Increased intracranial pressure must be carefully managed, and the use of corticosteroids is indicated. Initial antibiotic therapy should include four drugs. Rifampin, streptomycin, and ethambutol penetrate into cerebrospinal fluid well only when meninges are inflamed. Isoniazid and pyrazinamide have good cerebrospinal fluid penetration.

References

American Academy of Pediatrics. Tuberculosis. In: Pickering LK, editor. Red book: 2009 report of the committee on infectious diseases. 28th ed. Elk Grove Village, IL: American Academy of Pediatrics; 2009. p. 680–701.

Centers for Disease Control and Prevention. Treatment of tuberculosis, American Thoracic Society, CDC, and Infectious Diseases Society of America. MMWR 2003;52(RR-11):1–77.

Lighter J, Rigaud M, Eduardo R, et al. Latent tuberculosis diagnosis in children by using the QuantiFERON-TB Gold In-Tube test. Pediatrics 2009;123:30–7.

Marais BJ, Gle RP, Schaaf HS, et al. Childhood pulmonary tuberculosis: old wisdom and new challenges. Am J Respir Crit Care Med 2006;173:1078–90.

Newton SM, Brent AJ, Anderson A, et al. Paediatric tuberculosis. Lancet Infect Dis 2008;8:498–510.

Prasad K, Volmink J, Menon GR. Steroids for treating tuberculous meningitis. Cochrane Database Syst Rev 2000;3:CD002244.

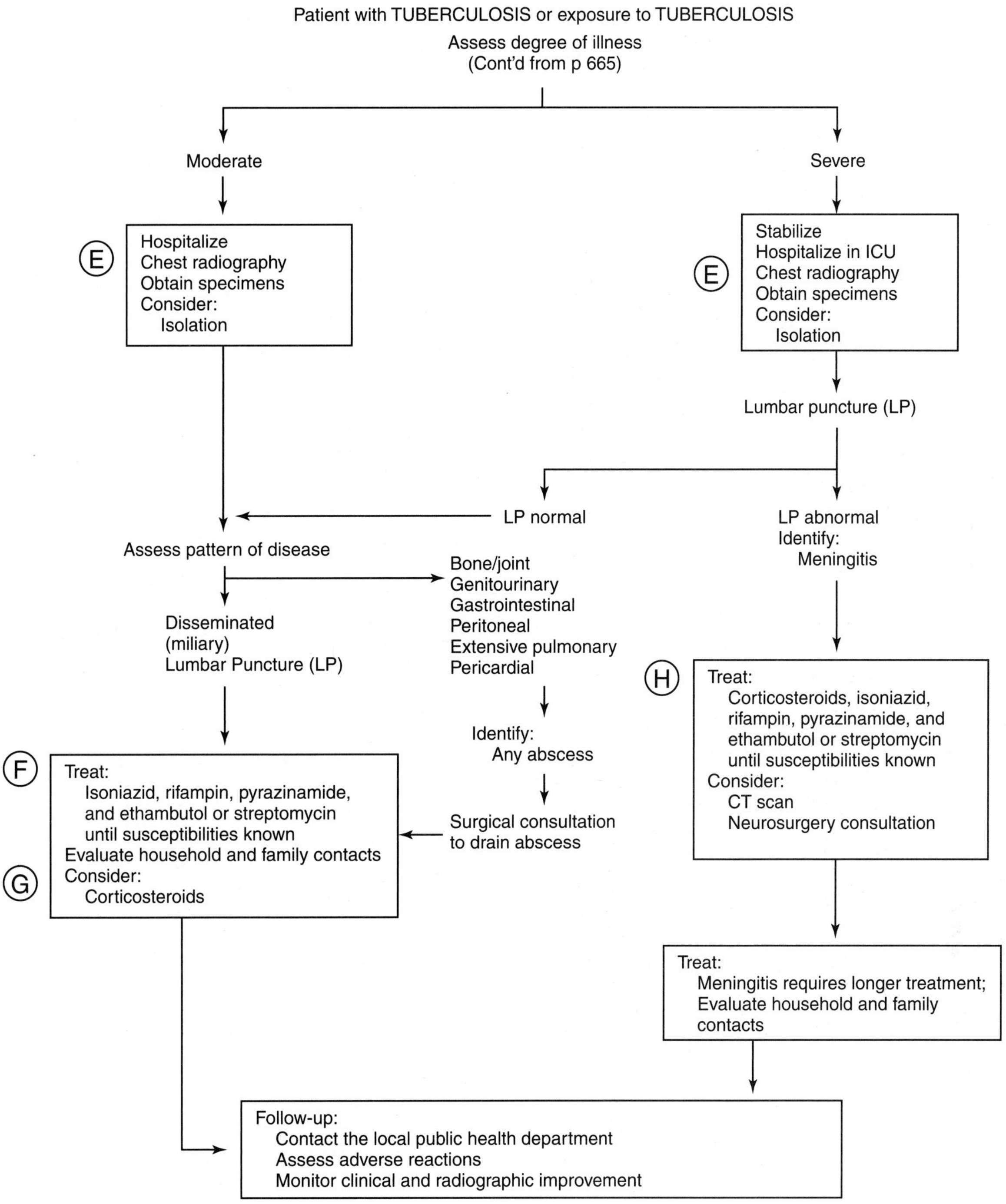
Patient with TUBERCULOSIS or exposure to TUBERCULOSIS
Assess degree of illness
(Cont'd from p 665)
Moderate
Severe
E
Hospitalize
Chest radiography
Obtain specimens
Consider:
Isolation
E
Stabilize
Hospitalize in ICU
Chest radiography
Obtain specimens
Consider:
Isolation
Lumbar puncture (LP)
LP normal
LP abnormal
Identify:
Meningitis
Assess pattern of disease
Disseminated
(miliary)
Lumbar Puncture (LP)
Bone/joint
Genitourinary
Gastrointestinal
Peritoneal
Extensive pulmonary
Pericardial
Identify:
Any abscess
Surgical consultation
to drain abscess
F
G
Treat:
Isoniazid, rifampin, pyrazinamide,
and ethambutol or streptomycin
until susceptibilities known
Evaluate household and family contacts
Consider:
Corticosteroids
H
Treat:
Corticosteroids, isoniazid,
rifampin, pyrazinamide, and
ethambutol or streptomycin
until susceptibilities known
Consider:
CT scan
Neurosurgery consultation
Treat:
Meningitis requires longer treatment;
Evaluate household and family
contacts
Follow-up:
Contact the local public health department
Assess adverse reactions
Monitor clinical and radiographic improvement

Metabolic and Genetic Disorders

Evaluation for a Genetic Disease

Birth Defects and Dysmorphic Features

Down Syndrome

Inborn Errors of Metabolism in the Neonate

Inborn Errors of Metabolism in the Acutely Ill Child

Evaluation for a Genetic Disease

Gunter H. Scharer, MD

Before birth and throughout life, genetic factors can cause or contribute to problems of growth, development, cognition, behavior, and general well-being. Knowledge of genetic disorders (single-gene defects), genomic imbalances (copy number variations), and abnormalities in gene regulation and gene interaction (epigenetics) plays an ever bigger role in modern medicine. Based on the correct diagnosis, potential complications can be recognized earlier and treated more effectively, adverse effects of existing and new treatments can be minimized, supportive therapies are optimized, and the prognosis for the individual may be predicted more accurately.

Although correct numbers vary, it is estimated that between 30% and 50% of all admissions to pediatric hospitals occur because of congenital malformations present at birth, or less obvious genetic causes including the contributions of an underlying genetic disorder to the patient's clinical presentation. Although our understanding of genetics and genetic disease mechanisms does increase rapidly, it will remain incomplete for the foreseeable future. Therefore, we have to rely not only on the results of an increasing number of diagnostic tools, but on the traditional clinical expertise of a dysmorphologist and the critical observations of the bedside clinician–researcher.

The more classic genetic diseases (major chromosome abnormalities, Mendelian or single-gene disorders) often have a recognizable pattern of prenatal/postnatal growth retardation (including abnormal head size), motor/cognitive delays, muscular hypotonia/hypertonia, and other unique physical features (dysmorphisms). Recognition of specific patterns of multiple birth defects (congenital anomalies) may aid in the diagnosis of the genetic syndrome; however, the majority of birth defects are caused by "multifactorial" interaction of genes and environmental factors.

These patterns are often missing in the more nonspecific presentations of global developmental delays, intellectual disabilities, behavioral problems, mental illness, and chronic disease typically encountered in pediatric medicine and increasingly in the adult medical practice as well. A carefully obtained family history can yield clues to a possible genetic/metabolic causative factor in some patients, but in the majority of cases, the clinical suspicion has to be followed up by screening tests or functional studies (Table 1).

The spectrum of diagnostic genetic testing has expanded rapidly in the first decade of the 21st century, especially since the completion of the Human Genome Project, with the availability of automated DNA sequencing assays, and the easy access to online genetic databases. More recently, emerging molecular tools for detection of genomic imbalances (array-based comparative genomic hybridization [aCGH] microarrays) have resulted in new insights in genetic processes and identification of new candidate genes linked to previously only clinically described syndromes. In the near future, the technologies for whole-genome sequencing will become available on a clinical basis. Because of the multitude of test options and the associated significant cost to the health care system, it is more important than ever to consult a clinical geneticist or metabolic specialist before embarking on an extended journey in the vastness of genetic tests. The issue is at times complicated by the ambiguous results of genetic testing. More often than not the findings of genetic testing do not allow the physician to arrive at a genetic diagnosis with the desired certainty. In general, genetic testing should not be used to rule out a genetic cause, but rather to confirm a diagnostic hypothesis. The still limited number of well-defined genes compared with known cDNAs, the few proven genotype–phenotype correlations, and the presence of genetic variation and novel mutations make the interpretation of test results often challenging even to the experienced geneticist. In addition, it is most important to understand that an inherited genetic disorder, once identified by a positive test result, may not manifest itself in the patient in the same way as the affected sibling, parents, or relative who carries the same mutation.

Still, even extended genetic testing is justified in cases where anticipated results do impact on the patient's medical management and clinical outcome, that is, expanded newborn screening or adverse reaction to pharmacologic treatment. Prenatal testing for known or suspected genetic disorders, assessing the individual risk for future disease or dependency, on the other hand, may require a more balanced approach involving the patient or parents, the primary care physician, a geneticist, other medical specialists, and possibly an expert in ethics. Society as a whole is needed to provide guidelines and consensus criteria for genetic testing, and has to protect the individual from discrimination based on the person's genetic profile.

A. Begin by obtaining a comprehensive medical history with one focus being the perinatal history, including any teratogenic exposures, maternal illness, fetal growth/movement, and neonatal presentation (Apgar scores). Be aware that conditions with prenatal manifestation can cause altered Dubowitz and Apgar scores. The general health history and feeding history can provide clues to disorders presenting with impaired growth, altered immune status, and metabolic deficiencies (see Inborn Errors of Metabolism in the Neonate, p. 684). Specifically, assess the progression of any neurodevelopmental abnormality, that is, improvement of early hypotonia is seen in Prader–Willi syndrome, whereas developmental regression or slowing, or increases in severity of neurologic symptoms can indicate a more severe and possibly degenerative genetic/metabolic disorder. A skin rash, birthmarks, abnormal hair, or delayed tooth eruption can aid as well in making a rapid diagnosis or raising

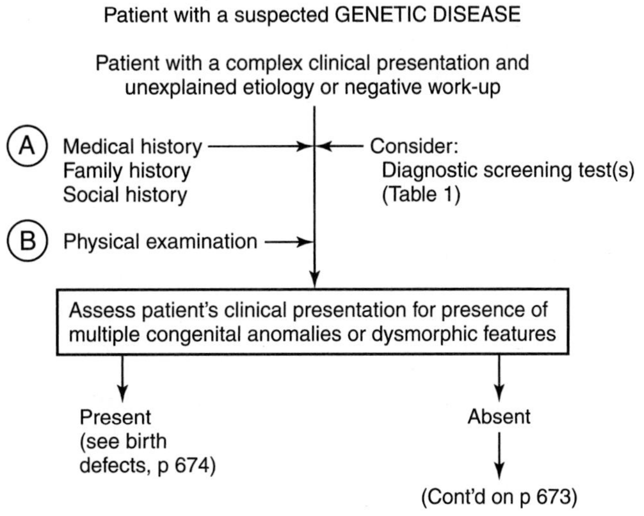
Patient with a suspected GENETIC DISEASE
Patient with a complex clinical presentation and unexplained etiology or negative work-up
A
Medical history
Family history
Social history
Consider:
Diagnostic screening test(s) (Table 1)
B
Physical examination
Assess patient's clinical presentation for presence of multiple congenital anomalies or dysmorphic features
Present (see birth defects, p 674)
Absent
(Cont'd on p 673)

Table 1. **Tests to Be Considered in Genetic Screening and Evaluation**

DNA microarray study, oligo-aCGH or SNP array (blood, other tissue)
Consider five-cell screen karyotype (blood, skin, other tissue)
Imaging (e.g., MRI, CT scan, bone films)
Functional studies (e.g., EEG, ECG/echocardiography)
DNA analysis for specific gene or genetic pathway (blood, other tissue)
Biochemical assays: metabolites
Blood: comprehensive metabolic panel, CPK, cholesterol, uric acid, ketones, acylcarnitine profile, amino acids, carnitine, lactate/pyruvate, ammonia very long chain fatty acids, serum transferrin by IEF, copper/ceruloplasmin
Urine: organic acids, amino acids, mucopolysaccharides, oligosaccharides
CSF: glucose, protein, lactate, amino acids, neurotransmitters
Biochemical assays: enzymes (blood, skin, liver, muscle)
Histology (e.g., blood [smear], muscle, other tissues)
Parental studies (e.g., confirm carrier status, verify DNA microarray results)

CPK, creatine phosphokinase; *CSF,* cerebrospinal fluid; *CT,* computed tomography; *ECG,* electrocardiography; *EEG,* electroencephalography; *IEF,* isoelectric focusing; *MRI,* magnetic resonance imaging; *oligo-aCGH,* oligonucleotide array-based comparative genomic hybridization; *SNP,* single nucleotide polymorphism.

suspicion for a genetic disorder. More important than ever is the need for obtaining a behavioral history of the patient in the context of the social environment at home and at school (attention-deficit disorder, autism spectrum disorder). Finally, a genetic pedigree (at least two to three generations) is essential for identifying inherited traits, predispositions, and known/suspected inherited diseases within a family. In evaluating a child with growth, developmental, and/or behavioral problems, ask about family history of miscarriages, birth defects, cognitive/learning disabilities, any neurodevelopmental deficits, and early childhood death. Ask about prevalence of cancer, diabetes, heart disease, mental illness, asthma/allergies, or other chronic conditions. In some cases, the presenting complaint is the parent's concern that a child may have or develop a condition that is present in other family members. The question of possible consanguinity of the parents should not be omitted, but carefully addressed. Remember, a negative or unremarkable family history does not exclude the possibility of a genetic disorder in the patient.

B. Perform a careful physical examination. Although a complete dysmorphology evaluation should be reserved to the experienced geneticist, every physician should be able to recognize asymmetries and to assess growth parameters correctly. Abnormal growth velocity or head size can point toward an easily identifiable diagnosis (e.g., achondroplasia), may need rapid intervention (e.g., macrocephaly caused by hydrocephalus), or can be familial traits that require simply careful monitoring. Other objective measurements to be considered include eye distance, arm span, and finger/hand length or penile length (e.g., in a male patient with hypoplastic genitalia). In general, careful attention to details is needed, because simple observations such as the nature of a birthmark (e.g., café-au-lait spots) may provide a clue to the patient's diagnosis (e.g., neurofibromatosis); see Birth Defects and Dysmorphic Features chapter (p. 674) for physical examination of a child. Presence of an organomegaly (e.g., liver, spleen) may indicate a possible metabolic disorder (e.g., storage disorder), especially if increase in size is progressive and associated with neurologic abnormalities in the patient. Hypertonia in the neonatal period and hypotonia after age 1 year, progressive ataxia, or a movement disorder is often linked to a genetic or metabolic disorder. Typically limited to the specialist, a careful eye examination is important for patients with suspected genetic/metabolic conditions; however, an abnormal light reflex, an iris colobomas, or heterochromia should be easily recognizable. For patients with deficits in coordination and hypotonia, a simple run up and down the clinical hallway can result in a genetic diagnosis. Finally, and if possible, do examine the child and the parents, especially in regard to behavioral problems, because these interactions are vital for assessment of appropriate parental response.

C. If the clinical evaluation (medical history and physical examination) and/or the family history provide obvious clues to the presence of a detectable or known genetic disorder in the patient, then confirmatory/diagnostic testing should be considered or the patient referred to the clinical geneticist. An increasing number of genetic reference laboratories can be found on the Internet, and information on sample collection and shipping conditions is often readily available online. It is recommended to contact the reference laboratory to ask for minimum sample requirements, especially in very young children and infants, because these patients often undergo multiple laboratory studies and total blood draw volume may be limited. Remember, whole-blood transfusion or organ transplantation can introduce donor DNA and can interfere with genetic testing. It is advisable to contact a clinical geneticist before pursuing genetic testing, because his/her expertise can be invaluable in minimizing unnecessary genetic testing, and to arrange for follow-up of genetic test results or genetic counseling for the family. Parents often may be interested in having carrier testing or predictive genetic testing performed on their children. The American Society of Human Genetics and the American Academy of Pediatrics suggest that such testing be deferred until the individual can give consent, unless there is a possibility of identifying a condition for which treatment or monitoring should begin already in childhood. Always consider the risk for discovery of nonpaternity when genetic testing is offered to family members of an individual with a genetic condition.

D. The presence of specific or recognizable neurologic abnormalities (e.g., developmental regression, progressive ataxia or muscle weakness, neonatal onset epilepsy) is a matter of grave concern. Although screening tests and functional studies may aid in establishing the correct diagnosis, contacting (or consulting) a neurologist and a clinical geneticist or metabolic expert should have priority. Before regression of developmental milestones becomes obvious, there is often a period of developmental slowing. It may be difficult to distinguish irreversible regression from the loss of developmental milestones because of severe and poorly controlled seizures or high-dose multiple anticonvulsant medications. The differential diagnosis of developmental regression is limited to specific groups of genetic/metabolic disorders (e.g., Rett syndrome, lysosomal storage disorders, energy metabolism deficiencies); malignancy and environmental factors need to be considered as well (e.g., poisoning, accidental exposure to toxins, and increased intracranial pressure because of trauma or infection). Screening tests for developmental regression can include a brain MRI/CT scan, a spinal tap, complete blood cell count (CBC)/comprehensive metabolic panel, a metabolic workup (serum amino acids, acylcarnitine profile, lactate/pyruvate ratio, very long chain fatty acids, lysosomal enzymes, and urine organic acids, urine mucopolysaccharides/oligosaccharides), and DNA testing for all forms of Rett syndrome, especially if acquired microcephaly and epilepsy is present. Specific neurologic signs (e.g., hypotonia) are often found in combination with developmental delays or dysmorphic features. In these cases, screening tests can be as simple as a serum creatine phosphokinase level or more inclusive, for example, oligonucleotide aCGH (oligo-aCGH).

E. The most commonly encountered patient suspicious for an underlying genetic disorder is the individual with global developmental delays and/or behavioral anomalies, with nonspecific neurologic signs, absent dysmorphic features, and often normal growth. In this case, a formal developmental and/or behavioral evaluation often yields the initial diagnostic clues. Contacting a clinical geneticist or pursuing genetic screening tests can equally be considered. DNA microarrays (oligo-aCGH) have emerged as the most powerful tools, because many of the patients owe their clinical presentation to an underlying genomic imbalance (microdeletion/duplication). Still, a DNA test for Fragile X syndrome in male patients needs to be included in the workup, as well as mutation analysis in the *PTEN* gene for patients with isolated macrocephaly. Interestingly, the same screening tests are recommended for patients with autism spectrum disorder, plus metabolic screening tests (Bratton–Marshal test and 7- and 8-dehydrocholesterol in serum).

Patient with a suspected GENETIC DISEASE

Patient with a complex clinical presentation and
unexplained etiology or negative work-up

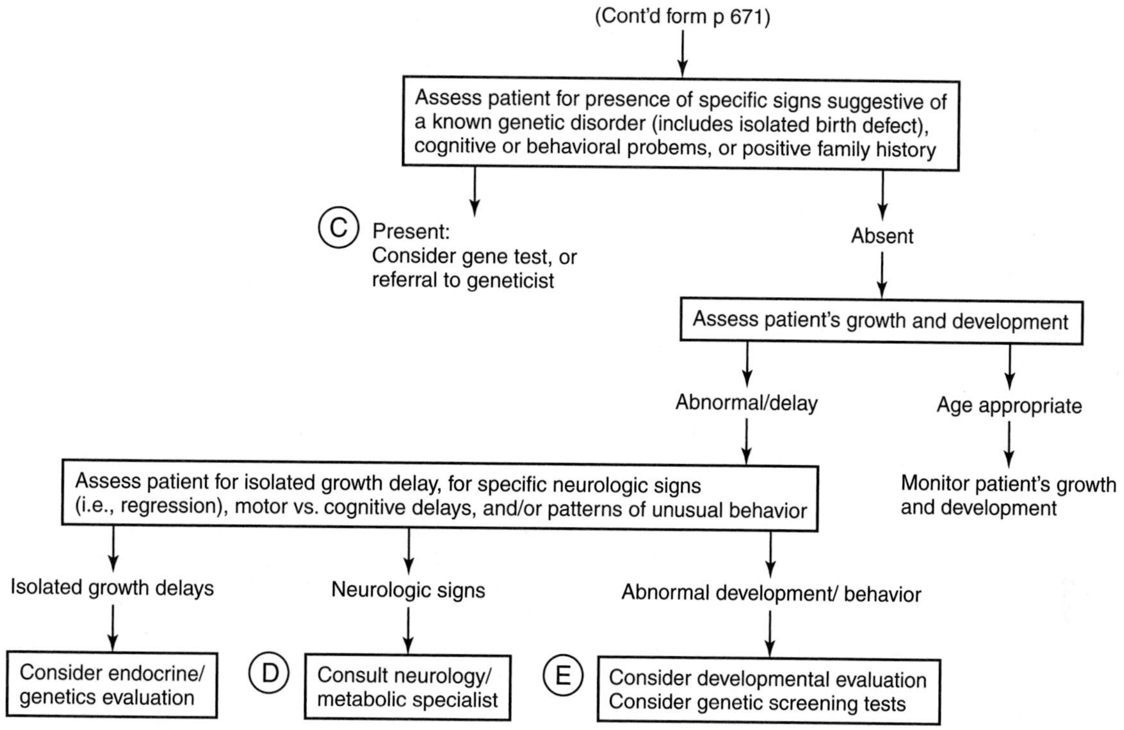
(Cont'd form p 671)
Assess patient for presence of specific signs suggestive of a known genetic disorder (includes isolated birth defect), cognitive or behavioral probems, or positive family history
C
Present:
Consider gene test, or referral to geneticist
Absent
Assess patient's growth and development
Abnormal/delay
Age appropriate
Monitor patient's growth and development
Assess patient for isolated growth delay, for specific neurologic signs (i.e., regression), motor vs. cognitive delays, and/or patterns of unusual behavior
Isolated growth delays
Neurologic signs
Abnormal development/ behavior
Consider endocrine/ genetics evaluation
D
Consult neurology/ metabolic specialist
E
Consider developmental evaluation
Consider genetic screening tests

References

Greene CL, Thomas JA, Goodman SI. Inborn errors of metabolism. In: Hay WW, Hayward AR, Levin MJ, Sondheimer JM, editors. Pediatric diagnosis and treatment. 15th ed. Norwalk, CT: Appleton & Lange; 2001. p. 881.

Knight SJ, Regan R, Nicod A, et al. Subtle chromosomal rearrangements in children with unexplained mental retardation. Lancet 1999;354: 1676–81.

Miller DT, Adam MP, Aradhya S, et al. Consensus statement: Chromosomal microarray is a first-tier clinical diagnostic test for individuals with developmental disabilities or congenital anomalies. Am J Genet 2010 May 14; 86(5):749–64. Review. PMID: 20466091.

Sujansky E, Stewart JM, Manchester DK. Genetics and dysmorphology. In: Hay WW, Hayward AR, Levin MJ, Sondheimer JM, editors. Pediatric diagnosis and treatment. 15th ed. Norwalk, CT: Appleton & Lange; 2001. p. 904.

Birth Defects and Dysmorphic Features

Anne Chun-Hui Tsai, MD, MSc, FAAP, FACMG

Birth defects or congenital anomalies are structural defects present at birth as the result of abnormal tissue differentiation or abnormal tissue and organ interaction during embryonic and fetal development. The incidence rate is 3% to 5% in liveborn infants and 15% to 20% in stillbirths. About one third of pediatric inpatients are hospitalized because of congenital abnormalities. Dysmorphology is a word coined by Dr. David W. Smith in 1966 to describe the study of human congenital defects—abnormalities of body structure that originate before birth. Dysmorphic anomalies can occur in any part of the body, and most arise during the first 3 months of intrauterine life. Some dysmorphic features may be of no clinical significance, whereas others may indicate increased risk for problems with growth, development, and health that can be predicted and managed. There may also be issues of recurrence risk.

Classification of birth defects or dysmorphic features can be made in different ways. By severity and the degree of involvement, these may include major versus minor anomalies and isolated versus multiple anomalies. Based on pathogenesis, these may include malformation, deformation, disruption, and dysplasia. Based on causative factors, multiple birth defects may be identified as sequence, syndrome, and association. Understanding such terms is helpful in approaching clinical dysmorphology. Terminology is discussed as follows.

Malformations may result from somatic cell mutation, aberrant cell migration, deficient or excess abundant cell divisions, and failure of tissue-specific cell interactions. In the absence of compelling evidence that exposure to a drug, toxin, or other exogenous element caused the malformation, there is usually slightly increased risk for recurrence for other family members. Prenatal diagnosis and occasionally prenatal management may be available for certain major malformations.

Deformations result from mechanical forces that cause unusual pressure on the developing fetus. Examples include fetal positioning, torticollis, and plagiocephaly. The sources of the mechanical forces can be extrinsic to the fetus (e.g., uterine anomaly, multiple pregnancies) or intrinsic (e.g., severe abdominal distention from urogenital anomalies causing a prune belly). Insufficient amniotic fluid allows compression of the fetus by the uterine wall.

Oligohydramnios can result from fetal renal hypoplasia or maternal fluid leak from infection or idiopathic reasons. If there is no intrinsic abnormality of the fetus that led to the deformation, the prognosis is usually excellent, and the distorted tissues usually normalize over time with growth.

Disruption results when extrinsic agents cause unscheduled cell death during development. Causes of disruption include processes that interfere with cellular metabolism (e.g., drugs), mechanical events (e.g., amniotic bands), vascular accidents (jejunal atresia and some unilateral limb reduction), and intrauterine viral infections (e.g., rubella, cytomegalovirus). The actual destruction of tissue is localized, and the adjacent structures are often unaffected. Recurrence risk is low.

Dysplasia results from the abnormal organization of cells into tissue. Alterations in one general tissue type can have widespread effects. The classic example is achondroplasia, which is caused by fibroblast growth factor receptor 3 mutations. Even though the dysplastic effect is of single origin, the resulting clinical anomalies are multiple. For example, individuals with achondroplasia present with multiple anomalies secondary to the bone dysplasia, including macrocephaly, midface hypoplasia, short stature, and spinal stenosis. Dysmorphic features caused by dysplasia may not be obvious at birth, but affect tends to be progressive over time.

In assessing a child with birth defects, the physician may be perplexed and unsure how to proceed. The diagnosis process is not mysterious, and the main diagnostic "tools" needed are familiar to practicing pediatricians: the ability to take a complete history, perform a meticulous physical examination, and discriminate between the normal (in all its variability) and truly abnormal. Only the emphasis is changed.

A. In the patient's history, ask about prenatal gestational, perinatal, medical, developmental, and family events. Specific elements of each category are listed in Table 1.

B. In the physical examination, particular attention should be paid to the detection of minor structural anomalies and spectrum variants because these may be valuable diagnostic clues. In many cases, the physical growth of various parts of the body is diagnostically significant, and careful measurements of these structures should be taken. Excellent compendia showing techniques for performing such measurements and providing normal growth grids for comparison and interpretation are available. Table 2 summarizes the tips for dysmorphologic examinations.

C. Reviewing past records of the patient is essential to gather information that may have been previously unavailable to the family and to verify accuracy of the information the family has reported. Genetic diseases are less common and often complicated; therefore, a family can be confused by the diagnosis. It is also important to verify how the diagnosis was made, such as by molecular testing or by clinical criteria. Information about diagnosis or clinical presentation might have been altered in transmission, and information that was correctly transmitted needs to be re-evaluated in light of increased knowledge about genetics and teratology, as well as current information about the family. It is

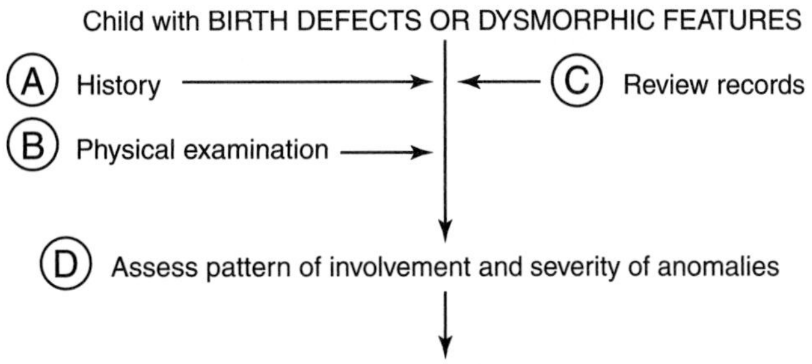
Child with BIRTH DEFECTS OR DYSMORPHIC FEATURES
A History
B Physical examination
C Review records
D Assess pattern of involvement and severity of anomalies

(Cont'd on p 677)

Table 1. **Elements of a Dysmorphologic History**

Prenatal History

- Maternal illness (e.g., hypertension, seizure disorder, and diabetes)
- Complications (e.g., bleeding, high fever, rash)
- Onset and quality of fetal movement
- Presence of oligohydramnios or polyhydramnios
- Fetal presentation: vertex or breech
- Fetal ultrasound abnormalities
- Teratogenic exposures to alcohol, tobacco, and toxic chemicals

Perinatal History

- Birth height, weight, and head circumference
- Delivery difficulties
- Apgar scores
- Hospital course
- Physical maturity at birth

Medical History

- Hospitalization
- Trauma and accidents
- Hearing and vision
- Feeding, diet, and bowel movement
- Sleeping pattern
- Behavior concerns
- Medications
- Review of systems

Developmental History

- Major milestones
- Pattern of growth and development throughout life
- Height, weight, head size
- Record of psychodevelopmental evaluation
- Denver developmental assessment
- Individual Education Program (IEP)-school assessment of development

Family History

Pedigree is the main component of family history. Pearls of taking pedigrees include the following:

- Give simple instructions to the patient regarding information desired.
- Use clearly defined symbols with a key for interpretation.
- Identify the informant, the historian, and the date of the interview.
- Start in the middle of page for expansion.
- Ascertain the ages of living persons and dates and causes of death for deceased family members.
- Obtain the maiden name of woman in the family (particularly helpful for X-linked conditions).
- Obtain data from both sides of family.
- Ask about spontaneous abortions, stillbirths, infertility, children relinquished for adoption, and deceased individuals. (Such details are essential for understanding conditions that are lethal or are associated with reproductive losses.)
- Ask for details such as place of birth, size of towns, and the presence of consanguinity. (These help to define recessive conditions and suspect certain disease more frequent in particular ethnic backgrounds.)
- In the course of taking the family history, one may find information that is not relevant in elucidating the cause of the patients' problem but indicate a risk for other important health concerns. Such information should be appropriately followed and addressed.

important to always obtain written permission from the individual. Documentation may be sought from hospital medical records departments, physicians, coroners' records, or other institutions. For an adopted individual, medical information is often available on biologic relatives from the appropriate private agency or state facility. Records that are most helpful in the records include reports of autopsy and surgical procedures, discharge summaries, and laboratory investigations such as chromosome studies. Family photographs are helpful when trying to assess physical characteristics or judge whether another family member was affected.

D. Assess the pattern of involvement and severity of the anomalies. Determine whether it is an isolated anomaly or is associated with other anomalies that suggest a syndromic cause. Most congenital anomalies are isolated—that is, present in an otherwise well-formed individual. The cause of isolated anomaly is believed to be multifactorial inherence, defined as the interaction between multiple genes and environmental factors with the recurrence risk range of 2% to 5%. Certain isolated major anomalies can cause early death or long-term disability and may have increased risk for recurrence. Adequate management and prenatal diagnosis can be offered if diagnosed promptly. A syndrome is defined as a cluster of findings that form a pattern that is recognizable. A syndromic cause usually indicates an increased recurrence risk and more of a genetic component in the pathogenesis. A genetic evaluation is required for children with multiple anomalies. Identifying a syndromic diagnosis helps to better understand the cause and prognosis. Isolated congenital defects can be subdivided into major and minor categories, as described in detail later.

Table 2. **Elements of Dysmorphology Examination**

Visual Assessment

Before touching the patient, observe the overall presentation.
- Is the individual behaving in an age-appropriate manner?
- Does the individual have peculiar movements, facial expressions, or limitations in movement?
- All examinations should be done with the patient disrobed, although this may be done in a progressive fashion.

Measurement

- Head circumference, height, and weight
- Measurements (should be compared with published standards for age, sex, and if possible, racial origin)
  - Inner canthal distance
  - Interpupillary distance
  - Ear length
  - Hand length
  - Middle finger length
  - Foot length
  - Penis length
  - Specific ratios of body portions with respect to different diseases, such as upper/lower segment ratio and arm span/height ratio in Marfan syndrome
- Family comparisons are essential
  - Finding similar values outside the normal range is usually reassuring (e.g., a child with a large head may have many normal family members with macrocephaly).
  - However, similar findings in child and parent could also indicate a genetic disease (e.g., parent and child with macrocephaly caused by dominant gene for neurofibromatosis).
- The child's features should be analyzed over time by examining earlier photographs

Extended Family

- If the diagnosis is unclear, examination of other affected or potentially affected family members may help.
- Clinical criteria for Marfan syndrome, neurofibromatosis, and tuberous sclerosis include positive family history as one criterion.
  - For example, if a child is suspected of having tuberous sclerosis, the family cannot be adequately counseled regarding recurrence risks unless the parents have been examined.

Important findings should be documented:
- By diagrams, clinical photographs, or videotape, particularly when the pattern of movement is a distinguishing feature.

E. A minor anomaly is found in less than 4% of the general population and usually has only cosmetic significance. Examples include frontal bossing, toe syndactyly, tapering fingers, and pre-auricular pit. Table 3 lists other common minor anomalies. Some of the minor abnormalities may run through the family as an autosomal dominant trait. However, they may be helpful diagnostic clues particularly when more than two occur together. Down syndrome is a typical example of diagnosing a condition based on a group of the minor anomalies without knowing any major anomaly; the pattern of flat nasal bridge, Brushfield spots, epicanthal folds, small, round, posteriorly rotated ears, and single palmar creases is recognizable as Down syndrome. Likewise, both anteverted nostrils and two and three toe syndactyly can be minor anomalies with no significance; however, when they occur together and are associated with developmental delay, Smith–Lemli–Opitz syndrome should be considered. As the number of minor anomalies increases, the chance for the occurrence of a major malformation increases. Table 4 summarizes the incidence and the chance of occurrence of major anomalies.

F. Major anomalies are arbitrarily defined as anomalies that, unless corrected, result in impairment of body function or shortening of life span. Examples include heart defect, abnormal brain, cleft lip and palate, and limb reduction defect. Examinations of major malformations can be accomplished through ultrasound studies of the brain, heart, and kidney, radiographs of the skeletal structure, and cranial computed tomographic/magnetic resonance imaging (CT/MRI) scan for brain structure and myelination. In evaluating a patient who has a major malformation, aggressive search for other anomalies should be performed. About one third of such patients will have other anomalies and be considered as having a malformation syndrome. For instance, individuals with midline cleft palate can have up to a 56% chance to have a syndromic cause. A genetic consult is usually recommended in the event of a major malformation unless such anomaly can be determined absolutely to be isolated. An isolated major anomaly is usually of multifactorial inheritance but could be caused by chromosomal anomalies and single-gene disorders such as seen in specific brain malformations such as dandy walker malformation and lissencephaly. To this end, microarray analysis and gene specific molecular analysis is crucial.

Using the most obvious, frequent, or rarest pivotal abnormalities can help in syndrome recognition and diagnosis. Upon diagnosis, "gene review" (http://www.genetests.org) can be a useful resource for each specific genetic syndrome. Each topic was written by invited authors who are most recognized in that field. Each topic covers medical management, genetic information, counseling and anticipatory guidance for a specific condition.

(Continued on page 678)

Child with BIRTH DEFECTS OR DYSMORPHIC FEATURES

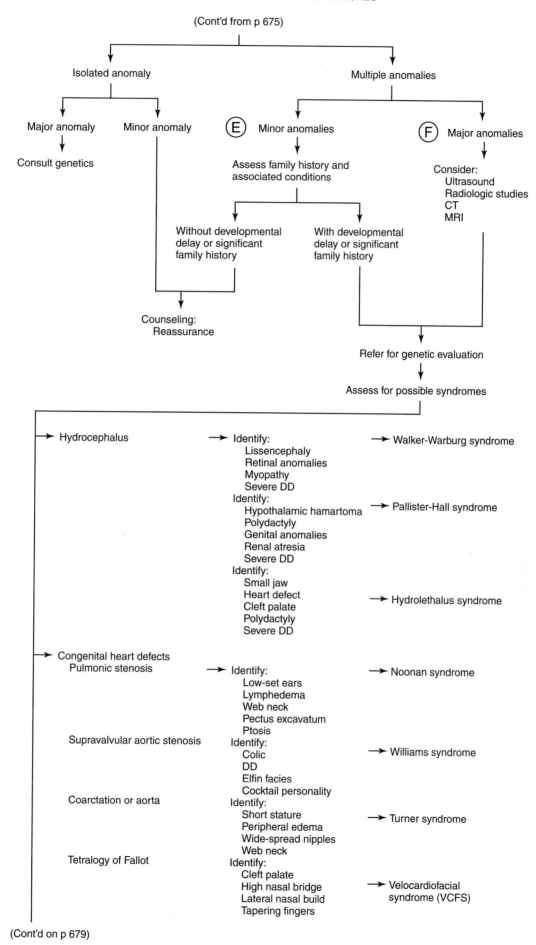

(Cont'd from p 675)

- Isolated anomaly
  - Major anomaly → Consult genetics
  - Minor anomaly → Counseling: Reassurance
- Multiple anomalies
  - (E) Minor anomalies → Assess family history and associated conditions
    - Without developmental delay or significant family history → Counseling: Reassurance
    - With developmental delay or significant family history → Refer for genetic evaluation
  - (F) Major anomalies → Consider: Ultrasound, Radiologic studies, CT, MRI → Refer for genetic evaluation

Refer for genetic evaluation → Assess for possible syndromes

- Hydrocephalus
  - Identify: Lissencephaly, Retinal anomalies, Myopathy, Severe DD → Walker-Warburg syndrome
  - Identify: Hypothalamic hamartoma, Polydactyly, Genital anomalies, Renal atresia, Severe DD → Pallister-Hall syndrome
  - Identify: Small jaw, Heart defect, Cleft palate, Polydactyly, Severe DD → Hydrolethalus syndrome
- Congenital heart defects
  - Pulmonic stenosis → Identify: Low-set ears, Lymphedema, Web neck, Pectus excavatum, Ptosis → Noonan syndrome
  - Supravalvular aortic stenosis → Identify: Colic, DD, Elfin facies, Cocktail personality → Williams syndrome
  - Coarctation or aorta → Identify: Short stature, Peripheral edema, Wide-spread nipples, Web neck → Turner syndrome
  - Tetralogy of Fallot → Identify: Cleft palate, High nasal bridge, Lateral nasal build, Tapering fingers → Velocardiofacial syndrome (VCFS)

(Cont'd on p 679)

Table 3. **Examples of Minor Anomalies and Common Syndromes That Can Present with Each**

Minor Anomaly	Common Syndrome Associated
Scalp defect	Trisomy 13, 4p deletion
Confluent eyebrow (synophrys)	Cornelia de Lange syndrome
Ptosis	Saethre–Chotzen syndrome, Noonan syndrome
Preauricular tags	Goldenhar syndrome, Townes–Brocks syndrome
Cleft uvula	22q deletion syndrome
Inverted nipples	Weaver syndrome, Congenital disorders of glycosylation (CDG)
Extra nipples	Simpson–Golabi–Behmel syndrome
Tapering fingers	Velocardiofacial syndrome, Cohen syndrome
Fifth finger clinodactyly	Down, fetal alcohol, and Russell–Silver syndromes
Fingernail hyperconvexity	Turner syndrome
Deep-set eyes	Smith–Magenis syndrome
Lacy/stellate irides	Williams syndrome

Table 4. **Incidence and Association of Major and Minor Anomalies**

Number of Minor Malformations	Incidence in General Population	Chance of Major Malformation (%)
0		1.4
1	Up to 13%	3
2	1%	11
3	1/2000	90

References

Aase JM. Diagnostic dysmorphology. New York: Plenum Medical Book Co.; 1990.

Aase JM. Dysmorphologic diagnosis for the pediatric practitioner. In: Hall JG, editor. Pediatric clinics of North America. Medical genetics, vol. 1. Philadelphia: WB Saunders; 1992.

Curry CM. An approach to clinical genetics. In: Rudolph AM, Kamei RK, Overby KJ, eds. Rudolph's fundamentals of pediatrics. 2nd ed. Norwalk, CT: Appleton & Lange; 1999. p. 147–80.

Gorlin RJ, Cohen MM Jr, Hennekam R. Syndromes of the head and neck. 4th ed. New York: Oxford University Press; 2001.

Graham JM. Clinical approach to human structural defects. Semin Perinatol 1991;15:2–15.

Graham JM. Smith's recognizable patterns of human deformation. 3rd ed. New York: Elsevier Health Sciences; 2007.

Hall JG, Allanson JE, Gripp KW, Slavotinek AM. Handbook of physical measures. 2nd ed. New York: Oxford University Press; 2007.

Jones KL, editor. Smith's recognizable patterns of human malformation. 6th ed. Philadelphia: Elsevier Saunders; 2006.

Leppig KA, Werler MM, Cann CI, et al. Predictive value of minor anomalies. I. Association with major malformations. J Pediatr 1987;110:531–7.

McKusick VA. Mendelian inheritance in man. <http://www.omim.org>; [accessed 11.05.11].

Saal HM. A prospective analysis of cleft palate: Associated syndromes and malformations [abstract]. Proceedings of the Greenwood Genetic Center 2001;78(20).

Saul RA, Skinner SA, Stevenson RE, et al. Growth references from conception to adulthood. Proceedings of the Greenwood Genetic Center. Greenwood, SC: Greenwood Genetic Center; 1998.

Child with BIRTH DEFECTS OR DYSMORPHIC FEATURES

Assess for possible syndromes
(Cont'd from p 677)

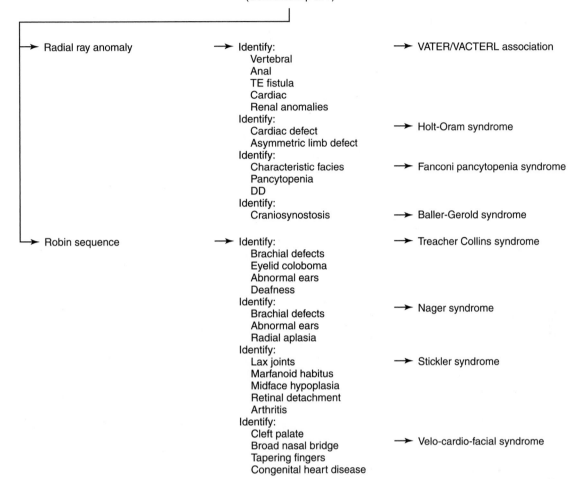

- → Radial ray anomaly
  - → Identify: Vertebral, Anal, TE fistula, Cardiac, Renal anomalies → VATER/VACTERL association
  - Identify: Cardiac defect, Asymmetric limb defect → Holt-Oram syndrome
  - Identify: Characteristic facies, Pancytopenia, DD → Fanconi pancytopenia syndrome
  - Identify: Craniosynostosis → Baller-Gerold syndrome
- → Robin sequence
  - → Identify: Brachial defects, Eyelid coloboma, Abnormal ears, Deafness → Treacher Collins syndrome
  - Identify: Brachial defects, Abnormal ears, Radial aplasia → Nager syndrome
  - Identify: Lax joints, Marfanoid habitus, Midface hypoplasia, Retinal detachment, Arthritis → Stickler syndrome
  - Identify: Cleft palate, Broad nasal bridge, Tapering fingers, Congenital heart disease → Velo-cardio-facial syndrome

Down Syndrome

Karen L. Kelminson, MD, Ellen Roy Elias, MD,
and Edward Goldson, MD

Down syndrome is the most common chromosomal abnormality. It results from the presence of extra genetic material from chromosome 21. This extra chromosomal material can come about in three ways: (1) trisomy 21, which occurs in 95% of children with Down syndrome; (2) translocation between chromosome 21 and another acrocentric chromosome, which occurs in 3% to 4% of children with Down syndrome; and (3) mosaicism, the presence of both normal and trisomy 21 cell lines, which occurs in the remaining 1% to 2% of children. The prevalence rate of Down syndrome is 1 per 770 live births. It is important to recognize the considerable range in the phenotypic characteristics, associated conditions, and degree of intellectual and cognitive disability, with mosaicism at the mildest end of the spectrum.

A. Initial Counseling: The primary counseling visit with the parents of a child diagnosed with Down syndrome occurs before or soon after the infant's delivery. Although it is important in this initial meeting not to overwhelm parents with information, the provider should clarify misunderstandings or misinformation regarding Down syndrome. The provider should also begin to prepare the family for issues and problems that may occur, especially during the child's first months and years. It may be necessary to meet with the family on several occasions early on to adequately answer questions and address concerns. During these meetings, the provider should explain how the diagnosis of Down syndrome is made using karyotype information and other studies. It is important to review the risk for recurrences in subsequent pregnancies; the recurrence risk for trisomy 21 is 1 in 100, plus the risk of maternal age. The provider should inquire about other family members with Down syndrome or other developmental disabilities. Families with translocations or mosaicism should be referred for genetic counseling to discuss the mechanism of occurrence and recurrence risk in these cases.

B. Associated Conditions: Medical services should address the early identification and treatment of a wide range of conditions associated with Down syndrome (Figure 1). These conditions include congenital heart disease (44%); gastrointestinal anomalies (5%), including atresias and Hirschsprung disease; atlantoaxial instability or subluxation (15%); eye disease, such as cataracts, strabismus, nystagmus, and visual impairment (60%); ear disease and hearing impairment (75%); hypothyroidism (15%); celiac disease (5%–10%); and leukemia (<1%).

(Continued on page 682)

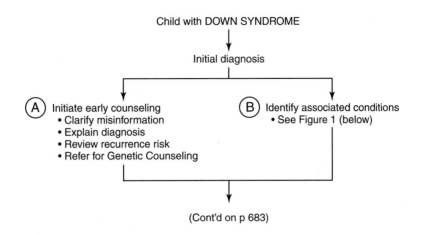

Child with DOWN SYNDROME

↓

Initial diagnosis

(A) Initiate early counseling
- Clarify misinformation
- Explain diagnosis
- Review recurrence risk
- Refer for Genetic Counseling

(B) Identify associated conditions
- See Figure 1 (below)

↓

(Cont'd on p 683)

Associated medical conditions

↓

Yes

Condition	Evaluation	Consult
<u>Cardiac</u> Congenital heart disease	Chest radiograph ECG Echocardiogram	Consult: Cardiology
<u>Gastrointestinal</u> Atresia Hirschsprung disease Constipation GERD Celiac disease	Radiology studies	Consult: Gastroenterology Surgery
<u>Musculoskeletal</u> Hypotonia Hip dysplasia Atlantoaxial subluxation	Radiology studies	Consult: Orthopedics Physical therapy
<u>Endocrine</u>	Thyroid function tests Birth, 6 mo, annual	Consult: Endocrinology
<u>Otolaryngology</u> Otitis media Sinusitis Sensorineural-hearing loss	Pneumococcal vaccine Annual hearing screen Close follow-up	Consult: ENT Audiology
<u>Ophthalmology</u> Cataracts Strabismus Nystagmus Refractive errors	Vision screening	Consult: Ophthalmology

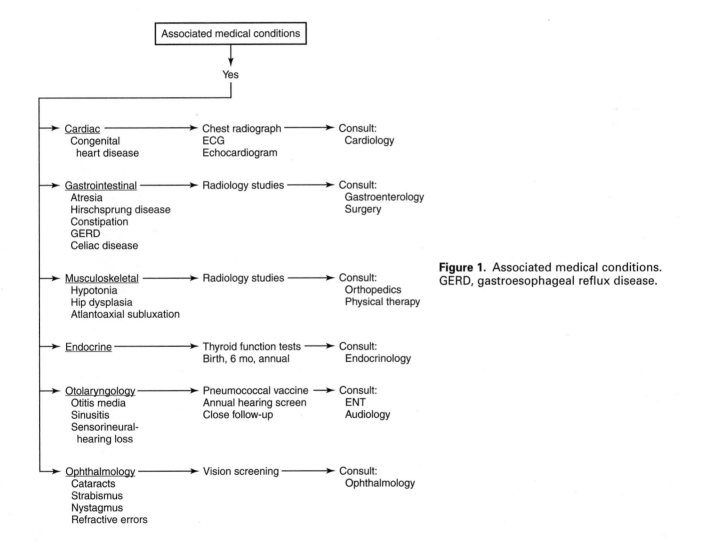

Figure 1. Associated medical conditions. GERD, gastroesophageal reflux disease.

C. The Newborn Period: After birth, the infant with Down syndrome should have a karyotype sent, an echocardiogram performed to assess for cardiac anomalies, a newborn screen including thyroid function panel, a complete blood cell count (CBC), and a newborn hearing evaluation. Surgical issues caused by cardiac, gastrointestinal, or other anomalies should be immediately addressed. The provider should complete a physical examination, noting the features of Down syndrome, which may include hypotonia, brachycephalic head, epicanthic folds, flat nasal bridge, upward slanting palpebral fissures, mottled spots on the iris (Brushfield spots), large-appearing tongue, small ears, excess skin at the nape of the neck, single transverse palmar crease, wide space between the first and second toes, and short fifth fingers with clinodactyly (curving of the finger). A thorough cardiac examination should be done, noting the presence of cyanosis, murmurs, and signs of congestive heart failure. The provider should assess for abdominal distention, which could be an indication of abnormalities of the intestinal tract. During infancy, feeding problems should be assessed, and growth should be carefully monitored using Down syndrome–specific growth charts. Vision testing and ophthalmology referral should be performed if the infant has evidence of eye abnormalities, including congenital cataracts. Children with Down syndrome should be referred for physical, occupational, and speech therapies early on. An emphasis on improving developmental processes can optimize outcomes of these children.

D. Childhood: Throughout childhood, the primary care provider is charged with providing preventive care and coordinating the services given by medical subspecialists, surgeons, and other health care professionals. Children with Down syndrome require health maintenance appropriate for all children including immunizations, growth, and nutrition. Growth should continue to be monitored on Down syndrome–specific growth charts. Special attention must be given to obesity prevention, because children with Down syndrome are at high risk for becoming overweight. At each visit the provider should emphasize diet and exercise to maintain a healthy weight. Children with Down syndrome should have annual hearing and vision screening, together with yearly thyroid function tests. Between age 3 and 5 years, children with Down syndrome are recommended to have cervical spine radiographs to assess for atlantoaxial instability or subluxation. A change of more than 5 mm in the atlantodens space between flexion and extension on lateral C-spine films suggests abnormality and magnetic resonance imaging of the cervical spine should be obtained. Careful examination of the deep tendon reflexes should be performed at each visit to identify findings of atlantoaxial instability to suggest need for imaging. In addition, signs of leukemia or lymphoma should be noted, especially toward the end of the first decade of life. These signs include pallor, easy bruising or bleeding, lymphadenopathy, and organomegaly. Next, the provider should review the child's behavior and, if needed, develop a plan for behavior management, socialization, and recreational skills. Families should be presented with options for preschool programs for children with developmental disabilities. In early childhood, the provider should begin the discussion of appropriate school placement. Once the child is in school, it is important to assess options to promote the development of prevocational skills.

E. Adolescence: Preventive health care measures as described earlier with the emphasis on obesity prevention should be continued in adolescents with Down syndrome. Yearly hearing and vision screening, annual thyroid function tests, and attention on physical examination to signs of atlantoaxial abnormalities and leukemia should be continued in this group. The provider should continue to discuss education with emphasis on the appropriateness of school placement and vocational training within the curriculum. Behavior and mental health issues in the adolescent with Down syndrome should be identified. Depression and signs of early-onset Alzheimer disease may present in late adolescence. As adolescents mature, it is also important to discuss psychosocial development and sexuality with patients and their families. In teenage girls, the provider should address menstrual hygiene and management. Although fertility is reduced in patients with Down syndrome, it is still important, as for all teenagers with disabilities, to review sexual education and birth control options. In late adolescence and early adulthood, it is important to discuss group homes, workshop settings, and other community-supported employment opportunities. At this time the provider should address transition of medical care to an adult setting.

F. Identify Family Needs and Support Services: At each visit the provider should inquire about the needs of the family and help identify resources for support, including other family members, friends, and clergy. Families should be provided with resources available to parents of children with Down syndrome, including community-based Down syndrome support groups. The benefits of participation in these communities should be reviewed often. The provider should implement a long-term planning process that anticipates issues such as financial planning, future guardianship, family relationships, and eventual transition to adulthood. It is important to frequently review financial support options, including Title V programs and high-risk insurance programs supplemented by the state. Families may consider Supplemental Social Security income benefits. The provider should advocate for the family when the patient has difficulty accessing needed health services because of obstacles with their health insurance plan.

G. Develop a Care Plan: The provider should work with the family and patient to develop a care plan that includes information about the patient's diagnoses, prescription medications, referrals to and recommendations from subspecialists, required health maintenance needs including immunizations and screening tests, and follow-up plans. The care plan should be reviewed and updated at each health maintenance visit. Periodic multidisciplinary staffing is often required to monitor the care plan and to make necessary adjustments.

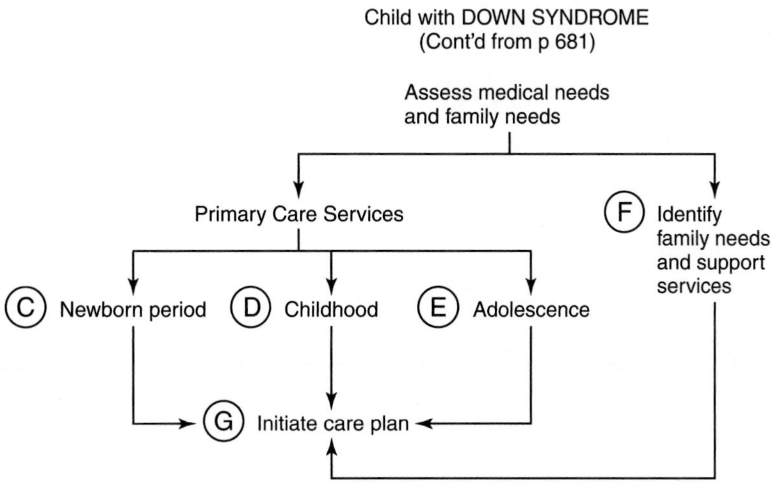
Child with DOWN SYNDROME
(Cont'd from p 681)
Assess medical needs
and family needs
Primary Care Services
F Identify family needs and support services
C Newborn period
D Childhood
E Adolescence
G Initiate care plan

References

American Academy of Pediatrics, Committee on Genetics, Health Supervision for children with Down syndrome. Pediatrics 2001;107:442–9.

Davidson MA. Primary care for children and adolescents with Down syndrome. Pediatr Clin N Am 2008;55:1099–111.

Roizen NJ, Patterson D. Downs syndrome. Lancet 2003;361:1281–9.

Inborn Errors of Metabolism in the Neonate

Renata C. Gallagher, MD, PhD, and Carol L. Greene, MD

Although each individual inborn error of metabolism (IEM) is rare, taken as a group they are an important cause of neonatal morbidity and mortality. Prompt identification of a possible inborn error, and the institution of appropriate treatment, may prevent severe neurologic injury or death for some infants. Even when the affected neonate does not survive, the identification of an inborn error, genetic counseling regarding the possibility of another affected child, and testing in a subsequent pregnancy, if available, may greatly aid the family.

A. In the neonatal period, IEM can present with nonspecific signs, initially suggestive of neonatal sepsis. The most common symptoms in neonates are poor feeding, lethargy, and irritability. These may be followed by progressive neurologic symptoms, including seizures and obtundation. Physical examination findings suggestive of an inborn error include altered mental status, hypertonia or hypotonia, hyperreflexia, apnea, and tachypnea. Tachypnea may result from respiratory compensation in metabolic acidosis, or from hyperammonemia, which stimulates respiration, causing a primary respiratory alkalosis. Other suggestive findings include hepatomegaly, jaundice, and unusual odors (e.g., maple syrup in maple syrup urine disease, sweaty feet in isovaleric acidemia). Unusual physical findings that may provide specific diagnostic clues include macrocephaly and cataracts. Positive findings on family history may be a clue to the presence of an inborn error. It is important to ask specifically about parental consanguinity, as well as a family history of mental retardation, seizures, recurrent emesis or altered mental status, and early death (especially neonatal deaths or sudden infant death syndrome).

B. Standard laboratory evaluations, once performed, should be reviewed for signs of an inborn error. These laboratory tests include electrolytes, glucose, a blood gas, a complete blood cell count (CBC), liver function tests, and a urinalysis. The anion gap should be reviewed or calculated if not provided. A profound anion gap acidosis in a newborn is strongly suggestive of either an organic acidemia or a congenital lactic acidosis. Marked acidosis in a very young infant is unlikely to be a physiologic response. The presence of hypoglycemia may indicate an inborn error. Anemia, neutropenia, and thrombocytopenia could indicate sepsis or bone marrow suppression caused by an organic acidemia. A CBC with an increased white blood cell count suggestive of infection does not rule out an inborn error, because inborn errors can co-occur with infection. A primary respiratory alkalosis is suggestive of a urea cycle defect. Increased aspartate aminotransferase (AST), alanine transaminase (ALT), and/or bilirubin may be signs of an inborn error. Newborns do not make ketones with poor feeding, but they can be elevated in organic acidurias; the presence of urine ketones in an ill neonate strongly suggests an inborn error. The presence of one or more of the earlier abnormal findings may warrant further testing for an inborn error.

C. Initial laboratory testing may have included other routine chemistries that are helpful in assessing the likelihood of an inborn error. These include lactate, ammonia, creatine kinase, coagulation studies, and urine for reducing substances. If these were not obtained, and there are concerning history, physical, or laboratory findings as discussed earlier, these should be ordered. A total plasma homocysteine should be obtained if the infant has seizures or thrombosis. An ammonia level should be ordered if there is unexplained altered mental status, vomiting, progressive neurologic symptoms, a marked metabolic acidosis, or a primary respiratory alkalosis. Blood for an ammonia level should be obtained from a free-flowing sample, placed on ice immediately, and processed rapidly to minimize false elevations; heelstick ammonia is unacceptable. Hyperammonemia in the neonate is a medical emergency. A markedly increased ammonia level in a neonate may result in irreversible brain injury or death. Levels can increase to the thousands within hours. It is critical to contact a specialist in management of IEMs as soon as a high ammonia level is identified. Increased AST, increased ALT, coagulopathy, cholestasis, increased creatine kinase, cardiac dysfunction, and/or an abnormal brain MRI image may be signs of an inborn error. Positive urine-reducing substances may indicate glucose, galactose, fructose, or other compounds, including drugs; therefore, it is important to obtain the urine sample for reducing substances before antibiotic treatment is administered. Urine-reducing substances may be negative in classic galactosemia if the child is not receiving galactose at the time of the test. This is also true in hereditary fructose intolerance if the child is not taking fructose. The clinical history and pattern of laboratory abnormalities may point to one or more possible inborn errors requiring further specialized biochemical testing for diagnosis (see later). If the routine chemistry laboratories are not concerning for an inborn error, but suspicion remains, obtain plasma (2–3 ml in a lithium or sodium heparin [green top] tube) and urine, and freeze for possible later biochemical analysis. These samples are best obtained before full resuscitation but should be taken at a later time if there is a concern for a possible inborn error.

D. Hyperammonemia and/or severe metabolic acidosis require obtaining the results of specialized biochemical laboratories rapidly, within 12 to 24 hours, if possible. Determining which are the appropriate biochemical laboratory studies to be ordered, and having them run

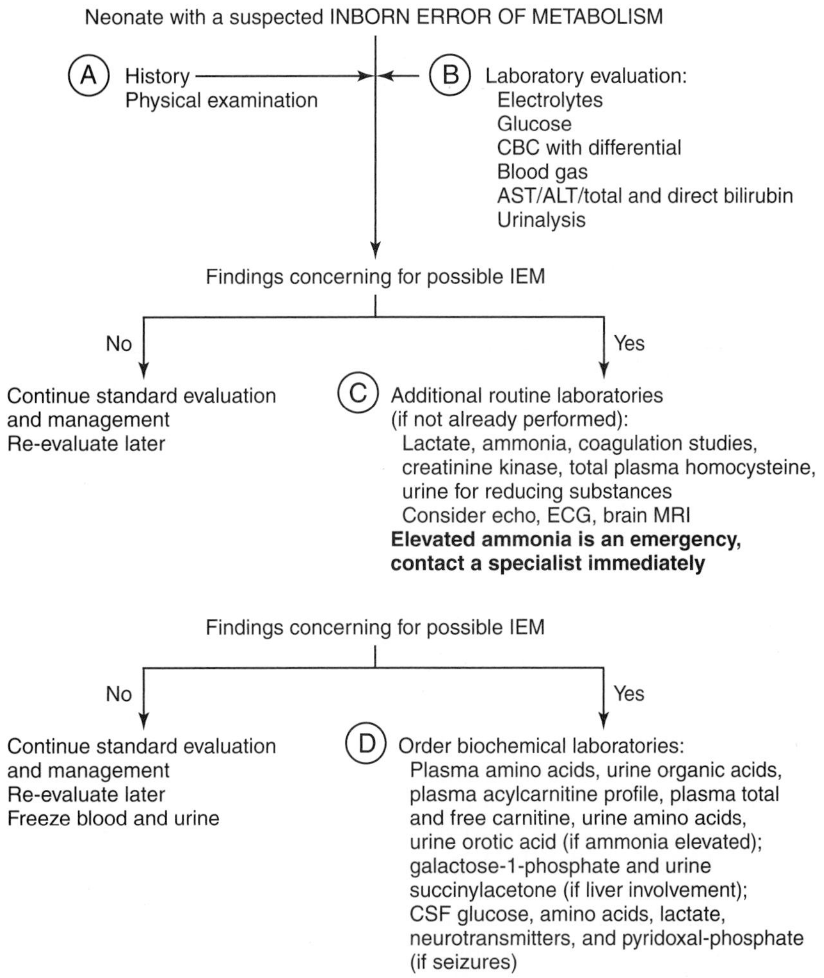
Neonate with a suspected INBORN ERROR OF METABOLISM
A
History
Physical examination
B
Laboratory evaluation:
Electrolytes
Glucose
CBC with differential
Blood gas
AST/ALT/total and direct bilirubin
Urinalysis
Findings concerning for possible IEM
No
Yes
Continue standard evaluation and management
Re-evaluate later
C
Additional routine laboratories (if not already performed):
Lactate, ammonia, coagulation studies, creatinine kinase, total plasma homocysteine, urine for reducing substances
Consider echo, ECG, brain MRI
Elevated ammonia is an emergency, contact a specialist immediately
Findings concerning for possible IEM
No
Yes
Continue standard evaluation and management
Re-evaluate later
Freeze blood and urine
D
Order biochemical laboratories:
Plasma amino acids, urine organic acids, plasma acylcarnitine profile, plasma total and free carnitine, urine amino acids, urine orotic acid (if ammonia elevated); galactose-1-phosphate and urine succinylacetone (if liver involvement); CSF glucose, amino acids, lactate, neurotransmitters, and pyridoxal-phosphate (if seizures)

(Cont'd on p 687)

as quickly as possible, requires consultation with a clinician experienced in the diagnosis and management of inborn errors, and contact with the biochemical genetics laboratory. A diagnosis can often be made within hours if there is a local biochemical laboratory. This allows rapid institution of the most appropriate therapy. High ammonia levels in a neonate may be caused by disorders of protein or fat metabolism. These are diagnosed through plasma amino acids, urine organic acids, and an acylcarnitine profile. Orotic acid is increased in certain urea cycle defects and should be ordered if there is hyperammonemia. Urine amino acids will identify specific or generalized renal transport defects and should be abnormal in homocystinurias. If the neonate has seizures or apnea, the listed CSF studies should be performed, in addition to the standard testing for glucose, cell count, and protein. It is important that, concurrent with the corresponding CSF studies, plasma glucose and plasma amino acids be obtained for evaluation of glucose transporter defect and glycine encephalopathy, respectively. CSF for neurotransmitters and for pyridoxal-phosphate require special tubes and handling; the testing laboratory should be contacted for information regarding these before the lumbar puncture. Newborn screening for some inborn errors is done in most states. The state newborn screening laboratory should be contacted if the results have not yet been reported or are unavailable. If the screen is abnormal, this may aid in diagnosis. A "normal" newborn screen does not rule out an inborn error, and diagnostic testing should always be ordered if there is a clinical concern. If there is reasonable suspicion for an inborn error based on the clinical presentation and routine laboratory studies, the listed biochemical laboratories should be performed. Other laboratory tests may be recommended by the consulting specialist(s).

E. Withholding potentially toxic precursors (protein, fat, galactose, fructose) to limit exogenous intoxication is critical if there is a high suspicion for an inborn error. Limitation of endogenous intoxication is facilitated by treatment with intravenous glucose, which will help decrease breakdown of endogenous protein and fat for energy. This treatment will also supply needed energy in disorders associated with reduced fasting tolerance such as fatty acid oxidation disorders, glycogen storage diseases, and gluconeogenesis defects. Only a few neonates (those with severe primary lactic acidosis because of pyruvate dehydrogenase deficiency or a mitochondrial respiratory chain defect) will become worse with intravenous glucose. Glucose should be given at 8 to 12 mg/kg/min. Protein should be held for 12 to 24 hours if there is a possible protein metabolism disorder (aminoacidopathy, organic acidemia, or urea cycle defect), but should not be withheld for a prolonged period or the infant will break down endogenous protein, worsening the clinical course. Fat should be withheld until a disorder of fat metabolism is ruled out. The infant should be switched to a soy formula if galactosemia is a possibility. Fructose is a component of some formulas and should be withheld if symptoms developed after the institution of a fructose-containing formula, or if there are other clinical and laboratory findings suggestive of this disorder. Vitamin cofactors are recommended in specific situations, such as vitamin B_{12} for possible B_{12}-responsive methylmalonic acidemia or thiamine for possible thiamine-responsive maple syrup urine disease. Intravenous carnitine is recommended for a suspected organic acidemia and may be lifesaving in primary carnitine deficiency. It should be used with caution in possible long-chain fatty acid oxidation disorders, because long-chain acylcarnitines may be arrhythmogenic. The recommended dose should be determined in consultation with a specialist. Other specific treatments include pyridoxine for possible pyridoxine-dependent epilepsy, and pharmacologic therapy for a possible urea cycle defect. Management of an inborn error should be directed by a specialist experienced in the evaluation and treatment of these disorders.

F. If ammonia levels are greater than can be brought down by pharmacologic therapy, if there is marked acidosis, or if there is hyperleucinemia (in maple syrup urine disease), dialysis may be indicated. This requires a coordinated effort by the neonatal intensive care unit (NICU), surgery, nephrology, and metabolic teams. Early transfer may be indicated if dialysis is not available at the local hospital.

G. If support is withdrawn because of a poor prognosis, or the failure of medical therapy, and no diagnosis has been established, consideration should be given to rapidly obtaining and freezing skeletal and cardiac muscle, liver, kidney, and brain in a metabolic autopsy. This may also include biochemical testing on blood, bile, and urine, if not performed before death. It is also recommended that skin be obtained for fibroblast culture, and that DNA be made and held for possible DNA sequencing in the event that a specific diagnosis is suggested by other studies.

References

Burton BK. Inborn errors of metabolism: the clinical diagnosis in early infancy. Pediatrics 1987;79:359.

Ernst LM, Sondheimer N, Deardorff MA, et al. The value of the metabolic autopsy in the pediatric hospital setting. J Pediatr 2006;148: 779–83.

Goodman SI, Greene CL. Metabolic disorders of the newborn. Pediatr Rev 1994;15:9.

Greene CL, Thomas JA, Goodman SI. Inborn errors of metabolism. In: Hay WW, Hayward AR, Levin MJ, Sondheimer JM, editors. Pediatric diagnosis and treatment. 15th ed. Norwalk, CT: Appleton & Lange; 2001. p. 881.

Prietsch V, Lindner M, Zschocke J, et al. Emergency management of inherited metabolic diseases. J Inherit Metab Dis 2002;531–46.

Surtees R, Leonard JV. Acute metabolic encephalopathy: a review of causes, mechanisms and treatment. J Inherit Metab Dis 1989;12(suppl 1):42.

Zschocke J, Hoffmann GF. Vademecum metabolicum. In: Manual of metabolic paediatrics. 2nd ed. Friedrichsdorf, Germany: Schattauer; 2004.

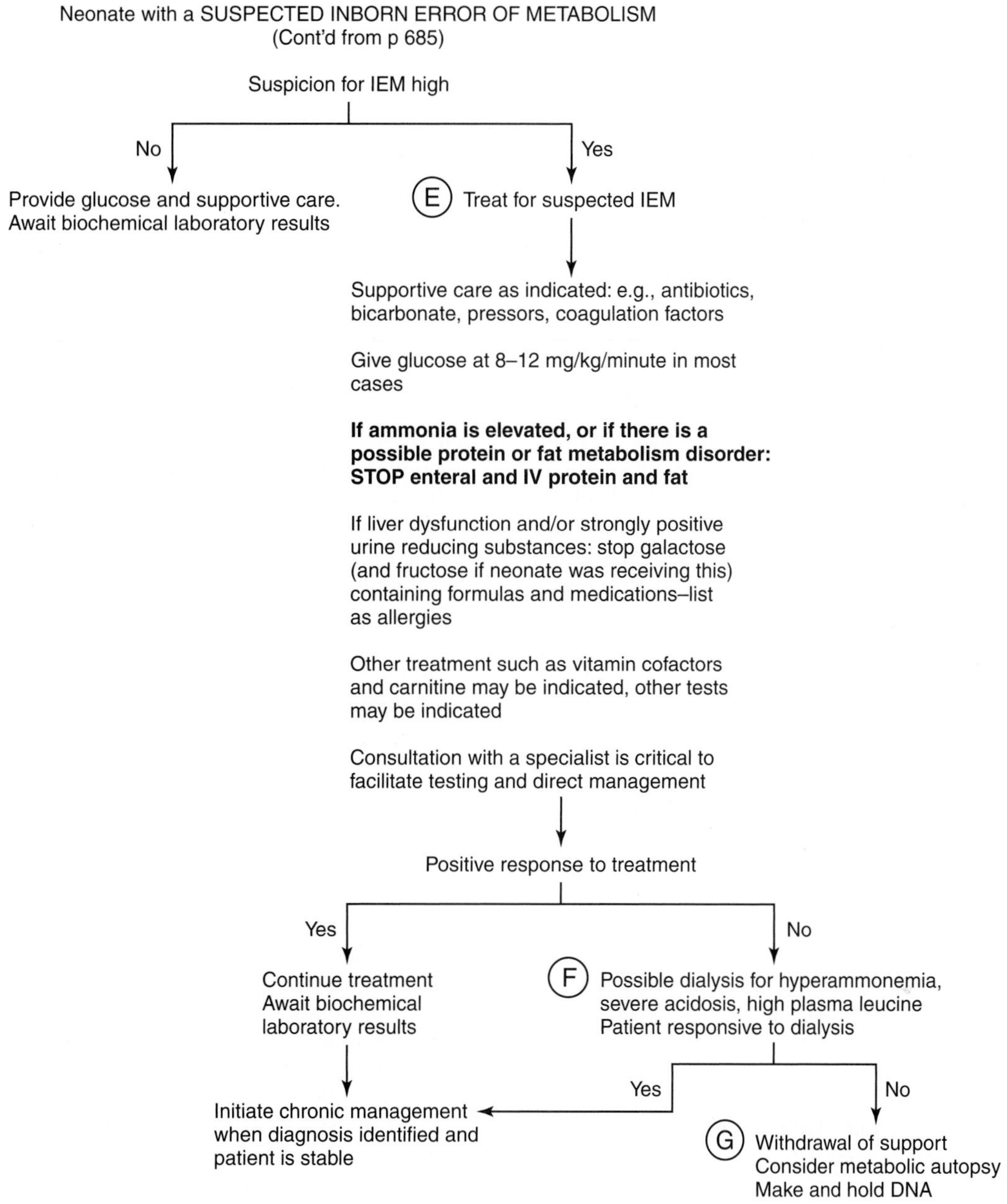
Neonate with a SUSPECTED INBORN ERROR OF METABOLISM
(Cont'd from p 685)
Suspicion for IEM high
No
Provide glucose and supportive care.
Await biochemical laboratory results
Yes
E
Treat for suspected IEM
Supportive care as indicated: e.g., antibiotics, bicarbonate, pressors, coagulation factors
Give glucose at 8–12 mg/kg/minute in most cases
If ammonia is elevated, or if there is a possible protein or fat metabolism disorder: STOP enteral and IV protein and fat
If liver dysfunction and/or strongly positive urine reducing substances: stop galactose (and fructose if neonate was receiving this) containing formulas and medications–list as allergies
Other treatment such as vitamin cofactors and carnitine may be indicated, other tests may be indicated
Consultation with a specialist is critical to facilitate testing and direct management
Positive response to treatment
Yes
Continue treatment
Await biochemical laboratory results
Initiate chronic management when diagnosis identified and patient is stable
No
F
Possible dialysis for hyperammonemia, severe acidosis, high plasma leucine
Patient responsive to dialysis
Yes
No
G
Withdrawal of support
Consider metabolic autopsy
Make and hold DNA

Inborn Errors of Metabolism in the Acutely Ill Child

Renata C. Gallagher, MD, PhD, and Carol L. Greene, MD

An acute presentation of an inborn error of metabolism may occur at any age. Although this chapter refers to a child, the algorithm may be applied to adults as well. An affected individual may have been previously healthy, though recurrent episodes of emesis, altered mental status, or other symptoms such as hypoglycemia or acidosis increase the likelihood of an inborn error, as does the presence of neurologic symptoms such as seizures, hypotonia, or developmental delay. For certain disorders, individuals presenting after the neonatal period may have milder biochemical defects with some residual enzyme activity, and may respond fairly well to acute and chronic management. Delay in diagnosis and treatment can result in irreversible neurologic damage and death. High suspicion for an inborn error is more likely to result in an accurate diagnosis, allowing early institution of the appropriate treatment and the best chance for an optimal outcome.

Inborn errors are due to defects in enzymes or transport proteins that result in blocks of biochemical pathways. There are multiple classes of inborn errors including lysosomal storage disorders, glycogen storage disorders, disorders of mitochondrial energy metabolism, neurotransmitter disorders, and disorders of protein, fat, and carbohydrate metabolism. Symptoms vary and include organomegaly, developmental delay, developmental regression, seizures, organ dysfunction, and acute metabolic decompensation with acidosis, hyperammonemia, and/or hypoglycemia. The inborn errors that are most likely to manifest as acute illness are the disorders of protein, fat, or carbohydrate metabolism, including glycogen storage disorders. In these disorders, symptoms are generally due to intoxication (e.g., from increased ammonia in urea cycle disorders) or reduced fasting tolerance (e.g., from hypoglycemia in fatty acid oxidation disorders). Inborn errors of metabolism may cause altered mental status, acidosis, or hypoglycemia. Because symptoms may be provoked by intercurrent illness, the diagnosis of an inborn error may be missed if the symptoms are attributed to infection alone; laboratory findings may be mistakenly attributed to dehydration or asphyxia. An inborn error should be considered when the clinical symptoms or laboratory abnormalities are greater than expected for the clinical history. Inborn errors should be considered in children with preexisting neurologic symptoms, progressive neurologic symptoms, unexplained altered mental status or emesis, and in those who require disproportionate intervention for control of acidosis or who exhibit marked hypoglycemia. It is important to note that the absence of acidosis or hypoglycemia does not rule out an inborn error. These abnormalities may be late findings in some disorders and are not typical in individuals with urea cycle defects or maple syrup urine disease, in which symptoms of altered mental status, ataxia, or emesis are due to hyperammonemia and hyperleucinemia, respectively.

A. The child's medical history may reveal previous episodes of emesis, altered mental status, ataxia, or dehydration. A history of failure to thrive, macrocephaly or microcephaly, seizures, developmental delay, or regression should increase the suspicion for an inborn error. The dietary history is important and may reveal a recent dietary change. Changes that may provoke symptoms in an affected individual include the introduction of lactose, which contains galactose (e.g., switch from lactose-free soy formula to cow's milk formula); introduction of fructose from juices, fruits, or certain formulas; or introduction of increased protein because of a switch from breast milk, which is low in protein, to infant formula or milk. Clarification of the duration of fasting before the onset of symptoms is also important. This may identify an increased duration of fasting because of a longer period of sleep with increasing age and/or decreased intake in illness. A history of abuse, neglect, or nonaccidental trauma may accompany inborn errors because affected children may have feeding difficulties or irritability and parenting may be difficult. It is also important to be aware that the organic acid disorder glutaric aciduria type 1 is a mimic of nonaccidental trauma. Children with apparent nonaccidental trauma should be evaluated for this disorder, particularly if the skeletal survey is negative. Physical examination findings suggestive of an inborn error include altered mental status, hypertonia or hypotonia, hyper-reflexia, apnea, and tachypnea. Tachypnea may result from respiratory compensation in metabolic acidosis or from hyperammonemia, which stimulates respiration, causing a primary respiratory alkalosis. Other suggestive findings include hepatomegaly, jaundice, and unusual odors (e.g., maple syrup in maple syrup urine disease, sweaty feet in isovaleric acidemia). Unusual physical findings that may provide specific diagnostic clues include macrocephaly and cataracts. Positive findings on family history may be a clue to the presence of an inborn error. It is important to ask specifically about parental consanguinity, as well as a family history of mental retardation, seizures, recurrent emesis or altered mental status, and early death (especially neonatal deaths or sudden infant death syndrome).

B. Standard laboratory evaluations, once performed, should be reviewed for signs of an inborn error. These laboratories include electrolytes, glucose, a blood gas, a complete blood cell count (CBC), liver function tests, and a urinalysis. The anion gap should be reviewed or calculated if not provided. An anion gap acidosis is suggestive of an inborn error. The presence of hypoglycemia may indicate an inborn error. A CBC with an increased white blood cell count suggestive of infection

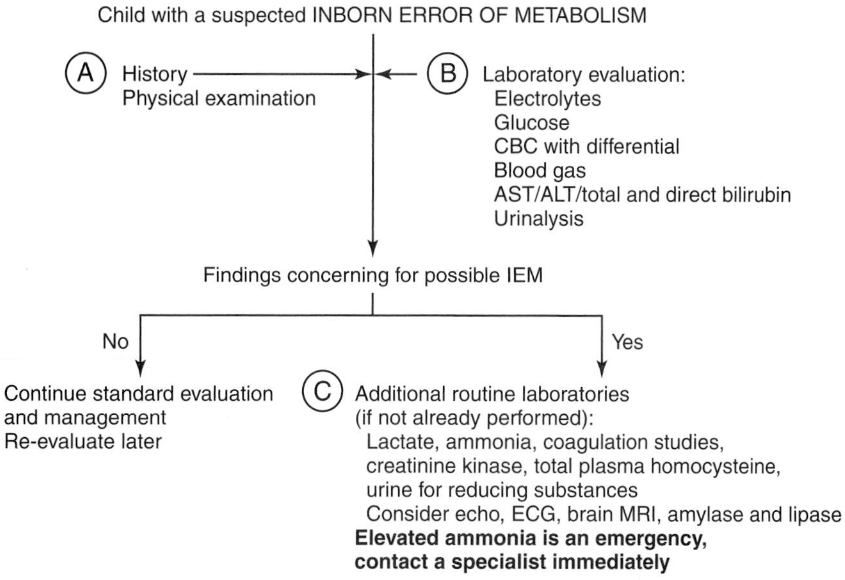
Child with a suspected INBORN ERROR OF METABOLISM
A
History
Physical examination
B
Laboratory evaluation:
Electrolytes
Glucose
CBC with differential
Blood gas
AST/ALT/total and direct bilirubin
Urinalysis
Findings concerning for possible IEM
No
Yes
Continue standard evaluation and management
Re-evaluate later
C
Additional routine laboratories (if not already performed):
Lactate, ammonia, coagulation studies, creatinine kinase, total plasma homocysteine, urine for reducing substances
Consider echo, ECG, brain MRI, amylase and lipase
Elevated ammonia is an emergency, contact a specialist immediately

(Cont'd on p 691)

does not rule out an inborn error, because inborn errors can co-occur with infection. Anemia, neutropenia, and/or thrombocytopenia may reflect marrow suppression, which may be seen in multiple classes of inborn errors. An increased mean corpuscular volume (MCV) may be seen in disorders of B_{12} metabolism, as well as other inborn errors. A primary respiratory alkalosis is suggestive of a urea cycle defect. Increased aspartate aminotransferase (AST), alanine aminotransferase (ALT), and/or bilirubin may be signs of an inborn error. The presence of urine ketones in an individual with hypoglycemia does not exclude an inborn error because patients with disorders of fatty acid oxidation may make some ketones in response to fasting. Insufficient ketone production for the degree of hypoglycemia may indicate an inborn error (though hyperinsulinism is also associated with low ketones). The presence of one or more of the earlier abnormal findings may warrant further testing for an inborn error.

C. Initial laboratory testing may have included other routine chemistries that are helpful in assessing the likelihood of an inborn error. These include lactate, ammonia, creatine kinase, coagulation studies, and urine for reducing substances. If these were not obtained, and there are concerning history, physical, or laboratory findings as discussed earlier, these should be ordered. A total plasma homocysteine should be obtained if the individual has seizures or thrombosis. An ammonia level should be ordered if there is unexplained altered mental status, vomiting, progressive neurologic symptoms, a marked metabolic acidosis, or a primary respiratory alkalosis. Blood for an ammonia level should be obtained from a free-flowing sample, placed on ice immediately, and processed rapidly to minimize false elevations; heelstick ammonia is unacceptable. Hyperammonemia is a medical emergency. A markedly increased ammonia level may result in irreversible brain injury or death. It is critical to contact a specialist in management of inborn errors of metabolism as soon as a high ammonia level is identified. Increased AST, increased ALT, coagulopathy, cholestasis, increased creatine kinase, cardiac dysfunction, and/or an abnormal brain MRI may be signs of an inborn error. A high lactate level in a patient with good peripheral perfusion and normal blood pressure is suggestive of a primary lactic acidosis. Some disorders are associated with pancreatitis, therefore amylase and lipase should be considered. Positive urine-reducing substances may indicate glucose, galactose, fructose, or other compounds, including drugs; therefore, it is important to obtain the urine sample for reducing substances before antibiotic treatment is administered. Urine-reducing substances may be negative in classic galactosemia if the individual is not receiving galactose at the time of the test. This is also true in hereditary fructose intolerance if the individual is not taking fructose. The clinical history and pattern of laboratory abnormalities may point to one or more possible inborn errors requiring further specialized biochemical testing for diagnosis (see later). If the routine chemistry laboratories are not concerning for an inborn error but suspicion remains, obtain plasma (2–3 ml in a lithium or sodium heparin [green top] tube) and urine, and freeze for possible later biochemical analysis. These samples are best obtained before full resuscitation, but should be taken at a later time if there is a concern for a possible inborn error.

D. If there is unexplained marked hyperammonemia, the results of specialized biochemical laboratories should be obtained rapidly, within 24 hours, if possible. This is also recommended for unexplained severe metabolic acidosis if there are other findings suggestive of an inborn error. Determining which are the appropriate biochemical laboratory studies to be ordered, and having them run as quickly as possible, requires consultation with a clinician experienced in the diagnosis and management of inborn errors and contact with the biochemical genetics laboratory. A diagnosis can often be made within hours if there is a local biochemical laboratory. This allows rapid institution of the most appropriate therapy. High ammonia levels may be associated with liver failure, the use of valproate, or may be caused by inborn errors of protein or fat metabolism. Mitochondrial energy metabolism disorders may also be associated with hyperammonemia. Please note that the presence of liver failure or valproate use does not exclude an underlying urea cycle disorder, and testing for urea cycle disorders may be indicated. Inborn errors of protein or fat metabolism are diagnosed through plasma amino acids, urine organic acids, and an acylcarnitine profile. Orotic acid is increased in certain urea cycle defects and should be ordered, particularly if there is hyperammonemia. Urine amino acids will identify specific or generalized renal transport defects and should be abnormal in homocystinurias. If the individual has seizures, the listed cerebrospinal fluid (CSF) studies should be considered in addition to the standard testing for glucose, cell count, and protein. It is important that, concurrent with the corresponding CSF studies, plasma glucose and plasma amino acids be obtained for evaluation for glucose transporter defect and for glycine encephalopathy, respectively. CSF for neurotransmitters and for pyridoxal-phosphate requires special tubes and handling; the testing laboratory should be contacted for information regarding these before the lumbar puncture. Newborn screening for some inborn errors is done in most states. The newborn screen results should be reviewed if possible, if there is a concern for an inborn error. The screen is not fully sensitive for all disorders, and results close to the cutoff values may suggest an underlying diagnosis. A "normal" newborn screen does not rule out an inborn error, and diagnostic testing should always be ordered if there is a clinical concern. If there is a reasonable suspicion for an inborn error based on the clinical presentation and routine laboratory studies, the listed biochemical laboratories should be performed. Other laboratories may be recommended by the consulting specialist(s).

E. Withholding potentially toxic precursors (protein, fat, galactose, fructose) to limit exogenous intoxication is critical if there is a high suspicion for an inborn error. Limitation of endogenous intoxication is facilitated by treatment with intravenous glucose, which will help decrease breakdown of endogenous protein and fat for energy. This treatment will also supply needed energy in disorders associated with reduced fasting tolerance such as fatty acid oxidation disorders, glycogen storage diseases, and gluconeogenesis defects. Only a few individuals (those with severe primary lactic acidosis caused by pyruvate dehydrogenase deficiency or a mitochondrial respiratory chain defect) will become worse with intravenous glucose. Glucose should be given at 6 to 10 mg/kg/min. Protein should be held for 12 to 24 hours if there is a possible protein metabolism disorder (aminoacidopathy, organic acidemia, or urea cycle defect) but should not be withheld for a prolonged period or the individual will break down endogenous protein, worsening the clinical course. Fat should be withheld until a disorder of fat metabolism is ruled out. A young child or infant should be switched to a soy formula if galactosemia is a possibility. Fructose is a component of some formulas and should be withheld if symptoms developed after the institution of a fructose-containing formula, juice, or fruit, or if there are other clinical and laboratory findings suggestive of this disorder. Vitamin cofactors are recommended in specific situations such as vitamin B_{12} for possible B_{12}-responsive methylmalonic acidemia, or thiamine for possible thiamine-responsive maple syrup urine disease. Intravenous carnitine is recommended for a suspected organic acidemia and may be lifesaving in primary carnitine deficiency. It should be used with caution in possible long-chain fatty acid oxidation disorders, because long-chain acylcarnitines may be arrhythmogenic. The recommended dose should be determined in consultation with a specialist. Other specific treatments include pyridoxine for possible pyridoxine-dependent epilepsy, and pharmacologic therapy for a possible urea cycle defect. Management of an inborn error should be directed by a specialist experienced in the evaluation and treatment of these disorders.

F. If ammonia levels are greater than can be brought down by pharmacologic therapy, if there is marked acidosis, or if there is marked hyperleucinemia (in maple syrup urine disease), dialysis may be indicated. This requires a coordinated effort by the intensive care unit, surgery, nephrology, and metabolic teams. Early transfer may be indicated if dialysis is not available at the local hospital.

G. If support is withdrawn because of a poor prognosis, or the failure of medical therapy, and no diagnosis has been established, consideration should be given to rapidly obtaining and freezing skeletal and cardiac muscle, liver, kidney, and brain in a metabolic autopsy. This may also include biochemical testing on blood, bile, and urine, if not performed before death. It is also recommended that skin be obtained for fibroblast culture, and that DNA be made and held for possible DNA sequencing in the event that a specific diagnosis is suggested by other studies.

Child with a suspected INBORN ERROR OF METABOLISM
(Cont'd from p 689)

Findings concerning for possible IEM

- No → Continue standard evaluation and management
  Re-evaluate later
  Freeze blood and urine
- Yes → (D) Order biochemical laboratories:
  Plasma amino acids, urine organic acids, plasma acylcarnitine profile, plasma total and free carnitine, urine amino acids, urine orotic acid; galactose-1-phosphate and urine succinylacetone (if liver involvement);
  CSF glucose, amino acids, lactate, neurotransmitters, pyridoxal-phosphate, and 5-methyltetrahydrofolate (if seizures)

Suspicion for IEM high

- No → Provide glucose and supportive care.
  Await biochemical laboratory results
- Yes → (E) Treat for suspected IEM
  ↓
  Supportive care as indicated: e.g., antibiotics, bicarbonate, pressors, coagulation factors

  Give glucose at 6–10 mg/kg/minute in most cases

  If ammonia is elevated, or if there is a possible protein or fat metabolism disorder: STOP enteral and IV protein and fat

  If liver dysfunction and/or strongly positive urine reducing substances: stop galactose (and fructose if neonate was receiving this) containing formulas and medications–list as allergies

  Other treatment such as vitamin cofactors and carnitine may be indicated, other tests may be indicated

  Consultation with a specialist is critical to facilitate testing and direct management
  ↓

Positive response to treatment

- Yes → Continue treatment
  Await biochemical laboratory results
  ↓
  Initiate chronic management when diagnosis identified and patient is stable
- No → (F) Possible dialysis for hyperammonemia, severe acidosis, very high plasma leucine
  Patient responsive to dialysis
  - Yes → Initiate chronic management when diagnosis identified and patient is stable
  - No → (G) Withdrawal of support
    Consider metabolic autopsy
    Make and hold DNA

References

Arens R, Gozal D, Williams JC, et al. Recurrent apparent life-threatening events during infancy: a manifestation of inborn errors of metabolism. J Pediatr 1993;123:415.

Calvo M, Artuch R, Macia E, et al. Diagnostic approach to inborn errors of metabolism in an emergency unit. Pediatr Emerg Care 2000;16(6):405–8.

Ernst LM, Sondheimer N, Deardorff MA, et al. The value of the metabolic autopsy in the pediatric hospital setting. J Pediatr 2006;148:779–83.

Goodman SI, Greene CL. Metabolic disorders of the newborn. Pediatr Rev 1994;15:359.

Greene CL, Blitzer MG, Shapira E. Inborn errors of metabolism and Reye syndrome: differential diagnosis. J Pediatr 1988;113:156.

Greene CL, Thomas JT, Goodman SI. Inborn errors of metabolism. In: Hay WW, Hayward AR, Levin MJ, Sondheimer JM, editors. Pediatric diagnosis and treatment. 15th ed. Norwalk, CT: Appleton & Lange; 2001. p. 881.

Prietsch V, Lindner M, Zschocke J, et al. Emergency management of inherited metabolic diseases. J Inherit Metab Dis 2002;25:531–46.

Rowe PC, Valle D, Brusilow SW. Inborn errors of metabolism in children referred with Reye's syndrome: a changing pattern. JAMA 1988;260:3167.

Surtees R, Leonard JV. Acute metabolic encephalopathy: a review of causes, mechanisms and treatment. J Inherit Metab Dis 1989;12(Suppl):42.

Waber L. Inborn errors of metabolism. Pediatr Ann 1990;19:105, 107.

Zschocke J, Hoffmann GF, editors. Vademecum metabolicum. Manual of metabolic paediatrics. 2nd ed. Friedrichsdorf, Germany: Schattauer; 2004.

Musculoskeletal Disorders

Evaluation of Musculoskeletal Disorders and Overuse Syndromes

Evaluation of the Active Athlete

Juvenile Idiopathic Arthritis

Osteomyelitis

Septic Arthritis

Evaluation of Musculoskeletal Disorders and Overuse Syndromes

Greg Gutierrez, MD, and Simon J. Hambidge, MD, PhD

A. History: In the patient's history, determine whether the injury is chronic (over 4–6 weeks) or acute.

For an acute injury, this history should give the provider a mental picture of the mechanism of injury. It should detail the immediate and delayed symptoms, focusing on the position of the body and injured site during and after the injury. The velocity of the patient (or projectile) and what impacted the site (e.g., ground, another person, ball) is important in assessing the severity of the injury. Ask whether the patient heard or felt a "pop." Was there swelling of a joint, and if so, how soon after the injury? Was the child or adolescent able to move the extremity or bear weight on an injured lower extremity? Has the patient sustained a similar injury in the past?

Immediate swelling, hearing a "pop" (especially in the knee), and inability to move the injured site or bear weight indicate more severe injury and should prompt referral. Referral options include the emergency department, a musculoskeletal specialist such as a sports medicine physician, and an orthopedist when surgical intervention may be needed. Many minor musculoskeletal injuries can be managed in the primary care setting with appropriate attention to rehabilitation and return to play precautions (see Evaluation of the Active Athlete, p. 702).

For a chronic injury, ask about systemic factors, as well as those pertaining to the specific area of musculoskeletal involvement. Note any precipitating factors, such as trauma, systemic illness, infections, activity change, and overuse. Assess predisposing conditions, such as malignancy, immunodeficiency, hemoglobinopathy, and steroid use. The duration of symptoms and their change over time are important, especially the way they vary with activities. Overuse syndromes may be painful only with activity. Changes in gait or a limp may not be painful to the patient and may be noticed only by family members (see section D).

B. Physical Examination: The physical examination should be performed with the child or adolescent sitting, reclining, and walking or running as appropriate.

Observation: If there is a deformity, determine what is causing it: a displaced fracture, a foreign body, a large hematoma, an abscess or other fluid collection, or a tumor. Skin that is red and warm may be indicative of cellulitis. Pale, cool skin may indicate neurovascular compromise. Lacerations and other breaks in the skin should be assessed for depth. Breaks in the skin associated with a nearby fracture should be considered an open fracture and the patient referred to an orthopedist. Rashes and pigment changes should be noted.

Palpation: The provider should attempt to localize the pain to specific anatomic structures: bone, muscle, joint, ligament, tendon, and other soft tissue. Palpate deformities for consistency, pain, and temperature. Palpate towards the injury from all directions.

Range of Motion: Joints above and below the injury should be moved through full range of motion both actively (by the patient) and passively (by the examiner). Note any limits in range of motion, as this will guide progress during rehabilitation. Also assess strength of the injured extremity against resistance (from the examiner) in all ranges of motion.

Neurovascular: In addition to movement, assess for specific functions (such as hand grip) and ability to sense light touch. Ensure that distal pulses and capillary refill are normal.

The physical examination for systemic disease should screen for muscle weakness, abnormal neurologic reflexes, jaundice, enlarged liver or spleen, lymphadenopathy, rashes, heart murmurs, and multiple bruises or fractures. Spasticity, hyper-reflexia, and clonus accompany cerebral palsy and other causes of upper motor neuron lesions, such as head trauma or spinal cord tumors. Unilateral bone pain at night may suggest malignancy, as opposed to growing pains, which are more commonly bilateral. Early-onset knee effusions (<12 hours) occur with intra-articular injury such as anterior cruciate ligament rupture. Signs of nonaccidental trauma include unusual bruising (especially age-inappropriate bruising), unexplained burns, and multiple fractures, especially of different ages.

C. Imaging: Plain radiographs are often indicated as adjunct to the initial evaluation after a careful history and physical examination, and will often be sufficient for diagnostic purposes. At times, additional imaging modalities may be needed, usually in consultation with a musculoskeletal specialist. Magnetic resonance imaging (MRI) allows visualization of both bone and soft tissue, especially the cartilage of the knee and tumors. Ultrasonography is useful for evaluating instability of the newborn hip and for cystic lesions. MRI or a nuclear bone scan may be indicated for stress fractures or to evaluate the entire body for multifocal sites of bony change. Computed tomographic scanning can provide good bony detail but should be used sparingly because of the greatly increased exposure to ionizing radiation. Other useful tests in evaluating musculoskeletal disorders may include blood cultures, synovial fluid analysis, electromyography, and nerve conduction studies.

(Continued on page 696)

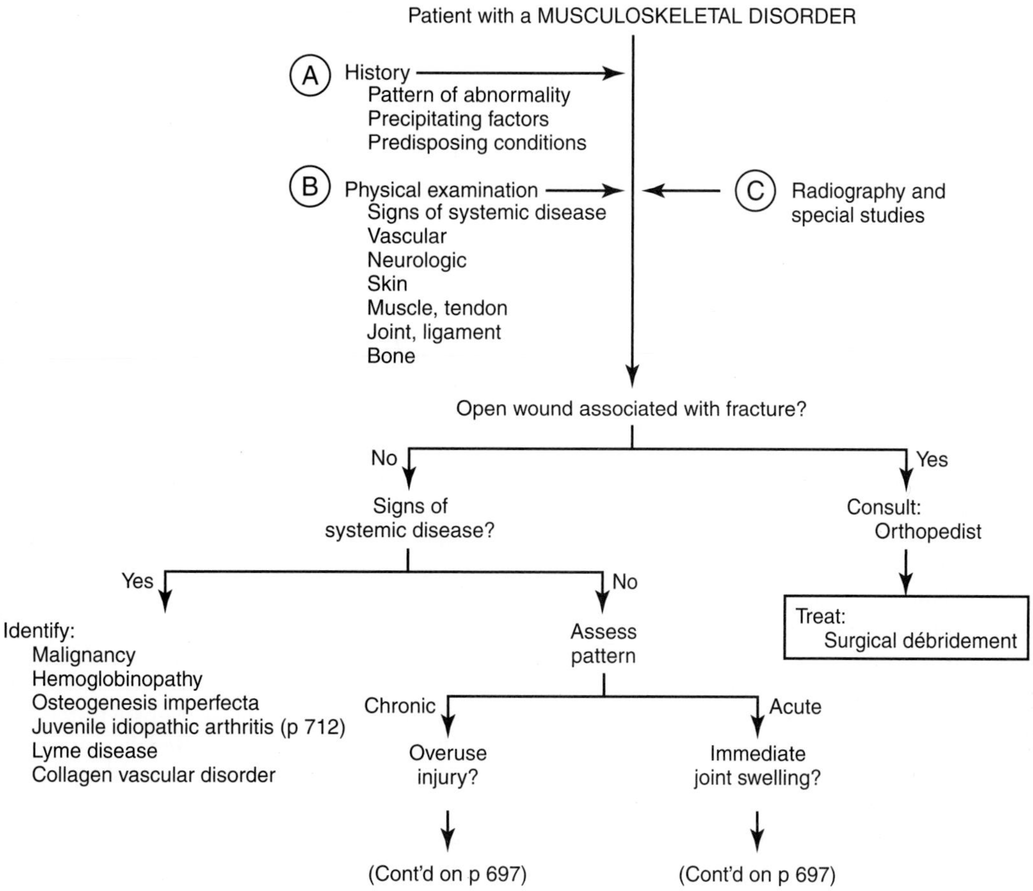
Patient with a MUSCULOSKELETAL DISORDER
A History
Pattern of abnormality
Precipitating factors
Predisposing conditions
B Physical examination
Signs of systemic disease
Vascular
Neurologic
Skin
Muscle, tendon
Joint, ligament
Bone
C Radiography and special studies
Open wound associated with fracture?
No
Yes
Signs of systemic disease?
Consult: Orthopedist
Treat: Surgical débridement
Yes
No
Identify:
Malignancy
Hemoglobinopathy
Osteogenesis imperfecta
Juvenile idiopathic arthritis (p 712)
Lyme disease
Collagen vascular disorder
Assess pattern
Chronic
Acute
Overuse injury?
Immediate joint swelling?
(Cont'd on p 697)
(Cont'd on p 697)

D. Overuse Syndromes: See Tables 1 and 2 and Figures 1 and 2 for specific syndromes. Overuse syndromes have become more common in children and adolescents as sport specialization and year-round training has become available. The common mechanism of overuse injuries is repetitive microtrauma to tissue, where the ability of the tissue to repair itself is outpaced by repetition of the insult.

In the patient's history, in addition to the earlier questions, it is important to determine when the symptoms first started, and what makes the pain better or worse. Is there pain at night, and if so, is it unilateral or bilateral? Has the pattern of pain changed over time? Are there associated systemic symptoms? The pain from overuse syndromes progresses from pain after activity to pain with activity, which begins to affect performance, and finally to pain at rest. Poor performance, fatigue, and vague pain may be the first signs of overuse problems that adults may need to be aware of in younger children.

The young skeleton is more vulnerable to overuse injury than the adult. Growth plates in young bone are weaker than surrounding bone and tendon attachments, and can be exposed to either traction or compression forces. These forces can cause a tendonitis, bursitis, muscle strain, or growth plate injury, such as an apophysitis or stress fracture.

Skeletal growth spurts cause inflexibility and tightness of muscle and tendon around joints, exposing them to increased traction forces throughout the muscle-tendon unit and its bony attachment. In "Little League Shoulder" repetitive throwing causes excessive traction forces on the proximal humeral growth plate growth, resulting in a stress fracture through the growth plate.

Growth plates at the end of bones such as the distal radius, distal femur, and proximal tibia are exposed to compressive forces. Irreversible damage to the growing cells in growth plates can cause growth disturbances such as the "gymnast's wrist." A gymnast landing on outstretched hands exposes the distal radius growth plate to repetitive compressive forces, which can result in early closure of the growth plate. The shortened radius changes the mechanics of the wrist and can lead to chronic wrist pain and arthritic changes.

Growth plate injury on radiograph often appears as a widened physis; images of the noninjured extremity may be needed for comparison. A long period of rest from weeks to months, rehabilitation, and adjustments of modifiable factors are the basis of treatment. Modifiable risk factors include improper technique, training errors, poorly fitting equipment (especially shoes), muscle weakness, and imbalance. Children with overuse injuries may need to have rehabilitation guided by a physical therapist. Return to play decisions should be guided by a team including a physical therapist, a musculoskeletal (MSK) physician, parents, coach, and the child.

E. Chronic Pain with No Overuse History: Chronic pain in the absence of a clear overuse history may be indicative of serious disease. Red flags include fevers and night sweats (malignancy, juvenile idiopathic arthritis), nightly unilateral bone pain (neoplasm, osteomyelitis), groin pain (hip joint disease), and difficulty breathing or chest pain (exercise-induced asthma, pneumothorax, chest mass, cardiac or pulmonary disease). Screening studies to consider with such symptoms include complete blood cell count (CBC), erythrocyte sedimentation rate (ESR), C-reactive protein (CRP), and plain radiographs or MRI.

(Continued on page 698)

Patient with a MUSCULOSKELETAL DISORDER

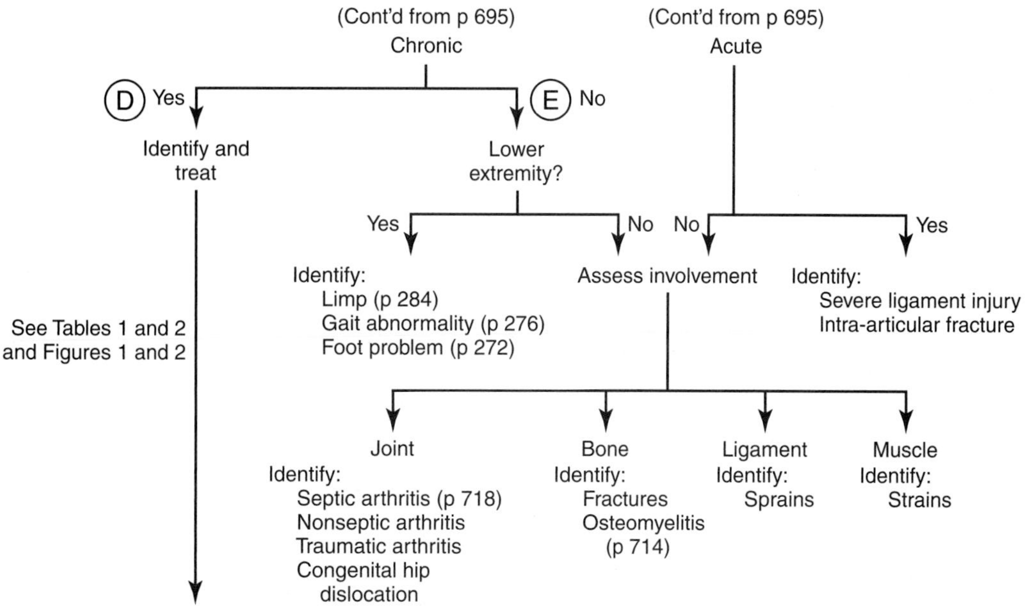

(Cont'd from p 695)
Chronic
(Cont'd from p 695)
Acute
D
Yes
E
No
Identify and treat
See Tables 1 and 2 and Figures 1 and 2
Lower extremity?
Yes
No
Identify:
Limp (p 284)
Gait abnormality (p 276)
Foot problem (p 272)
Assess involvement
No
Yes
Identify:
Severe ligament injury
Intra-articular fracture
Joint
Identify:
Septic arthritis (p 718)
Nonseptic arthritis
Traumatic arthritis
Congenital hip dislocation
Bone
Identify:
Fractures
Osteomyelitis (p 714)
Ligament
Identify:
Sprains
Muscle
Identify:
Strains

Patient with a MUSCULOSKELETAL DISORDER Algorithm

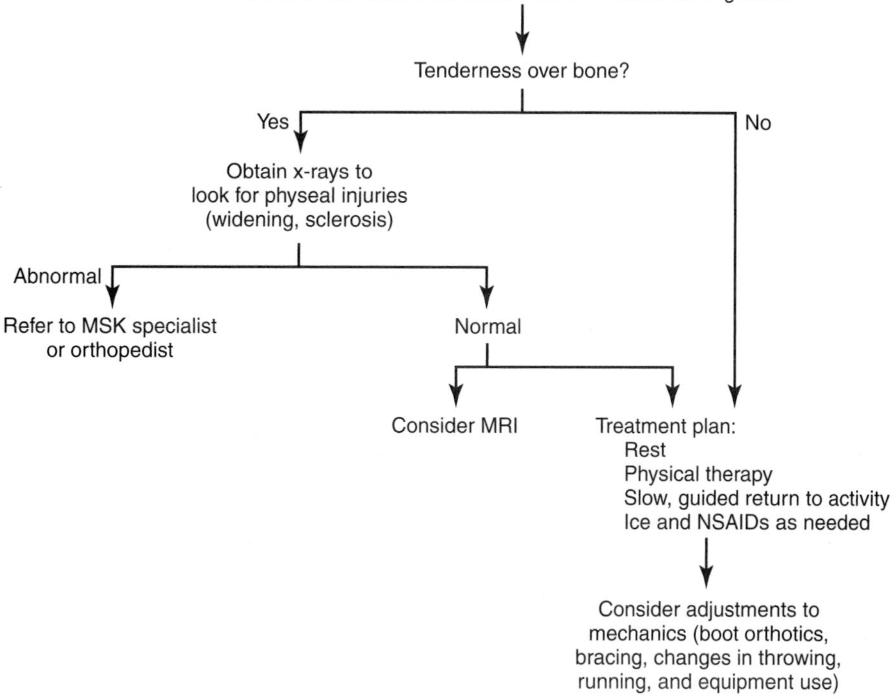

Tenderness over bone?
Yes
No
Obtain x-rays to look for physeal injuries (widening, sclerosis)
Abnormal
Refer to MSK specialist or orthopedist
Normal
Consider MRI
Treatment plan:
Rest
Physical therapy
Slow, guided return to activity
Ice and NSAIDs as needed
Consider adjustments to mechanics (boot orthotics, bracing, changes in throwing, running, and equipment use)

Table 1. **Upper Extremity Overuse Syndromes**

	History	Examination Findings	X-ray (anteroposterior, outlet, axillary)	Treatment
Shoulder				
Rotator cuff injury	Slow onset Deep shoulder pain Hurts at night Pain increased with use	Hawkins sign Neer sign Supraspinatus sign	Normal bony anatomy	Rest, ice, NSAIDs PT
Little League shoulder	Repetitive throwing Proximal arm pain	Pain over lateral shoulder	Widening of proximal humeral growth plate Comparison views needed	Rest, ice, NSAIDs PT
Glenohumeral instability	Subluxation or dislocation Joint laxity in other joints	Apprehension test Sulcus sign	Hill–Sachs or Bankart lesions with dislocations	PT, surgical consult
Distal clavicle Osteolysis	Pain on top of shoulder, young adult Weight-lifting history	Acromioclavicular (AC) joint pain	Osteolysis of distal clavicle	Rest, ice
Labral injury/Superior Labrum from Anterior to Posterior (SLAP)	Painful "clunks or catching"	O'Brien sign	Normal bony anatomy MRI with contrast to diagnosis	Surgical consultation
Elbow				
Panner disease	Repetitive throwing	Tender lateral epicondyle	AVN of capitellum	Rest, ice, NSAIDs PT
Lateral epicondylitis (tennis elbow)	Lateral elbow hurts with gripping, throwing, opening jars or doors	Pain increased with resisted hand and finger extension	Normal bony anatomy	Rest, ice, NSAIDs PT
Osteochondritis desiccans	Chronic elbow pain	Bony tenderness	Distal humerus, intra-articular areas of OCD	Surgical consultation
Medial epicondylitis	Medial symptoms similar to lateral epicondylitis	Pain increased with resisted wrist flexion	Normal bony anatomy	Rest, ice, NSAIDs PT
Little League elbow (medial apophysitis)	Repetitive throwing	Medial elbow tenderness	Widening of medial apophysis	Rest for up to 2 months
MCL strain	Repetitive throwing or acute valgus mechanism	+ Valgus stress test	Normal bony anatomy	Rest, ice, NSAIDs PT
Olecranon apophysitis	Overuse of triceps muscle, pain increased with pushing	Resisted extension of elbow increases pain Pain at olecranon tip	Possible widening of apophysis	Rest, ice, NSAIDs PT
Olecranon impingement	Hyperextension injury or repetitive hyperextension of elbow	Pain increased with hyperextension of elbow	Normal bony anatomy	Rest, ice, NSAIDs PT Elbow bracing to prevent hyperextension
Triceps tendonitis	Repetitive pushing or elbow extension	Triceps tendon tenderness at insertion on olecranon Pain with resisted elbow extension	Normal bony anatomy	Rest, ice, NSAIDs PT
Hand/Wrist				
Distal radius physeal stress injury (gymnast's wrist)	Repetitive landing on hands	Pain over distal radius	Widening of distal radial growth plate	Prolonged rest, ice, NSAIDs PT
deQuervain tenosynovitis	Pain in "snuff box" area of wrist with use of thumb	+ Finkelstein maneuver	Normal bony anatomy	Rest, ice, NSAIDs PT, thumb spica brace
Wrist flexor/extensor tendonitis	Wrist pain with use or movement	Pain on tendons with resisted flexion/extension	Normal bony anatomy	Rest, ice, NSAIDs PT

AVN, avascular necrosis; *MCL*, medial collateral ligament; *NSAID*, nonsteroidal anti-inflammatory drugs; *OCD*, osteochondritis desiccans; *PT*, physical therapy.

Table 2. **Lower Extremity Overuse Syndromes**

	History	Exam Findings	X-ray (anteroposterior, outlet, axillary)	Treatment
Knee Overuse Syndromes				
Patellofemoral pain syndrome	Anterior knee pain, dull radiation to popliteal area; slow onset, hurts with bending, going up/downstairs, after sitting long periods; can ache at night; occurs during period of rapid growth	Poor quad tone; tight quads, hams, ITB, and adductors; very tender patellofemoral joint; pain can be diffuse with joint line tenderness	Sunrise view usually shows laterally tilted patellae, otherwise normal bony anatomy	Ice, PT evaluation,* NSAIDs, consider temporary bracing with neoprene sleeve or hinged brace
Sinding–Larsen–Johansson • Patellar apophysitis at origin of patellar tendon	Anterior knee pain; Hx of knee overuse activity like running, jumping; occurs during period of rapid growth	Tight thigh musculature like in patellofemoral pain syndrome. Tender at inferior pole of patella	Apophysis of inferior pole of patella may have some irregularity	Ice, PT evaluation, NSAIDs, consider temporary bracing with neoprene sleeve or hinged brace Consider patellar tendon band
Runner's knee • ITB tendonitis	Pain on lateral knee just below joint line; can come and go with activity; dull to sharp bony ache; Hx of overuse of knee	Tight ITB (+ Ober sign); may be tender at insertion of ITB on lateral tibial prominence (Gerdy tubercle)	Severe cases may mimic a medial meniscus injury If no improvement with usual therapy, an MRI can be performed to r/o meniscal injury	PT evaluation, NSAIDs
Osgood–Schlatter disease • Tibial tuberosity apophysitis	Anterior knee pain at tibial tubercle; Hx of knee overuse; occurs during period of rapid growth	Tight thigh musculature like in patellofemoral pain syndrome; tender on tibial tubercle—insertion point of patellar tendon	Apophysis of tibial tubercle may have some irregularity Acute severe injury may show avulsion	Ice, PT evaluation, NSAIDs, consider patellar tendon band
Leg Overuse Syndrome				
Shin splints • Medial tibial syndrome	Pain up and down front of leg; increased with running	Tenderness up and down medial border of tibia; point tenderness could be stress fx	No bony abnormality; X-rays should be done to rule out stress Fx if clinically suspicious	Ice, PT evaluation, NSAIDs
Foot and Ankle Overuse Syndromes				
Sever disease • Calcaneal apophysitis	Heel pain hurts with activity, better with rest; can be bilateral; associated with lots of running and jumping	Tender heel at insertion of Achilles' tendon; tight calf musculature; associated with flat feet, pronated heels	Possible irregularities of apophysis at calcaneus	Ice, PT evaluation, NSAIDs, calf stretches, arch support, supportive footwear
Achilles tendonitis	Similar to Sever disease Pain in heel and lower leg	Tender Achilles tendon; tight calf muscles	X-ray films usually not necessary	Ice, PT evaluation, NSAIDs, calf stretches, arch support, supportive footwear, heel lift
Plantar fasciitis	Pain on bottom of foot, especially with first steps in the morning; overuse Hx; poor foot support in shoes	With ankle maximally dorsiflexed, the plantar fascia will be tight and very tender when palpated Associated with tight calf muscles, flat feet, high arches, pronated heels	X-ray films usually not necessary	Ice, PT evaluation, NSAIDs, calf stretches, arch support, supportive footwear
Peroneal tendonitis	Pain on lateral ankle; overuse Hx; can be associated with ankle sprains; subluxing peroneal tendons can "pop or snap"	Pain behind lateral malleolus up the peroneal tendons; pain with resisted foot eversion	X-ray films usually normal but may show bone abnormalities from old injuries	Ice, PT evaluation, NSAIDs
Base of fifth metatarsal apophysitis	Overuse Hx; pain on lateral side of foot, increased with running and jumping	Pain at base of the fifth metatarsal where peroneus brevis inserts; pain increased with resisted eversion	X-rays should be done to look for stress (Jones) Fx in the metaphysis	Rest, ice, PT evaluation, NSAIDs
Midfoot pain syndromes • Midfoot sprain • Tarsal stress Fx	Overuse Hx, especially long-distance running	Pain in midfoot when twisting forefoot with one hand and holding calcaneus steady with the other May have direct tenderness over tarsal with stress Fx	X-ray to rule out stress Fx of tarsals, especially navicular Consider CT or MRI	Rest, PT evaluation, arch support, supportive footwear

Continued

Table 2. **Lower Extremity Overuse Syndromes—cont'd**

	History	Exam Findings	X-ray (anteroposterior, outlet, axillary)	Treatment
Forefoot pain syndromes • Metatarsalgia • Turf toe • Metatarsal stress Fx	Overuse Hx, especially long-distance running Running with cutting may cause turf toe	Pain in fore foot on metatarsals with stress Fx; first MTP tenderness with turf toe Pain on metatarsal head with metatarsalgias	X-rays to look for stress Fx of metatarsals. Consider CT or MRI	Rest, PT evaluation, arch support, supportive footwear, metatarsal pad
Pelvic Overuse Syndromes				
Iliac apophysitis	Overuse Hx, especially running	Tenderness on iliac crest	X-ray films usually normal	PT evaluation, ice, NSAIDs
ITB tendonitis • Pain over lateral epicondyle of knee • Greater trochanteric bursitis	Pain starts at distal ITB insertion lateral to patella; more severe cases involve the entire ITB fascial plane along the lateral thigh and the greater trochanter on the outside of the hip	Pain lateral to patella + Ober sign of hip	Normal bony anatomy	Ice, NSAIDs, PT evaluation
Iliopsoas tendonitis • Snapping hip	Hx of deep snapping in groin; overuse in dancers, runners	Patients may reproduce snap: while standing, have patient forward flex hip and rotate out to side	Normal hip and pelvic bony anatomy	NSAIDs, PT evaluation
• Adductor tendonitis	Overuse Hx of lower extremity involving adduction: running, cutting, skating	Increased tenderness at area of strain with adductor stretching—"doing the splits"	Normal anatomy; acute injuries should have x-rays to rule out avulsion Fx	NSAIDs, PT evaluation

*PT evaluation should include treatment of acute pain and dysfunction, evaluation of mechanics, prescription of appropriate stretches, balance and strength exercises, equipment/shoe wear evaluation, and a maintenance program.

Fx, fracture; *Hx,* history; *ITB,* iliotibial band; *NSAIDs,* nonsteroidal anti-inflammatory drugs; *PT,* physical therapy.

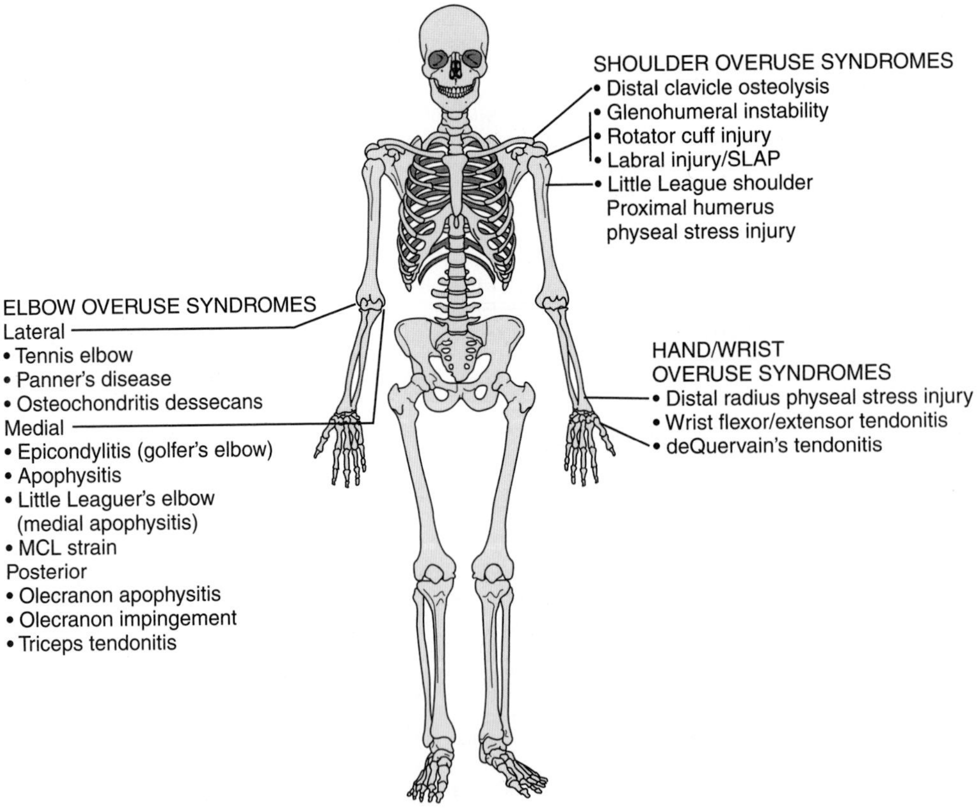
SHOULDER OVERUSE SYNDROMES
• Distal clavicle osteolysis
• Glenohumeral instability
• Rotator cuff injury
• Labral injury/SLAP
• Little League shoulder Proximal humerus physeal stress injury
ELBOW OVERUSE SYNDROMES
Lateral
• Tennis elbow
• Panner's disease
• Osteochondritis dessecans
Medial
• Epicondylitis (golfer's elbow)
• Apophysitis
• Little Leaguer's elbow (medial apophysitis)
• MCL strain
Posterior
• Olecranon apophysitis
• Olecranon impingement
• Triceps tendonitis
HAND/WRIST OVERUSE SYNDROMES
• Distal radius physeal stress injury
• Wrist flexor/extensor tendonitis
• deQuervain's tendonitis

Figure 1. Upper extremity overuse syndromes. *MCL,* medial collateral ligament; *SLAP,* Superior Labrum from Anterior to Posterior.

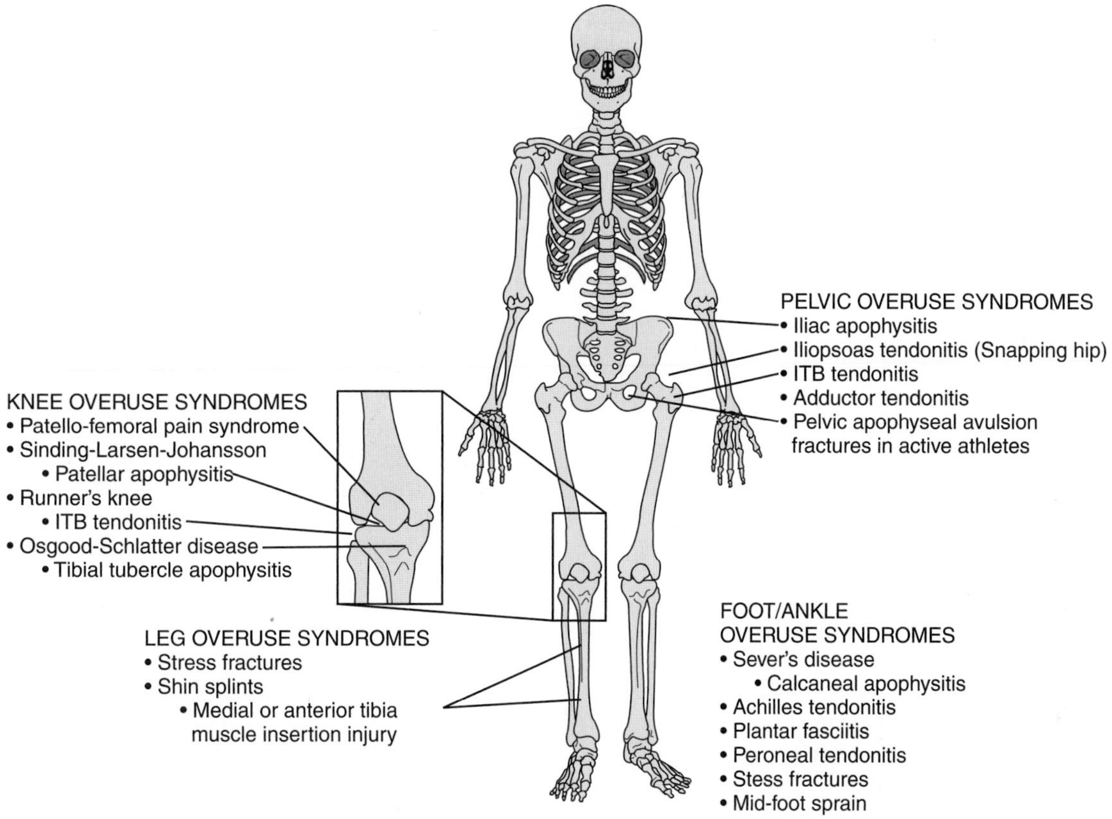
PELVIC OVERUSE SYNDROMES
• Iliac apophysitis
• Iliopsoas tendonitis (Snapping hip)
• ITB tendonitis
• Adductor tendonitis
• Pelvic apophyseal avulsion fractures in active athletes
KNEE OVERUSE SYNDROMES
• Patello-femoral pain syndrome
• Sinding-Larsen-Johansson
• Patellar apophysitis
• Runner's knee
• ITB tendonitis
• Osgood-Schlatter disease
• Tibial tubercle apophysitis
LEG OVERUSE SYNDROMES
• Stress fractures
• Shin splints
• Medial or anterior tibia muscle insertion injury
FOOT/ANKLE OVERUSE SYNDROMES
• Sever's disease
• Calcaneal apophysitis
• Achilles tendonitis
• Plantar fasciitis
• Peroneal tendonitis
• Stess fractures
• Mid-foot sprain

Figure 2. Lower extremity overuse syndromes. *ITB,* iliotibial band.

References

Brenner JS, American Academy of Pediatrics Council on Sports Medicine and Fitness. Overuse injuries, overtraining, and burnout in child and adolescent athletes. Pediatrics 2007;119:1242–5.

Caine D, DiFiori J, Maffulli N. Physeal injuries in children's and youth sports: reasons for concern? Br J Sports Med 2006;40:749–60.

Kerssemakers SP, Fotiadou AN, de Jonge MC, et al. Sport injuries in the paediatric and adolescent patient: a growing problem. Pediatr Radiol 2009;39:471–84.

Kocher MS, Sucato DJ. What's new in pediatric orthopaedics. J Bone Joint Surg Am 2006;88:1412–21.

Patel DR, Moore MD, Greydanus DE. Musculoskeletal diagnosis in adolescents. Adolesc Med State Art Rev 2007;18:1–10.

Soprano JV. Musculoskeletal injuries in the pediatric and adolescent athlete. Curr Sports Med Rep 2005;4:329–34.

Van Dijk CN. Physical examination is sufficient for the diagnosis of sprained ankles. J Bone Joint Surg Br 1996;78-B:958–62.

Evaluation of the Active Athlete

K. Brooke Pengel, MD

More than 30 million children and adolescents are involved in organized sports in the United States. Most states mandate that these athletes have a preparticipation sports examination (PPE) before the season. The PPE is not necessarily the same as a comprehensive health maintenance visit, where a variety of topics are covered that may not be specifically related to the sports participation.

The primary goal of the PPE is to maximize safe participation for the athlete. Identification of conditions that could lead to further injury from athletic activity is of paramount importance. Additional objectives are to diagnose previously undetected medical conditions that require treatment before and during participation; to identify and rehabilitate previously sustained musculoskeletal injuries; to remove unnecessary restrictions on participation; to counsel athletes as to appropriate sports in which to participate; and to identify and counsel athletes regarding risk-taking behaviors, such as smoking, substance abuse, and sexuality-related problems.

There have been recent attempts to standardize the components of the PPE. The American Academy of Pediatrics, together with the American Academy of Family Physicians, The American College of Sports Medicine, the American Orthopaedic Society for Sports Medicine, and the American Osteopathic Academy of Sports Medicine, developed a consensus statement regarding a standardized approach to the PPE. The recommendations are detailed in the fourth edition of the Preparticipation Physical Evaluation monograph published in 2010.

A. A detailed, accurate history is one of the most important aspects of the PPE, because the history alone can identify many of the problems that the athlete may face. The use of the standardized form from the PPE monograph is a reliable method of obtaining a comprehensive history. Free PPE forms can be downloaded from http://ppesportsevaluation.org/body.html (accessed May 7, 2011). Input should be obtained from both the athlete and the parent to increase the reliability of the history. In the patient's history, ask about cardiovascular disease for the family (history of sudden death in relatives younger than 50 years) and the participant (dizziness, syncope, chest pain, palpitations, shortness of breath, or fatigue with exercise; Table 1). Question the athlete regarding bleeding disorders, previous heat illness, asthma, previous seizures, headaches, head trauma, eye injuries, and current medications. Note past spinal and musculoskeletal injuries and their treatment.

B. The physical examination should include both a general evaluation and a specific musculoskeletal evaluation. Measure height, weight, and blood pressure. Assess vision. Blood pressure needs to be assessed using an appropriately sized cuff to avoid false readings. Abnormal readings should be repeated. A pressure greater than 140/85 mm Hg requires further evaluation. The physical examination should be approached systematically, and the use of the PPE physical examination form for the monograph can aid in assuring a comprehensive examination. Cardiovascular screening includes evaluation of the blood pressure, assessment of pulses, and auscultation of the heart. Pulmonary examination includes auscultation to evaluate for wheezing, prolonged expiratory phase, or significant coughing or wheezing after forced expiration. The gastroenterology examination is used to detect abdominal tenderness and enlarged organs. Dermatologic screening can be done throughout the examination to evaluate for signs of contagious infections. A musculoskeletal evaluation should be performed based on current symptoms, as well as prior injuries, and should focus on joint mobility, strength, and signs of injury.

C. Absolute disqualifying conditions include carditis, hypertrophic cardiomyopathy, a single coronary artery, and current fever. Other conditions require additional evaluation before athletic participation (Table 2). These include heart murmurs and dysrhythmias, structural heart defects, diarrhea, bleeding disorders, poorly controlled seizures, obesity and other eating disorders, organ transplants, sickle cell disease, malignant disease, and C1-2 spinal instability. Blood pressure greater than 130/75 mm Hg in patients younger than 12 years or 140/85 mm Hg in patients 12 years and older needs further evaluation. Patients with previous eye injuries, one functional eye, or one functional kidney should seek consultation before participating in contact sports (Table 3). Musculoskeletal abnormalities should be individually assessed. Patients with well-controlled asthma or diabetes mellitus should not be excluded from athletic participation.

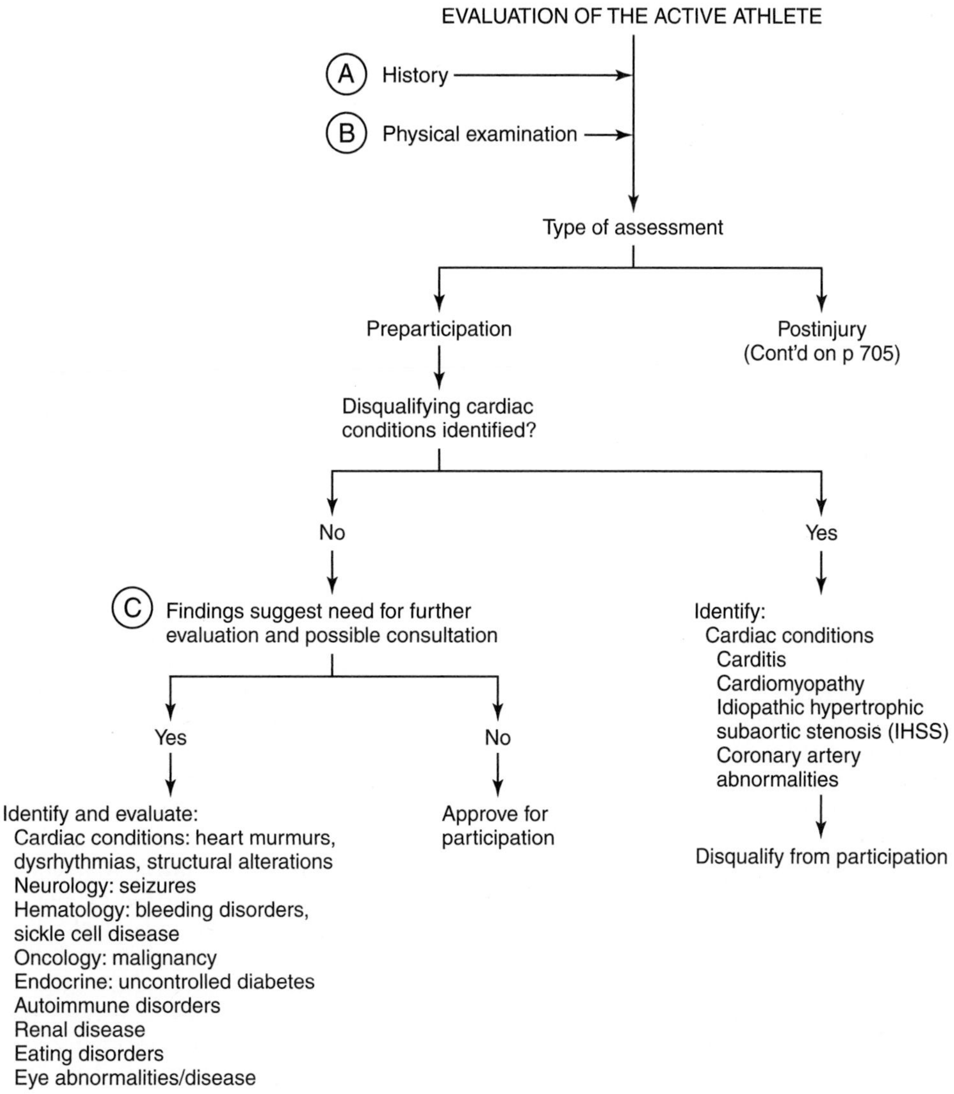

EVALUATION OF THE ACTIVE ATHLETE
A History
B Physical examination
Type of assessment
Preparticipation
Postinjury
(Cont'd on p 705)
Disqualifying cardiac conditions identified?
No
Yes
C Findings suggest need for further evaluation and possible consultation
Identify:
Cardiac conditions
Carditis
Cardiomyopathy
Idiopathic hypertrophic subaortic stenosis (IHSS)
Coronary artery abnormalities
Disqualify from participation
Yes
No
Identify and evaluate:
Cardiac conditions: heart murmurs, dysrhythmias, structural alterations
Neurology: seizures
Hematology: bleeding disorders, sickle cell disease
Oncology: malignancy
Endocrine: uncontrolled diabetes
Autoimmune disorders
Renal disease
Eating disorders
Eye abnormalities/disease
Approve for participation

Table 1. **American Heart Association Recommendations to Identify Risk for Sudden Cardiac Death in Athletes**

Screening Review of Systems
Does the athlete experience chest pain, shortness of breath, or abnormal heartbeats during exercise?
Has the athlete ever experienced syncope or near syncope during or after exercise?
Is there a recent history of unexplained exercise intolerance (a change in the ability to normally keep up with peers)?
Screening History
Does the athlete have any history of heart murmur or hypertension or any cardiac conditions?
Has the athlete ever had any cardiac testing including electrocardiogram or echocardiogram?
Is there a family history of sudden or unexplained death in relative younger than age 50?
Is there anyone in the family younger than age 50 with heart disease?
Is there anyone in the family with known heart conditions, including hypertrophic cardiomyopathy, Marfan syndrome, long QT, or other arrhythmogenic disorders?
Screening Physical Examination
Take sitting blood pressure.
Auscultate heart in two positions (supine and seated/standing).
Check femoral pulses.
Evaluate for physical signs of Marfan syndrome

Adapted from with permission from: Rice SG, American Academy of Pediatrics Council on Sports Medicine and Fitness. Medical conditions affecting sports participation. Pediatrics 2008; 121(4):841-848.

D. Injuries may be either acute (from a single event) or chronic (from overuse). Acute injuries involving the head and neck require immediate evaluation and appropriate treatment. Patterns of extremity injuries are related to the age of the child and to the specific sport. The injuries can occur to soft tissues (tendon, muscle, and ligament) and bone.

E. Concussions are the most common type of head trauma in sports. The management of sport-related concussion is one of the most controversial issues in sports medicine. Most sports medicine physicians rely heavily on the recommendations from the third conference regarding Concussion in Sport (published in 2009). The recommendations emphasize the importance of individualized management and a graduated return to play protocol after concussion. Young athletes are treated more conservatively because the immature brain is thought to be different in terms of healing. The previous grading system for concussion has fallen out of favor because the severity of a concussion can only be determined in retrospect once the total burden of the injury on the athlete can be determined. The cornerstone of concussion management involves reducing both physical and cognitive demands in order to facilitate recovery and to avoid further injury. Input from a multi-disciplinary team that includes the medical provider, parent, school, and athletic trainer/coach is valuable to evaluate the progress of the recovery. Return to play is based on the complete resolution of symptoms and the ability to progress through a graded protocol of activity successfully.

F. A stinger or burner, also known as transient brachial plexopathy, results from a blow to the head or shoulder and is felt as pain or tingling radiating down the arm that may be accompanied by a sensory deficit or motor weakness. Symptoms are always unilateral and can last from a few minutes to several days. A detailed cervical spine and neurologic examination is important in the management of this condition. Play can be resumed when all the sensory symptoms have cleared and the athlete has full range of motion, strength, and function. Recurrent injuries require a full cervical spine evaluation.

G. When a suspected soft-tissue injury occurs, assess the degree of soft-tissue injury. Mild injuries have diffuse, poorly localized pain without effusion or hemarthrosis. Moderate injuries have small and slowly developing effusions, minimal ecchymosis or swelling, no gross deformity, and pain and tenderness specific to the site of injury. Severe injuries are characterized by deformity, rapid onset of hemarthrosis or effusion, ligament laxity, or lack of joint motion. Gross deformity, point tenderness, and painful motion indicate a fracture. Treat acute soft-tissue injuries with rest, ice, elevation, and mild compression. A thorough evaluation should be performed before return to the activity. Patients with mild injuries may resume play when the injured part is fully functional without pain. A rehabilitation program should be implemented as soon as the acute symptoms allow. This includes active range-of-motion exercise, muscle strengthening, and stretching activities. Moderate or severe injuries may require additional evaluation and specialized treatment.

H. Overuse injuries that occur from repetitive motion activities are becoming increasingly prevalent in young athletes. Overuse injuries that involve soft tissue include tendinitis and bursitis. These usually improve with rest and changes in activity. Bone injury occurs as stress fractures in long bones and as compression or tension injuries to epiphyseal plates. The history often includes changes in the intensity or duration of an activity and pain during or shortly after use. Focal tenderness is usually present. Radiographic studies can be normal early. In later stages, the radiographs may show periosteal reaction with or without a definite fracture line. Tumor and infection should be ruled out. A bone scan will be abnormal sooner than the radiograph. Magnetic resonance imaging has been shown to be a reliable method for early diagnosis and offers the advantage of no extra radiation after plain radiographs have been used for screening. Specific overuse injuries are discussed in the chapters on the Evaluation of Musculoskeletal Disorders and Overuse Syndromes. Table 4 lists the common sports-related stress fractures. Treatment in general is aimed at reducing the activity level below the pain threshold, modifying the training program to increase activities gradually, and returning the athlete to play when symptom free at full performance.

(Continued on page 706)

EVALUATION OF THE ACTIVE ATHLETE

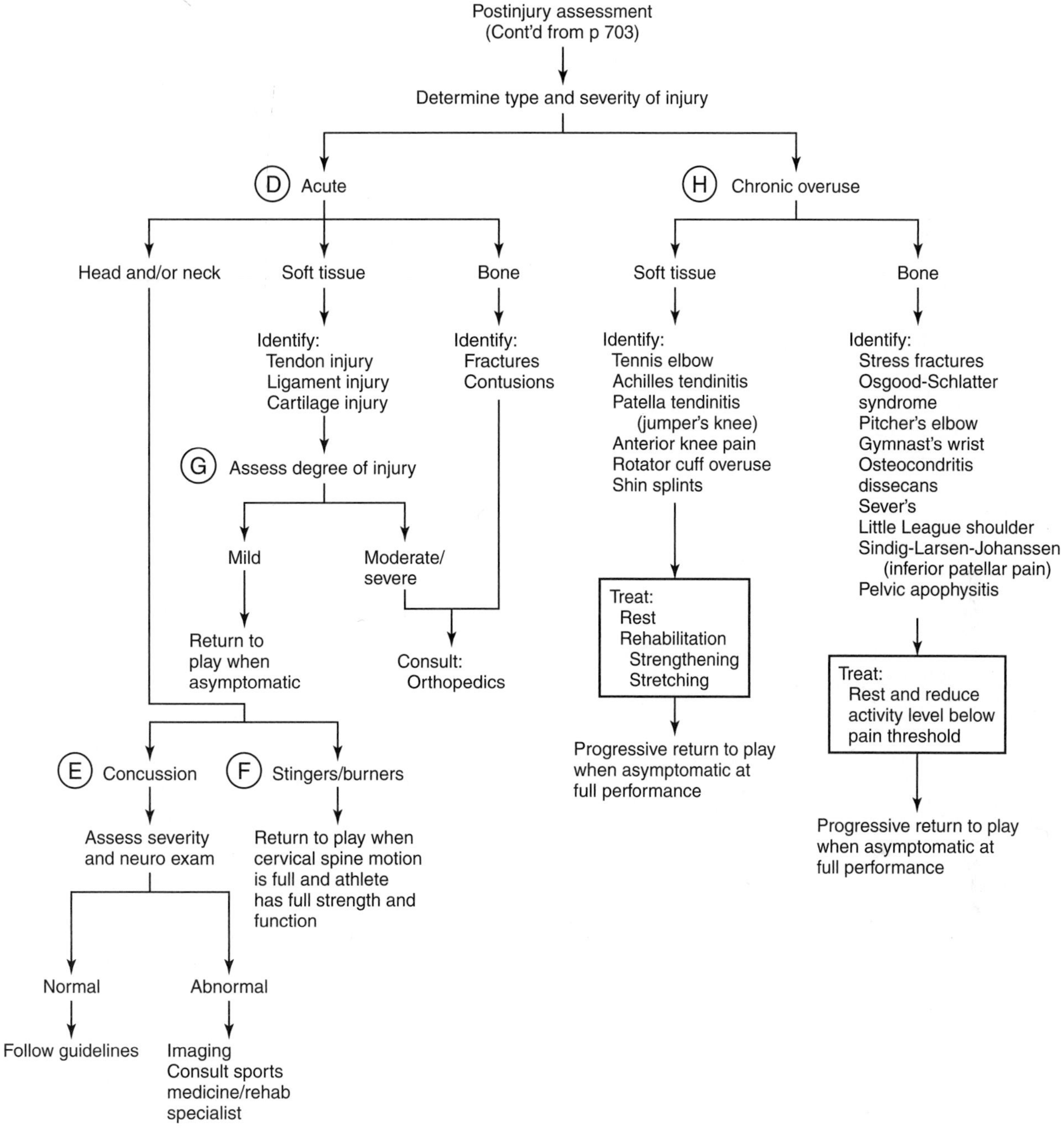
Postinjury assessment
(Cont'd from p 703)
Determine type and severity of injury
D Acute
H Chronic overuse
Head and/or neck
Soft tissue
Bone
Soft tissue
Bone
Identify:
Tendon injury
Ligament injury
Cartilage injury
Identify:
Fractures
Contusions
Identify:
Tennis elbow
Achilles tendinitis
Patella tendinitis
(jumper's knee)
Anterior knee pain
Rotator cuff overuse
Shin splints
Identify:
Stress fractures
Osgood-Schlatter
syndrome
Pitcher's elbow
Gymnast's wrist
Osteocondritis
dissecans
Sever's
Little League shoulder
Sindig-Larsen-Johanssen
(inferior patellar pain)
Pelvic apophysitis
G Assess degree of injury
Mild
Moderate/
severe
Return to
play when
asymptomatic
Consult:
Orthopedics
Treat:
Rest
Rehabilitation
Strengthening
Stretching
Progressive return to play
when asymptomatic at
full performance
Treat:
Rest and reduce
activity level below
pain threshold
Progressive return to play
when asymptomatic at
full performance
E Concussion
F Stingers/burners
Assess severity
and neuro exam
Return to play when
cervical spine motion
is full and athlete
has full strength and
function
Normal
Abnormal
Follow guidelines
Imaging
Consult sports
medicine/rehab
specialist

Table 2. **Medical Conditions and Sports Participation**

Condition	May Participate
Atlantoaxial instability (instability of the joint between cervical vertebrae 1 and 2) *Explanation:* Athlete (particularly if he or she has Down Syndrome or juvenile rheumatoid arthritis with cervical involvement) needs evaluation to assess risk of spinal cord injury during sports participation, especially when using a trampoline.	Qualified yes
Bleeding disorder *Explanation:* Athlete needs evaluation	Qualified yes
Cardiovascular disease	
Carditis (inflammation of the heart) *Explanation:* Carditis may result in sudden death with exertion.	No
Hypertension (high blood pressure) *Explanation:* Those with severe hypertension (>.99th percentile for age plus 5 mm Hg) should avoid heavy weight and power lifting, bodybuilding, strength training, and high-static component sports (Figure 5-1). Those with sustained hypertension (>95th percentile for age) need evaluation. The National High Blood Pressure Education Program working group report defined prehypertension and stage 1 and stage 2 hypertension.	Qualified yes
Congenital heart disease (structural heart defects present at birth) *Explanation:* Consultation with a cardiologist is recommended. Those with mild forms may participate fully in most cases; those with moderate or severe forms or who have undergone surgery need evaluation. The 36th Bethesda Conference defined mild, moderate, and severe disease for common cardiac lesions.	Qualified yes
Dysrhythmia (irregular heart rhythm) Long QT syndrome Malignant ventricular arrhythmias Symptomatic Wolff-Parkinson-White syndrome Advanced heart block Family history of sudden death or previous sudden cardiac event Implantation of a cardioverter-defibrillator *Explanation:* Consultation with a cardiology is advised. Those with symptoms (chest pain, syncope, near syncope, dizziness, shortness of breath, or other symptoms of possible dysrhythmia) or evidence of mitral regurgitation (leaking) on physical examination need evaluation. All others may participate fully.	Qualified yes
Heart murmur *Explanation:* If the murmur is innocent (does not indicate heart disease), full participation is permitted. Otherwise, the athlete needs evaluation (see congenital heart disease, structural heart disease [especially hypertrophic cardiomyopathy and mitral valve prolapse]).	Qualified yes
Structural/acquired heart disease	
Hypertrophic cardiomyopathy	Qualified no
Coronary artery anomalies	Qualified no
Arrhythmogenic right ventricular cardiomyopathy	Qualified no
Acute rheumatic fever with carditis	Qualified no
Ehlers-Danlos syndrome, vascular form	Qualified no
Marfan syndrome	Qualified yes
Mitral valve prolapse	Qualified yes
Anthracycline use *Explanation:* Consultation with a cardiologist is recommended. The 36th Bethesda Conference provided detailed recommendations. Most of these conditions carry a significant risk of sudden cardiac death associated with intense physical exercise. Hypertrophic cardiomyopathy requires a thorough workup and repeated evaluations, because disease may change manifestations during later adolescence. Marfan syndrome with an aortic aneurysm can also cause sudden death during intense physical exercise. An athlete who has ever received chemotherapy with anthracyclines may be at increased risk for cardiac problems because of the cardiotoxic effects of the medications, and resistance training in this population should be approached with caution; strength training that avoids isometric contractions may be permitted. Athlete needs evaluation.	Qualified yes
Vasculitis/vascular disease Kawasaki disease (coronary artery vasculitis) Pulmonary hypertension *Explanation:* Consultation with a cardiologist is recommended. Athlete needs individual evaluation to assess risk on the basis of activity of disease, pathologic changes, and medical regimen.	Qualified yes
Cerebral palsy *Explanation:* Athlete needs evaluation to assess functional capacity to perform sports specific activity.	Qualified yes
Diabetes mellitus *Explanation:* All sports can be played with proper attention to diet, blood glucose concentration, hydration, and insulin therapy. Blood glucose concentration should be monitored before exercise, every 30 minutes during continuous exercise, 15 minutes after completion of exercise, and at bedtime.	Yes

Diarrhea, Infectious *Explanation:* Unless symptoms are mild and the athlete is fully hydrated no participation is permitted, because diarrhea may increase risk for dehydration and heat illness. See fever.	Qualified no
Eating disorders *Explanation:* Athlete with an eating disorder needs medical and psychiatric assessment before participation.	Qualified yes
Eyes Functionally one-eyed athlete Loss of an eye Detached retina or family history of retinal detachment at a young age High myopia Connective tissue disorder, such as Marfan or Stickler syndromes Previous intraocular eye surgery or serious eye injury *Explanation:* A functionally one-eyed athlete is defined as having a best-corrected visual acuity of less than 20/40 in the eye with worse acuity. Such an athlete would suffer significant disability if the better eye were seriously injured, as would an athlete with loss of an eye. Specifically boxing and full-contact martial arts are not recommended for functionally one-eyed athletes because eye protection is impractical and-or not permitted. Some athletes who previously have undergone intraocular eye surgery or had a serious eye injury may have an increased risk of injury because of weakened eye tissue. Availability of eye guards approved by the American Society for Testing and Materials and other protective equipment may allow participation in most sports, but this must be judged on an individual basis.	Qualified yes
Conjunctivitis, infectious *Explanation:* An athlete with active infectious conjunctivitis should be excluded from swimming	Qualified no
Fever *Explanation:* Fever can increase cardiopulmonary effort, reduce maximum exercise capacity, make heat illness more likely, and increase orthostatic hypertension during exercise. Fever may rarely accompany myocarditis or other conditions that may make exercise dangerous.	No
Gastrointestinal Malabsorption syndromes (celiac disease, cystic fibrosis) *Explanation:* Athlete needs individual assessment for general malnutrition or specific deficits resulting in coagulation or other defects, with appropriate treatment, these defects can be adequately related to permit normal activities. Short bowel syndrome or other disorders requiring specialized nutritional support including parenteral or enteral nutrition. *Explanation:* Athlete needs individual assessment for collision, contact, or limited contact sports. Presence of a control or peripheral indwelling venous catheter may require special considerations for activities and emergency preparedness for unexpected trauma to the device(s).	Qualified yes
Heat illness, history of *Explanation:* Because of the likelihood of recurrence, the athlete needs individual assessment to determine the presence of predisposing conditions and to develop a prevention strategy, which includes sufficient acclimation, conditioning, hydration, and salt intake as well as other effective measures to improve heat tolerance and reduce heat injury risk.	Qualified yes
Hepatitis, infectious (primarily hepatitis C) *Explanation:* All athletes should have received Hep B Vaccination prior to participation. Because of the apparent minimal risk to others, all sports may be played that the athlete's state of health allows. In all athletes, skin lesions should be covered properly and athletic personnel should use universal precautions when handling blood or body fluid with visible blood.	Yes
Human immunodeficiency virus infection *Explanation:* Because of the apparent minimal risk to others, all sports may be played that the athlete's state of health allows (especially if the viral load is undetectable or very low). In all athletes, skin lesions should be covered properly, and athletic personnel should use universal precautions when handling blood or body fluids with visible blood. However, certain sports (such as wrestling or boxing) may create a situation that may favor viral transmission (likely bleeding plus-skin breaks). If a viral load is detectable these athletes should be advised to avoid such high contact sports.	Yes
Kidney, absence of one *Explanation:* Athlete needs individual assessment for contact, collision, and limited contact sports. Protective equipment may reduce risk of injury to the remaining kidney efficiently to allow participation in most sports, providing such equipment remains in place during activity.	Qualified yes
Liver, enlarged *Explanation:* If the liver is acutely enlarged, participation should be avoided because of risk of rupture. If the liver is chronically enlarged, individual assessment is needed before collision, contact, or limited-contact sports are played. Patients with chronic liver disease may have changes in liver function that may affect stamina, mental status, coagulation, or nutritional status.	Qualified yes
Malignant neoplasm *Explanation:* Athlete needs individual assessment	Qualified yes
Musculoskeletal disorders *Explanation:* Athlete needs individual assessment	Qualified yes

(Continued)

Neurologic disorders	
History of serious head or spine trauma or abnormality including craniotomy, epidural bleeding, subdural hematoma, intracranial hemorrhage, second impact syndrome, vascular malformation, and neck fracture. *Explanation:* Athlete needs individual assessment for collision, contact, or limited contact sports.	Qualified yes
History of simple concussion (mild traumatic brain injury), multiple simple concussions, and or complex concussion. *Explanation:* Athlete needs individual assessment. Research supports a conservative approach to concussion management, including no athletic participation while symptomatic or when deficits in judgment or cognition are detected; followed by a graduated, sequential return to full activity.	Qualified yes
Myopathic *Explanation:* Athlete needs individual assessment	Qualified yes
Recurrent headaches *Explanation:* Athlete needs individual assessment	Yes
Recurrent plexopathy (burner or stinger) and cervical cord neuropraxia with persistent defects *Explanation:* Athlete needs individual assessment for collision, contact or limited contact sports, regaining normal strength is an important benchmark for return to play.	Qualified yes
Seizure disorder, well controlled *Explanation:* Risk of seizure during participation is minimal.	Yes
Seizure disorder, poorly controlled *Explanation:* Athlete needs individual assessment for collision, contact, or limited contact sports. The following noncontact sports should be avoided: archery, riflery, swimming, wright or power lifting, strength training, or sports involving weights, in these sports occurrence of a seizure during the activity may pose a risk to self or others.	Qualified yes
Obesity *Explanation:* Because of the increased risk of heat illness, the obese athlete particularly needs careful acclimatization, sufficient hydration, and potential activity and recovery modifications during competition and training.	Yes
Organ transplant recipient (end those taking immunosuppressive medications) *Explanation:* Athlete needs individual assessment for contact, collision, and limited contact sports. In addition to the potential risk of infections, some medications: (eg, prednisone) may increase tendency for bruising.	Qualified yes
Ovary, absence of one *Explanation:* Risk of severe injury to the remaining ovary is minimal.	Yes
Pregnancy/postpartum *Explanation:* Athlete needs individual assessment. As pregnancy progresses, modifications to usual exercise routines will become necessary. Activities with a high risk of falling or abnormal trauma should be avoided. Scuba diving and activities	Qualified yes
Respiratory conditions	
Pulmonary compromise, including cystic fibrosis *Explanation:* Athlete needs individual assessment, but generally, all sports may be played if oxygenation remains satisfactory during a graded exercise test. Athletes with cystic fibrosis need acclimatization and good hydration to reduce the risk of heat illness.	Qualified yes
Asthma *Explanation:* With proper medication and education, only athletes with the most severe asthma will need to modify their participation. For those using inhalers, recommend having a written action plan and using a peak flow meter daily. Athletes with asthma may encounter risks when scuba diving.	Yes
Acute upper respiratory infection *Explanation:* Upper respiratory obstruction may affect pulmonary function. Athlete needs individual assessment for all but mild disease. See fever.	Qualified yes
Rheumatologic disease	
Juvenile rheumatoid arthritis *Explanation:* Athletes with system or polyarticular juvenile rheumatoid arthritis and history of cervical spine involvement need radiograph of vertebrae C1-C2 to assess risk of spinal cord injury. Athletes with systemic or HLA B27 associated arthritis require cardiovascular assessment for possible cardio complications during exercise. For those with micrognathia (open bite and exposed teeth), mouth guards are helpful if uveitis is present, the risk of eye damage from trauma is increased, ophthalmologic assessment is recommended and if visually impaired, guidelines for functionally one eye athletes should be followed.	Qualified yes
Juvenile dermatomyositis (JDM), idiopathic myositis Systemic lupus erythernatosis (SLE) Raynaud phenomenon *Explanation:* Athlete with JDM or SLE with cardiac involvement requires cardiology assessment before participation. Athletes on system corticosteroids are at higher risk of osteoporotic fractures and avascular necrosis, which should be assessed before clearance; those on immunosuppressive medication are at higher risk of serious infection. Sports activity should be avoided when myositis is active. Rhabdomyolysis during intensive exercise may cause renal injury in athletes with idiopathic myositis and other myopathies. Because of photosensitivity with JDM and SLE, sun protection is necessary during outdoor activity. With Raynaud phenomenon exposure to the cold presents risks to hands and feet.	Qualified yes

Sickle cell disease *Explanation:* Athlete needs individual assessment. In general, if status of the illness permits, all sports may be played; however, any sport or activity that entails overexertion, overheating, dehydration, and chilling should be avoided. Participation at high altitude, especially when not acclimatized, also poses risk of sickle cell crisis.	Qualified yes
Sickle cell traits *Explanation:* Athletes with sickle cell trait generally do not have an increased risk of sudden death or other medical problems during athletic participation under normal environmental conditions. However, when high exertion activity is performed under extreme conditions of heat and humidity or increased altitude, such catastrophic complications have occurred rarely. Athletes with sickle cell trait, like all athletes, should be progressively acclimatized to the environment and to the intensity and duration of activities and should be sufficiently hydrated to reduce the risk of exertional heat illness and/or rhabdomyolysis. According to NIH management guidelines, sickle cell trait is not a contraindication to participation in competitive athletics and there is no requirement for screening prior to participation. More research is needed to fully assess potential risks and benefits of screening athletes for sickle cell trait.	Yes
Skin infections Herpes simplex, molluscum contagiosum, verrucae (warts), staphylococcal and streptococcal infection (furuncle [boils], carbuncle, impetigo, methicillin-resistant Staphylococcus aureus [cellulitis, abscess, necrotizing fasciitis]), scabies, tinea *Explanation:* During contagious period, participation in gymnastics with mats, martial arts; wrestling; or other collision, contact or limited-contact sports is not allowed.	Qualified yes
Spleen, enlarged *Explanation:* If the spleen is acutely enlarged, participation should be avoided out of risk of rupture if the spleen is chronically enlarged individual assessment is needed before collision, contact, or limited contact sports are played.	Qualified yes
Testicle, undescended or absence of one *Explanation:* Certain sports may require a protective cup.	Yes

[a]Adapted with permission from: Rice SG, American Academy of Pediatrics Council on Sports Medicine and Fitness. Medical conditions affecting sports participation. Pediatrics. 2008; 121(4):841-848

[b]This table is designed for use by medical and nonmedical personnel. "Needs evaluation" means that a physician with appropriate knowledge and experience should assess the safety of a given sport for an athlete with the listed medical condition. Unless otherwise noted, this need for special consideration is because of the severity of the disease, the risk of injury for the specific sports listed in Box 5-1, or both.

Table 3. **Classification of Sports by Contact**

Contact or Collision	Limited Contact	Noncontact
Basketball	Adventure racing[a]	Badminton
Boxing[b]	Baseball	Body building[d]
Cheerleading	Bicycling	Bowling
Diving	Canoeing or kayaking (white water)	Canoeing or kayaking (flat water)
Extreme sports[d]	Fencing	Crew or rowing
Field hockey	Field events	Curling
Football, tackle	High jump	Dance
Gymnastics	Pole vault	Field events
Ice hockey[e]	Floor hockey	Discus
Lacrosse	Football, flag or touch	Javelin
Martial arts[f]	Handball	Shot put
Rodeo	Horseback riding	Golf
Rugby	Martial arts	Orienteering[g]
Ski jumping	Racquetball	Power lifting[c]
Skiing, downhill	Skating	Race walking
Snow boarding	Ice	Riflery
Soccer	In-line	Rope jumping
Team handball	Roller	Running
Ultimate Frisbee	Skiing	Sailing
Water polo	Cross-country	Scuba diving
Wrestling	Water	Swimming
	Skateboarding	Table tennis
	Softball	Tennis
	Squash	Track
	Volleyball	
	Windsurfing or surfing	

Adapted with permission from: Rice SG, American Academy of Pediatrics Council on Sports Medicine and Fitness. Medical conditions affecting sports participation. Pediatrics 2008;121(4):841-8.

[a]Adventure racing is defined as a combination of 2 or more disciplines, including orienteering and navigation, cross-country running, mountain biking, paddling, and climbing and rope skills.

[b]The American Academy of Pediatrics opposes participation in boxing for children, adolscents, and young adults.

[c]The American Academy of Pediatrics recommends limiting bodybuilding and power lifting until the adolescent achieves sexual maturity rating 5 (Tanner stage V).

[d]Extreme sports has been added since the previous statement was published.

[e]The American Academy of Pediatrics recommends limitng the amount of body checking allowed for hockey players 15 years and younger to reduce injuries.

[f]Martial arts can be subclassified as judo, karate, kung fu, and tae kwon do. Some forms are contact sports and others are limited-contact sports.

[g]Orienteering is a race (contest) in which competitors use a map and a compas to find their way through unfamiliar territory.

Table 4. **Sports-Specific Stress Fractures**

Sport	Injury
Running	Tibia, navicular, fibula, hip/femur
Marching	Second metatarsal
Golfing	Rib
Bowling	Ulna
Weight lifting	Ribs, clavicle, ulna
Gymnastics	Foot, acromion, distal radius, spine (pars interarticularis)
Basketball	Fibula, foot (fifth metatarsal, navicular), proximal tibia
Football	Metatarsals
Dancing	Metatarsals
Rowing	Rib

From Beaty JH, editor. The medical care of athletes. Orthopaedic Knowledge Update. Rosemont, IL: American Academy of Orthopaedic Surgeons; 1998.

References

American Academy of Family Physicians, American Academy of Pediatrics, American College of Sports Medicine, American Medical Society for Sports Medicine, American Orthopaedic Society for Sports Medicine, American Osteopathic Academy of Sports Medicine. Bernhardt DT, Roberts WO, eds. Preparticipation physical evaluation. 4th ed. New York: McGraw-Hill; 2010.

American Academy of Orthopaedic Surgeons and American Academy of Pediatrics. Sarwark JF, ed. Essentials of musculoskeletal care. 4th ed. Rosemont, IL: American Academy of Orthopaedic Surgeons; 2010.

Anderson SJ, Sullivan JA, eds. Care of the young athlete. 2nd ed. Rosemont, IL: American Academy of Pediatrics, American Academy of Orthopaedic Surgeons; 2009.

Beaty JH, editor. The medical care of athletes. In: Orthopaedic knowledge update. Rosemont, IL: American Academy of Orthopaedic Surgeons; 1998.

Maron BJ, Zipes DP. 36th Bethesda Conference eligibility recommendations for competitive athletes with cardiovascular abnormalities: November 6, 2004. J Am Coll Cardiol 2005;45:1317–75. <http://www.csmfoundation.org/36th_Bethesda_Conference_-_Eligibility_Recommendations_for_Athletes_with_Cardiac_Abnormalities.pdf>; 2005 [accessed 07.05.11].

McCrory P, Meeuwisse W, Johnston K, et al. Consensus Statement on Concussion in Sport: 3rd International Conference on Concussion in Sport held in Zurich, November 2008. Clin J Sports Med 2009;19(3):185–200.

Rice SG, American Academy of Pediatrics Council on Sports Medicine and Fitness. Medical conditions affecting sports participation. Pediatrics 2008;121:841–8.

Rice SG. Medical conditions affecting sports participation. Pediatrics 2008;121:841.

Juvenile Idiopathic Arthritis

Jennifer B. Soep, MD

Juvenile idiopathic arthritis (JIA) is diagnosed in children with pain, swelling, warmth, tenderness, and/or decreased range of motion in one or more joints, lasting for longer than 6 weeks. History, physical examination, and laboratory screening assist in sorting children into one of five primary forms of JIA: oligoarticular, polyarticular, systemic, enthesitis associated, and psoriatic arthritis. JIA is a diagnosis of exclusion; therefore, it is necessary to rule out other possible causative factors including orthopedic, oncologic, and infectious agents. There is no diagnostic test for JIA, and normal laboratory tests do not exclude this diagnosis.

A. The oligoarticular form includes children with arthritis involving four or fewer joints. Arthritis is usually in an asymmetric pattern. Asymptomatic uveitis is most frequently associated with this type of JIA, particularly in patients who are antinuclear antibody (ANA) positive.

B. The polyarticular form is defined as arthritis involving five or more joints, usually in a symmetric distribution. Polyarticular JIA is further divided into rheumatoid factor (RF)-negative and RF-positive disease. The latter is associated with more chronic, erosive arthritis and the presence of rheumatoid nodules.

C. Systemic JIA is characterized by arthritis, an evanescent, salmon pink, macular rash, spiking fever (daily or twice-daily fever to ≥39° C with rapid decrease to normal or subnormal temperatures), hepatosplenomegaly, lymphadenopathy, pericarditis, cervical spine involvement, and significantly increased markers of inflammation.

D. Enthesitis-associated arthritis most commonly occurs in male individuals older than 10 years. Patients often have lower extremity, large-joint arthritis, enthesitis (inflammation of tendinous insertions), and sacroiliitis. Carriage of HLA-B27 antigen is associated with this subtype. Nail or skin abnormalities may be the initial clinical manifestation of psoriatic arthritis, which is often associated with asymmetric joint involvement and dactylitis.

E. Physical and occupational therapy are important in the management of JIA to focus on range of motion, stretching, strengthening, and gait. In addition to exercises, other modalities including heat, water therapy, and ultrasound may be used. Splints, orthotics, and shoe lifts may also be indicated.

F. Nonsteroidal anti-inflammatory drugs are the mainstay of initial therapy. A wide range of agents are available, but only a few are approved for use in children, including naproxen (10 mg/kg twice daily), ibuprofen (40 mg/kg/day divided into three to four doses), and meloxicam (0.125 mg/kg once daily). Symptomatic improvement usually occurs in 1 month, but in some patients, improvement is not seen for 8 to 12 weeks.

G. Patients with oligoarticular disease require routine monitoring by an ophthalmologist to screen for uveitis. If present, topical steroids and dilating drops are initial treatment. If the uveitis persists, then sub-Tenon steroid injections and/or systemic medications such as methotrexate, cyclosporine, or infliximab may be indicated.

H. For patients with JIA who do not respond successfully to nonsteroidal anti-inflammatory drugs, methotrexate (0.5–1 mg/kg/wk PO or SC) is the second-line treatment. A complete blood cell count and liver function tests should be obtained every 2 to 3 months to monitor for bone marrow suppression and hepatotoxicity. Other potential side effects include nausea, vomiting, hair loss, and stomatitis.

I. Systemic steroids are usually reserved for patients with severe forms of arthritis or systemic manifestations. When treating arthritis, low doses of prednisone (~5 mg daily) are generally effective. High doses of oral prednisone (2 mg/kg/day) or intravenous methylprednisolone (30 mg/kg with a maximum of 1 g) may be necessary for the initial management of systemic JIA, followed by a slow taper. Local steroid joint injections, using a long-acting steroid such as triamcinolone hexacetonide, may be helpful in patients who have arthritis in one or a few joints.

J. Biologic agents have been developed to manage more severe forms of arthritis. Medications that inhibit tumor necrosis factor (etanercept, infliximab, and adalimumab) are generally quite effective at controlling the arthritis and preventing cartilage and bone damage that may be associated with chronic joint inflammation. Anakinra, an interleukin-1 receptor antagonist, is particularly effective in patients with systemic JIA. Thalidomide is also used in patients with recalcitrant systemic JIA and requires special oversight by the Food and Drug Administration. Newer biologic agents, including rituximab and abatacept, have demonstrated preliminary efficacy in patients who have not responded successfully to other treatments.

References

American Academy of Pediatrics, Section on Rheumatology and Section on Ophthalmology. Guidelines for the ophthalmologic examinations in children with juvenile rheumatoid arthritis. Pediatrics 1993;92:295.

Goldmuntz EA, White PH. Juvenile idiopathic arthritis: a review for the pediatrician. Pediatr Rev 2006;27:e24.

Hashkes PJ, Laxer RM. Medical treatment of juvenile idiopathic arthritis. JAMA 2005;294:1671.

Hofer M. Spondyloarthropathies in children—are they different from those in adults? Best Pract Res Clin Rheumatol 2006;20:315.

Ravelli A, Martini A. Juvenile idiopathic arthritis. Lancet 2007;369:767.

Wagner-Weiner L. Laboratory evaluation of children with rheumatic disease. Pediatr Ann 2002;31:362–71.

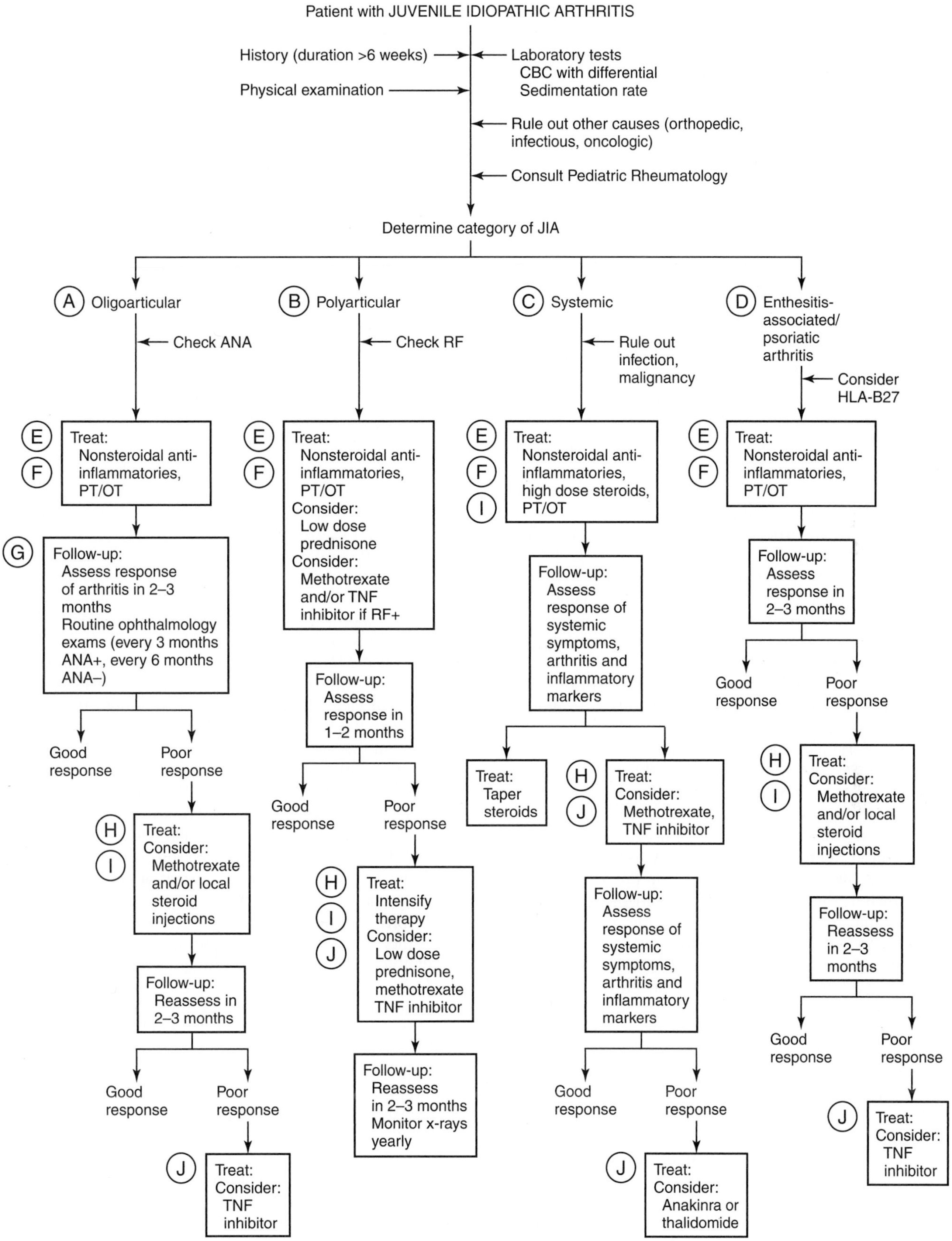

Patient with JUVENILE IDIOPATHIC ARTHRITIS
History (duration >6 weeks)
Physical examination
Laboratory tests
CBC with differential
Sedimentation rate
Rule out other causes (orthopedic, infectious, oncologic)
Consult Pediatric Rheumatology
Determine category of JIA
A Oligoarticular
Check ANA
E F Treat: Nonsteroidal anti-inflammatories, PT/OT
G Follow-up: Assess response of arthritis in 2–3 months Routine ophthalmology exams (every 3 months ANA+, every 6 months ANA–)
Good response
Poor response
H I Treat: Consider: Methotrexate and/or local steroid injections
Follow-up: Reassess in 2–3 months
Good response
Poor response
J Treat: Consider: TNF inhibitor
B Polyarticular
Check RF
E F Treat: Nonsteroidal anti-inflammatories, PT/OT Consider: Low dose prednisone Consider: Methotrexate and/or TNF inhibitor if RF+
Follow-up: Assess response in 1–2 months
Good response
Poor response
H I J Treat: Intensify therapy Consider: Low dose prednisone, methotrexate TNF inhibitor
Follow-up: Reassess in 2–3 months Monitor x-rays yearly
C Systemic
Rule out infection, malignancy
E F I Treat: Nonsteroidal anti-inflammatories, high dose steroids, PT/OT
Follow-up: Assess response of systemic symptoms, arthritis and inflammatory markers
Treat: Taper steroids
H J Treat: Consider: Methotrexate, TNF inhibitor
Follow-up: Assess response of systemic symptoms, arthritis and inflammatory markers
Good response
Poor response
J Treat: Consider: Anakinra or thalidomide
D Enthesitis-associated/ psoriatic arthritis
Consider HLA-B27
E F Treat: Nonsteroidal anti-inflammatories, PT/OT
Follow-up: Assess response in 2–3 months
Good response
Poor response
H I Treat: Consider: Methotrexate and/or local steroid injections
Follow-up: Reassess in 2–3 months
Good response
Poor response
J Treat: Consider: TNF inhibitor

Osteomyelitis

Sean T. O'Leary, MD, Jason Child, PharmD, and Sarah Parker, MD

Osteomyelitis is inflammation of bone and is most commonly caused by a bacterial infection. It is one of the most common invasive bacterial infections in children and is one of the most frequent reasons for prolonged antibiotic administration. It is commonly divided into acute and chronic forms. In children, acute osteomyelitis is primarily hematogenous in origin (AHO); this chapter focuses on this form. Other forms of osteomyelitis, including alternate forms of bacterial introduction (including trauma, postsurgical and contiguous spread), chronic osteomyelitis, recurrent osteomyelitis, and osteomyelitis in special hosts (neonates, immunocompromised, sickle cell disease, unusual exposures) are more complicated, and consultation with orthopedic and infectious disease specialists should be considered.

AHO is primarily a disease of young children because of the increased vascular supply needed for bony growth; about half of all cases occur in children younger than 5. In children younger than 18 months, a transphyseal vessel is usually present, providing a connection between the metaphysis, which is usually the first site of infection, and the epiphysis. As a result, these children are at risk not only for epiphyseal spread, but spread to the contiguous joint space. The long bones are most commonly involved (femur > tibia > humerus). The pelvis is involved in 9% and presents a unique clinical challenge. Multifocal osteomyelitis is uncommon except in neonates.

The bacteria most commonly involved is somewhat age dependent: *Staphylococcus aureus* predominates in all age groups, but in children younger than 3 years old, *Kingella kingae* is an increasingly recognized cause, and in some studies predominates. The rapid emergence of community-acquired, methicillin-resistant *Staphylococcus aureus* (CA-MRSA) as a common pathogen in the United States and elsewhere has significantly changed the approach to empiric management of AHO. *Streptococcus pyogenes* and *Streptococcus pneumoniae* are also common pathogens. Since the introduction of the conjugate *Haemophilus influenzae* type b vaccine (Hib), osteomyelitis secondary to this organism is quite rare.

A. Typically, in AHO, symptoms have been present for less than 2 weeks and include fever, pain at the site of the infection, and a tendency to avoid use of the affected extremity. Less commonly, there is anorexia, generalized malaise, or vomiting. Often, children appear otherwise quite well, though shock in association with osteomyelitis is also described. On physical examination, the most common findings are localized swelling, tenderness, warmth, and erythema. Range of motion of adjacent joints is usually not exquisitely painful in AHO and, if present, should raise suspicion for septic arthritis (see p. 718).

B. Standard markers of inflammation (white blood cell count [WBC], C-reactive protein [CRP], and erythrocyte sedimentation rate [ESR]) are usually increased in AHO. The CRP is almost always increased, whereas the ESR can lag 1 to 3 days. The CRP also tends to decline first in response to effective therapy. A blood culture will be positive in as many as 60% of cases. Plain films of the affected area often show soft-tissue swelling early, but usually do not show bony changes until at least 7 days into the course of the disease. In certain circumstances, further imaging such as technetium bone scan or magnetic resonance imaging (MRI) may be considered. Bone scan is particularly useful if the site of infection is poorly localized or if multifocal osteomyelitis is a concern. MRI is particularly useful for pelvic, vertebral, and small bone osteomyelitis, and additionally evaluates for adjacent muscle involvement (myositis). These considerations must be weighed against the potential disadvantages, though, which include cost and the need for sedation in younger children.

C. If a blood culture is positive shortly after presentation, this may obviate the need for a bone aspirate unless there is an abscess identified or if the child is younger than 18 months, and thus rupture into the epiphysis or contiguous joint is imminent. However, in the current era of CA-MRSA, identification of a micro-organism is of utmost importance in guiding therapy. A bone aspirate will yield a positive culture in about 90% of patients with AHO, assuming there was no pretreatment with antibiotics. However, pretreatment should not preclude attempts at isolating an organism, because cultures are often still positive. Pus, if available, should be sent to the microbiology laboratory in lieu of swabs, which have a lower microbiologic yield. Pathology is useful in differentiating acute from chronic osteomyelitis and can give clues to unusual organisms or alternative diagnoses.

D. Empiric antibiotic coverage while awaiting culture results is dependent on several factors: the degree of illness of the patient, the age of the patient, and the rate of MRSA isolates in the community. There is significant variation on recommendations for empiric coverage and, indeed, several approaches are reasonable. Because *S. aureus* is the most common pathogen across age groups, initial empiric coverage should include effective antistaphylococcal antibiotic. In children younger than 3 years, empiric coverage for *Kingella* spp. is also indicated. In critically ill patients, broad coverage including vancomycin and a third-generation cephalosporin is warranted while awaiting results of cultures. The decision on whether to use an agent effective against CA-MRSA should take into account the frequency with which such infections are seen in a community. Many experts recommend such coverage if the percentage of MRSA is greater than 10% to 15%. Vancomycin and clindamycin are generally considered the drugs of choice.

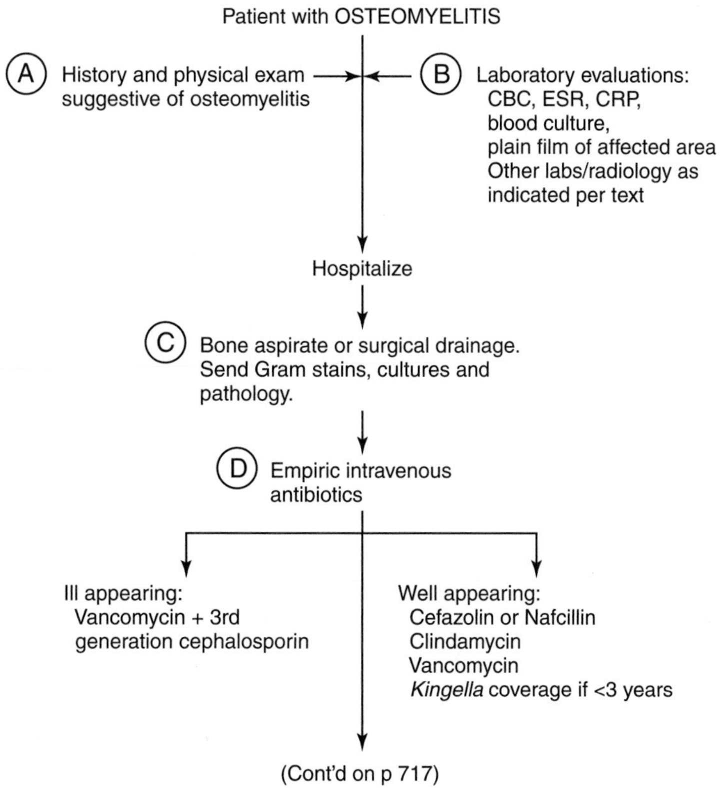
Patient with OSTEOMYELITIS
A
History and physical exam suggestive of osteomyelitis
B
Laboratory evaluations:
CBC, ESR, CRP,
blood culture,
plain film of affected area
Other labs/radiology as indicated per text
Hospitalize
C
Bone aspirate or surgical drainage. Send Gram stains, cultures and pathology.
D
Empiric intravenous antibiotics
Ill appearing:
Vancomycin + 3rd generation cephalosporin
Well appearing:
Cefazolin or Nafcillin
Clindamycin
Vancomycin
Kingella coverage if <3 years
(Cont'd on p 717)

However, rates of clindamycin resistance vary throughout the country from 10% to 50%. These antibiotics do not have activity against *Kingella* spp., and *Kingella* should be covered in those younger than 3 years. Empiric therapy with vancomycin without a specimen or if cultures are negative is problematic because there is no equivalent oral alternative. Anaerobes are unusual in AHO, except when associated with Lemierre syndrome. See Table 1 for a summary of antibiotic choices and doses.

E. Indicators of improvement include resolution of fever, clinical progress, and decreasing inflammatory markers. Lack of these features usually indicates a complication, such as abscess, or inadequate antibiotic coverage; repeat imaging, surgical intervention, and/or change in empiric therapy should be considered. In uncomplicated osteomyelitis with early signs of improvement, transition to oral therapy is reasonable when fever is gone, there is clinical improvement, and a decrease inflammatory parameters is observed, which usually takes 3 to 7 days.

F. See Table 1 for oral antibiotic choices. If the patient was persistently bacteremic, bony involvement is extensive, an abscess could not be débrided, or the organism is unusual, prolonged IV therapy is indicated. In addition, persistent bacteremia or multifocality indicates that an endovascular focus of infection should be considered.

G. Follow-up of a patient with osteomyelitis includes physical examination, interim history, follow-up radiographs, and laboratory evaluations both to follow infection and for antibiotic adverse effects (see Table 1). The examination and clinical signs should progressively improve. The CRP typically returns to normal within 7 to 10 days of appropriate therapy, and the ESR within 3 to 4 weeks; if this does not occur, or condition worsens, repeat imaging looking for abscess/sequestra and/or surgical intervention for débridement and pathology may be indicated. The recommended total duration of therapy for AHO is 4 to 6 weeks, but it should be guided by clinical scenario, clinical improvement, and normalized inflammatory markers.

Table 1. **Antibiotics for Pediatric Osteomyelitis**

	Nafcillin (IV)	Dicloxacillin (PO)	Cefazolin (IV)	Cephalexin (PO)	Cefotaxime (IV)	Ceftriaxone (IV)	Vancomycin (IV)	Clindamycin (IV or PO)
Dose, mg/kg/day	150–200 divided q6	100 divided q6	100 divided q6	100 divided q6	150 divided q6–8	100 divided q12–24	60 divided q6	40 divided q6–8
Dose, maximum single (mg)	2000	500	2000	1000	2000	2000	2000	1200 (div) and 600 (po)
Adverse effect								
Diarrhea, including *Clostridium difficile* colitis	+	+	+	+	+	+	+	+
Bone marrow suppression	+	+	+	+	+	+	+	+
Rash	+	+	+	+	+	+	+	+
Stevens–Johnson syndrome	+	+	+	+	+	+	+	+
Drug fever	+	+	+	+	+	+	+	+
Nephrotoxicity							+	
Interstitial nephritis	+	+	+	+	+	+		
Increased transaminases						+		+
Laboratory tests*								
CBC, ESR, CRP	BUN, Cr, UA micro	BUN, Cr, UA micro	BUN, Cr, UA micro	BUN, Cr, UA micro	BUN, Cr, UA micro	BUN, Cr, UA micro, LFTs	BUN, Cr, UA micro, vanc peak, trough†	LFTs
Organism								
MSSA	+	+	+	+	‡	‡	+	+
MRSA							+	+§
Streptococcus pyogenes (group A strep)	+	+	+	+	+	+	+	+
Streptococcus pneumoniae	+	+	+	+	+	+	+	+
Kingella kingae	+/−	+	+	+	+	+		

*All patients on antibiotics for osteomyelitis should be followed with a weekly complete blood cell count (CBC), erythrocyte sedimentation rate (ESR), and C-reactive protein (CRP). The laboratory tests listed are additional labs specific to the antibiotic.

†Although cefotaxime and ceftriaxone are often listed as having activity against methicillin-sensitive *Staphylococcus aureus* (MRSA), in general, antistaphylococcal penicillins (such as nafcillin) or first-generation cephalosporins (such as cefazolin) are the preferred therapy.

‡The use of clindamycin for methicillin-resistant *Staphylococcus aureus* (MRSA) depends on local susceptibility patterns and, if available, susceptibility testing. In general, if the local susceptibility pattern shows less than 10% resistance of MRSA to clindamycin, it is reasonable to use it as empiric therapy. It is important that the microbiology laboratory perform a "D-test" for inducible clindamycin resistance. Other possible oral alternatives include trimethoprim sulfamethoxazole, linezolid, and levofloxacin plus rifampin. The taste of clindamycin is not well tolerated and can be covered with chocolate syrup.

§For vancomycin levels, trough is drawn as it is associated with toxicity. Higher peaks theoretically should correlate with higher bone levels. If dosing has been established, levels do not necessarily need to be checked unless serum creatinine changes or therapy is prolonged.

BUN, blood urea nitrogen; *Cr*, creatine; *IV*, intravenously; *LFT*, liver function test; *PO*, orally; *UA*, urinalysis.

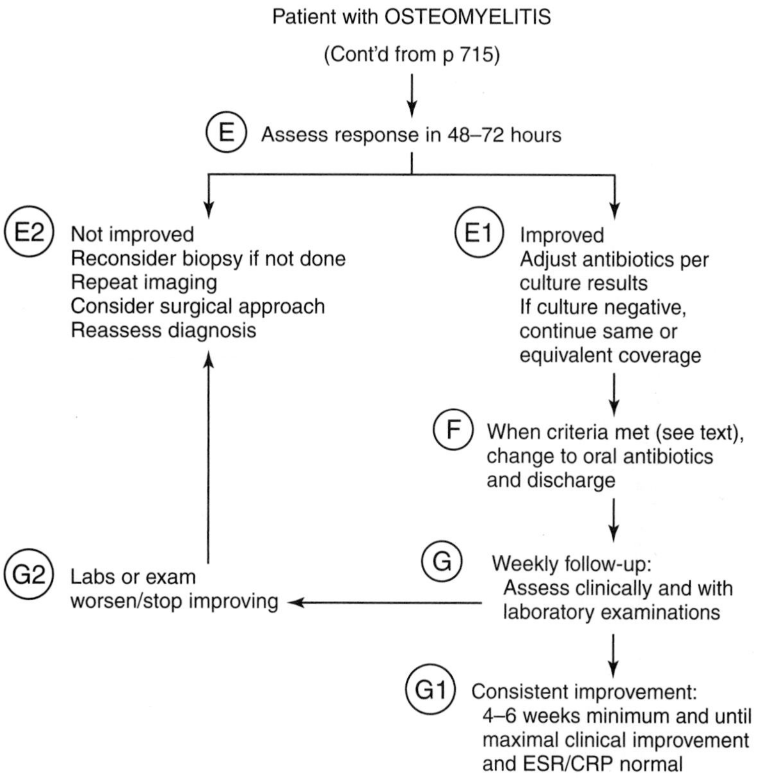
Patient with OSTEOMYELITIS
(Cont'd from p 715)
E Assess response in 48–72 hours
E2 Not improved
Reconsider biopsy if not done
Repeat imaging
Consider surgical approach
Reassess diagnosis
E1 Improved
Adjust antibiotics per culture results
If culture negative, continue same or equivalent coverage
F When criteria met (see text), change to oral antibiotics and discharge
G2 Labs or exam worsen/stop improving
G Weekly follow-up:
Assess clinically and with laboratory examinations
G1 Consistent improvement:
4–6 weeks minimum and until maximal clinical improvement and ESR/CRP normal

References

Arnold SR, Elias D, Buckingham SC, et al. Changing patterns of acute hematogenous osteomyelitis and septic arthritis: emergence of community-associated methicillin-resistant Staphylococcus aureus. J Pediatr Orthop 2006;26(6):703–8.

Bowerman SG, Green NE, Mencio GA. Decline of bone and joint infections attributable to haemophilus influenzae type b. Clin Orthop Relat Res 1997;(341):128–33.

Bradley JS, Kaplan SL, Tan TQ, et al. Pediatric pneumococcal bone and joint infections. The Pediatric Multicenter Pneumococcal Surveillance Study Group (PMPSSG). Pediatrics 1998;102(6):1376–82.

Darville T, Jacobs RF. Management of acute hematogenous osteomyelitis in children. Pediatr Infect Dis J 2004;23(3):255–7.

Ibia EO, Imoisili M, Pikis A. Group A beta-hemolytic streptococcal osteomyelitis in children. Pediatrics 2003;112(1 Pt 1):e22–6.

Kaplan SL. Osteomyelitis in children. Infect Dis Clin North Am 2005;19(4):787–97, vii.

Kiang KM, Ogunmodede F, Juni BA, et al. Outbreak of osteomyelitis/septic arthritis caused by Kingella kingae among child care center attendees. Pediatrics 2005;116(2):e206–13.

Martinez-Aguilar G, Avalos-Mishaan A, Hulten K, et al. Community-acquired, methicillin-resistant and methicillin-susceptible Staphylococcus aureus musculoskeletal infections in children. Pediatr Infect Dis J 2004;23(8):701–6.

Stott NS. Review article: paediatric bone and joint infection. J Orthop Surg (Hong Kong) 2001;9(1):83–90.

Unkila-Kallio L, Kallio MJ, Eskola J, Peltola H. Serum C-reactive protein, erythrocyte sedimentation rate, and white blood cell count in acute hematogenous osteomyelitis of children. Pediatrics 1994;93(1):59–62.

Yagupsky P, Proshe E, and St. Geme JW. Kingella Kingae: An emerging pathogen in young children. Pediatrics 2011;127(3):557–65.

Septic Arthritis

Sean T. O'Leary, MD, Jason Child, PharmD,
and Sarah Parker, MD

Septic arthritis is microbial invasion of the joint space with a subsequent inflammatory response, and is most commonly caused by a bacterial infection. Acute septic arthritis is a medical, and often surgical, emergency. In children younger than 18 months, septic arthritis is often secondary to osteomyelitis, which has eroded through the boney cortex. Pediatric acute septic arthritis is primarily hematogenous in origin (AHO); this chapter focuses on this form. Other forms of septic arthritis, including alternate forms of bacterial introduction (including trauma and postsurgical), chronic septic arthritis, septic arthritis with unusual pathogens (fungal, mycobacterial), and septic arthritis in special hosts (neonates, immunocompromised, sickle cell disease, unusual exposures) are more complicated, and consultation with orthopedic and infectious disease specialists should be considered.

Septic arthritis is primarily a disease of children, with more than half of cases occurring before age 20, and the peak incidence before age 3. Boys are affected twice as commonly as girls. The most commonly affected joints are in the lower extremity, the knee being most common, followed by the hip and ankle. The bacteria most commonly involved is somewhat age dependent: *Staphylococcus aureus* predominates in all age groups, but in children younger than 3 years old, *Kingella kingae* is an increasingly recognized cause, and in some studies predominates. The rapid emergence of community-acquired methicillin-resistant *Staphylococcus aureus* (CA-MRSA) as a common pathogen in the United States and elsewhere has significantly changed the approach to empiric management of septic arthritis. *Streptococcus pyogenes* and *Streptococcus pneumoniae* are also common pathogens. *Neisseria meningitis, Neisseria gonorrhoea,* and *Salmonella* spp. are less common. Since the introduction of the conjugate *Haemophilus influenzae* type b vaccine (Hib), septic arthritis secondary to this organism is quite rare.

A. In septic arthritis, pain in the affected joint occurs early in the course. Usually fever is present, and there is a tendency to avoid use of the affected extremity. Less commonly, there is anorexia, generalized malaise, or vomiting. On physical examination, the most common findings are localized swelling, tenderness, warmth, and erythema. Range of motion of the affected joint is usually decreased and often exquisitely painful. Diagnosis of septic arthritis of the hip requires a high index of suspicion, because swelling and erythema are usually not present. Signs and symptoms of a septic hip joint in younger children are often nonspecific.

B. Standard markers of inflammation (white blood cell [WBC] count, C-reactive protein [CRP], and erythrocyte sedimentation rate [ESR]) are markedly increased in greater than 90% of cases of septic arthritis. The CRP is almost always increased initially, whereas the ESR can lag 1 to 3 days. The CRP also tends to decline first in response to effective therapy. A blood culture will be positive in as many as 40% of cases. Plain films of the affected area often show soft-tissue swelling and widening of the joint space early, and occasionally an adjacent osteomyelitis is evident. Adjacent osteomyelitis should be assumed in those younger than 18 months. If clinically concerning, care should not be delayed by further imaging, but in certain circumstances, further imaging such as ultrasound, technetium bone scan, or magnetic resonance imaging (MRI) may be considered. Bone scan may be useful for evaluation of deeper joints, such as the hip or sacroiliac joint. MRI may be useful in the following circumstances: (1) in evaluation of small joints, (2) in identifying periarticular abscesses, and (3) in evaluation for potential adjacent osteomyelitis and/or pyomyositis. These considerations must be weighed against the potential disadvantages, though, which include cost and the need for sedation in younger children.

C. Joint aspiration is indicated for all children with possible septic arthritis, both for diagnostic purposes and decompression of the affected joint. Fluid should always be sent for cell count and culture, even if "clear." In the current era of CA-MRSA, identification of a micro-organism is of utmost importance in guiding therapy. A blood culture will be positive in about 40% of patients with septic arthritis, and synovial fluid will be positive in about 50% to 60%, assuming there was no pretreatment with antibiotics. However, pretreatment should not preclude attempts at isolating an organism, because cultures are often still positive. Pus, if available, should be sent to the microbiology laboratory in lieu of swabs, which have a lower microbiologic yield.

D. The hip joint essentially always requires open surgical drainage and irrigation because the joint capsule attaches below the ball of the femur. A similarly built joint is the shoulder joint, which also is usually surgically drained. Another indication for surgery on any joint is symptoms longer than 4 days or lack of improvement after aspiration and 24 hours of antibiotics. Synovial fluid should be sent for cultures and cell counts, and if surgery is performed, consideration should be given to a synovial biopsy. Pathology is

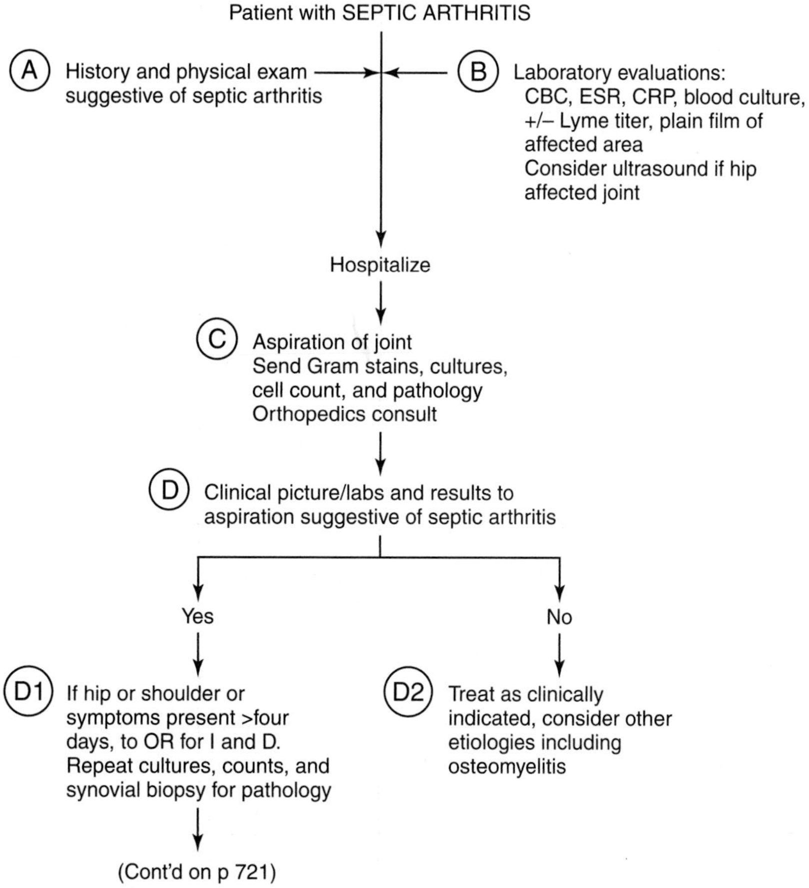
Patient with SEPTIC ARTHRITIS
A History and physical exam suggestive of septic arthritis
B Laboratory evaluations: CBC, ESR, CRP, blood culture, +/– Lyme titer, plain film of affected area
Consider ultrasound if hip affected joint
Hospitalize
C Aspiration of joint
Send Gram stains, cultures, cell count, and pathology
Orthopedics consult
D Clinical picture/labs and results to aspiration suggestive of septic arthritis
Yes
No
D1 If hip or shoulder or symptoms present >four days, to OR for I and D.
Repeat cultures, counts, and synovial biopsy for pathology
D2 Treat as clinically indicated, consider other etiologies including osteomyelitis
(Cont'd on p 721)

useful in differentiating acute from chronic septic arthritis and can give clues to unusual organisms or alternative diagnoses. The cell count is useful in helping distinguish septic arthritis from other causes. The WBC count in septic arthritis is usually greater than 50,000 cells per mL with a predominance of neutrophils. Rarely, other conditions such as Lyme arthritis or systemic-onset juvenile arthritis may have WBC counts greater than 50,000. Transient synovitis (or viral arthritis) typically has a WBC count of 5000 to 15,000, and is almost always less than 50,000. Unusual pathogens, such as *Mycobacteria* spp. and *Brucella* spp., generally have cell counts less than 100,000. Alternative diagnoses for septic arthritis include transient synovitis, reactive arthritis, osteomyelitis with sympathetic joint effusion, hemarthrosis, traumatic effusion, arthritis of acute rheumatic fever, juvenile idiopathic arthritis (all types), tumors, slipped capital femoral epiphysis, and avascular necrosis of the femoral head (Legg–Calve–Perthes disease).

E. Empiric antibiotic coverage while awaiting culture results is dependent on several factors: the degree of illness of the patient, the age of the patient, and the rate of MRSA isolates in the community. There is significant variation on recommendations for empiric coverage, and indeed, several approaches are reasonable. Because *S. aureus* is the most common pathogen across age groups, initial empiric coverage should include effective antistaphylococcal antibiotic. The decision whether to use an agent effective against CA-MRSA should take into account the frequency with which such infections are seen in a community. Many experts recommend such coverage if the percentage of MRSA is greater than 10% to 15%. Vancomycin and clindamycin are generally considered the drugs of choice. However, rates of clindamycin resistance vary throughout the country from 10% to 50%. These antibiotics do not have activity against *Kingella* spp., and *Kingella* should be covered in those younger than 3 years. In critically ill patients, broad coverage including vancomycin and a third-generation cephalosporin is warranted while awaiting results of cultures. Empiric therapy with vancomycin without a specimen or if cultures are negative is problematic because there is no equivalent oral alternative. Anaerobes are unusual in septic arthritis, except when associated with Lemierre syndrome. Empiric therapy for other pathogens based on exposure history may be warranted; for example, *N. gonorrhoeae* should be considered in the sexually active adolescent, and *Salmonella* spp. considered in those with reptiles as pets. There is no role for intra-articular instillation of antibiotics because this can produce chemical irritation and inflammation. See Table 1 in Osteomyelitis chapter (p. 714) for a summary of antibiotic choices and doses. A Gram stain of synovial fluid may help broaden therapy but should never be relied on to narrow therapy. Recent studies have suggested benefit from corticosteroids (0.15 mg/kg/dose intravenously every 6 hours for 4 days), in addition to antibiotics, in the treatment of uncomplicated pediatric septic arthritis.

F. Indicators of improvement include resolution of fever, clinical progress, and decreasing inflammatory markers. Lack of these features usually indicates a complication, such as adjacent osteomyelitis, myositis, abscess formation, incomplete surgical drainage, or inadequate antibiotic coverage; repeat imaging, surgical intervention, and/or change in empiric therapy should be considered. In uncomplicated septic arthritis with early signs of improvement, transition to oral therapy is reasonable when fever is gone and there is clinical improvement and a decrease inflammatory parameters, which usually takes 3 to 7 days. See Table 1 in Osteomyelitis chapter (p. 714) for oral antibiotic choices. If the patient was persistently bacteremic, there is adjacent osteomyelitis, the organism is unusual, or there is concern with compliance, prolonged IV therapy is indicated. In addition, persistent bacteremia or multifocality indicates that an endovascular focus of infection should be considered.

G. Follow up of a patient with septic arthritis includes physical examination, interim history, follow-up radiographs, and laboratory evaluations both to follow infection and for antibiotic adverse effects (see Table 1 in Osteomyelitis chapter, p. 714). The examination and clinical signs should progressively improve. The CRP typically returns to normal within 7 to 10 days of appropriate therapy, and the ESR within 3 to 4 weeks; if this does not occur or condition worsens, repeat imaging looking for adjacent osteomyelitis or abscess and/or surgical intervention for drainage, débridement, and pathology may be indicated. Relapse of symptoms may also indicate a complication such as aseptic necrosis. The recommended total duration of therapy for uncomplicated septic arthritis is 3 to 4 weeks, but should be guided by clinical scenario, clinical improvement, and normalized inflammatory markers.

References

Arnold SR, Elias D, Buckingham SC, et al. Changing patterns of acute hematogenous osteomyelitis and septic arthritis: emergence of community-associated methicillin-resistant Staphylococcus aureus. J Pediatr Orthop 2006;26(6):703–8.

Bowerman SG, Green NE, Mencio GA. Decline of bone and joint infections attributable to haemophilus influenzae type b. Clin Orthop Relat Res 1997;(341):128–33.

Bradley JS, Kaplan SL, Tan TQ, et al. Pediatric pneumococcal bone and joint infections. The Pediatric Multicenter Pneumococcal Surveillance Study Group (PMPSSG). Pediatrics 1998;102(6):1376–82.

Brown MD. Test characteristics of C-reactive protein (CRP) for pediatric septic arthritis. J Pediatr Orthop 2004;24(3):344.

Browne LP, Mason EO, Kaplan SL, et al. Optimal imaging strategy for community-acquired Staphylococcus aureus musculoskeletal infections in children. Pediatr Radiol 2008;38(8):841–7.

Dohin B, Gillet Y, Kohler R, et al. Pediatric bone and joint infections caused by Panton-Valentine leukocidin-positive Staphylococcus aureus. Pediatr Infect Dis J 2007;26(11):1042–8.

Gene A, Garcia-Garcia JJ, Sala P, et al. Enhanced culture detection of Kingella kingae, a pathogen of increasing clinical importance in pediatrics. Pediatr Infect Dis J 2004;23(9):886–8.

Harel L, Prais D, Bar-On E, Livni G, Hoffer V, Uziel V, Amir J. Dexamethasone therapy for septic arthritis in children: Results of a randomized double-blind placebo-controlled study. J Pediatr Orthop 2011;31:211–5.

Kiang KM, Ogunmodede F, Juni BA, et al. Outbreak of osteomyelitis/septic arthritis caused by Kingella kingae among child care center attendees. Pediatrics 2005;116(2):e206–13.

Kocher MS, Zurakowski D, Kasser JR. Differentiating between septic arthritis and transient synovitis of the hip in children: an evidence-based clinical prediction algorithm. J Bone Joint Surg Am 1999;81(12):1662–70.

Lee SK, Suh KJ, Kim YW, et al. Septic arthritis versus transient synovitis at MR imaging: preliminary assessment with signal intensity alterations in bone marrow. Radiology 1999;211(2):459–65.

Martinez-Aguilar G, valos-Mishaan A, Hulten K, et al. Community-acquired, methicillin-resistant and methicillin-susceptible Staphylococcus aureus musculoskeletal infections in children. Pediatr Infect Dis J 2004;23(8):701–6.

Odio CM, Ramirez T, Arias G, et al. Double-blind, randomized, placebo controlled study of dexamethasone therapy for hematogenous septic arthritis in children. Pediatr Infect Dis J 2003;22(10):883–8.

Stott NS. Review article: paediatric bone and joint infection. J Orthop Surg (Hong Kong) 2001;9(1):83–90.

Yagupsky P, Dagan R, Howard CW, et al. High prevalence of Kingella kingae in joint fluid from children with septic arthritis revealed by the BACTEC blood culture system. J Clin Microbiol 1992;30(5):1278–81.

Zamzam MM. The role of ultrasound in differentiating septic arthritis from transient synovitis of the hip in children. J Pediatr Orthop B 2006;15(6):418–22.

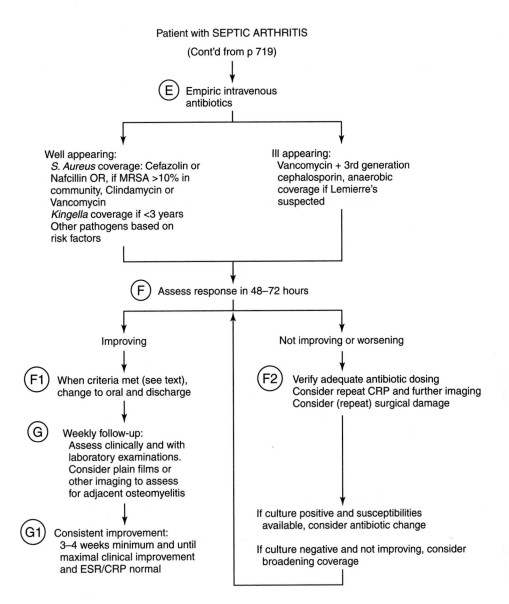

Patient with SEPTIC ARTHRITIS

(Cont'd from p 719)

(E) Empiric intravenous antibiotics

Well appearing:
S. Aureus coverage: Cefazolin or Nafcillin OR, if MRSA >10% in community, Clindamycin or Vancomycin
Kingella coverage if <3 years
Other pathogens based on risk factors

Ill appearing:
Vancomycin + 3rd generation cephalosporin, anaerobic coverage if Lemierre's suspected

(F) Assess response in 48–72 hours

Improving

(F1) When criteria met (see text), change to oral and discharge

(G) Weekly follow-up:
Assess clinically and with laboratory examinations.
Consider plain films or other imaging to assess for adjacent osteomyelitis

(G1) Consistent improvement:
3–4 weeks minimum and until maximal clinical improvement and ESR/CRP normal

Not improving or worsening

(F2) Verify adequate antibiotic dosing
Consider repeat CRP and further imaging
Consider (repeat) surgical damage

If culture positive and susceptibilities available, consider antibiotic change

If culture negative and not improving, consider broadening coverage

Neonatal Disorders

Necrotizing Enterocolitis

Neonatal Herpes Simplex Infections

Newborn Delivery Room Resuscitation

Necrotizing Enterocolitis

Pamela A. Zachar, MD

A. Necrotizing enterocolitis (NEC) can be a devastating and fatal disease in neonates, but early recognition and aggressive management can limit morbidity and mortality. Most infants (90%) who experience development of NEC are born prematurely. Age at onset is inversely related to gestational age at birth; thus, NEC presents in the convalescent stage of a preterm infant's course but usually within 2 or 3 days of birth in a term infant. The risk remains high in preterm infants until they reach 35 to 36 weeks of age.

B. Proven risk factors for NEC include prematurity, formula feeding, maternal cocaine use, and histamine-2 receptor blocker therapy. Other factors that have been associated with NEC include presence of a patent ductus arteriosus, intrauterine growth retardation, perinatal asphyxia, and ethnicity, with black infants being at particularly high risk.

C. Many aspects of infant feeding have been investigated as risk factors for the development of NEC. Breastfeeding is the only factor that has been clearly shown to reduce the risk for the development of NEC. No specific feeding regimen has been proved to prevent NEC, but most experts recommend cautious rates of feeding advancement in premature infants.

D. Early presenting signs of NEC include abdominal distension, feeding intolerance with increased gastric residuals, emesis, grossly bloody stools, and, less often, diarrhea. Infants may exhibit nonspecific systemic symptoms such as lethargy, temperature instability, and an increase in apnea and bradycardia. Common physical examination findings include abdominal distension, tenderness, mass, and, in severe cases, discoloration of the abdominal wall (erythema or a bluish cast). Severe cases may be accompanied by signs of shock, such as diminished pulses and perfusion, tachycardia, and hypotension. When disseminated intravascular coagulation (DIC) is present, oozing from the umbilical stump or puncture sites may occur.

E. Initial laboratory evaluation should include complete blood count (CBC) with differential, blood chemistries and blood gases, and cultures of blood and urine. Common findings include leukopenia or leukocytosis and thrombocytopenia, glucose instability, metabolic acidosis, and electrolyte abnormalities. Other tests such as lumbar puncture, stool studies, and coagulation profiles may be considered based on the clinical scenario.

F. Radiologic imaging is essential to the diagnosis of NEC. Abdominal radiography should include anteroposterior and left lateral decubitus or cross-table lateral views, because a single view is inadequate to detect the subtle signs of perforation (pneumoperitoneum). Early x-ray findings may include intestinal dilatation, thickened intestinal walls, and air–fluid levels. Other findings more specific to NEC include intramural air (pneumatosis intestinalis), portal venous air, and pneumoperitoneum. A fixed or persistent dilated loop of bowel that remains unchanged for 24 to 36 hours often represents a necrotic intestinal loop.

G. NEC may be indolent or fulminant. At presentation, patients can be stratified into groups based on the modified Bell stages of disease. Stage I (suspected NEC) includes infants with mild systemic symptoms, nonspecific abdominal symptoms, and radiographs either normal or with mild ileus. Stage II (mild-to-moderate definite NEC) includes infants with mild-to-moderate systemic symptoms that can include mild acidosis and thrombocytopenia, more prominent abdominal distension, and tenderness. In stage II, radiographs show pneumatosis. Stage III (advanced NEC) includes infants who are severely ill with respiratory failure, signs of shock and/or DIC, and those with evidence of perforation.

H. NEC stage I can represent either the earliest stages of a process that would have developed into more serious disease without treatment, or it can represent other, more benign, clinical entities. Initial treatment should be the same regardless of the stage at presentation. Differential diagnosis for NEC stage I includes septicemia, slow intestinal motility and simple feeding intolerance, milk allergy, and intestinal infections including rotavirus.

I. Initial treatment includes discontinuation of feeding, placement of large-bore orogastric or nasogastric tube (OG/NG) to suction, and initiation of antibiotic therapy with intravenous antibiotics. Choice of antibiotics will depend on the resistance patterns and common flora of the nursery, but will most likely include either ampicillin or vancomycin and an aminoglycoside or cephalosporin (Table 1).

J. In general, radiographs should be repeated every 6 to 8 hours, and blood gases, blood counts, and electrolytes should be followed at least every 12 to 24 hours until the condition stabilizes.

K. In a clinically stable infant with NEC stage I, measurement of serial C-reactive protein (CRP) levels can aid in the differentiation of true NEC from other entities. One recent study demonstrated that following a serum CRP level every 12 hours for three measurements was a strong marker for absence of NEC when all three levels were normal.

L. Consultation with a neonatologist should begin when the diagnosis of NEC is strongly suspected. In general, when NEC stage II or III is confirmed, consultation with pediatric surgery should also be initiated. These cases should be managed at a center where pediatric surgery is immediately available.

M. Very severely ill patients should receive ventilatory assistance before respiratory failure ensues. Apnea,

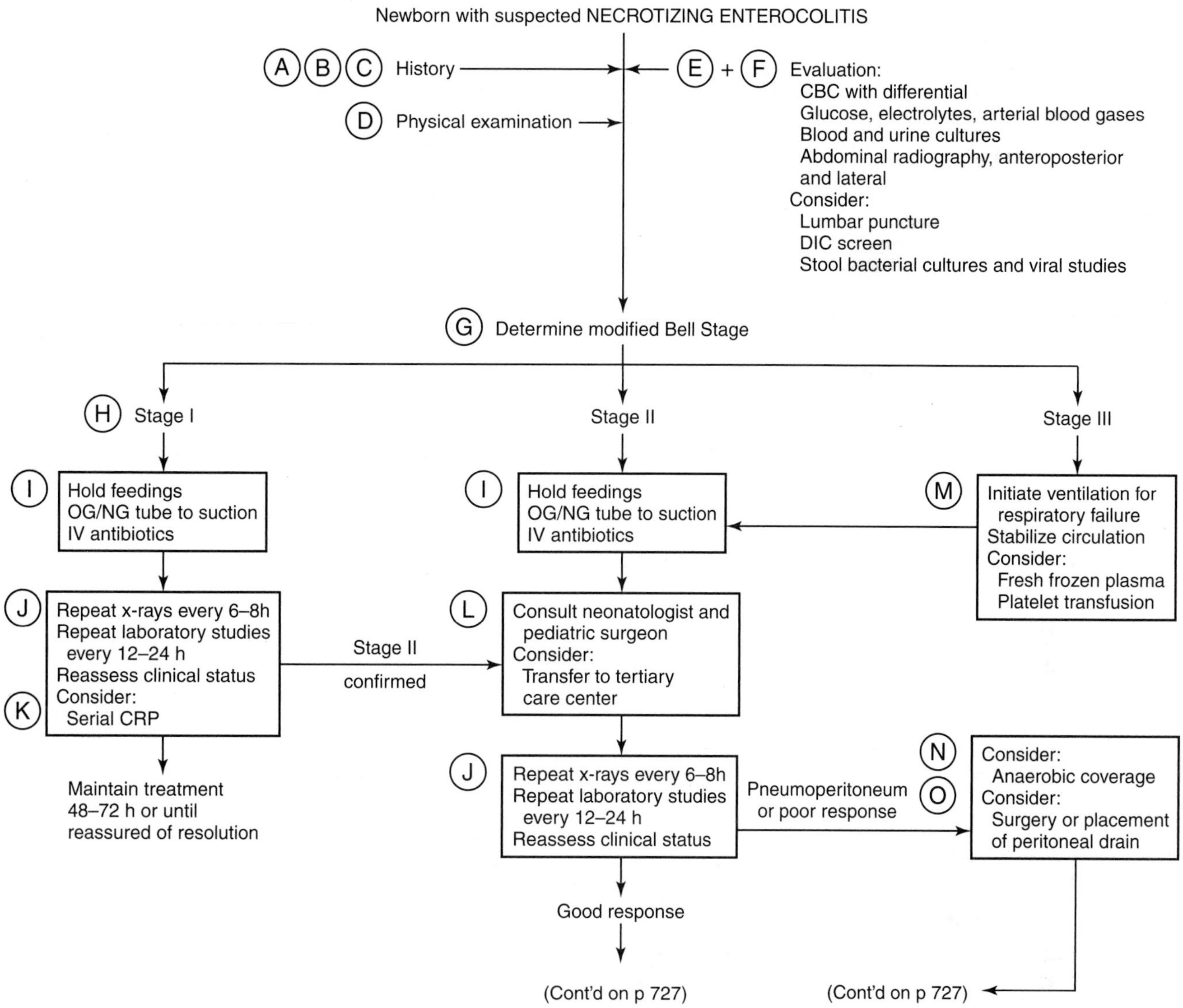
Newborn with suspected NECROTIZING ENTEROCOLITIS
A B C History
D Physical examination
E + F Evaluation:
CBC with differential
Glucose, electrolytes, arterial blood gases
Blood and urine cultures
Abdominal radiography, anteroposterior and lateral
Consider:
Lumbar puncture
DIC screen
Stool bacterial cultures and viral studies
G Determine modified Bell Stage
H Stage I
Stage II
Stage III
I Hold feedings
OG/NG tube to suction
IV antibiotics
I Hold feedings
OG/NG tube to suction
IV antibiotics
M Initiate ventilation for respiratory failure
Stabilize circulation
Consider:
Fresh frozen plasma
Platelet transfusion
J Repeat x-rays every 6–8h
Repeat laboratory studies every 12–24 h
Reassess clinical status
K Consider:
Serial CRP
Stage II
confirmed
L Consult neonatologist and pediatric surgeon
Consider:
Transfer to tertiary care center
Maintain treatment 48–72 h or until reassured of resolution
J Repeat x-rays every 6–8h
Repeat laboratory studies every 12–24 h
Reassess clinical status
Pneumoperitoneum or poor response
N Consider:
Anaerobic coverage
O Consider:
Surgery or placement of peritoneal drain
Good response
(Cont'd on p 727)
(Cont'd on p 727)

respiratory acidosis, and hypoxemia are specific indicators for assisted ventilation. Intestinal capillary leak may deplete circulating fluid volume and protein, and DIC and gastrointestinal hemorrhage may lead to significant blood loss. Maintenance fluids should be provided at 100% to 150% of baseline with additional crystalloid and packed red blood cells as indicated. DIC and significant thrombocytopenia should be treated with fresh frozen plasma and platelet transfusions.

N. If intestinal perforation is suspected, addition of clindamycin or metronidazole to antibiotic coverage should be considered. (Refer to most recent edition of The Harriet Lane Handbook for recommended dosing based on age and weight.) Although many experts recommend coverage for anaerobic pathogens, one small, randomized, controlled trial using clindamycin showed an increase in bowel strictures.

O. Surgical indications include pneumoperitoneum, presence of a fixed loop on serial radiographs, and clinical deterioration despite maximal medical management. Other relative indications include portal venous air, abdominal wall erythema, abdominal mass, unremitting metabolic acidosis, and hyperkalemia or severe DIC. Paracentesis has been shown to be useful at predicting presence of bowel necrosis. Primary peritoneal drainage may be considered rather than open laparotomy, although studies have not conclusively demonstrated which approach is superior.

P. Infants diagnosed with NEC stage II or beyond should be treated with antibiotics and kept NPO for 7 to 14 days. NEC stage I may be treated with shorter courses of antibiotics depending on clinical course and rate of resolution of symptoms. Parenteral nutrition should be initiated promptly by peripheral vein. After 24 hours of antibiotic therapy, central line placement should be considered.

Q. Once treatment is complete, enteral feedings can be introduced with unfortified breast milk or formula. Volume and strength should be increased slowly while tapering parenteral nutrition. A contrast study is indicated if signs of intestinal obstruction develop during refeeding, because strictures are not an uncommon sequela of NEC.

References

Bell MJ, Ternberg JL, Feidin MD, et al. Neonatal necrotizing enterocolitis. Therapeutic decisions based upon clinical staging. Ann Surg 1978;87:1–7.

Dimmitt RA, Moss RL. Clinical management of necrotizing enterocolitis. NeoReviews 2001;2:110–7.

Johns Hopkins Hospital, Arcara K, Tschuddy M. The Harriet Lane Handbook. 19th ed. Philadelphia: Elsevier Mosby; 2011.

Kosloske AM. Indications for operation in necrotizing enterocolitis revisited. J Pediatr Surg 1994;29(5):663–6.

Lin PW, Stoll BJ. Necrotising enterocolitis. Lancet 2006;368:1271–83.

Lucas A, Cole TJ. Breast milk and neonatal necrotizing enterocolitis. Lancet 1990;336:1519–23.

Neu J. Neonatal necrotizing enterocolitis: an update. Acta Paediatr 2005;94(Suppl 449):100–5.

Pourcyrous M, Korones SB, Yang W, et al. C-reactive protein in the diagnosis, management, and prognosis of neonatal necrotizing enterocolitis. Pediatrics 2005;116:1064–9.

Rees CM, Eaton S, Kiely EM, et al. Peritoneal drainage or laparotomy for neonatal bowel perforation? a randomized controlled trial. Ann Surg 2008;248(1):44–51.

Newborn with suspected NECROTIZING ENTEROCOLITIS

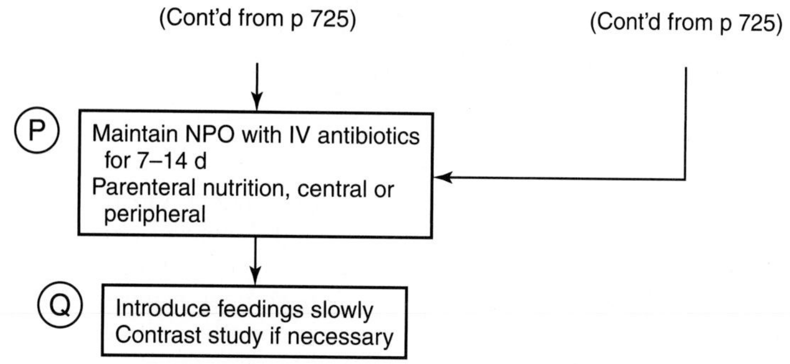
(Cont'd from p 725)
(Cont'd from p 725)
P
Maintain NPO with IV antibiotics for 7–14 d
Parenteral nutrition, central or peripheral
Q
Introduce feedings slowly
Contrast study if necessary

Neonatal Herpes Simplex Infections

John W. Ogle, MD

Neonatal herpes simplex virus (HSV) infections are uncommon but potentially devastating. No comprehensive maternal screening strategy can predict infants at risk, so early recognition and treatment are the keys to reducing morbidity and mortality.

A. Approximately 70% of neonates with HSV infection are born to mothers with no history of genital lesions. Most neonatal cases result from primary maternal HSV infection at delivery. The mother often lacks a distinguishing clinical picture; she may have a nonspecific febrile illness or be entirely asymptomatic. The risk for HSV infection in infants born to mothers with recurrent disease and specific immunoglobulin G antibody is no more than one tenth that of infants whose mothers have infection during pregnancy but lack type-specific antibody. The risk for neonatal infection resulting from delivery during an episode of primary maternal herpes is estimated to be 33% to 50%, and the risk for infection in the setting of recurrent maternal disease is probably 3% to 5%.

B. Nonspecific clinical signs (fever, lethargy, irritability, respiratory distress, poor feeding, poor tone) are probably more common than typical skin lesions. Because initial symptoms are rarely diagnostic for HSV, include this cause in the differential diagnosis of the sick infant. Search for the characteristic papulovesicular lesions, which are characteristically grouped 2- to 3-mm vesicles on an erythematous base. The lesions may be pustular and are often located at sites of minor abrasions (scalp electrodes). On the oral mucosa, the vesicles rupture and shallow ulcers may be seen.

C. Management of an asymptomatic infant who might have been exposed to HSV varies by maternal history. If a mother with documented recurrent genital herpes has no signs or symptoms at delivery, her infant does not require isolation and may simply be observed. An infant born to a mother with active lesions at delivery requires contact isolation. The infant should room with the mother, who must practice good handwashing and cover lesions. If the delivery is vaginal, culture specimens should be obtained at 24 to 48 hours (conjunctiva, oral or nasopharynx, and rectal) and the infant observed. Allow breast-feeding unless there are lesions on the breast. Defer circumcision. In cases of primary maternal infection, delivery by cesarean section is preferred; obtain culture specimens and observe the infant. If delivery is vaginal, consider prophylactic acyclovir pending culture results. When the type of maternal disease is unknown, guidelines for primary infection should be followed.

D. An asymptomatic infant who is not being treated may be discharged routinely if reliable follow-up is ensured. If prophylactic treatment is given, continue for 48 hours of negative cultures. Follow-up in both groups should include heightened vigilance for new rashes or symptoms of HSV until the patient is 4 to 6 weeks of age. If cultures are positive, further evaluation is needed. Treat for 14 to 21 days and arrange close follow-up.

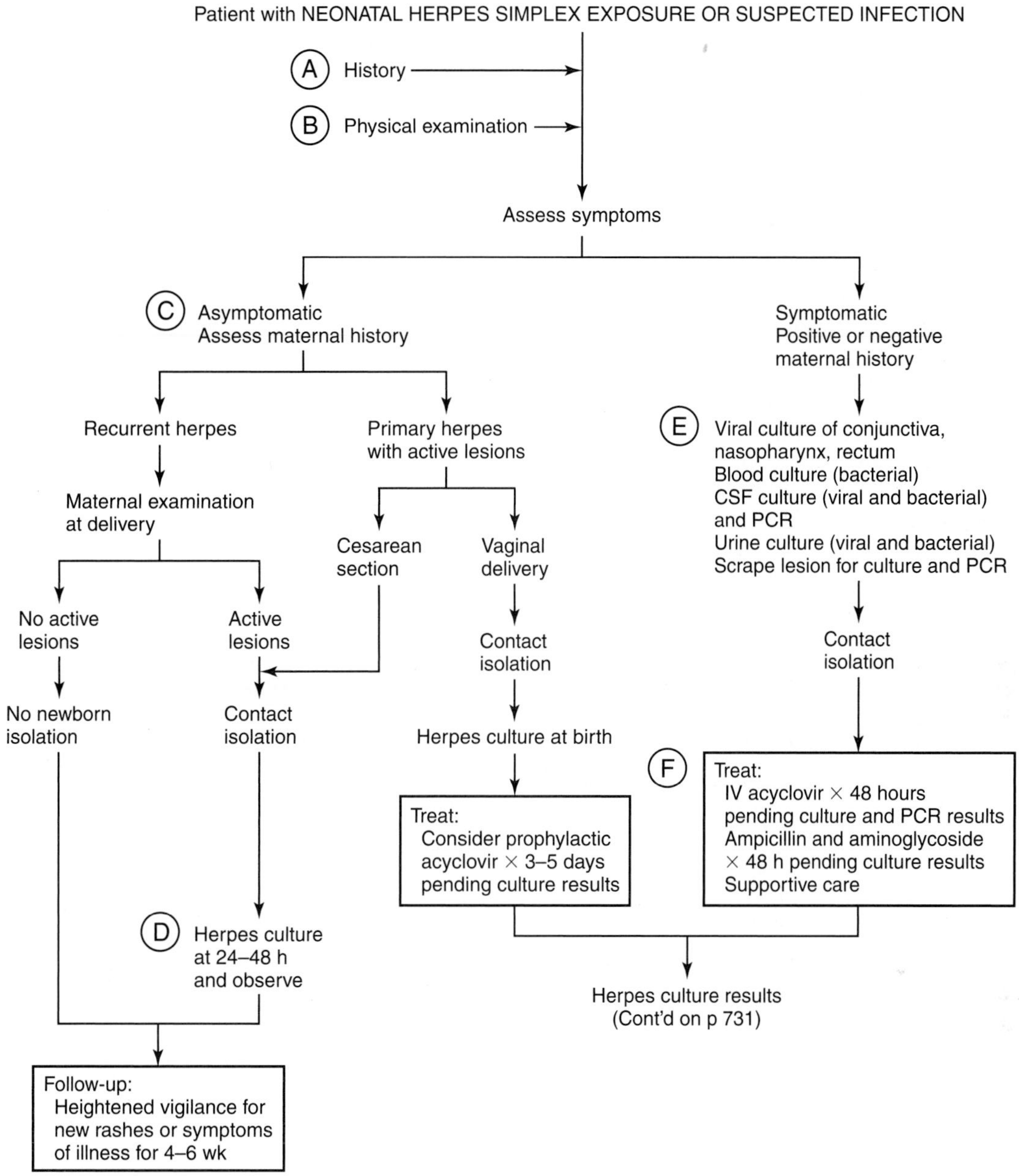
Patient with NEONATAL HERPES SIMPLEX EXPOSURE OR SUSPECTED INFECTION
A
History
B
Physical examination
Assess symptoms
C
Asymptomatic
Assess maternal history
Symptomatic
Positive or negative
maternal history
Recurrent herpes
Primary herpes
with active lesions
E
Viral culture of conjunctiva,
nasopharynx, rectum
Blood culture (bacterial)
CSF culture (viral and bacterial)
and PCR
Urine culture (viral and bacterial)
Scrape lesion for culture and PCR
Maternal examination
at delivery
Cesarean
section
Vaginal
delivery
No active
lesions
Active
lesions
Contact
isolation
Contact
isolation
No newborn
isolation
Contact
isolation
Herpes culture at birth
F
Treat:
IV acyclovir × 48 hours
pending culture and PCR results
Ampicillin and aminoglycoside
× 48 h pending culture results
Supportive care
Treat:
Consider prophylactic
acyclovir × 3–5 days
pending culture results
D
Herpes culture
at 24–48 h
and observe
Herpes culture results
(Cont'd on p 731)
Follow-up:
Heightened vigilance for
new rashes or symptoms
of illness for 4–6 wk

E. Symptomatic infants with nonspecific signs or characteristic evidence of herpes infection require complete evaluation for viral and bacterial sepsis. Include herpes cultures of conjunctiva, nasopharynx, rectum, and any lesions; blood cultures; and viral and bacterial cultures of urine and cerebrospinal fluid. Reserve an aliquot of cerebrospinal fluid for herpes polymerase chain reaction (PCR) analysis. Shell-vial centrifugation and immunoperoxidase staining of culture specimens may provide information in 24 hours; nearly 100% of routine cultures show positivity by 2 days. Either culture or PCR of skin lesions is reliable. Cost and availability determines whether culture or PCR is preferable.

F. Anticipate the need for intensive care in symptomatic patients. Impaired consciousness, respiratory distress, disseminated intravascular coagulation, and prematurity are significantly associated with mortality. Mechanical ventilation, fluid and pressor support, and access to advanced diagnostic facilities are often required. Maintain contact isolation. Pending cultures, begin therapy with antibiotics for presumed bacterial sepsis and initiate intravenous acyclovir (Table 1).

G. Assess the clinical pattern of HSV infection to guide management and aid in prognosis. Infants may have localized cutaneous (skin, eye, mucosa) infection, disseminated disease, or central nervous system (CNS; meningoencephalitis) disease. Localized skin lesions may spread or progress to disseminated disease. CNS involvement may be demonstrated by altered consciousness, focal or multifocal seizures, or paresis. Consider computed tomography and electroencephalography to define the degree of involvement. Disseminated disease often includes jaundice, hepatomegaly, shock, and disseminated intravascular coagulation. Pneumonitis coupled with hepatitis suggests HSV. Obtain an ophthalmology consultation to identify eye involvement; HSV causes keratoconjunctivitis and chorioretinitis.

H. The prognosis for neonates is far better with localized mucocutaneous disease than with other forms. Survival is the rule; approximately 30% of these children experience development of neurologic impairment, which may not be evident in the neonatal period. Approximately 15% of survivors have multiple cutaneous recurrences, a risk factor for subsequent abnormal development. Disseminated disease is fatal in 50% to 60% of cases, even with antiviral treatment. Meningoencephalitis is fatal in 14% to 18% of cases despite treatment. Nearly two thirds of survivors of CNS or disseminated disease develop abnormally. Because there is concern for relapse in the CNS, as well as spread to the CNS from cutaneous relapse, some experts administer long-term (3–6 months) suppressive therapy with oral acyclovir.

Table 1. **Antiviral Therapy for Neonatal Herpes Simplex Infection**

Drug	Dosage
Acyclovir	20 mg/kg/dose 24 hours intravenously every 8 hours for 14–21 days

References

American Academy of Pediatrics. Herpes simplex. In: Pickering LK, editor. Red book: 2009 report of the Committee on Infectious Diseases. 28th ed. Elk Grove Village, IL: American Academy of Pediatrics; 2009. p. 363–73.

Caviness AC, Demmler GJ, Almendarez Y, Selwyn BJ. The prevalence of neonatal herpes simplex virus infection compared with serious bacterial illness in hospitalized neonates. J Pediatr 2008;166:164–9.

Caviness AC, Demmler GJ, Swint M, Cantor SB. Cost-effectiveness analysis of herpes simplex virus testing and treatment strategies in febrile neonates. Arch Pediatr Adolesc Med 2008;162(7):665–74.

Kimberlin DW. When should you initiate acyclovir therapy in a neonate? J Pediatr 2008;153:155–67.

Long SS. In defense of empiric acyclovir therapy in certain neonates. J Pediatr 2008;153:157–8.

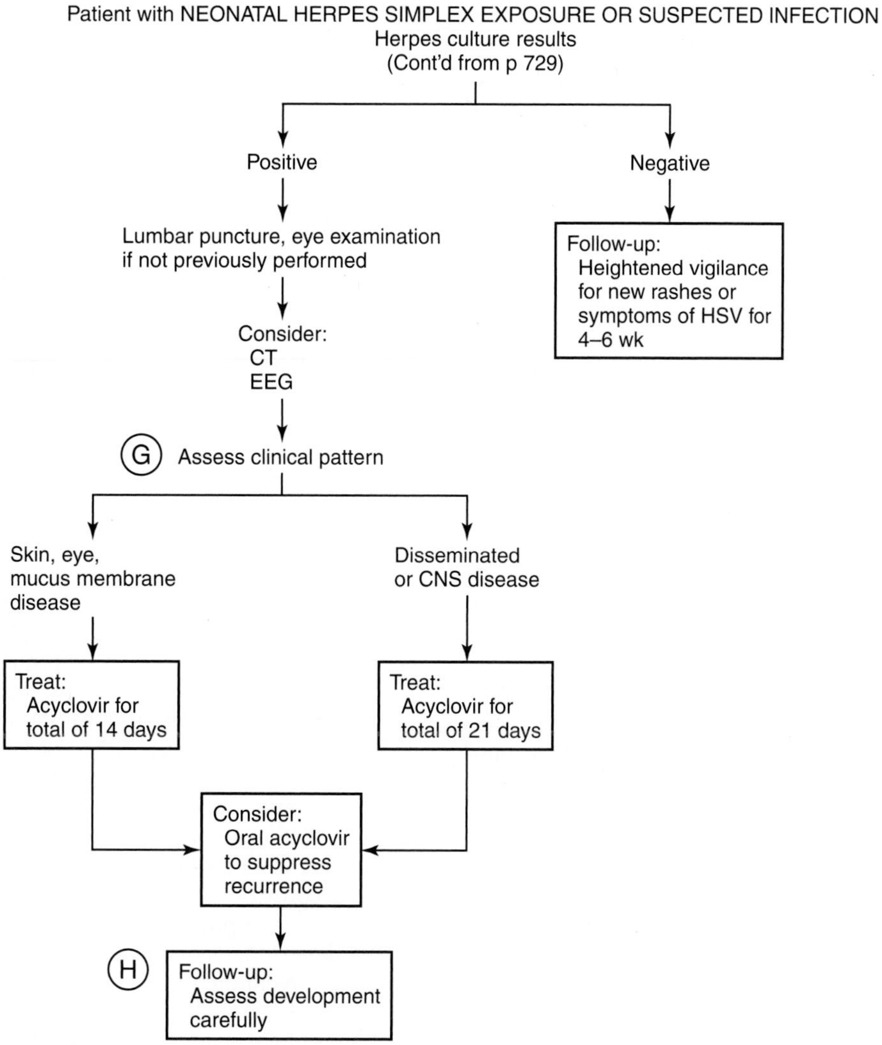
Patient with NEONATAL HERPES SIMPLEX EXPOSURE OR SUSPECTED INFECTION
Herpes culture results
(Cont'd from p 729)
Positive
Negative
Lumbar puncture, eye examination if not previously performed
Follow-up: Heightened vigilance for new rashes or symptoms of HSV for 4–6 wk
Consider: CT EEG
G Assess clinical pattern
Skin, eye, mucus membrane disease
Disseminated or CNS disease
Treat: Acyclovir for total of 14 days
Treat: Acyclovir for total of 21 days
Consider: Oral acyclovir to suppress recurrence
H Follow-up: Assess development carefully

Newborn Delivery Room Resuscitation

James S. Barry, MD

Neonatal resuscitation is a critical skill necessary to assist the newborn's transition from a fluid-filled intrauterine environment dependent on maternal-placental function to an independent existence in an air-filled extrauterine environment. Usually, this transition is successful; however, 10% of neonates require support during this time, and at least 1 of 100 newborns requires extensive assistance. Therefore, it is critical that personnel skilled in the evaluation and resuscitation of the newborn be immediately available at birth to prevent injury from a poor or incomplete transition. Effective resuscitation requires the presence of at least one person skilled in all aspects of neonatal resuscitation and responsible only for the newborn. At least two personnel responsible for the newborn should be present at "high-risk" deliveries, with one specifically skilled at intubation and drug administration. Other requirements include the immediate presence of the proper equipment and supplies, appropriate anticipation, timeliness of the neonatal resuscitation team, and advanced preparation of policies and procedures specific to neonatal resuscitation.

At delivery, a rapid assessment should include these four questions: Is the baby full term? Is the amniotic fluid clear of meconium? Is the baby breathing or crying? Is the muscle tone good? This rapid assessment assists in determining whether a newborn receives routine care (oral and nasopharyngeal suctioning, proper airway positioning, drying, stimulating, and warming) and can remain with mother, or whether a more extensive resuscitation is required. The initial steps of resuscitation are altered when a depressed newborn (ineffective respirations or apnea, poor muscle tone, or a heart rate (HR) less than 100 beats/min) with meconium-stained amniotic fluid presents at delivery. Instead of initially drying and stimulating, one should perform endotracheal (ET) intubation with direct tracheal suctioning immediately after birth and before respirations or stimulation have occurred. The rapid assessment and initial resuscitation steps (suctioning, positioning, drying, stimulating, and warming) are performed nearly simultaneously with the evaluation of breathing, HR, and tone within the first 30 seconds.

A. Assess respirations visually and by auscultation. Provide brief tactile stimulation to a gasping or apneic newborn. If this brief stimulation does not increase the rate and depth of respirations, initiate positive-pressure ventilation with supplemental oxygen (21%–100%) using an appropriate-sized mask and bag. Currently, data indicate that resuscitation with an oxygen concentration ranging from room air to 100% is acceptable. Continuing to provide tactile stimulation to a newborn without effective respirations or whose HR is less than 100 beats/min is of no benefit and only delays appropriate intervention.

B. Determine HR by palpation of umbilical cord pulsations or by auscultation. If the HR is less than 100 beats/min, positive-pressure ventilation is required, even if the infant has spontaneous respirations.

(Continued on page 734)

NEWBORN DELIVERY ROOM RESUSCITATION

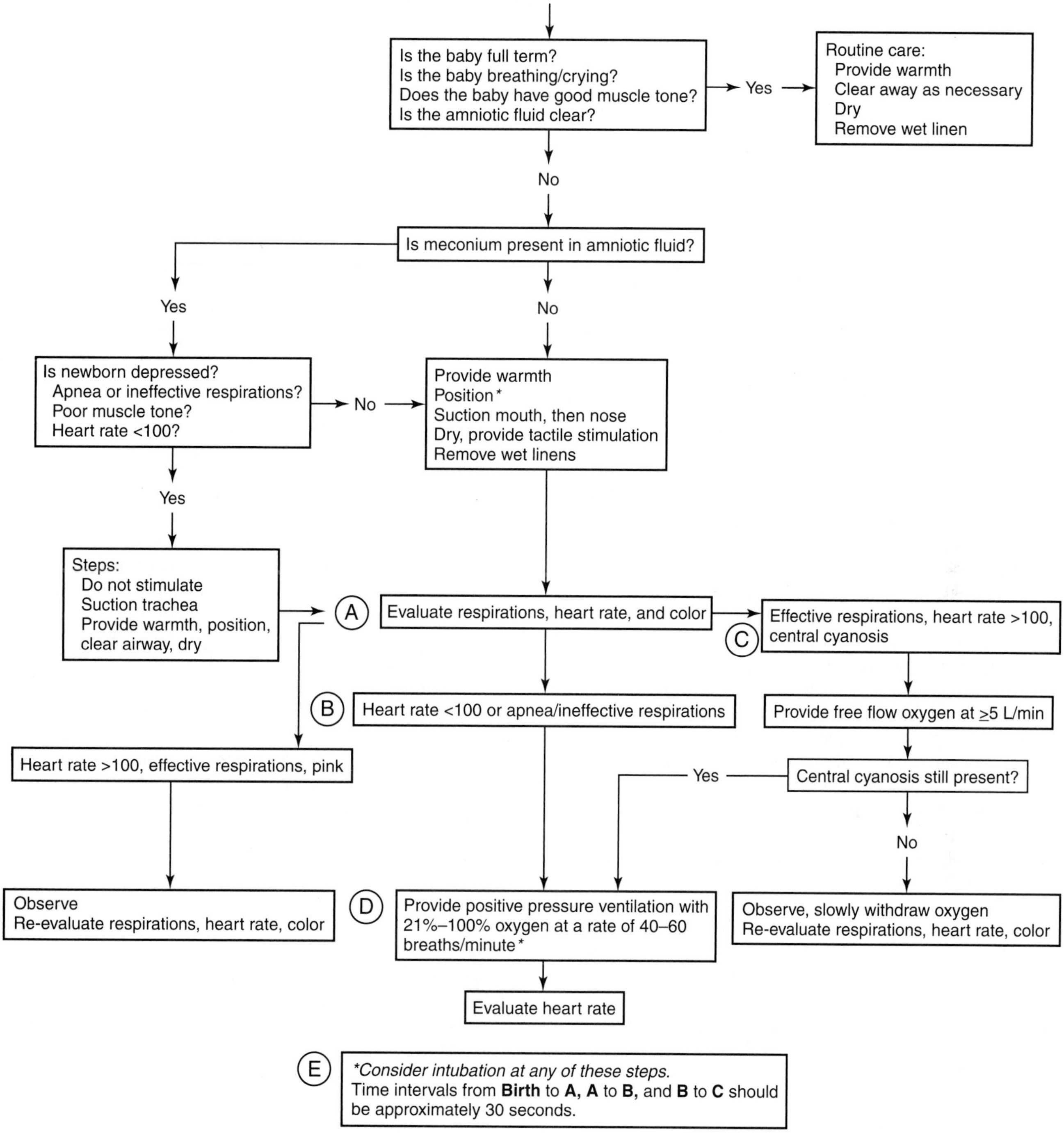
Is the baby full term?
Is the baby breathing/crying?
Does the baby have good muscle tone?
Is the amniotic fluid clear?
Yes
Routine care:
Provide warmth
Clear away as necessary
Dry
Remove wet linen
No
Is meconium present in amniotic fluid?
Yes
No
Is newborn depressed?
Apnea or ineffective respirations?
Poor muscle tone?
Heart rate <100?
No
Provide warmth
Position*
Suction mouth, then nose
Dry, provide tactile stimulation
Remove wet linens
Yes
Steps:
Do not stimulate
Suction trachea
Provide warmth, position, clear airway, dry
A
Evaluate respirations, heart rate, and color
Effective respirations, heart rate >100, central cyanosis
C
B
Heart rate <100 or apnea/ineffective respirations
Provide free flow oxygen at ≥5 L/min
Heart rate >100, effective respirations, pink
Yes
Central cyanosis still present?
No
Observe
Re-evaluate respirations, heart rate, color
D
Provide positive pressure ventilation with 21%–100% oxygen at a rate of 40–60 breaths/minute*
Observe, slowly withdraw oxygen
Re-evaluate respirations, heart rate, color
Evaluate heart rate
E
*Consider intubation at any of these steps.
Time intervals from Birth to A, A to B, and B to C should be approximately 30 seconds.

(Cont'd on p 735)

C. Assess for central cyanosis. Central cyanosis (lips, mucous membranes, trunk) indicates hypoxemia and requires the provision of free-flow, blended oxygen delivered by mask or tubing held cupped to the newborn's face at ≥5 L/min if the newborn is spontaneously breathing and has a HR greater than 100 beats/min. Positive-pressure ventilation with blended oxygen is indicated for a newborn with persistent central cyanosis despite administration of free-flow oxygen, ineffective respirations, or with a HR less than 100 beats/min.

D. Ventilation of the lungs is the most effective step in the resuscitation of a compromised newborn. Ventilation can be performed using a self-inflating bag, a flow-inflating bag, or with a T-piece device. Positive-pressure ventilation may be administered through an appropriately sized mask or ET tube attached to a resuscitation bag capable of delivering 21% to 100% oxygen and equipped with a manometer or an appropriate pressure release valve. Because fetal lungs are fluid filled, initial breaths may require higher pressures than subsequent breaths to inflate the lungs. Occasionally, this requires peak inspiratory pressures greater than 30 cm water, but care should be taken because high lung volumes and airway pressures may cause lung injury, especially in preterm newborns. The lowest inflation pressure that achieves an adequate breath should be used. Breaths should be delivered at a rate of 40 to 60 breaths/min to produce symmetric breath sounds and nonexcessive chest wall excursion. Intubation may be necessary for ineffective bag mask ventilation, prolonged positive-pressure ventilation without clinical improvement, administration of ET epinephrine, in cases of known or suspected congenital diaphragmatic hernia, in extremely preterm newborns, or for tracheal suctioning in depressed newborns with meconium-stained amniotic fluid.

E. ET tube placement should be confirmed by the presence of chest wall movement, audible breath sounds generated bilaterally, the presence of condensation within the ET tube, and the detection of exhaled carbon dioxide. In newborns with poor cardiac output, insufficient exhaled CO_2 levels may not be reliably detected with colorimetric or capnograph devices despite correct tracheal positioning of the ET tube.

F. Effectiveness of resuscitation is determined by assessing improvement in breathing, HR, color, and muscle tone. Most neonates improve with adequate lung inflation and ventilation. If ventilation is not effective, one should check that the mask seal is adequate, that the airway is not obstructed by secretions or incorrect positioning, and that adequate pressure is being provided. Uncommonly, chest compressions and epinephrine/volume administration may be necessary to improve cardiac output, to increase tissue perfusion, and to restore acid–base balance. Using the two-thumb method (preferred) or two-finger method, chest compressions (90 compressions per minute, ratio of 3:1 chest compressions to ventilation) are administered if the HR is less than 60 beats/min despite 30 seconds of positive-pressure ventilation. The chest should be compressed approximately one third of the anterior-posterior chest diameter. At 30-second intervals, the HR should be determined by counting the heartbeats in 6 seconds and then multiplying by 10 to determine beats per minute. Chest compressions can be discontinued when the HR is greater than 60 beats/min.

G. Medications are rarely indicated during neonatal resuscitation because bradycardia normally improves with appropriate ventilation using 100% oxygen. However, if the HR is less than 60 beats/min despite 30 seconds of positive-pressure ventilation and 30 seconds of positive-pressure ventilation in coordination with chest compressions (total 60 seconds), epinephrine is indicated. Epinephrine should preferably be given intravenously through a low-lying umbilical venous catheter or into the trachea through an ET tube (see Table 1) and readministered every 3 to 5 minutes if the HR remains less than 60 beats/min. If the HR remains less than 100 beats/min, consider use of a volume expander if there is evidence of acute blood loss or signs of hypovolemia.

H. Secondary medications are rarely indicated. Sodium bicarbonate may be considered in a prolonged resuscitation after other standard interventions have been unsuccessful and only after maintenance of effective ventilation. Naloxone, a narcotic antagonist, may be considered when respiratory depression is persistent after positive-pressure ventilation has restored a normal HR, acyanotic central color, and there is a history of recent (≤4 hours), nonchronic, maternal narcotic administration. Of note, the effects of naloxone may be shorter than the narcotic effects; therefore, the newborn should be monitored closely for any signs of recurrent narcotic-induced respiratory depression.

I. Newborns that require positive-pressure ventilation or more extensive resuscitation are at risk for deterioration even if they are seemingly stable after resuscitation. Postresuscitation management includes monitoring and evaluation of vital signs, oxygen saturation, acid–base balance, metabolic derangements, neurologic status, and end-organ perfusion. Ongoing ventilatory support, intravenous fluids, narcotic antagonists, buffering medications, and/or vasoactive agents are sometimes necessary. Avoidance of hyperthermia is important for newborns, especially those who may have had an episode of hypoxia and ischemia.

J. Special resuscitation considerations exist for preterm newborns. As very-low-birth-weight newborns (less than 1500 g) are at risk for hypothermia, additional warming techniques should be used to maintain normothermia, such as increasing the temperature in the delivery room and wrapping the newborn in food-grade, heat-resistant plastic and placing the newborn under a radiant heat source or on a portable warmer. Care should be taken with oxygen administration because preterm neonates are at an increased risk for oxygen-induced injury. Oxygen saturations, measured via pulse oximetry, should not be greater than 95% for prolonged periods (target saturations, 85%–95%). Preterm newborns may benefit from a continuous positive airway pressure (usually at 4–6 cm water) when they have spontaneous, but labored breathing and a HR greater than 100 beats/min. Preterm newborns are at an increased risk for brain injury. To decrease the risk for brain injury in the preterm neonate, handle gently, do not position in Trendelenburg, avoid excessive airway pressure, and do not administer rapid or hypertonic fluid infusions.

NEWBORN DELIVERY ROOM RESUSCITATION
(Cont'd from p 733)

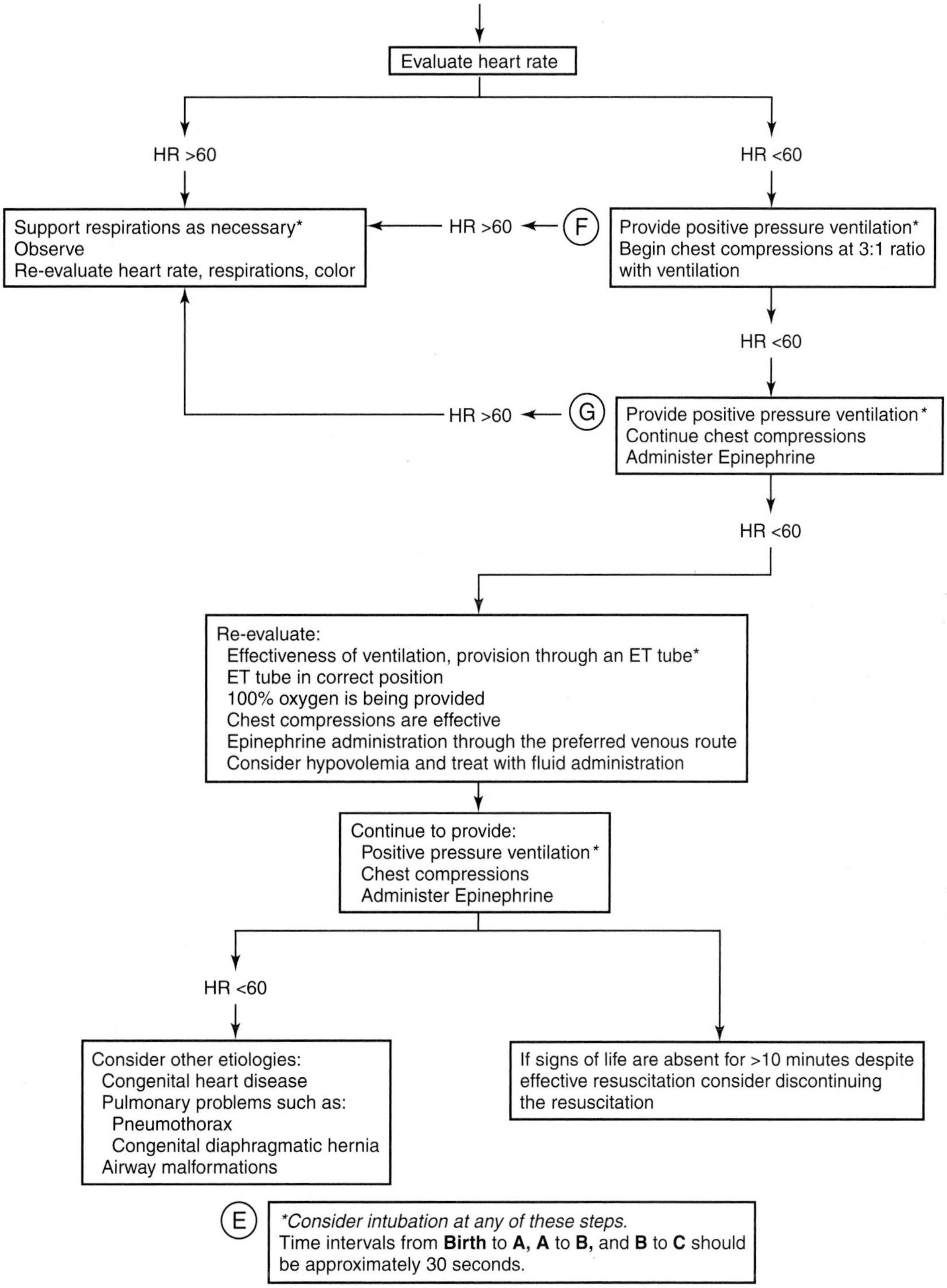
Evaluate heart rate
HR >60
HR <60
Support respirations as necessary*
Observe
Re-evaluate heart rate, respirations, color
HR >60
F
Provide positive pressure ventilation*
Begin chest compressions at 3:1 ratio with ventilation
HR <60
HR >60
G
Provide positive pressure ventilation*
Continue chest compressions
Administer Epinephrine
HR <60
Re-evaluate:
Effectiveness of ventilation, provision through an ET tube*
ET tube in correct position
100% oxygen is being provided
Chest compressions are effective
Epinephrine administration through the preferred venous route
Consider hypovolemia and treat with fluid administration
Continue to provide:
Positive pressure ventilation*
Chest compressions
Administer Epinephrine
HR <60
Consider other etiologies:
Congenital heart disease
Pulmonary problems such as:
Pneumothorax
Congenital diaphragmatic hernia
Airway malformations
If signs of life are absent for >10 minutes despite effective resuscitation consider discontinuing the resuscitation
E
*Consider intubation at any of these steps.
Time intervals from Birth to A, A to B, and B to C should be approximately 30 seconds.

K. When determined gestational age, weight, or congenital anomalies are associated with almost certain death or an unacceptably high rate of serious morbidity, noninitiation of resuscitation may be indicated. Such cases may include a confirmed gestational age of less than 23 weeks, a birth weight of less than 400 g, anencephaly, and chromosomal anomalies such as trisomy 13 and 18. Prenatal diagnosis aids in family counseling and informed decisions that may guide delivery room and intensive care unit (ICU) care. In cases of uncertain short- and long-term outcomes, parental desires for resuscitation should be supported.

L. If no signs of life are present (no HR, no respiratory effort), despite 10 minutes of continuous resuscitation, ceasing resuscitation is justified because outcomes after this period are universally poor.

Table 1. **Medications and Fluids For Neonatal Resuscitation**

Medication/Fluid	Concentration	Route	Dose	Administration	Interval
Primary					
Epinephrine	1:10,000	ET* IV (preferred)	ET: 0.3–1 ml/kg IV: 0.1–0.3 ml/kg	Give rapidly	q3–5min
Normal saline or Ringer lactate	0.9% NaCl	IV	10 ml/kg	Over 5–10 minutes	As needed
O, Rh-negative blood		IV	10 ml/kg	Over 10 minutes to 4 hours	As needed
Secondary					
Naloxone	1 mg/ml	IV (preferred) IM	0.1 mg/kg	Give rapidly	As needed
Sodium Bicarbonate	0.5 mEq/ml (4.2%)	IV	2 mEq/kg	Slowly, no faster than 1 mEq/kg/min	As needed

*Endotracheal (ET) epinephrine has unpredictable pulmonary absorption and, therefore, unreliable effect.
IM, intramuscularly; *IV,* intravenously; *SC,* subcutaneously.

References

American Heart Association and American Academy of Pediatrics. 2005 American Heart Association (AHA) guidelines for cardiopulmonary resuscitation (CPR) and emergency cardiovascular care (ECC) of pediatric and neonatal patients: neonatal resuscitation guidelines. Pediatrics 2006;117:e1029–38.

Kattwinkel J, editor. Textbook of neonatal resuscitation. 5th ed. Elk Grove Village, IL: American Academy of Pediatrics and American Heart Association; 2006.

Saugstad OD. Practical aspects of resuscitating asphyxiated newborn infants. Eur J Pediatr 1998;157:s11–6.

Wiswell T. Delivery room management of the meconium-stained newborn. J Perinatol 2008;28:s19–26.

Pulmonary Disorders

Asthma

Monica J. Federico, MD

Asthma is a chronic inflammatory disease of the airway that leads to recurrent episodes of airflow limitation, and respiratory symptoms including cough, shortness of breath and chest tightness, wheeze, and airway hyper-responsiveness that is at least partially reversible with an inhaled beta-agonist. The diagnosis can be made in any child who displays these symptoms as long as all other possible causes of recurrent airflow obstruction have been ruled out. Exacerbations of bronchospasm that lead to acute episodes of asthma are characterized by wheeze, increased work of breathing, and occasionally, hypoxemia. The cause of asthma is most likely multifactorial and may be specific to each patient. Unfortunately, there is no test to determine which children will have significant long-term morbidity and airway remodeling caused by asthma.

The basic concepts of asthma management include: (1) diagnosing asthma appropriately and determination of asthma severity and achieving control; (2) comprehensive pharmacologic therapy that includes medications to prevent and reverse underlying airway inflammation, and to relieve bronchospasm; (3) environmental measures to control factors that precipitate attacks; (4) educating the patient and family about the diagnosis and treatment of asthma; (5) fostering a partnership between the patient, family, and provider; and (6) objective measurement of lung function to assess the severity of asthma and to monitor the course of therapy.

The goals of asthma therapy are to control chronic symptoms (including nighttime symptoms), to maintain normal activity (no exercise limitation, no school absences), to prevent acute episodes (no emergency department [ED] visits or hospitalizations), to maintain normal or nearly normal pulmonary function, to maintain normal growth, to avoid adverse effects of medications, and to meet the patient's and family's expectations and satisfaction with their care.

MANAGEMENT OF AN ACUTE ASTHMA EPISODE

Acute asthma episodes have a variety of infectious, allergic, and nonspecific triggers. The respiratory pathogens most often associated with exacerbations in childhood are rhinovirus, respiratory syncytial virus, influenza virus, parainfluenza virus, and *Mycoplasma pneumoniae.* Bacterial respiratory infections such as sinusitis, otitis, and pneumonia may trigger asthma in certain individuals. Inhaled allergic triggers include cockroach, animal hair, dander, and dust. Nonspecific triggers include airway irritants (smoke, air pollution, perfumes, chemicals), weather changes, cold air, vigorous exercise, medications (salicylates), gastroesophageal reflux, and emotional stress.

A. In the patient's history, document the age of asthma diagnosis. You will need to know how many times the child has had illnesses with wheezing. Document the severity of the illnesses and how many times the child has been hospitalized, admitted to intensive care, and/or intubated for asthma or for wheezing with illnesses. Include questions about pneumonia or bronchiolitis treated with albuterol. Document the last time the child was hospitalized. Try to understand whether this is a typical episode. Ask what medications the child has been taking and how often, including daily medications. Try to understand the baseline asthma control by asking how frequently the child has cough, trouble breathing, or chest tightness when he or she is not sick. Ask what triggers symptoms or an attack. Finally, determine whether the child is atopic. In addition, work through a comprehensive differential and include questions about foreign body aspiration; pneumonia or infection indicated by fevers and chest pain; a mass or lymphadenopathy causing airway compression as indicated by weight loss, night sweats, positional trouble breathing, or poor response to bronchodilators; or a different chronic illness as indicated by chronic increased work of breathing and hypoxemia. Ask about sinusitis, headaches, bad breath, facial pain, and fever. Evaluate the family situation; note the availability of a telephone and transportation, and the family's ability to manage the child at home including their ability to fill the medications.

B. In the physical examination, take a full set of vital signs including oxygen saturation and note signs of respiratory distress, including tachypnea, retractions, dyspnea, nasal flaring, use of accessory muscles, ability to talk, wheezing, prolongation of the expiratory phase, forced expiratory phase, and decreased breath sounds. Signs of severe respiratory distress include markedly decreased or absent breath sounds, cyanosis, and increased pulsus paradoxus (exaggeration of the normal variation of cardiac output with the respiratory cycle). An altered mental status (lethargy, restlessness, disorientation, and air hunger) indicates severe hypoxia.

C. Treat acute asthma in the office or ED with oxygen to keep the oxygen saturation greater than 95%. Begin inhaled albuterol combined with ipratropium bromide either by nebulizer or metered-dose inhaler with spacer. Nebulized treatments with a mask work best for young children (albuterol dosing: 0.15 mg/kg minimum dose 2.5 mg). Older children using a metered-dose inhaler with a valved holding chamber may require 4 to 10 puffs per treatment. Nebulized treatments may also be preferable in older children who have more severe respiratory distress. Repeat inhaled treatments every 20 minutes for up to 3 treatments. For further dosing recommendations and alternative agents, please refer to the 2007 National Asthma Education and Prevention Program guidelines listed in the references.

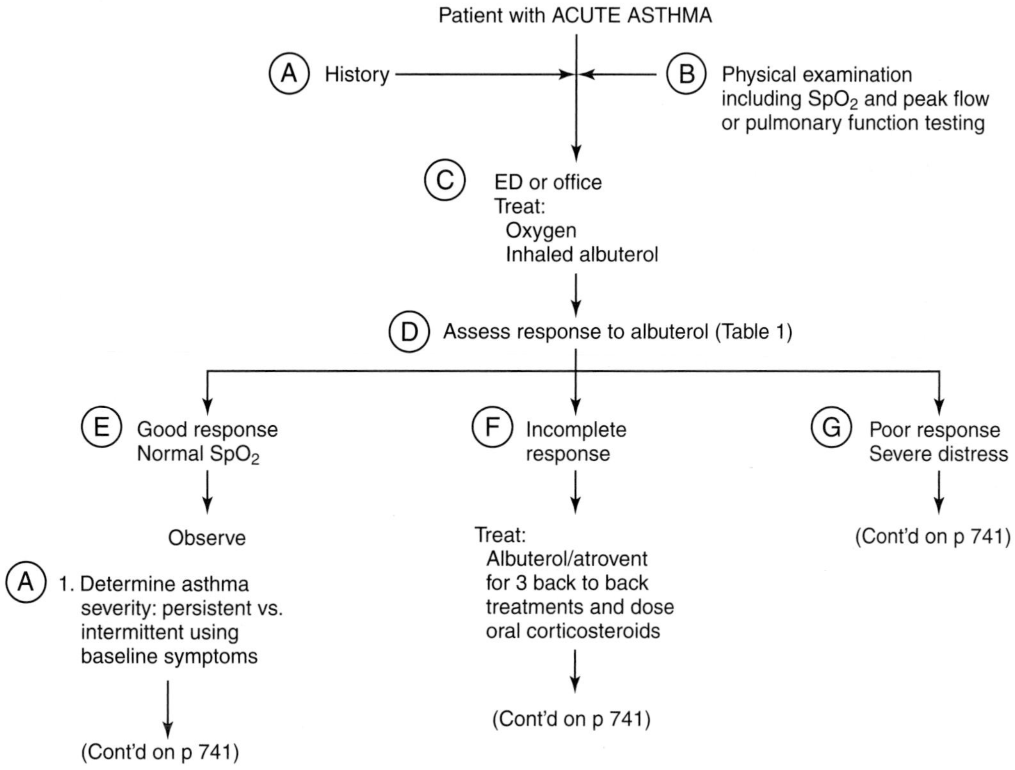
Patient with ACUTE ASTHMA
A History
B Physical examination including SpO_2 and peak flow or pulmonary function testing
C ED or office
Treat:
Oxygen
Inhaled albuterol
D Assess response to albuterol (Table 1)
E Good response
Normal SpO_2
F Incomplete response
G Poor response
Severe distress
Observe
A 1. Determine asthma severity: persistent vs. intermittent using baseline symptoms
(Cont'd on p 741)
Treat:
Albuterol/atrovent for 3 back to back treatments and dose oral corticosteroids
(Cont'd on p 741)
(Cont'd on p 741)

D. Assess the response to the initial inhaled albuterol treatment according to clinical signs of respiratory distress and oxygen saturation (Table 1).

E. If there is a good response without clinical signs of respiratory distress, observe the child for at least an hour before discharge home. Home medications should be resumed and inhaled albuterol can be administered every 3 to 4 hours if necessary. Consider a 5-day course of oral corticosteroids if this therapy was required in the past or if the initial degree of respiratory distress was significant. The recommended prednisone dose is 2 mg/kg per day with a maximum dose of 80 mg/kg/day for acute exacerbations.

F. When the response to inhaled albuterol is incomplete with signs of continued moderate respiratory distress, continue administering nebulized albuterol every 20 minutes for a total of three doses and begin corticosteroids. The recommended prednisone dose is 2 mg/kg per day with a maximum dose of 80 mg/kg/day for 5 days for an acute exacerbation. Assess the response to another hour of therapy. When there is a good response, observe the child for at least an hour before discharge home. Hospitalize patients who worsen despite therapy or who continue to have an incomplete response after 2 to 3 hours of therapy. Consider the use of adjunct therapies including continuous nebulization with a beta-agonist in patients with an incomplete response to bronchodilators before admission. Give patients admitted to the ward frequent or continuous nebulized treatments with albuterol (for dosing please refer to the 2007 guidelines). The frequency of the treatments can be decreased with improvement. Inhaled ipratropium may help. Continue a course of systemic corticosteroids given every 12 hours for 5 days. The maximum recommended dosage is 80 mg/day. The patient should be weaned to the outpatient doses of pharmacologic therapies before discharge.

G. When the response to inhaled albuterol is poor with signs of continued severe or very severe respiratory distress, administer continuous albuterol nebulizations. Consider injectable terbutaline or epinephrine if there is poor air exchange or a poor response to inhaled agents. These injected medications tend to produce more adverse effects (tachycardia, headache, tremor) than inhaled agents. Other therapies to consider in a child with impending respiratory failure include intravenous magnesium given over 30 minutes (see the 2007 guidelines for dosing). Some small studies indicate that heliox may be helpful with the hypoxemia. Noninvasive ventilation may also help prevent intubation.

H. Regarding asthma education, provide written instructions including a plan for daily medications and for escalation of care in the setting of worsening distress or symptoms (asthma action plan), and arrange a follow-up plan to include a telephone contact in 24 to 48 hours and a revisit in 1 week with the primary care provider. A known asthmatic patient can usually resume previous asthma medications in addition to the oral corticosteroid. Begin maintenance anti-inflammatory therapy if the patient has had two or more ED or office visits for acute attacks in the previous 6 months or three or more in the previous year, or if the history is consistent with persistent asthma (see Chronic Asthma Management section later in this chapter). Finally, notify the primary care physician treating the asthma of the visit and any changes in therapy.

I. Consider a chest radiograph if the examination is asymmetrical or the response to bronchodilators is incomplete. Obtain an arterial blood gas (ABG) analysis when the response is poor. Assess the severity of respiratory distress by clinical criteria, ABGs, pulse oximetry, and peak expiratory flow rate (Table 4). If the PCO_2 is greater 40 mm Hg and there is poor air exchange, very severe distress, or low oxygen saturation despite oxygen therapy, admit to the pediatric intensive care unit. If the PCO_2 is no more than 35 mm Hg and there is good air exchange, admit to the ward. Be cautious, because a PCO_2 of 35 to 50 mm Hg may indicate impending respiratory failure. Patients with a PCO_2 greater 50 mm Hg are at high risk for respiratory failure requiring mechanical ventilation.

J. Other comorbid illnesses including viral illnesses, pneumonia, sinusitis, otitis media, gastroesophageal reflux disease, and allergies or eczema.

(Continued on page 742)

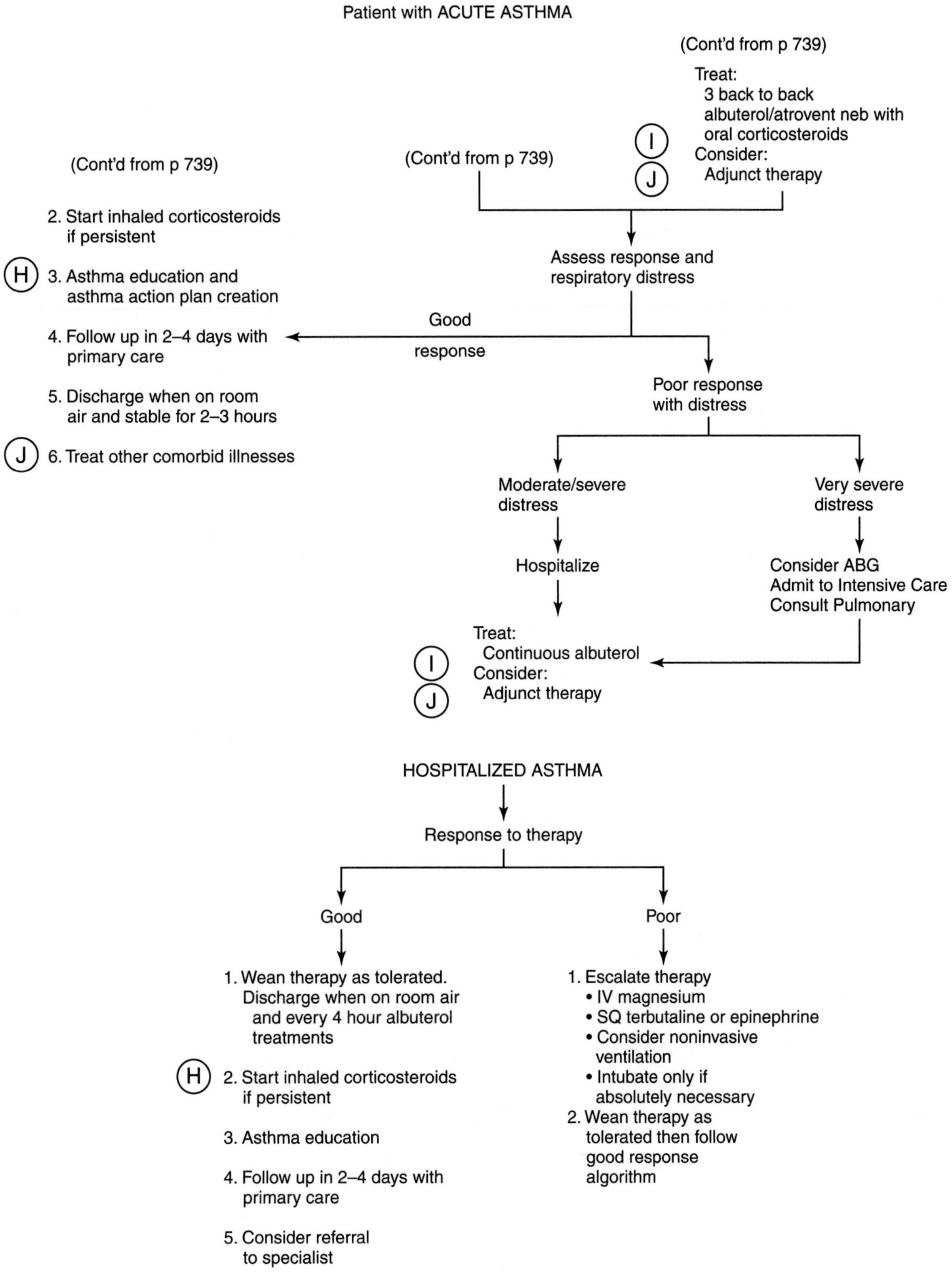
Patient with ACUTE ASTHMA
(Cont'd from p 739)
Treat:
3 back to back
albuterol/atrovent neb with
oral corticosteroids
Consider:
Adjunct therapy
I
J
(Cont'd from p 739)
(Cont'd from p 739)
2. Start inhaled corticosteroids
if persistent
H
3. Asthma education and
asthma action plan creation
4. Follow up in 2–4 days with
primary care
5. Discharge when on room
air and stable for 2–3 hours
J
6. Treat other comorbid illnesses
Assess response and
respiratory distress
Good
response
Poor response
with distress
Moderate/severe
distress
Very severe
distress
Hospitalize
Consider ABG
Admit to Intensive Care
Consult Pulmonary
Treat:
Continuous albuterol
Consider:
Adjunct therapy
I
J
HOSPITALIZED ASTHMA
Response to therapy
Good
Poor
1. Wean therapy as tolerated.
Discharge when on room air
and every 4 hour albuterol
treatments
H
2. Start inhaled corticosteroids
if persistent
3. Asthma education
4. Follow up in 2–4 days with
primary care
5. Consider referral
to specialist
1. Escalate therapy
• IV magnesium
• SQ terbutaline or epinephrine
• Consider noninvasive
ventilation
• Intubate only if
absolutely necessary
2. Wean therapy as
tolerated then follow
good response
algorithm

MANAGEMENT OF CHRONIC ASTHMA

Once the diagnosis of asthma has been made, asthma severity should be determined. A child who has daytime symptoms two or more times a week, or nighttime symptoms two or more times a month, or uses albuterol two or more times a week, or any exercise limitation, or has abnormal lung function testing showing airway obstruction, or asthma exacerbations requiring systemic corticosteroids two or more times in a year has persistent asthma. If he or she has fewer symptoms, then the severity is classified as intermittent asthma. Children with persistent asthma need to be on a daily medication to control airway inflammation. Severity should be determined when the child is not on a daily controller medication such as inhaled corticosteroids or a leukotriene receptor antagonist. The specific criteria for asthma severity for children ages 0–4, 5–11, and older than 12 years can be found in the 2007 National Asthma Education and Prevention Program Guidelines (see references at the end of the chapter). The management of chronic asthma is as follows:

A. When taking the history, document the age at diagnosis. Ask about the frequency and severity of symptoms such as cough, wheeze, chest tightness, exercise limitation, or shortness of breath. Determine the number of total exacerbations and how many the child has had in the last year that required systemic corticosteroids. The provider also needs to determine the history of hospitalizations and ED visits. Document any admissions to the intensive care unit and intubations. Determine what triggers an attack and whether the child has an allergy symptoms or a history of eczema. Ask medicine he or she is taking, the dose, how often, and what route (inhaler, home nebulizer, oral)? Ask about comorbid illnesses such as allergies, sinusitis, and gastroesophageal reflux disease. Evaluate the family situation; note the availability of a telephone and transportation, and the family's ability to manage the child at home.

B. In the physical examination, note signs of respiratory distress, including tachypnea, retractions, dyspnea, nasal flaring, use of accessory muscles, inability to talk, wheezing, prolongation of the expiratory phase, forced expiratory phase, and decreased breath sounds. Signs of severe respiratory distress include markedly decreased or absent breath sounds, cyanosis, and increased pulsus paradoxus (exaggeration of the normal variation of cardiac output with the respiratory cycle).

C. Educate the family and child (to the extent appropriate) about prevention, environmental controls with an emphasis on avoidance of allergens and other triggers (e.g., smoke, air pollution, chemicals), minimizing exposure to respiratory viruses, use of influenza vaccine, and allergy therapy when appropriate. Review the medications and how to use the medication delivery device. When the child with moderate or severe asthma is old enough to be taught the correct technique of doing accurate peak flow measurements, use peak flows to guide treatment. Develop with the family a plan for the home management of acute asthma episodes (asthma action plan). The plan should include information about how to evaluate and treat these episodes, as well as when to call for telephone advice and come to the ED. Provide written guidelines for administering treatments. For example, 4 puffs of albuterol may be repeated every 20 minutes for up to 1 hour. If there is a good response, continue with the beta-agonist every 3 to 4 hours and resume the usual medications. When the response remains incomplete after the three doses of albuterol or worsens at any time, call to have the child seen at either the office or the ED. It may be advisable to begin an oral steroid (prednisone, 1–2 mg/kg with a maximum dose of 60 mg per day for the treatment of outpatient exacerbations) at this point.

D. The approach to the management of asthma can be classified into three phases: achieving control, ongoing maintenance, and quick relief.

1. The goals of achieving control are to reduce signs and symptoms of the chronic disease so that the child can sleep through the night, stay in school, and be as active as he or she wants to be. When a child is on the appropriate therapy, and well controlled, he or she should have symptoms consistent with intermittent asthma. The first choice for a controller medication in all patients with asthma is a low-dose inhaled corticosteroid. Controller medication dosing increases according to symptoms as shown in Figure 1.

   Response to the medication should be reassessed within 4 to 6 weeks. After evaluating for compliance with the medication and environmental triggers, medications doses can be stepped up to achieve control. Ongoing pharmacologic management of persistent asthma uses a stepwise approach to incrementally change the potency of anti-inflammatory agents or to add complementary agents to control symptoms and restore functional and physiologic outcomes. If the child requires doses greater than medium dose to control her asthma, then the provider should consider referring the child to a specialist. Consider referral to an asthma specialist (pediatric allergist or pulmonologist) for the following reasons: concern about another diagnosis because of atypical signs or symptoms; inadequate response to therapy resulting in repeated steroid bursts, repeated ED visits, or repeated hospitalizations; life-threatening episodes; mechanical ventilation; or desire to improve education of the patient and family.
2. Ongoing maintenance: Once the child's asthma is well controlled, the child should be seen every 3 to 6 months. Lung function should be re-evaluated at least every year or with any clinical changes.
3. Quick relief should be used to control an acute increase in symptoms. See the algorithm for the management of an acute asthma episode for further direction.

(Continued on page 745)

Patient with CHRONIC ASTHMA

↓

Diagnose asthma in any child with recurrent symptoms of airway obstruction (e.g., cough, wheeze, shortness of breath) that is at least partially reversible with a bronchodilator **and** other possible etiologies have been ruled out.

(A) History →

(B) Physical examination →

↓

Determine asthma severity
Intermittent vs. Persistent
Persistent Asthma Criteria:

1. Daytime symptoms more than 2 days per week
OR
2. Awakening at night from asthma more than two nights per month
OR
3. Albuterol use more than 2 days a week **OR**
4. Any limitation of activities, despite pretreatment for exercise induced asthma **OR**
5. More than two steroid bursts in one year **OR**
6. FEV1 <80% predicted **OR** FEV1/FVC below 0.85 in children under 18 years (for older children, please refer to http://www.healthteamworks.org/guidelines/asthma.html.)

Intermittent asthma

↓

(C) Asthma education

and

Therapy: inhaled beta-agonist as needed

↓

(D) Follow regularly to evaluate for asthma control

Persistent asthma

↓

(C) Asthma education

and

(D) Therapy: Controller medication per Figure 1 and inhaled beta-agonist as needed

↓

(D) Follow regularly to evaluate asthma control

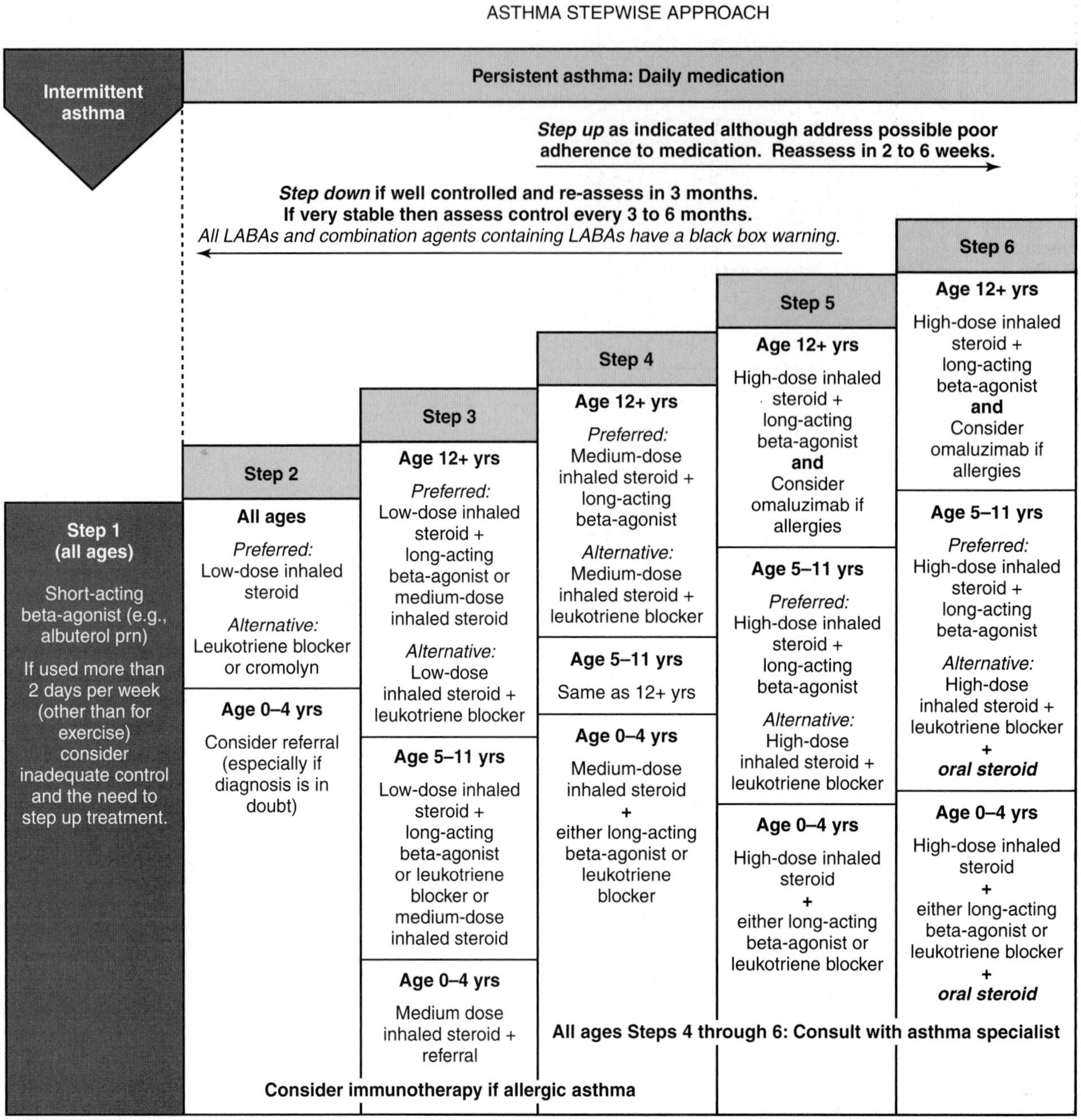
ASTHMA STEPWISE APPROACH
Intermittent asthma
Persistent asthma: Daily medication
Step up as indicated although address possible poor adherence to medication. Reassess in 2 to 6 weeks.
Step down if well controlled and re-assess in 3 months.
If very stable then assess control every 3 to 6 months.
All LABAs and combination agents containing LABAs have a black box warning.
Step 1 (all ages)
Short-acting beta-agonist (e.g., albuterol prn)
If used more than 2 days per week (other than for exercise) consider inadequate control and the need to step up treatment.
Step 2
All ages
Preferred: Low-dose inhaled steroid
Alternative: Leukotriene blocker or cromolyn
Age 0–4 yrs
Consider referral (especially if diagnosis is in doubt)
Step 3
Age 12+ yrs
Preferred: Low-dose inhaled steroid + long-acting beta-agonist or medium-dose inhaled steroid
Alternative: Low-dose inhaled steroid + leukotriene blocker
Age 5–11 yrs
Low-dose inhaled steroid + long-acting beta-agonist or or leukotriene blocker or medium-dose inhaled steroid
Age 0–4 yrs
Medium dose inhaled steroid + referral
Step 4
Age 12+ yrs
Preferred: Medium-dose inhaled steroid + long-acting beta-agonist
Alternative: Medium-dose inhaled steroid + leukotriene blocker
Age 5–11 yrs
Same as 12+ yrs
Age 0–4 yrs
Medium-dose inhaled steroid + either long-acting beta-agonist or leukotriene blocker
Step 5
Age 12+ yrs
High-dose inhaled steroid + long-acting beta-agonist **and** Consider omaluzimab if allergies
Age 5–11 yrs
Preferred: High-dose inhaled steroid + long-acting beta-agonist
Alternative: High-dose inhaled steroid + leukotriene blocker
Age 0–4 yrs
High-dose inhaled steroid + either long-acting beta-agonist or leukotriene blocker
Step 6
Age 12+ yrs
High-dose inhaled steroid + long-acting beta-agonist **and** Consider omaluzimab if allergies
Age 5–11 yrs
Preferred: High-dose inhaled steroid + long-acting beta-agonist
Alternative: High-dose inhaled steroid + leukotriene blocker + ***oral steroid***
Age 0–4 yrs
High-dose inhaled steroid + either long-acting beta-agonist or leukotriene blocker + ***oral steroid***
All ages Steps 4 through 6: Consult with asthma specialist
Consider immunotherapy if allergic asthma

Figure 1. Asthma stepwise approach. This guideline is designed to assist the clinician in the management of asthma. This guideline is not intended to replace the clinician's judgment or establish a protocol for all patients with a particular condition. *Adapted from the National Asthma Education and Prevention Program 3* for the Colorado Clinical Guidelines Collaborative, which is now Health Team Works: http://www.healthteamworks.org/guidelines/asthma.html.

Table 1. **Response to Therapy**

Good Response	Incomplete Response	Poor Response
No wheezing, good air wheezing, exchange	Mild-to-moderate wheezing, good air exchange	Severe poor air exchange
No accessory muscle use	Moderate accessory muscle use	Severe accessory muscle
Minimal or no dyspnea	Moderate dyspnea	Severe dyspnea
Decreased HR and RR	Increased HR and RR	Increased HR and RR
Pulsus paradoxus <10 mm Hg	Pulsus paradoxus 10–15 mm Hg	Pulsus paradoxus >15 mm Hg
PEFR >70% baseline	PEFR 40%–70% baseline	PEFR <40% baseline
Oxygen saturation >95%	Oxygen saturation 90%–95%	Oxygen saturation <90%

HR, heart rate; *PEFR*, peak expiratory flow rate; *RR*, respiratory rate.

References

Beers SL, Abramo TJ, Bracken A, Wiebe RA. Bilevel positive airway pressure in the treatment of status asthmaticus in pediatrics. Am J Emerg Med 2007;25(1):6–9.

Bisgaard H. Use of inhaled corticosteroids in pediatric asthma. Pediatr Pulmonol 1997;15:27–33.

Ciarallo L, Brousseau D, Reinert S. Higher-dose intravenous magnesium therapy for children with moderate to severe acute asthma. Arch Pediatr Adolesc Med 2000;154:979–83.

Cockcroft DW. Therapy for airway inflammation in asthma. J Allergy Clin Immunol 1991;87:914–9.

Drazen JM, Israel E, O'Byrne PM. Treatment of asthma with drugs modifying the leukotriene pathway. N Engl J Med 1999;340:197–206.

Gelfand EW. Pediatric asthma: a different disease. Proc Am Thorac Soc 2009;6(3):278–82.

Guidelines for the Diagnosis and Management of Asthma. National Asthma Education Program, Expert Panel Report 3. Bethesda, MD: U.S. Department of Health and Human Services, Public Health Service, National Institutes of Health, National Heart, Lung, and Blood Institute; 2007.

Larsen GL. Asthma in children. N Engl J Med 1992;326:1540–5.

Lofdahl CG, Reiss TF, Leff JA, et al. Randomised, placebo controlled trial of effect of a leukotriene receptor antagonist, montelukast, on tapering inhaled corticosteroids in asthmatic patients. BMJ 1999;319:87–90.

Panettieri RA Jr, Covar R, Grant E, et al. Natural history of asthma: persistence versus progression-does the beginning predict the end? J Allergy Clin Immunol 2008;121(3):607–13.

Patterson R. Goals in the management of asthma. Chest 1992;101:403S-4.

Provisional Committee on Quality Improvement. Practice parameter: the office management of acute exacerbations of asthma in children. Pediatrics 1994;93:119–26.

Robinson PD, Van Asperen P. Asthma in childhood. Pediatr Clin North Am 2009;56:191–226.

Szefler SJ. Early intervention for childhood asthma: inhaled glucocorticoids as the "preferred" medication. J Allergy Clin Immunol 1998;102:719–21.

Bronchiolitis

Lalit Bajaj, MD, MPH

Bronchiolitis is a clinical syndrome of infants and young children characterized by wheezing, retractions, and tachypnea. Inflammation of the bronchioles or small airways produces exudate, edema, necrosis, and bronchospasm, which results in air trapping, atelectasis, and ventilation-perfusion mismatch. The most common infectious agent causing bronchiolitis is respiratory syncytial virus. Other pathogens include human metapneumovirus, parainfluenza virus, influenza virus, rhinovirus, adenovirus, bocavirus, and *Mycoplasma pneumoniae*.

A. In the patient's history, ask when the cold and cough began. Is there fast breathing? Is it difficult for your child to breathe? Does the chest move in (chest indrawing) when your child breathes? Has your child stopped breathing or turned blue? Is your child too weak to eat or play? Has your child been vomiting? Has your child wheezed at other times? Does your child have asthma or heart or lung disease? Was your child born prematurely? Ask about access to a telephone and transportation.

B. In the physical examination, look and listen. Count the respirations for 1 minute. In patients with bronchiolitis, the respiratory rate correlates well with oxygenation. Respiratory rates greater than 70 per minute are concerning for poor oxygenation and ventilation. Risk for respiratory failure is also greater at rates more than 70 per minute. Look for retractions, cyanosis, pallor, and nasal flaring. Listen for grunting, wheezing, hoarseness, stridor, prolonged expiratory phase (the normal inspiration-to-expiration ratio is 1:2), poor air exchange, and rales (may be caused by atelectasis or pneumonia). Note signs of cardiac disease. Note signs of dehydration. With use of a pneumatic otoscope, note tympanic membrane color, landmarks, and mobility.

C. Pulse oximetry is a noninvasive technique to determine oxygen saturation. Patients with signs of moderate-to-severe respiratory distress should be studied (Table 1). Infants should be monitored before, during, and after feedings. Oxygen saturation less than 90% at sea level or 88% at 5000 feet indicates a need for supplemental oxygen therapy. Continuous pulse oximetry is not recommended for stable patients older than 3 months because small changes in oxygen saturation do not have clinical relevance but may result in frequent oxygen supplementation changes.

D. Obtain chest films in patients with severe disease to identify pneumonia or atelectasis. Patients with mild-to-moderate disease and who fit the diagnosis of bronchiolitis do not require chest radiograph (CXR). The radiologic findings of bronchiolitis include hyperexpansion with flattened diaphragm, peribronchial thickening, and patchy atelectasis with or without perihilar infiltrate. Lobar pneumonia on radiography may indicate a mixed viral-bacterial infection, although CXR has not been shown to be a reliable test to distinguish viral from bacterial disease.

E. There is no clinical value in obtaining specimens for identifying viral pathogens in children without severe respiratory distress or in those not at high risk because of an underlying condition. In severe disease, identification of respiratory syncytial virus may influence treatment decisions. Rapid viral diagnostic techniques are available. These include immunofluorescent staining and enzyme-linked immunosorbent assay (ELISA). These are performed with use of nasopharyngeal secretions that can be obtained by aspiration with either a DeLee tube or a small feeding tube attached to a syringe.

F. The many noninfectious causes of airway obstruction and wheezing include asthma, foreign body aspiration, tracheoesophageal fistula, neuromuscular disorders, gastroesophageal reflux, structural airway defects (tracheobronchomalacia, tracheal or bronchial stenosis), and extrinsic compression of the airway such as by vascular rings and slings, and malformation of the lungs (sequestrations, bronchogenic cysts, and teratomas). Children with chronic lung diseases, such as cystic fibrosis, bronchopulmonary dysplasia, and bronchiectasis, may have wheezing without infection.

G. Home measures include encouraging the child to drink liquids and to eat normally. Educate parents to return if their child develops fast breathing, chest indrawing (retractions), blue color (cyanosis), or fever, or becomes too weak to eat or drink.

H. Data assessing the effectiveness of albuterol and other β_2-agonists in treatment of bronchiolitis are conflicting, and there has not been any consistent inpatient or outpatient benefit shown. Less than half of children with viral bronchiolitis seem to respond to this therapy. Some patients clearly do worse (more tachypnea, hypoxia), so patients with mild-to-moderate bronchiolitis should not routinely be given albuterol. Some studies show racemic epinephrine to be more effective than albuterol in bronchiolitis. It is important to assess each child individually for signs of improvement, such as decreased wheezing, decreased retractions, better air exchange, decrease in respiratory rate, increased oxygen saturation, and a more comfortable appearance. There are little data to support the use of nebulized bronchodilators past the initial phase of treatment (i.e., one to two doses). Corticosteroids have not been shown to be effective. Mist tents provide no benefit and impede interaction with and evaluation of the patient. Do not routinely administer antibiotics to children with bronchiolitis.

I. Apnea may be a presenting sign of bronchiolitis. It usually occurs early in the course of the infection. Infants younger than 3 months who were born prematurely are at the greatest risk. The mechanism of the apnea is

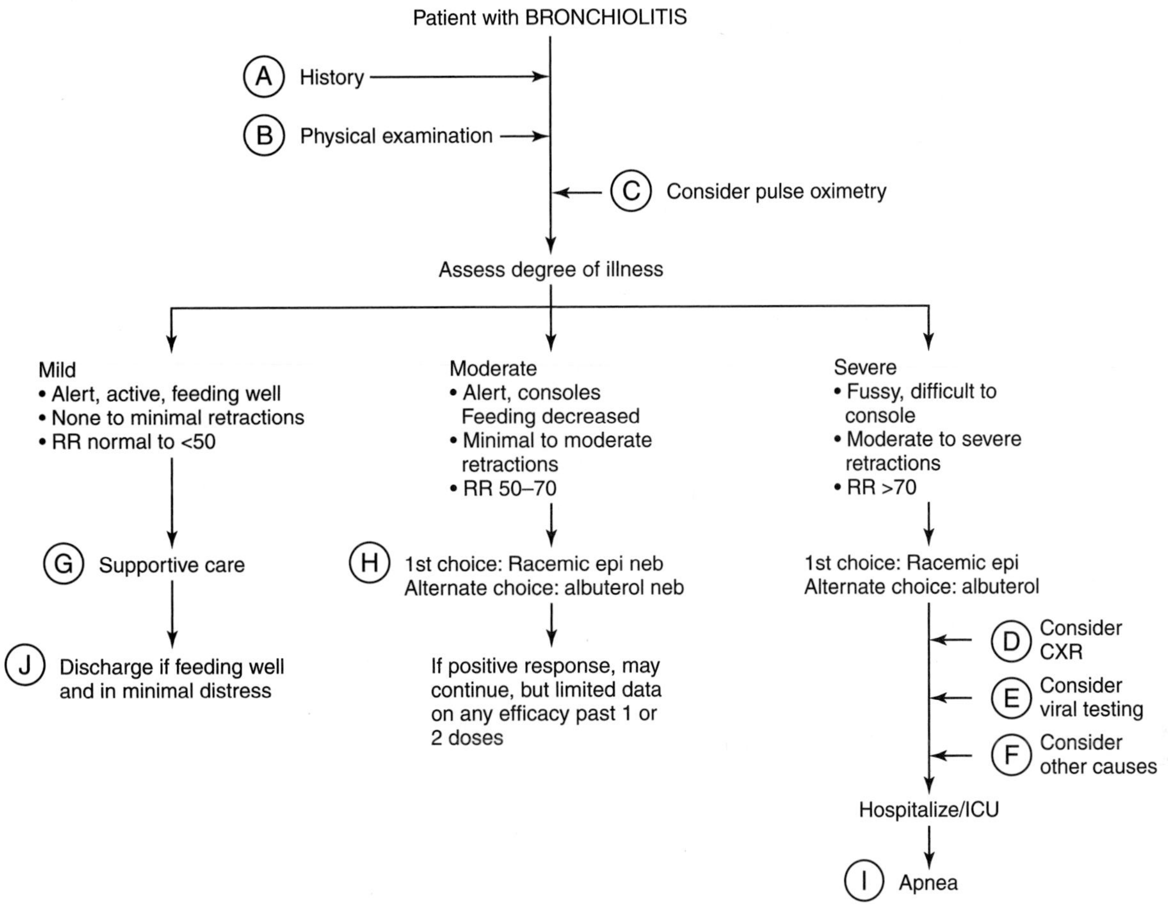

Patient with BRONCHIOLITIS
A History
B Physical examination
C Consider pulse oximetry
Assess degree of illness
Mild
• Alert, active, feeding well
• None to minimal retractions
• RR normal to <50
Moderate
• Alert, consoles
Feeding decreased
• Minimal to moderate retractions
• RR 50–70
Severe
• Fussy, difficult to console
• Moderate to severe retractions
• RR >70
G Supportive care
H 1st choice: Racemic epi neb
Alternate choice: albuterol neb
1st choice: Racemic epi
Alternate choice: albuterol
J Discharge if feeding well and in minimal distress
If positive response, may continue, but limited data on any efficacy past 1 or 2 doses
D Consider CXR
E Consider viral testing
F Consider other causes
Hospitalize/ICU
I Apnea

unclear, although it appears to correlate with the degree of hypoxia in some infants. The presence of secretions triggering a laryngeal chemoreflex has been hypothesized as a cause. In other infants, it appears before other clinical symptoms or signs of disease. Recurrent or prolonged apnea may occur without obvious signs of respiratory distress but still require intubation and assisted ventilation for 24 to 48 hours.

J. Children may be discharged from the hospital when respiratory distress has resolved. Consider discharge with home oxygen when oxygen saturations remain low but the patient is afebrile, eating well, and appropriately active. A follow-up visit should be scheduled 24 to 48 hours after discharge. Parents should be taught to call the physician immediately if signs of respiratory distress (fast breathing or chest indrawing) return.

Table 1. **Degree of Illness in Bronchiolitis**

Mild	Moderate	Severe	Very Severe
Respiratory rate below thresholds (60 <2 months: 50, 2–12 months; 40, >12 months) *and* Good air exchange *and* Minimal or no retractions *and* No signs of dehydration	Respiratory rate elevated above thresholds *or* Moderate retractions *or* Prolonged expiratory phase with decreased air exchange	High-risk patients* *or* Respiratory rate >70/min *or* Marked retractions *or* Minimal (poor) air exchange *or* Grunting respirations *or* Oxygen saturation <94% at sea level or <90% at 5000 feet *or* Signs of dehydration or systemic toxicity	Apnea or respiratory arrest *or* Cyanosis with oxygen *or* Inability to maintain Pa_{O_2} >50 mm Hg with Fi_{O_2} >80% *or* Inability to maintain P_{CO_2} <55 mm Hg *or* Signs of shock

*High-risk patients are premature infants younger than 12 weeks (postnatal) and children with congenital heart disease, bronchopulmonary dysplasia, other chronic lung disease, neuromuscular condition, or immunodeficiency disorder.

References

American Academy of Pediatrics Subcommittee on Diagnosis and Management of Bronchiolitis. Diagnosis and management of bronchiolitis. Pediatrics 2006;118(4):1774–93.

Zorc J, Breese-Hall C. Bronchiolitis: recent evidence of diagnosis and management. Pediatrics 2010;125(2):342–9.

Bronchopulmonary Dysplasia in the Premature Infant

Christopher D. Baker, MD, and Vivek Balasubramaniam, MD

Bronchopulmonary dysplasia (BPD) in preterm infants was first described in 1967 in infants with severe respiratory distress at birth requiring mechanical ventilation and high inspiratory oxygen levels. Now BPD is defined as a need for supplemental oxygen with signs of respiratory distress and an abnormal chest radiograph at 28 days of life or 36 weeks of postconceptional age. Associated symptoms are signs of respiratory insufficiency, including tachypnea, increased work of breathing, cough, audible wheeze, rhonchi, rales, expiratory grunting, and increased anterior-posterior diameter of the chest. The incidence rate of this complication is about 30% in infants who weighed 1000 g or less at birth. The cause of BPD is multifactorial. Prenatal factors include chorioamnionitis, fetal infections, smoking, drug use, as well as genetic factors that are not fully understood. In the immediate postnatal period, trauma from mechanical ventilation, hyperoxia, infection, and airway inflammation contribute to the development of BPD. Together, these factors cumulate in impaired lung alveolar and vascular growth, which leads to decreased lung function later in life.

A. Perform a complete physical assessment of respiratory status before initial hospital discharge and at each clinic visit. Note respiratory rate, presence of suprasternal and intercostal retractions, character of lung auscultation, and presence of expiratory grunting.

B. Before hospital discharge, obtain a baseline chest radiograph and screen for hypoventilation by blood gas assessment. Assess baseline oxygen saturation in room air and with required supplemental oxygen.

C. Assess the degree of illness to differentiate between mild, moderate, and severe BPD on the basis of clinical criteria in Table 1. Significant respiratory distress, persistent hypoxemia, or retention of carbon dioxide suggest poorly compensated or chronic respiratory failure. The infant may benefit from mechanical ventilation via tracheostomy until they recover from BPD. This decision should be made in consultation with a pediatric pulmonologist.

D. Outpatient management of the infant with BPD begins with the planning of the nursery discharge. This should begin well in advance of the intended day of release to allow time for teaching and arrangement of necessary equipment and services. Selection of a primary care provider and consultation with a pediatric pulmonologist are strongly recommended before hospital discharge. Infants who cannot maintain consistent oxygen saturations of 92% or greater while they are awake, feeding, and sleeping will require continuous supplemental oxygen by nasal cannula. Decisions about home cardiorespiratory monitoring depend on the presence of apnea and bradycardia spells and the degree of oxygen desaturation in room air. Infants who continue to exhibit spontaneously resolving episodes of bradycardia are safe for hospital discharge but should be released on a cardiorespiratory monitor. Before prescribing supplemental oxygen at home, the physician should make sure that the child remains stable on room air without apnea, bradycardia, or marked desaturation (<85%).

E. Primary care services for these patients cannot be separated from specifics of management related to their prematurity and BPD. Well-child visits should initially take place every 2 weeks after hospital discharge to assess nutritional progress and growth, assess respiratory status, review development, discuss family dynamics in caring for a child with chronic disease, and coordinate services and subspecialty visits. Both growth and development should be "corrected" for prematurity until 2 years of age. When the child is sufficiently stable, visits can be monthly and eventually spaced out to the frequency of regular well-child visits suggested by the American Academy of Pediatrics. Nutrition is a critical concern for these infants. Infants with BPD have increased calorie demands proportional to the severity of underlying lung disease. In addition, in some infants, a diminished intake because of fatigue, oral motor incoordination, or nipple aversion may also complicate matters. Breast-fed infants may require continued use of pumped milk fortified to 24 calories per ounce. Formula-fed babies should take at a minimum 22-calorie preterm transitional formulas, such as EnfaCare and NeoSure. These can be mixed to 24 calories per ounce, if additional calories are needed. Infants may be sensitive to large fluid loads and require restricted intake of higher caloric density feeds. Ensure an adequate intake (usually 110–130 calories/kg/day) to allow growth along a consistent percentile as the minimum acceptable rate of growth. At 1 year of age, consider nutritional supplements such as PediaSure. Growth can also be impaired by inadequate oxygenation (see section F) and gastroesophageal reflux. Gastroesophageal reflux, if present, should be aggressively managed with positioning and reduction of acid production, at a minimum, with ranitidine, 2 to 3 mg/kg PO twice a day, or omeprazole, 1 mg/kg once or twice a day. Infants who remain symptomatic during acid blockade should undergo formal swallow evaluation. In addition, the practitioner should consider the efficacy of gastrostomy tube placement with Nissen fundoplication. Reflux and silent aspiration may contribute to prolonged respiratory difficulties and impair recovery from neonatal lung injury.

F. There is no urgency to wean an infant with BPD from supplemental oxygen. Respiratory symptoms will be lessened and growth enhanced with oxygen. Oxygen

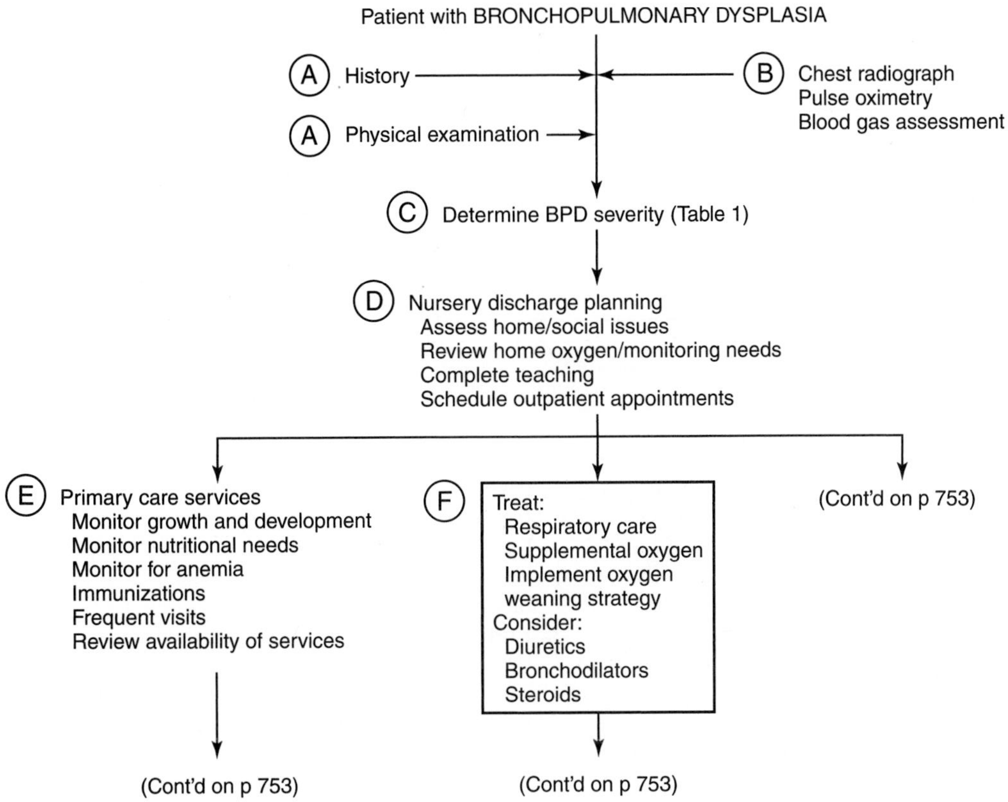
Patient with BRONCHOPULMONARY DYSPLASIA
(A) History
(A) Physical examination
(B) Chest radiograph
Pulse oximetry
Blood gas assessment
(C) Determine BPD severity (Table 1)
(D) Nursery discharge planning
Assess home/social issues
Review home oxygen/monitoring needs
Complete teaching
Schedule outpatient appointments
(E) Primary care services
Monitor growth and development
Monitor nutritional needs
Monitor for anemia
Immunizations
Frequent visits
Review availability of services
(F) Treat:
Respiratory care
Supplemental oxygen
Implement oxygen
weaning strategy
Consider:
Diuretics
Bronchodilators
Steroids
(Cont'd on p 753)
(Cont'd on p 753)
(Cont'd on p 753)

saturations should be kept greater than 92%. If saturations are 98% or greater on the usual oxygen flow rate, the amount of cannula flow can be slowly decreased. Wean oxygen gradually over a period of several weeks by increasing the time off while the child is awake. Discontinue supplemental oxygen during sleep only after a nighttime oximetry study in room air demonstrates oxygen saturations greater 92% for more than 90% of the time. During the weaning phase, parents should closely monitor the child's color, respiratory rate, work of breathing, and quality of feeding. They should watch for increased fatigue and irritability. Office visits should be frequent during oxygen weaning to assess weight gain and to evaluate for the symptoms described. Stop cardiorespiratory monitors when there are no further apnea or bradycardia spells. Infants with more severe disease may require diuretic therapy for accumulated lung water. The drug of choice is hydrochlorothiazide at 1 to 2 mg/kg once or twice a day. Furosemide at 1 to 2 mg/kg per dose can also be used, but it causes calcium wasting in the urine and increases the risk for osteopenia and nephrocalcinosis. Assess serum electrolytes periodically in infants receiving diuretics. Care should be taken to balance the goal of diuretic therapy with adequate weight gain. Consider the use of other medications, such as inhaled steroids (fluticasone, 44 mg/puff, or beclomethasone, 42 mg/puff, usually 2 puffs twice a day), systemic prednisone (1 mg/kg daily or every other day), and inhaled bronchodilators such as albuterol (1.25–2.5 mg by nebulizer or 2 puffs two to three times a day by HFA metered-dose inhaler) or ipratropium bromide (250–500 mg). Infants requiring diuretic or steroid therapy should be followed by a specialist in pediatric pulmonology.

Table 1. **Definition of Bronchopulmonary Dysplasia: Diagnostic Criteria**

Gestational Age	<32 wk	≥32 wk
Time point of assessment	36 weeks PMA or discharge to home, whichever comes first	>28 days but <56 days postnatal age or discharge to home, whichever comes first
	Treatment with oxygen >21% for at least 28 d plus	
Mild BPD	Breathing room air at 36 wk PMA or discharge, whichever comes first	Need* for <30% oxygen at 56 days postnatal age or discharge, whichever comes first
Severe BPD	Need* for >30% oxygen and/or positive pressure (PPV or NCPAP) at 36 weeks PMA or discharge, whichever comes first	Need* for ≥30% oxygen and/or positive (PPV or NCPAP) at 56 days postnatal age or discharge, whichever comes first

*A physiologic test confirming the oxygen requirement at the assessment time point remains to be defined. This assessment may include a pulse oximetry saturation range.
BPD, bronchopulmonary dysplasia; *NCPAP*, nasal continuous positive airway pressure; *PMA*, postmenstrual age; *PPV*, positive-pressure ventilation.
From Jobe AH, Bancalari E. Bronchopulmonary dysplasia. Am J Respir Crit Care Med 2001;163:1723–9.

G. The final cornerstone of respiratory management is prevention of intercurrent respiratory infections with the hope of avoiding rehospitalization. More than half of these infants are readmitted to the hospital within the first year of nursery discharge. Use influenza vaccine in infants older than 6 months and respiratory syncytial virus prophylaxis with palivizumab according to American Academy of Pediatrics guidelines.

H. Reactive airways disease is not uncommon in this population and should be managed as described on the algorithm in the Asthma chapter (see p. 738). As children get older, if significant symptoms persist or reactive airways disease is a problem, perform pulmonary function testing and refer for a pulmonary subspecialty consultation. Although most children are asymptomatic with normal levels of activity by school age, abnormalities may be uncovered by spirometry and/or cardiopulmonary exercise testing.

I. Cardiac complications associated with BPD include both systemic and pulmonary hypertension. Systemic hypertension is usually high renin in origin and should be treated with captopril at a dose titrated between 0.1 and 0.5 mg/kg (maximum: 6 mg/kg/day) two to three times per day. After several months with good blood pressure control, the drug can usually be slowly weaned because most of these infants become normotensive over time. Infants with severe disease should be monitored for the development of pulmonary hypertension. Screening for pulmonary hypertension and an estimate of its severity can be obtained using echocardiography. This should be performed every 3 to 6 months in all infants with BPD who demonstrate a prolonged oxygen requirement. Although oxygen therapy is the treatment of choice, patients with pulmonary hypertension should be followed by a pediatric pulmonologist or cardiologist as other medications may be indicated.

J. Preterm survivors with BPD may be at increased risk for neurodevelopmental conditions compared with comparable preterm infants without BPD. Monitor their developmental progress carefully and refer when progress is delayed and of concern.

K. Stridor is not a common symptom in infants with BPD but merits evaluation if it is present. Prolonged intubation for ventilator therapy can result in subglottic stenosis. If obstructive airway symptoms are clinically important, consult a pulmonary specialist for a bronchoscopy.

References

Allen J, Zwerdling R, Ehrenkranz R, et al. Statement on the care of the child with chronic lung disease of infancy and childhood. Am J Respir Crit Care Med 2003;168:356–96.

Bancalari E, Claure N. Definitions and diagnostic criteria for bronchopulmonary dysplasia. Semin Perinatol 2006;30:164–70.

Baraldi E, Filippone M. Chronic lung disease after premature birth. N Engl J Med 2007;357:1946–55.

Ehrenkranz RA, Walsh MC, Vohr BR, et al. Validation of the National Institutes of Health consensus definition of bronchopulmonary dysplasia. Pediatrics 2005;116:1353–60.

Jobe AH, Bancalari E. Bronchopulmonary dysplasia. Am J Respir Crit Care Med 2001;163:1723–9.

Northway WH Jr, Rosan RC, Porter DY. Pulmonary disease following respirator therapy of hyaline-membrane disease. Bronchopulmonary dysplasia. N Engl J Med 1967;276:357–68.

Patient with BRONCHOPULMONARY DYSPLASIA

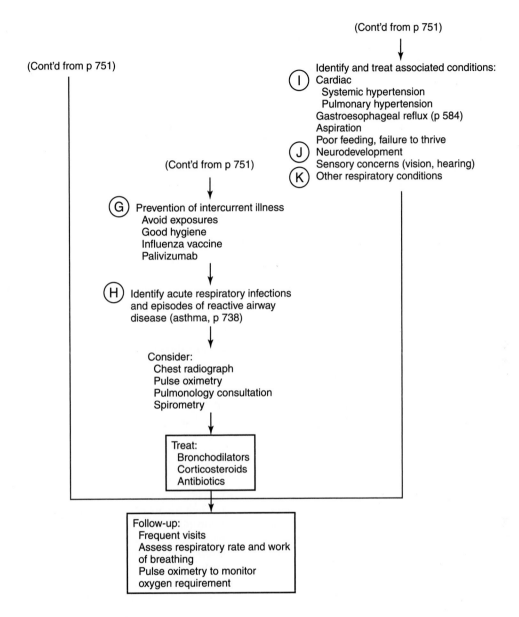

(Cont'd from p 751)

(Cont'd from p 751)

(I) Identify and treat associated conditions:
- Cardiac
  - Systemic hypertension
  - Pulmonary hypertension
- Gastroesophageal reflux (p 584)
- Aspiration
- Poor feeding, failure to thrive
- (J) Neurodevelopment
- Sensory concerns (vision, hearing)
- (K) Other respiratory conditions

(Cont'd from p 751)

(G) Prevention of intercurrent illness
- Avoid exposures
- Good hygiene
- Influenza vaccine
- Palivizumab

↓

(H) Identify acute respiratory infections and episodes of reactive airway disease (asthma, p 738)

↓

Consider:
- Chest radiograph
- Pulse oximetry
- Pulmonology consultation
- Spirometry

↓

Treat:
- Bronchodilators
- Corticosteroids
- Antibiotics

↓

Follow-up:
- Frequent visits
- Assess respiratory rate and work of breathing
- Pulse oximetry to monitor oxygen requirement

Pneumonia

Jeffrey S. Wagener, MD

Pneumonia in children typically presents with tachypnea (rapid breathing), fever, and cough. Viral infections are the most frequent cause of childhood pneumonia, particularly in preschool ages; however, bacterial infection and other causes should be considered (Table 1). The care provider can usually diagnose the cause and determine the appropriate therapy based on the history and physical examination, with occasional laboratory assistance.

A. History includes duration and degree of symptoms, as well as potential exposure to causative agents. Assess for rapid breathing, fever, and cough. Most pneumonias have a rapid onset unless they represent exacerbations of another underlying chronic condition (i.e., cystic fibrosis, tuberculosis, immune deficiency). Importantly, bacterial pneumonia can represent a complication of a prior viral infection, presenting as a child with a viral upper respiratory infection for 1 to 3 days suddenly developing worsening symptoms with fever and respiratory distress. Higher fevers (≥39° C) are more suggestive of bacterial pneumonias. Cough is not always present, but if productive of sputum is more indicative of a bacterial infection. A "staccato" cough in infants suggests *Chlamydia* infection, and a paroxysmal cough should always raise concern for pertussis. Other symptoms of pneumonia include poor feeding, lethargy, irritability, risk for aspiration, and occasionally skin rash. History of exposures to other people with similar infections, either at home or in school, helps define cause. Finally, immunization and chronic medication history, as well as information on conditions at home, such as exposure to tobacco smoke, may aid with the diagnosis.

B. Individuals at high risk for having a bacterial pneumonia include young infants; patients with chronic illnesses such as cystic fibrosis, malnutrition, or sickle cell anemia; or patients who are immunocompromised.

C. Physical examination includes both systemic and lung-specific signs of infection. Tachypnea can be defined as a respiratory rate more than two standard deviations above normal for age (Table 2). In infants, a high respiratory rate often indicates low oxygen, as does cyanosis in any age child. Work of breathing, assessed by high respiratory rate and the presence of nasal flaring and suprasternal and intercostal retractions, is a strong indicator of more severe disease. The child's activity level also reflects disease severity, and lethargy or poor fluid intake is a particularly concerning sign. Lung examination should include observation (signs of increased work of breathing, hyperinflation, or asymmetry), percussion (particularly looking for complications such as a pleural effusion), and auscultation (crackles are suggestive of bacterial pneumonia, whereas wheezing is more indicative of viral). Localized, decreased breath sounds suggest a complication such as effusion, consolidation, or foreign body aspiration and always necessitate further evaluation. Finally, other body systems should be examined for helpful diagnostic clues including conjunctivitis, otitis media, rhinitis, pharyngitis, cervical adenopathy, cardiac murmur, hepatosplenomegaly, arthritis, digital clubbing, and skin infections or rash.

D. Laboratory tests are usually not necessary for the diagnosis of community-acquired pneumonias because most children can be diagnosed using a good history and examination (Table 3). However, additional information may need to be obtained to evaluate for complications or to aid with specific therapy. Oxygen saturation (measured conveniently with a pulse oximeter) is normally 95% or above at sea level (≥93% at 5000 feet). Values less than 88% to 90% indicate more severe pneumonia and the need for supplemental oxygen. Arterial or capillary blood gases can be used to measure carbon dioxide levels in children with an increased work of breathing. A white blood cell (WBC) count with differential, C-reactive protein (CRP) level, and blood culture can be helpful in separating bacterial from viral disease. Sputum cultures are difficult to obtain in children; however, rapid diagnostic tests for some bacteria (group A streptococcus) and many viruses (respiratory syncytial virus, influenza, etc.) can be obtained from throat or nasal swabs. A chest radiograph (both anteroposterior and lateral) is necessary when a complicated pneumonia is suspected and also helps to separate viral and bacterial disease. Diffuse disease with hyperinflation, with or without areas of atelectasis, is typical of viral disease, whereas lobar consolidation and/or pleural effusion are most indicative of bacterial pneumonia. If an effusion is suspected, obtaining a lateral decubitus chest radiograph (with the child lying on the side of the effusion) will help determine whether the fluid is free flowing and can be easily sampled. Obtaining a cell count with differential and a culture with smear from this fluid is extremely valuable for determining therapy. Chest computed tomographic (CT) scanning is rarely, if ever, needed in uncomplicated pneumonia.

(Continued on page 756)

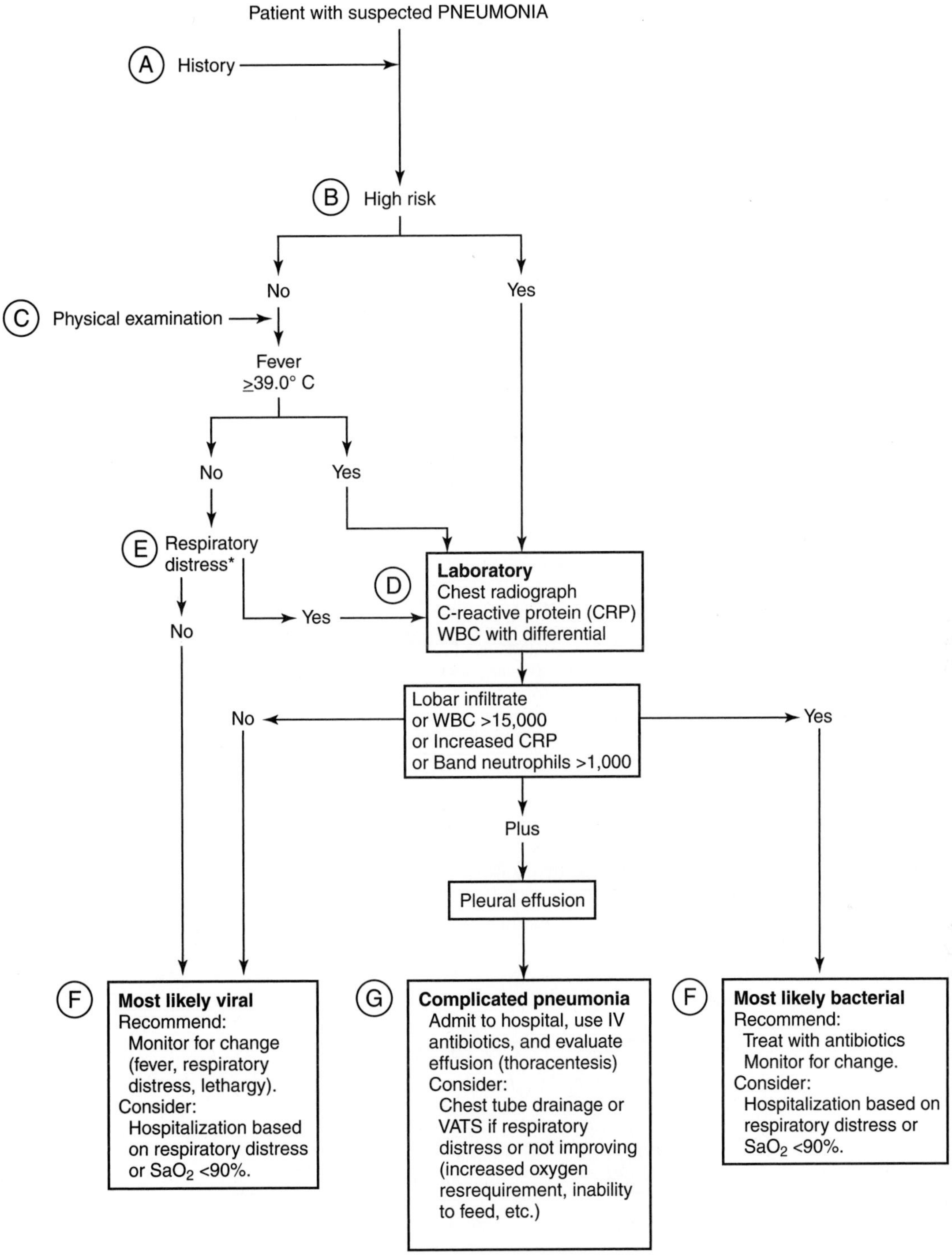
Patient with suspected PNEUMONIA
A History
B High risk
No
Yes
C Physical examination
Fever ≥39.0° C
No
Yes
E Respiratory distress*
No
Yes
D Laboratory
Chest radiograph
C-reactive protein (CRP)
WBC with differential
Lobar infiltrate
or WBC >15,000
or Increased CRP
or Band neutrophils >1,000
No
Yes
Plus
Pleural effusion
F Most likely viral
Recommend:
Monitor for change (fever, respiratory distress, lethargy).
Consider:
Hospitalization based on respiratory distress or SaO2 <90%.
G Complicated pneumonia
Admit to hospital, use IV antibiotics, and evaluate effusion (thoracentesis)
Consider:
Chest tube drainage or VATS if respiratory distress or not improving (increased oxygen resrequirement, inability to feed, etc.)
F Most likely bacterial
Recommend:
Treat with antibiotics
Monitor for change.
Consider:
Hospitalization based on respiratory distress or SaO2 <90%.

*Respiratory distress is indicated by an abnormal respiratory rate, increased work of breathing, intercostal and suprasternal retractions, use of accessory muscles of breathing, nasal flaring, grunting, and change in mental status.

E. Respiratory distress is indicated by an abnormal respiratory rate, increased work of breathing, intercostal and suprasternal retractions, use of accessory muscle, nasal flaring, grunting, and change in mental status.

F. Therapy can be separated by age groups and should be based first on the degree of illness, assessed primarily by the work of breathing, and second on the possible cause (Table 4). Infants younger than 3 weeks should always be admitted to the hospital and treated with intravenous (IV) antibiotics because of the risk for sepsis. Children 3 weeks to 4 months old with possible pneumonia should always be evaluated for fever, low oxygen saturation, and possible bacterial infection, usually requiring hospitalization and close observation. Outpatient management is not recommended for these children if a bacterial pneumonia is suspected (high fever or low oxygen saturation). For children older than 4 months with suspected viral pneumonia (low-grade fever, mild or no increased work of breathing, diffuse lung disease, and able to take fluids well), no therapy other than adequate fluids, observation, and possibly antipyretics for fever are needed. Children

Table 1. **Common Causes of Pneumonia in Childhood**

Age Group	Viral	Bacterial	Other
Birth to 3 weeks	Cytomegalovirus	Group B streptococci, gram-negative bacteria, *Listeria monocytogenes*	Congenital anomalies
3 weeks to <4 months	RSV, Parainfluenza viruses	*Chlamydia trachomatis, Streptococcus pneumoniae, Bordetella pertussis,* and *Staphylococcus aureus* (complicating viral infections)	Congenital anomalies, milk aspiration
4 months to 4 years	RSV, parainfluenza viruses, influenza A and B, metapneumovirus, adenovirus, rhinovirus	*Streptococcus pneumoniae, Haemophilus influenzae, Mycoplasma pneumoniae,* group A streptococcus, and *Staphylococcus aureus* (complicating viral infections)	Cystic fibrosis, foreign body aspiration, hypersensitivity, chronic aspiration
4 to 21 years	Influenza, adenovirus, rhinovirus, metapneumovirus	*Mycoplasma pneumoniae, Streptococcus pneumoniae,* group A streptococcus, *Chlamydia pneumoniae,* and *Staphylococcus aureus* (complicating viral infections)	Asthma, cystic fibrosis, hypersensitivity, aspiration, *Mycobacterium tuberculosis*

RSV, respiratory syncytial virus.

Table 2. **Respiratory Rates in Children**

Age	Normal	Abnormal
Birth	30	>60
2 years	25	>40
10 years	20	>30
18 years	15	>25

Table 3. **Separating Viral from Bacterial Pneumonia in Childhood**

Symptom or Sign	Viral	Bacterial
Tachypnea	++	+++
Fever	+	+++
Cough	++	++
Lethargy	+	+++
Work of breathing	+	++
Crackles	+ (Diffuse)	+++ (Localized)
Wheezing	+++	+
Grunting respirations	+	++
Conjunctivitis	+	++
Otitis media	++	+++
Hypoxia	++	++
Abnormal chest radiograph	Diffuse	Localized
Hyperinflation	+++	−
Atelectasis	++	±
Consolidation	±	+++
Pleural effusion	−	++++

Table 4. **Antibiotic Choices by Age Group**

Age Group	Oral	Intravenous
Birth to 3 weeks	Not recommended (admit to hospital)	Ampicillin plus cefotaxime (or aminoglycoside) plus MRSA coverage
3 weeks to <4 months	Generally not recommended Macrolide (if mild)	Ampicillin or cefotaxime Macrolide (if afebrile)
4 months to 4 years	Amoxicillin (high dose), or Augmentin, or cefuroxime, or macrolide	Ampicillin or cefuroxime or cefotaxime Add clindamycin or MRSA coverage if complicated pneumonia
4 to 21 years	Macrolide or amoxicillin (high dose) or Augmentin	Macrolide plus ampicillin, cefuroxime, or cefotaxime Add clindamycin or MRSA coverage if complicated pneumonia

MRSA, methicillin-resistant *Staphylococcus aureus.*

older than 4 months with suspected noncomplicated bacterial pneumonia (higher fever but only mild increased work of breathing, localized lung disease [crackles], and able to take fluids well) can be treated with oral antibiotics and watched at home for adequate fluid intake and improving symptoms. Importantly, children with respiratory distress (moderate to severe increased work of breathing), poor fluid intake, excessive irritability, or lethargy should be admitted to the hospital for care and monitoring, unrelated to the cause of the pneumonia. Only children with a suspected bacterial pneumonia, and select patients with influenza infection, require antibiotics (Table 5). Patients with uncomplicated pneumonia do not need follow-up chest radiographs if they have full resolution of respiratory symptoms.

G. Complicated pneumonias always need antibiotic therapy, and these patients usually need to be cared for in the hospital, particularly if they have low oxygen saturation or moderate-to-severe increased work of breathing. Pleural effusions should be cultured and always drained if the child is in respiratory distress. Obtaining the culture early, before antibiotic therapy if possible, provides the best opportunity to identify the bacterial causative agent. Video-assisted thoracoscopic surgery can be helpful if the fluid does not layer on the lateral decubitus chest radiograph, but generally is not needed if the effusion is drained early in the course of the pneumonia. Patients with complicated pneumonias need close follow-up and should not be discharged from the hospital until they are clinically improving, are taking adequate nutrition, can complete a minimum 14 days of antibiotics, have an improving chest radiograph, and are assured close follow-up. Long-term follow-up for patients with complicated pneumonia, including a chest radiograph several months later, is valuable for detecting patients at risk for recurrent problems.

Prevention of some pneumonias can be achieved through routine immunization for *Bordetella pertussis, Haemophilus influenza* type b, some strains of *Streptococcus pneumoniae,* and seasonal influenza. Children at risk for *Streptococcus pneumoniae* infections should receive additional vaccination after age 2. In addition, premature infants should be considered for passive immunity with palivizumab. Spread of infection can be reduced by proper isolation including good hand washing and avoiding contact with infected patients.

Table 5. **Antibiotic Doses for Treating Bacterial Pneumonia**

Antibiotic	Dosage	Comment
Oral		
Amoxicillin (high dose)	75–90 mg/kg/24 hours divided every 12 hours; maximum: 2–3 g/24 hours	First choice for community acquired or aspiration pneumonia
Amoxicillin with clavulanate (Augmentin)	<40 kg: 80–90 mg (amoxicillin component)/kg/24 hours of the extra strength concentration of 600 mg/5 ml >40 kg: 250–500 mg every 8 hours or 875 mg every 12 hours; maximum: 2 g/24 hours	Provides added coverage of MSSA
Cefuroxime	30 mg/kg/24 hours in two divided doses; maximum: 1 g/24 hours	Second-generation cephalosporin
Clindamycin	10–30 mg/kg/24 hours in 3–4 divided doses; maximum: 1.8 g/24 hours	For anaerobic and gram-positive bacteria
Doxycycline	2–5 mg/kg/24 hours in 1–2 divided doses; maximum: 200 mg/24 hours	Use only in patients >8 years old
Linezolid	≤11 years old: 10 mg/kg every 8 hours ≥12 years old: 600 mg every 12 hours	For MRSA
Macrolides		For mycoplasma and chlamydia infections
Azithromycin	12 mg/kg/24 hours once daily; maximum: 500 mg/24 hours	
Clarithromycin	15 mg/kg/24 hours divided every 12 hours; maximum: 1 g/24 hours	
Erythromycin	30–50 mg/kg/24 hours in four divided doses every 6 hours; maximum: 4 g/24 hours	
Quinolones		
Levofloxacin	<5 years old: 10 mg/kg twice a day >5 years old: 10 mg/kg every 24 hours; maximum 750 mg/24 hours	For suspected *Pseudomonas aeruginosa* infection or if ≥18 years old
Ciprofloxacin	20–40 mg/kg/24 hours in two divided doses; maximum: 2 g/24 hours	
Trimethoprim (TMP) with sulfamethoxazole	6–10 mg TMP/kg/24 hours in divided doses every 12 hours Serious infections: 15–20 mg TMP/kg/24 hours in divided doses every 6 hours	For mild to moderate *Staphylococcus aureus* infection
Oral Antiviral		
Oseltamivir	≤15 kg: 30 mg twice daily >15 to ≤23 kg: 45 mg twice daily >23 to ≤40 kg: 60 mg twice daily >40 kg: 75 mg twice daily	For some influenza infections
Intravenous		
Aminoglycosides		Monitor levels
Gentamicin	Neonates: 3.5 mg/kg every 24 hours Children: 2.5 mg/kg every 8 hours	For infant sepsis
Tobramycin	<7 days old: 2.5 mg/kg every 12 hours 7 days to one year old: 2.5 mg/kg every 8 hours >1 year old: 10 mg/kg every 24 hours	For *Pseudomonas aeruginosa*
Ampicillin	100–200 mg/kg/24 hours in four to six divided doses; maximum: 8–12 g/24 hours	First choice for community acquired and aspiration pneumonia
Ampicillin with sulbactam	100–400 mg ampicillin/kg/24 hours divided every 6 hours; maximum: 12 g ampicillin/24 hours	Provides added coverage for MSSA
Azithromycin or erythromycin	Azithromycin: same as oral Erythromycin: 20–40 mg/kg/24 hours divided every 6 hours, maximum: 4 g/24 hours	For mycoplasma and chlamydia infections
Cefuroxime	75–150 mg/kg/24 hours divided every 8 hours; maximum: 6 g/24 hours	Second-generation cephalosporin
Cefotaxime	100–200 mg/kg/24 hours in three to four divided doses; maximum: 12 g/24 hours	Third-generation cephalosporin
Ceftazidime	30–50 mg/kg/dose every 8 hours; maximum: 6 g/24 hours	For suspected *Pseudomonas aeruginosa*
Ceftriaxone	50–100 mg/kg/24 hours in one to two divided doses; maximum: 4 g/24 hours	Third-generation cephalosporin
Clindamycin	25–40 mg/kg/24 hours divided every 6–8 hours; maximum: 4.8 g/24 hours	For anaerobes and gram-positive stains
Meropenem	60–120 mg/kg/24 hours divided every 8 hours; maximum: 6 g/24 hours	Broad spectrum coverage
Nafcillin	100–200 mg/kg/24 hours in divided doses every 4–6 hours; maximum: 12 g/24 hours	For MSSA
Vancomycin	10–15 mg/kg every 6–8 hours; maximum: 2 g/24 hours	Monitor levels For MRSA

MRSA, methicillin-resistant *Staphylococcus aureus*; *MSSA*, methicillin-sensitive *Staphylococcus aureus*.

References

Kabra SK, Lodha R, Pandey RM. Antibiotics for community acquired pneumonia in children. Cochrane Database Syst Rev 2006;(3):CD004874.
McIntosh K. Community-acquired pneumonia in children. N Engl J Med 2002;346:429–37.
Michelow IC, Olsen K, Lozana J, et al. Epidemiology and clinical characteristics of community-acquired pneumonia in hospitalized children. Pediatrics 2004;113:701–7.
Nelson JD. Community-acquired pneumonia in children: guidelines for treatment. Pediatr Infect Dis J 2000;19:251–3.
Schultz KD, Fan LL, Pinsky J, et al. The changing face of pleural empyemas in children: epidemiology and management. Pediatrics 2004;113:1735–40.
Sinaniotis CA, Sinaniotis AC. Community-acquired pneumonia in children. Curr Opin Pulm Med 2005;11:218–25.
Wacogne I, Negrine RJS. Are follow-up chest x-ray examinations helpful in the management of children recovering from pneumonia? Arch Dis Child 2003;88:4057–8.

Sleep Disordered Breathing in Children

Naveen Kanathur, MBBS, and Ann C. Halbower, MD

Obstructive sleep apnea syndrome (OSA) is a common disorder in the pediatric population. The spectrum of sleep disordered breathing includes simple snoring, upper airway resistance syndrome, and OSA.

EPIDEMIOLOGY

Based on a recent review of multiple studies, prevalence rate of parent-reported snoring by any definition is believed to be around 7.45%, and estimated prevalence rate of OSA by diagnostic studies between 1% and 4%. OSA is more common between ages 2 and 8 years and tends to be more common in boys, in heavier children, and among African Americans.

PATHOPHYSIOLOGY

During sleep, neuromuscular tone allows patency of the pharynx for breathing, but factors such as decreased neuromuscular tone, altered ventilatory drive, and mechanical obstruction from adenotonsillar hypertrophy, craniofacial, or soft-tissue abnormalities leads to a tendency toward upper airway collapse. This results in partial or complete reduction in airflow on a recurrent basis and is accompanied with gas-exchange abnormalities (oxygen desaturation, hypercapnia) and arousals (sleep fragmentation).

Consequences of untreated OSA in children include failure to thrive and neuropsychological and behavioral problems such as inattention, aggression, restlessness, depression, and cardiovascular problems (systemic and pulmonary hypertension, and increased inflammatory markers of cardiovascular risk). OSA is believed to play a significant role in the increase of insulin resistance in obese children. Significant improvements in lipid profile and C-reactive protein have been seen after treatment of OSA in both nonobese and obese children.

A. In the patient's history, ask about snoring, restless sleep, unusual sleep positions, mouth breathing, paradoxical breathing, nocturnal enuresis, daytime hyperactivity, or sleepiness. See Table 1 for daytime and nighttime clinical features of sleep disordered breathing. See Table 2 for risk factors of sleep disordered breathing in children.

B. In the physical examination, look for tonsillar hypertrophy, crowded oropharynx, craniofacial abnormalities, dental malocclusion, nasal obstruction, adenoid face, obesity, Down syndrome, and Prader–Willi syndrome.

C. In making the diagnosis, clinical history or questionnaires are not sufficient to differentiate OSA from habitual snoring. A normal nocturnal oximetry study does not rule out significant sleep disordered breathing. Laboratory-based polysomnogram (PSG; sleep study) is the gold standard. A PSG includes information on airflow at the nose and mouth, work of breathing by chest and abdominal movements, blood gas values, arousals from sleep, cardiac rhythm, and body movements. Respiratory events recorded by PSG include obstructive or hypopnea events (complete or partial airflow reduction, respectively), central apnea (lack of airflow during lack of breathing effort), and arousals from sleep that can be caused by respiratory events. The apnea–hypopnea index (AHI) is the number of events scored per hour. The International Classification of Sleep Disorders (ICSD-2) criteria require PSG documentation of at least one event per hour of sleep for a diagnosis of pediatric OSA. The differential diagnosis for persistent sleepiness includes narcolepsy, delayed sleep phase syndrome, and drug use. Gas exchange abnormalities stem from multiple diagnoses including central hypoventilation and may require follow-up with a pulmonologist.

D. In treatment of mild OSA, intranasal steroids alone and in combination with leukotriene antagonists have been shown to reduce the severity of mild OSA (AHI <5) and the magnitude of adenoid hypertrophy, and should be considered as an initial option in mild OSA.

E. Tonsillectomy and adenoidectomy (T&A) involves removal of adenoids and tonsils and is the recommended initial treatment in pediatric OSA. The success rate of T&A in published literature is highly variable. A recent meta-analysis of 23 studies involving 1079 patients (mean age, 6.5 years) when "cure" defined as an AHI less than 1 suggested that the treatment success rate with T&A was only 66.3%. The failure rate is greater in high-risk groups such as patients with morbid obesity, high preoperative AHI, Down syndrome, craniofacial syndromes, and neuromuscular disorders. Children younger than 3 years are at a greater risk for postoperative complications after T&A and require close observation after the surgery. Children sent for T&A without prior PSG may require a postoperative PSG to determine cure, especially those in high-risk groups or with persistent symptoms.

F. For children with persistent OSA (AHI >5) after T&A, continuous positive airway pressure therapy (CPAP) is an option. CPAP is an FDA-approved therapy for children older than 2 years, but studies have shown that it is effective even in younger children and infants. Surgical procedures such as inferior turbinate reduction and septoplasty attempt to decrease nasal obstruction and may help

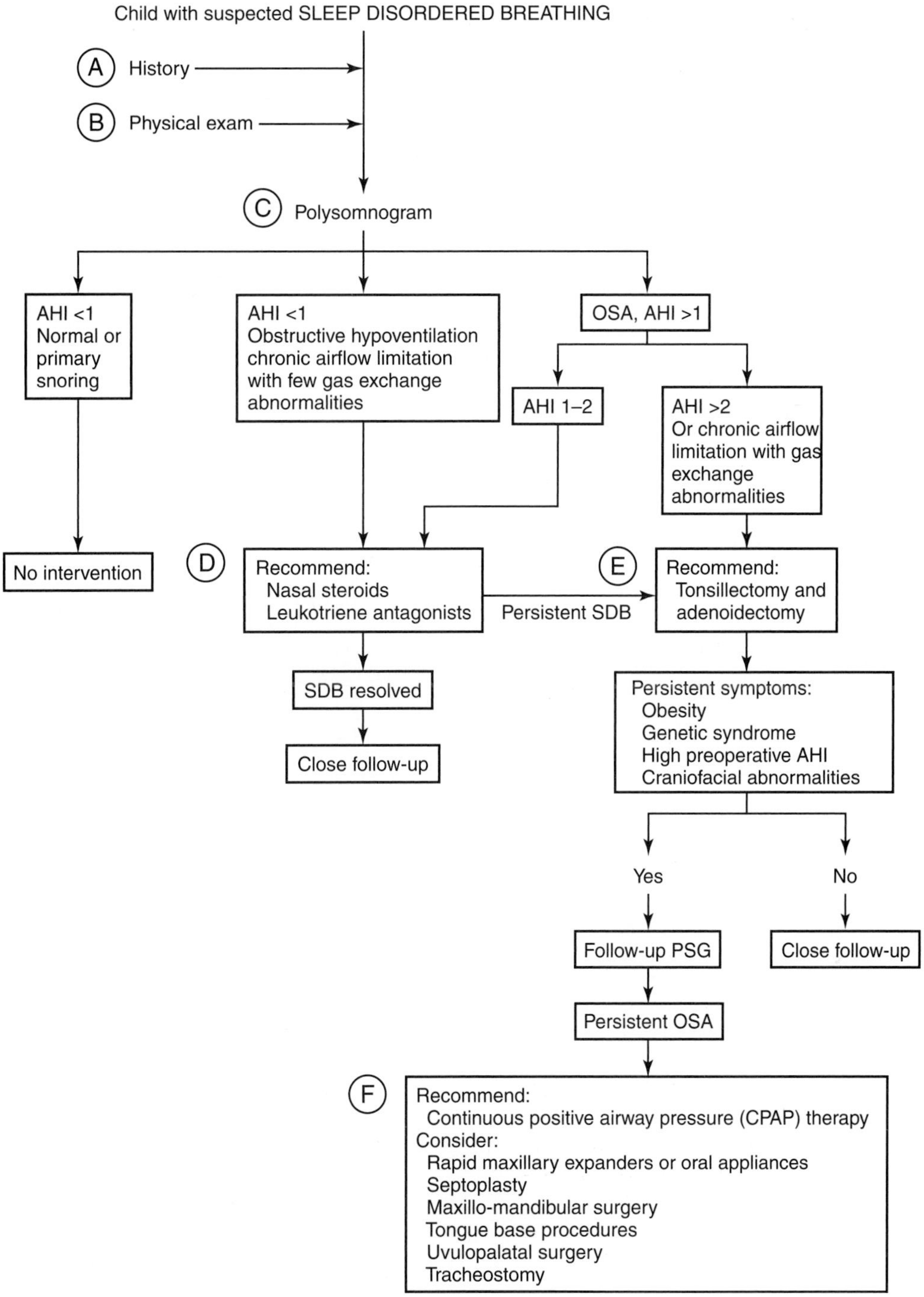
Child with suspected SLEEP DISORDERED BREATHING
A History
B Physical exam
C Polysomnogram
AHI <1
Normal or primary snoring
AHI <1
Obstructive hypoventilation chronic airflow limitation with few gas exchange abnormalities
OSA, AHI >1
AHI 1–2
AHI >2
Or chronic airflow limitation with gas exchange abnormalities
No intervention
D
Recommend:
Nasal steroids
Leukotriene antagonists
Persistent SDB
E
Recommend:
Tonsillectomy and adenoidectomy
SDB resolved
Close follow-up
Persistent symptoms:
Obesity
Genetic syndrome
High preoperative AHI
Craniofacial abnormalities
Yes
No
Follow-up PSG
Close follow-up
Persistent OSA
F
Recommend:
Continuous positive airway pressure (CPAP) therapy
Consider:
Rapid maxillary expanders or oral appliances
Septoplasty
Maxillo-mandibular surgery
Tongue base procedures
Uvulopalatal surgery
Tracheostomy

children with residual OSA after T&A. Similarly, rapid maxillary expanders increase nasal cavity volume and decrease nasal resistance, and should be considered in children with high arched palates or crowded dentition. Major surgical interventions such as mandibular distraction, maxillomandibular advancement, and tracheotomy may be necessary in life-threatening OSA or in patients with craniofacial anomalies.

Table 1. **Clinical Features of Sleep Disordered Breathing in Children**

Nighttime	Daytime
Snoring/noisy breathing: worse during upper respiratory infection or allergic rhinitis	Grogginess in morning
Mouth breathing	Headache, dry mouth, or sore throat on awakening
Neck hypertension during sleep	Behavioral changes: hyperactive behavior (young children <8 years)
Restless sleeper	Learning, attention, and executive function deficits
Excessive perspiration	Daytime sleepiness
Witnessed apneas (less frequent than in adults)	Mouth breathing during wakefulness
Nocturnal enuresis	
Sleepwalking, sleep talking, and night terrors	

Table 2. **Risk Factors of Sleep Disordered Breathing in Children**

Age 2–8 years: peak adenotonsillar hypertrophy relative to the upper airway size
Chronic nasal obstruction
Craniofacial abnormalities
Prader–Willi syndrome
Obesity
Hypothyroidism
Down syndrome
Pierre–Robin syndrome
Sickle cell disease
Cleft palate after surgery
Choanal atresia
Brainstem disorders: Chiari malformation, syringobulbia

References

American Academy of Sleep Medicine. The AASM Manual for the Scoring of Sleep & Associated Events. Darien, IL: American Academy of Sleep Medicine; 2007.

Friedman M, Wilson M, Lin HC, Chang HW. Updated systematic review of tonsillectomy and adenoidectomy for treatment of pediatric obstructive sleep apnea/hypopnea syndrome. Otolaryngol Head Neck Surg 2009;140(6):800–8.

Gozal D, Capdevila OS, Kheirandish-Gozal L. Metabolic alterations and systemic inflammation in obstructive sleep apnea among nonobese and obese prepubertal children. Am J Respir Crit Care Med 2008;177:1142–9.

Halbower AC, Ishman SL, McGinley BM. Childhood obstructive sleep-disordered breathing. Chest 2007;132:2030–41.

Hoban T, Chervin R. Sleep-related breathing disorders of childhood: description and clinical picture, diagnosis and treatment approaches. Sleep Med Clin 2007;2(3):445–62.

Kheirandish-Gozal L, Gozal D. Intranasal budesonide treatment for children with mild obstructive sleep apnea syndrome. Pediatrics 2008;122:e149–55.

Lumeng J, Chervin R. Epidemiology of pediatric obstructive sleep apnea. Proc Am Thorac Soc 2007;5:242–52.

Renal and Urologic Disorders

Clinical Presentation and Evaluation of Acute versus Chronic Renal Disease

Nimisha Amin, MD, and Joshua J. Zaritsky, MD, PhD

When a patient is newly diagnosed with renal failure, many clues may help the physician determine whether the onset is acute or chronic. This distinction is important to make, for both diagnostic and therapeutic reasons. Both situations warrant supportive care and possibly renal replacement therapy, but hydration, removal of inciting agents, aggressive immunosuppression, or plasmapheresis may greatly improve the course of certain causes of acute renal failure. This chapter focuses on important components of the history, physical, laboratory evaluation, and relevant imaging studies that can help differentiate acute from chronic renal failure (see Table 1).

A. History: The physical manifestations of both acute and chronic renal failure may include generalized fatigue, lack of appetite and nausea (with or without vomiting), pallor, decreasing urine output, or edema. A progressive worsening of these symptoms over a period of weeks to months often suggests chronic renal failure, whereas acute renal failure will often manifest in a matter of days. The intensity of these symptoms may also be less striking in the setting of chronic renal failure, as the body has had time to acclimate to worsening uremia. Specific extrarenal symptoms may also point toward an acute onset, such as severe and persistent vomiting and/or diarrhea (dehydration-induced acute tubular necrosis), bloody diarrhea (hemolytic uremic syndrome), hemoptysis (Wegener's granulomatosis or Goodpasture's syndrome), and rash or joint pain (lupus nephritis).

A recent history of infection, exposures, or medication use may also be related to an acute onset of renal failure. Postinfectious glomerulonephritis is a potential, but infrequent, cause of acute renal failure, associated with tea-colored urine and hypertension. Sweet-smelling toxins such as toluene (from glue and paint thinner) or ethylene glycol (found in antifreeze) are known to cause acute renal failure and serve as attractive hazards for small children. A substance abuse history should be obtained in adolescent patients, because amphetamines, "ecstasy," and heroin can also induce renal failure. In pediatrics, medication-induced acute renal failure often occurs in the setting of multiple renal insults, such as dehydration, sepsis, or the concurrent use of multiple nephrotoxic medications.

Pertinent aspects of the past medical history may provide insight into chronic causes of renal failure. A history of low birth weight is associated with reduced renal mass and an increased incidence of chronic renal failure. Recurrent nonspecific febrile illnesses or recurrent urinary tract infections throughout childhood may suggest undiagnosed reflux nephropathy. Patients with long-term enuresis or significant delays in toilet training may have a concentration defect, as seen in nephronophthisis or multicystic dysplastic kidneys. Certain prolonged infections, such as human immunodeficiency virus (HIV), may also cause chronic renal failure. Failed hearing screens or a confirmed hearing loss may correlate with Alport syndrome. Finally, developmental delay or poor school performance is often seen in conjunction with chronic renal failure.

Family history should include inquiry about any family member with chronic renal disease, congenital hearing loss, autoimmune disorders, or need for renal replacement therapy (dialysis or kidney transplant). Detailed questioning is important here, because many patients may not consider a family member with a kidney transplant to have renal disease "anymore."

B. Physical Examination: Interesting physical findings can be found on the patient with both acute and chronic renal failure. Documentation of height and growth percentile is crucial in making this distinction. Chronic renal failure impairs growth by a variety of mechanisms. Short stature may be the only clue on physical examination to suggest a chronic cause of renal failure. Blood pressure is important to note for management purposes but can be significantly elevated in both circumstances. However, hypertensive retinopathy on funduscopic examination or a displaced point of maximal impact (PMI) on cardiac examination (suggestive of dilated cardiomyopathy) may suggest long-term hypertension consistent with chronic renal failure. Signs of fluid overload, such as peripheral edema, diminished breath sounds, or rales, can be appreciated in both acute and renal failure. Cardiac murmurs (often secondary to anemia) may be present in both situations as well. Careful palpation of the abdomen is also important in any case of renal failure, specifically looking for a mass, which could represent enlarged kidneys from cystic disease, hydronephrosis, or tumor. Certain skin findings may be more consistent with acute renal failure (such as pallor and petechiae in hemolytic uremic syndrome) or chronic renal failure (such as heavy bruising from uremia-induced platelet dysfunction). Rashes and joint pain/swelling may be suggestive of lupus nephritis, which can cause acute or chronic renal failure. Finally, bony abnormalities such as genu varum/valgum or the windswept deformity may be secondary to renal osteodystrophy, as seen with chronic renal failure.

C. Laboratory Workup: In both acute and chronic renal failure, one expects to see an increased blood urea nitrogen (BUN) and creatinine. If the BUN/creatinine ratio is

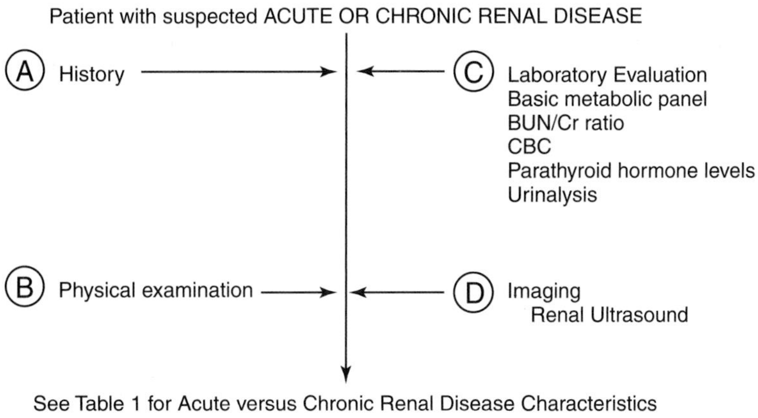
Patient with suspected ACUTE OR CHRONIC RENAL DISEASE
(A) History
(B) Physical examination
(C) Laboratory Evaluation
Basic metabolic panel
BUN/Cr ratio
CBC
Parathyroid hormone levels
Urinalysis
(D) Imaging
Renal Ultrasound
See Table 1 for Acute versus Chronic Renal Disease Characteristics

greater than 20, a prerenal cause (such as dehydration) may be the cause of acute renal failure. Metabolic disturbances found in either form of renal failure include hyperkalemia, metabolic acidosis (with or without an anion gap), hypocalcemia, and hyperphosphatemia. The latter two abnormalities tend to be more pronounced in chronic renal failure. Anemia is another finding that can be seen in both circumstances, but again tends to be much more significant (with hemoglobin levels <8 g/dL) and better compensated (for lack of tachycardia or shortness of breath) in chronic renal failure. Parathyroid hormone levels, which very roughly correlate with the degree of renal osteodystrophy, will be increased only in chronic renal failure. Urinalyses tend to be bland in chronic disease, whereas acute renal failure secondary to a potentially treatable glomerulonephritis may demonstrate proteinuria, hematuria, or both. If a significant amount of protein or blood is found in the urine, the algorithms provided in the Hematuria and Proteinuria chapters should be followed for a more comprehensive evaluation.

D. Imaging: Renal ultrasound is the most useful imaging modality in differentiating between acute and chronic renal failure. Kidneys that are small, shrunken, dysplastic, or cystic suggest chronic renal failure, whereas normal- or large-sized kidneys, usually with abnormal corticomedullary differentiation, are usually more reflective of an acute process. If there is a history of recurrent urinary tract infections, a voiding cystourethrogram (VCUG) may confirm vesicoureteral reflux. In addition, a dimercaptosuccinic acid (DMSA) scan may also reveal areas of renal scarring from previous episodes of pyelonephritis. In any patient with renal failure and hypertension, an echocardiogram is also useful, because the presence of left ventricular hypertrophy suggests long-standing hypertension and, thus, chronic renal failure.

More invasive testing, such as a renal biopsy, is most frequently performed when the aforementioned workup is suggestive of acute renal failure and ultrasound reveals normal-sized kidneys.

Table 1. **Important Aspects in the Evaluation of Renal Failure and Association of Each Item with Acute versus Chronic Onset**

	Acute	Chronic
History		
Onset of symptoms	Days	Months
Constitutional symptoms	+	+ (± Less intense)
Extrarenal symptoms	+	−
Preceding infection	+ (PIGN)	− (Unless acute on chronic)
Toxins/medications	+	−
Low birth weight	−	+
Recurrent urinary tract infections/fevers	−	+
Chronic enuresis	−	+
Hearing loss/developmental delay	−	+
Family history	−	+
Physical Examination		
Short stature	−	+
Hypertension	+	+
Hypertensive retinopathy	−	+
Displaced PMI	−	+
Rales	+	+
Peripheral edema	+	+
Abdominal mass	−	+
Skin findings	+ (Petechiae, pallor)	+ (Bruising)
Joint pain/tenderness	+	+
Bony deformities	−	+
Laboratory Workup		
Increased BUN	+	+
Increased creatinine	+	+
Hyperkalemia	+	+
Metabolic acidosis	+	+
Hypocalcemia	+	++
Hyperphosphatemia	+	++
Hyperparathyroidism	−	+
Anemia	+	++
Urinalysis	Protein/blood	Bland
Imaging		
Renal ultrasound	Normal size	Shrunken, cystic, dysplastic
VCUG	−	+ In reflux nephropathy
DMSA scan	−	+ In reflux nephropathy
Echocardiogram	−	Left ventricular hypertrophy

BUN, blood urea nitrogen; *DMSA,* dimercaptosuccinic acid; *PIGN,* postinfectious glomerulonephritis; *PMI,* point of maximal impact; *VCUG,* voiding cystourethrogram.

References

Vikse BE, Irgens LM, Leivestad T, et al. Low birth weight increases risk for end stage renal disease. J Am Soc Nephrol 2008;19(1):151–7.

Webb N, Postlethwait R. Clinical paediatric nephrology. 3rd ed. New York: Oxford University Press; 2003.

Proteinuria

Nimisha Amin, MD, and Joshua J. Zaritsky, MD, PhD

Proteinuria can be a common finding within a general pediatric practice. The purpose of this chapter is to review the definition, common causes, evaluation, and management of proteinuria, with particular emphasis placed on nephrotic syndrome. This chapter also provides guidelines as to when a referral to a pediatric nephrologist is warranted.

Within the discussion of proteinuria, nephrotic syndrome deserves special consideration, because it is the most frequent clinical manifestation of symptomatic isolated proteinuria in a young child. The syndrome itself is defined by the presence of significant proteinuria, hypoalbuminemia, edema, and hypercholesterolemia. See later in this chapter for further details about cause and management.

DEFINITION

Urine dipstick analysis, which largely measures urinary albumin, is the most common method for initial detection of proteinuria. True proteinuria is defined as ≥1+ proteinuria when the specific gravity (SG) of the urine sample is ≤1.015, or ≥2+ proteinuria when the SG of the sample is >1.015. Typically, these findings need to be present in two of three specimens, obtained at least 1 week apart. Proteinuria can also be defined on the basis of a spot urinary protein/creatinine (Cr) ratio, which measures all forms of urinary protein. Normal values for this ratio are less than 0.5 for children age 6 months to 2 years, and less than 0.2 for all children older than 2 years.

The gold standard for detection and quantification of proteinuria is a 24-hour urine collection for protein and Cr. Less than 4 $mg/m^2/hr$ protein is considered normal, whereas 4 to 40 $mg/m^2/hr$ defines proteinuria, and greater than 40 $mg/m^2/hour$ is usually present during nephrotic syndrome (see later). Cr measurements should also be evaluated. A 24-hour urine Cr that is less than normal is suggestive of an inaccurate collection with an insufficient volume of urine. This results in a falsely decreased amount of urinary protein that has been quantified for the 24-hour period. Normal 24-hour Cr measurements are as follows: 8 to 10 mg/kg/day for newborns, 10 to 12 mg/kg/day for children, 12 to 15 mg/kg/day for female adults, and 15 to 20 mg/kg/day for male adults.

CAUSATIVE FACTORS

Proteinuria occurs secondary to increased permeability of the glomerular basement membrane or renal tubule to serum proteins. This can occur on a transient basis, often related to exercise, fever, infection, dehydration, or congestive heart failure. Proteinuria can also be detected on urinalysis during a urinary tract infection.

Benign orthostatic proteinuria refers to a process in which there is increased urinary protein excretion in the upright position only. This can be detected by a 24-hour split urinary collection (separating daytime voids from nighttime voids), which typically reveals the majority of urinary protein isolated to the daytime collection. Of note, if the total 24-hour urinary protein (regardless of allocation between daytime and nighttime voids) exceeds 1 g, consultation with a pediatric nephrologist is warranted. Otherwise, orthostatic proteinuria is considered a benign process in which no further evaluation is needed.

The most common glomerular causes of isolated proteinuria include minimal change disease, focal and segmental glomerulosclerosis, and membranous nephropathy. Minimal change disease is the most common cause of nephrotic syndrome is children age 1 to 6 years. Focal and segmental glomerulosclerosis and membranous nephropathy can be asymptomatic initially or present similar to minimal change disease. Diagnosis of these latter two conditions must be made via renal biopsy. Both can be idiopathic in nature, but have been seen in the setting of infection, namely, hepatitis B, hepatitis C, and human immune deficiency virus (HIV).

Genetic causes for isolated proteinuria can manifest at any time between infancy and adulthood, and are also glomerular in origin. Causes of congenital nephrotic syndrome include Finnish type congenital nephrotic syndrome, diffuse mesangial sclerosis, Pierson syndrome, or Galloway syndrome. There are also a wide variety of genetic mutations responsible for later-onset focal and segmental glomerulosclerosis.

Proteinuria in conjunction with significant hematuria (as defined as greater than 20 RBC/high-power field [hpf] on urinalysis) should be cause for alarm, because it may be reflective of malignant renal pathology. Further evaluation of proteinuria with hematuria should be performed promptly, using guidelines here as well as in the Hematuria chapter. A number of glomerulonephritides are responsible for proteinuria with hematuria, including postinfectious glomerulonephritis, membranoproliferative glomerulonephritis, IgA nephropathy, Henoch-Schönlein purpura, or systemic lupus erythematosus.

Finally, renal tubular dysfunction can also cause proteinuria. Recall that tubular proteinuria may not be detected on routine dipstick analysis (which largely measures urinary albumin), but can be measured by way of urinary β_2-microglobulin, retinol binding protein, or a urinary protein/Cr ratio. Examples of such tubular disorders include interstitial nephritis, tubular injury (by way of acute tubular necrosis, nephrotoxic medications, or heavy metal toxicity), or Fanconi syndrome (as seen in cystinosis, Lowe syndrome, α1-antitrypsin deficiency, etc).

EVALUATION

A. The evaluation of proteinuria begins with the history and physical. Inquiry about clinical manifestations of fever, edema, frothy urine, abdominal symptoms, medical history (including exposures), and family history of renal disease should be performed.

B. Physical examination should be comprehensive, paying close attention to blood pressure, evaluation of edema (peripheral, periorbital, labial/scrotal or ascites), auscultation of the lungs (for diminished breath sounds consistent with a pleural effusion), and abdominal examination (looking for ascites or rebound/guarding).

C. Urinary studies evaluating proteinuria include urinalysis, urine culture, urine protein/Cr ratio, and 24-hour urine protein collection, as noted earlier. These studies are often performed before obtaining blood work, depending on acuity of the patient's clinical presentation. Important blood tests to obtain in the evaluation of persistent and pathologic proteinuria include electrolytes, albumin, blood urea nitrogen (BUN)/Cr, complete blood cell count (CBC), and cholesterol. Additional studies such as C3, C4, antinuclear antibody (ANA), hepatitis serologies, and HIV testing should be considered especially when minimal change disease appears unlikely.

In patients who present with nephrotic syndrome, a chest radiograph will typically demonstrate evidence of intravascular fluid depletion (somewhat dark lung fields) and a small, elongated heart. Pleural effusions are also a common and expected finding with nephrotic syndrome. The presence of pulmonary edema or an enlarged heart are worrisome and unexpected findings, in which case, great caution is needed before moving forward with treatment.

Renal ultrasound is usually the only imaging modality needed during evaluation of proteinuria. Ultrasound is often normal in the setting of isolated proteinuria but may provide insightful information about renal size, echogenicity, or evidence of hydronephrosis related to vesicoureteral reflux. Renal biopsy is reserved for complex cases, after consultation with a pediatric nephrologist. It is rarely performed in the straightforward case of nephrotic syndrome in a child age 1 to 6 years, because minimal change disease is the most likely diagnosis.

MANAGEMENT

Given the high incidence of minimal change disease in pediatric patients with nephrotic syndrome, and its high propensity for steroid responsiveness, it is entirely appropriate for the general practitioner to initiate treatment of a routine case of minimal change disease. Prednisone, 2 mg/kg/day given as a single dose every morning, for 1 month is the mainstay of treatment (maximum dose: 60 mg/day). Of note, it is recommended that documentation of a recent negative tuberculin skin test (TST) be obtained before initiating therapy.

After treatment has begun, remission can be expected in 70% of patients within 2 weeks and 95% of patients within 1 month. Assuming that remission has been achieved during the initial month of therapy, dosing is subsequently weaned to 2 mg/kg every other day for 1 month, followed by discontinuation of treatment. If remission is not achieved within the first month, 2 mg/kg/day should be continued for 1 additional month and then weaned. Six months after prednisone has been discontinued, approximately 44% of patients will not have relapsed, 22% will have had one relapse, 31% will have had two or more relapses, and 3% will become steroid nonresponders. If the patient remains nephrotic after 2 consecutive months of therapy, begins to relapse during the taper period, or frequently relapses after withdrawal of treatment, referral to a pediatric nephrologist is indicated.

Although the majority of patients with minimal change disease can be managed as outpatients, hospital admission for intravenous albumin (and furosemide) administration is necessary under certain circumstances, including patients with the following:

1. Serum albumin level <2 g/dL
2. Severe symptomatic edema (scrotal/labial or edema with skin breakdown)
3. Nausea/vomiting and an inability to tolerate oral prednisone
4. Atypical findings such as hypertension, increased BUN/Cr, pulmonary edema, or enlarged heart on chest radiograph.

Inpatient management should always be performed in consultation with a pediatric nephrologist.

One other management aspect of minimal change disease is close monitoring for known complications, including thrombosis (secondary to loss of anticoagulant proteins in the urine) and spontaneous bacterial peritonitis (usually secondary to encapsulated organisms, i.e., *Streptococcus pneumoniae*).

Indications for referral to a pediatric nephrologist for proteinuria include hypertension, presence of concomitant hematuria (>20 RBC/hpf), increased BUN/Cr, findings consistent with pathology beyond minimal change syndrome on laboratory workup, lack of response to prednisone after 2 months, relapse during weaning of prednisone, frequent relapses after withdrawal of treatment (two or more relapses in 6 months), or need for hospitalization. Renal biopsy will likely be performed in many of these circumstances, followed by initiation of additional immunosuppression pending biopsy results.

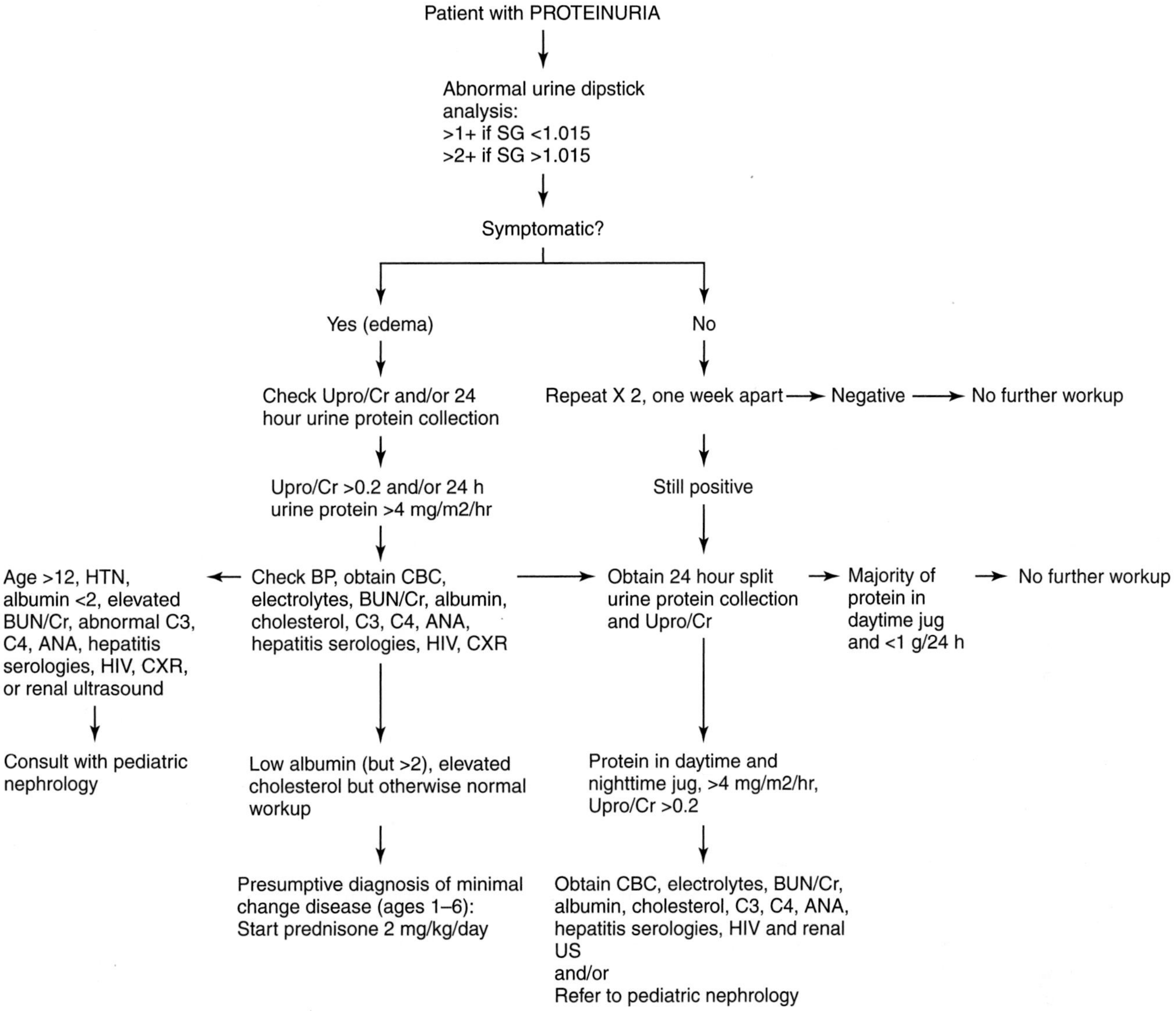
Patient with PROTEINURIA
Abnormal urine dipstick analysis: >1+ if SG <1.015 >2+ if SG >1.015
Symptomatic?
Yes (edema)
No
Check Upro/Cr and/or 24 hour urine protein collection
Repeat X 2, one week apart
Negative
No further workup
Upro/Cr >0.2 and/or 24 h urine protein >4 mg/m2/hr
Still positive
Age >12, HTN, albumin <2, elevated BUN/Cr, abnormal C3, C4, ANA, hepatitis serologies, HIV, CXR, or renal ultrasound
Check BP, obtain CBC, electrolytes, BUN/Cr, albumin, cholesterol, C3, C4, ANA, hepatitis serologies, HIV, CXR
Obtain 24 hour split urine protein collection and Upro/Cr
Majority of protein in daytime jug and <1 g/24 h
No further workup
Consult with pediatric nephrology
Low albumin (but >2), elevated cholesterol but otherwise normal workup
Protein in daytime and nighttime jug, >4 mg/m2/hr, Upro/Cr >0.2
Presumptive diagnosis of minimal change disease (ages 1–6): Start prednisone 2 mg/kg/day
Obtain CBC, electrolytes, BUN/Cr, albumin, cholesterol, C3, C4, ANA, hepatitis serologies, HIV and renal US
and/or
Refer to pediatric nephrology

References

Ettenger R. The evaluation of the child with proteinuria. Pediatr Ann 1994;23:486–94.

Hogg RJ, Portman RJ, Milliner D, et al. Evaluation and management of proteinuria and nephrotic syndrome in children: recommendations from a pediatric nephrology panel established at the National Kidney Foundation Conference on Proteinuria, Albuminuria, Risk, Assessment, Detection and Elimination (PARADE). Pediatrics 2003;105:1242–9.

Quigley R. Evaluation of hematuria and proteinuria: how should a pediatrician proceed? Curr Opin Pediatr 2008;20:140–4.

Tarshish P, Tobin JN, Bernstein J, Edelmann CM Jr. Prognostic significance of the early course of minimal change nephrotic syndrome: report of the International Study of Kidney Disease in Children. J Am Soc Nephrol 1997;8:769–76.

The primary nephrotic syndrome in children. Identification of patients with minimal change nephrotic syndrome from an initial response to prednisone. A report of the International Study of Kidney Disease in Children. J Pediatr 1981;98:561–4.

The Undescended Testis

Garrett Pohlman, MD, and Jeffrey B. Campbell, MD

The undescended testis (UDT) is one of the most common congenital anomalies of the male genitalia, affecting approximately 30% of premature infants and 2% to 5% of those born at term. The incidence rate declines to approximately 1% by 1 year of age. This has been attributed to the postnatal testosterone surge that occurs during the first few months of life. The majority of undescended testes are unilateral, with the right more commonly affected than the left. Although most undescended testes are palpable, approximately 20% are nonpalpable. In such cases, the testis may be intra-abdominal, atrophic, or absent.

A. The physical examination is of paramount importance in the evaluation of the child with a UDT. The examination should be performed in a warm, nonthreatening environment with the child supine. A UDT can often be identified by sweeping the second and third fingers from just above the inguinal canal onto the scrotum. The examiner will often feel a "pop" as the testis springs back to its original position. A helpful technique is to use soapy water on the fingertips or a water-based lubricant on the skin to reduce friction. If unable to identify the testis, ectopic locations (suprapubic, lateral or inferior to the scrotum, contralateral hemiscrotum) should be carefully examined.

B. A child with a UDT should be re-evaluated around 6 months of age, as approximately two thirds of undescended testes will descend during the first few months of life. Should the testis remain undescended, referral to a pediatric urologist is indicated.

C. Patients with nonpalpable testes (bilateral) warrant special consideration, because this finding may be associated with a disorder of sexual differentiation (DSD). In such cases, a karyotype should be obtained, with further evaluation and management to be determined in consultation with a pediatric urologist.

Radiographic imaging is usually not indicated in the evaluation of a UDT, given its low overall accuracy and impact on management.

D. Surgical correction should be performed at 6 to 12 months of age in an effort to minimize the progressive, deleterious effect of cryptorchidism on spermatogenesis. This is of particular importance in those patients with undescended testes (bilateral). Men with a history of a UDT surgically corrected in a timely fashion have a similar paternity rate to those with fully descended testes (89% and 93%, respectively), whereas men with a history of undescended testes (bilateral) have a significantly lower paternity rate (65%). A UDT also conveys an increased risk for the development of testicular cancer (approximately fourfold increase). Surgical correction reduces the risk for malignancy and places the testis within the scrotum, facilitating routine testicular self-examination.

An inguinal or scrotal orchiopexy is performed for a palpable UDT. In such cases, an indirect inguinal hernia is often identified and ligated. In patients with a nonpalpable testis, diagnostic laparoscopy is typically performed. Findings include an intra-abdominal testis, an atrophic testis, and an absent/vanishing testis (approximately 50%, 30%, and 20%, respectively). In such cases, a laparoscopic orchiopexy or orchiectomy is typically performed.

E. Care must be taken to differentiate a UDT from a retractile testis. A careful history and physical examination are of paramount importance in making this distinction. A retractile testis is a fully descended testis that intermittently ascends from the scrotum because of an overactive cremasteric reflex. This is a normal finding in young boys and does not convey an increased risk for infertility or testicular carcinoma. There is often a history of fully descended testes on previous examinations, and parents often report having seen both testes within the scrotum when in a warm, relaxing environment such as a bath. The examination should be performed in a warm, nonthreatening environment with the child supine. The scrotum is observed for the presence of testes, which often retract on palpation. A retractile testis can be manipulated into the dependent portion of the scrotum, where it remains on fatigue of the cremasteric fibers. An UDT will immediately return to its original position on release. Although a retractile testis does not require surgical intervention, it should be re-evaluated annually during childhood, as approximately one third of retractile testes will ascend (i.e., become a UDT). Secondary ascent is a rare phenomenon thought to be due to failure of the spermatic cord to elongate as the child grows. In such cases, referral to a pediatric urologist is indicated.

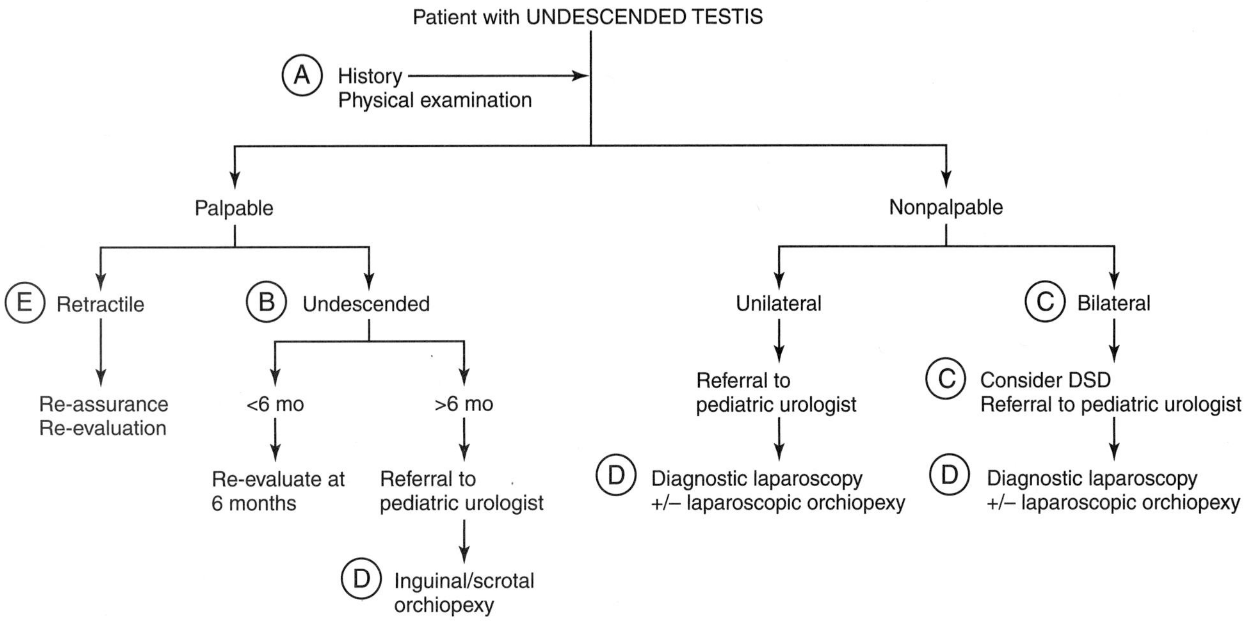
Patient with UNDESCENDED TESTIS
A History
Physical examination
Palpable
Nonpalpable
E Retractile
B Undescended
Unilateral
C Bilateral
Re-assurance
Re-evaluation
<6 mo
>6 mo
Referral to
pediatric urologist
C Consider DSD
Referral to pediatric urologist
Re-evaluate at
6 months
Referral to
pediatric urologist
D Diagnostic laparoscopy
+/– laparoscopic orchiopexy
D Diagnostic laparoscopy
+/– laparoscopic orchiopexy
D Inguinal/scrotal
orchiopexy

References

Cortes D, Throop JM, Visfeldt J. Cryptorchidism: aspects of fertility and neoplasms. Horm Res 2001;55:21–7.

Elder JS. Abnormalities of the genitalia in boys and their surgical management. In: Wein AJ, Kavoussi LR, et al, editors. Campbell's urology. 9th ed. Philadelphia: WB Saunders; 2007. p 3763–87.

Lee PA, Couglin MT. Fertility after bilateral cryptorchidism. Horm Res 2001;55:28–32.

Madden NP. Testis, hydrocele and varicocele. In: David T, Duffy PG, Rickwood A, editors: Essentials of paediatric urology. London: Informa Healthcare; 2008. p. 247–57.

Pettersson A, Richiardi L, Nordenskjold A, et al. Age at surgery for undescended testis and risk of testicular cancer. N Engl J Med 2008;356:1835–41.

Walsh TJ, Dall'Era MA, Croughan MS, et al. Prepubertal orchiopexy for cryptorchidism may be associated with lower risk of testicular cancer. J Urol 2007;178:1440–6.

Index

Note: Page numbers followed by f indicate figures; t, tables; b, boxes.

D

N

U

V

W

X

Z

Acronyms and Their Definitions

A1AT alpha-1 antitrypsin
AA Alcoholics Anonymous; amino acids
AAP American Academy of Pediatrics
ABCs airway, breathing, and circulation
ABG arterial blood gas
ABPA allergic bronchopulmonary aspergillosis
Abx antibiotics
ACE angiotensin-converting enzyme
ACE-I angiotensin-converting enzyme inhibitor
ACL anterior cruciate ligament
ACTH adrenocorticotropic hormone
ADEM acute disseminated encephalomyelitis
ADHD attention-deficit/hyperactivity disorder
AED automated external defibrillator
AFP α-fetoprotein
AHI apnea-hypopnea index
AIDS acquired immunodeficiency syndrome
ALT alanine aminotransferase
ANA antinuclear antibody
AOM acute otitis media
AP anteroposterior
aPTT activated partial thromboplastin time
ARDS acute respiratory distress syndrome
ASD autism spectrum disorder
ASO antistreptolysin O
AST aspartate aminotransferase
AV arteriovenous; atrioventricular
AXR abdominal x-ray
BAL blood alcohol level; bronchoalveolar lavage
BC blood culture
BEARS *b*edtime problems, *e*xcessive daytime sleepiness, *a*wakenings at night, *r*egularity and duration of sleep, and *s*leep-disordered breathing
BFNC benign familial neonatal convulsion
BINC benign infantile neonatal convulsion
BMI body mass index
BMP basic metabolic panel
BP blood pressure
BPD bronchopulmonary dysplasia
BS bag specimen
BUN blood urea nitrogen
C and S culture and sensitivity
CAH congenital adrenal hyperplasia
CBC complete blood cell count
CC clean catch
CF cystic fibrosis
CHD cyanotic heart disease
CHF congestive heart failure
CK creatine kinase
CL/CP cleft lip and/or cleft palate
CMP comprehensive metabolic panel
CMV cytomegalovirus
CN cranial nerve
CNS central nervous system
CPAP continuous positive airway pressure
CPP central precocious puberty
CPR cardiopulmonary resuscitation
CPS child protective services
CRP C-reactive protein
CSF cerebrospinal fluid
CSHCN children with special health care needs
CSVT cerebral sinovenous thrombosis
CT computed tomography
CTA computed tomography angiography
CTV computed tomography venography
c/w consistent with
Cx culture
CXR chest x-ray
DA ductus arteriosus
D/C discharge
DD developmental delay
DDAVP 1-deamino-8-D-arginine vasopressin
DFA direct fluorescent antibody
DH dermatitis herpetiformis
DHE dihydroergotamine
DHEA-S dehydroepiandrosterone sulfate
DHT dihydrotestosterone
DI diabetes insipidus
DIC disseminated intravascular coagulation
DKA diabetic ketoacidosis
DM diabetes mellitus
DNA deoxyribonucleic acid
dRVVT dilute Russell viper venom time
DSD disorder of sexual differentiation
dsDNA double-stranded DNA
DSM-IV-TR *Diagnostic and Statistical Manual of Mental Disorders*, 4th Edition, Text Revision
DTP diphtheria-tetanus-pertussis vaccine
DUB dysfunctional uterine bleeding
DVT deep venous thrombosis
DWI diffusion-weighted imaging
E_2 estradiol
EACA ϵ-aminocaproic acid
EB epidermolysis bullosa
EBV Epstein-Barr virus
EC ejection click
ECG electrocardiogram
ECMO extracorporeal membrane oxygenation
ED emergency department
EEG electroencephalogram
ELISA enzyme-linked immunosorbent assay
EMS emergency medical services
ENT ear, nose, and throat
ESR erythrocyte sedimentation rate
ET endotracheal
FAST focused abdominal sonography in trauma
FFP fresh frozen plasma
FSH follicle-stimulating hormone
FTT failure to thrive
F/U follow-up
G6PD glucose 6-phosphate dehydrogenase
GAS group A streptococcus
GBS group B streptococcus
GCS Glasgow Coma Scale
GER gastroesophageal reflux
GERD gastroesophageal reflux disease
GGT γ-glutamyl transferase
GH growth hormone
GnRH gonadotropin-releasing hormone

GU genitourinary
H_2RA histamine$_2$ receptor antagonist
HAV hepatitis A virus
HB_eAg hepatitis B e antigen
HB_sAg hepatitis B surface antigen
HCG human chorionic gonadotropin
HCT hematocrit
HCV hepatitis C virus
HDL high-density lipoprotein
HEV hepatitis E virus
HFOV high-frequency oscillatory ventilation
HIDA hepato-iminodiacetic acid
HIT heparin-induced thrombocytopenia
HIV human immunodefeciency virus
HMG 3-hydroxy-3-methylglutaryl
HPF high-power field
HR heart rate
HSP Henoch-Schönlein purpura
HSV herpes simplex virus
HTN hypertension
HUS hemolytic-uremic syndrome
I&D incision and drainage
IBD inflammatory bowel disease
ICP intracranial pressure
ICU intensive care unit
IEM inborn error of metabolism
IEP individualized educational plan
IGF insulin-like growth factor
INR international normalized ratio
IO intraosseous
IP inpatient
ITB iliotibial band
ITP idiopathic thrombocytopenic purpura
IUP intrauterine pregnancy
IV intravenous
IVIG intravenous immunoglobulin
JIA juvenile idiopathic arthritis
JRA juvenile rheumatoid arthritis
KOH potassium hydroxide
LCL lateral collateral ligament
LCP Legg–Calvé–Perthe disease
LDH lactate dehydrogenase
LDL low-density lipoprotein
LFT liver function test
LH luteinizing hormone
LMWH low-molecular-weight heparin
LP lumbar puncture
LTRA leukotriene receptor antagonist
LUQ left upper quadrant
LVH left ventricular hypertrophy
MAO monoamine oxidase
MCKD multicystic kidney disease
MCL medial collateral ligament
MCV mean corpuscular volume
MIBG metaiodobenzylguanidine
MRA magnetic resonance angiography
MRI magnetic resonance imaging
MRSA methicillin-resistant *Staphylococcus aureus*
MRV magnetic resonance venography
MS mental status
MSK musculoskeletal
MSW medical social worker
mTBI mild traumatic brain injury
MVC motor vehicle collision
NA Narcotics Anonymous
NAFLD nonalcoholic fatty liver disease
NAT nonaccidental trauma
NCS nerve conduction study
NCV nerve conduction velocity
NG nasogastric; nasogastric tube
NGT nasogastric tube
NJ nasojejunal
NM neuromuscular
NMDA *N*-methyl-D-aspartate
NO nitric oxide
NOS not otherwise specified
NS normal saline
NSAID nonsteroidal anti-inflammatory drug
OA organic acid
OCB oligoclonal bands
OCD obsessive-compulsive disorder; osteochondritis dissecans
OG orogastric
17-OHP 17-hydroxyprogesterone
OM otitis media
OMA opsoclonus-myoclonus-ataxia
OME otitis media with effusion
OMV outer membrane vesicles
OP outpatient
OR operating room
ORS oral rehydration solution
OS opening snap
OSA obstructive sleep apnea
OT occupational therapy
PAC premature atrial contraction
PALS pediatric advanced life support
PAS periodic acid–Schiff
PCD primary ciliary dyskinesia
PCKD polycystic kidney disease
PCL posterior cruciate ligament
PCOS polycystic ovary syndrome
PCP primary care physician
PCR polymerase chain reaction
PD persistent diarrhea
PDA patent ductus arteriosus
PE physical examination; pulmonary embolus
PED paroxysmal exertion-induced dyskinesia
PET pneumatic equalization tube; positron emission tomography
PFA platelet function analyzer
PFPS patellofemoral pain syndrome
PGE_1 prostaglandin E_1
PI protein intolerance
PID pelvic inflammatory disease
PKD paroxysmal kinesigenic dyskinesia
PKND paroxysmal non-kinesigenic dyskinesia
PPD purified protein derivative
PPHN persistent pulmonary hypertension
PPI proton-pump inhibitor
PPP peripheral precocious puberty
PSG polysomnogram
PT physical therapy; prothrombin time